MEDICAL ASPECTS OF DISABILITY *for the* REHABILITATION PROFESSIONAL

Alex Moroz, MD, is associate professor, Department of Rehabilitation Medicine, New York University School of Medicine, and was an editor and contributing author to the fourth edition of *Medical Aspects of Disability for the Rehabilitation Professional.* He continues to build an impressive journal article publication resume (more than 40 articles); has received multiple grants including the Hartford Foundation, American Geriatrics Society grant to develop a geriatrics curriculum for physical medicine and rehabilitation residents; and is a four-time Teaching Excellence Award winner (2001, 2008, 2011, 2015) from the graduating resident class.

Steven R. Flanagan, MD, is the chairman, Department of Rehabilitation Medicine, New York University School of Medicine, and medical director, Rusk Rehabilitation, New York University–Langone Medical Center. Dr. Flanagan is widely published with over 50 journal articles and book chapters and has researched the impact and treatment of brain injury. He is a frequent guest in multimedia venues and has lectured both nationally and internationally on topics related to brain injury and rehabilitation.

Herb Zaretsky, PhD, is currently clinical professor of Rehabilitation Medicine at the New York University School of Medicine and has also served for many years as the administrator, Department of Rehabilitation Medicine, Rusk Institute, New York University–Langone Medical Center. He received his PhD from Adelphi University. He has published extensively in the field of rehabilitation in such areas as psychological aspects of disability, geriatric rehabilitation, learning and conditioning with the neurologically impaired and spinal cord injured, rehabilitation psychology and long-term care of the chronically ill, chronic pain management, and behavioral medicine applications in rehabilitation. Dr. Zaretsky is a fellow of the American Psychological Association (APA), past president of APA's Division of Rehabilitation Psychology, and recipient of APA's Distinguished Contributions to Rehabilitation Psychology Award. He is a long-serving member of the board of directors of the national and international Commission on Accreditation of Rehabilitation Facilities (CARF) and currently is chair of the CARF board. Dr. Zaretsky was also formerly president of the board of directors of the American Cancer Society's (ACS) Eastern Division (New York and New Jersey) and the recipient of the St. George Medal, a national award from ACS in recognition of outstanding contributions to the control of cancer.

MEDICAL ASPECTS OF DISABILITY *for the* REHABILITATION PROFESSIONAL

Fifth Edition

Alex Moroz, MD
Steven R. Flanagan, MD
Herb Zaretsky, PhD

Editors

SPRINGER PUBLISHING COMPANY
NEW YORK

Springer Publishing Company, LLC
11 West 42nd Street
New York, NY 10036
www.springerpub.com

Acquisitions Editor: Sheri W. Sussman
Compositor: Exeter Premedia Services Private Ltd.

ISBN: 9780826132277
e-book ISBN: 9780826132284

Instructors Materials: Qualified instructors may request supplements by e-mailing textbook@springerpub.com.
Instructors Manual: 9780826133182
Instructors PowerPoints: 9780826133199

16 17 18 19 20 / 5 4 3 2 1

Library of Congress Cataloging-in-Publication Data

Names: Moroz, Alex, editor. | Flanagan, Steven R., editor. | Zaretsky, Herbert H., editor.
Title: Medical aspects of disability for the rehabilitation professional / [edited by] Alex Moroz, Steven R. Flanagan, and Herb Zaretsky.
Other titles: Medical aspects of disability
Description: Fifth edition. | New York, NY: Springer Publishing Company, LLC, [2017] | Preceded by Medical aspects of disability: a handbook for the rehabilitation professional / Steven R. Flanagan, Herb Zaretsky, Alex Moroz, editors. 4th edition. 2011. | Includes bibliographical references and index.
Identifiers: LCCN 2016035331 | ISBN 9780826132277 | ISBN 9780826132284 (e-book) | ISBN 9780826133182 (instructors manual) | ISBN 9780826133199 (instructors PowerPoints)
Subjects: | MESH: Disabled Persons—rehabilitation | Disability Evaluation | Rehabilitation—methods
Classification: LCC RM930 | NLM WB 320 | DDC 617/.03—dc23
LC record available at https://lccn.loc.gov/2016035331

Printed in the United States of America by McNaughton & Gunn.

With gratitude for my family, teachers, and students.
—Alex Moroz

Many thanks to my friends and family, especially Lou, for their inspiration and support. In particular, a debt of gratitude is extended to Linda Yuen-Moy for her persistence, determination, and hard work, without which this text would not have been possible.
—Steven R. Flanagan

To my wife, Diane, for her love, inspiration, extraordinary support, and cherished friendship; to my daughter, Lauren; my son, Andrew; my son-in-law, Lee; my daughter-in-law, Brooke; and to my grandchildren, Alec, Will, Jake, and Kinley, each of whom is a constant source of joy and love in my life.
—Herb Zaretsky

Contents

PART III: SPECIAL TOPICS

Contributors

Steven B. Abramson, MD
Frederick H. King Professor and Chair
Department of Medicine
New York University School of Medicine
New York, New York

Jung Ahn, MD
Clinical Professor of Rehabilitation Medicine
New York University School of Medicine
New York, New York

Kirill Alekseyev, MD, MBA
Resident Physician
Kingsbrook Rehabilitation Institute
Brooklyn, New York

Stefanie Auer, PhD
Professor for Dementia Studies
Department for Clinical Neurosciences and Preventive Medicine
Danube University
Krems, Austria
Scientific Director
MAS Alzheimerhlife
Bad Ischl, Austria

Steve M. Aydin, DO
Assistant Clinical Professor of Physical Medicine and Rehabilitation
Hofstra–Northwell Health School of Medicine
Manhasset, New York
Director of Musculoskeletal Medicine
Manhattan Spine & Pain Medicine
New York, New York

Raymona Baldwin, BA
Assistive Technology Specialist
Bellevue College
Bellevue, Washington

Matina Balou, PhD, CCC-SLP, BCS-S
Assistant Professor
Department of Otolaryngology and Rehabilitation Medicine
New York University School of Medicine
New York, New York

Reema Batra, MD
Medical Oncologist and Hematologist
San Diego, California

Claribell Bayona, OTR/L
Senior Occupational Therapist
New York University–Langone Medical Center Rusk Rehabilitation–Occupational Therapy Department
New York, New York

Aleksandar Beric, MD, DSc
Professor of Neurology, Neurosurgery Rehabilitation Medicine and Orthopedic Surgery
Director
Clinical Neurophysiology
New York University School of Medicine
New York, New York

Jeffrey Berliner, DO
Director Outpatient SCI Medicine
Craig Hospital
University of Colorado
Englewood, Colorado

Frederick A. Bevelaqua, MD
Clinical Assistant Professor of Medicine
New York University School of Medicine
New York, New York

Amandeep Bhandal, MD
Aging and Dementia Clinical Research Center
Fisher Alzheimer's Disease Program
Center for Cognitive Neurology
New York University–Langone Medical Center
New York, New York

Sushma Bhusal, MD
Fellow in Nephrology
New York University School of Medicine
New York, New York

Gary R. Bond, PhD
Senior Research Associate
IPS Employment Center
Westat
Lebanon, New Hampshire

Brian J. Boon, PhD
President/CEO
CARF International, Inc.
Tuscon, Arizona

Christopher Boudakian, DO
Stanford School of Medicine
Palo Alto, California

Andrew Brash, BS
State University of New York
Stonybrook School of Medicine
Great Neck, New York

Susanne M. Bruyère, PhD, CRC
Professor of Disability Studies and Director
K. Lisa Yang and Hock E. Tan Institute on Employment and Disability
Cornell University
ILR School
Ithaca, New York

Tamara Bushnik, PhD, FACRM
Director of Rehabilitation Research and Associate Professor
New York University School of Medicine
New York, New York

Efren Caballes, DO
Department of Rehabilitation Medicine
New York University School of Medicine
New York, New York

Antonia M. Carbone, Pharm D, BCPS, BCACP
Clinical Assistant Professor of Pharmacy Practice
Fairleigh Dickinson University School of Pharmacy
Florham Park, New Jersey
Ambulatory Care Pharmacist
Overlook Family Medicine
Summit, New Jersey

Jeffrey M. Cohen, MD
Clinical Professor of Rehabilitation Medicine
New York University School of Medicine
New York, New York

Roy Gordon Cole, OD, FAAO
Director of Vision Program Development
Lighthouse Guild
Adjunct Professor of Optometric Science
Columbia University Medical Center
New York, New York

John R. Corcoran, PT, DPT, MS
Site Director for Rehabilitation Therapy Services
Clinical Assistant Professor
Rusk Rehabilitation
New York University–Langone Medical Center
New York, New York

Adrian Cristian, MD, MHCM
Chairman
Department of Rehabilitation Medicine
Northwell Health–Glen Cove Hospital
Glen Cove, New York

Laurentiu I. Dinescu, MD
Pain Management
Kingsbrook Jewish Medical Center
New York, New York

Joan E. Edelstein, MA, PT, FISPO
Special Lecturer
Columbia University
New York, New York

Marcia Epstein, MD, FIDSA, FACP
Associate Professor of Medicine
Hofstra North Shore–LIJ School of Medicine
Manhasset, New York

Elsa Escalera, MD, MPH
Chief Medical Officer
Medical Services
Lighthouse Guild
New York, New York

Emile Franssen, MD
Research Associate Professor
Department of Psychiatry
New York University School of Medicine
New York, New York

Heidi N. Fusco, MD
Clinical Instructor of Rehabilitation Medicine
New York University School of Medicine
New York, New York

Christopher Gharibo, MD
Associate Professor of Anesthesiology and Orthopedics
Department of Anesthesiology
Perioperative Care and Pain Medicine
New York University–Langone Hospital for Joint Diseases
New York University School of Medicine
New York, New York

Joan T. Gold, MD
Clinical Professor of Rehabilitation Medicine
New York University School of Medicine
New York, New York

Thomas P. Golden, EdD, CRC
Executive Director
K. Lisa Yang and Hock E. Tan Institute on Employment and Disability
Cornell University
ILR School
Ithaca, New York

Stuart Green, DMH, LCSW
Associate Director
Overlook Family Medicine Residency
Overlook Medical Center
Clinical Assistant Professor of Family and Community Medicine at Sidney Kimmel Medical College at Thomas Jefferson University
Summit, New Jersey

Ilana Grunwald, PhD
Clinical Assessment Coordinator–Psychology
Clinical Assistant Professor of Rehabilitation Medicine
Department of Psychology
Rusk Rehabilitation
New York University School of Medicine
New York, New York

Francoise Guillo-Benarous, MD
Research Clinician
New York University Alzheimer's Disease Research Center
New York University–Langone Medical Center
New York, New York

Andrew J. Haig, MD
Vice President for Accountable Care and Medical Informatics
Mary Free Bed Rehabilitation Hospital
Grand Rapids, Michigan
Professor Emeritus
University of Michigan
Ann Arbor, Michigan

Geoffrey W. Hall, FACHE, MBA, MSW, LCSW
Department Administrator
Rusk Rehabilitation
New York University School of Medicine
New York, New York

Mary R. Hibbard, PhD, ABPP(RP)
Professor of Rehabilitation Medicine
New York University School of Medicine
New York, New York

Joan Y. Hou, MD
TBI/Polytrauma Fellow
Hunter Holmes McGuire VA Medical Center/VCU
Kingsbrook Jewish Medical Center
Brooklyn, New York

Abraham P. Houng, MD, MSE, FACS
Assistant Professor of Surgery
Weill Cornell Medical College
New York Presbyterian Hospital–Weill Cornell Medical Center
New York, New York

Matthew B. Huish, MBA
Administrative Director Physical Medicine and Rehabilitation
University of Utah
School of Medicine
Salt Lake City, Utah

Natalie Hyppolite, DO
Hofstra–Northwell School of Medicine
Department of Physical Medicine and Rehabilitation
Manhasset, New York

Armando Iannicello, MD, PGY-2
Kingsbrook Jewish Medical Center
Brooklyn, New York

Brian Im, MD
Assistant Professor of Rehabilitation Medicine
New York University School of Medicine
New York, New York

Koto Ishida, MD
Assistant Professor of Neurology
New York University School of Medicine
New York, New York

Glenn R. Jacobowitz, MD
Professor of Surgery and Vice Chair for Clinical Operations
Department of Surgery
New York University–Langone Medical Center
New York, New York

Parul Jajoo, DO
Clinical Instructor of Rehabilitation Medicine
New York University School of Medicine
New York, New York

Khurram S. Janjua, MD
Clinical Research Intern
New York University Alzheimer's Disease Center
Aging and Dementia Clinical Research Center
Fisher Alzheimer's Disease Program
Center for Cognitive Neurology
New York University–Langone Medical Center
New York, New York

Annalee V. Johnson-Kwochka, BA
Research Assistant
IPS Employment Center
Westat
Lebanon, New Hampshire

Sunnie Kenowsky, DVM
Co-Director
Zachary and Elizabeth M. Fisher Alzheimer's Disease Education and Resources Program at the New York University School of Medicine
Clinical Instructor and Senior Public Educator
Aging and Dementia Clinical Research Center
Department of Psychiatry
New York University–Langone Medical Center
New York, New York

Asma Khizar, MD
Clinical Research Intern
New York University Alzheimer's Disease Center
Aging and Dementia Clinical Research Center and Fisher Alzheimer's Disease Program
Center for Cognitive Neurology
New York University–Langone Medical Center
New York, New York

Charles Kim, MD, CAC
Assistant Professor of Rehabilitation Medicine and Anesthesiology
New York University School of Medicine
New York, New York

Christopher J. Kort, CPO
President/CEO
Prosthetics in Motion, Inc.
New York, New York

Sicy H. Lee, MD
Clinical Assistant Professor
Department of Medicine
New York University School of Medicine
New York, New York

Jaime M. Levine, DO
Clinical Assistant Professor of Rehabilitation Medicine
New York University School of Medicine
New York, New York

Richard J. Lin, MD
Clinical Fellow in Hematology Oncology
New York University School of Medicine
Laura and Isaac Perlmutter Cancer Center
New York, New York

Mary Anne Loftus, MS, RN, CRRN, NEA-BC
Director of Nursing for Rusk Rehabilitation and Ambulatory Care Services
Hospital for Joint Diseases
New York University–Langone Medical Center
New York, New York

Athena M. Lolis, MD
Assistant Professor
Division of Clinical Neurophysiology
Department of Neurology
New York University School of Medicine
New York, New York

Jerome Lowenstein, MD
Professor
Department of Medicine
Nephrology Division
New York University School of Medicine
New York, New York

Anthony Steven Lubinsky, MD
Assistant Professor of Medicine
New York University School of Medicine
New York, New York

Amy Miano, MSW, LCSW, C-ASWCM
Social Worker
Care Management Department
Overlook Medical Center
Summit, New Jersey

Ana Mola, PhD, RN, ANP-C, MAACVPR
Director of Care Transitions and Population Health Management
Department of Care Management
New York University–Langone Medical Center
New York, New York

Richard J. Morris, PhD
Professor Emeritus of School Psychology
University of Arizona
Tucson, Arizona

Yvonne P. Morris, PhD
Licensed Psychologist
Tucson, Arizona

Kotresha Neelakantappa, MD, FACP
Chief of Nephrology
New York Methodist Hospital
Brooklyn, New York

Alexandra Nielsen, MD
Fellow
Brain Injury Medicine
Department of Rehabilitation Medicine
New York University School of Medicine
New York, New York

Bryan O'Young, MD
Medical Director of Physiatric Pain Management
Department of Physical Medicine and Rehabilitation, Geisinger Health System
Clinical Professor of Rehabilitation Medicine
New York University School of Medicine
Adjunct Clinical Professor of Rehabilitation Medicine
Weill Cornell Medical College
New York, New York

Nnabugo Ozurumba, MD
Kingsbrook Jewish Medical Center
Brooklyn, New York

Kate Parkin, PT, DPT, MA
Clinical Assistant Professor
Department of Physical Medicine and Rehabilitation
Sr. Director of Rehabilitation Therapy Services
Rusk Rehabilitation
New York University–Langone Medical Center
New York, New York

Hersh Patel, MD, MBA
Chief Resident
New York University School of Medicine
New York, New York

Komal G. Patel, DO
Resident Physician
Physical Medicine and Rehabilitation
Hofstra–Northwell School of Medicine
Hempstead, New York

Aleksandra Policha, MD
Division of Vascular Surgery
New York University–Langone Medical Center
New York, New York

Bruce G. Raphael, MD
Clinical Professor of Medicine
New York University School of Medicine
New York, New York

Mary Regina Reilly, MS, CCC-SLP
Director of Speech Language Pathology
New York University–Langone Medical Center
New York, New York

Barry Reisberg, MD
Professor, Department of Psychiatry
Director, Fisher Alzheimer's Disease Program
Clinical Director, Aging and Dementia Research Center
Emeritus Director, Clinical Core, NYU Alzheimer's Disease Center
New York University School of Medicine
New York, New York

Kirk S. Roden, MBA, FACHE
Director
Management Operations
Departments of Neurology and Physical Medicine and Rehabilitation
McGovern Medical School
University of Texas Health Science Center
Houston, Texas

Bruce P. Rosenthal, OD, FAAO
Chief of Low Vision
Lighthouse Guild
Adjunct Professor
Department of Ophthalmology
Mt. Sinai Hospital
Adjunct Distinguished Professor
College of Optometry
State University of New York
New York, New York

Pamela B. Rosenthal, MD
Assistant Professor
Department of Medicine
New York University School of Medicine
New York, New York

Matt Saleh, PhD, JD
Research Associate
K. Lisa Yang and Hock E. Tan Institute on Employment and Disability
Cornell University
ILR School
Ithaca, New York

David H. Salsberg, PsyD, DABPS
Pediatric Neuropsychologist
Director of Pediatric Assessment, Learning and Support
Clinical Instructor
Department of Pediatrics
New York University School of Medicine
Adjunct Clinical Assistant Professor of Neuropsychology
Department of Neurological Surgery
Weill Cornell Medical College
New York, New York

Romi G. Shah, MD
Fisher Alzheimer's Disease Program
Aging and Dementia Clinical Research Center
New York University Medical Center
New York, New York

Umang Shah, MD, MPH
Clinical Research Intern
Aging and Dementia Clinical Research Center
Fisher Alzheimer's Disease Program
New York University Alzheimer's Disease Center
Center for Cognitive Neurology
New York University Medical Center
New York, New York

Matthew Shatzer, DO
Residency Program Director
Physical Medicine and Rehabilitation
Hofstra–Northwell School of Medicine
Chief
Physical Medicine and Rehabilitation
North Shore University Hospital
Assistant Professor
Hofstra–Northwell School of Medicine
Department of Physical Medicine and Rehabilitation
Hempstead, New York

Anna Shor, MD
Assistant Professor
Division of Clinical Neurophysiology
Department of Neurology
New York University School of Medicine
New York, New York

Anuradha Singh, MD
Clinical Associate Professor of Neurology
New York University School of Medicine
New York, New York

Satneet Singh, MD
New York University Alzheimer's Disease Center
Aging and Dementia Clinical Research Center and Fisher Alzheimer's Disease Program
Center for Cognitive Neurology
New York University–Langone Medical Center
New York, New York

Liduïn E. M. Souren, RN, MSN
Research Assistant Professor
Department of Psychiatry
New York University School of Medicine
New York, New York

Steven A. Stiens, MD, MS
Attending Physician Spinal Cord Injury Unit
Veterans Affairs Puget Sound Health Care System
Associate Professor
Department of Rehabilitation Medicine
University of Washington
Seattle, Washington

Angela Stolfi, PT, DPT
Clinical Instructor
Department of Physical Medicine and Rehabilitation
Director of Physical Therapy
Rusk Rehabilitation
New York University–Langone Medical Center
New York, New York

Dale C. Strasser, MD
Professor of Rehabilitation Medicine
Emory University Medical School
Atlanta, Georgia

Gregory Sweeney, PT, DPT, CCS
Clinical Instructor of Rehabilitation Medicine
New York University School of Medicine
New York, New York

Patrick T. Swift, PhD
Clinical Neuropsychologist
Robert Wood Johnson Barnabas Health
Newark, New Jersey

Bryn N. Thatcher, MEd
Bowling Green State University
Bowling Green, Ohio

Kristin C. Thompson, PhD
University of Arizona
Tucson, Arizona

Jose Torres, MD
Assistant Professor of Neurology
New York University School of Medicine
New York, New York

Stephen Trevick, MD
Senior Resident
Department of Neurology and Psychiatry
New York University School of Medicine
New York, New York

Joseph Tribuna, MD
Director
Overlook Family Medicine Residency Program
Overlook Medical Center
Summit, New Jersey
Clinical Assistant Professor of Family and Community Medicine
Sidney Kimmel Medical College at Thomas Jefferson University
Philadelphia, Pennsylvania

Patricia A. Tufaro, OTR/L, CLT
Supervisor of Hand and Occupational Therapy
New York Presbyterian/Weill Cornell Hospital
New York, New York

Sandra W. Veigne, MD
New York University Alzheimer's Disease Center
Aging and Dementia Clinical Research Center and Fisher Alzheimer's Disease Program
Center for Cognitive Neurology
New York University–Langone Medical Center
New York, New York

Lynn Videka, PhD, BSN, AM
Collegiate Professor and Dean
University of Michigan School of Social Work
Ann Arbor, Michigan

Elfie Wegner, MSN, APN, CDE
Nurse Practitioner
Overlook Family Medicine
Summit, New Jersey

Jonathan H. Whiteson, MD
Assistant Professor of Rehabilitation Medicine
New York University Medical Center
New York, New York

Mark Young, MD, MBA, FACP
Chair
Physical Medicine and Rehabilitation
The Workforce and Technology Vocational Rehabilitation Center
State of Maryland
Division of Rehabilitation (DORS)
Faculty
The Johns Hopkins School of Medicine Physical Medicine and Rehabilitation
Baltimore, Maryland

Preface

The delivery of medical and rehabilitative care is in continuous and rapid flux. Shrinking resources, growing regulatory pressures, and novel technologies are only some of the factors that significantly impact all health care. Parallel to increasing efforts to establish evidence-based rehabilitation practices, economic and political forces continue to challenge the delivery of care to people with disabilities. This fifth edition of *Medical Aspects of Disability for the Rehabilitation Professional* has been substantially updated to reflect advancements in medical care for specific disabling conditions as well as changes in forces that impact the delivery of that care. In particular, reviews of relevant legislature, quality improvement frameworks, accreditation systems, and trends in payments for rehabilitation and other health care services complement the core areas of medical conditions and clinical care for people with disabilities. Chapters in the fifth edition have been either substantially updated by previous authors or rewritten by new contributors. New chapter authors, among the most widely respected authorities in their respective fields, include Aleksandar Beric (neuromuscular disorders), Heidi N. Fusco and Koto Ishida (stroke), Mary Anne Loftus (rehabilitation nursing), and Charles Kim (integrative medicine), among others. Our primary goal in this latest edition is to provide health care professionals, teachers, and students with a comprehensive guide that addresses the conditions and topics impacting people with physical, developmental, and cognitive disabilities.

Alex Moroz, MD

CHAPTER

Introduction

Kate Parkin, John R. Corcoran, and Angela Stolfi

THE HISTORY OF REHABILITATION

In the ancient world, people with disabilities were summarily excluded from everyday life (Conti, 2014). The notion that disabilities were punishments from the gods and deities was widely accepted. Disabilities were assumed to be the direct result of one's moral failings, sins, or acts against the gods. People with disabilities were thus prescribed complete removal from society. Unfortunately, this provides us with little information about disabilities of the time—the disabled were hidden away to live a life of reclusion and banishment. Individuals unfortunate enough to be suffering from a physical affliction were left to their own resources and often labeled as cripples, invalids, or worse. Because people were not widely treated for disabilities but were rather removed from society, the treatments for disabilities did not advance for thousands of years.

The first known medical document was discovered in Egypt and dates back to 2000 BCE. This document is known as *The Edwin Smith Surgical Papyrus* (named after the American Egyptologist who purchased the treatise in 1862). The treatise describes the general sentiment of how most disabilities were treated, which could be summarized as sparse at best. For example, when describing spinal cord injuries, this injury was often deemed "an ailment not to be treated" because treatment options were nonexistent (Donovan, 2007).

A seismic shift occurred when Hippocrates (460–370 BCE), the father of modern medicine, started to categorize illness and disability in terms of physiology as opposed to divine affliction. This, coupled with the Greek focus on physical abilities and conditioning as the Olympic games were becoming of paramount importance in society, helped to usher in an era and culture of physical training and interest in the effects of exercise and rehabilitation for peak performance. Soldiers and athletes were considered precious commodities, and they provided numerous subjects for case studies.

As power shifted from Greece to Rome, so did the medical leaders with the resources to study disability. The famed physician Galen (130–200) in the first century CE recognized the association between physical activity and medical outcomes. Because of the numerous Roman military campaigns at the time, Galen had ample soldiers as subjects to work with. He researched medical rehabilitation of the war injuries that were common at the time. As we shall see, wars tragically continue to provide fodder for research advances in rehabilitation.

Wars often produce many injuries and conditions that require rehabilitation. A common war injury is amputation. The French surgeon Paré (1510–1590) is credited with inventing modern lower limb prostheses (Conti, 2014). In the Middle Ages, prostheses were made of metal. These early prostheses were very heavy and, as the reader can easily imagine, very uncomfortable. Paré was also credited with establishing that phantom limb pain (a condition in which a limb that is no longer present continues to provide the sensation of pain) was of cerebral origin.

The Renaissance brought advancements in the technical study and understanding of disability and disease especially in terms of anatomy and the study of kinetics (Conti, 2014). In addition, the Renaissance period also put forward the practice and idea of disability prevention using "medical gymnastics." Medical gymnastics was the term used at the time to describe therapeutic exercises designed with the aim of helping patients recover from a physical disability or impairment.

One monumental advancement in the history of rehabilitation was by the Swiss physician Joseph Clément Tissot (1747–1826). He proposed early mobilization for surgical patients. Traditionally, bedrest was prescribed for almost all surgical and nonsurgical patients. Tissot proposed moving or mobilizing patients and getting them out of bed quickly. This proved to be beneficial, and his principles are still being slowly advanced to this day (Kress, 2014).

It was the Swedish teacher of "medical gymnastics," Pehr Henrik Ling (1776–1839), who put forth the direct link between medical rehabilitation and functional recovery. Function refers to one's ability to engage with one's surroundings and the environment. It was a fight indeed, as light exercise and gentle massage were the standard of care (Conti, 2014). Ling realized that more aggressive rehabilitation often resulted in better outcomes for patients. It is interesting because even when we fast-forward to today, we have not found the ceiling effect in terms of how far we can and should progress patients in terms of the intensity of the rehabilitation program.

Despite these pockets of advances in the history of rehabilitation (and with the slowly growing notion that disabilities were not caused by divine punishment), most patients with disabilities were treated by their families or in religious establishments until the latter part of the 20th century (Ohry, 2004). In fact, General George Patton (1885–1945), who is famous for many highly successful campaigns in World War II, sustained a spinal cord injury shortly after returning from the war. It is said that he was well aware (likely from seeing injured soldiers firsthand) that there were no cures or efficacious treatments available, and thus he refused all treatments. Patton died as a result of his injuries in the hospital on December 21, 1945 (Donovan, 2007). It was Alexander Fleming's discovery of penicillin that greatly decreased deaths from infections, including those seen in spinal cord injury care, and a host of other disabilities that revolutionized all of medicine, including physical medicine and rehabilitation (PM&R; Donovan, 2007).

It was not until the early 1900s that rehabilitation as a profession started to gain prominence, even though it was initially viewed in large part as quackery (Folz, Opitz, Gelfman, & Peters, 1997). The struggle for legitimacy continued during much of the early years as the field developed.

Two icons in the field who transformed and essentially established rehabilitation as a profession were Frank H. Krusen, MD, and Howard A. Rusk, MD. Drs. Krusen and Rusk were instrumental in creating the scope of the field as it is known today. Dr. Krusen's (1898–1973) interest in rehabilitation was shaped by personal experience. While working in his first year of surgical residency training, he was infected with tuberculosis (Folz et al., 1997). He spent 5 months in a sanitarium, during which time he recognized that he and other patients were becoming physically deconditioned, causing them to become increasingly more dependent on the institution for care. It was then that he came up with the idea of physical rehabilitation with an emphasis on social reintegration, physical reconditioning, and vocational rehabilitation as essential components of convalescence, which ultimately became his life's work.

The American Medical Association (AMA) did not initially view physical rehabilitation favorably. It was not until 1939 that the first scientific paper on rehabilitation was accepted in a medical journal (Folz et al., 1997). Dr. Krusen experienced great resistance from several groups that organized against him. His most significant opponents were from the fields of orthopedics and pediatrics as well as from the National Foundation for Infantile Paralysis (Peters, Gelfman, Opitz, & Folz, 1997). Many were concerned about the use of the word "rehabilitation" in this developing specialty because it was felt to have a place in many other disciplines.

Dr. Howard Archibald Rusk (1901–1989) had a similar insight as Dr. Krusen. Although he is often mistaken for a physiatrist, Howard Rusk was an internist who organized comprehensive medical rehabilitation departments in Army Air Corps hospitals during World War II (Peters et al., 1997). While working in medical rehabilitation, he noticed that the soldiers were becoming deconditioned and listless during their convalescence. Rusk organized academic classwork and physical exercise during the soldiers' hospitalization. He also emphasized interdisciplinary teams and psychosocial functioning in addition to physical and vocational rehabilitation (Peters et al., 1997). Through his work, soldiers regained physical fitness and were able to return to active duty at a faster pace while experiencing significantly lower rates of hospital readmission (an important concept that is still being analyzed and studied today). He also included military training as part of the academic coursework provided to the soldiers to enhance their performance when they returned to active duty. For example, he organized small replicas of German planes to cycle over the soldiers' hospital beds to assist in identifying them when they returned to the battlefield (Rusk, 1977).

Rusk was also a pioneer in the concept and implementation of early mobilization after illness or injury. He conducted experiments to analyze the impact of returning to activity quickly after surgery, and the initial findings were favorable. This success spurred further research, and like the earlier work of Joseph Clément Tissot, research into early mobilization is continuing to take shape and advance today.

When Dr. Rusk completed his military service, he petitioned the AMA to start residencies in medical rehabilitation. The AMA deferred to the Council on Physical Medicine because of the similarities of the two fields (Peters et al., 1997). Dr. Krusen also recognized the close association, and with their backing, the AMA Council on Physical Medicine approved a motion to change the residencies to a combination of physical medicine and rehabilitation (Peters et al., 1997). Dr. Rusk, who is generally recognized as the "father of comprehensive rehabilitation," went on to teach and train physicians across the United States and throughout the world, including Russia, Korea, China, and Vietnam.

Just as World War II shaped Rusk's views and thoughts on rehabilitation, the wars in Afghanistan and Iraq have also profoundly influenced the field in more recent times. Many soldiers have returned from combat with amputations, traumatic brain injuries (TBI), multisystem blast injuries, and posttraumatic stress disorder (PTSD). There has been an increase in research and development in these areas because of the prevalence of these injuries and the desire to help the soldiers return to productive, functional, and meaningful lives. As described throughout this book, the reader will learn of recent advances in the care and rehabilitation for people with conditions such as limb loss and TBI resulting from these conflicts and other more common causes (e.g., motor vehicle accidents) of disability.

DEFINITIONS AND EPIDEMIOLOGY

"Physical rehabilitation in its essence is the preservation and restoration of function" (anonymous; Haig, Nagy, Lebreck, & Stein, 1995). A significant portion of the U.S. population lives with physical disabilities. Rehabilitation is a process aimed at enabling people with disabilities to reach and maintain their optimal physical, sensory, intellectual, psychological, vocational, social, and functional potential. Rehabilitation provides people with disabilities the tools they need to attain greater independence. In 2013, the World Health Organization (WHO) estimated that 12.6% of the world's population experienced some form of disability or impairment. The number of people with disabilities is increasing due to population growth, aging, emergence of chronic diseases, increasing motor vehicle use, and medical advances that preserve and prolong life. The most common causes of impairment and disability include chronic diseases such as diabetes, cardiovascular disease, cancer, traumatic injuries, mental impairments, birth defects, malnutrition, HIV/AIDS, and other communicable diseases. These conditions are creating overwhelming demands for health and rehabilitation services (WHO, 2014). Managing these conditions is one of the biggest challenges our health care system faces as we move through the 21st century. People are living longer, yet the percentage of those living with chronic diseases has increased significantly over the past two decades. Between 110 million and 190 million adults worldwide have significant difficulties in functioning. With proper care, the onset and progression of these diseases can be better contained and controlled for many years. In addition to the suffering and early death they can cause, "these chronic conditions cost a staggering $1.7 trillion yearly" (www.barackobama.com, 2009 and WHO December 2014).

According to the U.S. Census Bureau American Community Survey (ACS), the Disability Statistics Annual Report classifies disability into one or more of six categories (hearing, visual, cognitive, ambulatory, self-care, independent living). The 2013 annual report indicates that 12.6% of the entire population has a disability (one or more of the six listed categories of disability). However, the percentage of disability increases over time as individuals age:

Disability Rate	*Age*
0.8%	Less than 4 years old
5.3%	5 to 15 years old
5.6%	16 to 20 years old
10.8%	21 to 64 years old
25.8%	65 to 74 years old
50.7%	Greater than 75 years old

People with disabilities have less access to health care services and therefore experience unmet health care needs. Rehabilitation provides people with disabilities the tools they need to attain greater independence through the continuum.

> While some health conditions associated with disability result in poor health and extensive health care needs, others do not. However all people with disabilities have the same general health care needs as everyone else, and therefore need access to mainstream health care services. Article 25 of the UN Convention on the Rights of Persons with Disabilities (CRPD) reinforces the right of persons with disabilities to attain the highest standard of health care, without discrimination. (www.un.org/en/universal-declaration-human-rights)

The International Classification of Functioning, Disability and Health (ICF) defines disability as an umbrella term for impairments, activity limitations, and participation restrictions. Disability is the interaction between individuals with a health condition (e.g., cerebral palsy, Down's syndrome, and depression) and personal and environmental factors (e.g., negative attitudes, inaccessible transportation and public buildings, and limited social supports).

In the 66th World Health Assembly (May 2013), it was recognized that disability is a human rights issue and a development issue. The UN General Assembly has continued focused work in these two key areas around the world.

REHABILITATION TEAM

As the health care system changes and the ability to provide care across a long continuum is being remolded, effective communication between rehabilitation team members becomes increasingly essential. Thus, the medical rehabilitation model consists of a core group of medical professionals who comprise a comprehensive team to evaluate and treat people to best meet these people's needs, with communication between members occurring on a regular basis. The interdisciplinary team involves a large number of disciplines, which are led by rehabilitation physicians (Figure 1.1). The physician usually determines which team members should be involved in the care of a particular patient, noting that all disciplines are not always required or involved at the same time. Each discipline plays an integral role in the patient's recovery and includes:

- Child life therapist
- Creative art therapist
- Horticultural therapist
- Nutritionist
- Occupational therapist (OT)
- Pastoral care
- The patient himself or herself
- Physiatrist/physician
- Physical therapist (PT)
- Psychologist
- Rehabilitation engineer
- Rehabilitation nurse (RN)
- Social worker (SW)
- Speech-language pathologist (SLP)
- Therapeutic recreational specialist (TRS)
- Vocational rehabilitation counselor (VRC)

The following text consists of a brief description of the most common team members.

The *patient* is by far the most important member of the interdisciplinary team and should be involved in all decisions regarding his or her care. If the patient (or the designee, if the patient is incapable of participation) is not included or is not in agreement with the plan of treatment, rehabilitation is unlikely to succeed.

OTs are licensed professionals who help promote health and enhance independence in the performance of activities of daily living (ADLs) for

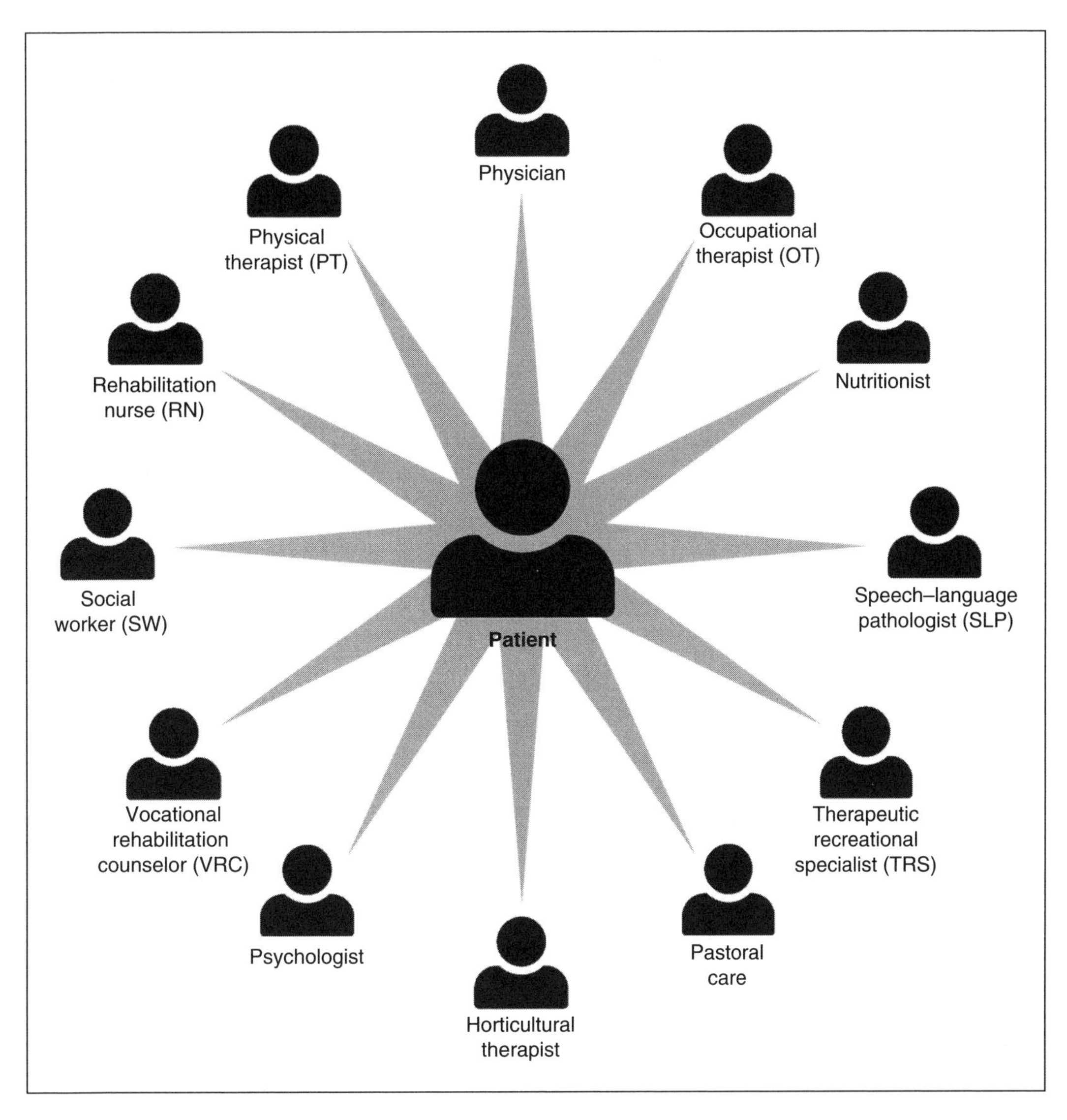

FIGURE 1.1 Patient-centered interdisciplinary team approach.

people with disabilities. OTs assess people's skills and limitations regarding ADLs and use meaningful and purposeful activities in addition to specialized equipment and adaptive aids to promote independent function.

PTs are licensed professionals who provide services to patients with physical impairments, functional limitations, disabilities, or changes in function and health resulting from injury or disease. PTs assess and treat bed mobility, the ability to move from place to place (e.g., wheelchair to bed), ambulation skills, balance, strength, range of motion, and function.

Physiatrists are physicians specializing in the field of PM&R and lead the rehabilitation team. After reviewing the history and performing the physical examination, the physiatrist prescribes the rehabilitation program and provides medical treatment to people with disabilities.

Psychologists are licensed professionals who assess patients' cognitive status and mental health. Psychologists help emotionally distressed patients adjust to life that has changed due to injury or illness and provide therapy to improve cognitive performance when necessary.

TRSs are trained and certified to provide treatment, education, and recreational services to help people with illnesses and disabilities develop leisure activities that enhance their health, functional abilities, independence, and quality of life.

RNs are licensed professionals responsible for monitoring patients' medical status including, but not limited to, vital signs, skin integrity, and sleep status. RNs also evaluate the patient's mental state, medication usage and effectiveness, pain, and bowel and bladder function, and provide essential education to both patients and their families. Many rehabilitation units have RNs who have a specialty certification in rehabilitation (Certified Rehabilitation Registered Nurse [CRRN]).

SLPs are licensed professionals who assess the patient's ability to communicate by both spoken and written language in addition to evaluating swallowing ability, which is often impaired following brain injury. They provide treatment to improve both communication skills and the ability to safely swallow food and liquids.

SWs are licensed professionals who assess patients' psychosocial status, including their living situations, support system, and financial status. They assist patients by helping them cope with social issues that impact their life, particularly as the issues pertain to their disability, in addition to dealing with patients' personal and professional relationships.

VRCs assess patients' ability to return to work or to activities they enjoyed prior to the commencement of their disability. VRCs determine the jobs that are best suited to their patients via interviews, evaluation of their abilities, and selected tests.

The historical culture in most health care settings has traditionally been hierarchical, which is a model that has been described as potentially hindering care (Paradis et al., 2013). Team leaders in a hierarchical system may have positive attitudes toward teamwork, but may be undecided in sharing decision-making roles in an interprofessional team, which may be due to lack of clear understanding of potential roles of the team members (Klinar et al., 2013). Recently, a move toward interprofessional collaborative practice has been occurring in health care because it has been shown to lead to efficiencies in care. In rehabilitation settings, some of the traditional hierarchical cultures exist; however, as previously discussed, the nature of the work favors a team-based culture. This positions rehabilitation professionals to lead the way in developing a successful model for interprofessional collaborative practice.

PATIENT EXPERIENCE

Patients, depending on many factors (e.g., age, level of ability, access to services), have varied experiences as they interact with the health care system. A patient's experience depends on the setting in which the rehabilitation is being provided. "Patient experience" is defined as the sum of all interactions, shaped by an organization's culture, that influence patient perceptions across the continuum of care. There has been a rapid expansion in the use of the term "patient experience" in general health care, both in clinical practice and in research (Locatelli, Turcios, & LaVela, 2014).

Patients, being at the front and center of their experience, have helped the shift in both public policy as well as providers recognizing the impact this can have on outcomes. This is now a top priority for health care leaders. For example, services provided acutely after injury in an acute inpatient rehabilitation hospital, subacute rehabilitation (SAR) facility, or outpatient venue have unique characteristics and regulations that dictate the type and intensity of treatment provided. Services can also vary within each setting, with individual rehabilitation centers often offering highly specialized programs to meet the needs of the patients they serve. After the onset of an adverse medical event (e.g., stroke, cardiac event, or neurologic event), patients will usually be taken to an acute care hospital. Once patients are medically stabilized, they are discharged from the acute care hospital and may be transferred to an acute rehabilitation facility if they can participate and benefit from intensive therapy.

A common element for patients destined for acute rehabilitation is that their lives have been altered physically, psychologically, and often spiritually by the experience. Imagine for a moment that your ability to walk, dress, and even comprehend a loved one's speech has been suddenly lost because of an acute medical event such as a stroke or TBI. Now you find yourself in a medical center with a team of individuals working with you to restore what previously was taken for granted.

This scenario is quite typical for patients in need of acute rehabilitation following a sudden illness or injury and outlines some key points. In most acute inpatient rehabilitation facilities (IRFs), bedside rounds attended by representatives of the team occur daily. This is a time to review daily progress, receive updates on medical status and medication changes, review issues that occurred overnight, and answer questions from the patients or their significant others. This is also an opportunity to get the patient's feedback, review team goals, discuss discharge planning, and get information on the patient's preferences.

The team conference is a gathering of the various disciplines that are working with the patient and typically occurs weekly in acute inpatient settings. This conference, usually led by the physician, will include updates on the patient's medical condition, functional changes, progress toward patient goals, unusual occurrences, discharge planning, and modification of desired or expected goals. In addition to setting individual goals that are specific to each discipline, the team will create and review goals that cross disciplines, such as community mobility that requires the use of mass transportation. Discussions will also focus on planning for discharge, which may include the need for continued medical, nursing, and rehabilitation care. Potential barriers to discharge will be reviewed, including access to and within the patient's home and the availability of others to assist in the patient's care once in the community. Ongoing rehabilitation is often needed after discharge, which may be provided at home, as an outpatient, or at a subacute facility. SAR is provided in a skilled nursing facility (SNF), but at a lower intensity with about 1 hour of therapy given daily, as opposed to acute rehabilitation where at least 3 hours of daily therapy is provided.

Family meetings are typically arranged by the SW or case coordinator and include the physician and many of the team members. The psychologist is often present at these meetings as family dynamics are often explored. When possible and appropriate, the patient is included in these meetings. This is a good opportunity for problem solving of discharge planning issues and making arrangements for the next level of care. Many factors are considered, such as the availability and adequacy of family and community support and the provision of continued needed care.

Conditions seen for rehabilitation include, but are not limited to, persons who have suffered from the following:

- TBI
- Stroke
- Multiple sclerosis
- Limb loss
- Sports injury
- Vestibular disorders
- Spinal cord injuries
- Developmental delay
- Parkinson's disease
- Muscular dystrophy
- Cerebral palsy
- Amyotrophic lateral sclerosis

Patients requiring rehabilitation often have complex medical, psychological, and social needs that warrant a coordinated and interdisciplinary approach. The definition of the interdisciplinary team "refers to activities performed towards a common goal by individuals from a group of different disciplines" (Melvin, 1980). The members of the interdisciplinary team need to be skilled not only in their specific discipline but in others as well to be effective interdisciplinary team members. The goal should be "to accomplish an outcome which is greater than each functioning separately" (Keith, 1991). This also requires considerable education for the patients, their families, and significant others.

CONTINUUM OF CARE

The delivery of services provided throughout the continuum of care is continually changing as health care reform progresses. The current model in the United States can provide all aspects of rehabilitation care in various settings, noting that the intensity of services in these practice settings varies. Most rehabilitation professionals are available throughout the continuum of care that is described in the following. National, state, and local laws dictate who is authorized to provide these services. In considering the patients' experience through the continuum, the mantra of "nothing about me without me" in health care has fostered professionals to engage patients and families in the overall care delivery and the importance of engagement and partnership at a more robust level

The Patient Protection and Affordable Care Act (PPACA), commonly called the Affordable Care Act (ACA), is the U.S. federal statute signed into law by President Barak Obama on March 23, 2010. Together with the Health Care and Education Reconciliation Act amendment, it represents the most significant regulatory overhaul of the U.S. health care system since the passage of Medicare and Medicaid in 1965. Under the act, hospitals and physicians are to transform their practices financially, technologically, and clinically to ensure better health outcomes, lower costs, and improve their methods of distribution to ensure accessibility. Since its inception, there have been multiple mechanisms to ensure accessibility to all. In March 2015, the Centers for Disease Control and Prevention (CDC) reported that the average number of uninsured during the period from January to September 2014 was 11.4 million fewer than in 2010 (Alonso-Zaldivar, 2015; Pear, 2015).

Rehabilitation is involved in all levels of the continuum of care.

> The core of the law expands coverage, consistency within care, providing structures and accountable cost-efficient, higher quality care. The pressure on PM&R is to develop uniform standards across the post-acute continuum to cope with providing services to 32 million more insured lives and to report numerous quality metrics. (American Medical Rehabilitation Providers Association [AMRPA], 2015)

The opportunity to participate in the full continuum is significant. Several of the areas that PM&R is already actively participating in are the discussion of the CARE tool (Continuity Assessment Record and Evaluation) and implications for practical use across all levels of care, bundled payment initiatives, as well as value-based purchasing and value-based medicine and implications for PM&R to affect cost and care.

The triple aim, described by Institute for Healthcare Improvement, is a framework to navigate health care reform to allow for the optimization of individuals and systems. The three dimensions of the triple aim include population health (better health for the population), experience of care (better care for individuals), and per capita cost (lower cost through improvement). Defining the continuum of care and rehabilitation's involvement in each is critical to understand it as a patient-centered approach to care along with the legislative requirements to manage through each.

The levels of care described in the following text are based on the U.S. health care model.

Acute Care

Acute care is provided in a hospital setting. The patient is typically admitted following an acute injury, medical occurrence, or for a surgical procedure. Length of acute hospitalization varies but is often only a few days, and patients are routinely discharged to another level of care or to their homes when medically stable.

Acute Inpatient Rehabilitation Facility

Patients admitted to acute rehabilitation facilities require around-the-clock medical care but do not require the level of medical service provided in an acute care hospital. Patients are usually transferred to IRF centers after medical stability has been achieved in an acute hospital. These patients must be able to tolerate at least 3 hours of therapy services daily (working with a PT, OT, and/or SLP), require both acute nursing care and physician availability 24 hours a day, and have the ability to make timely functional improvements.

Subacute Rehabilitation

SAR provides care that is less intense than in acute rehabilitation, but patients continue to manifest the potential to improve their functional skills through rehabilitation. Patients are generally required to tolerate only 1 to 2 hours of daily therapy, but will still require acute nursing care 24 hours a day and periodic physician care.

Skilled Nursing Facility

These facilities have distinct beds that allow patients the opportunity to recuperate for an extended period of time, with some therapy services on a daily basis. These designated beds can also be within a freestanding acute licensed rehabilitation hospital, a freestanding long-term care facility, or a freestanding skilled rehabilitation hospital. Patients treated in this setting have fewer acute medical needs than either acute rehabilitation or SAR. It is typically targeted at older, postacute patients who may not be able to tolerate the intensity of acute rehabilitation but who have the capacity for functional recovery.

Home-Based Therapy

Home therapy is provided to patients who need continued rehabilitation but no longer require care within a hospital, subacute facility, or SNF. Patients are typically considered homebound and are therefore incapable of participating in outpatient rehabilitation programs.

Outpatient Therapy

Outpatient services are provided to those patients who no longer require hospital-based therapies and who are not homebound. Services are designed to provide either general rehabilitation to a wide group of individuals or more specialized care to specific groups of patients. Depending on the individual needs of the person being served and the specific discipline prescribed, outpatient therapy is typically provided two to three times per week per discipline. The number of sessions and frequency of treatment depend on the amount of treatment needed and the patient's progress.

Wellness and Prevention Centers

These are centers that are often within community fitness centers, health clubs, or health care facilities. Their goal is to educate, instruct, and promote the practices of wellness and the prevention of illness or injury. A physiatrist and other rehabilitation professionals often refer individuals to these centers after they have had a course of a more traditional rehabilitation. These services are currently very rarely covered by health insurance and are a self-pay option for individuals. The goal of these programs is to support and encourage community reintegration and maintenance of functional outcomes attained during formal rehabilitation services.

Comprehensive Day Treatment Programs

Comprehensive day rehabilitation programs have the goal of preventing long-term institutionalization while providing a daily program of activities. Some comprehensive day rehabilitation programs provide restorative services and are geared toward achieving specific therapeutic end points within a defined period of time, with the goal of living a more independent life in the community. Some common types of day treatment programs include brain injury day treatment programs, adult day treatment programs, and dementia day treatment programs. These programs often provide some degree of respite for full-time care providers of severely disabled individuals. If these programs were otherwise not available, it would necessitate that many individuals be institutionalized due to the level of care they require.

In addition to the various settings designed to assist the patients in recovery, there are also organizations that work on a large scale to improve the lives of people who require rehabilitation services. Most states have governing bodies to assist in policy interpretation and regulations as supportive groups to all levels of health care operations. National organizations such as the AMRPA and the American Congress of Rehabilitation Medicine (ACRM) are bodies within the United States that work to improve rehabilitation care for people with disabilities. WHO is an international leader providing resources and support to hospitals, communities, and individuals with disability. To enhance the quality of life and to promote and protect the rights and dignity of people with disabilities, the key focus is the following:

- Advocacy
- Data collection
- Medical care and rehabilitation
- Community-based rehabilitation
- Assistive devices/technologies
- Capacity building
- Policies

DISABLEMENT MODELS

WHO and other groups have been instrumental in creating models to understand function and disability, which are better known as "disablement models." One of the earliest theories in rehabilitation, and the most familiar, concerns the consequences of disease and injury, that is, disablement, and how they integrate the medical and social models of practice. In the *medical model*, disability is viewed as a "characteristic or attribute of the person, which is directly caused by disease, trauma, or other health condition and requires some type of intervention provided by professionals to 'correct' or 'compensate' for the problem" (Jette, 2006). In the *social model*, disability is viewed as a "socially created problem and not as an attribute of the person." In the social model of disability, the underlying problem is created by an unaccommodating or inflexible environment brought about by the attitudes or features of the social and physical environment itself, which calls for a political and physical response or solution (Jette, 2006). The combination of the medical and social model subsequently is the biopsychosocial model. It attempts to integrate both models of disability. This is the key framework of the disablement model that is widely used today.

Rehabilitation medicine experts had struggled with the concepts and language that describe disablement for decades. Nagi in the 1960s and WHO in the 1980s were among the major contributors to the literature of rehabilitation medicine (Table 1.1).

The World Health Assembly developed a common language and framework to understand and describe similar concepts of rehabilitation. WHO's model of the International Classification of Impairments, Disabilities, and Handicaps (ICIDH; Jette, 2006) was completed in the early 1980s and differentiated health conditions into *impairments, disabilities*, and *handicaps*. Each model works to try to provide a language and a structure to define disablement (Figure 1.2).

The WHO model, currently known as the International Classification of Functioning, Disability and Health (ICF), was not endorsed by the World Health Assembly at the United Nations until 2001, after major revisions from the initial document were made. The intent in the development of the ICF as a disablement model was to provide professionals in the field of rehabilitation medicine a universal, standardized disablement language. One of its goals is to provide a scientific basis for understanding and studying health and health-related disability throughout the world. This common language was designed to help with research, care, and provision of services. The ICF

> provides a standard language and framework for the description of health and health related states. . . . It is a classification of health-related domains—domains that help us to describe changes in body function and structure, what a person with a health condition can do in a standard environment (level of capacity) as well as what they actually do in their usual environment (level of performance). (www.cdc.gov/nchs/data/icd/icfoverview_finalforwho10sept.pdf)

The ICF also lists environmental factors that interact with all these components: "It is the prevailing

TABLE 1.1

DISABLEMENT CONCEPTS AND DEFINITIONS	
Nagi	**International Classification of Functioning, Disability and Health (ICF)**
• *Active pathology*—interruption or interference with normal processes and effort of the organism to regain normal state • *Impairment*—anatomical, physiological, mental, or emotional abnormalities • *Functional limitation*—limitation in performance at the level of the whole organism or person • *Disability*—limitation in performance of socially defined roles and tasks within a sociocultural and physical environment	• *Health conditions*—diseases, disorders, and injuries • *Body function*—physiological functions of body systems • *Body structures*—anatomical parts of the body • *Impairments*—problems in body functions or structure • *Activity*—the execution of a task or an action by an individual • *Activity limitation*—difficulties an individual may have in executing activities • *Participation*—involvement in a life situation • *Participation restriction*—problems an individual may experience in involvement in life situations

Source: Reprinted from the World Health Organization (2001), with permission.

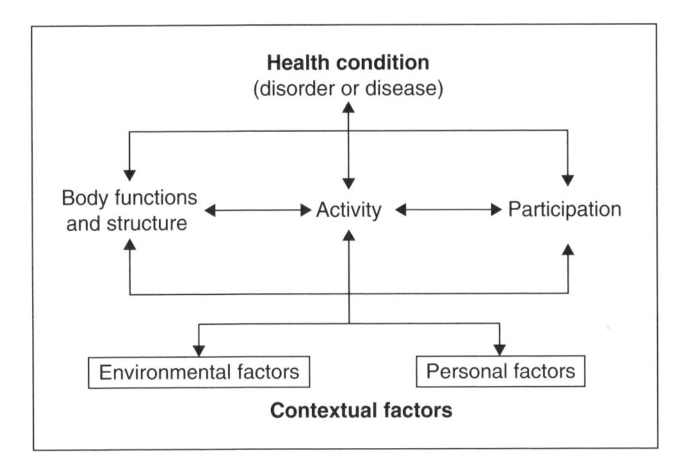

FIGURE 1.2 The International Classification of Functioning, Disability and Health (ICF).

Source: Reprinted from the World Health Organization (2001), with permission.

method of describing disability in the framework of health and function rather than disability" (www.cdc.gov/nchs/data/icd/icfoverview_finalforwho10sept.pdf).

Stineman and Streim (2010) have proposed yet another new model that introduces "Health Environment Integration" or HEI into our health care models. They believe that the current ICF framework does not completely address the needs of the medically complex and environmentally challenged populations that PM&R specialists care for (Stineman & Streim, 2010).

The current disablement model supports the biopsychosocial approach. Stimeman and Streim's approach includes the ecological principles and their impact on disability. We may hear more on this approach in the years to come.

RESEARCH

This is an exciting time for research in rehabilitation. Many challenging unanswered questions need to be resolved. It is always a challenge to conduct a well-designed study, and in rehabilitation, there are several added hurdles. First, there are many team members with overlapping responsibilities. Second, there are many types of disabilities and a multitude of different treatments occurring simultaneously (e.g., surgical, pharmaceutical, various therapies, and medical management). In addition, it is also difficult to isolate how much of an impact rehabilitation has versus the effect of time alone on recovery.

Disease-specific research in rehabilitation holds great promise. For example, what is the etiology of Parkinson's disease and multiple sclerosis? Can these and other conditions be prevented? If we understand the disease process better, we can develop more effective interventions or prevent them altogether. Additionally, research about the efficacy of specific treatment interventions can assist us with providing the most appropriate and effective care for patients in the least amount of time, which can have a favorable effect on the overall cost of health care. With health care reform, access to health care and cost to individuals is changing annually. The goal is to have strong, equal access to care for all.

A specific type of research relates to outcomes achieved by a group of patients receiving care from a defined group of health practitioners. Outcomes data are becoming a more common means of assessing the effectiveness of health care including medical rehabilitation. Outcome measures allow an organization to chart its performance over time and compare its performance with others in the region and the nation.

Many types of outcomes, such as patient satisfaction, can be assessed. These data points are used to analyze how patients report their overall satisfaction with those health care professionals and organizations that provided their care. For example, Press Ganey® is a popular and widely used patient satisfaction tool. This and other similar tools have been found to be valid and reliable and allow comparisons of patient satisfaction between medical centers throughout the country, which use the same tool. However, one difficulty with these types of data is that they are obtained by patients voluntaring to complete a survey, which often includes a majority of those who are either highly satisfied or highly dissatisfied, potentially skewing the results.

Another commonly used outcome assessment in inpatient rehabilitation is the Functional Independence Measure (FIM®), which quantifies a patient's progress and burden of care. The FIM is considered a PM&R industry standard and measures a patient's improvement (or regression) across several standardized domains such as length of inpatient rehabilitation, abilities in locomotion, transfers, dressing, bathing, cognition, and bowel and bladder function. FIM data can be combined among specific diagnostic groups within a particular rehabilitation organization and can be compared with similar patients in other organizations. This type of benchmarking provides a means to compare the magnitude of outcomes a particular rehabilitation organization has on a specific group of patients against others in their immediate area, their state, or even the country. This information can then be used to highlight exemplary care or identify problem areas that may be addressed through quality improvement initiatives.

Although the FIM is the most widely used instrument to measure outcomes, it does have some limitations. For example, one limitation relative to using the FIM in evaluating survivors of TBI is that it is not diagnosis specific. Although found to be reliable and valid, the scale has few cognitive, behavioral, and communication-related functional items relevant to assessing persons with TBI (Center for Outcome Measurement in Brain Injury, 2016). The FIM is a tool that reflects the level of care or assistance a patient needs to perform functional tasks and thus does not necessarily reflect a patient's true functional abilities. For this reason, the collection of additional data such as ambulation distance in addition to the FIM score can provide a more accurate picture of a patient's function (Cournan, 2012).

Outcomes data have led to a critical assessment of inpatient length of stay. Length of stay is a measure of how long a patient remains in the hospital or other setting. Currently, there is a lack of good-quality scientific data to show what the ideal length of stay should be to benefit patients most efficiently with various diagnoses and conditions. To further complicate matters when trying to predict the ideal length of stay, there are individual factors that may influence a patient's rehabilitation course. Patients are unique and thus the patient's age, severity of disability, presence of comorbid conditions, ability to participate in rehabilitation, and intensity of services provided in a particular setting can all have an effect on the length of stay. A patient's progress and change in functional status give important individual information when determining length of stay, but the ideal length of stay for various conditions and presentations remains largely unknown.

Length of stay for inpatient rehabilitation has continually decreased over the past two decades. For example, in the early 1990s, many patients had more than 30 days of continual inpatient care. Today, the average adult patient stays in the inpatient rehabilitation setting for only 12.4 days (Dobson DeVanzo & Associates, 2014). Until optimal length of stay data are clearly delineated, it is likely that inpatient rehabilitation lengths of stay will continue to decrease. Whereas it is certainly initially less costly to have shorter lengths of stay, it remains unclear whether patients receive maximum benefit, or if an early discharge potentially leads to greater disability and cost over time. The current fiscal climate appears to beckon for continued length of stay reductions and this will likely continue until research can show that there is a point of diminishing returns whereby patients with shorter lengths of stay begin to experience worse outcomes as compared with those who experienced a longer length of stay.

Increased regulation in health care has also led to some changes in patients who qualify for admission to inpatient rehabilitation. Certain diseases and conditions are now considered to be best managed at other settings within the continuum of care. This, coupled with the previously mentioned trend toward shorter lengths of stay in inpatient rehabilitation, has caused a shift toward more rehabilitation in the acute care setting, outpatient rehabilitation, SAR, and home-based therapy services for patients who would have previously been accepted into IRFs. We are starting to explore the effects of limiting the patients who qualify for inpatient rehabilitation on outcomes. There is some evidence to support that patients who are admitted to inpatient rehabilitation settings have better outcomes, including lower mortality, fewer readmissions, and more days at home than those who have rehabilitation in SNFs (Dobson DeVanzo & Associates, 2014). This warrants further exploration as it could influence changes in health care regulations.

One example where outcomes data have supported the role of rehabilitation and have had an effect on the delivery of care is in the acute care setting. Recent efforts to study the intensity of services provided by therapists to critically ill patients while in the hospital have yielded promising results. It has been demonstrated that by increasing the amount of rehabilitation provided by therapists in the acute care setting, the overall length of the hospital stay and costs associated with providing care have been reduced. An additional benefit is that patients who receive more intensive rehabilitation in acute care are also more likely to be discharged to home-based and outpatient services rather than facility-based care (Needham, 2010). Outcomes data such as these need to be further explored for all settings, they have implications for health care policy and are critical in establishing the importance of rehabilitation as we all move toward achieving the triple aim in health care.

There are many exciting research questions to answer in the next decade. The answers to these and many other questions that we have not even begun to explore will have a profound influence on rehabilitation care and quality of life for generations to come. Chapter 33 in this book provides additional insight into the important role research plays in the future of health care.

ACCREDITATION

To accredit means to "certify as meeting certain set standards" (Webster's New World College Dictionary, 2004). The accreditation process for a rehabilitation hospital involves review of conformance to written standards outlining best practice principles from a third-party regulatory body. The most widely known rehabilitation accrediting entity is the Commission on Accreditation of Rehabilitation Facilities (CARF©).

CARF was formed in 1966 and is an international independent, nonprofit accreditor of health and human service entities (CARF, 2015). CARF outlines a series of best practice standards, which are created with input from experts in the field across a broad spectrum of the industry.

CARF takes a consultative approach to the accreditation process and focuses on patients' experience and considers patients as its "moral owners" (CARF, 2015). CARF also looks for new and innovative practices in the field, which are considered exemplary. Exemplary practices are groundbreaking and have the potential to profoundly and positively affect the experience of the persons served (the term CARF uses to refer to patients and clients). These new exemplary practices are then shared with the rehabilitation community at large in a process of continuous quality improvement. The goal is that all rehabilitation hospitals and institutes will have access to these new and innovative methods of service delivery. In short, the CARF accreditation process is a systematic means of ensuring quality, value, and optimal outcomes (CARF, 2015). Much more is learned about CARF and other regulatory bodies in Chapter 35 in this textbook.

NEW AREAS OF REHABILITATION AND CURRENT CONCEPTS

Assistive Devices/Technologies

Assistive devices and technologies such as wheelchairs, prostheses, mobility aids, hearing aids, visual aids, and specialized computer software and hardware improve mobility, hearing, vision, and communication capacities. With the aid of technology, people with a loss in functioning are able to enhance their abilities and are better able to live independently and participate in their communities.

In many low-income and middle-income countries, only 5% to 15% of people who require assistive devices and technologies have access to them because their production is low and often of limited quality. There is a scarcity of personnel trained to manage the provision of such devices and technology, especially at the provincial and district levels. In many settings where access might be possible, costs are prohibitive (Eldi & Parkin, 2005).

The U.S. Assistive Technology Act of 1998 defines these devices as "any item, piece of equipment, or product system, whether acquired commercially, modified, or customized, that is used to increase, maintain, or improve the functional capabilities of individuals with disabilities" (Eldi & Parkin, 2005). Accessing this equipment and technology is often a critical component to successfully reintegrating many individuals with their communities, home, school, and work lives.

The CRPD (Articles 20 and 26), the World Health Assembly resolution (WHA58.23), and the UN Standard Rules on the Equalization of Opportunities for Persons with Disabilities all highlight the importance of assistive devices. States are requested to promote access to assistive devices and technologies at an affordable cost and facilitate training for people with disabilities and for professionals and staff working in habilitation and rehabilitation services (Violence and Injury Prevention, 2009).

Safe Patient Handling

Safe patient handling has very recently become a much more mainstream and accepted concept in health care. According to the U.S. Department of Labor's (DOL) Bureau of Labor Statistics, health care occupations rank among the highest in the incidence of work-related musculoskeletal disorders and days away from work resulting from an injury (DOL, 2015). Rehabilitation professionals, in the course of performing their daily work tasks, encounter many opportunities to sustain work-related musculoskeletal injuries. These injuries typically occur during the course of manually assisting patients to move and perform functional tasks. Safe patient handling is a term used to describe the use of assistive equipment to reduce manual patient handling. Adoption of safe patient handling practices, such as the use of mobile lifts, ceiling lifts, and transfer aids, has been shown to reduce the risk of injuries among health care workers (Powell-Cope, 2014), and most hospitals now have a safe patient handling program with staff and technology to support it.

Although safe patient handling techniques have been shown to decrease injury rates for both patients and staff, there are some who have been slow to adopt safe patient handling practices. There are those in rehabilitation who have not been historically as proactive in using safe patient handling equipment as their colleagues from nursing. PTs and OTs have traditionally been slower to adopt safe patient handling, citing concerns that using technology in order to move patients could interfere with their progress with respect to rehabilitation. Research suggests that this is not true. Incorporating safe patient handling practices into treatment has been shown to lead to similar outcomes in rehabilitation (Darragh, Shiyko, Margulis, & Campo, 2014).

To date, 11 states have enacted safe patient handling laws or regulations, and 10 states require a comprehensive program in health care facilities in which there is established policy and guidelines for securing appropriate equipment and training, collection of data, and evaluation (American Nurses Association [ANA], 2015). Although the legislation regarding safe patient handling is similar, there is still some variation in legislation by state, and there is some evidence to suggest that health care facilities rely more on standards of regulatory agencies such as CARF, the Leapfrog group, and the Joint Commission, than they do on legislation to improve safety (Devers, Pham, & Liu, 2004).

Rehabilitation professionals have a unique role in the care of patients and are experts in patient handling. In the future, rehabilitation professionals should focus on establishing themselves as leaders in safe patient handling by developing unique ways to use existing safe patient handling equipment to enhance treatment and consult with companies to design equipment to meet patients' needs.

Disasters, Disability, and Rehabilitation

Disasters are times of great stress and challenge for all people. This is just as true of natural disasters (e.g., hurricanes, tornadoes, floods, earthquakes, volcanic activity) as it is with man-made disasters (e.g., acts of terrorism, industrial accidents, blackouts). For people with disabilities, a disaster of any kind often presents exponential challenges. As was witnessed during Super Storm Sandy in 2012 as flooding reached the east side of Manhattan, able-bodied patients in a hospital walked down the stairs to evacuate when the power failed and the elevators stopped operating. Those who were bedbound, wheelchair dependent, or who needed assistance required alternative means of evacuation (e.g., Med Sleds®).

Hospitals have special resources and are equipped to respond to many types of emergencies. This may not be the case for people with disabilities residing in their home. Planning well in advance of a disaster by both able-bodied people and those with disabilities is an essential component of ensuring safety. For example, having a "Go Bag" ready at all times with essential items (e.g., flashlights, extra batteries, medications, medical supplies, medical contact information, water, and nonperishable food items [Ready New York, 2015]) will help ensure access to needed resources. It is also important for people with disabilities to alert local emergency services (e.g., fire department, emergency medical services [EMS]) about their needs prior to and during an emergency (e.g., requiring emergency generator power for medical devices during a blackout or other causes of loss of electricity). Emergency services may also be able to provide resources if elevators and/or lifts stop operating during a disaster and an individual needs assistance to exit the home to a more secure area.

Many governmental bodies and organizations now provide resources for people with disabilities before, during, and after a disaster (e.g., Red Cross, WHO, and Federal Emergency Management Agency [FEMA]).

> Disasters have an impact on disability, by disproportionately affecting persons with existing disabilities and by creating a new generation of persons with disabilities who will be in need of rehabilitation services. In settings where resources are limited, the impact of disasters on these groups of people can be long term and far reaching. (www.barackobama.com [2009]; www.who.int/violence_injury_prevention [2009])

Local and institutional emergency preparedness has become more of a recognized need, the resolution of which rehabilitation professionals are actively involved.

In addition, it is important that people with disabilities be part of the planning committees for designing resources, plans, and educational materials for emergency management (National Organization on Disability, 2015). As issues arise, the impact on individuals with disabilities can be addressed by rehabilitation professionals who are readily available to aid them. Some issues significantly affecting those with a disability during a disaster may include the following:

- Persons with disabilities are often more at risk of injury or abandonment.
- Many persons with disabilities lose their assistive devices, including prostheses, crutches, hearing aids, and glasses.

Rehabilitation infrastructure is often disrupted during a disaster because care providers are often diverted, cannot reach the individuals in need whom they care for, or are injured themselves. Therefore, individuals with special needs are left in even greater need.

Preparation is the key to being able to sustain oneself during an emergency or natural disaster. Many important lessons have been learned during recent devastating natural disasters such as the earthquakes in Nepal, Haiti, and Pakistan, Super Storm Sandy, and the tsunami in Japan. We also have learned repeatedly that much more needs to be done to prepare for future disasters and the larger impact disasters have on people with disabilities.

Technology and Innovation in Rehabilitation

Technology is continuously being developed to assist with solving everyday problems encountered in all areas of health care, and it is becoming more prevalent in rehabilitation. Robotics is an area that has seen tremendous growth recently. Advancements are being made in the implantation of cerebral electrodes in patients with spinal cord injury as an area of future interest and promise (Blakeslee, 2009).

The use of computer chips embedded in people's bodies and brains may sound like science fiction, but the technology is already here. Computer chips or microelectrodes embedded in the cerebral cortices of the human brain are currently allowing some people with paralysis to control robotic arms (Hiremath, 2015). The technology, known as brain–computer interface (BCI) connects the human brain to robotic components. Now some individuals with paralysis can not only move a robotic arm but they can "sense" the actions and reactions of the robotic arm as well. BCI research is very likely to expand much further and be refined to enhance its utility. It is also likely that the use of robotic arms will expand to the use of robotic legs, and people with amputations or paralysis will exert sophisticated and more coordinated control of robotic components with their thoughts.

On a more macroscopic scale, we are also already seeing the use of implanted mechanical heart assists (e.g., left ventricle assist device—an implanted mechanical assist device that replaces the work of the failing left ventricle). The use of robotic gait systems and robotic upper extremity devices in rehabilitation after a loss of function now enables patients to move their affected extremities in normal physiologic patterns to increase muscle strength and range of motion. We are seeing better and lighter exoskeletons that help patients with spinal cord injuries to walk and even negotiate stairs. These devices are now being further developed so that one day they will be used with patients who have had strokes, brain injuries, or other diagnoses. We are also seeing this technology start to expand beyond the rehabilitation setting and enter the home. Although initially exoskeletons were only available to those who were having rehabilitation in inpatient or outpatient facilities, some are currently approved by the U.S. Food and Drug Administration (FDA) and available for people living with spinal cord injury to use on a daily basis in their homes and the community.

This merging of technologies and the pace at which innovation in health care technology is moving are very exciting to the rehabilitation community. The merging of robotics and biology are exciting frontiers in rehabilitation. Computer technology is also empowering patients in rehabilitation. The use of technology to help with communication is upcoming. Many patients whose illness precluded or limited communication (e.g., being mechanically ventilated or having a severe stroke) will now have several options to restore communication via various computer applications. This is critical, as many patients have reported the loss of the ability to communicate as one of the most frightening situations to experience in a hospital setting.

As devices become more mainstream and clinicians become more familiar with using technology, even greater innovation will be possible. Makerspaces associated with hospitals and rehabilitation centers are beginning to be developed where people can work to come up with solutions for everyday problems encountered in health care. A makerspace, also known as a hackerspace or an innovation lab, is a physical space where people have access to technology, including three-dimensional printers, electronics, and other supplies, and can create devices to be used for patient care. Development of such spaces where rehabilitation professionals can collaborate with engineers and other technological specialists is an important step in the future of rehabilitation innovation and technology.

Rehabilitation should be at the forefront of prevention. For a variety of reasons, prevention is not prominently promulgated or incentivized in the United States. The reasons for this disconnect are variable (e.g., the high value placed on independence and free choice, insurance companies with little or no structured programs for rewards to embark on a healthy lifestyle). Building incentives for an active, healthy lifestyle may decrease the burden of type 2 diabetes, stroke, some forms of cancer, and so forth. In addition, some diseases and future disabilities can be predicted and possibility averted. For example, based on changes in gait speed and simple balance testing, it can be predicted who will likely fall in the near future. An annual wellness visit to a rehabilitation professional may highlight these areas of concern, prompting the initiation of treatment that possibly decreases the occurrence of falls. This model of prevention has the potential for saving a great deal of individual pain and suffering, reducing overall disabilities, and decreasing health care dollars by reducing the need for emergency medical procedures (e.g., corrective surgery after an injury from a fall and resultant hospitalization).

Rehabilitation is entering a renaissance period. Nearly all research studies on outcomes in the field have shown favorable results. Rehabilitation has been shown to decrease length of stay, decrease delirium, improve function, improve cognition, increase quality of life, assist with individuals staying at home/in their communities rather than in health care facilities, and decrease health care costs overall. The Institute of Medicine has defined health care quality as "the degree to which health services for individuals and populations increase the likelihood of desired health outcomes and are consistent with current professional knowledge." Rehabilitation fosters function. The more we study function in a systematic fashion, the more it is evident that function transcends everything. "As we function, so shall we live" (Granger & Kishner, 2015). Rehabilitation naturally interfaces with nearly every element of the hospital and almost all medical specialties. It has been shown that the added staffing costs of adding rehabilitation services to a hospital is offset by decreased average direct costs, medication use, medical–surgical supplies, and decreased length of stay (Lord et al., 2013). At some point, nearly all of us will need rehabilitation services. As we enter this renaissance period of rehabilitation, people will begin to receive optimal value, outcomes, and benefit from these services.

REFERENCES

Alonso-Zaldivar, R. (2015). *Uninsured down more than 11 million since passage of Obama's health care law, CDC reports*. Associated Press.

American Nurses Association. (2015). Safe Patient Handling and Mobility (SPHM). Retreived from http://www.nursingworld.org/MainMenuCategories/Policy-Advocacy/State/Legislative-Agenda-Reports/State-SafePatientHandling

American Medical Rehabilitation Providers Association. (2015, September). Volume 18, No.9

Blakeslee, S. (2009). Researchers train minds to move matter. *The New York Times*, p. 6.

CARF. (2015). *Medical Rehabilitation Standards Manual July 1, 2015–July 30, 2015*. Tucson, AZ: Commission on Accreditation of Rehabilitation Facilities.

Center for Outcome Measurement in Brain Injury. (2016). Introduction to the Functional Assessment Measure. Retrieved from http://www.tbims.org/combi/FAM

Conti, A. A. (2014). Western medical rehabilitation through time: A historical and epistemological review. *The Scientific World Journal, 2014*, 1–5.

Cournan, M. (2012). Use of the functional independence measure for outcomes measurement in acute inpatient rehabilitation. *Rehabilitation Nursing, 36*(3), 111–117.

Darragh, A. R., Shiyko, M., Margulis, H., & Campo, M. (2014). Effects of a safe patient handling and mobility program on patient self-care outcomes. *American Journal of Occupational Therapy, 68*(5), 589–596.

Devers, K. J., Pham, H. H., & Liu, G. (2004). What is driving hospitals' patient safety efforts. *Patient Safety, 23*(2), 103–115.

Dobson DeVanzo & Associates. (2014). Assessment of patient outcomes of rehabilitative care provided in inpatient rehabilitation facilities (IRFs) and after discharge. Retrieved from https://www.amrpa.org/newsroom/Dobson%20DaVanzo%20Final%20Report%20-%20Patient%20Outcomes%20of%20IRF%20v%20%20SNF%20-%207%2010%2014%20redated.pdf

Donovan, W. H. (2007). Spinal cord injury: Past, present and future. *The Journal of Spinal Cord Medicine, 30*, 85–100.

Eldi, H., & Parkin, C. (2005). *Expanding assistive technology services for the departments of physical therapy and occupational therapy at NYU Medical Center* (Unpublished manuscript).

Folz, T. J., Opitz, J. L., Peters, D. J., & Gelfman, R. (1997). The history of physical medicine and rehabilitation as recorded in the diary of Dr. Frank Krusen: Part 2. Forging ahead (1943–1947). *Archives of Physical Medicine & Rehabilitation, 78*, 446–450.

Granger, C. V., & Kishner, S. (2015, October 16). Quality and outcome measures for rehabilitation programs. *Medscape*.

Haig, A. J., Nagy, A., Lebreck, D. B., & Stein, G. L. (1995). Outpatient planning for persons with physical disabilities: A randomized prospective trial of physiatrist alone versus a multidisciplinary team. *Archives of Physical Medicine and Rehabilitation, 76*, 341–348.

Hiremath, S. V., Chen W., Wang, W., Foldes, S., Yang Y., Tyler-Kabara E. C., . . . Boninger, M. L. (2015). Brain computer interface learning for systems based on electrocorticography and intracortical microelectrode arrays. *Frontiers in Integrative Neuroscience*, *9*, 40.

Jette, A. M. (2006). Toward a common language for function, disability, and health. *Physical Therapy, 86*, 726–734.

Keith, R. (1991). The comprehensive treatment team in rehabilitation. *Archives of Physical Medicine and Rehabilitation, 72*, 269–274.

Klinar, I., Ferhatovic, L., Banozic, A., Raguz, M., Kostic, S., Sapunar, D., & Puljak, L. (2013). Physicians' attitudes about interprofessional treatment of chronic pain: Family physicians are considered the most important collaborators. *Scandinavian Journal of Caring Sciences*, *27*(2), 303–310.

Kress, J. P., & Hall, J. B. (2014). CU-acquired weakness and recovery from critical illness. *New England Journal of Medicine*, *370*(17), 1626–1635. doi:10.1056/NEJMra1209390

Locatelli, S. M., Turcios, S., & LaVela, S. L. (2014). Veterans' experiences of patient-centered care: Learning from guided tours. *Patient Experience Journal*, *1*(1), 88–94.

Lord, R. K., Mayhew, C. R., Korupolu, R., Mantheiy, E. C., Friedman, M. A., Palmer, J. B., & Needham, D. M. (2013). ICU Early physical rehabilitation programs: Financial modeling of cost savings. *Critical Care Medicine, 41*(3), 717–724.

Melvin, J. L. (1980). Interdisciplinary and multidisciplinary activities and the ACRM. *Archives of Physical Medicine & Rehabilitation, 61*, 379–380.

National Organization on Disability. (2015). Retrieved from www.nod.org

Needham, D. M., Korupolu, R., Zanni, J. M., Pradhan, P., Colantuoni, E., Palmer, J. B., . . . Fan, E. (2010). Early physical medicine and rehabilitation for patients with acute respiratory failure: A quality improvement project. *Archives of Physical Medicine & Rehabilitation*, *91*(4), 536–542.

Ohry, A. (2004). Clinical commentary—people with disabilities before the days of modern rehabilitation medicine: Did they pave the way? *Disability & Rehabilitation, 26*, 546–548.

Paradis, E., Leslie, M., Gropper, M. A., Aboumater, H. J., Kitto, S., & Reeves, S. (2013). Interprofessional care in intensive care settings and the factors that impact it: Results from a scoping review of ethnographic studies. *Journal of Critical Care*, *28*(6), 1062–1067.

Pear, R. (2015). Number of uninsured has declined by 15 million since 2013, administration says. *The New York Times*, A11.

Peters, D. J., Gelfman, R., Folz, T. J., & Opitz, J. L. (1997). The history of physical medicine and rehabilitation as recorded in the diary of Dr. Frank Krusen: Part 4. Triumph over adversity (1954–1969). *Archives of Physical Medicine & Rehabilitation, 78*, 562–565.

Powell-Cope, G., Toyinbo, P., Patel, N., Rugs, D., Elnitsky, C., Hahm, B., . . . Hodgson, M. (2014). Effects of a national safe patient handling program on nursing injury incidence rates. *Journal of Nursing Administration*, *44*(10), 525–534.

Ready New York. (2015). Retrieved from www1.nyc.gov

Rusk, H. A. (1977). *A world to care for–the autobiography of Howard A. Rusk, MD*. New York, NY: Random House/Reader's Digest Association.

Stineman, M. G., & Streim, J. E. (2010). The biopsycho-ecological paradigm: A foundational theory for medicine. *PM&R: The Journal of Injury, Function, and Rehabilitation*, *2*(11), 1035–1045.

U.S. Department of Labor. (2015). Bureau of Labor Statistics: Nonfatal occupational injuries and illnesses requiring days away from work. Retrieved from http://www.bls.gov/news.release/osh2.nr0.htm

Violence and Injury Prevention. (2009). Retrieved from www.who.int/violence_injury_prevention

Webster's New World College Dictionary 4th Edition. (2004). *M. Agnes, editor in chief; D.B. Guralnik, editor in chief (1951–1985)*. Cleveland, OH: Wiley Publishing.

World Health Organization. (2001). *International classification of functioning, disability and health: ICF*. Geneva, Switzerland.

World Health Organization. (2014). *Disability and rehabilitation WHO action plan 2014–2021*. Retrieved from http://www.who.int/disabilities/about/action_plan/en

CHAPTER

Disabling Conditions Seen in AIDS and HIV Infection

Komal G. Patel, Natalie Hyppolite, Matthew Shatzer, and Marcia Epstein

A clinician should view HIV infection as a spectrum of illnesses ranging from the primary infection to the most advanced stage known as AIDS. HIV is caused by one of two retroviruses, HIV-1 or HIV-2, the former being more common worldwide and leading to a hastier decline in immune function. Both viruses share a common mode of transmission via sexual exposure, through contact with blood or other bodily fluids, vertically from mother to child during birth, or via breast milk.

The Centers for Disease Control and Prevention (CDC) estimates the prevalence of people living with HIV/AIDS in the United States at more than 1.2 million, with an incidence of greater than 50,000 new infections annually (CDC, 2013). The number of newly HIV-infected patients is highest in the 25- to 34-year-old range (CDC, 2013). Major risk groups continue to be men who have sex with other men and African Americans (Cohen, Hellmann, Levy, DeCock, & Lange, 2008). The burden of HIV infections falls disproportionally on minority populations, in particular, African Americans who comprise 54% of the total living cases, on the basis of the 2011 data (CDC, 2013). This being said, high-risk heterosexual contacts did account for 32% of transmitted HIV infections in 2007 (CDC, 2013).

The hallmark of HIV disease is a profound immunodeficiency that results from a progressive quantitative and qualitative deficiency in the subset of T lymphocytes known as T-helper, or cluster of differentiation 4+ (CD4+), cells (González-Scarano & Martín-García, 2005). Theoretically, any cell in the body that expresses the CD4+ molecule on its cell surface has the potential to get infected with the HIV virus; however, two other major coreceptors, C-C chemokine receptor 5 (CCR5) and C-X-C chemokine receptor 4 (CXCR4), need also to be present to promote efficient HIV passage through the T-cell membrane.

The CDC has recently updated its guidelines on how to test for HIV. Testing begins with a combination immunoassay that detects HIV-1 and HIV-2 antibodies and HIV-1 p24 antigen (fourth-generation HIV immunoassay). All specimens that are reactive on this initial assay undergo supplemental testing with an immunoassay that differentiates HIV-1 from HIV-2 antibodies. Specimens that are reactive on the initial immunoassay and nonreactive or indeterminate on the antibody differentiation assay proceed to HIV-1 nucleic acid testing (HIV-1 NAT) for resolution.

For HIV-infected patients, measurement of the CD4+ T-cell count and the level of plasma HIV RNA replication (also known as viral load) are considered part of routine evaluation and monitoring. The CD4+ T-cell count provides information about the current immunological status of the patient, prognosticating which complications an infected individual is at the greatest risk of developing and helping to guide which prophylactic medications a given patient should be on to help prevent opportunistic infections. The viral load, on the other hand, predicts the likely future immunological health of the patient. The viral load also assesses a patient's compliance with and the effectiveness of a given antiretroviral regimen. The goal of therapy is to maximally suppress the measurable plasma HIV to below the lower limit of detection of the viral load assay with the utilization of highly active antiretroviral therapy (HAART). Medications have improved over the years in order to reduce the side effect profile and to more directly target the virus.

Severe and disabling conditions associated with HIV become more common as the patient's CD4+ count declines and the illness progresses. The key elements in treating complications of HIV disease are simultaneously achieving control of HIV replication through the use of combination antiretroviral therapy (ART) and implementing therapies directed at curing or mitigating the disabling HIV-associated conditions.

The remainder of this chapter reviews specific conditions that may create disability in persons infected with HIV.

PERIPHERAL NEUROPATHIES

Peripheral nerve damage is the most common neurological complication for individuals with HIV/AIDS. It is estimated that nearly one third of the people with HIV/AIDS acquire this complication, making it the most common neurological complication in these patients.

There are a host of mechanisms underlying the pathophysiology of peripheral neuropathy in HIV/AIDS patients. The virus itself, the medications used to treat HIV/AIDS, and opportunistic infections all play a role in the damage of peripheral nerves. Peripheral neuropathy typically presents as abnormal sensation in the distal extremities, often described as burning, stiffness, prickling, tingling, pins and needles, or numbness. Patients often note a loss of feeling in their toes and soles of their feet. More commonly, the peripheral nerves of the feet are affected, but those in the fingers, hands, and wrists can also be involved. This distribution of symptoms is referred to as a "stocking–glove" pattern, which is characteristic of peripheral neuropathy. Symptoms may progress proximal to the ankles or wrists, indicating more severe nerve damage.

Distal Symmetric Peripheral Neuropathy

The most common form of peripheral neuropathy in this patient population is distal symmetric peripheral neuropathy (DSPN). There are two categories of DSPN (Cornblath & McArthur, 1988). The first type is associated with the HIV organism damaging the peripheral nerves directly. Increased viral loads and immunosuppression puts the patient at a higher risk of developing DSPN. This mechanism of neuropathic injury was by far the most common cause of peripheral neuropathy in the era prior to powerful antiretroviral medications (Ferrari et al., 2006). With the advancement in HIV treatment, the second type of DSPN, antiretroviral-induced toxic peripheral neuropathy, has become the more common cause of nerve damage in these patients (Barohn et al., 1993). Didanosine and stavudine, drugs previously used to treat HIV, are no longer recommended because of their potent neurotoxic effects (Cherry et al., 2006).

DSPN, like most peripheral neuropathies, typically produces complaints of painful or uncomfortable paresthesias. Symptoms may include allodynia, which is a painful response to a stimulus that is not typically painful. Other descriptions may be those of a sensation of pins and needles, burning, and/or numbness, all of which typically begin distally and progress proximally (Cornblath & McArthur, 1988). DSPN has been found to be more common in the late stages of HIV disease, when generalized wasting and cachexia may also be present.

The clinical presentation of antiretroviral-induced neuropathy is similar to the symptoms of DSPN. Although the exact pathophysiology is unclear, the underlying mechanism is thought to be related to mitochondrial toxicity caused by these therapeutic agents (Lehmann, Chen, Borzan, Mankowski, & Hoke, 2011). Among the pharmacological treatments, nucleoside analogs, such as abacavir, didanosine, lamivudine, and stavudine, are most commonly associated with this type of neuropathy.

The decrease in sensation due to neuropathy places the individual at risk of injury to the skin, soft tissue, and/or underlying bone of the affected area, thus increasing the likelihood of related infections, such as cellulitis and osteomyelitis. In addition, lack of sensation increases the risk of falls and related injuries, resulting from decreased proprioception (knowing where one's limb is in space) as well as the patient having difficulty sensing obstacles in his or her path.

Prior to beginning treatment, the medical practitioner should first evaluate for alternative etiologies underlying the peripheral neuropathy. This may include nutritional or metabolic deficiencies, such as depleted stores of vitamin B12 or folate, which may be the cause of or a contributing factor to the development of neuropathy. Treatment is primarily symptomatic and may include various medications to dampen the intensity of the uncomfortable sensations. These include tricyclic antidepressants (TCAs), anticonvulsants, and other typical and atypical pain medications. Gabapentin, an anticonvulsant, and duloxetine, a TCA, are two other commonly prescribed medications. Experimentally, pathogenesis-based approaches have shown promising results, such as HAART (Dwyer, Mayer, & Lee, 1992). Recombinant human nerve growth factor has also been used experimentally with significant improvement in the patient's pain (Engsig et al., 2009).

Necrotizing Vasculitis–Associated Neuropathy

Necrotizing vasculitis has been described in patients with HIV (Garstang, 2002). This condition is an immunologically induced process causing an inflammatory response resulting in necrosis of the vasa nervorum—the blood vessels that nourish the peripheral nerves. The clinical syndromes that arise from vascular damage include a distal symmetrical neuropathy or a mononeuritis multiplex, which is damage or death of multiple individual nerves. Distal neuropathy, the most common clinical manifestation of vasculitic neuropathy, usually presents with pain, weight loss, and myalgias. CD4+ counts are usually below 600/mL in patients who are affected. This form of neuropathy is relatively rare, affecting only 0.1% to 0.3% of patients with AIDS. The clinical course can be monophasic, but patients often have relapses. In many patients, there is an overlap with hepatitis B or C and cryoglobulinemia diseases. An evaluation for opportunistic infections associated with vasculitides, such as cytomegalovirus (CMV), *Mycobacterium tuberculosis*, and fungal parasitic infections, should be performed.

The gold standard in diagnosing necrotizing vasculitic neuropathy is by nerve and muscle biopsies that reveal inflammatory cell infiltrates and necrosis of blood vessels. Therapy presents a peculiar problem, as most immunosuppressive or cytotoxic agents regularly used to treat vasculitides are contraindicated in patients with HIV. Options for treatment include corticosteroids, intravenous γ-globulin, and plasmapheresis, which have been used successfully in combination with antiretroviral treatment (Gonzalez-Duarte, Robinson-Papp, & Simpson, 2008).

MUSCLE DISORDERS

Severe muscle wasting from repeated infections, malignancy, malabsorption, and nutritional deficiency often accounts for weakness and disability seen in patients with HIV/AIDS. Such wasting is characterized by loss of lean body muscle mass and is associated with muscle weakness. Although weakness may be associated with nervous system involvement from infections or immunologically mediated neuropathies, the possibility of a primary skeletal muscle disease should not be excluded, as several musculoskeletal disorders causing weakness have been identified in HIV-infected patients.

Myopathy

A review of nearly 5,000 HIV-infected patients demonstrated a 0.2% prevalence of myopathy (Griffiths, 2004). The affected individuals generally present with myalgias and symmetric proximal muscle weakness, with a predilection for the lower extremities. Rarely, patients encounter myopathy as their presenting manifestation of HIV infection. It may, however, occur in the setting of already established AIDS. Unlike neuropathy, the development of myopathy does not correlate with the degree of immunosuppression or CD4+ T-cell levels. The pathogenesis of HIV myositis is not well understood, but there are two theories—direct invasion of HIV itself into the muscle and cell-mediated immunological response by the virus. HIV myositis tends to have a good prognosis, responding well to immunosuppressive therapy (Johnson, Williams, Kazi, Dimachkie, & Reveille, 2003).

HIV-associated myopathies include polymyositis and dermatomyositis, zidovudine (AZT) myopathy, rhabdomyolysis, nemaline rod myopathy, inclusion body myositis, myasthenia gravis, HIV wasting syndrome, myopathy associated with local neoplasm, and myopathy associated with local infection (Lyons, Venna, & Cho, 2011). Opportunistic muscle infections are encountered in untreated patients, whereas treated patients are more likely to develop inflammatory myopathies or drug-induced muscle involvement.

In early HIV infection, polymyositis, dermatomyositis, and nemaline rod myopathy may occur. Polymyositis and dermatomyositis are immune mediated and are similar in presentation to patients who do not have HIV. Symptoms include generalized and progressive muscle weakness that develops gradually and tends to target proximal muscles such as those in the shoulders, hips, thighs, and neck. Nemaline rod myopathy, although rare, is characterized by slowly progressive weakness and muscle wasting, which may be autoimmune in nature (Haas et al., 2004). Later in the disease process, AZT-related myopathy may occur once therapy for HIV has begun (Hall et al., 2008). Patients with this condition present with proximal muscle weakness, myalgias of the calves and thighs, and easy fatigability. In the later stages of HIV disease, myopathy may be caused by a local infection, such as toxoplasmosis, or from neoplasm, such as non-Hodgkin's lymphoma or Kaposi's sarcoma. In the setting of an infection, affected muscles become painful and swollen, with variable presence of fever and fatigue. There have been a few reported cases of myasthenia gravis in patients with HIV, but it is unclear whether this is a coincidence or an immunologically mediated process. In most of these cases, the symptoms of myasthenia gravis were transient.

Treatment of HIV-related myopathy is based on its etiology. Just as polymyositis and dermatomyositis patients without HIV are treated with corticosteroids, so are HIV-infected individuals. Responders to corticosteroid therapy generally improve in strength within 1 to 2 months. Patients who are unresponsive to steroids are often treated with an alternative immunosuppressant, such as azathioprine, cyclosporine, or methotrexate, but these medications must be used with caution (Reveille & Williams, 2006). Intravenous immunoglobulin treatments may help some people who are also unresponsive to other immunosuppressants. Patients with nemaline rod myopathy also respond to corticosteroid treatment (Horberg et al., 2008). In AZT myopathy, the offending medication is discontinued and alternative treatment initiated. Muscle enzymes and muscle strength usually return to normal within a few months after AZT is discontinued. Opportunistic infections that cause myositis, such as toxoplasmosis, respond well to antibiotic therapy. The treatment of choice for extrapulmonary toxoplasmosis is a combination of pyrimethamine and sulfadiazine.

HIV-Associated Neuromuscular Wasting Syndrome

This syndrome includes neuromuscular clinical manifestations such as progressive myopathy and a rapidly progressing sensorimotor polyneuropathy. In HIV-associated neuromuscular wasting syndrome (HANWS), patients present with progressive weakness, weight loss, and metabolic abnormalities such as elevated serum lactate and liver function tests. Neurological manifestations vary, as there is a spectrum of pathologies. Many patients exhibit clinical features of demyelination, which results in slowing of nerve conduction as myelin normally surrounds neuronal axons to increase the speed of signal transmission. However, the majority of patients have primary axonal pathology, caused by direct involvement of the nerve. The axonal form of this syndrome carries a worse prognosis than the demyelinating type. When elevated serum lactate develops in the setting of therapy with nucleoside reverse transcriptase inhibitors, there is a high likelihood that HANWS will develop. Systemic symptoms may include nausea, vomiting, abdominal distention, weight loss, and hepatomegaly, which are associated with a rapidly ascending motor weakness that develops over days to weeks. This syndrome may mimic Guillain-Barré syndrome, which is an autoimmune process directed against peripheral nerves, and can result in respiratory failure and death (Griffiths, 2004).

The pathogenesis of HANWS in HIV-infected patients is likely to be multifactorial and may result from a combination of mitochondrial and immunological mechanisms caused by HIV disease, although HAART therapy may contribute as well. Although a majority of patients present with alterations in their axonal structure, intravenous immunoglobulin or plasmapheresis could be considered as possible treatment options if demyelination is felt to be a contributing factor. The treatment of HANWS is controversial, because it is a potentially fatal syndrome that requires the interruption of HAART therapy. The reintroduction of HAART then becomes quite challenging, requiring that other therapeutic options be considered.

SPINAL CORD DISEASES

Vacuolar Myelopathy

Vacuolar myelopathy (VM) is the most common disease afflicting the spinal cord in those infected with HIV and has been found in up to 50% of

AIDS-infected individuals at autopsy (Dal Pan, Glass, & McArthur, 1994). Clinical manifestations are seen in advanced pathologic states and approximately a quarter of the patients with VM display symptoms during life. It is a slowly progressive painless spastic paraparesis, with proprioceptive impairment, sensory ataxia, and neurogenic bladder and bowel. Changes in the manner in which electrical activity is transmitted in the sensory nerves during electrodiagnostic testing may precede clinical symptoms. The specific cause of VM is unknown but is thought to be related to an abnormal transmethylation process activated by the virus or other immunopathologic by-products. Histopathologically, VM is a demyelinating condition characterized by prominent vacuolar changes in the myelin sheaths of tracts of the dorsal columns and dorsal half of the lateral columns of the spinal cord, with a particular affinity for the thoracic region (Figure 2.1). This type of myelopathy is only clinically symptomatic in about 5% to 10% of AIDS patients. Most patients who develop this disease die within 6 months of developing related symptoms. This typically occurs during the later stages of HIV infection, when other neurological problems may be present as well, including peripheral neuropathies, dementia, and opportunistic central nervous system (CNS) and peripheral nervous system infections or malignancies. VM is not typically fatal but rather a cause of significant disability (Jose, Saravu, Jimmy, & Shastry, 2007).

There is no specific treatment that has been proven to be effective for VM, but the use of aggressive antiretroviral regimens to manage viral load may help with symptom improvement. Treatments are symptomatic and aimed at relief from spasticity, managing neurogenic bladder and bowel, and improving function with multidisciplinary rehabilitation.

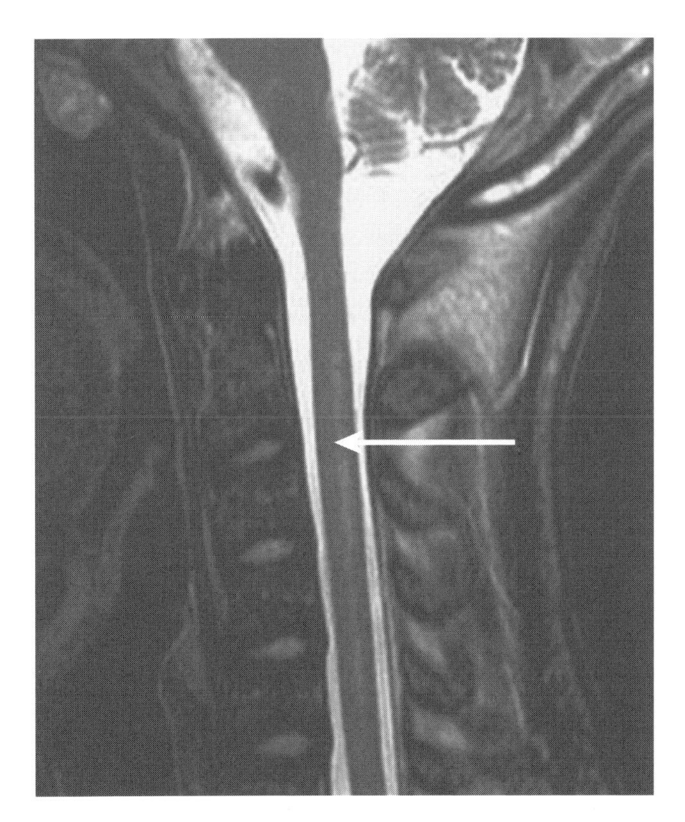

FIGURE 2.1 Sagittal T2-weighted MRI scan of the cervical spinal cord in a patient with vacuolar myelopathy. There is increased signal in the spinal cord noted by arrow.

Source: Courtesy of Rona Woldenberg.

Infectious Myelitis

Infectious myelitis in patients with HIV may result from a variety of different etiologies. The involvement of the spinal cord in patients with HIV can be caused by either HIV itself or other opportunistic infections. These infections may be bacterial, viral, or fungal in nature.

Varicella zoster is one of the viruses associated with HIV in many cases. Varicella zoster myeloradiculitis in patients with HIV sometimes coexists with encephalitis as well. Varicella myelitis usually involves the dorsal horns of the spinal cord because the infection spreads from the dorsal root ganglia through the posterior roots (Figure 2.2).

Patients often note burning pain and hypersensitive skin, which is then followed by the characteristic rash. The blistering rash follows a dermatomal pattern (representing the sensory distribution of a particular nerve), which appears as a bandlike pattern on the skin. The lesions will eventually crust over and

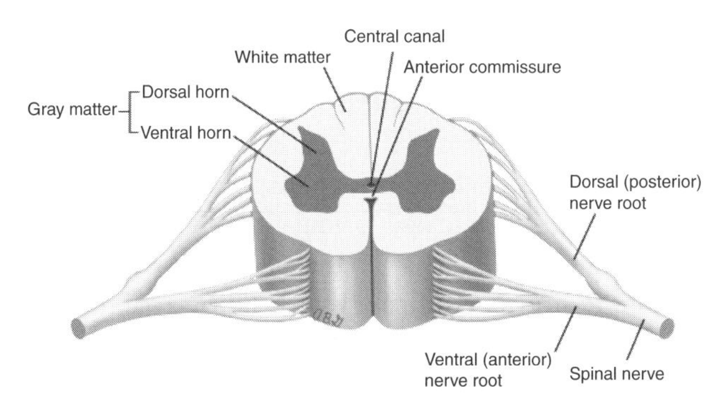

FIGURE 2.2 Basic anatomy of spinal cord, representing the dorsal (posterior) and ventral (anterior) horns and nerve roots.

heal. The duration of a typical outbreak lasts 3 to 4 weeks prior to full resolution. Motor weakness may accompany the typical sensory symptoms. Treatment includes pain medications as well as antiviral agents and oral corticosteroids (Di Rocco, 1999).

Bacterial infections causing myelitis tend to be rare in HIV patients, with *M. tuberculosis* being the most common pathogen. Tuberculosis (TB) is the most common opportunistic infection worldwide affecting HIV-infected persons and is the most common cause of death in these patients. Involvement of the spine by TB is known as Pott's disease. The signs and symptoms of Pott's disease include back pain, fever, night sweats, weight loss, focal neurological deficits determined by the level of spinal cord involvement, and paraspinal masses. In adults, the lumbar region is the most commonly involved. Treatment includes long-term multidrug antituberculous therapy. Surgery may occasionally be indicated to prevent progressive neurological decline or spinal deformity. Overall, the prognosis for recovery is excellent with a recovery rate of more than 90% with appropriate treatment (Kalichman, Heckman, Kochman, Sikkema, & Bergholte, 2000).

HTLV-1 Myelopathy

Human T-cell lymphotropic virus type 1 (HTLV-1) is commonly found in tropical climates such as the Caribbean, South America, Melanesian islands, central and southern Africa, Papua New Guinea, the Middle East, and southern Japan. It is rarely found in North America and Europe and occurs more commonly in women than men. It is transmitted through sexual, parenteral, and maternal routes; thus, risk factors for infection include intravenous drug use, promiscuous sexual activity, and the presence of HIV disease. HTLV-1 myelopathy is found in a small percentage of patients infected with the virus and causes pyramidal, spinocerebellar, and spinothalamic tract inflammation, with less involvement of the posterior columns. The clinical manifestations of HTLV-1 myelopathy include a slowly progressive spastic paraparesis, segmental sensory abnormalities, urinary dysfunction, and back pain. HTLV-1 is diagnosed based on clinical suspicion and is confirmed with laboratory testing demonstrating HTLV-1 antibodies in the serum and cerebrospinal fluid (CSF; Geraci et al., 2000). Magnetic resonance imaging of the spinal cord may show abnormalities in the periventricular white matter and atrophy of the thoracic cord. There is no long-term disease-altering treatment available for this disease, noting that corticosteroids, cyclophosphamide, AZT, and vitamin C have been ineffective. Plasmapheresis has also been tried with minimal success (Kalichman et al., 2000). The mainstay of treatment, as with VM, involves the symptomatic treatment of associated conditions, prevention of secondary complications such as falls, pressure ulcers, and urinary tract infections, and the rehabilitation interventions to maximize function and preserve independence for as long as possible.

BRAIN DISORDERS

Progressive Multifocal Leukoencephalopathy

Progressive multifocal leukoencephalopathy (PML) is a fatal viral disease characterized by progressive inflammation of the white matter of the brain at multiple locations. This disease typically occurs in patients who are immunocompromised, most commonly in patients with HIV or AIDS with T-cell counts <200 per mm^3. PML is caused by the John Cunningham (JC) virus. Although antibodies to the JC virus are found in 86% of the general adult population, the virus typically remains latent in the kidneys and lymphoid tissues and is harmless in individuals who are not immunocompromised.

The JC virus produces disease only when the immune system is severely compromised. Once reactivated, the virus causes lytic infection of the oligodendrocytes within the CNS. Research has shown that HIV enables viral activation in the brain, which results in the clinically detrimental effects. The symptoms and signs of PML result from the loss of white matter throughout the brain (Figure 2.3). PML is a demyelinating disease, which results in a slowing of nerve conduction. Patients experience symptoms that include weakness or paralysis, dysarthria, impaired vision, and cognitive dysfunction. Patients with PML typically deteriorate very rapidly, with average survival being about 6 months after diagnosis in most cases. There is no known cure for PML; however, patients have been able to survive longer when treated with HAART (Power, Boisse, Rourke, & Gill, 2009). Other antiviral medications have also been studied as possible treatment options; however, more research is required in this area.

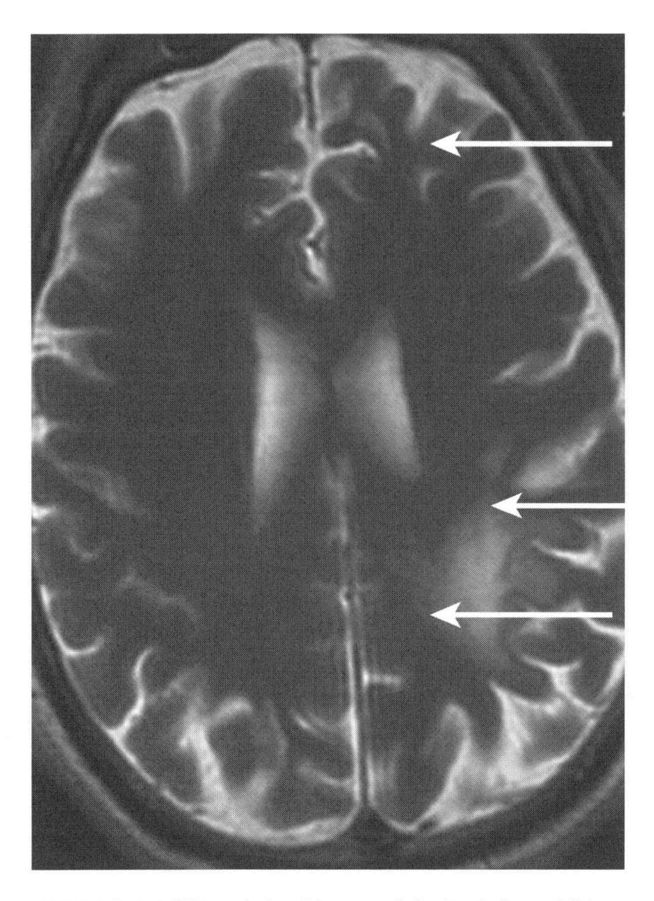

FIGURE 2.3 Axial T2-weighted image of the brain in an HIV-infected patient with progressive multifocal leukoencephalopathy who presented with behavioral changes as the initial manifestation of HIV infection. Arrows indicate multiple areas of abnormal signal change within the brain.

Source: Courtesy of Rona Woldenberg.

CMV Encephalitis

CMV belongs to the family of herpes viruses. It typically occurs in patients with a CD4 count <50 cells/mcL. CMV encephalitis is typically diagnosed on clinical suspicion in HIV-infected patients who have a history of infection with CMV disease. These patients present with altered mental status and a clinically progressive encephalopathy. Imaging studies often reveal evidence of ventriculitis. MRI or CT of the brain with contrast are the preferred imaging studies in order to exclude other potential neurological conditions such as PML, toxoplasmosis, or lymphomas. The diagnosis is then confirmed with polymerase chain reaction (PCR) testing and CSF cultures revealing presence of the virus. CSF-PCR is the diagnostic test of choice.

CMV encephalitis, when associated with HIV infection, can vary in the way in which it presents clinically. Patients who have ventriculoencephalitis suffer an acute onset and rapid deterioration characterized by confusion and lethargy. The cranial nerves may also be affected, causing focal neurological deficits. Other medical problems that may be associated with CMV encephalitis include myelitis, retinitis, esophagitis, neuropathy, and adrenal insufficiency.

If CMV encephalitis is not treated, it typically progresses to death in a period of days to weeks. The treatment consists of antiviral medications such as ganciclovir, foscarnet, or cidofovir. Patients are usually treated with induction doses initially and then continued on maintenance doses of medication (Robinson-Papp & Simpson, 2009). Since the arrival of ART, the incidence of CMV neurological disease has decreased and the survival rate following infection has increased.

Dementia

HIV-associated dementia produces a wide spectrum of disabilities that range from reduced work efficiency and quality of life to complete dependence for self-care. The HIV virus enters the CNS very early in the disease process. HIV-associated dementia is thought to arise from an HIV-induced defect in immune cellular signaling that produces neuronal damage in the brain (Said & Lacroix, 2005).

The clinical syndrome known as the AIDS dementia complex (ADC) is one of the most common and clinically important CNS complications of late HIV infection. Risk factors include high CSF viral load, illicit drug use, female sex, advanced age, and low educational level (McArthur et al., 1997). ADC includes behavioral changes, cognitive dysfunction, or brain-related motor impairment that is not directly attributable to a specific etiologic agent such as PML or CMV. It is quite common for patients with HIV to have deficits in cognition, including in areas such as memory, concentration, problem solving, and mood. These symptoms may be present in different stages of severity. Because ADC is a diagnosis of exclusion, it is important to consider multiple etiologic possibilities, including the possibility of cognitive impairment caused by medications. For example, efavirenz has been associated with multiple CNS side effects, including impaired concentration (Simpson & Bender, 1988).

Prior to the advent of treatment with HAART, dementia was associated with a high mortality and was seen in many patients before their death.

The incidence of dementia in HIV has declined with HAART treatment; however, the prevalence has remained the same, as persons with HIV live longer. Treatment with HAART has even been found to reverse some of the neurological deficits caused by HIV. HAART also delays the onset of dementia in HIV, although it does not seem to prevent the onset of cognitive impairment.

The treatment of HIV-associated dementia is with HAART combined with aggressive treatment of related psychiatric disorders that may also be present. For example, patients who present with depression along with dementia should be evaluated for the need for antidepressant medications. The commonly used antidepressants in patients with HIV include citalopram, escitalopram, fluoxetine, paroxetine, and sertraline. The treatment of concomitant depression results in not only improvement of mood but also better adherence to the patient's antiretroviral medication regimen (Simpson, Citak, Godfrey, Godbold, & Wolfe, 1993).

BONE DISEASE

As therapies to treat HIV infection continue to improve and extend the life span of individuals infected with the virus, these patients begin to develop additional ailments at a higher rate than the general population. This is especially true in regard to bone pathology. Those with HIV treated with ART are more likely to lose bone mineral density, leading to osteopenia and osteoporosis (Borderi, 2009). There are several reasons for these complications. Causative factors for the development of osteopenia and osteoporosis include the more sedentary lifestyle of those with HIV, increased tobacco and alcohol use, decreased amount of calcium and vitamin D intake, and ART, which causes greater bone mineral density loss. Tenofovir has been associated with a modest initial bone loss that eventually levels off. Protease inhibitors, such as atazanavir, are associated with significantly more mineral density loss in the spine than in the hip (McComsey et al., 2011; Stellbrink et al., 2010). The significance of bone loss is extremely important as noted by studies that have found that patients with HIV have an overall fracture prevalence of 2.87 per 100 persons as compared to the general population, whose overall fracture prevalence is 1.77 per 100 persons (Triant, Brown, Lee, & Grinspoon, 2008). In the prospective HIV Outpatient Study (HOPS), over 5,000 HIV-infected patients across 10 clinics in the United States had age-adjusted fracture rates 1.89 to 3.69 greater than those of the general population (Young et al., 2011). Another study concluded that HIV patients are almost nine times more likely to develop a hip fracture than noninfected individuals (Prieto-Alhambra, 2014).

With the significant increase in fracture prevalence in this population, it is vital to implement remedies to help prevent significant bone loss. This includes therapies that are similar to those for patients who are without HIV. Lifestyle changes including smoking cessation and weight-bearing exercises, in addition to medications including calcium, vitamin D, and bisphosphonates, have shown to improve bone strength in patients with and without HIV.

Despite ART causing increased loss of bone mineral density in these patients, it has not been shown to be an independent risk factor in another common bone manifestation in these immunodeficient patients, avascular necrosis (AVN). In HIV-infected patients, AVN is seen most commonly at the femoral head. Additionally, HIV-infected patients on corticosteroids, lipid-lowering agents, or testosterone were noted to have an even higher incidence of osteonecrosis (Miller et al., 2002). Bone disease can be a debilitating setback for those infected with HIV; therefore, it is crucial to diagnose and manage these conditions in a timely fashion.

PSYCHOLOGICAL CONDITIONS

Neuropsychiatric conditions in the HIV/AIDS population are related to numerous factors including, but not limited to, effects of the virus itself, preexisting comorbid psychiatric conditions, personal response to societal views, and the environment in which patients live after the diagnosis is made. The most common psychological conditions affecting this group include delirium, depression, HIV-associated dementia, schizophrenia, bipolar disorder, substance abuse or addiction, post-traumatic stress disorder (PTSD), and minor cognitive and motor disorders that impair attention, memory, organizational, and simple task skills. One study showed that patients with psychiatric disorders who received HAART improved their overall survival rate by remaining on the therapy (Himelhoch, Moore, Treisman, & Gebo, 2004).

Another facet affecting this population is pain. It is a contributor to a patient's quality of life and often underdiagnosed and undertreated in this population. Pain is a contributing cause of psychological distress in the general population and can also be applied to the HIV/AIDS population. The introduction of HAART changed the lives of patients with HIV dramatically. Before HAART treatment was available, patients with HIV suffered from extremely poor health characterized by a downward spiral of negative medical events, which dramatically affected life span, as well as quality of life. Patients often became very depressed as they began to lose their jobs and sources of income because of the severity of their illness. With the introduction of HAART, the life expectancy for patients with HIV has been prolonged, and their overall health has improved, which has obvious psychological benefits. Occasionally, the disease is less likely to result in disability. However, the importance of psychologists and mental health professionals remains critical in patients with HIV. Patients with HIV often experience social and psychological distress and require mental health intervention to address these important issues. Patients may suffer from various psychological conditions, including depression, anxiety, panic attacks, and adjustment disorders. The stigma associated with HIV infection alone is a psychological burden for those individuals with the disease. These patients, as a result, often have higher rates of suicide when compared with the general population. In one study that evaluated the psychological status of HIV patients in New York City, significantly more persons with HIV disease exhibited suicidal behavior as compared with patients with an unknown HIV status (Wu, Zhao, Tang, Zhang-Nunes, & McArthur, 2007). It is critical to address the psychiatric component of the HIV disease process as this may affect compliance with ART regimen. Depression, in particular, often goes underdiagnosed and undertreated in the general population, let alone in those with chronic medical conditions including HIV/AIDS. Psychological support is therefore critical for HIV patients, and families and friends should be included as part of the support system. It is important for mental health providers to allow the patients to share their feelings and experiences in order to help them remain optimistic and maintain hope throughout the course of the disease. The different services that should ideally be available for these patients include crisis intervention, individual psychotherapy, family interventions and support, support groups, and treatment for those with substance abuse. Those who counsel these patients should have a good understanding of the different psychosocial aspects involved with HIV and the social aspects involved with HIV-associated disability.

As HIV patients survive longer with improved therapies, we continue to see more of the secondary pathologies, both related to the virus itself as well as the treatments we provide. Living with HIV is proving to be a disabling ailment, and with a better understanding of how the virus affects the human body and the side effects of medications we use to treat it, we can help these patients live a more functional life. In summation, this provides a brief overview of the disabling nature of AIDS/HIV.

REFERENCES

Barohn, R., Gronseth, G., LeForce, B., McVey, A., McGuire, S., Butzin, C., & King, R. (1993). Peripheral nervous system involvement in a large cohort of human immunodeficiency virus-infected individuals. *Archives of Neurology, 50*(2), 167–171.

Borderi, M., Gibellini, D., Vescini, F., De Crignis, E., Cimatti, L., Biagetti, C., . . . Re, M. C. (2009). Metabolic bone disease in HIV infection. *AIDS, 23*(11), 1297.

Cherry, C., Skolasky, R., Lal, L., Creighton, J., Hauer, P., Raman, S., . . . McArthur, J. (2006). Antiretroviral use and other risks for HIV-associated neuropathies in an international cohort. *Neurology, 66*, 867–873.

Cohen, M., Hellmann, N., Levy, J., DeCock, K., & Lange, J. (2008). The spread, treatment, and prevention of HIV-1: Evolution of a global pandemic. *The Journal of Clinical Investigation, 118*(4), 1244–1254.

Cornblath, D. R., & McArthur, J. C. (1988). Predominantly sensory neuropathy in patients with AIDS and AIDS-related complex. *Neurology, 38*, 794–796.

Dal Pan, G. J., Glass, J. D., & McArthur, J. C. (1994). Clinicopathologic correlations of HIV-1-associated vacuolar myelopathy: An autopsy-based case-control study. *Neurology, 44*, 2159.

Di Rocco, A. (1999). Diseases of the spinal cord in human immunodeficiency virus infection. *Seminar Neurology, 19*, 151.

Dwyer, B. A., Mayer, R. F., & Lee S. C. (1992). Progressive nemaline (rod) myopathy as a presentation of human immunodeficiency virus infection. *Archives of Neurology, 49*, 440.

Engsig, F. N., Hansen, A. B., Omland, L. H., Kronborg, G., Gerstoft, J., Laursen, A. L., . . . Obel, N. (2009). Incidence, clinical presentation and outcome of progressive multifocal leukoencephalopathy in HIV-infected patients during the highly active antiretroviral therapy era: A nationwide cohort study. *Journal of Infectious Diseases, 199*, 77–83.

Ferrari, S., Vento, S., Monaco, S., Cavallaro, T., Cainelli, F., Rizzuto, N., & Temesgen, Z. (2006). Human immunodeficiency virus-associated peripheral neuropathies. *Mayo Clinic Proceedings, 81*(2), 213–219.

Garstang, S. V. (2002). Infections of the spine and spinal cord. In S. Kirshblum, D. I. Campagnolo, & J. A. DeLisa (Eds.), *Spinal cord medicine* (pp. 498–512). Philadelphia, PA: Lippincott Williams and Wilkins.

Geraci, A., Di Rocco, A., Liu, M., Werner, P., Tagliati, M., Godbold, J., . . . Morgello, S. (2000). AIDS myelopathy is not associated with elevated HIV viral load in cerebrospinal fluid. *Neurology, 55*, 440.

Gonzalez-Duarte, A., Robinson-Papp, J., & Simpson, D. M. (2008). Diagnosis and management of HIV-associated neuropathy. *Neurologic Clinics, 26*, 821–832.

González-Scarano, F., & Martín-García, J. (2005). The neuropathogenesis of AIDS. *Nature Reviews Immunology*, *5*, 69.

Griffiths, P. (2004). Cytomegalovirus infection of the central nervous system. *Herpes, 11*, 95A–104A.

Haas, D. W., Ribaudo, H. J., Kim, R. B., Tierney, C., Wilkinson, G. R., Gulick, R. M., . . . Acosta, E. P. (2004). Pharmacogenetics of efavirenz and central nervous system side effects: An adult aids clinical trials group study. *AIDS, 18*, 2391–2400.

Hall, H. I., Ruiguang, S., Rhodes, P., Prejean, J., An, Q., Lee, L. M., . . . Janssen, R. S. (2008). Estimation of HIV incidence in the United States. *Journal of the American Medical Association, 300*, 520–529.

Himelhoch, S., Moore, R., Treisman, G., & Gebo, K. (2004). Does the presence of a current psychiatric disorder in AIDS patients affect the initiation of antiretroviral treatment and duration of therapy? *Journal of Acquired Immune Deficiency Syndrome*, *37*(4), 1457.

Horberg, M. A., Silverberg, M. J., Hurley, L. B., Towner, W. J., Klein, D. B., Bersoff-Matcha, S., . . . Kovach, D. A. (2008). Effects of depression and selective serotonin reuptake inhibitor use on adherence to highly active antiretroviral therapy and on clinical outcomes in HIV-infected patients. *Journal of Acquired Immune Deficiency Syndrome, 47*, 384–390.

Johnson, R., Williams, F., Kazi, S., Dimachkie, M., & Reveille, J. (2003). Human immunodeficiency virus–associated polymyositis: A longitudinal study of outcome. *Arthritis Care and Research, 49*(2), 172–178.

Jose, J., Saravu, K., Jimmy, B., & Shastry, B. A. (2007). Distal sensory polyneuropathy in human immunodeficiency virus patients and nucleoside analogue antiretroviral agents. *Annals of Indian Academy of Neurology, 10*, 81–87.

Kalichman, S. C., Heckman, T., Kochman, A., Sikkema, K., & Bergholte, J. (2000). Depression and thoughts of suicide among middle-aged and older persons living with HIV-AIDS. *Psychiatric Services, 51*, 903–907.

Lehmann, H., Chen, W., Borzan, J., Mankowski, J., & Hoke, A. (2011). Mitochondrial dysfunction in distal axons contributes to human immunodeficiency virus sensory neuropathy. *Annals of Neurology, 69*(1), 100–110.

Lyons, J., Venna, N., & Cho, T. (2011). Atypical nervous system manifestations of HIV. *Seminars of Neurology, 31*(3), 254–265.

McArthur, J., McClernon, D., Cronin, M., Nance-Sproson, T., Saah, A., St Clair, M., & Lanier, E. R. (1997). Relationship between human immunodeficiency virus-associated dementia and viral load in cerebrospinal fluid and brain. *Annals of Neurology, 42*(5), 689.

McComsey, G. A., Kitch, D., Daar, E. S., Tierney, C., Jahed, N. C., Tebas, P., . . . Sax, P. E. (2011). Bone mineral density and fractures in antiretroviral-naive persons randomized to receive abacavir-lamivudine or tenofovir disoproxil fumarate-emtricitabine along with efavirenz or atazanavir-ritonavir: Aids clinical trials group A5224s, a substudy of ACTG A5202. *Journal of Infectious Diseases*, *203*(12), 1791–1801.

Miller, K. D., Masur, H., Jones, E. C., Joe, G. O., Rick, M. E., Kelly, G. G., . . . Kovacs, J. A. (2002). High prevalence of osteonecrosis of the femoral head in HIV-infected adults. *Annals of Internal Medicine, 137*(1), 17.

Power, C., Boisse, L., Rourke, S., & Gill, M. J. (2009). NeuoAIDS: An evolving epidemic. *Canadian Journal of Neurological Sciences, 36*, 285–295.

Prieto-Alhambra, D., Güerri-Fernández, R., De Vries, F., Lalmohamed, A., Bazelier, M., Starup-Linde, J., . . . Vestergaard, P. (2014). HIV infection and its association with an excess risk of clinical fractures: A nationwide case-control study. *Journal of Acquired Immune Deficiency Syndromes*, *66*(1), 90.

Reveille, J., & Williams, F. (2006). Rheumatologic complications of HIV infection. *Clinical Rheumatology, 20*(6), 1159–1179.

Robinson-Papp, J., & Simpson, D. M. (2009). Neuromuscular diseases associated with HIV-1 infection. *Muscle & Nerve, 40*, 1043–1053.

Said, G., & Lacroix, C. (2005). Primary and secondary vasculitic neuropathy. *Journal of Neurology, 252*, 633–641.

Simpson, D. M., & Bender, A. N. (1988). Human immunodeficiency virus-associated myopathy: Analysis of 11 patients. *Annals of Neurology, 24*, 79–84.

Simpson, D. M., Citak, K. A., Godfrey, E., Godbold, J., & Wolfe, D. E. (1993). Myopathies associated with human immunodeficiency virus and zidovudine: Can their effects be distinguished? *Neurology, 43*, 971–976.

Stellbrink, H. J., Orkin, C., Arribas, J. R., Compston, J., Gerstoft, J., Van Wijngaerden, E., . . . Pearce, H. (2010). Comparison of changes in bone density and turnover with abacavir-lamivudine versus tenofovir-emtricitabine in HIV-infected adults: 48-week results from the ASSERT study. *Clinical Infectious Diseases, 51*(8), 963–972.

Triant, V. A., Brown, T. T., Lee, H., & Grinspoon, S. K. (2008). Fracture prevalence among human immunodeficiency virus (HIV)-infected versus non-HIV-infected patients in a large U.S. healthcare system. *Journal of Clinical Endocrinology & Metabolism, 93*(9), 3499.

Wu, Y.-C., Zhao, Y.-B., Tang, M.-G., Zhang-Nunes, S. X., & McArthur, J. C. (2007). AIDS dementia complex in China. *Journal of Clinical Neuroscience, 14*, 8–11.

Young, B., Dao, C. N., Buchacz, K., Baker, R., Brooks, J. T., & HIV Outpatient Study (HOPS) Investigators. (2011). Increased rates of bone fracture among HIV-infected persons in the HIV Outpatient Study (HOPS) compared with the US general population, 2000–2006. *Clinical Infectious Diseases, 52*(8), 1061–1068.

3

CHAPTER

Alzheimer's Disease

Barry Reisberg, Emile Franssen[†], Liduïn E. M. Souren, Sunnie Kenowsky, Khurram S. Janjua, Sandra W. Veigne, Francoise Guillo-Benarous, Satneet Singh, Asma Khizar, Umang Shah, Romi G. Shah, Amandeep Bhandal, and Stefanie Auer

Evidence suggests that approximately 10% to 15% of community-residing persons in the United States aged 65 years and older may be afflicted with Alzheimer's disease (AD) or closely related dementing illnesses of late life (Evans et al., 1989; Katzman, 1986). Presently, it is estimated that in the United States, more than 5 million persons aged 65 years and older have AD (Alzheimer's Association, 2015). Additionally, approximately 200,000 persons younger than age 65 years are estimated to have AD in the United States (Alzheimer's Association, 2015). At the other end of the demographic spectrum, about one third of persons older than age 85 years in the United States are believed to have AD (Alzheimer's Association, 2015). More specifically, in the United States, dementia, secondary to AD, in entirety or in part, affects about 30% of community-residing persons between 85 and 89 years of age, and about 50% of those in the community between 90 and 94 years of age. For community-residing U.S. persons 95 years or greater, nearly 75% are found to have dementia (Graves et al., 1996; Montine & Larson, 2009). Worldwide, it has been estimated that 26.6 million persons have AD (Bookmeyer, Johnson, Ziegler-Graham, & Arrighi, 2007). Alzheimer's Disease International (ADI) presently estimates that there are over 46 million persons worldwide living with dementia and that the majority of these persons have dementia associated with AD (ADI, 2015). The prevalence of AD approximately doubles every 5 years after the age of 65 in developed nations and every 7 years in developing nations (Larson & Langa, 2008; Lobo et al., 2000).

In the United States, AD is the sixth leading cause of death for all age groups, after heart disease, cancer, respiratory diseases, accidents, and stroke. AD is the single major cause of institutionalization of aged people in the United States and in many other industrialized nations in the world. Studies have indicated that a large majority of the approximately 1.4 million residents in nursing homes in the United States manifest a dementia syndrome generally associated with AD (Chandler & Chandler, 1988; Rovner, Kafonek, Filipp, Lucas, & Folstein, 1986). However, the current Centers for Disease Control and Prevention (CDC) data from 2013 report that 48.5% are diagnosed with Alzheimer's or other dementias (Harris-Kojetin, Sengupta, Park-Lee, & Valverde, 2013). Additionally, 44.3% of the 1.2 million persons in hospice care in the United States have AD and other dementias (Harris-Kojetin et al., 2013). Furthermore, the institutional or "semi institutional" burden of AD, depending upon the precise definition of institutionalization, is truly much greater. More than 735,000 persons in the United States reside in assisted living facilities, (2015 National Center for Assisted Living), which are "depicted as residential settings for cognitively intact older people with functional limitations" (Kaplan, 2005). The White House Conference on Aging in 2015 concluded that up to 70% of assisted living residents experience a diagnosable form of AD or another dementia evenly divided across the mild, moderate, and severe stages of disease (Kaskie, Nattinger, & Potter, 2015). In a study of 22 such facilities in Maryland, approximately two thirds of these persons have been

[†]Deceased

found to have dementia, and the great majority of these persons with dementia were found to have AD (Rosenblatt et al., 2004). The dimensions of the institutional burden associated with AD are even more striking when it is noted that well under 1 million persons are in U.S. hospitals at any particular time (American Hospital Association, 2015).

Pre-AD conditions add further to the true burden of the disease. For example, approximately 10% to 20% of persons aged 65 years and older in the United States have mild cognitive impairment (MCI; Alzheimer's Association, 2015). This condition, which is a precursor of overt AD, is associated with a decrease in performance in complex occupational and social tasks (also referred to as executive activities), as well as a generalized decrement in cognitive performance and an increased susceptibility to delirium (Gauthier et al., 2006). MCI is also associated with a decrease in balance and coordination (Franssen, Souren, Torossian, & Reisberg, 1999). These MCI-related disabilities likely have considerable economic, social, and medical consequences, the dimensions of which are largely uncharted. In addition, a pre-MCI condition termed subjective cognitive impairment (SCI) is now increasingly recognized as an early antecedent of eventual AD. Very subtle cognitive and functional changes appear to occur in this SCI stage of eventual AD, which have unknown consequences apart from heralding an eventual decline to MCI, and, ultimately, the dementia of AD (Mitchell, Beaumont, Ferguson, Yadegarfar, & Stubbs, 2014; Reisberg & Gauthier, 2008; Reisberg, Shulman, Torossian, Leng, & Zhu, 2010). However, it is clear that large proportions of older persons take a variety of medications, nutraceuticals, vitamins, and other substances in an effort to mitigate their perceived symptoms, and the economic costs associated with this self-prescribing are very considerable (Reisberg & Shulman, 2009; Reisberg, Franssen, Souren, Kenowsky, & Auer, 1998).

The course of AD has been described in increasing detail over the past decades. The cognitive, functional, and behavioral concomitants at each stage of the illness can presently be described in detail (see Figure 3.1). The clinically observable symptomatology of AD dramatically changes in form from the earliest manifest deficits to the most severe stage; therefore, recognition and differentiation of the stages of this illness are imperative for proper diagnosis, prognosis, management, and treatment. Progressive cognitive changes that occur are manifest in concentration, recent memory, past memory, orientation, functioning and self-care, language, praxis ability, and calculation, among other areas (Reisberg, London, Ferris, et al., 1983; Reisberg, Schneck, Ferris, Schwartz, & de Leon, 1983). Characteristic behavioral symptoms are also a frequent component of AD (Finkel, 1996; Finkel & Burns, 2000; Kumar, Koss, Metzler, Moore, & Friedland, 1988; Lyketsos et al., 2000; Reisberg, Franssen, Sclan, Kluger, & Ferris, 1989; Reisberg, Monteiro, Torossian, et al., 2014; Rubin, Morris, Storandt, & Berg, 1987). These behavioral symptoms peak in occurrence at various points in the course of AD and subsequently recede in magnitude and frequency with the progression of the disease. A comprehensive view of the nature and progression of these cognitive, functional, and behavioral changes is critical for the optimization of residual capacity, rehabilitation, and the identification and management of excess disability in these patients.

An outline of global cognitive, functional, and behavioral changes in normal aging and progressive AD is provided in the Global Deterioration Scale (GDS; Reisberg, Ferris, de Leon, et al., 1982) outlined in Table 3.1 and described in greater detail in the following text.

GLOBAL DESCRIPTION OF NORMAL BRAIN AGING AND AD

Seven major, clinically distinguishable global stages from normality to the most severe AD have been described with the GDS (Reisberg et al., 1982; Reisberg, Sclan, Franssen, et al., 2008). Functionally, the progressive course of brain aging and AD can be described in even greater detail with the Functional Assessment Staging procedure (FAST stages; Reisberg, 1988; Sclan & Reisberg, 1992). In this section, we focus on the GDS stages and their implications, which are as follows.

GDS Stage 1: No Cognitive Impairment (NCI); Diagnosis: Normal

No objective or subjective evidence of cognitive decrement is seen. A significant proportion, although possibly only a minority, of persons 65 or older, fall within this category (Blazer, Hays, Fillenbamn, & Gold, 1997; Brucki & Nitrini, 2008; Gagnon et al.,

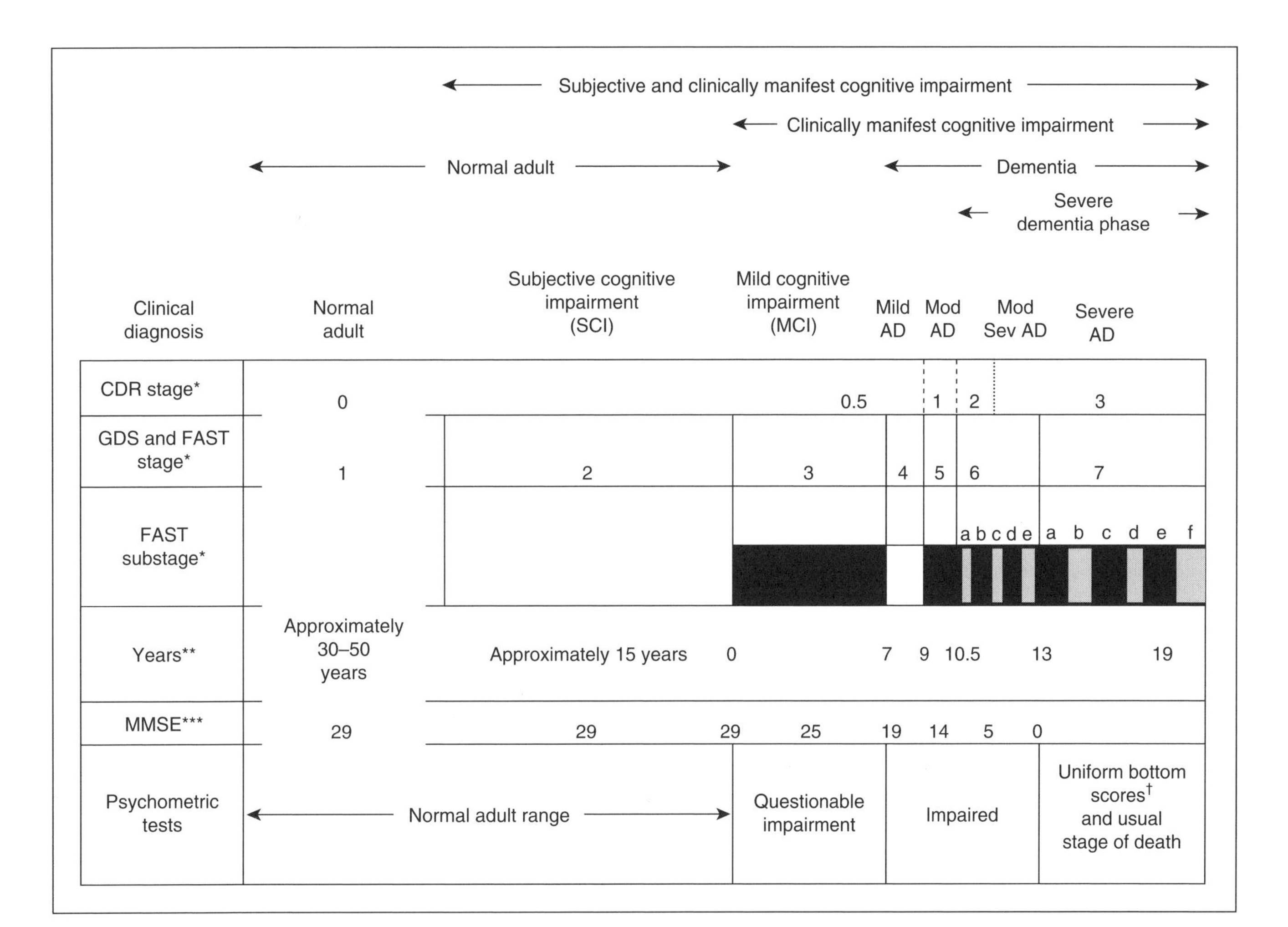

FIGURE 3.1 Typical time course of normal brain aging, subjective cognitive impairment, mild cognitive impairment associated with AD, and the dementia of AD.

*Stage range comparisons shown between the CDR and GDS/FAST stages are based upon published functioning and self-care descriptors.

**Numerical values represent time in years. For GDS and FAST stage 1, the temporal values are subsequent to the onset of adult life. For GDS and FAST stage 2, the temporal value is prior to onset of mild cognitive impairment symptoms. For GDS and FAST stage 3 and higher, the values are subsequent to the onset of mild cognitive impairment symptoms. In all cases, the temporal values refer to the evolution of AD pathology. All temporal estimates are based upon the GDS and FAST scales and were initially published based upon clinical observations in Reisberg (1986). These estimates have been supported by subsequent clinical and pathological cross-sectional and longitudinal investigations (e.g., Bobinski et al., 1995; Bobinski et al., 1997; Kluger, Ferris, Golomb, Mittelman, & Reisberg, 1999; Prichep et al., 2006; Reisberg & Gauthier, 2008; Reisberg, Ferris, Franssen, Shulman, Monteiro, et al., 1996; Reisberg et al., 2010; Wegiel et al., 2008). The spacing in the figure is approximately proportional to the temporal duration of the respective stages and substages, with the exception of GDS and FAST stage 1, for which the broken lines signify abbreviated temporal duration spacing for this normal adult condition, which lasts approximately 30 to 50 years.

***MMSE scores are approximate mean values from prior published studies.

†For typical adult psychometric tests.

AD, Alzheimer's disease; CDR, Clinical Dementia Rating (Hughes, Berg, Danziger, Coben, & Martin, 1982; Morris, 1993); FAST, Functional Assessment Staging (Reisberg, 1988; Sclan & Reisberg, 1992); GDS, Global Deterioration Scale (Reisberg, Ferris, de Leon, & Crook, 1982; Reisberg, Ferris, de Leon, et al., 1988); MMSE, Mini-Mental State Examination (Folstein, Folstein, & McHugh, 1975); Mod AD, moderate Alzheimer's disease; Mod Sev AD, moderately severe Alzheimer's disease.

Source: Copyright 2007, 2009 Barry Reisberg. All rights reserved.

1994; Jonker, Geerlings, & Schmand, 2000; Wang et al., 2000). The prognosis is excellent for continued adequate cognitive functioning (Geerlings, Jonker, Bouter, Ader, & Schmand, 1999; Kluger, Ferris, Golomb, Mittelman, & Reisberg, 1999; Mitchell, Beaumont, Ferguson, Yadegarfar, & Stubb, 2014; Reisberg, Shulman, Torossian, Leng, & Zhu, 2010).

TABLE 3.1

GLOBAL DETERIORATION SCALE (GDS) FOR AGE-ASSOCIATED COGNITIVE DECLINE AND ALZHEIMER'S DISEASE*

GDS Stage	Clinical Characteristics	Diagnosis
1	No subjective complaints of memory deficit. No memory deficit evident on clinical interview.	Normal
2	Subjective complaints of memory deficit, most frequently in following areas: (a) Forgetting where one has placed familiar objects. (b) Forgetting names one formerly knew well. No objective evidence of memory deficit on clinical interview. No objective deficit in employment or social situations. Appropriate concern with respect to symptomatology.	Subjective cognitive impairment
3	Earliest subtle deficits. Manifestations in more than one of the following areas: (a) Person may have gotten lost when traveling to an unfamiliar location. (b) Coworkers become aware of person's relatively poor performance. (c) Word and/or name-finding deficit become evident to intimates. (d) Person may read a passage or book and retain relatively little material. (e) Person may demonstrate decreased facility remembering names upon introduction to new people. (f) Patient may have lost or misplaced an object of value. (g) Concentration deficit may be evident on clinical testing. Objective evidence of memory deficit obtained only with an intensive interview. Decreased performance in demanding employment and social settings. Denial begins to become manifest in person. Mild to moderate anxiety frequently accompanies symptoms.	Mild cognitive impairment
4	Clear-cut deficit on careful clinical interview. Deficit manifest in following areas: (a) Decreased knowledge of current and recent events. (b) May exhibit some deficit in memory of one's personal history. (c) Concentration deficit elicited on serial subtractions. (d) Decreased ability to travel, handle finances, etc. Frequently no deficit in following areas: (a) Orientation to time and place. (b) Recognition of familiar persons and faces. (c) Ability to travel to familiar locations. Inability to perform complex tasks. Denial is dominant defense mechanism. Flattening of affect and withdrawal from challenging situations occur.	Mild Alzheimer's disease
5	Patient can no longer survive without some assistance. Patient is unable during interview to recall a major relevant aspect of current life, e.g., (a) Address or telephone number of many years. (b) The names of close members of the family (such as grandchildren). (c) The name of the high school or college from which the patient graduated. Frequently some disorientation to time (date, day of the week, season, etc.) or to place. An educated person may have difficulty counting back from 40 by 4s or from 20 by 2s. Persons at this stage retain knowledge of many major facts regarding themselves and others. They invariably know their own names and generally know their spouse's and children's names. They require no assistance with toileting or eating, but may have difficulty choosing the proper clothing to wear.	Moderate Alzheimer's disease

(*continued*)

TABLE 3.1 (*continued*)

GLOBAL DETERIORATION SCALE (GDS) FOR AGE-ASSOCIATED COGNITIVE DECLINE AND ALZHEIMER'S DISEASE*		
GDS Stage	**Clinical Characteristics**	**Diagnosis**
6	May occasionally forget the name of the spouse upon whom they are entirely dependent for survival. Will be largely unaware of all recent events and experiences in their lives. Retain some knowledge of their surroundings; the year, the season, etc. May have difficulty counting by 1s from 10, both backward and sometimes forward. Will require some assistance with activities of daily living. (a) May become incontinent. (b) Will require travel assistance but occasionally will be able to travel to familiar locations. Diurnal rhythm frequently disturbed. Almost always recall their own name. Frequently continue to be able to distinguish familiar from unfamiliar persons in their environment. Personality and emotional changes occur. These are quite variable and include: (a) Delusional behavior, e.g., patients may accuse their spouse of being an impostor; may talk to imaginary figures in the environment or to their own reflection in the mirror. (b) Obsessive symptoms, e.g., person may continually repeat simple cleaning activities. (c) Anxiety symptoms, agitation, and even previously nonexistent violent behavior may occur. (d) Cognitive abulla, e.g., loss of willpower because an individual cannot carry a thought long enough to determine a purposeful course of action.	Moderately severe Alzheimer's disease
7	All verbal abilities are lost over the course of this stage. Early in this stage, words and phrases are spoken but speech is very circumscribed. Later there is no speech at all—only babbling. Incontinent of urine; requires assistance toileting and feeding. Basic psychomotor skills (e.g., ability to walk) are lost with the progression of this stage. The brain appears to no longer be able to tell the body what to do. Generalized and cortical neurological signs and symptoms are frequently present.	Severe Alzheimer's disease

*When scoring the most appropriate stage is selected.

Source: Reisberg, Ferris, de Leon, et al. (1982).

GDS Stage 2: Subjective Cognitive Decline Only; Diagnosis: SCI

Many persons above age 65 have subjective complaints of cognitive decrement such as a subjective perception of forgetting names of people they know well or of forgetting where they placed familiar objects such as keys or jewelry. These subjective complaints may be elicited by comparing the persons' perceived abilities with their perceptions of their performance 5 to 10 years previously (Figure 3.2). A recent review has supported the primacy of the symptoms described in the preceding text in identifying this SCI stage. Rabin et al. identified 19 studies of self-report measures from eight countries (Rabin et al., 2015). A total of 34 self-report measures in five languages with 640 self-report items were identified. It was found that "items relating to memory for names of people and the placement of common objects were represented in the greatest percentage of measures (56% each)." Hence, to the extent a consensus regarding important items is identifiable at this time, the GDS stage 2 descriptions appear to have adumbrated them.

Apart from the occurrence of complaints of cognitive impairment with what appears to be seemingly "normal aging," these complaints may also occur with other, frequently more serious common conditions in the elderly, notably MCI, dementia, and depression. Persons with the comparatively benign complaints associated with this stage can

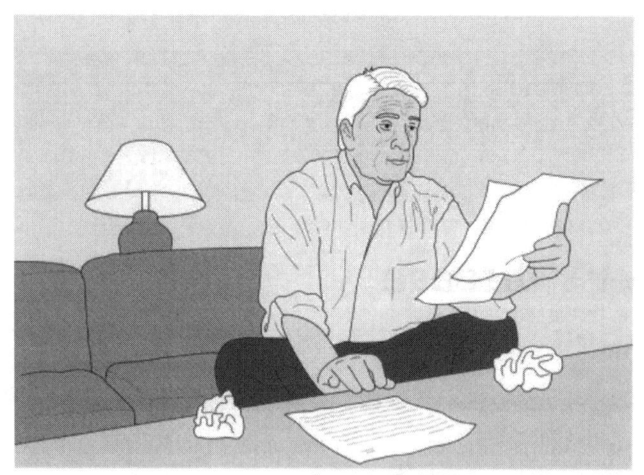

Copyright © 1999 Barry Reisberg, M.D.

FIGURE 3.2 GDS stage 2: Subjective cognitive impairment. "Why can't I remember where I put those papers? I used to remember where everything that I put away was located."
GDS, Global Deterioration Scale.

usually recall the names of two or more primary school teachers, classmates, or friends and are oriented to the time of day, date, day of week, month, season, and year (although, of course, occasional minor errors may occur). They also display normal recall when queried about recent events and normal concentration and calculation abilities, for example, when asked to perform serial subtractions of 7s from 100. The terminology *subjective cognitive impairment* has been suggested for this condition especially when it occurs in the absence of identifiable etiopathogenic factors apart from possible incipient AD (Reisberg, Prichep et al., 2008). In SCI persons, the clinical interview reveals no objective evidence of memory deficit, and there are no deficits in employment or social situations. However, physiologic studies have shown clear, significant decrements in persons with these symptoms in comparison with age-matched subjects free of subjective complaints. For example, a study found an 18% decrement in cerebral metabolism in a particular brain region, the parahippocampal gyrus, as well as significant metabolic decrements in some other brain regions in healthy older persons with SCI in comparison with age-matched subjects who were also healthy and free of SCI (Mosconi et al., 2008). Significant increases in urinary cortisol levels have also been reported in SCI subjects in comparison with age-matched control subjects (Wolf et al., 2005). Additionally, a large European study found that an abnormal Aβ42 to tau ratio was more common in SCI persons than in healthy older persons without SCI (Visser et al., 2009). They also found continuing increments in the percentages of persons with this abnormal Aβ-to-tau CSF ratio in nonamnestic MCI and amnestic SCI persons. Visser et al. (2009) concluded that "patients with SCI might be in the early stages of AD and that cognitive decline might become apparent only after longer follow-up" (i.e., longer than 3 years). Neuroanatomically, studies of the hippocampus and related brain regions were conducted by van Norden et al. (2008). They found that subjects with what they termed *subjective cognitive failures* and *subjective memory failures* and good objective cognitive performance had lower hippocampal volumes and that this finding was independent of white matter lesions (van Norden et al., 2008). In a small study, Jessen et al. found that the entorhinal cortex was significantly smaller in what they termed *subjective memory impairment* (*SMI*) subjects on the right side in comparison with no cognitive impairment (NCI) subjects. They found continuing reductions from SMI to MCI and AD (Jessen et al., 2006). Perrotin et al. (2012) studied brain amyloid deposition in relation to memory complaints in cognitively normal older persons (mean MMSE = 29). They found that subjects with high brain uptake of ^{11}C-PIB (Pittsburgh compound B) using positron emission tomographic imaging, indicating more brain amyloid deposition, rated their memory abilities as worse in comparison with their peers (Perrotin et al., 2012).

Apart from the evidence of physiologic changes in SCI persons in comparison with NCI persons, important prognostic differences have been demonstrated. In 2010, a study was published, which compared outcomes in terms of progression to MCI or dementia of otherwise healthy SCI (GDS stage 2) and NCI (GDS stage 1) persons (Reisberg et al., 2010). Subjects were followed over a mean of 7 years. It was found that after controlling for baseline demographic variables (age, gender, and formal education) and also for follow-up time, the hazard ratio of decline in SCI persons was 4.5 times that of NCI persons. Also, SCI persons declined more rapidly, at 60% of the rate of NCI subjects. The mean time to decline was 3.5 years longer for NCI than SCI subjects. Furthermore, current data from a prospective longitudinal study indicates that these subjective impairments are in most cases a harbinger of subsequently manifest cognitive impairments after an average of about 7.5 years (Prichep et al., 2006; Reisberg & Gauthier, 2008). The total duration of this stage has been estimated to be an average of about 15 years prior to the onset of more overtly manifest impairments such as those associated with MCI (Reisberg, 1986; Reisberg & Gauthier, 2008). Although medications, nutraceuticals, and nostrums are frequently taken for these perceived deficits, largely in order to prevent further decline, there is no convincing evidence of their efficacy in treating the symptoms of this stage at the present time.

GDS Stage 3: Mild Cognitive Decline; Diagnosis: MCI

This now widely recognized condition was first described, and subsequently named, in association with the GDS (Reisberg, Ferris, de Leon, Sinaiko, Franssen, et al., 1988; Reisberg, Ferris, Kluger, Franssen, Wegiel, et al., 2008). Various subsequent definitions of MCI have been proposed (e.g., Petersen et al., 1999; Petersen et al., 2001; Winblad et al., 2004); however, current consensus is consistent with the original GDS descriptions of the MCI entity (Gauthier et al., 2006; Winblad et al., 2004). MCI is a condition in which subtle deficits in cognition and cognition-associated functioning occur. Subtle evidence of objective decrement in complex occupational or social tasks may become evident in various ways. For example, the person may become confused or hopelessly lost when traveling to an unfamiliar location; relatively poorer performance may be noted by coworkers in a demanding occupation; persons may display overt word- and name-finding deficits; concentration deficits may be evident to family members and upon clinical testing; relatively little material may be retained after reading a passage from a book or newspaper; and/or an overt tendency to forget what has just been said and to repeat oneself may be manifest (Figure 3.3). A teacher who had routinely recalled the names of all of the students in his class by the end of a semester now may have difficulty recalling the names of any students. This same teacher may, for the first time, begin to miss important appointments. Similarly, a professional who had previously completed hundreds, perhaps thousands, of reports in the course of her lifetime, now, for the first time, may be unable to accurately complete a single report.

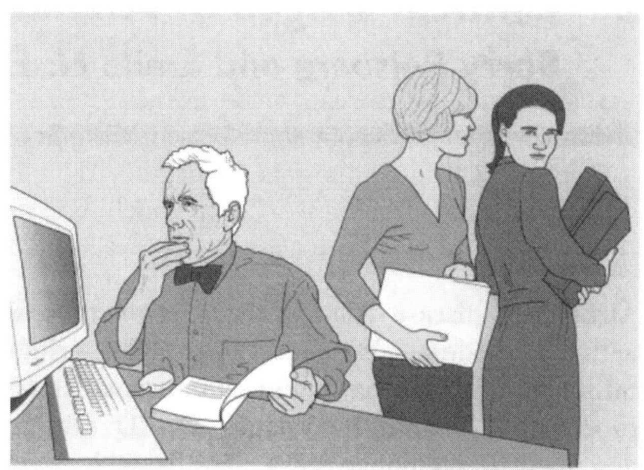

FIGURE 3.3 GDS stage 3: Mild cognitive impairment. In this stage, the ability to perform complex occupational and social tasks is compromised and the deficits may be noted by colleagues, coworkers, and/or family members.

GDS, Global Deterioration Scale.

The person may lose or misplace objects of value. Mild to moderate anxiety is frequently observed and is an appropriate reaction to the awareness of impairment.

The prognosis associated with these subtle but objectively identifiable symptoms varies. In some cases, these symptoms are the result of brain insults, such as small strokes, which may not be evident from the clinical history, neurological examination, or neuroimaging findings. In other cases, symptoms are due to subtle and perhaps not clearly identifiable psychiatric, medical, and neurological disorders of diverse etiology. These symptoms are benign in many of the subjects who report them. However, in most cases where other conditions have been ruled out in terms of etiology, these symptoms do represent the earliest symptoms of subsequently manifest AD. The mean true duration of this stage as a precursor of subsequently manifest mild AD has been estimated to be approximately 7 years (Reisberg, 1986). A review of 19 longitudinal studies found that the "overall conversion rate [of MCI subjects per annum] was 10%, with large differences between studies" (Bruscoli & Lovestone, 2004). They noted that self-selected, clinic attendees had the highest conversion rates. In a rigorous 4-year prospective study of otherwise healthy subjects fulfilling the exclusionary criteria for probable AD at baseline (except for the presence of dementia), MCI subjects declined at a rate of 17.8% per year to dementia, a rate quite similar to the 14.3%

per annum change, which would be anticipated for a stage that lasts approximately 7 years (Kluger, Ferris, Golomb, Mittelman, & Reisberg, 1999).

However, subjects commonly present with these symptoms well into this stage, and mild AD frequently becomes manifest after a much briefer period (Devanand, Folz, Gorlyn, Moesller, & Stern, 1997; Flicker, Ferris, & Reisberg, 1991; Morris et al., 2001; Petersen et al., 1999; Tierney et al., 1996). Presently, no pharmacologic agents have been approved for preventing further decline or in treating cognitive impairments in MCI.

GDS Stage 4: MCI; Diagnosis: Mild AD

Clinical interview reveals clearly manifest deficits in various areas, such as concentration, recent and past memory, orientation, calculation, and functional capacity. Concentration deficit may be of sufficient magnitude that the AD person may have difficulty subtracting serial 4s from 40. Recent memory may be affected to the degree that some major events of the previous week are not recalled, and there may be superficial or scanty knowledge of current events and activities. Detailed questioning may reveal that the spouse's knowledge of the AD person's past is superior to the AD person's own recall of his or her personal history, and the AD person may confuse the chronology of past life events. The AD person may mistake the date by 10 days or more but generally knows the year and the season. The AD person may manifest decreased ability to handle such routine activities as shopping or managing personal and household finances (Figure 3.4).

Psychiatric features that may be prominent in this stage include decreased interest in personal and social activities, accompanied by a flattening of affect and emotional withdrawal. These behavioral changes are related to the person's decreased cognitive abilities rather than to a depressed mood. However, they are frequently mistaken for depression. True depressive symptoms may also be noted but are generally mild, requiring no specific treatment. In cases where depressive symptoms are of sufficient severity to warrant treatment, a low dose of an antidepressant is frequently effective in reducing affective symptoms. At this stage, AD persons are still capable of independent community survival if assistance is provided with complex but essential activities such as bill paying and managing the AD person's bank account. Denial is the dominant defense mechanism protecting the AD person from the devastating consequences of the awareness of dementing illness.

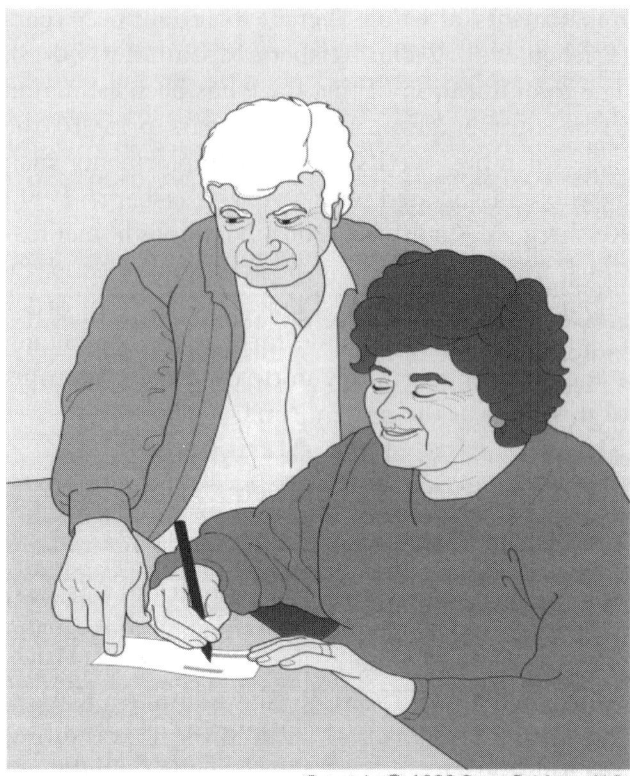

FIGURE 3.4 GDS stage 4: Mild AD. The characteristic functioning deficit in these persons is a decreased ability to manage instrumental (complex) activities of daily living. Examples of common deficits include decreased ability to manage personal finances, to prepare meals for guests, and to shop for oneself and one's family. The stage 4 person shown has difficulty writing the correct date and the correct amount on the check. Consequently, her husband has to supervise this activity. The mean duration of this stage is 2 years in otherwise healthy persons.

AD, Alzheimer's disease; GDS, Global Deterioration Scale.

The diagnosis of probable AD can be arrived at with confidence in this stage. It is possible to follow the person with AD through the course of this stage, the mean duration of which has been estimated to be approximately 2 years in persons who fulfill the McKhann et al. criteria for probable AD (McKhann et al., 1984; Reisberg, 1986; Reisberg, Ferris et al., 1996). Cholinesterase inhibitors (donepezil, rivastigmine and galantamine) have been approved for treating the symptoms of AD in this stage and have been demonstrated to slow cognitive and cognition-related functional decline to a modest extent. It is important to emphasize that these modest effects are symptomatic only. What this means is that (a) there is no demonstrated effect on the course of AD and (b) if the medication is removed, the effect of the medication is lost and the person with AD returns to a point where he or she would have been if he or she had not taken the medication.

GDS Stage 5: Moderately Severe Cognitive Decline; Diagnosis: Moderate AD

Cognitive and functional deficits are of sufficient magnitude that AD persons can no longer survive without assistance.

Persons at this stage can no longer recall major relevant aspects of their lives. They may not recall the name of the current national leader (e.g., president or prime minister), their correct current address or telephone number, or the names of schools they attended. Persons at this stage frequently do not recall the current year and may be unsure of the weather or season. Concentration and calculation deficits are generally of sufficient magnitude as to create difficulty in subtracting serial 4s from 40 and possibly even serial 2s from 20. Persons at this stage retain knowledge of many major facts regarding themselves and others and generally require no assistance with toileting or eating, but they may have difficulty choosing the appropriate clothing to wear for the season or the occasion and may begin to forget to bathe regularly unless reminded (Figure 3.5).

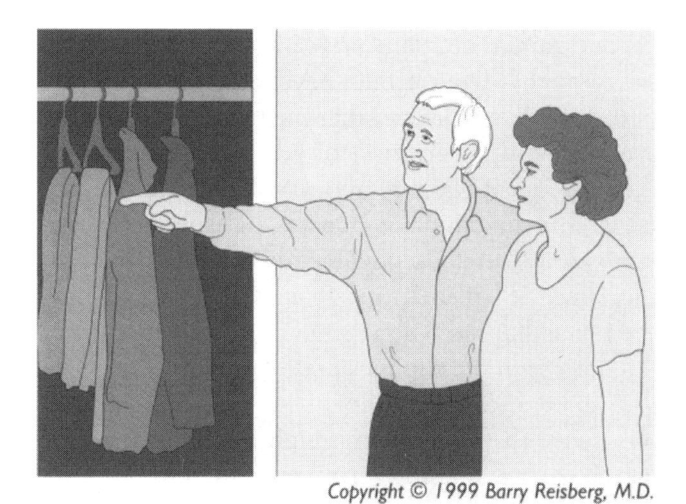

FIGURE 3.5 GDS stage 5: Moderate AD. In this stage, deficits are of sufficient magnitude as to prevent catastrophe-free, independent community survival. The characteristic functional change in this stage is incipient deficits in basic activities of daily life. This is manifest in a decrement in the ability to choose proper clothing to wear for the weather conditions and/or for the daily circumstances (occasions). Some AD persons begin to wear the same clothing day after day unless reminded to change. The spouse or other caregiver begins to counsel the AD person regarding the choice of clothing. The mean duration of this stage is 1.5 years in AD persons who fulfill the McKhann et al. criteria for probable AD.

AD, Alzheimer's disease; GDS, Global Deterioration Scale.

Psychiatric symptoms in this stage of moderate AD are in many ways similar, although generally more overt, than those noted in mild AD. The AD person's denial and flattening of affect tend to be more evident. True depressive symptoms, with mild to moderate mood dysphoria, may occur. Anger and other more overt behavioral symptoms of AD, such as anxieties, paranoia, and sleep disturbances, are frequently evident. Paranoid and delusional ideation peak in occurrence at this stage, with almost 75% of AD persons exhibiting one or more delusions. Such delusions as people stealing the AD person's belongings or money, that one's house is not one's home, or that one's spouse is an impostor, are common (Reisberg, Franssen et al., 1989). Aggressivity may include verbal outbursts, physical threats and violence, or general agitation. Depending on the nature and magnitude of the psychiatric symptomatology, treatment with an antipsychotic medication may be indicated. When this class of medication is used, the dictum for the treatment of behavioral and psychological symptoms of dementia (BPSD) applies: "Start low and go slow." We have recently extended this dictum to "Start low, go slow, stay low" (Reisberg, Monteiro, et al., 2014).

AD persons who are living alone in the community at this stage require at least part-time assistance for continued community survival. When additional community assistance, such as day care or home health aides, is not feasible or available, a more protective environment such as an assisted living facility may be required. AD persons who are residing with a spouse frequently resist additional assistance at this stage as an invasion of their privacy and home. The duration of this stage is approximately a year and one half (Reisberg, 1986; Reisberg, Ferris, Franssen, et al., 1996). Cholinesterase inhibitor medications have been approved for the treatment of AD symptoms at this stage. Another class of pharmacologic treatment that has been shown to be efficacious in improving the symptoms of AD in this stage is glutamatergic antagonist treatment. Memantine, the first and only medication in this relatively recently developed class of agents, is believed to reduce the glutamate-induced excitotoxicity caused by presynaptic neuronal injury. Memantine reversibly blocks glutamate transmission postsynaptically at the *N*-methyl-D-aspartate (NMDA) receptor. A pivotal study has indicated that memantine slowed the symptomatic progression of AD in this stage and the subsequent stage by about 50% in terms of cognitive and functional outcomes (Reisberg, Doody, et al., 2003). A subsequent study has indicated that the effects of memantine remain robust and may even be enhanced when memantine is given in combination with the cholinesterase inhibitor, donepezil (Tariot et al., 2004). It should be noted that, in common with the cholinesterase inhibitors, memantine is only a symptomatic treatment and does not alter the ultimate course of AD. Furthermore, like the cholinesterase inhibitors, if memantine treatment is stopped, the effects of the treatment are lost.

GDS Stage 6: Severe Cognitive Decline; Diagnosis: Moderately Severe AD

Cognitive and functional deficits are of sufficient magnitude as to require assistance with basic activities of daily living. Recent and remote memory are increasingly affected. AD persons at this stage frequently have no idea of the date and may occasionally forget the name of the spouse upon whom they are dependent for survival but usually continue to be able to distinguish familiar from unfamiliar persons in their environment. AD persons continue to know their own names until the final portion of this stage but frequently do not recall their correct address, although they may be able to recall some important aspects of their domicile, such as the street or town. AD persons at this stage have generally forgotten the schools they attended but recall some aspects of their early life, such as their birthplace, their former occupation, or one or both of their parents' names. Concentration and calculation deficits are of such magnitude that persons with moderately severe AD frequently have difficulty counting backward from 10 by 1s and may even begin to count forward in endeavoring to complete this task.

The functional deficits in this moderately severe AD stage are discussed in detail in the following section. However, briefly, in this stage, AD persons progressively lose the ability to put on their clothing without assistance, to bathe without assistance, to handle the mechanics of toileting, and subsequently, develop urinary and then fecal incontinence. These progressive deficits are shown in Figures 3.6 to 3.9.

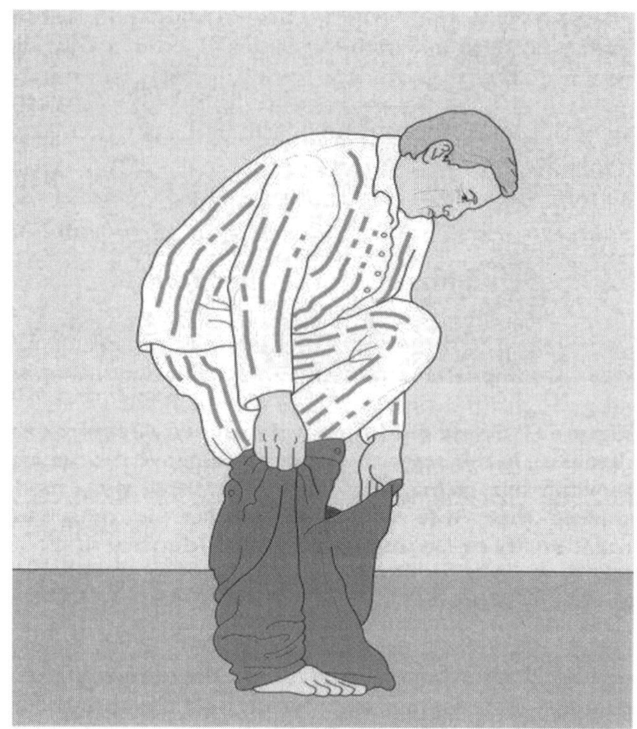

FIGURE 3.6 GDS stage 6, FAST stage 6a: Moderately severe AD. Decreased ability to put on clothing properly without assistance. In the stage of moderately severe AD, the cognitive deficits are of sufficient magnitude as to interfere with the ability of the AD person to carry out basic activities of daily life. Generally, the earliest such deficit noted in this stage is a decreased ability to put on clothing correctly without assistance. The total duration of this stage of moderately severe AD (from the beginning of FAST stage 6a to the end of FAST stage 6e) is approximately 2.5 years.

AD, Alzheimer's disease; FAST, Functional Assessment Staging; GDS, Global Deterioration Scale.

Agitation and even violence frequently occur in this stage. Language ability declines progressively so that by the end of this stage, speaking is impaired in obvious ways. At this point in the late sixth stage, stuttering and word repetition are common; patients who learned a second language in adulthood sometimes revert to a varying degree to their childhood language; other patients may use neologisms or nonsense words, interspersed to a varying degree in the course of their speech.

In this stage, emotional and behavioral problems generally become most manifest and disturbing, with 90% of patients exhibiting one or more behavioral symptoms (Reisberg, Franssen et al., 1989). A fear of being left alone or abandoned is frequently exhibited. Agitation, anger, sleep disturbances, physical violence, and negativity are examples of symptoms that commonly require treatment

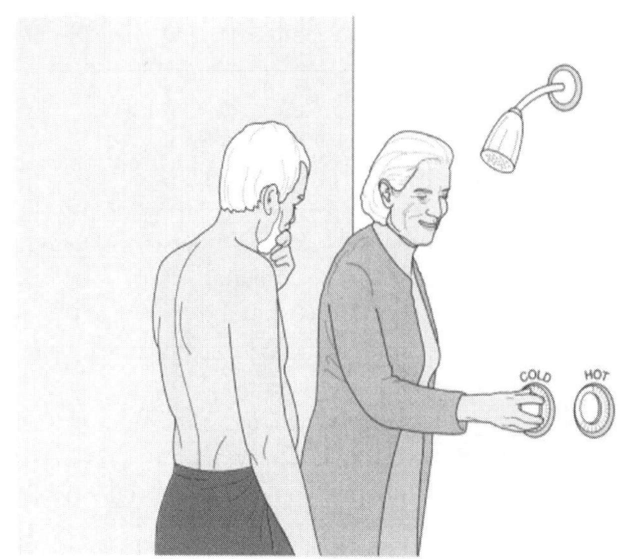

FIGURE 3.7 GDS stage 6, FAST stage 6b: Moderately severe AD. Requires assistance adjusting the temperature of the shower or bathwater. At approximately the same time as Alzheimer's persons begin to lose the ability to put on clothing properly without assistance but generally just a little bit later in the disease course, persons with Alzheimer's begin to require assistance in handling the mechanics of bathing. Difficulty in adjusting the water temperature of the shower and/or bathwater is the classical earliest deficit in bathing capacity.

AD, Alzheimer's disease; FAST, Functional Assessment Staging; GDS, Global Deterioration Scale.

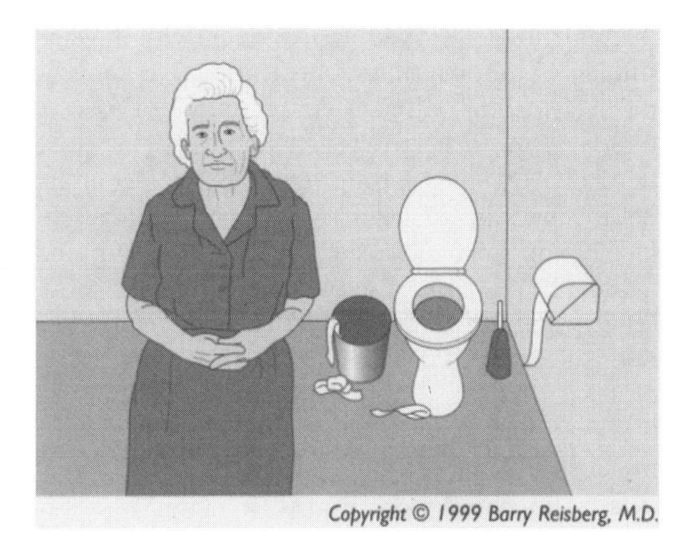

FIGURE 3.8 GDS stage 6, FAST stage 6c: Moderately severe AD. Requires assistance with the mechanics of toileting. After AD persons lose the ability to dress and bathe without assistance, they begin to have difficulties with the mechanics of toileting. A frequent initial deficit is forgetting to flush the toilet. Also, the AD person may begin to err in washing up properly after toileting.

AD, Alzheimer's disease; FAST, Functional Assessment Staging; GDS, Global Deterioration Scale.

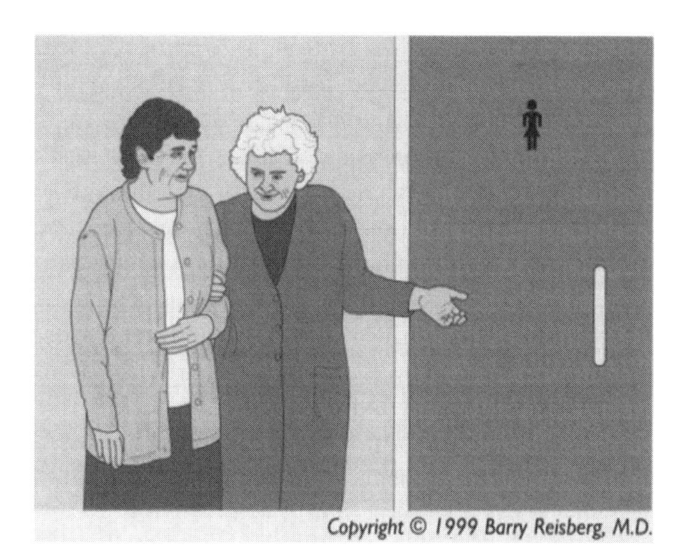

FIGURE 3.9 GDS stage 6, FAST stages 6d to 6e: Moderately severe AD. Development of urinary incontinence and, subsequently, fecal incontinence. After AD persons lose the ability to dress and bathe independently, and after they begin to require assistance with cleanliness in toileting, they develop incontinence. Generally, urinary incontinence precedes fecal incontinence. Strategies to prevent or minimize incontinence include frequent toileting.

AD, Alzheimer's disease; FAST, Functional Assessment Staging; GDS, Global Deterioration Scale.

at this point in the illness. Low doses of so-called atypical antipsychotics may be useful for many patients. Side effects can be avoided if the medication is titrated upward with intervals of weeks between dosage adjustments. Present efficacy data on the treatment of these symptoms are most compelling for the atypical antipsychotic risperidone (De Deyn et al., 2005).

Howcvcr, thc dosagc of antipsychotic medications given by clinicians and the titration schedules used by clinicians are frequently much higher and many times more rapid than those that are recommended herein and previously (Reisberg & Saeed, 2004; Reisberg, Monteiro, et al., 2014). For example, for risperidone, the current recommendation for treatment is as follows: In terms of pharmacological treatment of BPSD symptomatology, the clinical adage "Start low, go slow, stay low" applies (Reisberg, Monteiro, et al., 2014). For risperidone treatment, this rule translates into an optimal starting dose of half of a 0.25 mg tablet daily (because 0.25 mg is the lowest dosage currently manufactured, it is necessary to cut this tablet in half, resulting in a starting dosage of 0.125 mg daily). Although clinical circumstances dictate the schedule of dosage titration, an optimal clinical response is not achieved for a few weeks on any particular dosage of medication.

Also, extrapyramidal side effects may not peak until a patient has been on a particular dosage of medication for as long as 6 months (Stephen & Williamson, 1984). Therefore, ideally, the clinician should endeavor to leave a patient on a particular dosage of medication for weeks before further dosage adjustments. The exigencies of particular situations, of course, will frequently not permit this time luxury in dose adjustments, and clinicians will frequently need to make rapid dosage adjustments. However, the clinician should also be prepared to adjust medication dosage downward as well as upward in response to particular patient needs and the emergence of side effects. After some months of treatment, a steady-state dosage of approximately 0.125 or 0.25 mg of risperidone daily is frequently effective in controlling BPSD symptoms (updated information from Reisberg & Saeed, 2004; Reisberg, Monteiro, et al., 2014). A major problem with risperidone treatment is the side effect of akathisia. Akathisia means "an inability to sit still." This side effect can emerge with dosages >0.25 mg. Because akathisia frequently is indistinguishable from agitation, the clinician's response is frequently to increase the dosage of risperidone, resulting in increasing akathisia and, effectively, increasing agitation in the AD person. This cycle can be avoided by not going above 0.25 mg in the dose of risperidone. Also, it is important for the clinician to be knowledgeable regarding, and vigilant with respect to, the akathisia side effect.

In clinical trials of atypical antipsychotic medications in the treatment of BPSD in AD persons, dosages considerably greater than these recommended amounts, titrated over a much more rapid time interval, have been used. For example, in the study by Katz et al. (1999), dementia patients with BPSD were randomly assigned to treatment with placebo or 0.5 mg/day, 1.0 mg/day, or 2 mg/day of risperidone for 12 weeks. The mean age of the patients was 83 years, and 96% of the patients had moderately severe or severe AD as evidenced by FAST (Reisberg, 1988, see Table 3.2) scores of ≥6a and Mini-Mental State Examination (MMSE) (Folstein et al., 1975) mean scores of 6.6. When a meta-analysis was used to review the results of this and similar studies, an increased mortality was found to be associated with the use of atypical antipsychotic medication in dementia patients (Schneider, Dagerman, & Insel, 2005). This finding by Schneider et al. (2005) resulted in the U.S. Food and Drug Administration (FDA) "blackboxing" with a warning of "Increased Mortality in Elderly Patients with Dementia-Related Psychosis" for antipsychotic medications used for the treatment of BPSD. This warning states in part that "analyses of 17 placebo-controlled trials (modal duration of 10 weeks), largely in patients taking atypical antipsychotic drugs, revealed a risk of death in drug-treated patients of . . . 1.6 to 1.7 times the risk in placebo-treated patients" (PDR Network, 2009, p. 2683). The warning also notes that the increased mortality is due to varied causes, of which most were related to cardiovascular (heart failure or sudden death) or infectious (such as pneumonia) factors. The Schneider et al. (2005) study and subsequent studies (e.g., Wang et al., 2005) have also found an increased mortality associated with the treatment of BPSD (psychosis) in dementia patients with so-called typical antipsychotic medications (e.g., haloperidol). In general, the risk of mortality has been found to be greater for "typical" than so-called atypical (e.g., risperidone) antipsychotic medications, although one major study found no difference between the two classes of antipsychotic medication in terms of mortality (Kales et al., 2007).

Unfortunately, even more recently published studies of antipsychotic medications in dementia such as the Clinical Antipsychotic Trials of Intervention Effectiveness-Alzheimer's Disease (CATIE-AD) Study Group report (Schneider et al., 2006) continue to begin with higher dosages of medication than those suggested by Reisberg and Saeed (2004). For example, the Schneider et al. (2006) published study (which was embarked upon in April 2001) used a starting "low" dose of Risperdal, the brand form of risperidone, of 0.5 mg. This "low dose" is four times the starting dosage being recommended herein. The actual mean starting dosage in the CATIE-AD study was 0.7 mg of Risperdal. Dosages were adjusted upward or downward. For entry, in addition to AD, subjects had to have psychosis, aggression, or agitation. The subjects were followed for up to 36 weeks; however, the main outcome analysis was done at 12 weeks. The mean last dose of Risperdal in the CATIE-AD study was 1.0 mg. Schneider et al. found that significantly more subjects were discontinued from the placebo treatment because

TABLE 3.2

FUNCTIONAL ASSESSMENT STAGES (FAST)* AND TIME COURSE OF FUNCTIONAL LOSS IN NORMAL AGING AND ALZHEIMER'S DISEASE (AD)

FAST Stage	Clinical Characteristics	Clinical Diagnosis	Estimated Duration in Normal Adults, Normal Brain Aging, and AD[a]	Mean MMSE[b]
1	No decrement	Normal adult	50 years	29–30
2	Subjective deficit in word finding or recalling location of objects	Subjective cognitive impairment	15 years	29
3	Deficits noted in demanding employment settings	Mild cognitive impairment	7 years	24–27
4	Requires assistance in complex tasks, e.g., handling finances, planning dinner party	Mild AD	2 years	19–20
5	Requires assistance in choosing proper attire	Moderate AD	18 months	15
6a	Requires assistance in dressing	Moderately severe AD	5 months	9
b	Requires assistance in bathing properly		5 months	8
c	Requires assistance with mechanics of toileting (such as flushing, wiping)		5 months	5
d	Urinary incontinence		4 months	3
e	Fecal incontinence		10 months	1
7a	Speech ability limited to about a half dozen words	Severe AD	12 months	0
b	Intelligible vocabulary limited to a single word		18 months	0
c	Ambulatory ability lost		12 months	0
d	Ability to sit up lost		12 months	0
e	Ability to smile lost		18 months	0
f	Ability to hold head up lost		12 months or longer	0

[a]In subjects without other complicating illnesses who survive and progress to the subsequent deterioration stage.

[b]MMSE, Mini-Mental State Examination score (Folstein et al., 1975). Estimates based in part on published data summarized in Reisberg, Ferris, de Leon, et al. (1989) and obtained in Reisberg, Ferris, Torossian, Kluger, and Monteiro (1992).

*These stages are, in part, derived from, and are designed to be, optimally concordant with the corresponding Global Deterioration Scale (GDS) stages with the progression of subjective cognitive impairment, mild cognitive impairment, and dementia associated with AD. The FAST stage is the highest ordinal (successive) stage. Additional (nonordinal) stages or substages are noted, if present.

Source: Adapted from Reisberg (1986). Copyright 1984 by Barry Reisberg.

of perceived lack of efficacy than subjects from the blinded Risperdal treatment group. On the other hand, significantly more subjects discontinued the Risperdal treatment because of perceived side effects than subjects in the placebo group. At 12 weeks, there was little difference between the subjects in the Risperdal and the placebo groups on a main outcome measure, the Clinical Global Impression of Change (CGIC). However, only small percentages of either Risperdal-treated (28.6%) or placebo-randomized subjects (20.9%) reached this 12-week study evaluation point. Improvement was observed in 29% of the Risperdal-treated subjects and in 21% of the placebo-randomized subjects.

The conclusion of this study was that "adverse effects offset advantages of atypical antipsychotic drugs for the treatment of psychosis, aggression, or agitation in patients with Alzheimer's disease." We have suggested that much better results can be obtained if the "start low, go slow, stay low" recommendations that we have forwarded and continuously updated and extended (Reisberg & Saeed, 2004; Reisberg, Monteiro, et al., 2014; and the recommendations forwarded herein) are followed.

In addition to Risperdal (the brand is recommended because of sensitivities in dosing), other medications can be useful for treating agitation in AD persons. These other medications frequently have the disadvantages from the viewpoint of optimal treatment of the AD person in terms of being sedating. The goal of treatment should be to keep the AD person optimally functioning, not sedated. Examples of these alternative treatments for agitation in BPSD are the antipsychotic medication, quetiapine, and the antidepressant medication, trazodone. Apart from the sedating effect per se of these medications being a disadvantage in terms of optimizing the cognition of the AD person, a further disadvantage of the sedating effect is an increased risk of falling, to which AD persons are increasingly susceptible as the disease process advances.

In summary, with respect to the treatment of BPSD symptoms in persons with dementia (primarily persons with AD), current consensus has concluded that treatment with antipsychotic medications, approached judiciously, continues to be a necessary option. In the words of a 2008 consensus, "There is insufficient evidence to suggest that psychotropics other than antipsychotics represent an overall effective and safe, let alone better, treatment choice for psychosis or agitation in dementia" (Jeste et al., 2008).

Apart from medication treatment approaches to the treatment of AD, a very broad variety of other approaches to the treatment of persons with AD, and to those who share the burden of the AD person, have been tried and investigated. Traditionally, these other approaches have frequently been termed *nonpharmacologic therapies* (Olazarán et al., 2010). Recently, a terminology for these diverse interventions, which defines them by what they are, that is, *ecopsychosocial interventions*, not by what they are not, that is, *nonpharmacologic therapies*, is being suggested (Zeisel, Reisberg, Whitehouse, Woods, & Verheul., 2016).

Some of these ecopsychosocial approaches have been very successful. For example, multicomponent interventions for the caregiver have demonstrated very significant delays in institutionalization of mild to moderately severe AD persons (GDS stages 4 to 6), in comparison to usual care (Belle et al., 2006; Lawton, Brody, & Saperstein, 1989; Mittelman et al., 1993). In a pooled analysis, there was a 33% lower rate of institutionalization after 6 to 12 months in the intervention subject groups in comparison with control groups, which received usual care or minimal support.

For outcomes apart from institutionalization, such as the remediation of cognition, improved activities of daily living, improved behavioral disturbances, or improved mood, the magnitude of the effects with ecopsychosocial treatments have, in general, been comparable to the effect sizes seen with, for example, cholinesterase inhibitor medications (Luijpen, Scherder, Van Someren, Swaab, & Sergeant, 2003). However, these treatments, of course, should be viewed as additions to pharmacotherapies, not as alternatives to pharmacotherapy.

In the moderately severe AD stage, the magnitude of cognitive and functional decline, combined with disturbed behavior and affect, make caregiving especially burdensome to spouses or other family members. These family members frequently must devote their lives to helping persons with AD who often can no longer even recall their names, much less appreciate, in all the ways that may be desired, the kindness and care being provided to them.

The caregivers' burden may be alleviated, for example, through regular participation in a dementia caregiver support group, utilization of day care and respite centers for patients, or utilization of home health aides, either part time or full time. Clinical experience and research findings show that if behavioral disturbances are not successfully managed, they become the primary reason for institutionalization, and successful management of the disturbances can postpone this event. The mean duration of this stage is approximately 2.5 years (Reisberg, 1986; Reisberg, Ferris et al., 1996). Memantine has been approved for the treatment of AD in this stage and does appear to be useful in slowing the progression of cognitive and functional decline during the time AD persons remain on the medication (Reisberg, Doody, et al., 2003; Tariot et al., 2004; Winblad & Poritis, 1999). In 2006, donepezil became the first cholinesterase inhibitor to be FDA approved for treating symptoms in this stage. More recently, the rivastigmine patch has also been approved for treating symptoms (primarily cognition-related symptoms) in this stage.

Stage 7: Very Severe Cognitive Decline; Diagnosis: Severe AD

A succession of functional losses in this stage results in the need for continuous assistance in all aspects of daily living. During the course of FAST stage 6e, when AD persons are doubly incontinent, speech abilities begin to break down in the AD person. This occurs in various ways. For example, some AD persons develop verbigeration, repeating words and phrases over and over again (a phenomenon similar to stuttering). Other AD persons begin to make up new words (neologisms). Irrespective of how speech ability is lost, AD persons emerge in the final, seventh stage, with severely limited verbal abilities. In the early part of the seventh stage, verbal abilities appear to be limited to approximately a half dozen different intelligible words during the course of an average day, frequently interspersed with unintelligible babbling. Eventually, only a single word remains, commonly "yes," "no," or "OK." Subsequently, the ability to speak even this final single word is largely lost, although the person with AD may utter seemingly forgotten words and phrases in response to various circumstances for years after meaningful, volitional speech is lost. It is important to recognize that although the person with AD may no longer be capable of speaking, thinking capacity remains. Test measures originally developed for infants are able to demonstrate continuing thinking capacities of the AD person in the seventh stage (Auer, Sclan, Yaffee, & Reisberg, 1994). Although agitation can be a problem for some AD persons at this stage, psychotropic medication can generally be reduced as this stage progresses and ultimately discontinued.

Memantine has been approved for treating the symptoms (cognitive and functional) of AD persons in this stage. However, only one published memantine study has included these seventh-stage AD persons. That study (Winblad & Poritis, 1999) did investigate memantine's efficacy in institutionalized, primarily nursing home–residing AD persons. However, only 6% of these subjects were in the GDS stage 7. Therefore, there is very little current information regarding the role of memantine in this final stage of the disease.

Donepezil was the first cholinesterase inhibitor approved for the treatment of AD at this stage. Also, because rivastigmine was not studied in AD persons in this stage (see the following), donepezil is the only cholinesterase inhibitor with evidence of efficacy in this stage. The pivotal trial by Winblad et al. (2006) included 61 randomized and treated patients with a FAST stage of 7a or greater (25% of the study population). Hence, fully a quarter of the subjects in this pivotal trial had little or no remaining speech. Additionally, 23 randomized and treated subjects were losing the ability to ambulate independently (FAST stage 7c). Hence, the most robust pivotal trial data for any medication in the treatment of persons in this final stage of AD at the present time are that available for donepezil treatment. However, even this trial had a requirement of a minimum MMSE score of 1 at entry. Because most stage 7 subjects, even in the early part of stage 7, have MMSE scores of 0 (bottom), even this study by Winblad et al. (2006) included relatively cognitively less impaired final-stage AD subjects (Reisberg, 2007).

The rivastigmine transdermal system (Exelon patch) is approved for the treatment of "severe Alzheimer's disease." (See Exelon© Patch [rivastigmine transdermal system]. Initial U.S. approval 2000. Revised 02/2015.) However, "severe Alzheimer's disease," in this context, refers to what is termed "moderately severe Alzheimer's disease" in this chapter. This confusion is a result of the tendency of many clinicians and investigators to completely ignore the final seventh GDS and FAST stages of AD, comprising 7 or more potential years of the disease. A review of rivastigmine published in 2011 concluded that the "greatest treatment effects with rivastigmine patch and capsule were seen in patients with more advanced dementia" (Farlow, Grossberg, Meng, Olin, & Somogyi, 2011, Abstract, p. 1236). Subsequently, a study was published of what were termed "patients with severe Alzheimer's disease." However, these so-called severe AD persons had MMSE scores of 3 to 12. Hence, on the GDS, these AD persons would be in GDS stages 5 or 6. None of the subjects would have been in GDS stage 7. The study compared the low-dose rivastigmine patch (4.6 mg/24 hr) with the high-dose rivastigmine patch (13.3 mg/24 hr) and found greater efficacy for the high-dose patch (Farlow, Grossberg, Sadowsky, Meng, & Somogyi, 2013). Unfortunately, this study says nothing, apart from possible inferences about the treatment of AD persons in GDS stage 7.

Nursing homes or similar care facilities may be better equipped than spouses for the management of AD persons in this stage. If family members maintain the patient at home, round-the-clock health care assistance may be necessary to manage incontinence and basic activities of daily living such as bathing and feeding. Human contact continues to make a great difference in the quality of life of a person with AD, whether in the home or in an institution. A loving voice, attention, and gentle touch are important for the AD person's emotional and physical well-being. As described subsequently, movement and physical activity are particularly important.

AD persons who survive until some point in GDS stage 7 generally die from pneumonia, traumatic or decubital ulceration, or a less specific failure in the central regulation of vital functions. Although approximately half of all patients who reach this stage are dead within 2 to 3 years, patients may potentially survive for 7 years or longer in this final stage.

FUNCTIONAL CHANGES IN AD

Understanding the progression of AD from the standpoint of change and deterioration in functional abilities is of great importance to both clinicians and families. In terms of a primary diagnosis, as well as differential diagnosis, it is useful to determine whether the nature of the dementia is consistent with uncomplicated senile dementia of the Alzheimer type, because dementing processes associated with other causes frequently proceed differently from those of AD. Knowledge of the functional progression of AD can assist in this differential diagnostic process and, additionally, in identifying possible remediable complications of the illness. Furthermore, even the most severe AD patients can be assessed in terms of a functional level when all traditional mental status and psychometric assessment measures produce uniform bottom (0) scores (Reisberg, Franssen et al., 1996; Reisberg, Wegiel, Fransseen, Kadiyala, et al., 2006b). Functional assessment is presently capable of producing a detailed, meaningful map of the entire course of AD and, from the standpoint of physical rehabilitation, is extremely important in describing the AD patient's level of incapacity and areas of residual capacity.

Requirements for the management of AD fall into two categories: those relating to the patient and those relating to the primary caregiver. It is essential for the benefit of both that management advice be appropriate to each stage of the illness.

FUNCTIONAL DESCRIPTION OF AD

A practical diagnostic and assessment tool, the FAST (Reisberg, 1988; Sclan & Reisberg, 1992) permits identification of the stages of characteristic decline in functional activities in AD and their estimated duration (outlined in Table 3.2). Because of their utility, these FAST stages of AD are mandated for usage for certain purposes by the Center for Medicare & Medicaid Services in the United States, as well as in certain international jurisdictions (Health Care Financing Administration, 1988). Since 2008, the FAST stages of AD have also been mandated in association with AD medication prescribing by the U.S. Veterans Health Administration. These stages of functional deterioration in AD correspond optimally with the GDS stages described earlier. Table 3.2 indicates the approximate corresponding mean MMSE scores for each of the FAST stages and substages (Folstein et al., 1975). Research has indicated strong relationships between progressive functional deterioration assessed on the FAST and progressive cognitive deterioration in AD (e.g., Pearson correlation coefficients of ~0.8 or greater between MMSE and FAST scores have been reported [Reisberg, Ferris, Anand, et al., 1984; Sclan & Reisberg, 1992]). Therefore, the relationships shown between FAST and MMSE scores are approximations of likely findings in individual patients, although there is variability. Functionally, the late stages of AD can be subdivided into FAST stages 6a to 6e and FAST stages 7a to 7f. Consequently, a total of 16 functioning stages can be recognized that describe in detail the characteristic changes that occur with the progression of AD. In uncomplicated dementia of the Alzheimer's type, progression through each of the functional stages described in the following occurs in a generally ordinal (sequential) pattern (Sclan & Reisberg, 1992).

FAST Stage 1: No Objective or Subjective Functional Decrement

The aged subject's objective and subjective functional abilities in occupational, social, and other settings remain intact, compared with prior performance. The prognosis is excellent for continued adequate cognitive functioning.

FAST Stage 2: Subjective Functional Decrement but no Objective Evidence of Decreased Performance in Complex Occupational or Social Activities

The most common age-related functional complaints are forgetting names and locations of objects (Rabin et al., 2015). Subjective decrements are generally not noted by acquaintances or coworkers, and complex occupational and social functioning is not compromised.

When affective disorders, anxiety states, or other remediable conditions have been excluded, the older person with these symptoms can be reassured with respect to the relatively benign prognosis for persons with these subjective symptoms. However, currently recognized strategies for decreasing the risk of cognitive decline such as physical exercise, a healthy low-fat diet, and avoidance of obesity should be discussed.

FAST Stage 3: Objective Functional Decrement of Sufficient Severity to Interfere With Complex Occupational and Social Tasks

This is the stage at which persons may begin to forget important appointments, seemingly for the first time in their lives. Functional decrements may become manifest in complex psychomotor tasks, such as the ability to travel to new locations. Persons at this stage have no difficulty with routine tasks such as shopping, handling finances, or traveling to familiar locations, but they may stop participating in demanding occupational and social settings. These symptoms, although subtle clinically, can considerably alter lifestyle. When psychiatric, neurological, and medical concomitants apart from AD have been excluded, the clinician may advise withdrawal from complex, anxiety-provoking situations. Because persons at this stage can still perform all basic activities of daily living satisfactorily, withdrawing from demanding activities may result in complete symptom amelioration for a period of years.

FAST Stage 4: Deficient Performance in the Complex Tasks of Daily Life

Aspects of decreased functioning from former levels are apparent. At this stage, shopping for adequate or appropriate food and other items is noticeably impaired. The person may return with incorrect items or inappropriate amounts of a certain item. The individual may have difficulty preparing meals for family dinners and may display similar deficits in the ability to manage complex occupational and social tasks. Family members may note that the person is no longer able to balance the checkbook, no longer remembers to pay bills properly, and may make significant financial errors. Persons who are still able to travel independently to and from work may not recall names of clients or details of their employment duties. Because choosing clothing, dressing, bathing, and traveling to familiar locations can be adequately performed at this stage, persons may still function independently in the community, although supervision is often useful.

Maximizing the functioning of the person with AD at this stage is the goal of the family and health professionals. Financial supervision and structured or supervised travel should be arranged. Identification bracelets, ID cards, or clothing labels with a name, address, and telephone number may be useful for unusually stressful situations where anxiety or other factors further impair the person's capacities.

FAST Stage 5: Incipient Deficit in Performance of Basic Tasks of Daily Life

At this stage, persons with AD can no longer satisfactorily function independently in the community. The person not only requires assistance in managing financial affairs and shopping but also begins to require help in choosing the appropriate clothing for the season and the occasion. The person may wear obviously incongruous clothing combinations or wear the same clothing day after day unless supervision is provided.

At this stage, some persons with AD develop anxieties and fears about bathing. Another functional deficit that frequently becomes manifest at this stage is difficulty in driving an automobile. The person with AD may slow down or speed up the vehicle inappropriately or may go through a stop sign or traffic light. Occasionally, the person may have a collision with another vehicle for the first time in many years. The person with moderate AD may be sufficiently alarmed by these deficits to voluntarily discontinue driving. Sometimes, however, intervention and coercion are necessary from family members or even from the AD person's physician or licensing authorities. A useful strategy for the physician is to arrange for an automobile driving retest.

It is important that functional abilities be maximized. Persons at this stage are still capable of putting on their clothing with minimal guidance once it has been selected for them. They are also capable of bathing and washing themselves, even though they may have to be cajoled into performing these activities. A supportive environment that provides adequate stimulation, in addition to adequate protection, is desirable. It is important that these persons continue to engage in and practice skills in which they remain capable.

FAST Stage 6: Decreased Ability to Dress, Bathe, and Toilet Independently

Throughout the course of stage 6, which lasts for approximately 2.5 years and encompasses five substages, increasing deficits in dressing and bathing occur. In addition to not being able to choose the proper clothing, AD persons at early stage 6 develop difficulties in putting on their clothing properly (stage 6a). Other dressing difficulties include putting on street clothing over night clothing, putting clothing on backward or inside out, and putting on multiple and inappropriate layers of clothing. The AD person may also have difficulty zippering or buttoning their clothing or tying their shoelaces. More overt dressing difficulties develop as this stage progresses and the AD person requires increasing assistance in dressing.

A bathing difficulty that becomes apparent at this stage is a decreased ability to adjust the temperature of the shower or bathwater (substage 6b). Subsequently, taking a bath or shower without assistance becomes increasingly problematic, ultimately with difficulty getting into and out of the bathtub and washing properly. Fear of bathing may develop, combined with resistance to bathing. This fear of bathing sometimes precedes actual difficulties in handling the mechanics of bathing.

Later in the course of this stage, persons with AD begin to have difficulties with the mechanics of toileting. Initially, they may forget to flush the toilet, and/or the AD person may dispose of toilet tissue improperly. Furthermore, persons with AD at this stage may fail to clean themselves adequately (stage 6c).

Subsequently, urinary incontinence begins (stage 6d), followed by fecal incontinence (stage 6e), both of which appear to be the result of decreased cognitive capacity to respond appropriately to urinary or fecal urgency. Assisting the person with AD to use the toilet often helps to forestall and remediate incontinence. Anxieties regarding toileting are frequently noted in stage 6c prior to the actual development of incontinence. Persons with AD may go to the toilet repeatedly even in the absence of a true need for elimination.

Motor capacity deficits also become notable during stage 6. Walking becomes more halting and steps generally become smaller and slower, but the ability to ambulate is still maintained. Because orientation in space is affected, persons with moderately severe AD in FAST stage 6 may approach a chair and sit down with greater difficulty. AD persons may also require assistance in walking up and down a staircase.

Full-time home health care is frequently useful at this time, and it may be appropriate or necessary to discuss assisted living or nursing home placement with the caregiver and family members. Management strategies and supportive techniques must be utilized to assist the AD person in bathing, dressing, and toileting, as this stage evolves as well as in minimizing the emotional stress of both the AD person and the caregiver.

Stage 7: Loss of Speech and Locomotion

This final stage of AD is marked by decreased vocabulary and speech abilities. Speech becomes increasingly limited, from a vocabulary of a half dozen different intelligible, purposeful, and meaningful words (stage 7a) to, at most, a single distinguishable purposeful word that may be uttered repeatedly (stage 7b). Eventually, speech becomes limited to babbling, unintelligible utterances, and occasional, intelligible, random utterances.

Prior to the loss of ambulatory ability, persons with AD may exhibit a twisted gait (i.e., instead of walking directly forward, the person puts the right foot in front of the left foot and vice versa), take progressively smaller and slower steps, or lean forward, backward, or sideways while walking. Eventually, the ability to walk unassisted is lost with the progression of AD (stage 7c; Figure 3.10). It should be noted that after the loss of speech ability, the ability to walk is invariably lost. However, AD patients, for various reasons, especially including excess disability, are susceptible to the loss of ambulation from the beginning of the final 7th AD stage, as well as subsequently.

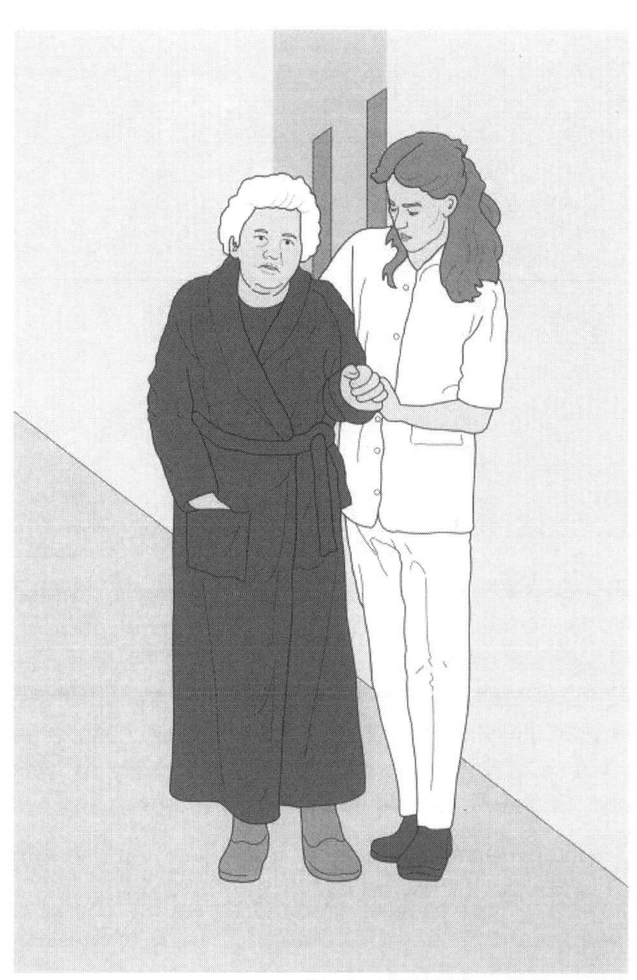

FIGURE 3.10 GDS stage 7, FAST stage 7c: Severe Alzheimer's disease. Loss of the ability to ambulate independently. Ambulatory ability is lost and the person requires assistance in walking.

FAST, Functional Assessment Staging; GDS, Global Deterioration Scale.

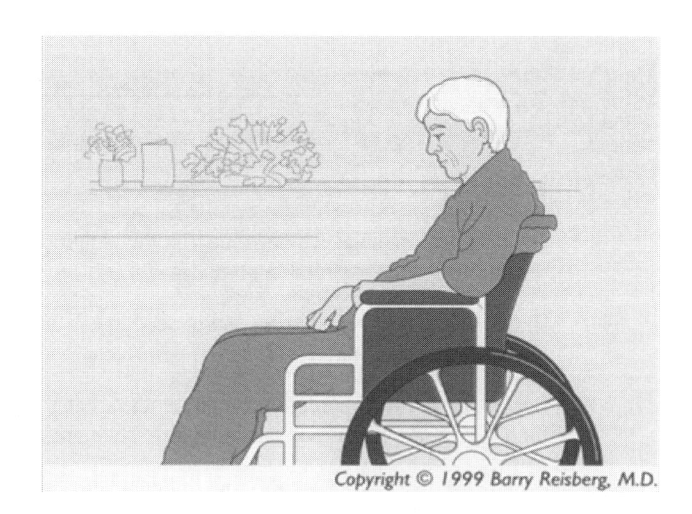

FIGURE 3.11 GDS stage 7, FAST stage 7d: Severe AD. Loss of the ability to sit up independently. After ambulatory ability is lost, with the progression of AD, the ability to sit up independently is lost. Without armrests on the chair, the person with AD would fall to the side.

AD, Alzheimer's disease; FAST, Functional Assessment Staging; GDS, Global Deterioration Scale.

Approximately a year after ambulatory ability is lost, the ability to sit up without assistance (such as lateral chair rests) is also lost (stage 7d). At this point, the AD person will require a chair with armrests (Figure 3.11).

Subsequently, the ability to smile (stage 7e) and to hold up the head independently (stage 7f) are also lost. At this point, babbling and grasping may still be observed, and AD persons can still move their eyes, although familiar persons or objects are apparently no longer recognized. Approximately 3 to 4 years after the onset of stage 7, generally after the loss of ambulatory ability, many persons with AD die. However, some persons with AD survive in this stage for 7 years or longer. Pneumonia, which is often associated with aspiration, is a frequent cause of death.

Full-time assistance at home or in an institution is a necessity at this final seventh stage, and as AD persons are increasingly well cared for, it is likely that more will survive to these final substages of the illness.

FEEDING CONCOMITANTS OF AD

Progressive changes in the ability to prepare meals and in feeding skills have been observed in AD patients and enumerated in accordance with the corresponding GDS and FAST stages (Reisberg, Pattschull-Furlan,

TABLE 3.3

FEEDING CONCOMITANTS OF ALZHEIMER'S DISEASE	
Stage*	**Clinical Characteristics**
1–2	No objective or subjective decrement in the ability to adequately prepare meals, order food and beverages in a restaurant setting, or in table etiquette
4	Decreased facility in preparing and/or serving relatively complex meals and/or decreased facility in ordering food and beverages in a restaurant setting
5	Decreased ability in preparing simple foods or beverages (e.g., coffee or tea); may occasionally make mistakes in eating food (e.g., improper use of seasoning or condiments)
6	(a) Occasional difficulty with proper manipulation or choice of eating utensils (b) Meat and similar foods must be cut up for the patient (c) No longer trusted to use a knife; may also eat foods that would have formerly been refused (d) No longer trusted to properly use a knife and decreased ability to use a fork, but can still properly use a spoon; may also display occasional misrecognition of dietary substances (pica) (e) Capable of going to the refrigerator or cupboard but has difficulty discerning and choosing food, may have difficulty chewing hard food
7	(a) Capable of picking up spoon or fork; will occasionally drop food or misutilize silverware (e.g., may attempt to drink soup or other liquids with a fork); capable of reaching for a cup when desirous of fluid (b) Must be assisted in actual feeding; generally, patients are not permitted to handle a knife or fork; may not be able to properly lift a cup (c) Can reach for and pick up food with hands; cannot properly pick up a fork or a spoon but can grasp a spoon or other utensil; must be spoon-fed, but can chew. (d) Cannot distinguish foods from nondietary substances; will reach out for objects, including food.

*Stages have been enumerated to be optimally concordant with the corresponding Global Deterioration Scale (GDS) and Functional Assessment Staging (FAST) stages in Alzheimer's disease. The most appropriate numerical stage is selected.

Source: Reisberg, Pattschull-Furlan, Franssen, et al. (1990). Copyright 1988 by Barry Reisberg.

Franssen, et al., 1990). These "feeding concomitants of Alzheimer's disease" are outlined in Table 3.3. The progression of these disturbances in meal preparation and self-feeding, as with the progression of deterioration in cognitive and functional abilities, appears to be characteristic of AD.

BALANCE AND COORDINATION

Although it is clear from the preceding description of functional losses in AD that balance and coordination are eventually lost with the progression of the illness process, these aspects are actually very early changes, coincident with the advent of MCI and mild AD. For example, a detailed study indicated that tandem walking, foot-tapping speed, hand pronation and supination speed, and finger-to-thumb apposition speed, all decreased significantly in MCI subjects in comparison with normal elderly controls (Franssen, Souren, Torossian, et al., 1999). Additional decrements were noted in mild AD subjects.

Another study has demonstrated that complex motor and fine motor measures can be just as robust markers of MCI and mild AD as a cognitive psychometric battery (Kluger, Gianutsos, Golomb, et al., 1997). These observations of motor and equilibrium changes in MCI and AD are consistent with neuropathologic observations of strong clinicopathologic correlations with cerebellar atrophy in AD (Wegiel, Wisniewski, Dziewiatkowski, et al., 1999).

RIGIDITY AND CONTRACTURES

In the latter stages of AD, rigidity becomes increasingly manifest (Franssen, 1993; Franssen, Kluger, Torossian, & Reisberg, 1993; Franssen, Reisberg, Kluger, Sinaiko, & Boja, 1991). Initially, this rigidity is of a paratonic type, that is, elicited in response to an irregular motion of an extremity, such as an irregular movement of an elbow. Later, the rigidity becomes increasingly evident. Figure 3.12 depicts the emergence of paratonic rigidity in AD. Although infrequently manifest in persons with mild AD (i.e., GDS stage 4), approximately 50% of the persons with moderate AD (GDS stage 5), 75% of persons with moderately severe AD (GDS stage 6), and virtually all persons with severe AD (GDS stage 7) manifest at least a mildly detectable form of paratonic rigidity. Figure 3.12 shows the methodology for the elicitation of this paratonic rigidity by the clinician.

One probable result of this increasing rigidity is the development of contractures (Figure 3.13). Contractures are irreversible deformities of joints, limiting range of motion. In a study by Souren et al. (Souren, Franssen, & Reisberg, 1995), a contracture was defined as a limitation of 50% or more of the passive range of motion of a joint, secondary to permanent muscle shortening, ankylosis, or both. Souren and associates found that contractures meeting this definition were present in 10% of moderately severe AD patients with incipient incontinence (i.e., AD patients at FAST stages 6d and 6e). In severe AD, contractures are very common. Forty percent of incipient averbal AD patients (FAST stages 7a and 7b) manifested contractures and 50% of incipient nonambulatory AD patients (FAST stage 7c) manifested these deformities. By late stage 7, that is, in the immobile category (FAST stages 7d to f), 95% of AD patients manifested these deformities. Furthermore, at all stages, when contractures occurred, they generally were present in more than one extremity. Specifically, in the great majority of patients with contractures (69%), all four extremities were involved. All but one of the 39 patients found to have contractures (97%) had at least two limbs affected. By limiting mobility, contractures predispose patients to further morbidity, such as decubital ulcerations. One third of the patients with contractures in the study by Souren et al. (1995) had decubital ulcerations, either noted by direct patient observation or in the patient's medical record.

There is evidence based upon patient observations that contractures may be prevented until very late in the course of AD by the maintenance of patient activities, stretching, other movements, and, especially, frequent specific range of motion exercises of all joints including the hands and fingers.

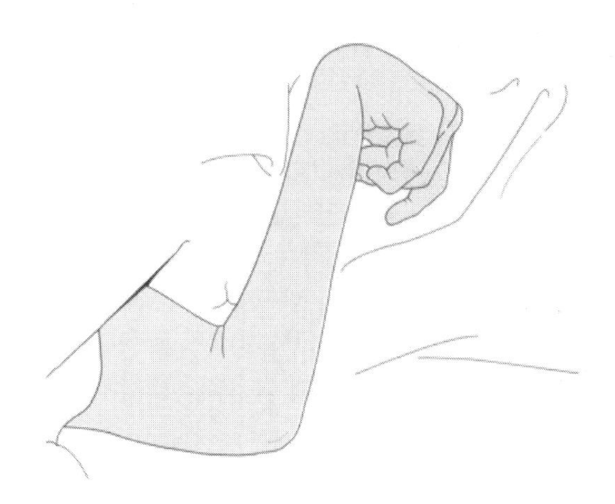

FIGURE 3.13 Contractures of the elbow, wrist, and fingers. Contractures in Alzheimer's persons are irreversible deformities of the joints. They are found to occur in 10% of AD persons in FAST stages 6d and 6e and become increasingly common in AD persons with the progression of GDS and FAST stage 7. These deformities are largely preventable by range of motion exercises in late-stage AD persons.

AD, Alzheimer's disease; FAST, Functional Assessment Staging; GDS, Global Deterioration Scale.

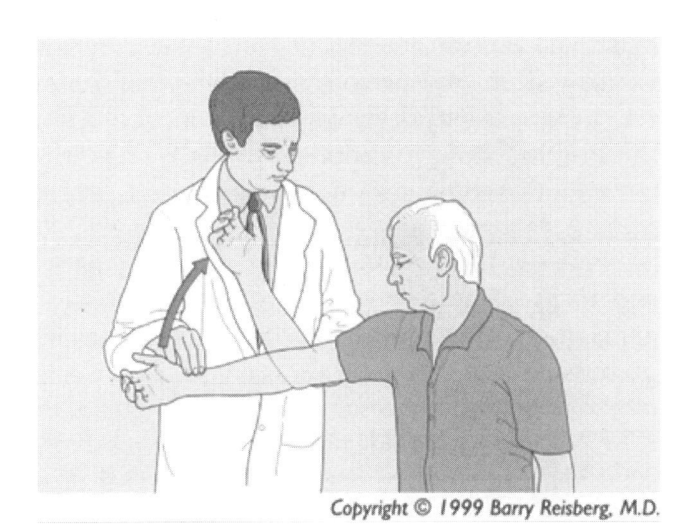

FIGURE 3.12 Paratonic rigidity. As the process of Alzheimer's disease (AD) advances, persons manifest increasing paratonic rigidity. This is elicited by asking the person with AD to hold out the arm and to relax, and by holding the outstretched arm just above the elbow with one hand and by moving the forearm with the other hand, while continuing to ask the AD person to relax.

DIFFERENTIAL DIAGNOSTIC IMPLICATIONS OF THE CHARACTERISTIC FUNCTIONAL COURSE OF AD

Cognitive and functional deficits in persons with AD characteristically follow the progression outlined in the preceding sections. However, other disorders frequently associated with the presence of dementia do not necessarily follow this characteristic pattern. It has been observed that the characteristic pattern of functional loss in AD is useful in differential diagnosis (Reisberg, 1986; Reisberg, Ferris, & Franssen, 1985). Common functional presentations of non-AD dementing disorders are outlined in Table 3.4. For example, normal pressure hydrocephalus (NPH) commonly presents with gait disturbance as the earliest symptom, antedating any overt cognitive disturbance. In NPH, this ambulatory disturbance is commonly followed by urinary incontinence. Only subsequently, after the advent of ambulatory disturbance and urinary incontinence in NPH, may cognitive disturbances become manifest. As summarized in Table 3.2, the sequence of functional loss in AD is very different. In AD, overt cognitive disturbance precedes urinary incontinence, which, in turn, precedes ambulatory loss.

Creutzfeldt-Jacob disease is a rare form of rapidly progressive dementia that presents with ambulatory disturbance as the earliest symptom in approximately one third of the cases. In AD, the ambulatory disturbance is a much later event. The two conditions also may be distinguished temporally. The course of AD extends over many years, as outlined in Table 3.2, and is frequently much slower than the relatively rapid course of the acute and subacute forms of Creutzfeldt-Jacob disease.

Multi-infarct dementia, or dementia associated with an overt, large infarction, may produce speech disturbance as the only symptom. Alternatively, the infarction may produce urinary incontinence as the major overt manifestation. Commonly, ambulatory loss may be the major sequela of a stroke. Clearly, the evolution of functional losses in AD follows a very different and much more stereotyped pattern (as outlined in Table 3.2). As shown in Table 3.4, the evolution of functional disturbance in dementia associated with multiple infarctions may follow a very different course from that which is characteristic of AD.

Depression is a psychiatric disturbance associated with mood dysphoria and other symptoms. Among these other symptoms are negativity and subjective complaints of cognitive impairment. Occasionally, the depression produces a dementia-like syndrome that is potentially reversible when the underlying mood disturbance is treated. This potentially reversible dementia syndrome of depression, formerly called pseudodementia, does not necessarily follow the functional course outlined in Table 3.2. For example, as outlined in Table 3.4, depression may be accompanied by a refusal to dress and bathe as a result of the patient's negativity. However, the patient may be able to point to exactly the clothes he or she wishes to wear. In AD, the loss of ability to pick out clothing properly precedes the loss of ability to put on one's clothing properly.

As outlined in Table 3.4, dementia associated with hyponatremia or other electrolyte disturbances, central nervous system (CNS) metastases, and other conditions all may follow a course markedly at variance with the course of AD as outlined in the FAST.

In a person with AD, a variety of coexisting conditions may result in functional disturbances that may occur prematurely or nonordinally (i.e., out of sequence) in terms of the FAST predictions. Examples of conditions that may be associated with premature (i.e., nonordinal) functional losses in an AD person are outlined in Table 3.5. For example, if an AD person is at GDS stage 5 and FAST stage 5 and develops urinary incontinence, this incontinence may, at this early point in AD, be a remediable complication, perhaps secondary to a urinary tract infection.

Similarly, if a person with AD at GDS stage 5 and FAST stage 5 develops loss of independent ambulation, this may be the result of a stroke or possibly the result of a variety of potentially treatable conditions common in the elderly, such as medication-induced parkinsonian symptoms, arthritis, a fracture, and so forth. Table 3.5 provides an extensive list of causes of premature functional losses in an AD person, many of which are potentially remediable.

The relationship between the FAST and the GDS or the FAST and the MMSE is also useful in the identification of excess functional disability that may be remediable. Specifically, if an AD person

TABLE 3.4

FUNCTIONAL LOSS IN NON-ALZHEIMER DISORDERS ASSOCIATED WITH PROGRESSIVE OR GRADUAL ONSET OF DEMENTIA AND FAST (FUNCTIONAL ASSESSMENT STAGING) CHARACTERISTICS IN AD

Functional Loss in Non-AD Disorders			FAST AD Distinctions		
Disorder	**Pathology or Presumed Etiology**	**Functional Loss in Non-AD Disorder****	**Equivalent FAST Stage***	**Functional Loss in AD per FAST***	**FAST Stages in AD***
Normal Pressure Hydrocephalus	Dilated cerebral ventricles	1. Gait disturbance	7c	1. Loss of ability to perform complex tasks	4
		2. Urinary incontinence	6d	2. Urinary incontinence	6d
		3. Loss of ability to perform complex tasks	4	3. Ambulatory (gait) disturbance	7c
Creutzfeldt-Jakob Disease	Prion	1. Gait disturbance	7c	1. Loss of ability to perform complex tasks	4
		2. Loss of ability to perform complex tasks	4	2. Gait (ambulatory) disturbance	7c
Multi-Infarct Dementia	Multiple cerebral infarctions	1. Loss of speech	7a–7b	1. Loss of ability to perform complex tasks	4
		2. Loss of urinary continence	6d	2. Loss of ability to pick out clothing properly	5
		3. Loss of ability to put on clothing	6a	3. Loss of ability to put on clothing without assistance	6a
		4. Loss of ability to bathe without assistance	6b	4. Loss of ability to bathe without assistance	6b
		5. Loss of ambulatory capacity	7c	5. Loss of urinary continence	6d
		6. Loss of ability to perform complex tasks	4	6. Loss of fecal continence	6e
		7. Loss of ability to pick out clothing properly	5	7. Loss of speech	7b
		8. Fecal incontinence	6e	8. Loss of ambulatory capacity	7c
Dementia Syndrome of Depression ("Pseudodementia")	Affective disorder associated with neurotransmitter imbalance	1. Loss of ability to perform complex tasks	4	1. Loss of ability to perform complex tasks	4
		2. Refusal to put on clothing (associated with negativity)	6a	2. Loss of ability to pick out clothing properly	5
		3. Refusal to bathe (associated with negativity)	6b	3. Loss of ability to put on clothing without assistance.	6a
		4. Loss of ability to pick out clothing properly	5	4. Inability to bathe without assistance	6b

(*continued*)

TABLE 3.4 (*continued*)

FUNCTIONAL LOSS IN NON-ALZHEIMER DISORDERS ASSOCIATED WITH PROGRESSIVE OR GRADUAL ONSET OF DEMENTIA AND FAST (FUNCTIONAL ASSESSMENT STAGING) CHARACTERISTICS IN AD					
Functional Loss in Non-AD Disorders			**FAST AD Distinctions**		
Disorder	**Pathology or Presumed Etiology**	**Functional Loss in Non-AD Disorder****	**Equivalent FAST Stage***	**Functional Loss in AD per FAST***	**FAST Stages in AD***
Dementia Associated With Hyponatremia	Electrolyte disturbance	1. Loss of ability to perform complex tasks	4	1. Loss of ability to perform complex tasks	4
		2. Loss of ability to pick out clothing properly	5	2. Loss of ability to pick out clothing properly	5
		3. Loss of ability to dress, bathe, and toilet independently	6a–6c	3. Loss of ability to dress, bathe, and toilet independently	6a–6c
		4. Loss of ambulation capacity	7c	4. Loss of urinary and fecal continence	6d–6e
		5. Loss of urinary and fecal continence	6d–6e	5. Loss of speech	7a–7b
		6. Loss of speech	7a–7b	6. Loss of ambulatory capacity	7c
Dementia Associated With Diffuse CNS Metastasis	Neoplastic diffuse cerebral trauma	1. Loss of ability to perform complex tasks	4	1. Loss of ability to perform complex tasks	4
		2. Loss of ability to dress, bathe, and toilet independently	6a–6c	2. Loss of ability to dress, bathe, and toilet independently	6a–6c
		3. Loss of ambulation capacity	7c	3. Loss of urinary and fecal continence	6d–6e
		4. Loss of urinary and fecal continence	6d–6e	4. Loss of speech	7a–7b
		5. Loss of speech	7a–7b	5. Loss of ambulatory capacity	7c

*Functional Assessment Staging (FAST) in Normal Aging and Alzheimer's Disease, copyright 1984 by Barry Reisberg. All rights reserved.

**The sequences of functional loss shown are typical for normal pressure hydrocephalus and Creutzfeldt-Jakob disease; the sequence for multi-infarct dementia is one of various common presentations; the sequences in the dementia syndrome of depression, dementia associated with hyponatremia, and dementia associated with diffuse CNS metastasis are previously observed examples of the presentation of these dementias. It should be noted that in some of the non-AD disorders, particularly multi-infarct dementia, the "sequence" described may appear abruptly, rather than over an extended time interval.

AD, Alzheimer's disease; CNS, central nervous system.

Source: Reisberg, Pattschull-Furlan, Franssen, et al. (1990).

is notably more impaired functionally, in comparison with the magnitude of the cognitive impairment (e.g., a GDS stage 5 person who is at stage 6d on the FAST), this is an indication of the likely presence of excess functional disability. For example, the person may have coexisting arthritis and AD. As a result of the combination of arthritis and dementia, in addition to not being able to handle finances and to pick out clothing without assistance (deficits that occur only because of the person's AD), the person may be unable to dress, bathe, and toilet without assistance, the latter resulting in occasional urinary incontinence. The arthritis may or may not be remediable. Similarly, the excess functional disability may or may not be remediable. Interestingly, when excess functional disability

TABLE 3.5

DIFFERENTIAL DIAGNOSTIC CONSIDERATIONS IN CASES OF DEVIATIONS FROM FAST*

Stage	FAST Characteristics	Differential Diagnostic Considerations (Particularly if FAST Stage Occurs Prematurely in the Evolution of Dementia)
1	No functional decrement, either subjectively or objectively, manifest	
2	Complains of forgetting location of objects; subjective work difficulties	Anxiety disorder, depression
3	Decreased functioning in demanding employment settings evident to coworkers, difficulty in traveling to new locations	Depression, subtle manifestations of medical pathology
4	Decreased ability to perform complex tasks such as planning dinner for guests, handling finances, and marketing	Depression, psychosis, focal cerebral process (e.g., Gerstmann's syndrome)
5	Requires assistance in choosing proper clothing, may require coaxing to bathe properly	Depression
6	(a) Difficulty putting on clothing properly (b) Requires assistance in bathing, may develop fear of bathing (c) Inability to handle mechanics of toileting (d) Urinary incontinence (e) Fecal incontinence	(a) Arthritis, sensory deficit, stroke, depression (b) Arthritis, sensory deficit, stroke, depression (c) Arthritis, sensory deficit, stroke, depression (d) Urinary tract infection, other causes of urinary incontinence (e) Infection, malabsorption syndrome, other causes of fecal incontinence
7	(a) Ability to speak limited to one to five words (b) Intelligible vocabulary lost (c) Ambulatory ability lost (d) Ability to sit up independently lost (e) Ability to smile lost (f) Ability to hold up head lost	(a) Stroke, other dementing disorder (e.g., diffuse space-occupying lesions) (b) Stroke, other dementing disorder (e.g., diffuse space-occupying lesions) (c) Parkinsonism, neuroleptic-induced or other secondary extrapyramidal syndrome, Creutzfeldt-Jakob disease, normal pressure hydrocephalus, hyponatremic dementia, stroke, hip fracture, arthritis, overmedication (d) Arthritis, contractures (e) Stroke (f) Head trauma, metabolic abnormality, other medical abnormality, overmedication, encephalitis, other causes

*FAST, Functional Assessment Staging in normal aging and Alzheimer's disease.

Source: From Reisberg (1986).

occurs in AD persons, it tends to occur "along the lines of the FAST." It appears that AD predisposes to functional losses outlined on the FAST. When an insult occurs, the closer the AD person is to the inevitable point of loss of a functional ability on the FAST, the more predisposed the AD person is to the premature loss of that capacity on the FAST. Not only illnesses but psychological stressors may also produce these premature losses. For example, if an AD person at GDS stage 6 and FAST stage 6c is moved to an unfamiliar environment, the person may develop urinary and fecal incontinence that remits when the AD person is returned to familiar surroundings. Subsequently, these capacities will, tragically, be lost with the advance of AD.

Knowledge of the FAST progression of AD, in conjunction with the global concomitants, feeding concomitants, and other aspects, also provides invaluable information on the potential for the treatment of disability, even in AD that is uncomplicated by the presence of additional pathology. For example, strategies for forestalling incontinence can be contemplated in FAST stage 6c. In FAST stage 6d or 6e, treatment of incontinence requires different strategies, such as frequent toileting. With the advance of deficits in FAST stage 7, strategies and goals for the management of incontinence need to be modified.

Other symptoms in AD, notably symptoms associated with the behavioral syndrome as outlined in Table 3.6, also require treatment. These symptoms are commonly treated with neuroleptics or other psychotropic medications. It should be noted that treatment of these symptoms may also be related to the treatment of functional disabilities. For example, it has been observed that AD persons with excess functional disability in relation to the magnitude of their cognitive disturbances

TABLE 3.6

BEHAVIORAL AND PSYCHOLOGICAL PATHOLOGIC SYMPTOMATOLOGY IN ALZHEIMER'S DISEASE (AD)
Paranoid and Delusional Ideation *The "people are stealing things" delusion.* Alzheimer's patients can no longer recall the precise whereabouts of household objects. This is probably the psychological explanation for what apparently is the most common delusion of AD patients—that someone is hiding or stealing objects. More severe manifestations of this delusion include the belief that persons are actually speaking with or listening to the intruders. *The "house is not one's home" delusion.* As a result of their cognitive deficits, AD patients may no longer recognize their home. This appears to account, in part, for the common conviction of the AD patient that the place in which they are residing is not their home. Consequently, while actually at home, AD patients commonly request that their caregiver "take me home." They may also pack their bags for their return home. More disturbing to the caregiver, and of great potential danger to the patient, are actual attempts to leave the house to go "home." Occasionally attempts to prevent the patient's departure may result in anger or even violence toward the caregiver, which is extremely upsetting to the spouse or other caregiver. *The "spouse (or other caregiver) is an impostor" delusion.* As cognitive deficit progresses, AD patients recognize their caregivers less well. Perhaps for this reason, a frequent delusion of the AD patient is that persons are impostors. In some instances, anger and even violence may result from this conviction. *The delusion of "abandonment."* With the progression of intellectual deficit in AD, patients retain a degree of insight into their condition. Although AD patients are largely aware of their cognitive deficits, denial protects them from their awareness. Similarly, they may be aware of the burden they have become. These insights are probably related to common delusions of abandonment, institutionalization, or of conspiracy or plot to institutionalize the patient. *The "delusion of infidelity."* The insecurities described previously are also related to the AD patient's occasional conviction that the spouse is unfaithful, sexually or otherwise. This conviction of infidelity may also apply to other caregivers. *Other suspicions, paranoid ideation, or delusions.* Although these delusions are the most commonly observed in AD, others may also be present (e.g., phantom boarder [strangers are living in the home], delusions that one still carries on activities in which one actually no longer participates [e.g., working, traveling]; delusions about former family members or the present status of family members [e.g., father is still alive; daughter is still a child]; delusions of doubles [e.g., there are two of the same person]). Suspicion and paranoid ideation may occur regarding strangers, people staring, people plotting to do harm, and so forth.
Hallucinations *Visual hallucinations.* These can be vague or clearly defined. Commonly, AD patients see intruders or dead relatives at home or have similar hallucinatory experiences. *Auditory hallucinations.* Occasionally, in the presence or absence of visual hallucinations, AD patients may hear dead relatives, intruders, or others whispering or speaking to them; sometimes voices are only heard when caregivers are not present. *Other hallucinations.* Less commonly, other forms of hallucinations may be observed in AD patients (e.g., smelling a fire or something burning; the patient perceiving imaginary objects, such as a piece of paper, which they offer the caregiver).
Activity Disturbances The decreased cognitive capacity of AD patients renders them less capable of channeling their energies in socially productive ways. Since motor abilities are not severely compromised until the final stage of illness, the patient may develop various psychological/motoric solutions for the need to channel their energies. A few of the most common examples are the following: *Wandering.* For a variety of reasons including inability to channel energies, anxieties, delusions such as those described, and the decreased cognitive abilities per se, AD patients frequently wander away from the home or caregiver. Restraints may be necessary and this, in turn, may provoke anger or violence in the patient.

(*continued*)

TABLE 3.6 (*continued*)

BEHAVIORAL AND PSYCHOLOGICAL PATHOLOGIC SYMPTOMATOLOGY IN ALZHEIMER'S DISEASE (AD)
Purposeless activity (cognitive abulla). As the condition advances, the AD patient loses the ability to complete or to carry out many of the activities in which he or she formerly engaged. This may be the basis in part of a variety of purposeless, frequently repetitive activities including opening and closing a purse or pocketbook; packing and unpacking clothing; repeatedly putting on and removing clothing; opening and closing drawers; incessant repetition of demands or questions; or simply pacing. In the absence of more productive, structured activities, these purposeless activities provide a means for AD patients to channel their energies and their need for movement. Among the most severe manifestations of this syndrome is repetitive self-abrading. *Inappropriate activities.* These occur primarily as a result of decreased cognitive capacities, increased anxieties and suspiciousness, and excess physical energies. They include storing and hiding objects in inappropriate places (e.g., throwing clothing in the wastebasket, putting empty plates in the oven). Attempts by the caregiver to prevent these inappropriate activities may be met by anger or even violence.
Aggressivity *Verbal outbursts.* As already noted, these may occur in association with many of the behavioral symptoms already described. They can also occur as isolated phenomena. For example, an AD patient may begin to use unaccustomed foul and abrasive language with intimates and/or with strangers. *Physical outbursts.* These also may occur as a part of the aforementioned syndromes or as an isolated manifestation. The AD patient may, in response to frustration or seemingly without cause, strike out at the spouse or caregiver. *Other agitation.* This includes anger, which is expressed nonverbally, for example, the patient's "stewing." Also common is negativity manifested by the patient's resistance to bathing, dressing, toileting, walking, or participating in other activities. Agitation may also be expressed as continuous and seemingly incessant talking (i.e., pressured speech), by panting (hyperventilation), banging, or in other ways.
Diurnal Rhythm Disturbance Sleep problems are a frequent and significant part of the behavioral syndrome of AD. They may, in part, be the result of decreased cognition (which upsets habitual and other diurnal cues), the energy and motoric changes occurring in the illness, and the neurochemical processes predisposing to agitation and false beliefs. *Day/night disturbance.* The most common sleep problem in AD patients is multiple awakenings in the course of the evening. These can occur in the context of an overall decrease in sleep or in association with increased daytime napping.
Affective Disturbance The depressive syndrome of AD is primarily reactive in nature; it tends to frequently become manifest somewhat earlier in the course of AD than many of the other symptoms already described and may be related to the pattern of insight and denial in the patient. *Tearfulness.* This predominant depressive manifestation generally occurs in brief periods. If queried as to the reason for the tearfulness, patients might respond that they are crying because "the person I once was is gone," or "of what is happening to me," or "I forgot the reason." This tearfulness frequently may be a precursor of more severe behavioral symptomatology. *Other depressive manifestations.* A depressive syndrome may coexist with early AD just as other illnesses may coexist with AD. The most common affective symptom in AD is the patient saying, "I wish I were dead" or uttering a similar phrase, frequently in a repetitive and manneristic fashion. These pessimistic commentaries of the patient are not accompanied by any more overt suicidal ideation or gestures.
Anxieties and Phobias These may be related to the previously described behavioral manifestations of AD or may occur independently. *Anxiety regarding upcoming events (Godot syndrome).* This common symptom appears to result from decreased cognition and, more specifically, memory disabilities in AD patients, and from the inability to channel remaining thinking capacity productively. Consequently, the patient will repeatedly query with respect to an upcoming event. These queries may be so incessant and persistent as to become intolerable to family and caregiver. *Other anxieties.* Patients commonly express previously nonmanifest anxieties regarding their finances, their future, their health (including their memory), and regarding previously nonstressful activities, such as being away from home. *Fear of being left alone.* This is the most commonly observed phobia in AD, but as a phobic phenomenon, it is out of proportion to any real danger. For example, the anxieties may become apparent as soon as the spouse goes into another room. Less dramatically, the patient may simply request of the spouse or caregiver, "Don't leave me alone." *Other phobias.* Patients with AD sometimes develop a fear of crowds, of travel, of the dark, or of activities such as bathing.

Source: Adapted from "Behavioral Pathology in Alzheimer's Disease (BEHAVE-AD)," copyright 1986 by Barry Reisberg. All rights reserved. Published in Reisberg, Borenstein, Salob, et al. (1987). See also, Reisberg, Borenstein, Franssen, et al., 1986.

may frequently have particularly marked behavioral disturbances. Conversely, marked behavioral disturbances may be associated with excess functional disability. This excess functional disability may be remediated in part by successful treatment of the behavioral symptoms.

OVERALL MANAGEMENT SCIENCE AND THE RETROGENESIS PROCESS IN AD

As shown in Table 3.7, a very interesting and important aspect of the functional progression of AD is that the order of losses on the FAST from stage 3 to stage 7f is a precise reversal of the order of acquisition of the same functions in normal human development (Reisberg, 1986; Reisberg, Ferris, & de Leon, 1985; Reisberg, Ferris, & Franssen, 1986).

Hence, as shown in Table 3.7, in MCI (FAST stage 3), persons begin to have difficulty with executive job functioning and equivalently complex social tasks. These abilities are acquired in normal human development during adolescence, approximately from 13 to 19 years of age. In mild AD (FAST stage 4), AD persons begin to have difficulties with instrumental (complex) daily life activities. These include management of personal financial matters. For example, the FAST stage 4 person may begin to write the wrong date and/or the wrong amount on their checks when paying their bills. These abilities are acquired in normal development from approximately 8 to 12 years of age. In FAST stage 5, persons with moderate AD begin to have difficulty choosing the proper clothing to wear for the weather conditions of the day and/or for the events of the day. This ability to select clothing properly, for example, for school, is acquired from about 5 to 7 years of age.

In moderately severe AD (FAST stage 6), a total of five successive substages are identifiable. These are, respectively, FAST stage 6a, in which the ability to put on clothing independently becomes compromised; FAST stage 6b, in which the ability to wash oneself independently is compromised (e.g., the ability to adjust the shower or bathwater temperature independently is compromised and assistance in this area is required); FAST stage 6c, in which cleanliness in toileting is compromised; FAST stage 6d, in which independent urinary continence is compromised; and FAST stage 6e, in which fecal continence is compromised. These abilities are acquired during normal human development from approximately 2 to 5 years of age. Of course, in normal human development, there are great differences between the 2-year-old child and the 5-year-old child. There are similarly great differences between the FAST 6e doubly incontinent AD person and the FAST stage 6a AD person who is having difficulty putting on clothing properly. Also, just as the ability to dress oneself independently is acquired at approximately the same time in normal development as is the ability to bathe oneself independently, these abilities are lost over approximately the same time period in the course of AD. Similarly, just as the acquisition of fecal continence and of urinary continence is closely temporally related in normal human development, the loss of these functions is quite closely related in the degenerative course of AD (Sclan & Reisberg, 1992).

In severe AD (FAST stage 7), a total of six successive substages are identifiable. These are, respectively, FAST stage 7a, in which speech ability appears to be severely limited to only approximately a half dozen or so words in the course of an intensive interview or in what appears to be an average day; FAST stage 7b, in which speech ability appears to be limited to, at most, a single, final, intelligible word; FAST stage 7c, in which the ability to ambulate independently is lost; FAST stage 7d, in which the ability to sit up independently is lost; FAST stage 7e, in which the ability to smile is lost; and FAST stage 7f, in which the ability to hold up the head independently is lost. These abilities are acquired in normal human development from approximately 1 month to 1.5 years of age. Of course, in normal development, there are great differences between the infant at 1 month of age and the child at 1.5 years. There are similarly great differences between the FAST stage 7f AD person who cannot hold up the head and the FAST stage 7a person, who can only speak a few words. However, just as the ability to speak a single word in infant development and the point at which the infant has the ability to speak a few words may be indistinguishable, similarly, the point at which the AD person in FAST stage 7 can speak only a few words and the point at which the AD person can only say a single word can be very close together and difficult to distinguish. Also, there are caveats to the developmental analogies

TABLE 3.7

Normal Development
Approximate Total Duration: 20 Years

Alzheimer's Degeneration
Approximate Total Duration: 20 Years

FUNCTIONAL LANDMARKS IN NORMAL HUMAN DEVELOPMENT AND ALZHEIMER'S DISEASE (AD)

Approximate Age		Approximate Duration in Development	Acquired Abilities	Lost Abilities	Alzheimer Stage	Approximate Duration in AD	Developmental Age of AD
Adolescence	13–19 years	7 years	Hold a job	Hold a job	3—incipient	7 years	19–13 years: adolescence
Late childhood	8–12 years	5 years	Handle simple finances	Handle simple finances	4—mild	2 years	12–8 years: late childhood
Middle childhood	5–7 years	2.5 years	Select proper clothing	Select proper clothing	5—moderate	1.5 years	7–5 years: middle childhood
Early childhood	5 years	4 years	Put on clothes unaided	Put on clothes unaided	6a—moderately severe	2.5 years	5–2 years: early childhood
	4 years		Shower unaided	Shower unaided	b		
	4 years		Toilet unaided	Toilet unaided	c		
	3–4.5 years		Control urine	Control urine	d		
	2–3 years		Control bowels	Control bowels	e		
Infancy	15 months	1.5 years	Speak 5–6 words	Speak 5–6 words	7a—severe	7 years or longer	15 months to birth: infancy
	1 year		Speak 1 word	Speak 1 word	b		
	1 year		Walk	Walk	c		
	6–10 months		Sit up	Sit up	d		
	2–4 months		Smile	Smile	e		
	1–3 months		Hold up head	Hold up head	f		

(Reisberg, Kenowsky, Franssen, Auer, & Souren, 1999; Reisberg, Franssen, Souren, Auer, Akram, & Kenowsky, 2002). These include the fact that AD persons have a total life history, which infants do not. Therefore, even very late in FAST stage 7, AD persons can speak seemingly forgotten words on occasion, whereas young infants do not have access to such words. Other caveats to the development stage analogies have been described in detail previously (Reisberg, Franssen, Souren, et al., 2002).

Subsequent work has indicated that AD also reverses normal development in terms of other functional parameters such as feeding abilities and figure drawings (Reisberg, Pattschull-Furlan, Franssen, et al., 1990). The approximate mean duration of the FAST stages in normal brain aging, SCI, MCI, and AD, which is not complicated by the presence of significant excess morbidities, is described in Table 3.2.

Figure 3.14 shows a plot of the temporal course of the acquisition of functions in the course of normal human development on the left-hand graph. It begins with the FAST stage 7e function (i.e., the acquisition of the ability to smile at about 2 months of age). It continues with the acquisition of the ability to sit up, to walk, to say a single word, to say a half dozen words, to achieve fecal continence, and so forth. The left-hand graph in Figure 3.14 ends with the ability to manage a complex occupational or social task independently at the beginning of adult life. It can be seen from Figure 3.14 that these abilities are acquired in normal human development over a period of approximately 18 years. Also shown in Figure 3.14 on the left-hand side is the plot of the ability to obtain other functions, specifically, praxis abilities (dotted line) and feeding abilities (broken line) to the extent that current knowledge permits these abilities to be temporally graphed in terms of chronologic age (Reisberg, Pattschull-Furlan, Franssen, et al., 1990).

The right-hand side of Figure 3.14 shows the temporal course of the loss of the same functions in the course of MCI (about 7 years), mild AD (about 2 years), moderate AD (about 1.5 years), moderately severe AD (about 2.5 years), and severe AD for persons who survive until the final 7f substage (about 6 years until FAST stage 7f). It can be seen that despite the fact that in the final stage 7 of AD, functions that are acquired in the course of normal human development over a period of only approximately a year and a half are lost in the course of

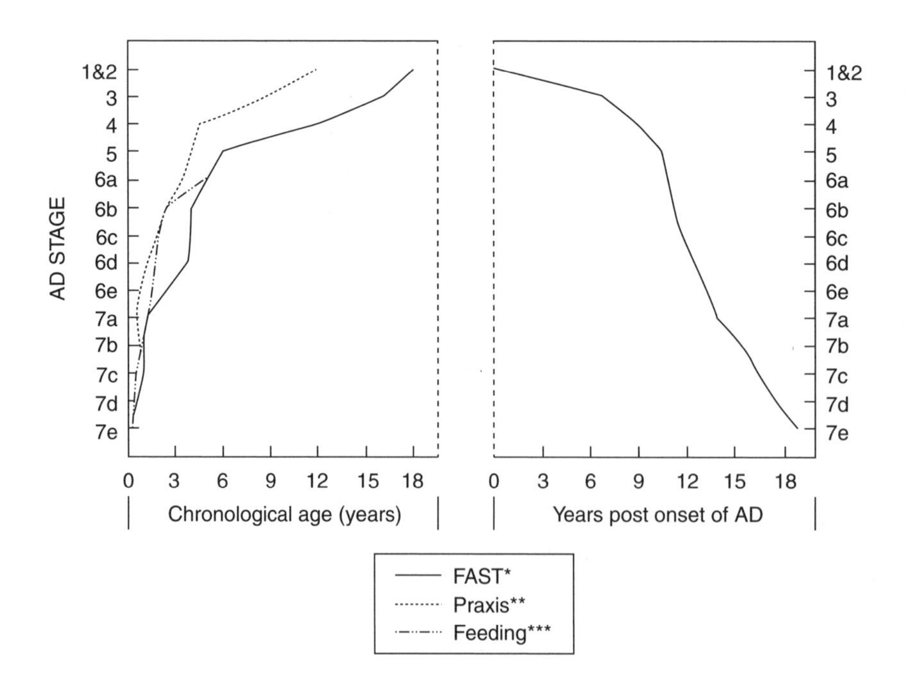

FIGURE 3.14 Relationship between the temporal course of acquisition of functional,* praxis,** and feeding*** capacities in normal human development and the typical temporal course of degeneration in Alzheimer's disease (AD).

*Functional Assessment Staging (FAST) in normal aging and AD.

**Praxis axis from the Brief Cognitive Rating Scale (BCRS): Parts 1 and 2, Copyright 1984, Barry Reisberg. All rights reserved.

***Feeding concomitants of AD.

Source: Copyright 1988, Barry Reisberg. All rights reserved.

FAST stage 7 over a period of 6 years (or even longer if stage 7f is included), there is a striking inverse symmetry between the temporal (as well as ordinal) course of acquisition of functions in normal human development and the loss of the same functions in the course of the process of MCI and AD. To the extent that current knowledge permits, mechanisms for this developmental reversal are discussed later in this chapter.

In addition to the AD process reversing normal development functionally, the course of the AD process also reverses normal human development cognitively (Auer et al., 1994; Ouvrier, Goldsmith, Ouvrier, & Williams, 1993; Sclan, Foster, Reisberg, Franssen, & Welkowitz, 1990; Shimada et al., 2003).

For example, the MMSE is a well-known and widely used cognitive assessment developed for the assessment of dementia patients (Folstein et al., 1975). The MMSE score has shown approximately as robust a relationship to the mental age of children as it has shown to any noncognitive measure of dementia pathology. Initially, in a study of Australian children, a 0.83 Pearson correlation of the MMSE score to the mental age of children was found (Ouvrier et al., 1993). A subsequent study, in Spanish children, found a 0.76 Pearson correlation between childhood mental ages and MMSE scores and a 0.80 correlation between MMSE scores and children's chronological ages (Rubial-Álvarez et al., 2007).

Conversely, a study was conducted in AD persons using a cognitive assessment measure specifically developed for infants and small children, the Ordinal Scales of Psychological Development (OSPD) assessment (Uzgiris & Hunt, 1975). This OSPD test was slightly modified for use in severe dementia persons. The resulting Modified-OSPD measurement of cognition (the M-OSPD) showed approximately the same relationship to the FAST stage in stage 6 and stage 7 AD persons (0.8 correlation) as is seen between the FAST functional stage and MMSE cognitive assessment in somewhat less severe AD persons who are testable with the MMSE (Auer et al., 1994; Reisberg, Ferris, Torossian et al., 1992).

Similarly, a widely used intelligence test measure for children, the Binet scale, has been applied to AD persons in FAST stages 5, 6, and 7. A Spearman's correlation of −0.85 between the Binet test measure basic age value and the FAST stage was found (Shimada et al., 2003). This is at least as robust as the relationship between the MMSE and the FAST assessment in dementia patients in the corresponding FAST range (Reisberg, Ferris, Torossian, et al., 1992).

The remarkable relationships between cognition and functioning in normal human development and the losses of these capacities in the course of brain aging and AD were recently illustrated in a comprehensive study conducted at centers in Spain (Rubial-Álvarez et al., 2013). Rubial-Álvarez and colleagues compared the performance of 181 children ranging in age from 4 to 12 years with that of 148 adults. The adults included cognitively normal persons (GDS stages 1 and 2), subjects with MCI (GDS stage 3), and persons with mild (GDS stage 4) to moderately severe (GDS stage 6) AD. It should be noted that the moderately severe AD persons in this study, at GDS stage 6, were relatively mildly impaired for this stage, because all were in FAST stages 6a or 6b. The study result, in terms of a cognitive measure, is illustrated in Figure 3.15, which shows the correspondence for MMSE scores.

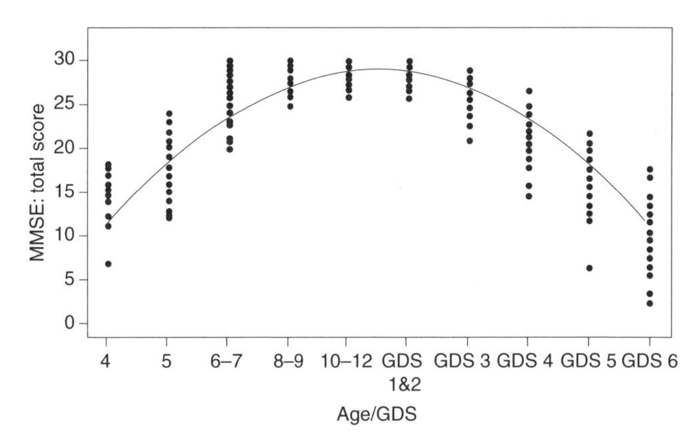

FIGURE 3.15 Comparison between MMSE scores in children from 4 to 12 years of age and adults with normal cognition, mild cognitive impairment, and mild to moderately severe Alzheimer's disease.

Total Mini-Mental status examination (MMSE) scores obtained by mentally and physically healthy children aged 4 to 12 years (n = 181) and elderly participants (≥65 y, n = 148) with normal cognition (control, GDS [Global Deterioration Scale] stages 1 and 2), mild cognitive impairment (GDS stage 3), mild dementia (GDS stage 4), moderate dementia (GDS stage 5), and moderately severe dementia (GDS stage 6 and FAST [Functional Assessment Staging] stage 6a and 6b) symptomatology. All dementia subjects had probable AD. Results indicate a substantial correspondence in cognitive status (MMSE total score) as a function of age (children) and GDS staging (adults), respectively. The curve represents the fit of a linear regression model with a quadratic term (R^2 = .83).

Source: Adapted from Rubial-Álvarez et al. (2013). Printed with permission from the corresponding author, Jordi Peña Casanova.

As described previously, the MMSE is a very widely used screening test for dementia, and the results show a substantial correspondence between the cognitive status as a function of age and the corresponding developmental age (DA)–based GDS stages. Similar patterns were observed for the functioning assessment studied by the investigators, for the vocabulary measure studied, and for an overall intelligence test score.

Table 3.7 illustrates that the FAST stages of AD can be expressed in terms of DAs. Remarkably, so-called developmental infantile reflexes appear to be equally good markers for the emergence of the stage of severe AD, corresponding to a DA of infancy, as the same reflexes are in marking the emergence from infancy in normal development (Franssen, Souren, Torossian, & Reisberg, 1997; see Figure 3.16). An illustration of this phenomenon is the grasp reflex shown in the GDS and FAST stage 7 AD person in Figure 3.17.

Similar to the findings with neurological reflexes, a leading investigator in neurometabolism has reported remarkable similarities between the pattern of brain metabolic activity in the late-stage AD patient and that in the normal infant brain (Phelps, 2000). These findings, obtained using PET scanning techniques, are very different from the metabolic patterns observed in the normal adult brain.

Yet another way in which the process of progressive brain change from normal aging, to MCI, to the progressive stages of AD reverses normal human development is in terms of brain electrophysiology. The electrical activity of the brain is commonly measured with the EEG. It has long

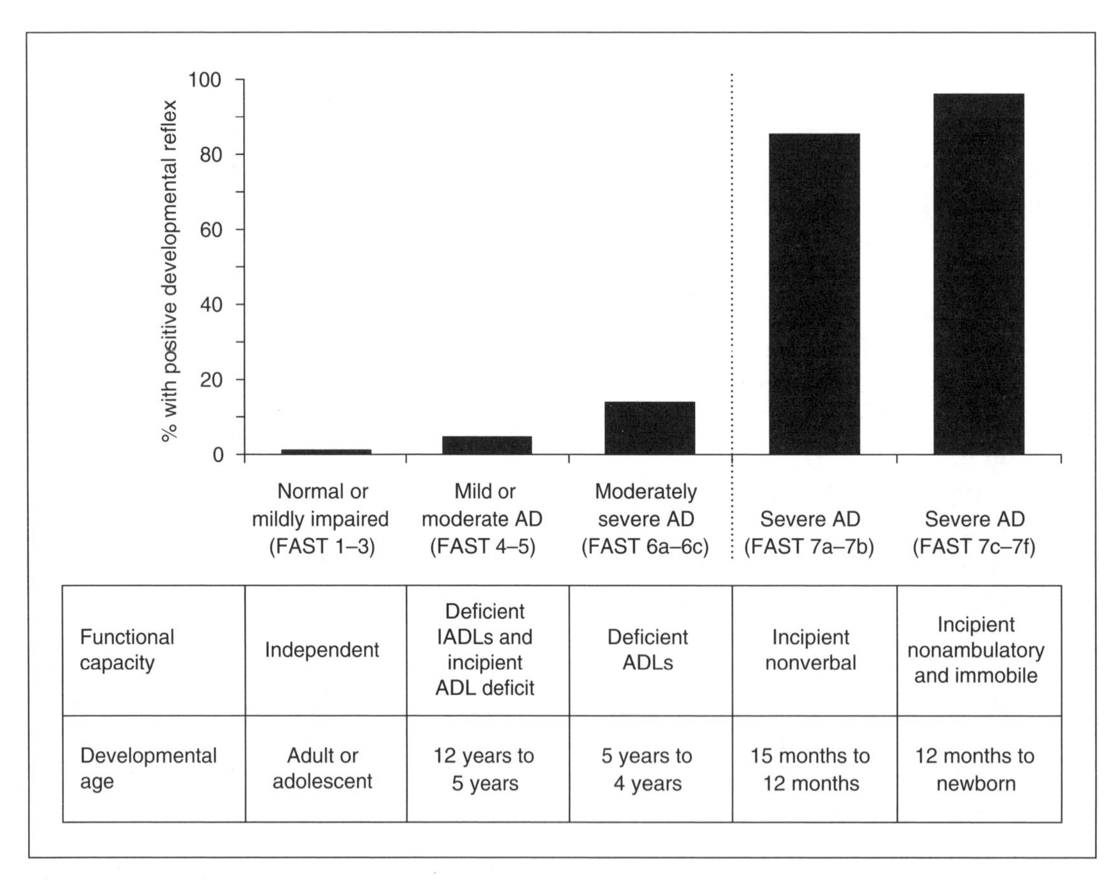

Functional capacity	Independent	Deficient IADLs and incipient ADL deficit	Deficient ADLs	Incipient nonverbal	Incipient nonambulatory and immobile
Developmental age	Adult or adolescent	12 years to 5 years	5 years to 4 years	15 months to 12 months	12 months to newborn

FIGURE 3.16 Neurological retrogenesis: the emergence of "infant reflexes" in advanced Alzheimer's disease. Percentages of patients with one or more of the following developmental reflexes (also known as primitive reflexes or frontal release signs) are shown: the tactile sucking reflex, the palmar grasp (hand grasp) reflex, the plantar grasp (foot grasp) reflex, and the plantar extensor (Babinski) reflex. All reflexes were elicited according to standard procedures and were assessed as being present when they were prominent and persistent, defined by a rating of ≥5 on the scale of Franssen (Franssen et al., 1991, 1993; Franssen, 1993; Franssen & Reisberg, 1997). For the three reflexes that were assessed bilaterally, specifically, the palmar grasp reflex, the plantar grasp reflex, and the plantar extensor reflex, a positive response on either side was assessed as positive. Subject samples were as follows: independent, subjective deficit, or mild impairment only (FAST stages 1 to 3), *n* = 314; deficient IADLs and incipient ADL deficit (FAST stages 4 to 5), *n* = 247; deficient ADLs (FAST stages 6a to 6c), *n* = 113; incipient nonverbal (FAST stages 7a to 7b), *n* = 29; incipient nonambulatory and immobile (FAST stages 7c to 7f), *n* = 32. IADLs are instrumental (complex) activities of daily life; ADLs are basic activities of daily life.

Source: Data and figure are adapted from Franssen, Souren, Torossian, and Reisberg (1997).

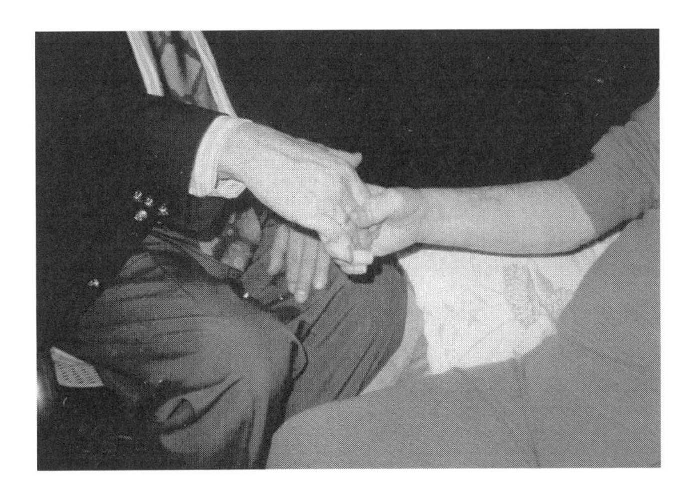

FIGURE 3.17 The emergence of a grasp reflex in this GDS and FAST stage 7 AD person.

FAST, Functional Assessment Staging; GDS, Global Deterioration Scale.

Source: Copyright 1994 by Barry Reisberg.

been recognized that the aging and dementia process is accompanied by a progressive slowing of the brain waves measured with the EEG. As the AD process advances, EEG slow waves, usually seen during sleep in the normal adult, become increasingly common during the waking state. Prichep and colleagues published these changes from GDS stage 1 to GDS stage 6 in 1994 (Prichep et al., 1994; see Figure 3.18). Twelve years later, Prichep and associates demonstrated that the slowing of EEG wave activity was so sensitive that it could be used to predict which SCI (GDS stage 2) persons would go on to decline at the time of follow-up, 7 to 9 years subsequently (Prichep et al., 2006).

To determine the precise relationship between EEG slowing in AD and the EEG changes seen in normal human development, Borza and colleagues did a meta-analysis of the world literature (Borza, Reisberg, Astarastoae, & Dascalu, 2010). They studied 30 publications from the scientific literature from 1949 until 2008. Fourteen of the publications reported data on the EEG activity of normal subjects from infancy to 29 years of age, and 16 of the publications reported data on the EEG activity of AD subjects at various stages. The findings are illustrated in Figure 3.19.

Figure 3.19 shows the findings for each of the major EEG wave bands, that is: (a) the delta wave band, which is the slowest EEG wave activity (about 1 to 3 cycles per second); (b) the theta wave band, which is the next slowest wave activity (about 4

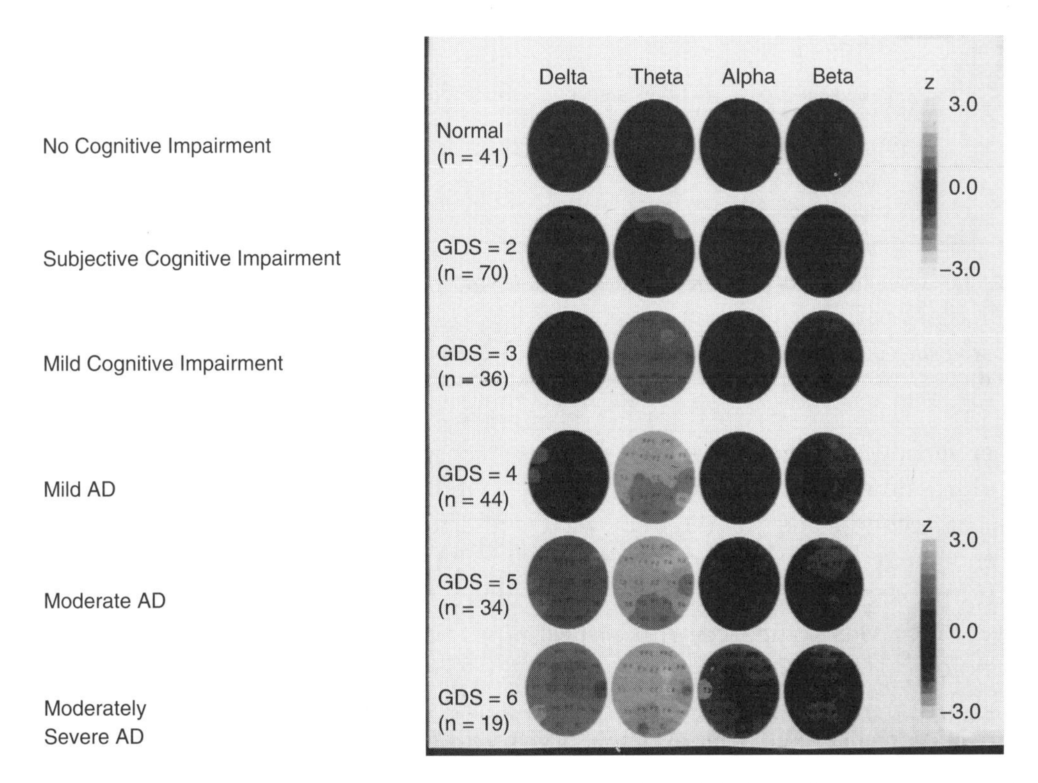

FIGURE 3.18 EEG wave frequencies in brain aging with no cognitive impairment (NCI, Global Deterioration Scale stage 1), subjective cognitive impairment (GDS stage 2), mild cognitive impairment (GDS stage 3), and mild, moderate, and moderately severe Alzheimer's disease (AD).

Source: Adapted from Prichep et al. (1994).

	Age in normal human development	Stages of AD and corresponding, functionally based, developmental age (DA) of AD (see also Table 3.7)			
	Chronologic age	Severe AD (DA = 0 to 2 years)	Moderately severe AD (DA = 2–5 years)	Moderate AD (DA = 5–7 years)	Mild AD (DA = 7 years–adolescence)
Delta waves (slowest EEG waves)	Birth to 2 years	No difference	*	**	***
	2–5 years	**	No difference	**	**
	5–7 years	***	***	No difference	***
	7 years to adolescence	***	***	***	No difference
Theta waves (2nd slowest EEG waves)	Birth to 2 years	No difference	No difference	**	**
	2–5 years	No difference	No difference	**	***
	5–7 years	***	***	No difference	***
	7 years to adolescence	***	***	***	No difference
Alpha waves (3rd slowest EEG waves)	Birth to 2 years	No difference	**	***	***
	2–5 years	***	No difference	***	***
	5–7 years	***	***	No difference	***
	7 years to adolescence	***	***	***	No difference
Beta waves (Fast EEG waves)	Birth to 2 years	No difference	*	**	**
	2–5 years	No difference	No difference	**	**
	5–7 years	**	**	No difference	***
	7 years to adolescence	**	**	***	No difference

FIGURE 3.19 EEG brain wave frequency patterns in normal development and in Alzheimer's disease (AD) severity stages.
*$p \leq .05$, **$p \leq .01$, ***$p \leq .001$.

Source: Adapted from data published in Borza, Reisberg, Astarastoae, and Dascalu (2010).

to 7 cycles per second); (c) the alpha wave band, which is the third slowest wave activity (about 8 to 15 cycles per second); and (d) the beta wave band, which encompasses fast wave activity (about 16 to 31 cycles per second). The activity on each of these wave bands was compared with respect to four chronological age groups (i.e., [a] birth to 2 years, [b] 2 to 5 years, [c] 5 to 7 years, and [d] 7 years to adolescence) and four AD severity groups (i.e., [a] severe AD, [b] moderately severe AD, [c] moderate AD, and [d] mild AD).

As already discussed in some detail, with respect to the FAST stages of AD, severe AD (FAST stage 7) corresponds to a DA of about birth to 2 years of age, moderately severe AD corresponds to a DA of about 2 to 5 years of age, moderate AD corresponds to a DA of about 5 to 7 years of age, and mild AD corresponds to a DA of about 7 years to adolescence. Therefore, the actual EEG findings in each DA group were compared with the corresponding AD stages. As can be seen in Figure 3.19, for each of the four EEG wave bands, there was no significant difference between chronologic age group and the corresponding DA-based AD stage group in terms of the level of EEG wave activity for any of the 16 relevant comparisons. In contrast, for the 48 comparisons in which a chronologic age group was compared with a noncorresponding DA group–based AD stage, 45 comparisons showed significant differences. Of the three remaining instances in which a chronologic age group showed a significant difference to a noncorresponding DA-based AD stage, in all instances they were to an adjacent DA group.

For example, with respect to delta wave activity, shown in the first row in Figure 3.19, there was no significant difference between the EEG activity of the subject group from birth to 2 years of age and the AD subjects with severe AD (corresponding to a DA from 0 to 2 years of age). However, there was a significant difference between the activity of the subject group from birth to 2 years of age and the moderately severe AD subjects ($p \leq .05$), the moderate AD subjects ($p \leq .01$), and the mild AD subjects ($p \leq .001$).

Collectively, the meta-analysis shown in Figure 3.19 indicates that electrophysiologically, in terms of EEG brain wave activity, AD also reverses normal human developmental patterns.

Neuroanatomic brain changes in AD have also been observed to mirror, in various ways, the brain changes in normal human development. In early studies of the neuropathology of AD, Brun and Gustafson concluded that "the pattern described may be related to ontogenic [developmental] features" (Brun & Gustafson, 1976). Subsequently, McGeer et al., noting the patterns of neuronal loss described by Brun and Englund (1981) and their own PET studies of neurometabolic changes in AD, concluded that the AD neurodegenerative process appears to relate to the pattern and process of brain myelination in normal development (McGeer et al., 1990). They observed that the areas of the brain that are the last to be myelinated in normal development (and that are therefore the most thinly myelinated; Flechsig, 1920) appear to be the areas that are the most vulnerable to the pathology of AD in terms of neuronal losses and decrements in cerebral metabolism (reviewed in Reisberg, Franssen, Hasan, et al., 1999). The pattern of neurofibrillary pathology in AD has also been related to the developmental pattern of myelinization of the brain in reverse (Braak & Braak, 1991; Braak & Braak, 1996). Raz has provided a numerical value for these anatomic relationships between myelinization in normal human development and myelin loss in the AD pathologic process as seen with neuroimaging. He noted that "the gradient of vulnerability seems to follow the rules of last (. . . ontogenetically) in–first out . . . the later a region completes its myelination, the greater age-related difference in volume it exhibits, $r = .60$, $p < .05$" (Raz, 1999). This process, by which the degenerative changes in AD and, to some extent, other dementias reverse the order of acquisition of capacities and processes in normal development has been termed *retrogenesis* (Reisberg, Franssen, Hasan, et al., 1999). The process of myelin loss, which is associated with the retrogenic process occurring in AD has been termed *arboreal entropy* (Reisberg, Franssen, Souren, et al., 2002).

> Just as the bark of a tree protects it from . . . injury and, to some extent, the thicker the bark, the greater the protection, the myelin protects the axon and its neuron. Hence, to some extent, . . . the thicker the myelin [and the earlier in development the neuron is myelinated], the greater the protection. (Reisberg, Franssen, Souren, et al., 2002)

The advent of diffusion tensor imaging (DTI) radiographic techniques permitted an objective examination of the myelination retrogenesis hypothesis. Therefore, in 2005, we published an initial study, which was found to support the retrogenesis-based hypothesis that the last brain regions to be myelinated would be the most vulnerable in the progression of AD (Choi, Lim, Monteiro, & Reisberg, 2005). Subsequently, other investigators conducted a study comparing AD patients and demographically matched healthy older adults targeting early myelinating and late myelinating fiber patterns (Stricker et al., 2009). They found that

> permutation-based, voxelwise analysis supported the retrogenesis model. There was significantly lower fractional anisotropy (FA) in AD patients compared to healthy older adults in late-myelinating but not early-myelinating pathways. . . . Consistent with the retrogenesis model, AD patients showed demonstrable changes in late-myelinating WM [white matter] fiber pathways. (Stricker et al., 2009)

In addition to the retrogenesis process having been observed for the brain's white matter in progressive AD, this process has also been observed in what has been called "the normal aging brain," presumably including GDS stages 1 to 3, corresponding to NCI, SCI, and MCI. Specifically, Raz et al. (1997) have found that "the myelinization order predicts vulnerability of cortical regions to aging." More specifically, Flechsig, in the early 20th century, described the myelinogenesis order for different brain regions (Flechsig, 1901). Raz et al. (1997) observed that the later the myelinization of a brain region, the stronger the association between age and the regional volume. It should be noted that in general, the later a brain region is myelinated, the thinner the myelin covering of the axon and, in accordance with the retrogenesis hypothesis, the greater the vulnerability of the axon to, among other forms of injury, the AD-related degenerative process.

Interestingly, the retrogenesis process can explain many of the other symptoms and findings in AD, such as the nature of patient behavioral disturbances (Reisberg, Auer, Monteiro, Franssen & Kenowsky, 1998) and the kind of symptoms, which are progressively and invariably lost, such as speaking and walking, in comparison with the kind of symptoms, which are more variable, such as the behavioral disturbances (Reisberg, Franssen, Souren, Auer, & Kenowsky, 1998). A summary of the major developmental functional, cognitive, neurological, neuroanatomic, electrophysiologic, neurometabolic, and psychologic processes manifesting the retrogenesis process is shown in Table 3.8.

Most importantly, the retrogenic process provides a rapid appreciation of the general care and management needs of the AD person at each stage of the disease (Reisberg, Kenowsky, Franssen, et al., 1999; Table 3.9).

An understanding of the retrogenic process in AD also provides the basis for a detailed management science (Reisberg, Franssen, Souren, et al., 2002). This science includes care axioms, care postulates, and care caveats. The care axioms apply to all human beings and to AD persons at all stages (Table 3.10). The postulates are testable hypotheses of AD persons' care based on the DA retrogenesis model (Table 3.11).

Finally, the caveats are based upon acknowledged differences between AD persons and their DA peers (Table 3.12). The combination of these care axioms, postulates, and caveats forms the nascent science of AD management.

TABLE 3.8

RETROGENESIS IN AD*
Definition of retrogenesis: The reversal of normal, developmental biologic processes in the course of disease.
Evidence for retrogenesis in Alzheimer's disease (AD):
1. The **functional progression** of AD reverses the functional progression of normal human development quite precisely.
2. **Cognitive measures** in AD reverse normal human development (a) **Praxis and figure drawing** (b) **Language** (c) The **MMSE** shows the same relationship to the mental age in normal children as it does to objective measures of dementia in the course of AD.
3. **Infantile reflexes** emerge in AD at the developmental age–appropriate point. These reflexes are just as powerful markers of the dementia stage of AD as they are of normal infant and child development.
4. The **neuropathologic changes** in myelination in AD appear to reverse normal developmental patterns.
5. **Electroencephalographic activity** with AD progression seems to reverse the normal developmental pattern.
6. **Neurometabolic activity** in AD, as measured with positron emission tomographic (PET) scans, seems to reverse the normal human developmental pattern.
7. **Emotional changes** in AD appear to be largely explainable using the corresponding developmental age.

*See text for further details and references.

MMSE, Mini-Mental State Examination.

Source: Copyright 2015 Barry Reisberg. All rights reserved.

TABLE 3.9

STAGES OF AGING AND ALZHEIMER'S DISEASE (AD) AND CORRESPONDING DEVELOPMENTAL AGES (DAs): CARE NEEDS AND CARE RECOMMENDATIONS

GDS Stage	Diagnosis	DA	Care Needs	Care Recommendations
1	Normal	Adult	None	None
2	Subjective cognitive impairment	Aged adult	None	Reassurance with respect to relatively benign prognosis
3	Mild cognitive impairment	Adolescence	None	"Tactical" withdrawal from situations that have become, by virtue of their complexity, anxiety provoking
4	Mild AD	Late childhood	Independent survival still attainable	Assistance toward goal of maximum independence with financial supervision; structured or supervised travel; identification bracelets and labels may be useful
5	Moderate AD	Middle childhood	AD person can no longer survive in the community without assistance; needs supervision with respect to travel and social behavior	Part-time home health care assistance can be very useful in assisting the patient's caregiver. Driving becomes hazardous and should be discontinued at some point over the course of this stage. Family may require guidance in handling the AD person's emotional outbursts
6	Moderately severe AD	Early childhood	AD person requires assistance with basic activities of daily life. Early in this stage, assistance with dressing and bathing is required. Subsequently, assistance with continence becomes necessary as well	Full-time home health care assistance is frequently very useful in assisting the AD person's caregiver. Strategies for assistance with bathing, toileting, and in the management of incontinence should be discussed with the family. Emotional stress in the caregiver should be minimized with supportive techniques
7	Severe AD	Infancy	Early in this stage, assistance with feeding as well as dressing, bathing, and toileting is required. Subsequently, assistance with ambulation and purposeful movement becomes necessary. Prevention of aspiration, contractures, and decubiti is a major issue in care	Full-time assistance in the community home residence or institutional setting is a necessity. Strategies for maintaining locomotion should be explored. The need for psychopharmacological intervention for behavioral disturbances decreases. Soft food or liquid diet is generally tolerated. AD persons must be fed and instructed and encouraged to maintain chewing and basic eating skills

Source: Copyright 2003, 2004 by Barry Reisberg. All rights reserved.

RELATIONSHIP BETWEEN AD CLINICAL COURSE AND MANAGEMENT AND THE OBSERVED PATHOLOGIC AND BIOMOLECULAR FEATURES OF AD

The classical observed brain pathology accompanying AD dementia is extracellular plaques containing a substance called amyloid and intraneuronal neurofibrillary tangles. The amyloid plaques are primarily composed of a protein called beta amyloid. The intracellular neurofibrillary tangles are derived from neuronal microtubules. There are generally 40 to 42 amino acids in the ß amyloid protein. This ß amyloid protein is itself derived from a much larger protein, the amyloid protein precursor (APP) protein. The APP protein is known as a transmembrane protein because it crosses the cell membrane of the neuron. The APP protein is normally cleaved

TABLE 3.10

ALZHEIMER'S DISEASE (AD) CARE AXIOMS	
Axiom I	All human beings avoid trauma and humiliation
Axiom II	All human beings seek a sense of accomplishment
Axiom III	All human beings seek a sense of dignity and self-worth
Axiom IV	All human beings are social organisms
Axiom V	All human beings seek praise and acceptance
Axiom VI	All human beings have the capacity to learn
Axiom VII	All human beings require love
Axiom VIII	All human beings have the capacity for happiness if basic needs are fulfilled
Axiom IX	All human beings have the need for physical movement
Axiom X	All human beings have the capacity to remember
Axiom XI	All human beings have the capacity to think
Axiom XII	All human beings seek to influence their environment
Axiom XIII	All human beings have a sense of "taste," i.e., likes and dislikes

Source: Copyright 2002, 2004 by Barry Reisberg. All rights reserved.

by an enzyme, alpha secretase, which cleaves the APP outside the cell membrane. When alpha secretase cleavage occurs, there is no amyloid beta produced. Alternatively, the APP is cleaved by another extracellular enzyme, the beta secretase enzyme. This beta secretase cleavage is followed by cleavage within the cell membrane by an enzyme known as gamma secretase. The result of this beta and gamma secretase cleavage is the amyloid beta (Aß) protein, which is in the plaques in AD. Both aging and AD are associated with increased amyloid beta protein in the brain (Näslund et al., 2000; Seubert et al., 1992).

The neurofibrillary tangles in AD, seen inside the neuron, are comprised of paired helical filaments (Kidd, 1963). The major constituent of these paired helical filaments is a protein known as "tau" (Kondo et al., 1988; Wischik et al., 1988; Wischik et al., 1988). Tau is believed to be a scaffolding molecule, which maintains the structural integrity of the microtubules in the neurons.

The relationship between the clinically observed "plaques and tangles" of AD (including the more recently discovered biomolecular constituents of the plaques and tangles) and the observed behavioral course of AD, described in the preceding sections of this chapter, can presently be elucidated.

As described in prior sections, remarkably similar patterns between the neurometabolic activity of a late-stage AD patient and those of the infant brain have been noted (Phelps, 2000). In 2002, Reisberg et al. hypothesized that these patterns could be explained if "the most metabolically active regions of the brain in AD . . . are the regions which are the most vulnerable in AD" (Reisberg, Franssen, Souren, et al., 2002). In 2005, it was found by Buckner et al. that, in fact, the pattern of deposition of amyloid plaques in the brain of AD patients appeared to occur in the regions of the brain that are the most active during the resting, so-called default state, when the brain is not focused upon any particular activity (Buckner et al., 2005). Hence, there appears to be a direct relationship between the metabolic activity of the brain and a major form of microscopically evident AD pathology, the amyloid plaques, containing beta amyloid.

In 1980, Ferris and associates reported, using the then new positron emission scanning techniques, that there is a continuous decrease in metabolism in

TABLE 3.11

ALZHEIMER'S DISEASE (AD) CARE POSTULATES	
Postulate I	The magnitude of care and supervision required by an AD person, at a developmental age (DA), is mirrored by the amount of care and supervision required by a child or infant at the corresponding DA
Postulate II	The kinds of activities enjoyed by an AD person, at a particular DA, are mirrored by the kinds of activities enjoyed by children at a corresponding DA
Postulate III	The capacity of an AD person to perform in an area of residual expertise is dependent on the AD person's DA
Postulate IV	Previous experiences may determine the kinds of activities enjoyed by an AD person
Postulate V	The emotional level of the AD person is dependent on the DA
Postulate VI	Life experiences appropriate to the DA become most relevant for the AD person at any particular stage
Postulate VII	Socialization of the AD person is dependent on the DA
Postulate VIII	Diversity in children's and infants' activities and interests is mirrored in diversity in the AD person's interests and activities at a corresponding DA
Postulate IX	The emotional changes that occur in AD at a DA are mirrored by the emotional changes observed in children at a corresponding DA
Postulate X	Care settings appropriate to AD persons at a DA are mirrored by care settings appropriate to children at the corresponding DA
Postulate XI	Vulnerability (emotional, physical, and cognitive) of the AD person at a DA is mirrored by the vulnerability of children at the corresponding DA
Postulate XII	The need of an AD person for physical movement is mirrored by the corresponding DA
Postulate XIII	Just as one judges development in an infant or child by what the infant or child can do and has achieved, not by what the infant or child cannot do, AD persons at any particular DA should be assessed in terms of their residual skills and accomplishments, what they have learned and relearned, not by what they cannot do
Postulate XIV	The developmental analogy is sufficiently strong to trigger DA-appropriate childhood memories, beliefs, and anxieties in the AD person
Postulate XV	The language changes of the AD person are mirrored by the DA

Source:

many brain regions with the advance of the behaviorally evident AD process (Ferris et al., 1980). These findings have been supported in numerous subsequent studies. This process of continuing neurometabolic loss in AD has been termed *neurometabolic entropy* (Reisberg, Wegiel, Franssen, Auer, et al., 2006). The continuing neurometabolic entropy, affecting first the most metabolically active brain regions, appears to provide an explanation for the observed neurometabolic retrogenesis seen in AD.

Recent studies have provided an understanding of the mechanisms underlying these metabolic changes in AD. The insulin receptor and the insulin-like growth factor receptor signaling pathway play a major role in controlling maximum life span and age-associated diseases in all species of multicellular organisms, which have been studied (Puglielli, 2008). Interestingly, a decrease in insulin-like growth factor 1 (IGF-1) blood levels occurs with normal aging in a retrogenic-like pattern. Specifically, there is a continuing increase in IGF-1 blood levels from infancy to about 15 years of age and this is followed by a continuing decrease in levels of IGF-1 in the blood, reaching an infant and early childhood level by about age 80 to 85 (Laboratory Corporation of America, accessed 2003; Reisberg, Wegiel, Franssen, Auer et al., 2006). These circulating blood changes in IGF-1 levels may be related to currently observed

TABLE 3.12

ALZHEIMER'S DISEASE (AD) CARE CAVEATS	
Caveat I	Development in infants and children is accompanied by increasing expectations, whereas AD at all stages is accompanied by progressively diminished expectations
Caveat II	AD persons experience developmentally analogous brain changes; however, they do not undergo developmentally analogous physical changes
Caveat III	AD persons can, to some extent, draw upon previously mastered skills, whereas infants and children may not have access to these skills
Caveat IV	AD persons can, to some extent, draw upon previously mastered knowledge, whereas infants and children may not have access to this knowledge
Caveat V	AD persons are older than their DA peers, and old age predisposes to various physical disabilities that influence the life and experience of an AD patient
Caveat VI	AD persons appear to be more prone to rigidity than their DA peers
Caveat VII	AD persons can potentially concentrate on a task longer than infants or children at a corresponding DA
Caveat VIII	AD persons appear to be less fascinated by the world and less inquisitive than infants and children at a corresponding DA

DA, developmental age.

Source:

changes in the IGF-1 insulin receptor in aging and AD. A decreased number of neurons have been reported to express the IGF-1 receptor in AD (Moloney et al., 2010). Also, Moloney et al. have reported that the IGF-1 receptor is aberrantly distributed in AD, particularly in neurons affected by neurofibrillary tangles, in that it is concentrated intracellularly rather than at the neuronal cell membrane. Related to this, Moloney et al. have reported decreased insulin receptor substrate levels in AD neurons, and these decrements are localized with the neurofibrillary tangles. Interestingly, in terms of the other major microscopically observed pathology in AD, the beta amyloid formed in part by gamma secretase cleavage, the same enzyme, gamma secretase, is also being related to the IGF-1 receptor. Specifically, gamma secretase has been reported to be involved in the proteolysis (breakdown) of the IGF-1 receptor (McElroy, Powell, & McCarthy, 2007).

In addition to direct relationships between the IGF-1 receptor and AD pathology, the insulin receptor has also been directly related to AD pathology. Soluble, amyloid beta (Townsend, Mehta, & Selkoe, 2007) as well as amyloid beta oligomers (Zhao, DeFelice, Fernandez et al., 2008) have been shown to impair insulin receptor function.

The net result of these changes in the IGF-1 receptor and in insulin receptor signaling is that the neurons that degenerate in AD may be more resistant to these signals (Moloney et al., 2010). This resistance has been widely observed, and AD is now frequently referred to as a type 3 diabetes (Hoyer, 1998; Steen et al., 2005). As with many changes in biology, the arrows, in terms of etiopathogenesis of metabolic deficits in the brain in AD, appear to point in both directions. The decrease in oxidative metabolism, which occurs in the brain in AD, has been observed to be associated with amyloid accumulation in several studies (Pluta, 2002; Popa-Wagner, Schröder, Walker, & Kessler, 1998; Sinigaglia-Coimbra, Cavalheiro, & Coimbra, 2002).

To fully understand the nature of the pathology in AD, together with associated pathogenic mechanisms and their relationship to the clinical manifestations of AD, an additional principle must be recognized and addressed. This is that there is a homeostatic, regenerative, developmental, physiologic response to the progressive pathology of AD. This regenerative physiologic response in AD has many elements, which notably include the following: (a) There is a reactivation of the cell cycle enzymes in terminally differentiated neurons in AD (reviewed in Reisberg, Franssen, Souren, et al., 2002); (b) there is an activation of neurogenesis (new neuron production) in a region of the hippocampus (the dentate gyrus) in AD; (c) the activation of the beta secretase enzyme appears to be associated with a myelin regeneration effect; (d) the activation of gamma secretase may also be associated with a regenerative effect; (e) the production of amyloid beta may be associated with injury repair in the brain; and (f) the reduction in IGF-1 signaling appears to delay age-associated protein-related toxicity (e.g., from toxic soluble and oligomeric forms of Aß).

For example, to the extent that the function of the beta secretase enzyme is known, apart from its role in the generation of amyloid beta, it plays an important role in cleavage associated with the production of myelin (Glabe, 2006; Willem et al. 2006). Interestingly, IGF-1 also plays a role in myelin production, causing the oligodendrocytes, the myelin-producing brain cells, to produce more myelin (Carson, Behringer, Brinster, & McMorris, 1993; Flores et al., 2008). Beta secretase knockout mice show decreased myelin production and decreased IGF-1 signaling (Hu et al., 2006). Therefore, the beta secretase response in AD appears to be a homeostatic compensation for the decreased IGF-1 activity with aging and AD. Nevertheless, as described earlier, there are continuing IGF-1 signaling abnormalities in AD and these can account for the observed myelin arboreal entropy and myelin retrogenesis seen in AD.

Gamma secretase activation also appears to be a developmental response to the pathology in AD, in addition to its role in the production of beta amyloid and in the protein breakdown of the IGF-1 receptor. For example, notch, an element of the gamma secretase complex, is involved in signaling, which is "crucial for long term memory." (Costa, Drew, & Silva, 2005). Also, "the notch pathway has been shown to regulate neurite growth and adult neurogenesis." (Breunig, Silbereis, Vaccarino, Sestan, & Rakic, 2007; Costa et al., 2005).

Amyloid beta itself appears to be involved in brain injury repair. Brody et al. have shown that there is an increase in amyloid beta in the brain interstitial fluid in the 72-hour period after a brain trauma associated with coma in persons who show signs of recovering from a coma. However, this increase in amyloid beta in the brain interstitial fluid is not seen in the persons with poor signs of coma recovery (Brody et al., 2008).

Additionally, the reduced insulin and IGF-1 signaling in AD appears to be, in part, a physiologic homeostatic response to toxic proteins produced by the AD process. For example, a study showed that reduction in IGF signaling in an Alzheimer mouse model decreased behavioral impairment, neuroinflammation, and neuronal loss (Cohen et al., 2009).

In addition to the role of IGF-1 signaling in AD pathogenesis, another IGF, which has been studied, may also play a role in AD pathogenesis. IGF-II is the most abundantly expressed IGF in the adult brain. The highest concentration of IGF-II is in the hippocampus, the "memory region of the brain." Hippocampal atrophy (Bobinski et al., 1995) and hippocampal neuronal loss (Bobinski et al., 1997) have been shown to correlate very strongly with AD progression. IGF II administration in the rodent model has been shown to enhance memory retention and to prevent forgetting. IGF-II injections into the hippocampus have been shown to promote long-term potentiation, which is the neuronal equivalent of "memory." Finally, IGF-II and the resultant IGF-II receptor signaling correlate with the activation of synaptic GSK-3β, which is tau protein kinase 1, the principal enzyme responsible for the hyperphosphorylation of tau and the resultant neurofibrillary tangles, which are a pathologic hallmark of AD and a strong correlate of AD progression (Bobinski et al., 1997; see Chen et al., 2011, for a review of the preceding).

Hence, there is a complex homeostatic, physiologic response to the behavioral and biomolecular changes associated with AD. This response can presently provide a good understanding of the nature of the changes seen in AD, including the retrogenic physiologic process and the consequent management needs in AD.

THE SCIENCE OF AD MANAGEMENT

Case History 1: Mrs. S.M.

S.M. was born on June 9, 1932. She and her future husband had met at the High School of Music and Art in New York City. In her senior year, S.M. went into architecture. Her husband went into advertising. After high school, S.M. went to Cooper Union College for one semester. She and her husband were married in 1952. Subsequently, in the early 1960s, S.M. enrolled in the High School of Visual Arts, where she took an advertising course. Afterwards, she worked in the advertising industry where she graphically created "ads." Contemporaneously, S.M. was painting at home.

Later, with a high-school friend, S.M. started a business doing textile designs. She did a line for a fabric company and worked on upholstery and drapery. Subsequently, S.M. designed dinnerware patterns for a famous company. Some years later, for another company, she did tableware design.

S.M. and her husband raised two successful sons. Her husband also became a successful designer. S.M. had been very physically fit and completed a marathon in 1984 when she was 52 years of age. Her only significant medical history prior to her initial evaluation was of a mitral valve prolapse "many years previously." Her husband stated that S.M. had "never been hospitalized," and that she "never had surgery."

■ Initial Evaluation: October 27, 2001. BCRS Scores 5, 5, 5, 5, FAST Stage 5, GDS Stage 5, and MMSE = 19

At this time, S.M. was 69 years of age and was brought to the office by her husband, J.M., who had been referred for a diagnostic consultation. S.M. was reported to have been experiencing problems with short-term memory since 1997. She was described as having "searched for thoughts." Her husband stated that there was "decreased processing of her information." At the time of the initial evaluation, S.M. had already completed diagnostic tests including standard blood tests and a thyroid function test. She also had completed a single-photon emission computed tomography (SPECT) scan and an MRI of the brain. An electroencephalographic study showed slowing and questionable spike activity. All of the test results were considered to have been compatible with AD, and S.M. had previously been treated with donepezil. Subsequently, the cholinesterase inhibitor treatment was changed to rivastigmine 6 mg twice daily.

At the time of her initial visit, S.M. was attending an "adult health care center," 3 days a week, for 6 hours each day. This facility was said to be for people with diverse problems.

During the initial evaluation, S.M. was assessed on the Brief Cognitive Rating Scale (BCRS). The BCRS (part 1) consists of seven rating point assessments of the level of cognitive functioning in the areas of: (a) concentration and calculation ability; (b) recent memory; (c) remote memory; (d) orientation; and (e) functioning and self-care (Reisberg & Ferris, 1988). The BCRS axes have been designed to be optimally concordant with each other and with the corresponding GDS stages. Studies have confirmed this optimal concordance (e.g., Reisberg & Ferris, 1988; Reisberg, Ferris, Torossian, et al., 1992; Reisberg, Franssen, Bobinski, et al., 1996). Furthermore, the FAST scale, already described herein in some detail (Table 3.2), is an expanded version of BCRS axis 5, with five successive substages within BCRS level 6 and six successive substages within BCRS level 7. At the time of the initial evaluation, S.M.'s scores on the first four BCRS "axes" were 5, 5, 5, 5, indicating that she was at the moderate dementia level in concentration and calculation ability, recent memory, remote memory, and orientation. The FAST, as already noted, is equivalent to BCRS axis 5. S.M.'s score on the FAST (Table 3.2) was also 5. This FAST score is also indicative of a moderate dementia baseline level of functioning and self-care. Accordingly, she was at GDS stage 5, also indicating moderate dementia. Her MMSE score was 17.

Complete laboratory testing, including several tests that had apparently not been conducted previously, was ordered. These included serum B12 and folate levels, a Venereal Disease Research Laboratory test (VDRL), and a serum Lyme titer, to test for the presence of Lyme's disease.

At the time of the initial evaluation, S.M.'s internist had been treating her with Exelon (rivastigmine) 6 mg twice daily, as well as with several hormonal "postmenopausal" medications and several vitamins and nutraceutical substances. These medications and substances were continued.

■ Second Evaluation: 2 Months Later: Mood and Behavior Assessment

S.M.'s second evaluation was on December 27, 2001. In the interim, she had been started on Paxil (paroxetine) 20 mg daily by her internist. Evaluation on December 27, 2001 on the Hamilton Depression Scale (Hamilton, 1960) indicated that the only "depression"-related symptom was a loss of interest in sexual activity. On the Behavioral Pathology in Alzheimer's Disease (BEHAVE-AD; Reisberg, Borenstein, Salob, et al., 1987) rating scale, S.M. was reported by her husband to have numerous symptoms. She thought that the day care center, which she was attending, was plotting to get rid of her. She also had accused her husband of having a girlfriend. Additionally, she had mild haptic hallucinations, finding imaginary things on her back and scratching her back. Several purposeless activities were also reported including opening and closing her pocketbook, asking the same questions over and over, and picking at her skin. She was reported to put dirty socks in the jewelry drawer. Additionally, S.M. had angry outbursts, which her husband referred to as "blowouts," which were directed at him. There was also tearfulness, as well as occasional statements such as "I wish I were dead." S.M. was found to be anxious about her future and her memory. She was afraid to be left alone. S.M. also avoided and wanted to leave "parties" and gatherings because she felt socially unacceptable. Her total score on the BEHAVE-AD (see Table 3.6 for symptoms surveyed) was 19. These symptoms were considered to be of moderate severity, and suspiciousness was judged to be the most important BPSD (Finkel, 2000; 2001; Finkel, Costa e Silva, Cohen, Miller, & Sartorius, 1996) problem, requiring treatment. The Empirical BEHAVE-AD (E-BEHAVE-AD) assessment (Auer, Monteiro, & Reisberg, 1996), based upon direct observation and a semistructured interview of S.M. at the time of the visit, confirmed the symptoms reported by her husband. Risperdal (risperidone) 0.25 mg in the morning was prescribed for the treatment of the BPSD symptoms described earlier.

■ Three Months After the Initial Evaluation: Remission of Most Behavioral Disturbances

At the subsequent visit on February 5, 2002, S.M.'s husband reported that she was "feeling very good" and that her "spirit is where it was before." S.M. was going to the "center" four times per week and returning home by herself. Also, her husband reported that "her paranoia has disappeared" and that "the issue of a girlfriend has disappeared." S.M.'s husband noted that his wife had begun to assist an "advanced AD" person at the center, Dorothy, who no longer had intelligible speech. S.M. was affectionate and helpful with Dorothy, who appreciated the help. At this visit, a variety of possible activities for S.M. were discussed with her husband. She already had a personal trainer. She "worked out" on the treadmill. S.M. and her husband also frequently had dinner out together. They went out to the theater and to the opera. At cocktail parties, S.M. would say, "Let's go home." S.M. was evidently uncomfortable in cocktail party settings where she would have to interact with various strangers and also with people whom she, perhaps, did not know as well as she should. Various possible additional activities were discussed.

■ Thirteen Months After the Initial Evaluation: BCRS Scores 5, 6, 6, 6, FAST Stage = 5 + 6b Nonordinal, MMSE = 11

Subsequently, S.M.'s condition gradually advanced. For example, on December 3, 2002, a little more than a year after the initial evaluation, she had advanced to a FAST stage 5 + 6b nonordinal, indicating that in addition to not being able to select her clothing properly for the events of the day and all of the preceding FAST deficits (see Table 3.2), she could no longer bathe herself independently. Her BCRS axis 1 to 4 scores were 5, 6, 6, 6, indicating decline to a moderately severe dementia level on recent memory, remote memory, and orientation, although her concentration and calculation abilities were still at the moderate dementia level (BCRS axis 1). Her MMSE score was 11. At this time, her husband had recently arranged for a companion 1 day per week. S.M. had previously been painting but had reportedly lost interest in painting at this time. She previously had been reading children's books but had lost interest in this activity. However, she was attending a "day care center" 4 days per week, for 5½ hours per day. Also, a physical trainer was working with her one morning per week. Weekends, she went shopping with her husband. Her husband noted that she was "constantly arranging things." For example, she would fold and refold a napkin. She would align utensils. Her husband noted that he had more success speaking with his wife in Italian. S.M. was born in the United States, however, the Sicilian Italian dialect was S.M.'s original language because it was spoken at home by her parents and her grandmother. However, S.M.'s schooling was always in English.

One and a Half Years After the Initial Evaluation: FAST Stage 6b Ordinal, MMSE = 12

On April 22, 2003, it was noted that S.M. had lost approximately 20 lb. in the prior year and weighed 135 lb. Her husband reported that she was complaining of feeling cold. S.M. was still going to the physical trainer once a week, doing 20 minutes on the treadmill as well as weight training. Additionally, S.M. had a professional home health aide 2 days per week. The aide took S.M. to "activities," such as movies and musicals. Also, S.M. continued to go to the "center" 3 days per week.

At this time, S.M. was very interested in puzzles, which she did on a daily basis. In general, she did puzzles designed for 3- to 4-year-old children. S.M. was reported to have approximately 10 puzzles in her home. Furthermore, S.M. went for "aroma therapy" in which "oil of lavender" was rubbed on her back. Also, Mrs. M. continued to go out shopping with her husband.

On April 22, 2003, Mrs. M was 6b ordinal on the FAST (Table 3.2), indicating that she could no longer manage her money, pick out her clothing, or dress independently, and she had also lost the ability to bathe without assistance. Her MMSE at this visit was 12. She continued to receive both risperidone and paroxetine. Her only behavioral symptoms on the BEHAVE-AD (see Table 3.6) were "anxieties and phobias" (category G). Specifically, S.M. would query repeatedly regarding upcoming events and ask, "When are we going?" Also, she expressed anxieties when she was away from home. Additionally, S.M. was afraid to be left alone and she was never left alone. For the first time, S.M. was reported to be afraid of crowds. On the E-BEHAVE-AD, some of these symptoms were observable in a brief 20-minute interview. For example, S.M. said repeatedly to the interviewer, "I want to go home." She also continued to get up from her chair to go look for her husband. Furthermore, she was talking loudly and rapidly to the interviewer and seemed to "stew" with anger at other times.

Of course, many of the symptoms displayed by S.M. are readily understood from the retrogenesis perspective. S.M. at the April 22, 2003 visit, was in FAST stage 6b. As shown in Table 3.7, this functional level is equivalent to a developmental age (DA) of 4 years. S.M. was interested in puzzles, which were said to have been designed for 3- to 4-year-old children. Like a 4-year-old child, she could not be left alone. Like a 4-year-old child attached to his or her mother, S.M. would repeatedly get up from her chair to go look for her husband.

Two Years and Five Months After the Initial Evaluation: BCRS Scores 6, 6, 6, 6, FAST Stage 6c, GDS Stage 6, MMSE = 6

On March 20, 2004, S.M. was at stage 6c on the FAST, indicating that she no longer was able to independently maintain cleanliness in toileting, in addition to the preceding FAST deficits (Table 3.2). She was also at level 6 on the first four BCRS axes and her MMSE score was 6. Disrupted sleep was her main behavioral problem. At this time, the professional caregiver was reading to S.M. and S.M. was reading to the professional caregiver. They also would play "flash cards," where they would name the picture in the cards. S.M. was noted to have a collection of children's books during this period. She would do simple puzzles at the 3- to 5-year-old child level and had a stuffed animal, which she talked to and rocked. The analogies of S.M.'s behavior to the behaviors of her DA peers, at approximately 4 years of age (see Table 3.7), are evident.

Almost a year later, in early 2005, Dr. Sunnie Kenowsky, a dementia care specialist, gave S.M. a line drawing of flowers. S.M. colored in the drawings of the flowers. During this period, Mrs. M. was reported to reject "silly cartoons" such as a picture of a "pussy cat." She was reported to have preferred the floral pictures. In her husband's words on May 7, 2005, "This has raised her up tremendously."

Four Years After the Initial Evaluation: BCRS Scores 7, 6, 6, 6, FAST Stage 6c, GDS Stage 6, MMSE = 5

In late 2005, S.M., at GDS stage 6, with BCRS axis 1 to 4 scores of 7, 6, 6, 6, an MMSE score of 5, and still at FAST stage 6c, colorized line drawings based on outlines from the famous French impressionist painter, Paul Cezanne. The colorization was entirely hers.

At this time, S.M. was reported by her husband to be reading children's books and doing puzzles, as well as colorizing the line drawings. That year, in late 2005, her husband sent out holiday cards featuring his wife's creations (Figure 3.20). About a

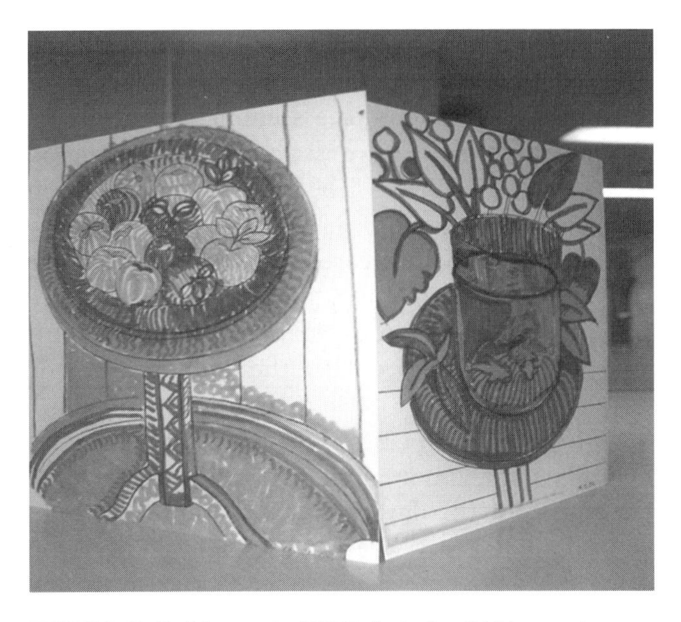

FIGURE 3.20 Holiday card of 2005, featuring S.M.'s recent colorized drawings.

Photograph by Barry Reisberg (card recipient).

Source: Photograph copyright 2006 Barry Reisberg.

year earlier, on September 28, 2004, *The New York Times* published a story about Marla Olmstead, a 4-year-old contemporary "developmental age peer" of S.M. who had sold 24 paintings of her abstract works for $40,000 (York, Michelle, "A Portrait of the Artist as a Young Girl: Early Ability on Abstracts: 4-Year-Old Paints With Flair," *The New York Times,* September 28, 2004, page B1).

Four Years and 10 Months After the Initial Evaluation: BCRS Scores 7, 7, 7, 6, FAST Stage 6c, GDS Stage 6, MMSE = 2

On August 22, 2006, S.M. was reported by her husband to be "sliding a bit." J.M. stated that his wife repeated what he said. J.M. also said that his wife's reply to everything is "No." J.M. said his wife would look through her hands like a lens. However, he said that his wife was still "drawing well." She was attending a "neighborhood house," working out with a personal trainer once a week, and seeing Dr. Kenowsky once a month. Furthermore, he and his wife went for 2-mile walks three days a week. J.M. said that his wife continued to be sociable with people. At that time, S.M. remained 6c ordinal on the FAST; however, her BCRS axis 1 to 4 scores were 7, 7, 7, 6. This indicated that S.M. had marked difficulty counting from 1 to 10 and had no evident knowledge of either recent or remote events; however, she still knew her own name. S.M.'s MMSE score was 2 out of 30. She was credited with knowing the town (New York) and being able to take a paper in her right hand. S.M. continued to take considerable satisfaction from her recent creations as can be seen from Figure 3.21, showing S.M. in her kitchen, which was decorated with her recent works. S.M. remained very creative, as can be seen from her freestyle watercolor of January 31, 2007, at which time S.M. remained at FAST stage 6c and her MMSE score was 2 (Figure 3.22). Her husband believes that his wife had not previously done artwork using this medium.

Eight Years and Six Months After the Initial Evaluation: BCRS Scores 7, 7, 7, 7, FAST Stage 7a, GDS Stage 7, MMSE = 0 for Approximately the Prior 2 Years

More than 3 years later, S.M. remained very sociable and, in many ways, she continued to enjoy life. For example, Figure 3.23 shows a picture of her when she was on an outing with her friends with AD. This picture was taken on April 23, 2010. At that time, her MMSE score had been 0 for approximately 2 years (since May 10, 2008). When this picture was taken, S.M. was in the final seventh stage in the GDS. Her BCRS axis 1 to 4 scores were

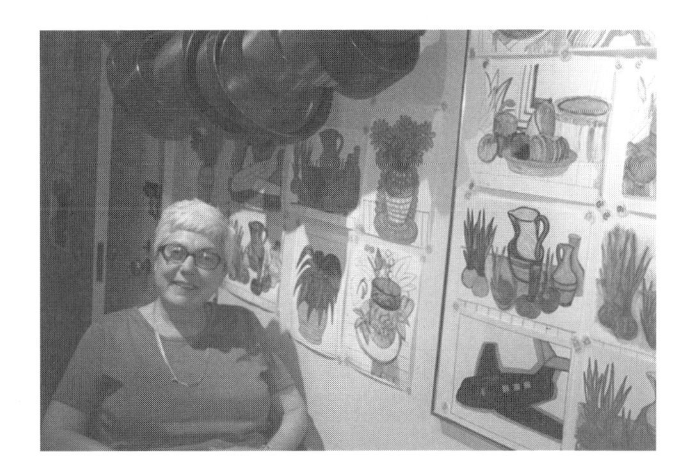

FIGURE 3.21 S.M. at age 74, in her kitchen, which is decorated with her recent artistic creations comprised of colorized line drawings. At this time, on August 22, 2006, S.M. was at Global Deterioration Scale (GDS) stage 6 and Functional Assessment Staging Scale (FAST) stage 6c (ordinal). Her Mini-Mental Status Examination (MMSE) score was 2 and her Brief Cognitive Rating Scale (BCRS) scores on Axes 1 to 4 were 7, 7, 7, 6.

Source: Photograph copyright 2006 Barry Reisberg.

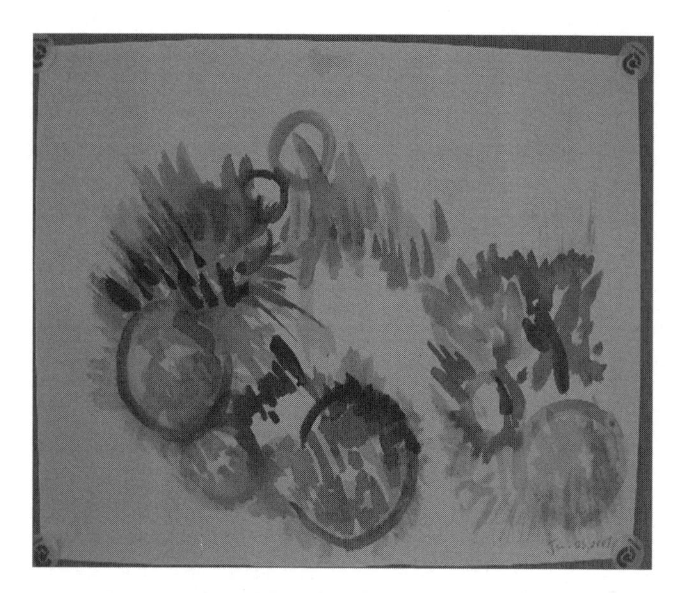

FIGURE 3.22 S.M.'s creation of January 31, 2007. At this time, S.M. was at Global Deterioration Scale (GDS) stage 6, and Functional Assessment Staging (FAST) stage 6c. Her Brief Cognitive Rating Scale (BCRS) axis I to IV scores were 7, 6, 6, 6, and her Mini Mental Status Examination (MMSE) score was 2 out of 30.

Source: Drawing used with permission from S.M.'s husband, Mr. J. M.

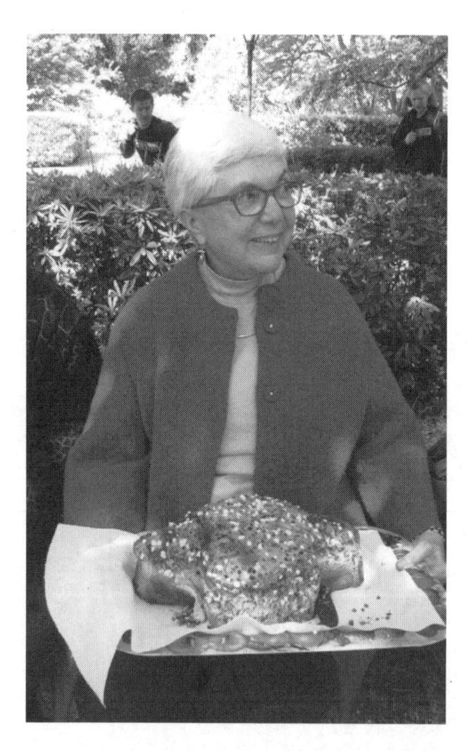

FIGURE 3.23 S.M. at an outing with her friends with AD on April 23, 2010. At this time S.M. was at FAST stage 7a, indicating that her intelligible speech was limited to only a half dozen or so words in an average day. Her MMSE score had been 0 (bottom) for approximately 2 years. However, S.M. was still, in many ways, continuing to enjoy life and socialization.

AD, Alzheimer's disease; FAST, Functional Assessment Staging; MMSE, Mini-Mental State Examination.

Source: Photograph used with permission from S.M.'s husband, Mr. J.M.

7, 7, 7, 7 and her FAST stage was 7a, indicating that S.M. continued to say some words in the context of an intensive interview or a seemingly typical day. During this time, J.M. described his wife's mood as "fabulous." He described her as waking up in the morning laughing. S.M.'s husband was very involved in his wife's care. He helped his wife to shower and with toileting. S.M. also had assistance from a home health aide. On the day of her medical evaluation (March 6, 2010), the home health aide had said to S.M., "You're a very pretty woman." S.M. replied, "Yes, I know." At this time, S.M. was beginning to get more reluctant going up and down the stairs. At the day care center, children would come in 1 day per week. Pets would come in on other days. A piano player would come in to sing and dance. S.M. danced with both the persons with dementia and with the accompanying aides.

S.M. was described by her husband as being very social with most people. As noted, in accordance with her reluctance going upstairs and downstairs, S.M. was reluctant to get off the bus when travelling (of course, always with an assistant). At approximately this time, while S.M. was in FAST stage 7a, she successfully and happily celebrated her high school reunion on July 24, 2010.

■ Eleven Years and 5 Months After the Initial Evaluation: BCRS Scores 7, 7, 7, 7, FAST Stage 7b, Feeding Axis Level 7c, GDS Stage 7, MMSE = 0 for Approximately 5 Years

Approximately 3 years later, on April 6, 2013, a major problem was preventing loss of ambulation. Although S.M. was not capable of maintaining continence independently, by being attentive to the patient's signals, and with frequent toileting and medication treatment, there were very infrequent problems with the maintenance of continence. With respect to medication treatment, a laxative (in this case, Miralax [polyethylene glycol]) was used, and a bladder smooth muscle relaxant medication Myrbetriq (mirabegron) was also prescribed. Both of these medications were given on a daily basis. With this regimen, actual episodes of urinary incontinence only occurred when S.M. developed urinary tract infections. These, in turn, may have been related to urinary retention from the mirabegron treatment.

At this time, S.M. did not speak every day. When she did speak, she usually said, "mmmm" or "yes" or "no." Reportedly she said "no" more often than "yes." It was estimated that there was approximately one intelligible word in an average day. If S.M. heard laughter, she would join in. Therefore, there was empathetic laughter. She would also laugh spontaneously. S.M. would pull her husband's hands to her lips and kiss his hands. On the FAST, S.M. was assessed as being at stage 7b ordinal. Earlier in this chapter, we presented the "Feeding Concomitants of Alzheimer's Disease" (Table 3.3). Particularly in the GDS/FAST stage 7 AD person, these descriptions can be very useful in describing residual capacities in the AD person. In common with the GDS, the BCRS, and the FAST, the most appropriate level in this Feeding axis is selected. Also in common with the GDS, the BCRS, and the FAST, the Feeding axis level is optimally concordant in level (stage) with the corresponding GDS, BCRS, and FAST stages. On April 6, 2013, S.M., as noted earlier, was still capable of walking independently; however, she was not capable of going to a refrigerator or cupboard and selecting food (Feeding axis stage 6e). She also was not capable of independently picking up a spoon or a fork, or a cup if she wanted to drink (Feeding axis stage 7a). In addition to being unable to select utensils, S.M. required assistance with feeding (Feeding axis 7b). However, S.M. did have residual feeding skills. For example, she was reported to be capable of reaching out for food and picking up food with her hands. She also was reported to be capable of distinguishing food from nondietary substances. Her level on this Feeding axis was 7c, which was quite close to her level on the FAST, which, as we have noted earlier, was 7b ordinal.

We should also note at this point, that there are also subtleties to the FAST assessment. S.M.'s FAST level was 7b ordinal. However, there were no actual episodes of urinary incontinence (FAST stage 6d) or fecal incontinence (FAST stage 6e). The reason she was judged to be beyond these stages was that she required assistance with toileting, both in terms of urination and in terms of defecation. Without this personal assistance, S.M. would be incontinent; therefore, she is assessed as incontinent in terms of her FAST staging.

As discussed previously, a major problem at this point in the evolution of AD is the occurrence of rigidity and the prevention of contractures. In the case of S.M., physical therapy and range of motion exercises of the extremities were emphasized. Despite this emphasis, a physical examination revealed considerable rigidity of the extremities. There was approximately 75% range of motion of the left arm and approximately 30% range of motion of the right arm. Also, S.M. held her head down. In addition to standard physical therapy, the patient's home health aide was instructed by Dr. B.R. in providing range of motion exercises of all four extremities, three times daily for S.M.

Key events and important insights from visits subsequent to April 6, 2013, are briefly summarized.

More Than 12 Years After the Initial Evaluation and 5.5 Years After the MMSE Score Bottomed Out, S.M. Reaches FAST Stage 7c

On her November 16, 2013, visit, S.M. had developed nighttime myoclonus. She was also having increasing problems with ambulation. There were episodes of collapse. J.M. got a seat belt for S.M.'s wheelchair. Also, S.M. was sleeping more, both during the day and at night. At that time, she was found to have lost independent ambulation and to have moved to FAST stage 7c. S.M.'s level in the Feeding axis was also 7c, the same level as 6 months previously, during the April 6, 2013, visit.

On March 1, 2014, it was noted that S.M. had shaking (tremors) of both hands and her left arm. Also, she was holding her head down. A trial of carbidopa/levodopa, 10/100 mg tablets, 1 tablet twice daily was initiated.

On March 14, 2014, J.M. called to say that his wife had collapsed several times and subsequently fell and dislocated her left tibia. A cast was placed on the left leg and Mrs. S.M. was in a hospital bed with a special mattress, which oscillated.

Subsequently, S.M. had a cast on her left leg for 6 weeks. On May 21, 2014, J.M. reported that he had gone away for a business trip for 3 days. When he returned, his wife started crying. S.M. had realized that her husband had been away, and she was happy, with tears, to see him return. J.M. stated, "It was very touching."

On June 14, 2014, it was noted that S.M.'s shaking had stopped on the carbidopa/levodopa regimen. However, it was also noted from Dr. B.R.'s physical examination that S.M.'s range of motion in the upper extremities was becoming very restricted. Therefore, physical therapy was ordered and the patient's surgeon was also contacted regarding the need for physical movement of S.M. to prevent the development of contractures. J.M. had understood the surgeon saying that S.M. "should not be moved." Contact with the surgeon confirmed that he had suggested only "that the left ankle should not be moved" not that S.M. "should not be moved" more generally. Dr. B.R. subsequently called J.M. and explained the misunderstanding and that J.M. should proceed with the physical therapies as ordered to prevent further rigidity and the development of contractures.

On June 30, 2014, it was confirmed that S.M. was receiving both physical therapy and also range of motion exercises from her home health aide. J.M reported that S.M. was less rigid. An additional issue at this time was S.M.'s sleep. A sedating "antidepressant" medication, trazodone, had been prescribed by Dr. B.R. to address J.M.'s concerns that his wife had difficulties sleeping during the night. This medication was stopped for 2 days and S.M. was noted to have become very restless during the night. Therefore, the trazodone at night was renewed. The initial dosage was 50 mg at night; however, this was increased to 100 mg on July 22, 2014, which worked ideally in terms of producing a restful sleep.

On September 13, 2014, S.M. had to be assisted in transfer from her automobile to a wheelchair by Dr. B.R. as well as by an assistant and J.M. She arrived at the office in her wheelchair. It was noted that S.M did not speak at all or say any words at this time, during these procedures, or, indeed, during the subsequent office visit, which lasted for a few hours. At this point, the left tibial dislocation had healed. S.M. could "walk" with one person assistance with great difficulty. J.M. and S.M. have two homes, one in the city and one in the countryside. At this time, they had hospital beds with mattresses to prevent decubiti. The mattresses in both homes had electrical motors, which permitted oscillations.

Examination indicated marked rigidity of S.M.'s hands and elbows. However, with some difficulty, Dr. B.R. was able to fully extend the hands and the arms. S.M.'s legs were relatively flexible. A neck brace was being used daily for about 45 minutes to keep S.M.'s neck up. Additionally, S.M.'s husband and aides were slowly and gently retracting her neck back several times per day. Apart from physical therapy and other treatments, Dr. B.R. ordered for S.M.'s husband and aides: complete extension of both hands, both arms, and both legs, every 3 hours when S.M is awake.

■ More Than 13 Years After the Initial Visit and More Than 6.5 Years After the MMSE Became 0: GDS stage 7, FAST stage 7c. Elements of Both 7c and of 7e on the Feeding Axis

Highlights of an office visit on December 20, 2014, included that S.M. appeared to be speaking more. The remaining words were "yes" or "no." Mr. J.M reported that he heard these words about three times per week. Also physical examination indicated almost complete return of range of motion of the hands, arms, and legs. J.M. commented on his views regarding his efforts to care for his wife.

> She's instinctive, she appreciates being cared for. I'm comfortable with it. I don't feel denied. I'm still working. I'm still designing furniture. I don't mind caring for her at all. I get up at 6 a.m. I prepare things for her. She has nighttime diapers that are wet and I put on fresh ones. She [S.M.] has a commode with wheels and is wheeled into the shower in the commode. On Fridays, I also give her breakfast, in addition to dressing and bathing her. In the evening, she has dinner with her nightgown on. She's changed before she goes to sleep. She cannot get on a toilet.

J.M stated,

> I don't feel denied. I don't get angry at her. Her life is still meaningful for me, absolutely. I care for her out of love, out of respect. I do not feel burdened by her condition. She is totally accepted by her family, for example, on Thanksgiving they are all together. When her 25-year-old granddaughter whom she knew before her dementia, kisses her, she reacts more positively than when her 12-year-old granddaughter, whom she doesn't remember as well, kisses her.

J.M also noted that he has home health aide assistance from 8:30 a.m. to 6 p.m. At this time, on December 20, 2014, S.M was at FAST stage 7c. On the Feeding axis, she had elements of both 7c and of 7e. For example, if S.M. had oatmeal for breakfast, she needed to be spoonfed; however, she could chew the food. For lunch and dinner, she was fed with a fork. However, S.M. also had elements of stage 7e on the Feeding axis (see Table 3.3). Specifically, apparently she could no longer distinguish food from nondietary substances. Also, she no longer attempted to reach out for objects.

■ Thirteen Years and 5 Months After the Initial Visit and 6 Years and 10 Months After the MMSE Reached Bottom (0), S.M. Is Described by Her Husband as "Doing Well." When Her Husband Asked S.M. "Are You OK?," S.M. Replied, "Sure." FAST Stage = 7c, GDS Stage 7

On March 21, 2015, S.M was seen with her husband who described her as "doing very well." S.M.'s physical therapist was reported to have said that she has become stronger. S.M. was able to stand if she held on to a grab bar or another steady object. Also S.M. was able to sit up independently. Her husband stated that she laughs on occasion. S.M.'s husband reported occasional words. For example, on March 6, 2015, he asked her, "Are you OK?" S.M. responded, "Sure." S.M. was still going to the AD center 2 days a week. Her home health aide accompanied her to the center where there was entertainment, such as the guitar player. The home health aide also was doing exercises with S.M, such as standing up and grabbing the bar. S.M. still had the neck brace and was sleeping "a lot," with naps during the day and also reportedly sleeping well at night. Her husband found her excessive sleep reminiscent of an infant's sleep.

At this time, on March 21, 2015, there was no agitation. S.M. ate small pieces of hard foods, such as steak and chicken as well as tuna salads, oatmeal, and so forth. When the home health aide would not come in, S.M.'s husband did everything for her. He noted that S.M does not resist care. J.M noted that

> I think [S.M.] senses that I'm not disturbed about caring for her, therefore she doesn't get agitated. She thinks my care for her is genuine. I don't feel any sense of denial. I still have a career. Instinctively she knows the care she's getting is genuine.

■ Most Recent Evaluation, 13 Years, 9 Months After the Initial Visit and More Than 7 Years After the MMSE Reached 0 (Bottom). FAST Stage = 7c + (?) 7f Nonordinal. Feeding Axis Stage 7c

The last time S.M was evaluated was on August 8, 2015, nearly 14 years after the initial visit. On examination, S.M. was found to have full range of motion of both elbows; however, there was marked resistance to this range of motion. Also, there was full extension of the hands and the fingers. S.M continued to receive formal physical therapy as well as a bedrail standing exercise. At this time, there was an ongoing change in the home health aide providers. Therefore, a regimen of full range of motion of arms, hands, and legs was reinstituted, 10 times each, twice daily. S.M. continued to use the neck brace, 1 hour daily, to hold her head up. Her FAST level was assessed as 7c ordinal and it was noted that she had elements of FAST stage 7f, in terms of her difficulties in holding her head up. On the Feeding axis, S.M. could grasp a spoon and she was said to be capable of chewing. However, she could not reach for or pick up food with her hands. She also could not pick up a fork or a spoon. She was assessed as being at Feeding level 7c.

Commentary on S.M.'s Progression

The estimated durations of the FAST stages in AD are described in Table 3.2. S.M. was at FAST stage 5 when first seen on October 27, 2001. At the last visit on August 8, 2015, S.M. was at FAST stage 7c. If we assume she was at the midpoint of FAST stage 5 on October 27, 2001, and that she was at the midpoint of FAST stage 7c when she was seen on August 8, 2015, then we would expect the transition to occur over (stage 5 = 18 months/2 = 9 months) + (stage 6 = 29 months) + (stage 7a = 12 months) + (stage 7b = 18 months) + (stage 7c = 12 months/2 = 6 months) = 74 months = 6.17 years. In actuality, S.M.'s transition (decline) occurred over approximately 13 years and 9 months (i.e., 165 months) or 223% longer than anticipated. It is likely that J.M.'s dedication and care and the love he continued to provide his wife helped lengthen the time course of her progression in the AD dementia process. Also, as we have seen, S.M. continued to participate as a member of her family, and her life continued to have meaning for her husband and her broader family. From a retrogenesis prospective, AD can be seen as the final stage of life, perhaps with some of the same meaning as the beginning of life. Just as the developmental milestones in the beginning of life can be attenuated or inhibited by poor care or illness, similarly, the progression of the AD process can be seemingly accelerated by poor care or general inattentiveness to the needs of the person with AD. Unfortunately, this poor care and inattentiveness is the rule, rather than the exception, in the final seventh stage of AD. Hopefully, S.M.'s story of exemplary care will assist in making such care more common.

Case History 2: Mr. L.K.

L.K. was born on August 27, 1926. He became a very successful businessman. He also married a very beautiful, well-read, and intelligent woman, J.K. Among other accomplishments, J.K. was a former fashion model in New York. Mr. and Mrs. K. (Figure 3.24) traveled very widely throughout the world.

Initial Evaluation: July 30, 2009. GDS Stage 6, FAST Stage 6b (Ordinal) + 6d Nonordinal, Questionably 7c Nonordinal, and MMSE = 5, With History of Brain Infarct and a Transient Ischemic Attack

L.K. was seen for an initial evaluation by Dr. B.R. on July 30, 2009, when he was 82 years of age. He was referred by a colleague in the Department of Psychiatry and by his internist. At the initial visit, he was seen with his wife, J.K., and a home health aide, D.B. who had been assisting L.K. since December 26, 2008, 6 days per week, 8 hours per day. His medical history included: (a) an episode of giardiasis contracted while visiting Russia in 1969; (b) glaucoma diagnosed in the 1970s; (c) trabeculectomy of the left eye for the treatment of the glaucoma in 1994; (d) prostate adenocarcinoma and prostatectomy in 1995; (e) liposarcoma of the kidney and left nephrectomy in 1996; (f) a right-sided brain infarct in the posterior limb of the internal capsule in 1998, with no apparent residua, and a transient ischemic attack in 2005; (g) cataract surgery of the right eye in 1999; and (h) decreased cognition, which was first evident in 2004. On June 25, 2004, his MMSE score was 26.

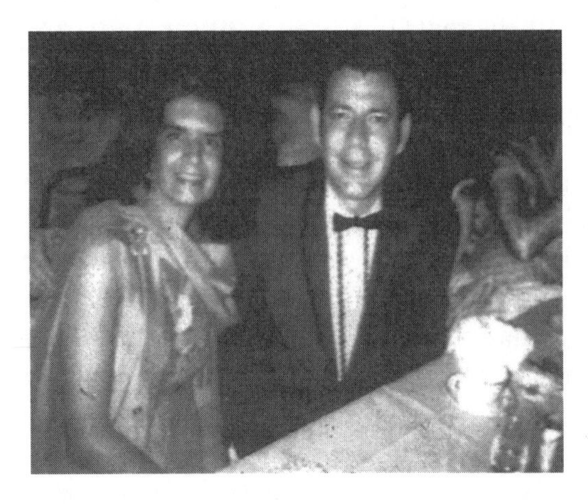

FIGURE 3.24 Mrs. J.K and Mr. L.K. in midlife at a reception.
Source: Photograph property of Mrs. J.K. used with permission.

L.K's medications at the time of the initial visit were: (a) memantine 10 mg twice daily (to optimize cognitive functioning); (b) donepezil (also to optimize cognitive function); (c) olanzapine 2.5 mg at night (for behavioral disturbances associated with the dementia); (d) clopidogrel 75 mg in the morning (to reduce platelet aggregation and blood clotting); (e) amlodipine 5 mg in the morning (to control hypertension); (f) atenolol 25 mg in the morning (also for control of hypertension); (g) three different, "as necessary" medications for episodes of agitation. These were alprazolam 0.25 mg, diazepam 5 mg, or Tylenol PM (acetaminophen/diphenhydramine).

An initial evaluation of L.K. found that the FAST stage was 6b ordinal. In addition, there were nonordinal FAST stage deficits of 6d, indicating urinary incontinence and, questionably, 7c, indicating a loss of the ability to walk. It was thought that both of these excess FAST disabilities might have been related to nondementia-related conditions or the medications. The MMSE score was 5.

In an effort to restore some functionality, the olanzapine dosage was decreased to 2.5 mg every other day.

Second Evaluation: August 13, 2009, Multiple Infarcts on the MRI of the Brain, BCRS Scores 6, 7, 7, 7.

At L.K.'s second evaluation, the recent MRI scan findings were reviewed. They indicated interval infarcts in the left and right parietal lobes, the left posterior frontal lobe, the right external capsule and the internal capsule, and chronic infarction in the right basal ganglia. L.K. was able to count from 1 to 10 forward, but not backward. He had no knowledge of recent events. He did not know his address, the weather conditions, or the name of the U.S. president. He also gave his wife's name in response to questions about his father's name or his mother's name. He could not correctly state his own name and had no idea of the year or season.

On this evaluation, L.K. moaned continuously. On the BEHAVE-AD, he was reported to manifest threatening behavior, to refuse to do things (negativity), and to be afraid to be left alone. He was quoted as saying, "Save me, I don't want to die."

On this visit, the olanzapine was stopped. Also, the alprazolam and diazepam were stopped. Doxepin 10 mg at night was prescribed for sleep. Sertraline 25 mg in the morning was prescribed for the alleviation of some of L.K.'s affective disturbances. Diagnostically, L.K. was believed to have dementia associated with AD, which was complicated by cerebrovascular disease as well as by some of the medications he was receiving and by other medical conditions.

L.K.'s subsequent course is very briefly summarized. On October 24, 2009, his FAST level was assessed as 6e ordinal + 7c nonordinal, indicating that he could not dress, bathe, or toilet properly, was doubly incontinent and, additionally, had lost the ability to walk independently. It was noted that he was given no daily activities and that his sleep was irregular. Physical therapy was ordered and a consult with a dementia activity care specialist, Dr. Sunnie Kenowsky, was arranged. Despite these efforts, on November 16, 2009, L.K. developed a decubitus in the lower vertebral region. This was treated and arrangements were made for L.K.'s aides to do regular range of motion exercises both during the day and at night. Also, daytime activities were emphasized.

Dr. Kenowsky helped to retrain L.K. to sit on a regular chair. Also, the home health aide assisted L.K. in walking using a "walker" device, which provided him with stability and which he could lift as he moved.

■ Six Months After the Initial Evaluation: January 24, 2010. BCRS 7, 7, 7, 7, FAST Stage 6d Ordinal + 7c Nonordinal

At this point, largely as a result of the guidance provided by Dr. Kenowsky, L.K. was walking with the walker and the aide's assistance. Earlier fecal incontinence had resolved. L.K. was said to be laughing more. He was also said to be enjoying reading the (children's) books and playing games. D.B., the primary aide, was doing physical therapy with L.K. on a daily basis. Examination indicated no resistance to range of motion of the arms or hands bilaterally.

■ Fours Years After the Initial Evaluation: July 11, 2013. GDS Stage 7, BCRS Scores 7, 7, 7, 7 (All Bottom Scores), FAST Stage 7c Ordinal + ? 7e Nonordinal, MMSE = 0

Despite the efforts described earlier, L.K.'s condition continued to advance along the lines of the progression of AD. Although there was a clear history of cerebrovascular disease evidenced by the neuroimaging findings, the impact of the cerebrovascular disease on L.K.'s presentation and symptomatology is unclear. In any event, as would be anticipated from the course of AD, L.K. lost all serviceable speaking ability. D.B. and the other aides continued to do range of motion exercises of L.K.'s arms and legs daily before lunch. At this time, the physical therapist had reportedly "given up" on the patient.

D.B., the home health aide, noted that when she spoke to someone else on the telephone, L.K. frequently squeezed her hand or wrist, seemingly out of jealousy.

Also, Dr. Kenowsky continued to read to L.K., as well as paint and draw with him. The paintings, which L.K. did were assisted by Dr. Kenowsky. She would ask him which color he preferred. Nonverbally, L.K. would indicate to Dr. Kenowsky the color he preferred. Dr. Kenowsky would place the paintbrush in his hand, pick his hand holding the brush up, and dip it in the paint. Subsequently, she would guide his hand to where he wanted to place it on the paper. L.K. would then put the brush on the paper with the color. An example of the paintings, which L.K. produced at this time when he could no longer speak or walk, is shown in Figure 3.25. L.K.'s DA at this point was about 12 months (1 year) of age (see Table 3.7). However, although there is a mental retrogenesis in AD, there is no physical involution. Hence, potentially, AD persons can be much more skilled than their DA peers because of residual motor skills. Similarly, AD persons are much larger and stronger than infants and small children, and hence they can, potentially, be more difficult to manage. However, the positive side of these differences between 12-month-old infants and an AD person at stage 7c is that an AD person can express himself or herself physically in some ways in which a 12-month-old infant cannot.

FIGURE 3.25 Artwork produced by L.K. on October 8, 2013. At this time, L.K. was stage 7c ordinal on the FAST. This is a point in the evolution of Alzheimer's disease at which persons need total assistance with dressing, bathing, and toileting, and can no longer speak in any serviceable manner. Intelligible words are infrequently heard (less than one per day on average). Furthermore, persons at this stage cannot walk independently. Because of the excellent care that L.K. was receiving, he could still use his hands. He had not developed the contractures, which many persons in his stage develop. Therefore, he could still put a brush on a paper. However, the dementia care specialist Dr. Kenowsky had to help him to choose the colors and hand L.K. the paintbrush. L.K. put the brush on the paper and created the pattern.

Source: Art work used with permission from L.K.'s wife, J.K.

■ Six Years After the Initial Evaluation: June 20, 2015. GDS Stage 7, BCRS Scores 7, 7, 7, 7, FAST Stage 7c Ordinal, Feeding Axis Stage 7c, MMSE = 0 for ~5 Years

L.K. came to the office with his caregiver Ms. D.B. He was in a wheelchair, which had been obtained from the physical medicine department. The wheelchair had several special features, which assisted with L.K.'s care needs. D.B. reported that L.K. was "eating, painting, and laughing." She also noted that L.K. was not walking.

During this visit, the caregiver elaborated that she often kissed L.K. She also said she "talks to Mr. K." Ms. D.B. reported that the other caregivers also spoke to and kissed L.K. often.

In accord with Dr. B.R.'s instructions, L.K. was receiving range of motion exercises of all extremities in the morning, while he was still in bed, at lunch, and also at bedtime. The exercises included leg raises as well as "stretching" of the wrists and fingers and the arms and legs. An examination by Dr. B.R. did not find evidence of contractures.

At this time, L.K. was in FAST stage 7c. Hence, in addition to all of the earlier FAST stage deficits, L.K. had lost the ability to say a single intelligible word in an average day. In fact, D.B., his primary caregiver, reported that there were "never any words." In addition, L.K. was unable to walk without assistance. However, L.K. was able to sit up without assistance. Also, as stated earlier, he laughed at times and he smiled, especially, in D.B.'s words "when he is playing games." L.K. continued to be able to hold up his head independently.

On the Feeding axis (Table 3.3), L.K. was also at level 7c (see Table 3.3). More specifically, L.K. could not properly pick up a fork or spoon; however, he could grasp a spoon. He needed to be spoonfed, but he could chew. However, L.K. could not reach for or pick up food with his hands. Hence, L.K.'s level (stage) was 7c, that is, he was able to accomplish some skills at this stage (level), but not others.

D.B. reported that L.K. would open his mouth for a kiss. Also, she stated that L.K. would push people away if he didn't want to be changed. D.B. said, "L.K. loves his vegetables and will say 'mmm' when eating them."

D.B. also reported that L.K. would open his eyes and listen to his wife when she spoke. Also, L.K. was said to not like being ignored, for example, when Dr. Kenowsky, his "painting mentor," spoke with his wife.

In terms of his painting, D.B. reported that Dr. Kenowsky would ask L.K. to "choose a color." Then she might say, "Here is the purple." Dr. Kenowsky then held L.K.'s hand and gave him the color, putting L.K.'s hand in the paint. L.K. subsequently "does his own stuff" (in terms of the painting).

L.K. became quite popular as a result of his paintings. For example, the doorman would tell him how much he liked L.K.'s paintings when L.K. would be wheeled into or out of his home. Also, L.K.'s paintings were exhibited by an Alzheimer's society and may be featured on an international TV program. Apart from painting, L.K. continued to enjoy going out to the park and to the store. Even in the park, L.K. became a celebrity and was featured with many others in a 2013 photography book. L.K. also enjoyed going to the grocery store. Apart from the paintings, when Dr. Kenowsky read stories to L.K. on the iPad, the characters moved and L.K. liked that.

In summary, L.K. continued to receive the love and attention, which are some of the essentials of life. As previously stated, from a retrogenesis perspective, AD can be viewed as a final stage in life. With proper care, including the absence of excess disability, L.K. can be viewed as "enjoying" and "succeeding in" this final stage of life.

CONCLUSIONS

AD is a very common condition primarily in older persons, marked by a characteristic cognitive and functional course of disability. Knowledge of this characteristic course is essential for the identification and treatment of excess functional disability and for many other aspects of AD person management and care. Proper management and care can alleviate and, indeed, even eliminate suffering in the person with AD and reduce burden for those who live with, care about, care for, and in other ways interact with the person with AD.

ACKNOWLEDGMENT

This work was supported in part by U.S. Department of Health and Human Services (DHHS) grants AG03051, AG08051, AG09127, and AG11505 from the National Institute on Aging and by grant MH43486 from the National Institute of Mental Health of the U.S. National Institutes of Health; by grants 90AZ2791, 90AM2552, and 90AR2160 from the U.S. DHHS Administration on Aging; by grant NCRRM01 RR00096 from the General Clinical Research Center Program and by Clinical and Translational Science Institute grant 1UL1RR029893 from the National Center for Research Resources of the U.S. National Institutes of Health; by grants from Mr. Zachary Fisher and Mrs. Elizabeth M. Fisher, and by the Fisher Center for Alzheimer's Research Foundation; by a grant from the Estate of Rosalind Cherry and a grant from Mr. William Silberstein; by the Leonard Litwin Fund for Alzheimer's Disease Research; by the Woodbourne Foundation; by the Hagedorn Fund, the Stringer Foundation, the Louis J. Kay and June E. Kay Foundation, and donations from Mrs. Miriam Glaubach and Dr. Felix Glaubach, and a Clinical Researcher Development Fund of the New York University School of Medicine.

REFERENCES

Alzheimer's Association. (2015). 2015 Alzheimer's disease facts and figures. *Alzheimer's & Dementia*, *11*, 332–384.

Alzheimer's Disease International. (2015). *World Alzheimer's Report 2015, The Global Impact of Dementia*. Retrieved from www.alz.co.uk/worldreport2015

American Hospital Association. (2015). *AHA Hospital Statistics, 2015*. Retrieved from http://www.aha.org/research/rc/stat-studies/fast-facts.shtml

Auer, S. R., Monteiro, I. M., & Reisberg, B. (1996). The empirical behavioral pathology in Alzheimer's disease (E-BEHAVE-AD) rating scale. *International Psychogeriatrics*, *8*, 247–266.

Auer, S. R., Sclan, S. G., Yaffee, R. A., & Reisberg, B. (1994). The neglected half of Alzheimer's disease: Cognitive and functional concomitants of severe dementia. *Journal of the American Geriatrics Society*, *42*, 1266–1272.

Belle, S. H., Burgio, L., Burns, R., Coon, D., Czaja, S. J., Gallagher-Thompson, D., . . . Resources for enhancing Alzheimer's caregiver health (REACH) II investigators. (2006). Enhancing the quality of life of dementia caregivers from different ethnic or racial groups: A randomized, controlled trial. *Annals of Internal Medicine*, *145*, 727–738.

Blazer, D. G., Hays, J. C., Fillenbaum, G. G., & Gold, D. T. (1997). Memory complaint as a predictor of cognitive decline: A comparison of African American and White elders. *Journal of Aging and Health*, *9*, 171–184.

Bobinski, M., Wegiel, J., Wisniewski, H. M., Tarnawski, M., Reisberg, B., Mlodzik, B., . . . Miller, D. C. (1995). Atrophy of hippocampal formation subdivisions correlates with stage and duration of Alzheimer disease. *Dementia*, *6*, 205–210.

Bobinski, M., Wegiel, J., Tarnawski, M., Reisberg, B., de Leon, M. J., Miller, D. C., & Wisniewski, H. M. (1997). Relationships between regional neuronal loss and neurofibrillary changes in the hippocampal formation and duration and severity of Alzheimer disease. *Journal of Neuropathology Experimental Neurology*, *56*, 414–420.

Bookmeyer, R., Johnson, E., Ziegler-Graham, K., & Arrighi, H. M. (2007). Forecasting the global burden of Alzheimer's disease. *Alzheimer's & Dementia*, *3*(3), 186–191.

Borza, L., Reisberg, B., Astarastoae, V., & Dascalu, C. (2010). An electrophysiologic model of retrogenesis. In M. Tsolaki (Ed.), *Proceedings of the 25th International Conference of Alzheimeir's Disease International. Thessaloniki [Greece], March 10-13, 2010* (pp. 25–29), Bologna: Pianoro.

Braak, H., & Braak, E. (1991). Neuropathological stageing of Alzheimer-related changes. *Acta Neuropathologica, 82*, 239–259.

Braak, H., & Braak, E. (1996). Development of Alzheimer-related neurofibrillary changes in the neocortex inversely recapitulates cortical myelogenesis. *Acta Neuropathologica, 92*, 197–201.

Breunig, J. J., Silbereis, J., Vaccarino, F. M., Sestan, N., & Rakic, P. (2007). Notch regulates cell fate and dendrite morphology of newborn neurons in the postnatal dentate gyrus. *Proceedings of the National Academy of Sciences of the United States of America, 104*, 20558–20563.

Brody, D. L., Magnoni, S., Schwetye, K. E., Spinner, M. L., Esparza, T. J., Stocchetti, N., . . . Holtzman, D. M. (2008). Amyloid-beta dynamics correlate with neurological status in the injured human brain. *Science, 321*, 1221–1224.

Brucki, S. M. D., & Nitrini, R. (2008). Subjective memory impairment in a rural population with low education in the Amazon rainforest: An exploratory study. *International Psychogeriatrics, 21*, 164–171.

Brun, A., & Englund, E. (1981). Regional pattern of degeneration in Alzheimer's disease: Neuronal loss and histopathological grading. *Histopathology, 5*, 549–564.

Brun, A., & Gustafson, L. (1976). Distribution of cerebral degeneration in Alzheimer's disease. *Archiv für Psychiatrie und Nervenkrankheiten, 223*, 15–33.

Bruscoli, M., & Lovestone, S. (2004). Is MCI really just early dementia? A systematic review of conversion studies. *International Psychogeriatrics*, *16*, 129–140.

Buckner, R. L., Snyder, A. Z., Shannon, B. J., LaRossa, G., Sachs, R., Fotenos, A. F., . . . Mintun, M. A. (2005). Molecular, structural, and functional characterization of Alzheimer's disease: Evidence for a relationship between default activity, amyloid, and memory. *The Journal of Neuroscience, 25*, 7709–7717.

Carson, M. J., Behringer, R. R., Brinster, R. L., & McMorris, F. A. (1993). Insulin-like growth factor I increases brain growth and central nervous system myelination in transgenic mice. *Neuron, 10*, 729–740.

Center for Disease Control and Prevention, National Vital Statistics Report. (2013). *Deaths: Final Data for 2013*. Retrieved from http://www.cdc.gov/nchs/data access/vitalstatsonline.htm

Chandler, J. D., & Chandler, J. E. (1988). The prevalence of neuropsychiatric disorder in a nursing home population. *Journal of Geriatric Psychiatry and Neurology, 1*, 71–76.

Chen, D. Y., Stern, S. A., Garcia-Osta, A., Saunier-Rebori, B., Pollonini, G., Bambah-Mukku, D., . . . Alberini, C. M. (2011). A critical role for IGF-II in memory consolidation and enhancement. *Nature, 469*, 491–497.

Choi, S. J., Lim, K. O., Monteiro, I., & Reisberg, B. (2005). Diffusion tensor imaging of frontal white matter microstructure in early Alzheimer's disease: A preliminary study. *Journal of Geriatric Psychiatry and Neurology, 18*, 12–19.

Cohen, E., Paulsson, J. F., Blinder, P., Burstyn-Cohen, T., Du, D., Estepa, G., . . . Dillin, A. (2009). Reduced IGF-1 signaling delays age-associated proteotoxicity in mice. *Cell, 139*, 1157–1169.

Costa, R. M., Drew, C., & Silva, A. J. (2005). Notch to remember. *Trends in Neurosciences, 28*, 429–435.

De Deyn, P. P., Katz, I. R., Brodaty, H., Lyons, B., Greenspan, A., & Burns, A. (2005). Management of agitation, aggression, and psychosis associated with dementia: A pooled analysis including three randomized, placebo-controlled double-blind trials in nursing home residents treated with risperidone. *Clinical Neurology and Neurosurgery, 107*, 497–508.

Devanand, D. P., Folz, M., Gorlyn, M., Moesller, J. R., & Stern, Y. (1997). Questionable dementia: Clinical course and predictors of outcome. *Journal of the American Geriatrics Society, 45*, 321–328.

Evans, V. D., Funkenstein, H., Albert, M. S., Soherr, P. A., Cook, N. R., Chown, M. J., . . . Taylor, J. O. (1989). Prevalence of Alzheimer's disease in a community population of older persons. *Journal of the American Medical Association, 262*, 2551–2556.

Farlow, M. R., Grossberg, G. T., Meng, X., Olin, J., & Somogyi, M. (2011). Rivastigmine transdermal patch and capsule in Alzheimer's disease: Influence of disease stage on response to therapy. *International Journal of Geriatric Psychiatry, 26*, 1236–1243.

Farlow, M. R., Grossberg, G. T., Sadowsky, C. H., Meng, X., & Somogyi, M. (2013). A 24-week, randomized, controlled trial of rivastigmine patch 13.3 mg/24 h versus 4.6 mg/24 h in severe Alzheimer's dementia. *CNS Neuroscience and Therapeutics, 19*(10), 745–752.

Ferris, S. H., de Leon, M. J., Wolf, A. P., Farkas, T., Christman, D. R., Reisberg, B., . . . Rampal, S. (1980). Positron emission tomography in the study of aging and senile dementia. *Neurobiology of Aging, 1*, 127–131.

Finkel, S. I. (Ed.). (1996). Behavioral and psychological signs and symptoms of dementia: Implications for research and treatment. *International Psychogeriatrics, 8*(Suppl. 3), 552 pp.

Finkel, S. I. (2000). Introduction to behavioural and psychological symptoms of dementia (BPSD). *International Journal of Geriatric Psychiatry, 15*(Suppl. 1), S2–S4.

Finkel, S. I. (2001). Behavioral and psychological symptoms of dementia: A current focus for clinicians, researchers, and caregivers. *The Journal of Clinical Psychiatry, 62*(Suppl. 2), 3–6.

Finkel, S., & Burns, A. (Eds.). (2000). Behavioural and psychological symptoms of dementia (BPSD): A clinical and research update. *International Psychogeriatrics*, *12*(Suppl. 1), 424 pp.

Finkel, S. I., Costa e Silva, J., Cohen, G., Miller, S., & Sartorius, N. (1996). Behavioral and psychological signs and symptoms of dementia: A consensus statement on current knowledge and implications for research and treatment. *International Psychogeriatrics/IPA*, *8*(Suppl. 3), 497–500.

Flechsig, P. (1901). Developmental (myelogenetic) localization of the cerebral cortex in the human subject. *The Lancet*, *158*(4077), 1027–1029.

Flechsig, P. (1920). *Anatomie des menschlichen Gehirns und Rückenmarks auf myelogenetischer Grundlage*. Leipzig: Thieme.

Flicker, C., Ferris, S. H., & Reisberg, B. (1991). Mild cognitive impairment in the elderly: Predictors of dementia. *Neurology*, *41*, 1006–1009.

Flores, A. I., Narayanan, S. P., Morse, E. N., Shick, H. E., Yin, X., Kidd, G., . . . Macklin, W. B. (2008). Constitutively active Akt induces enhanced myelination in the CNS. *The Journal of Neuroscience*, *28*, 7174–7183.

Folstein, M. F., Folstein, S. E., & McHugh, P. R. (1975). Mini-mental state: A practical method for grading the cognitive state of patients for the clinician. *Journal of Psychiatry Research*, *12*, 189–198.

Franssen, E. H. (1993). Neurologic signs in aging and dementia. In A. Burns & R. Levy (Eds.), *Aging and dementia: A methodological approach* (pp. 144–174), London, UK: Edward Arnold.

Franssen, E. H., & Reisberg, B. (1997). Neurologic markers of the progression of Alzheimer's disease. *International Psychogeriatrics*, *9*(Suppl. 1), 297–306.

Franssen, E. H., Kluger, A., Torossian, C. L., & Reisberg, B. (1993). The neurologic syndrome of severe Alzheimer's disease: Relationship to functional decline. *Archives of Neurology*, *50*, 1029–1039.

Franssen, E. H., Reisberg, B., Kluger, A., Sinaiko, E., & Boja, C. (1991). Cognition independent neurologic symptoms in normal aging and probable Alzheimer's disease. *Archives of Neurology*, *48*, 148–154.

Franssen, E. H., Souren, L. E. M., Torossian, C. L., & Reisberg, B. (1997). Utility of developmental reflexes in the differential diagnosis and prognosis of incontinence in Alzheimer's disease. *Journal of Geriatric Psychiatry and Neurology*, *10*, 22–28.

Franssen, E. H., Souren, L. E. M., Torossian, C. L., & Reisberg, B. (1999). Equilibrium and limb coordination in mild cognitive impairment and mild Alzheimer's disease. *Journal of the American Geriatrics Society*, *47*, 463–499.

Gagnon, M., Dartigues, J. F., Mazaux, J. M., Dequae, L., Letenneur, L., Giroire, J. M., & Barberger-Gateau, P. (1994). Self-reported memory complaints and memory performance in elderly French community residents: Results of the PAQUID Research Program. *Neuroepidemiology*, *13*, 145–154.

Gauthier, S., Reisberg, B., Zaudig, M., Petersen, R. C., Ritchie, K., Broich, K., . . . On behalf of the participants of the IPA Expert Conference on MCI. (2006). Mild cognitive impairment. *Lancet*, *367*, 1262–1270.

Geerlings, M. I., Jonker, C., Bouter, L. M., Ader, H. J., & Schmand, B. (1999). Association between memory complaints and incident Alzheimer's disease in elderly people with normal baseline cognition. *American Journal of Psychiatry*, *156*, 531–537.

Glabe, C. (2006). Biomedicine. Avoiding collateral damage in Alzheimer's disease treatment. *Science*, *314*, 602–603.

Graves, A. B., Larson, E. B., Edland, S. D., Bowen, J. D., McCormick, W. C., McCurry, S. M., . . . Uomoto, J. M. (1996). Prevalence of dementia and its subtypes in the Japanese American population of King County, Washington State: The Kame Project. *American Journal of Epidemiology*, *144*(8), 760–771.

Hamilton, M. (1960). A rating scale for depression. *Journal of Neurology, Neurosurgery & Psychiatry, 23*, 56.

Harris-Kojetin, L., Sengupta, M., Park-Lee, E., & Valverde, R. (2013). Long-term care services in the United States: 2013 overview. *National Health Center for Health Statistics, Vital Health Stat, 3*(37), 1–107.

Health Care Financing Administration. (1998). Hospice-determining terminal status in non-cancer diagnoses-dementia. *The Medicare News Brief/Empire Medical Services*, (MNB-98–7), 45–47.

Hoyer, S. (1998). Is sporadic Alzheimer disease the brain type of non-insulin dependent diabetes mellitus? A challenging hypothesis. *Journal of Neural Transmission*, *105*, 415–422.

Hu, X., Hicks, C. W., He, W., Wong, P., Macklin, W. B., Trapp, B. D., & Yan, R. (2006). Bace1 modulates myelination in the central and peripheral nervous system. *Nature Neuroscience*, *9*, 1520–1525.

Hughes, C. P., Berg, L., Danziger, W. L., Coben, L. A., & Martin, R. L. (1982). A new clinical scale for the staging of dementia. *British Journal of Psychiatry, 140*, 566–572.

Jessen, F., Feyen, L., Freymann, K., Tepest, R., Maier, W., Heun, R., . . . Scheef, L. (2006). Volume reduction of the entorhinal cortex in subjective memory impairment. *Neurobiology Aging*, *27*(12), 1751–1756.

Jeste, D. V., Blazer, D., Casey, D., Meeks, T., Salzman, C., Schneider, L., . . . Yaffe, K. (2008). ACNP White Paper: Update on use of antipsychotic drugs in elderly persons with dementia. *Neuropsychopharmacology*, *33*, 957–970.

Jonker, C., Geerlings, M. I., & Schmand, B. (2000). Are memory complaints predictive for dementia? A review of clinical and population-based studies. *International Journal of Geriatric Psychiatry, 15*, 983–991.

Kales, H. C., Valenstein, M., Kim, H. M., McCarthy, J. F., Ganoczy, D., Cunningham, F., & Blow, F. C. (2007). Mortality risk in patients with dementia treated with antipsychotics versus other psychiatric medications. *The American Journal of Psychiatry, 164*, 1568–1576.

Kaplan, A. (2005). High rates of dementia, psychiatric disorders found in assisted living facilities. *Psychiatric Times*, *22*(3), 1, 5–6.

Kaskie, B. P., Nattinger, M., & Potter, A. (2015). Special Issue: 2015 WHCOA, Policies to protect persons with dementia in assisted living; Déjà vu all over again? *The Gerontologist, 55*(2), 199–209.

Katz, I. R., Jeste, D., Mintzer, J. E., Clyde, C., Napolitano, J., & Brecher, M. (1999). Comparison of Resperidone and placebo for psychosis and behavioral disturbances associated with dementia: A randomized, double-blind trial. *Journal of Clinical Psychiatry*, *60*, 107–115.

Katzman, R. (1986). Alzheimer's disease. *New England Journal of Medicine*, *314*, 964–973.

Kidd, M. (1963). Paired helical filaments in electron microscopy of Alzheimer's disease. *Nature*, *197*, 192–193.

Kluger, A., Ferris, S. H., Golomb, J., Mittelman, M. S., & Reisberg, B. (1999). Neuropsychological prediction of decline to dementia in nondemented elderly. *Journal of Geriatric Psychiatry and Neurology*, *12*, 168–179.

Kluger, A., Gianutsos, J. G., Golomb, J., Ferris, S. H., George, A. E., Franssen, E., & Reisberg, B. (1997). Patterns of motor impairment in normal aging, mild cognitive decline and early Alzheimer's disease. *Journal of Gerontology: Psychological Sciences*, *52B*, P28–P39.

Kondo, J., Honda, T., Mori, H., Hamada, Y., Miura, R., Ogawara, M., & Ihara, Y. (1988). The carboxyl third of tau is tightly bound to paired helical filaments. *Neuron*, *1*, 827–834.

Kumar, A., Koss, E., Metzler, D., Moore, A., & Friedland, R. (1988). Behavioral symptomatology in dementia of the Alzheimer's type. *Alzheimer Disease and Associated Disorders*, *2*, 363–365.

Laboratory Corporation of America. (2003). *Holdings and Lexi-Comp Inc*. Retrieved from http://www.labcorp.com/datasets/labcorp/html/chapter/mono/sr003600.htm

Larson, E. B., & Langa, K. M. (2008). The rising tide of dementia worldwide. *The Lancet*, *372*, 430–432.

Lawton, M. P., Brody, E. M., & Saperstein, A. R. (1989). A controlled study of respite service for caregivers of Alzheimer's patients. *Gerontologist*, *29*, 8–16.

Lobo, A., Launer, L. J., Fratiglioni, L., Andersen, K., Di Carlo, A., Breteler, M. M., . . . Hofman, A. (2000). Prevalence of dementia and major subtypes in Europe: A collaborative study of population-based cohorts. Neurologic Diseases in the Elderly Research Group. *Neurology*, *54*, S4–S9.

Luijpen, M. W., Scherder, E. J., Van Someren, E. J., Swaab, D. F., & Sergeant, J. A. (2003). Non-pharmacological interventions in cognitively impaired and demented patients: A comparison with cholinesterase inhibitors. *Reviews Neuroscience, 14*, 343–368.

Lyketsos, C. G., Steinberg, M., Tschanz, J. T., Norton, M. C., Steffens, D. C., & Breitner, J. C. (2000). Mental and behavioral disturbances in dementia: Findings from the Cache County Study on Memory in Aging. *American Journal of Psychiatry*, *157*, 708–714.

McElroy, B., Powell, J. C., & McCarthy, J. V. (2007). The insulin-like growth factor 1 (IGF-1) receptor is a substrate for gamma-secretase-mediated intramembrane proteolysis. *Biochemical and Biophysical Research Communications*, *358*(4), 1136–1141.

McGeer, P. L., McGeer, E. G., Akiyama, H., Itagaki, S., Harrop, R., & Peppard, R. (1990). Neuronal degeneration and memory loss in Alzheimer's disease and aging. *Experimental Brain Research*, (Suppl. 21), 411–426.

McKhann, G., Drachman, D., Folstein, M., Katzman, R., Price, D., & Stadlan, E. M. (1984). Clinical diagnosis of Alzheimer's disease: Report of the NINCDS-ADRDA work group under the auspices of Department of Health and Human Services Task Force on Alzheimer's Disease. *Neurology, 34*(7), 939–944.

Mitchell, A. J., Beaumont, H., Ferguson, D., Yadegarfar, M., & Stubbs, B. (2014). Risk of dementia and mild cognitive impairment in older people with subjective memory complaints: Meta-analysis. *Acta Psychiatrica Scandinavica*, *130*(6), 439–451.

Mittelman, M. S., Ferris, S. H., Steinberg, G., Shulman, E., Mackell, J. A., Ambinder, A., & Cohen, J. (1993). An intervention that delays institutionalization of Alzheimer's disease patients: Treatment of spouse-caregivers. *Gerontologist*, *33*, 730–740.

Moloney, A. M., Griffin, R. J., Timmons, S., O'Connor, R., Ravid, R., & O'Neill, C. (2010). Defects in IGF-1 receptor, insulin receptor and IRS-1/2 in Alzheimer's disease indicate possible resistance to IGF-1 and insulin signaling. *Neurobiology of Aging*, *31*, 224–243.

Montine, T. J., & Larson, E. B. (2009). Late-life dementias: Does this unyielding global challenge require a broader view? *Journal of the American Medical Association*, *302*(23), 2593–2594.

Morris, J. C. (1993). The clinical dementia rating (CDR): Current version and scoring rules. *Neurology, 43*, 2412–2414.

Morris, J. C., Storandt, M., Miller, P., McKeel, D. W., Price, J. L., Rubin, E. H., & Berg, L. (2001). Mild cognitive impairment represents early-stage Alzheimer disease. *Neurology*, *58*, 397–405.

Mosconi, L., De Santi, S., Brys, M., Tsui, W. H., Pirraglia, E., Glodzik-Sobanska, L., . . . de Leon, M. J. (2008). Hypometabolism and altered cerebrospinal fluid markers in normal apolipoprotein E E4 carriers with subjective memory complaints. *Biological Psychiatry*, *63*, 609–618.

Näslund, J., Haroutunian, V., Mohs, R., Davis, K. L., Davies, P., Greengard, P., & Buxbaum, J. D. (2000). Correlation between elevated levels of amyloid ß-peptide in the brain and cognitive decline. *The Journal of the American Medical Association*, *283*, 1571–1577.

Olazarán, J., Reisberg, B., Clare, L., Cruz, I., Peña-Casanova, J., del Ser, T., . . . Muñiz, R. (2010). Nonpharmacological therapies in Alzheimer's disease: A systematic review of efficacy. *Dementia Geriatric Cognitive Disorders*, *30*, 161–178.

Ouvrier, R. A., Goldsmith, R. F., Ourvrier, S., & Williams, I. C. (1993). The value of the mini-mental state examination in childhood: A preliminary study. *Journal of Child Neurology*, *8*(2), 145–148.

PDR Network. (2009). *Physicians' desk reference* (p. 2683). Montvale, NJ: Author.

Perrotin, A., Mormino, E. C., Madison, C. M., Hayenga, A. O., & Jagust, W. J. (2012). Subjective cognition and amyloid deposition imaging: A Pittsburgh Compound B positron emission tomography study in normal elderly individuals. *Archives of Neurology*, *69*(2), 223–229.

Petersen, R. C., Smith, G. E., Waring, S. C., Ivnik, R. J., Tangalos, E. G., & Kokmen, E. (1999). Mild cognitive impairment: Clinical characterization and outcome. *Archives of Neurology*, *56*, 303–308.

Petersen, R. C., Stevens, J. C., Ganguli, M., Tangalos, E. G., Cummings, J. L., & DeKosky, S. T. (2001). Practice parameter: Early detection of dementia: Mild cognitive impairment (an evidence-based review). Report of the Quality Standards Subcommittee of the American academy of neurology. *Neurology*, *56*, 1133–1142.

Phelps, M. E. (2000). Positron emission tomography provides molecular imaging of biological processes. *Proceedings of the National Academy of Sciences of the United States of America*, *97*, 9226–9233.

Pluta, R. (2002). Astroglial expression of the beta-amyloid in ischemia-reperfusion brain injury. *Annals of the New York Academy of Sciences*, *977*, 102–108.

Popa-Wagner, A., Schröder, E., Walker, L. C., & Kessler, C. (1998). ß-Amyloid precursor protein and ss-amyloid peptide immunoreactivity in the rat brain after middle cerebral artery occlusion: Effect of age. *Stroke*, *29*(10), 2196–2202.

Prichep, L. S., John, E. R., Ferris, S. H., Rausch, L., Fang, Z., Cancro, R., Torossian, C., & Reisberg, B. (2006). Prediction of longitudinal cognitive decline in normal elderly using electrophysiological imaging. *Neurobiology of Aging*, *27*, 471–481.

Prichep, L. S., John, E. R., Ferris, S. H., Reisberg, B., Almas, M., Alper, K., & Cancro, R. (1994). Quantitative EEG correlates of cognitive deterioration in the elderly. *Neurobiology of Aging*, *15*(1), 85–90.

Puglielli, L. (2008). Aging of the brain, neurotrophin signaling, and Alzheimer's disease: Is IGF1-R the common culprit? *Neurobiology of Aging*, *29*, 795–811.

Rabin, L. A., Smart, C. M., Crane, P. K., Amariglio, R. E., Berman, L. M., Boada, M., . . . The Subjective Cognitive Decline Initiative (SCD-I) Working Group. (2015). Subjective cognitive decline in older adults: An overview of self-report measures used across 19 international research studies. *Journal of Alzheimer's Disease*, *48*, S63–S86.

Raz, N. (1999). Aging of the brain and its impact on cognitive performance: Integration of structural and functional findings. In F. I. M. Craik & T. A. Salthouse (Eds.), *Handbook of aging and cognition*. Mahwah, NJ: Erlbaum.

Raz, N., Gunning, F. M., Head, D., Dupuis, J. H., McQuain, J., Briggs, S. D., . . . Acker, J. D. (1997). Selective aging of the human cerebral cortex observed in vivo: Differential vulnerability of the prefrontal gray matter. *Cerebral Cortex*, *7*, 268–282.

Reisberg, B. (1986). Dementia: A systematic approach to identifying reversible causes. *Geriatrics*, *41*(4), 30–46.

Reisberg, B. (1988). Functional assessment staging (FAST). *Psychopharmacology Bulletin*, *24*, 653–659.

Reisberg, B. (2007). Global measures: Utility in defining and measuring treatment response in dementia. *International Psychogeriatrics*, *19*, 421–456.

Reisberg, B., Auer, S. R., Monteiro, I., Franssen, E., & Kenowsky, S. (1998). A rational psychological approach to the treatment of behavioral disturbances and symptomatology in Alzheimer's disease based upon recognition of the developmental age. *International Academy for Biomedical and Drug Research*, *13*, 102–109.

Reisberg, B., Borenstein, J., Franssen, E., Shulman, E., Steinberg, G., & Ferris, S. H. (1986). Remediable behavioral symptomatology in Alzheimer's disease. *Hospital and Community Psychiatry*, *37*, 1199–1201.

Reisberg, B., Borenstein, J., Salob, S. P., Ferris, S. H., Franssen, E., & Georgotas, A. (1987). Behavioral symptoms in Alzheimer's disease: Phenomenology and treatment. *Journal of Clinical Psychiatry*, *48*(Suppl. 5), 9–15.

Reisberg, B., Doody, R., Stöffler, A., Schmitt, F., Ferris, S., Möbius, H.-J., & The Memantine Study Group. (2003). Memantine in moderate-to-severe Alzheimer's disease, *New England Journal of Medicine*, *348*, 1333–1341.

Reisberg, B., & Ferris, S. H. (1988). The Brief Cognitive Rating Scale (BCRS). *Psychopharmacology Bulletin*, *24*, 629–636.

Reisberg, B., Ferris, S. H., & Franssen, E. (1985). An ordinal functional assessment tool for Alzheimer's-type dementia. *Hospital and Community Psychiatry*, *36*, 593–595.

Reisberg, B., Ferris, S. H., & Franssen, E. (1986). Functional degenerative stages in dementia of the Alzheimer's type appear to reverse normal human development. In C. Shagass, R. Josiassen, W. H. Bridger, K. Weiss, D. Stoff, & G. M. Simpson (Eds.), *Biological psychiatry*, 1985 (Vol. 7, pp. 1319–1321). New York, NY: Elsevier Science Publishing.

Reisberg, B., Ferris, S. H., Anand, R., de Leon, M. J., Schneck, M. K., Buttinger, C., & Borenstein, J. (1984). Functional staging of dementia of the Alzheimer's type. *Annals of the New York Academy of Sciences*, *435*, 481–483.

Reisberg, B., Ferris, S. H., & de Leon, M. J. (1985). Senile dementia of the Alzheimer type: Diagnostic and differential diagnostic features with special reference to functional assessment staging. In J. Traber & W. H Gispen (Eds.), *Senile dementia of the alzheimer type* (Vol. 2, pp. 18–37). Berlin, Germany: Springer-Verlag.

Reisberg, B., Ferris, S. H., de Leon, M. J., & Crook, T. (1982). The global deterioration scale for assessment of primary degenerative dementia. *American Journal of Psychiatry*, *139*, 1136–1139.

Reisberg, B., Ferris, S. H., de Leon, M. J., Kluger, A., Franssen, E., Borenstein, J., & Alba, R. (1989). The stage specific temporal course of Alzheimer's disease: Functional and behavioral concomitants based upon cross-sectional and longitudinal observation. In K. Iqbal, H. M. Wisniewski, & B. Winblad (Eds.), *Alzheimer's disease and related disorders: Progress in clinical and biological research* (Vol. 317, pp. 23–41). New York, NY: Alan R. Liss.

Reisberg, B., Ferris, S. H., de Leon, M. J., Sinaiko, E., Franssen, E., Kluger, A., . . . Cohen, J. (1988). Stage-specific behavioral, cognitive, and in vivo changes in community residing subjects with age-associated memory impairment and primary degenerative dementia of the Alzheimer type. *Drug Development Research*, *15*, 101–114.

Reisberg, B., Ferris, S. H., Franssen, E. H., Kluger, A., & Borenstein, J. (1986). Age-associated memory impairment: The clinical syndrome. *Developmental Neuropsychology*, *2*, 401–412.

Reisberg, B., Ferris, S. H., Franssen, E., Shulman, E., Monteiro, I., Sclan, S. G., . . . Laska, E. (1996). Mortality and temporal course of probable Alzheimer's disease: A five-year prospective study. *International Psychogeriatrics*, *8*, 291–311.

Reisberg, B., Ferris, S. H., Kluger, A., Franssen, E., Wegiel, J., & de Leon, M. J. (2008). Mild cognitive impairment (MCI): A historical perspective. *International Psychogeriatrics*, *20*, 18–31.

Reisberg, B., Ferris, S. H., Torossian, C., Kluger, A., & Monteiro, I. (1992). Pharmacologic treatment of Alzheimer's disease: A methodologic critique based upon current knowledge of symptomatology and relevance for drug trials. *International Psychogeriatrics*, *4*(Supp. 1), 9–42.

Reisberg, B., Franssen, E. H., Hasan, S. M., Monteiro, I., Boksay, I., Souren, L. E. M., . . . Kluger, A. (1999). Retrogenesis: Clinical, physiologic and pathologic mechanisms in brain aging, Alzheimer's and other dementing processes. *European Archives of Psychiatry and Clinical Neuroscience*, *249*(Suppl. 3), 28–36.

Reisberg, B., Franssen, E. H., Souren, L. E. M., Auer, S., & Kenowsky, S. (1998). Progression of Alzheimer's disease: Variability and consistency: Ontogenic models, their applicability and relevance. *Journal of Neural Transmission, 54*, 9–20.

Reisberg, B., Franssen, E. H., Souren, L. E. M., Auer, S. R., Akram, I., & Kenowsky, S. (2002). Evidence and mechanisms of retrogenesis in Alzheimer's and other dementias: Management and treatment import. *American Journal of Alzheimer's Disease, 17*, 202–212.

Reisberg, B., Franssen, E., Bobinski, M., Auer, S., Monteiro, I., Boksay, I., . . . Ferris, S. H. (1996). Overview of methodologic issues for pharmacologic trials in mild, moderate, and severe Alzheimer's disease. *International Psychogeriatrics*, *8*, 159–193.

Reisberg, B., Franssen, E., Sclan, S. G., Kluger, A., & Ferris, S. H. (1989). Stage specific incidence of potentially remediable behavioral symptoms in aging and Alzheimer's disease: A study of 120 patients using the BEHAVE-AD. *Bulletin of Clinical Neuroscience*, *54*, 95–112.

Reisberg, B., Franssen, E., Souren, L., Kenowsky, S., & Auer, S. (1998). Severity scales. In A. Wimo, B. Jönsson, G. Karlsson & B. Winblad (Eds.), *Health economics of dementia* (pp. 327–357). Chichester: John Wiley and Sons.

Reisberg, B., & Gauthier, S. (2008). Current evidence for subjective cognitive impairment (SCI) as the pre-mild cognitive impairment (MCI) stage of subsequently manifest Alzheimer's disease. *International Psychogeriatrics*, *20*, 1–16.

Reisberg, B., Kenowsky, S., Franssen, E. H., Auer, S. R., & Souren, L. E. M. (1999). President's report: towards a science of Alzheimer's disease management: A model based upon current knowledge of retrogenesis. *International Psychogeriatrics, 11*, 7–23.

Reisberg, B., London, E., Ferris, S. H., Borenstein, J., Scheier, L., & de Leon, M. J. (1983). the brief cognitive rating scale: Language, motoric, and mood concomitants in primary degenerative dementia. *Psychopharmacology Bulletin, 19*, 702–708.

Reisberg, B., Monteiro, I., Torossian, C., Auer, S., Shulman, M., Ghimire, S., . . . Xu, J. (2014). The BEHAVE-AD Assessment system: A perspective, commentary on new findings and historical review. *Dementia and Geriatric Cognitive Disorders*, *38*(1–2), 89–146.

Reisberg, B., Pattschull-Furlan, A., Franssen, E., Sclan, S. G., Kluger, A., Dingcong, L., & Ferris, S. H. (1990). Cognition related functional, praxis and feeding changes in CNS aging and Alzheimer's disease and their developmental analogies. In K. Beyreuther & G. Schettler (Eds.), *Molecular mechanisms of aging* (pp. 18–40). Berlin, Germany: Springer-Verlag.

Reisberg, B., Prichep, L., Mosconi, L., John, E. R., Glodzik-Sobanska, L., Boksay, I., . . . de Leon, M. J. (2008). The pre-mild cognitive impairment, subjective cognitive impairment stage of Alzheimer's disease. *Alzheimer's & Dementia*, *4*(Supp. 1), S98–S108.

Reisberg, B., & Saeed, M. U. (2004). Alzheimer's disease. In J. Sadovoy, L. F. Jarvik, G. T. Grossberg & B. S. Meyers (Eds.), *Comprehensive textbook of geriatric psychiatry* (3rd ed., pp. 449–509). New York, NY: W.W. Norton.

Reisberg, B., Schneck, M. K., Ferris, S. H., Schwartz, G. E., & de Leon, M. J. (1983). The brief cognitive rating scale (BCRS): Findings in primary degenerative dementia (PDD). *Psychopharmacology Bulletin*, *19*, 47–50.

Reisberg, B., Sclan, S., Franssen, E., de Leon, M. J., Kluger, A., Torossian, C., . . . Ferris, S. H. (2008). The GDS staging system: Global deterioration scale (GDS), Brief cognitive rating scale (BCRS), Functional assessment staging (FAST). In A. J. Rush, Jr., M. B. First, & D. Blacker (Eds.), *Handbook of psychiatric measures* (2nd ed., pp. 431–435). Washington, DC: American Psychiatric Publishing.

Reisberg, B., & Shulman, M. B. (2009). Commentary on "A roadmap for the prevention of dementia II: Leon Thal symposium 2008." Subjective cognitive impairment as an antecedent of Alzheimer's dementia: Policy import. *Alzheimer's & Dementia*, *5*(2), 154–156.

Reisberg, B., Shulman, M. B., Torossian, C., Leng, L., & Zhu, W. (2010). Outcome over seven years of healthy adults with and without subjective cognitive impairment. *Alzheimer's & Dementia*, *6*, 11–24.

Reisberg, B., Wegiel, J., Franssen, E., Auer, S., Shimada, M., Meguro, K., . . . Borza, L. (2006). Behavioral and neuropathophysiologic course of Alzheimer's disease (AD): A synthesis based on retrogenesis, arboreal and neurometabolic entropy and possible etiopathogenic events. In K. Iqbal, B. Winblad, & J. Avila (Eds.), *Alzheimer's Disease: New Advances* (pp. 219–222). Bologna: Medimond International Proceedings.

Reisberg, B., Wegiel, J., Franssen, E., Kadiyala, S., Auer, S., Souren, L., Sabbagh, M., & Golomb, J. (2006b). Clinical features of severe dementia: Staging. In A. Burns & B. Winblad (Eds.), *Severe dementia* (pp. 83–115). London, UK: John Wiley & Sons.

Rosenblatt, A., Samus, Q. M., Steele, C. D., Baker, A. S., Harper, M. G., Brandt, J., . . . Lyketsos, C. G. (2004). The Maryland assisted living study: Prevalence, recognition, and treatment of dementia and other psychiatric disorders in the assisted living population of central Maryland. *Journal of the American Geriatrics Society*, *52*, 1618–1625.

Rovner, B. W., Kafonek, S., Filipp, L., Lucas, M. J., & Folstein, M. F. (1986). Prevalence of mental illness in a community nursing home. *American Journal of Psychiatry*, *143*, 1446–1449.

Rubial-Álvarez, S., de Sola, S., Machado, M.-C., Sintas, E., Böhm, P., Sánchez-Benavides, G., . . . Peña-Casanova, J. (2013). The comparison of cognitive and functional performance in children and Alzheimer's disease supports the retrogenesis model. *Journal of Alzheimer's Disease*, *33*, 191–203.

Rubial-Álvarez, S., Machado, M.-C., Sintas, E., de Sola, S., Böhm, P., & Peña-Casanova, J. (2007). A preliminary study of the mini-mental state examination in a Spanish child population. *Journal of Child Neurology*, *22*, 1269–1273.

Rubin, E., Morris, J., Storandt, M., & Berg, L. (1987). Behavioral changes in patients with mild senile dementia of the Alzheimer's type. *Psychiatry Research*, *21*, 55–61.

Schneider, L. S., Dagerman, K. S., & Insel, P. (2005). Risk of death with atypical antipsychotic drug treatment for dementia: Meta-analysis of randomized placebo-controlled trials. *Journal of the American Medical Association*, *294*, 1934–1943.

Schneider, L. S., Tariot, P. N., Dagerman, K. S., Davis, S. M., Hsiao, J. K., Ismail, M. S., . . . The CATIE-AD Study Group. (2006). Effectiveness of atypical antipsychotic drugs in patients with Alzheimer's disease. *The New England Journal of Medicine*, *355*, 1525–1538.

Sclan, S. G., Foster, J. R., Reisberg, B., Franssen, E., & Welkowitz, J. (1990). Application of Piagetian measures of cognition in severe Alzheimer's disease. *Psychiatric Journal of the University of Ottawa*, *15*, 221–226.

Sclan, S. G., & Reisberg, B. (1992). Functional assessment staging (FAST) in Alzheimer's disease: Reliability, validity and ordinality. *International Psychogeriatrics*, *4*, 55–69.

Seubert, P., Vigo-Pelfrey, C., Esch, F., Lee, M., Dovey, H., Davis, D., . . . Schenket, D. (1992). Isolation and quantification of soluble Alzheimer's beta-peptide from biological fluids. *Nature*, *359*, 325–327.

Shimada, M., Hayat, J., Meguro, K., Oo, T., Jafri, S., Yamadori, A., . . . Reisberg, B. (2003). Correlation between functional assessment staging and the 'Basic Age' by the Binet scale supports the retrogenesis model of Alzheimer's disease: A preliminary study. *Psychogeriatrics*, *3*, 82–87.

Sinigaglia-Coimbra, R., Cavalheiro, E. A., & Coimbra, C. G. (2002). Postischemic hyperthermia induces Alzheimer-like pathology in the rat brain. *Acta Neuropathologica (Berlin)*, *103*(5), 444–452.

Souren, L. E. M., Franssen, E. M., & Reisberg, B. (1995). Contractures and loss of function in patients with Alzheimer's disease. *Journal of the American Geriatrics Society*, *43*, 650–655.

Steen, E., Terry, B. M., Rivera, E. J., Cannon, J. L., Neely, T. R., Tavares, R., . . . de la Monte, S. M. (2005). Impaired insulin and insulin-like growth factor expression and signaling mechanisms in Alzheimer's disease–is this type 3 diabetes? *Journal of Alzheimer's Disease*, *7*(1), 63–80.

Stephen, P. J., & Williamson, J. (1984). Drug-induced parkinsonism in the elderly. *The Lancet, 2*, 1082–1083.

Stricker, N. H., Schweinsburg, B. C., Delano-Wood, L., Wierenga, C. E., Bangen, K, J., Haaland, K. Y., . . . Bondi, M. W. (2009). Decreased white matter integrity in late-myelinating fiber pathways in Alzheimer's disease supports retrogenesis. *Neuroimage, 45*(1), 10–16.

Tariot, P. N., Farlow, M., Grossberg, G. T., Graham, S. M., McDonald, S., Gergel, I., & The Memantine Study Group. (2004). Memantine treatment in patients with moderate to severe Alzheimer Disease already receiving Donepezil. *Journal of the American Medical Association, 3*, 317–324.

Tierney, M. C., Szalai, J. P., Snow, W. G., Fisher, R. H., Nores, A., Nadon, G., . . . St.George-Hyslop, P. H. (1996). Prediction of probable Alzheimer's disease in memory-impaired patients: A prospective longitudinal study. *Neurology*, *46*, 661–665.

Townsend, M., Mehta, T., & Selkoe, D. J. (2007). Soluble Abeta inhibits specific signal transduction cascades common to the insulin receptor pathway. *Journal of Biological Chemistry*, *282*(46), 33305–33312.

Uzgiris, I., & Hunt, J. McV. (1975). *Assessment in infancy: Ordinal scales of psychological development.* Urbana: University of Illinois.

van Norden, A. G., Fick, W. F., de Laat, K. F., van Uden, I. W., van Oudheusden, L. J., Tendolkar, I., . . . de Leeuw, F. E. (2008). Subjective cognitive failures and hippocampal volume in elderly with white matter lesions. *Neurology, 71*(15), 1152–1159.

Visser, P. J., Verhey, F., Knol, D. L., Scheltens, P., Wahlund, L.-O., Freund-Levi, Y., . . . Blennow, K. (2009). Prevalence and prognostic value of CSF markers of Alzheimer's disease pathology in patients with subjective cognitive impairment or mild cognitive impairment in the DESCRIPA study: A prospective cohort study. *Lancet Neurology*, *8*(7), 619–627.

Wang, P. S., Schneeweiss, S., Avorn, J., Fischer, M. A., Mogun, H., Solomon, D. H., & Brookhart, M. A. (2005). Risk of death in elderly users of conventional vs. atypical antipsychotic medications. *The New England Journal of Medicine, 353*, 2335–2341.

Wang, P.-N., Wang, S.-J., Fuh, J.-L., Teng, E. L., Liu, C. Y., Lin, C. H., . . . Liu, H. C. (2000). Subjective memory complaint in relation to cognitive performance and depression: A longitudinal study of a rural Chinese population. *Journal of the American Geriatrics Society*, *48*, 295–299.

Wegiel, J., Dowjat, K., Kaczmarski, W., Kuchna, I., Nowicki, K., Frackowiak, J., . . . Hwang, Y.-W. (2008). The role of overexpressed DYRK1A protein in the early onset of neurofibrillary degeneration in Down syndrome. *Acta Neuropathologica*, *116*, 391–407.

Wegiel, J., Wisniewski, H. M., Dziewiatkowski, J., Badmajew, E., Tarnawski, M., Reisberg, B., . . . Miller, D. C. (1999). Cerebellar atrophy in Alzheimer's disease clinicopathological correlations. *Brain Research*, *819*, 41–50.

Willem, M., Garratt, A. N., Novak, B., Citron, M., Kaufmann, S., Rittger, A., . . . Haass, C. (2006). Control of peripheral nerve myelination by the beta-secretase BACE1. *Science*, *314*, 664–666.

Winblad, B., & Poritis, N. (1999). Memantine in severe dementia: results of the M-BEST Study (Benefit and efficacy in severely demented patients during treatment with memantine). *International Journal of Geriatric Psychiatry*, *14*, 135–146.

Winblad, B., Kilander, L., Eriksson, S., Minthon, L., Båtsman, S., Wetterholm, A.-L., . . . The Severe Alzheimer's Disease Study Group. (2006). Donepezil in patients with severe Alzheimer's disease: Double-blind, parallel-group, placebo-controlled study. *Lancet, 367*, 1057–1065.

Winblad, B., Palmer, K., Kivipelto, M., Jelic, V., Fratiglioni, L., Wahlund, L. O., . . . Petersen, R. C. (2004). Mild cognitive impairment–beyond controversies, towards a consensus: Report of the International working group on mild cognitive impairment. *Journal of Internal Medicine*, *256*, 240–246.

Wischik, C. M., Novak, M., Edwards, P. C., Klug, A., Tichelaar, W., & Crowther, R. A. (1988). Structural characterization of the core of the paired helical filament of Alzheimer disease. *Proceedings of the National Academy of Sciences of the United States of America*, *85*, 4884–4888.

Wischik, C. M., Novak, M., Thøgersen, H. C., Edwards, P. C., Runswick, M. J., Jakes, R., . . . Klug, A. (1988). Isolation of a fragment of tau derived from the core of the paired helical filament of Alzheimer disease. *Proceedings of the National Academy of Sciences of the United States of America*, *85*, 4506–4510.

Wolf, O. T., Dziobek, I., McHugh, P., Sweat, V., de Leon, M. J., Javier, E., & Convit, A. (2005). Subjective memory complaints in aging are associated with elevated cortisol levels. *Neurobiology of Aging*, *26*, 1357–1363.

Zeisel, J., Reisberg, B., Whitehouse, P., Woods, R., & Verheul, A. (2016). Ecopsychosocial interventions in cognitive decline and dementia: A new terminology and a new paradigm, *American Journal of Alzheimer's Disease & Other Dementias*, *31*(6), 502–507.

Zhao, W.-Q., De Felice, F. G., Fernandez, S., Chen, H., Lambert, M. P., Quon, M. J., . . . Klein, W. L. (2008). Amyloid beta oligomers induce impairment of neuronal insulin receptors. *Federation of American Societies for Experimental Biology Journal*, *22*(1), 246–260.

CHAPTER

Traumatic Brain Injury

Alexandra Nielsen, Brian Im, Mary R. Hibbard, Ilana Grunwald, and Patrick T. Swift

OVERVIEW

In this chapter, medical aspects of traumatic brain injury (TBI) are reviewed with attention paid to its epidemiology, etiology, mechanisms of injury, measurement of injury severity, and potential complications. The role of an interdisciplinary treatment team in addressing the unique cognitive and behavioral rehabilitation needs of individuals with varying severity of TBI in both the acute inpatient rehabilitation setting and in the community are discussed.

INTRODUCTION

A TBI often results in devastating and lifelong challenges that can impact a person's physical, cognitive, and psychological functioning. These challenges reveal the importance of understanding TBI and its impact on both persons who have experienced the injury and their family/friends. Although post-TBI physical impairments undoubtedly can hinder functional independence, the behavioral, cognitive, emotional, psychosocial, and personality changes associated with TBI frequently lead to even greater functional dependency. Although not all TBIs result in dysfunction in all of these domains, it is also not uncommon for some or all of these domains to be affected. As typical of many disabilities, the more functional domains that are impacted by the TBI, the more challenging the recovery course would be. When the cultural, social, and personality backgrounds of each individual are also considered, it is easy to see how all individuals with a TBI require a unique approach to their acute care management and their postacute rehabilitation efforts to optimize recovery.

Although there has been improved education in medical schools, professional training programs in rehabilitation interventions, and the public regarding the unique cluster of challenges that emerge after brain injury, more than superficial knowledge about the challenges faced by individuals following TBI and appropriate and targeted interventions have been slow to develop. Increased awareness on the part of clinical assessment teams will allow for appropriate referral of patients for either inpatient or outpatient rehabilitation services.

EPIDEMIOLOGY OF TBI

TBIs occur worldwide resulting in many deaths (i.e., mortality) as well as in significant disability and dysfunction (i.e., morbidity) within a subset of every nation's population. In 1996, one estimate attributed at least 10 million deaths or hospitalizations to TBIs worldwide, with an estimated 57 million people living who have been hospitalized with one or more TBIs. Undoubtedly, there are many more people who were never diagnosed or who never sought treatment after a TBI (Langlois, Rutland-Brown, & Wald, 2006), indicating that these figures underestimate the true burden of this condition.

Long-term outcomes after a TBI differ across nations significantly. In general, mortality secondary to TBI is greater in low- and middle-income countries, whereas disability rates after TBI are less in these countries when compared with high-income countries (De Silva et al., 2009). One probable reason for these findings is that high-income nations have developed better detection and acute care interventions for severe TBI resulting in more individuals surviving with significant disabilities.

In the United States, the Centers for Disease Control and Prevention (CDC) reported that in 2010, approximately 50,000 deaths, 280,000 hospitalizations, and 2.2 million emergency department visits occurred as a result of TBIs. High incidences of TBI in both the young and the elderly formed two peak age groups, with the highest risk of TBI occurring among 0- to 4-year-olds and 15- to 19-year-olds. However, later studies with modified age ranges revealed that the young adult and middle-aged populations were equally at an elevated risk of TBI. A significantly higher risk of severe TBI resulting in hospitalizations and mortality was identified in those older than 65 years. Men were one-and-a-half to two times as likely to experience a TBI as women, except in the elderly where the gender ratio is fairly even (Langlois et al., 2006).

Findings across select nations suggest that certain subgroups of individuals are at elevated risk of TBI. For example, multiple studies from Australia, New Zealand, and the United States reveal that more than half of the prisoners surveyed had sustained a TBI in their past (Schofield et al., 2006).

Based on CDC data from the 2015 report to Congress, it is estimated that 2.5 million TBIs occurred in the United States in 2010. Available CDC data probably underestimates the full impact of TBI, as many mild injuries remain undiagnosed (Powell, Ferraro, Dikmen, Temkin, & Bell, 2008), many people who experience a TBI do not seek treatment despite experiencing problems related to their injury, and many injuries are treated outside of a traditional hospital system such as in private clinics and/or doctors' offices (Langlois et al., 2006). Mild TBIs, even among individuals seen in emergency departments, often remain undetected, especially if the deficits are subtle enough not to interfere with basic functioning. This is particularly the case when an individual has experienced other life-threatening body trauma, which shifts the focus of acute care interventions to these injuries. Injuries resulting in a TBI may also go unreported in the work place if there is motivation by either the worker or employer not to report an injury.

Sports-related TBIs are notoriously underreported and underdiagnosed. This may be the result of numerous factors including a lack of understanding and recognition of concussions, a lack of proper personnel available with the understanding and training to fully evaluate the impact of a potential concussion, pressure among players and staff to minimize the severity of sports injuries, and/or an existing false belief that there are no long-term consequences from a concussion. The CDC estimates that 1.6 to 3.8 million sports-related concussions occur in the United States each year, with many of these athletes never seeking medical treatment beyond that given by a sideline medical specialist (Langlois et al., 2006). A majority of these injuries do not result in a loss of consciousness, further hindering detection (Guskiewicz, Weaver, Padua, & Garrett, 2000). Yet, even for those without loss of consciousness, a concussion can result in significant cognitive decline (Collins et al., 1999). Football is estimated to account for the majority of these injuries, with a significant number occurring among high-school athletes (McCrea, Hammeke, Olsen, Leo, & Guskiewicz, 2004). It is important to note that sports-related concussions are not limited to men and football; high incidences of concussions occur in other sports and recreational activities, even those not usually associated with high-impact collisions, for both men and women. The existing fallacy that there were no long-term consequences from a concussion is now being challenged by multiple studies showing that individuals can have residual cognitive deficits on neuropsychological testing for a significant period of time after concussion even when the patient reports being symptom-free (Broglio, Macciocchi, & Ferrara, 2007; Fazio, Lovell, Pardini, & Collins, 2007). Furthermore, individuals who have experienced one concussion are at a greater risk of having a second concussion (Guskiewicz et al., 2003).

Substance abuse often plays an indirect role in the onset of a TBI. By far, the most widely used substance is alcohol, with more than 50% of patients who experience a TBI found to have elevated blood alcohol levels at the time of injury (Levy et al., 2004; Kolakowsky-Hayner et al., 1999).

Another large source of underreporting in current databases is due to the lack of integration of data on individuals in the military who sustain TBIs. Although there is some controversy as to the exact number of military personnel who sustain a TBI due to potential misdiagnosing of post-traumatic stress disorder (PTSD) as TBI (Hoge, Goldberg, & Castro, 2009), it is undeniable that

TBI is a significant source of disability among injured soldiers and has been described as the signature injury of the Afghanistan/Iraq wars. Better protective equipment and improved acute care interventions in the field have increased the probability of survival from blast injuries in combat. Therefore, it is not unreasonable to expect that the number of nonfatal TBIs among soldiers will only continue to increase (Okie, 2005).

In much the same way that a prior concussion increases the risk of a subsequent concussion, a prior TBI of any severity also places an individual at an increased risk of a repeat TBI. This risk rises further with each subsequent TBI (Annegers, Grabow, Kurland, & Laws, 1980). Most TBI surveillance systems do not include these repeat TBIs in their data. When these varied sources of undetected TBI are combined with the known prevalence of TBI, it is clear that the incidence of TBI is much higher than reported in any one source.

COST OF TBI

The burden on the United States due to TBI is significant. The care and medical costs of a person with a severe TBI can easily surpass $1 million over a lifetime. In a study on the public health implications of TBI, approximately 3.17 million Americans were determined to be living with long-term disability related to TBI (Zaloshnja, Miller, Langlois, & Selassie, 2008). The cost to caretakers, both financially and emotionally, can be significant. Family members of individuals who suffer a TBI often need to leave their jobs or reduce their responsibilities at work in order to take care of their injured relative. Given that there are probably a significant number of TBIs that go undetected and even a seemingly mild TBI can lead to permanent disabilities, which limit a person's functional independence and/or capacity to maintain employment, this is undoubtedly a low estimate of the actual proportion of the population that is affected socioeconomically (Langlois et al., 2006). Consequently, the $60 billion was calculated to be the financial toll from medical expenses and lost productivity due to TBI in this country in the year 2000 (Finkelstein, Corso, & Miller, 2006) is likely underestimated.

CAUSES OF TBI

According to the CDC 2002 to 2010 data, falls are the leading cause of TBI overall, accounting for 40% of TBI from 2006 to 2010. This is followed by struck by/against events (where either intentional or unintentional contact is made between one person and another person/object or where a person is caught between two people/objects) or motor vehicle accidents dependent on whether the population is in the emergency department or hospitalized. Other researchers feel that motor vehicle accidents may be the leading cause of TBI, especially if all forms of transportation, and not just automobiles, are considered (Silver, McAllister, & Yudofsky, 2005).

When the causes of injury are examined with respect to specific subsets of the general population, there are differences as compared with the population as a whole. In young children (<4 years) and the elderly (>65 years), falls are the clear leading cause of TBI. Among hospitalized patients aged 15 to 44 years, motor vehicle accidents are the most common cause of TBI according to CDC data from 2006 to 2010. Sports- and bicycle-related injuries are also a leading cause of TBI, especially mild TBI, in children, teenagers, and young adults. Firearm use has been reported as one of the leading causes of death related to TBI, with a large percentage of these events being suicidal in nature (Langlois, Rutland-Brown, & Thomas, 2004). However, the most recent CDC report to Congress in 2015 suggests that motor vehicle accidents are the leading cause of death from TBI followed by suicide. Unlike in the civilian population, blast exposures are a common cause of TBI in active military personnel during combat operations. However, servicemen and servicewomen are also injured by the most common mechanisms found in the general population. Alcohol use has been shown to be present in a large percentage of TBIs. One study in patients presenting with mild traumatic brain injury (mTBI; Scheenen et al., 2016) reported that approximately 30% of the patients were intoxicated on presentation. A study in patients presenting with moderate to severe brain injury (Joseph et al., 2015) reported that approximately 60% of the patients were under the influence of alcohol on admission. Understanding the causes of TBIs within specific subsets of the population is crucial for developing focused and effective prevention programs.

MECHANISMS OF TBI

Mechanisms of TBI are typically described by either the timing of the injury in relationship to the inciting TBI event (primary vs. secondary injuries) or the characteristics of the traumatic event itself (open vs. closed injuries, blunt vs. sharp trauma, and penetrating vs. nonpenetrating injuries). Each mechanism is described in the following.

Primary injuries occur at the moment of impact directly due to the actual trauma. These injuries include contusions or bruises of the brain itself, lacerations or tears in the lining of the brain, diffuse axonal injury (DAI), rupture of blood vessels leading to hemorrhages, and cranial nerve injuries.

Secondary injuries occur as a consequence of the primary injury and can develop anywhere from hours to days after the initial injury. The mechanisms of secondary injuries include compression of brain structures, hypoxia (lack of oxygen to the brain), cerebral edema or swelling, and metabolic cellular damage. Causes of these injuries include intracranial hypertension, hypotension, intracranial or intraventricular hemorrhage or fluid collection, vasospasm (spasm of cerebral blood vessels), infection, electrolyte and metabolic disturbances, hyperthermia (elevated body temperature), anemia, endocrine disturbances, and seizures.

Closed injuries are those injuries where the skull and lining of the brain are left intact. Open injuries are those injuries where the intracranial vault is exposed to the outside environment. These injuries expose the patient to a higher risk of infection.

Nonpenetrating injuries are caused by a trauma that does not break the skin or enter the body. Penetrating injuries are those that do enter the body. In those penetrating injuries caused by a projectile such as a bullet, the velocity of the projectile directly influences the extent of brain damage that occurs. The velocity of the projectile is important to consider because the size of the fluid wave, which is dependent on how fast the projectile was traveling as it entered the brain, usually causes more widespread damage to the brain than the actual path of the projectile itself.

Blunt force trauma refers to impact against a relatively flat object or surface. Blunt trauma does not necessarily imply a closed head injury because blunt forces can cause skull fractures and soft tissue injury as well. Sharp force trauma is caused by an object with an edge or point and usually implies a penetrating injury.

Blast injuries such as those experienced by many military personnel do not necessarily fit completely into any of these categories because blast injuries typically result from acceleration–deceleration type forces on the brain as well as a unique mechanism of injury by which blast waves enter the brain itself causing neuronal damage (Courtney & Courtney, 2009).

The mechanism of injury does not necessarily indicate the severity of the TBI or its clinical presentation. Counterintuitively, open skull, sharp force, and penetrating injuries may lead to less brain damage than closed skull, blunt force, or nonpenetrating traumas if the skull fracture is nondisplaced and/or the penetration is minor. Fracturing the skull may actually lead to a dissipation of forces, lessening the movement of the brain and its impact against the skull.

TBI PATHOPHYSIOLOGY

Trauma to the brain can result in significant pathology. Typically, individuals identified as having experienced a TBI are seen in an emergency department and, along with a clinical examination, undergo immediate neuroradiological assessment, usually with a non-contrast head CT scan. Those with identified brain pathology on CT scans are typically admitted to a trauma or neurological/neurosurgical unit for close observation and needed interventions. Common pathology associated with TBI is discussed in this section.

Brain contusions, or bruises of the brain, occur due to impact of the brain against the bony ridges of the skull and are detected on head CT and MRI as areas of localized hemorrhages and/or different attenuation as compared to the rest of the brain. Two types of injury leading to contusions are coup and contrecoup injuries: Coup injuries refer to damage caused by the initial impact of the brain against the skull; contrecoup injuries occur at the opposite side of the brain as a result of the brain rebounding against the skull. These contusions manifest in a wide variety of neurological and behavioral dysfunction depending on the area of the brain impacted. The most common area affected in TBI is the lower frontotemporal region of the brain due to the bony anatomy at the base of the skull.

DAI results in shearing forces on the brain from acceleration–deceleration and rotational forces that are often associated with high-velocity impact, such as those occurring in a motor vehicle accident and/or blast injury. These shearing forces disrupt nerve cells in the brain, especially where the more freely moving portion meets the more fixed portion of the brain. DAI is a common underlying reason for the abrupt onset of neurological deficits in a significant proportion of patients with TBI. Patients can present with variable severity of cognitive deficits, from those detectable only under stressful situations to altered levels of consciousness, depending on the severity of injury. CT and MRI of the brain may reveal microhemorrhages in select areas of the brain (i.e., the corpus callosum, central white matter, and midbrain), but many times there are no discernible findings on imaging. As a result, the diagnosis of TBI is often based on clinical examination and subjective complaints of new-onset neurological symptoms, especially in those with mild injuries.

Intracranial hemorrhages or hematomas are caused by bleeding underneath the skull from ruptured blood vessels. They are most commonly described by the layer of the brain within which the bleeding occurs. The brain is lined by three layers of tissue: the dura mater, pia mater, and arachnoid mater.

Epidural hematomas are collections of blood between the skull and the outermost layer of the brain called the dura mater. This type of hematoma grows rapidly in size and can lead to death within a matter of hours if untreated. The presence of a lucid interval, where the patient appears to recover from the initial trauma for a short period of time soon after the event, often confuses the clinical presentation. In these situations, the patient's level of arousal rapidly declines after this brief lucid time interval.

Subdural hematomas are collections of blood between the dura and arachnoid mater layers of the brain. These bleeds are usually slower growing, and if they grow slow enough, they can increase for weeks or even months before obvious clinical symptoms of dysfunction are noted.

Subarachnoid hematomas occur between the pia mater and the arachnoid membrane, the former being the closest lining surrounding the brain. They often develop as a result of blood vessel abnormalities (i.e., rupture of an arteriovenous malformation or saccular aneurysm) but also occur as a result of trauma. The classic presentation is that of the patient describing "the worst headache of my life" followed by a sudden loss of consciousness.

Intracerebral or intraventricular hematomas are collections of blood within the brain or ventricles of the brain itself. As with the other hemorrhagic injuries, the patient can develop subsequent neurological deficits and can present with symptoms of increasing headaches, visual changes, nausea, vomiting, dizziness, confusion, weakness, difficulties with balance, and, ultimately, loss of consciousness and death. Although intracranial hemorrhages can lead to ischemia due to decreased blood supply to parts of the brain, pressure on the brain as the hematoma grows is usually the more life-threatening and devastating cause of neurological decline. In cases of ischemia, where there is cell death, treatment is aimed at reducing the extent of surrounding swelling and inflammation in an attempt to preserve nerve function.

Skull fractures themselves do not usually cause neurological deficits, but the potential complications associated with certain fractures can be significant. Depressed skull fractures are associated with worse neurological deficits and outcomes as opposed to nondepressed fractures, and any open injury will increase the risk of infection as mentioned earlier. With temporal bone fractures, there is an increased risk of epidural hematomas due to the vascularity of the area as well as injury to the facial nerve. Basilar skull fractures can damage the facial, acoustic (i.e., hearing), and vestibular (i.e., balance) nerves.

Cranial nerve damage can occur following more severe TBIs. The type of injury, such as compressive versus direct insult to the nerve, will also affect the nature of the deficit, the most appropriate treatment, and the prognosis for recovery. The most common cranial nerve injury after a TBI is to the olfactory nerve (cranial nerve I), leading to anosmia (i.e., a loss of the sense of smell and possible alterations in taste; Marion, 1999). A lack of awareness of this deficit can potentially lead to significant safety risks such as if the patient fails to detect smoke or a gas leak in the home. Depending on the nerve injured, cranial nerve damage can result in other deficits such as monocular blindness, diplopia, visual field deficits, blurring, blind spots, paralysis of the eyes, ptosis of the eyelid, abnormal dilation of the pupil, numbness of the face, decreased salivation, corneal drying, paralysis of the face, hypersensitivity to sound, ringing in the ears, hearing loss, positional vertigo, autonomic system dysfunction, tongue dysfunction, swallowing and speech difficulties, and shoulder muscle dysfunction.

CLASSIFICATION OF TBI

Historically, some definitions of TBI state that the diagnosis must involve a known traumatic impact to the head that has resulted in the disruption of brain functioning. This narrow view does not account for disrupted brain functioning caused by energy forces without a direct traumatic impact to the head such as shock waves from explosions (Zasler, Katz, & Zafonte, 2013) or acceleration—deceleration forces in motor vehicle collisions. Often, especially in milder TBIs, there is lack of documented physical evidence of the injury on either physical examination or brain imaging. Trauma can cause focal or diffuse injury in the brain. More diffuse and/or microscopic damage after TBI is often not visible on standard neuroradiological assessment tools such as head CT or brain MRI. In such cases, more advanced neuroradiological imaging such as PET, single-photon emission computed tomography (SPECT), diffusion tensor imaging (DTI), and susceptibility weighted imaging (SWI) scans may be of greater help in identifying neuronal damage secondary to trauma. However, the clinical history, neurological exam, and neuropsychological testing remain important diagnostic assessment tools.

TBIs are categorized along a continuum of severity: severe, moderate, and mild injury. The vast majority of TBIs are classified as mild in nature. Guidelines for classification typically consider factors such as the presence or absence of consciousness, the duration of the posttraumatic amnesia (PTA) state, and the initial level of function after injury. In general, the more severe the TBI, the more likely the patient is to have a longer recovery course and permanent functional deficits. However, the prognosis for any given individual after a TBI depends on multiple factors including, but not limited to, age, occupation, education, medical and surgical history, severity of injury, location of injury, medical complications of injury, and recovery course to date.

ALTERED LEVELS OF CONSCIOUSNESS

Consciousness, defined as the state of being alert, aware, and responsive to one's environment, is a function of the ascending reticular activating system. In the early phase of recovery after a TBI, a more severely injured patient typically presents with an altered level of consciousness. Altered states of consciousness are usually divided into coma, vegetative, and minimally conscious state, with coma representing the least responsive state. Once beyond the minimally conscious state, patients usually evolve through some combination of confused, agitated, and amnestic states before behaviors become appropriate. The duration of altered consciousness after an injury is indicative of the level of TBI severity. Some patients never progress beyond the lower levels of consciousness and ultimately require long-term care. Each level of altered consciousness requires differing acute and long-term rehabilitation interventions. Significant research has been done and continues to investigate these altered levels of consciousness and possible interventions, including medications and devices, to facilitate recovery from lowered levels of consciousness.

Coma

Coma is a state of unconsciousness from which the patient cannot be aroused. The eyes remain continuously closed, there is no spontaneous purposeful movement or communication, there is no ability to localize noxious stimuli, and there is no evidence of a sleep–wake cycle on EEG. Coma can occur acutely after a traumatic or non-TBI.

Vegetative State

The Multi-Society Task Force on persistent vegetative state (Multi-Society Task Force on PVS, 1994) defines vegetative state as an unawareness of the environment and self in conjunction with a preservation of sleep–wake cycles, hypothalamic function, and brainstem autonomic functions. The transition to vegetative state is apparent when the patient exhibits spontaneous arousal through eye opening, but there is no evidence of purposeful behavior or verbal or gestural communication. The defining characteristic of a vegetative state is intermittent wakefulness with the presence of a sleep–wake cycle on EEG. The vegetative state can be a phase in recovery as the patient becomes more interactive and aware of the environment. However, there is a subset of patients who remain in the vegetative state for an extended period of time, often termed persistent vegetative state.

The prognosis for emergence from the vegetative state is different for TBIs and non-TBIs. Recovery of consciousness within 12 months was reported in 52% of patients in a vegetative state after TBI. In contrast, for patients in a vegetative state after nontraumatic injury, only 11% had recovered consciousness 3 months after injury (The Multi-Society Task Force on PVS, 1994). The different timelines suggest that the usual period of most rapid recovery is longer following a TBI than in a non-TBI. For patients in a vegetative state after TBI, good recovery of function at 1 year, as defined by the Glasgow Outcome Scale, is poor, reported at only 7%. The remaining patients had either died (33%), remained in a persistent vegetative state (15%), or were left with moderate (17%) to severe (28%) disability (The Multi-Society Task Force on PVS, 1994).

Minimally Conscious State

The detection of visual tracking is indicative of the transition out of the vegetative state into the minimally conscious state. The Aspen Workgroup (Giacino et al., 2002) described the minimally conscious state as a state in which there is evidence of minimal, but definite, awareness of self or the environment. The patient is able to demonstrate inconsistent yet reproducible behaviors, such as simple command following, intelligible verbalization, gestural responses, or object manipulation. The Aspen Workgroup proposed that the patient has progressed beyond the minimally conscious state when there is demonstration of consistent command following, functional object use, and functional interactive communication.

ASSESSMENT TOOLS TO CLASSIFY TBI

Several standardized assessment measures are commonly used to assess the severity of TBI and to track patients' progress and recovery. Several of these measures are described in the following.

The Glasgow Coma Scale (GCS) is traditionally used by early response, emergency, and trauma teams to rapidly determine the level of responsiveness of a patient (Table 4.1). Although multiple factors should be considered when trying to classify the severity of a TBI, many times the GCS is used alone to make a simplified determination of severity. The GCS quickly assesses the depth of impaired consciousness across three categories: eye opening, verbal response, and motor response. Each category is scored and totaled to obtain a composite score between 3 and 15, with higher scores suggesting a greater level of responsiveness. Scores of 3 to 8 are considered an indicator of a severe TBI, 9 to 12 of a moderate TBI, and 13 to 15 of a mild TBI. Of the three items in the GCS, the motor response is the best acute predictor of long-term outcome. The best GCS score within the first 24 hours of recovery has been described as the best predictor of recovery (Jennett, 1979).

The Galveston Orientation and Amnesia Test (GOAT) is a standardized tool used to evaluate the duration of PTA. PTA is a state of acute

TABLE 4.1

GLASGOW COMA SCALE

Score	Best Motor Response	Best Verbal Response	Eye Opening
1	None	None	None
2	Decerebrate posturing (extension) to pain	Mutters unintelligible sounds	Opens eyes to pain
3	Decorticate posturing (flexion) to pain	Utters inappropriate words	Opens eyes to loud voice (verbal commands)
4	Withdraws limb from painful stimuli	Able to converse—confused	Opens eyes spontaneously
5	Localizes pain/ pushes away noxious stimuli	Able to converse—alert and oriented	
6	Obeys verbal commands		

Source: Adapted from Teasdate and Jennett (1974).

confusion marked by difficulty with perception, thinking, and concentration that occurs during the early stages of recovery after TBI. Patients often cannot form new memories (anterograde amnesia) or recall memories that were made just prior to the injury (retrograde amnesia). The duration of PTA is a common predictor of long-term outcome, with longer duration of PTA being an indication of a poorer prognosis. The GOAT includes evaluation of a person's orientation, ability to recall the events prior to and after the injury, and ability to describe the circumstances of the hospitalization. Scores can range from 0 to 100, with a score of 75 or higher for 2 consecutive days indicating that the patient is no longer in a state of PTA (Levin, O'Donnell, & Grossman, 1979).

The JFK Coma Recovery Scale-Revised (CRS-R) is a measure used to determine when a patient enters into, and progresses beyond, the minimally conscious state. The scale consists of six subscales that investigate the auditory, visual, motor, oromotor, communicative, and arousal functions of a patient with an altered level of consciousness. Evidence of purposeful activity with testing at any time indicates that a patient has entered into the minimally conscious state (Giacino, Kezmarsky, DeLuca, & Cicerone, 1991).

The Rancho Los Amigos Levels of Cognitive Function is an instrument used to categorize behavioral and cognitive patterns typically seen during acute brain injury recovery (Kay & Lezzak, 1990). The original eight stages range from a patient exhibiting no response (Level I) to a patient who exhibits purposeful/appropriate behavior (Level VIII). The levels between categorize a patient's response to stimuli, confusion, and behavior. There has been expansion of the original scale to include 10 levels, which further describe the level of assistance (minimum assist, standby assist, modified independent) required by those patients with appropriate behavior.

EARLY-ONSET COMPLICATIONS OF TBI

Medical complications occur fairly often during the acute phase of recovery after a TBI and can be life-threatening if not addressed in a timely fashion. The most common early-onset medical complications include the following.

Increases in intracranial pressure (ICP) due to cerebral edema or bleeding can cause compression of brain structures, cerebral ischemia from reduced cerebral blood perfusion, or herniation of the brain through the skull. Physicians can detect elevated ICPs by finding papilledema (swelling at the rear of the eye) on exam, evidence of brain compression on head CT scans, or elevated pressures with a lumbar puncture or ICP monitoring device. Clinically, a reduction in the patient's level of consciousness may occur with an elevated ICP, ultimately resulting in death if untreated. When this occurs, establishing an airway for breathing, or mechanical ventilation, and restoring adequate blood flow to the brain are the first steps in medical management. Declines in neurological functioning on follow-up examinations or evidence of worsening findings on serial head CT imaging are suggestive of delayed neurological compromise. Various intracranial surgeries may be needed to decrease ICP. One such surgery is a decompressive hemicraniectomy, although a reduction in morbidity and mortality after this surgery has not been definitively established (Braddom, 2011).

Posttraumatic hydrocephalus (PTH) is caused by blockage of normal cerebrospinal fluid (CSF) flow, overproduction of CSF, or insufficient absorption of CSF back into the body. If PTH is left untreated, there is an increased risk of morbidity and mortality (Mazzini et al., 2003). The first symptoms of PTH can also be intermittent headache, vomiting, confusion, drowsiness, and/or a functional plateau or decline in rehabilitation progress. CT imaging of the brain is helpful in determining whether PTH is present and to what extent. A surgically inserted ventricular drain may be indicated in some cases for the treatment of hydrocephalus. In more severe cases, a ventricular shunt emptying somewhere else in the body (usually into the abdominal cavity) may be permanently placed.

Posttraumatic agitation, described as a subtype of delirium, is marked by restlessness, impulsivity, aggression, emotional lability, disinhibition, and confusion usually occurring during early recovery. The first line of treatment is nonpharmacological, with a focus on reducing environmental stimulation and providing calm and reassuring cues. The protection of the patient from harming self or others is paramount and can be facilitated using nonpharmacological means such as de-escalation techniques, close monitoring, safety devices, and nonthreatening barriers. Assessing for and addressing potential medical issues such as pain, urinary issues, constipation, and infection are important because they can trigger or exacerbate agitation. When conservative interventions fail and/or the safety of the patient or others is jeopardized, there is a role for pharmacological intervention. The most commonly used agents are mood stabilizers, atypical antipsychotic medications, beta-blockers, and anxiolytic (antianxiety) medications. Neurostimulants have also been utilized to decrease agitation based on the principle that improving cognitive function may help the patient behave more appropriately. However, these medications should be used judiciously as these same medications may increase agitation or promote delirium in some patients. Certain medications used for agitation management in other situations, such as benzodiazepines, anticholinergic medications, or certain antipsychotics, are avoided as much as possible in the TBI population due to their sedating and cognitively impairing effects.

ONGOING COMPLICATIONS OF TBI

TBIs can be complicated by a wide variety of chronic physical, cognitive, and emotional sequelae that are discussed in the following. They often require lifelong medical and rehabilitation management.

Hypertension following a TBI often resolves spontaneously with time. Earlier generation beta-blockers such as propranolol are commonly mentioned to treat hypertension in TBI patients because they provide additional cardiovascular benefits and can help decrease anxiety and restlessness.

Headaches occur commonly after a TBI, both in patients with and without evidence of intracranial bleeding. Typically, these headaches will improve with time if it is a result of the TBI and not related to any other pathology or condition. However, a small proportion of TBI patients continue to have chronic headaches, especially under situations of stress or intense cognitive activity. Treatment includes addressing any other causes for the headache besides TBI, minimizing stress, avoiding other triggers if possible, and using analgesic medications.

Sleep disturbances are often seen in patients after a TBI. Early on, patients usually present with decreased sleep, poor-quality sleep, and/or altered sleep–wake cycles. These problems usually improve during the course of recovery. Measures taken to facilitate these improvements include fostering better sleep hygiene, decreasing stimuli during desired sleep hours, addressing any pain or medical issues that may be a source of irritation, and using medications that promote sleep. Although all sleep-promoting medications have a sedating effect by their very nature, those with longer lasting effects and those known to cause more cognitive inhibition such as benzodiazepines and anticholinergics are typically avoided. Long-term sleep disturbances may still exist and often shift to excessive sleepiness. In these cases, addressing any psychiatric disturbance such as depression is important. Furthermore, neurostimulant medications, psychological counseling, better sleep hygiene, and attempts to engage patients regularly in social interactions, activities, and hobbies may be beneficial.

Dysautonomia, also called autonomic dysfunction syndrome, can occur after a TBI as a result of damage to sections of the brain involved in regulating the autonomic system. Clinical symptoms may include fever, hypertension, rapid heartbeat, increased respiratory rate, agitation, sweating, pupillary dilatation, and extensor posturing. Treatment involves addressing both the symptoms as well as any underlying medical triggers for the dysautonomic episode. As a result, multiple classes of medications are used to treat dysautonomia.

Posttraumatic seizures can develop after a TBI. Seizures occurring in the first 24 hours after a TBI are classified as immediate, those in the first week are called early seizures, and those after that time period are late seizures (Temkin, Dikmen, & Winn, 1991). The American Academy of Physical Medicine and Rehabilitation and the American Association of Neurological Surgeons recommend that all TBI patients with postresuscitation GCS scores of less than 12 receive a course of antiseizure medication for 1 week. Most studies were originally performed with phenytoin (Teasell, Bayona, Lippert, Villamere, & Hellings, 2007), but clinically, levetiracetam is now the more common choice of antiepileptic medication. If the patient has an immediate or early-onset seizure, there is no substantial evidence that ongoing antiepileptic medication is necessary. However, a seizure in the late period may necessitate ongoing antiepileptic medications. Attention must be paid to the use of antiepileptic medications as certain medications such as phenytoin may impair cognitive recovery (Timble, 1987).

Deep venous thrombosis (DVT) is a common complication after a TBI and is associated with immobility, fractures, and soft tissue damage during the early stages of TBI recovery. Although DVTs can be painful and cause swelling, the more serious concern associated with having a DVT is that it increases the risk of developing a pulmonary embolus, a blood clot that travels to the lung vasculature that can be fatal. The most commonly used diagnostic tool for DVT detection is a Doppler ultrasound. Due to the serious health risk posed by pulmonary emboli, DVT prevention is important. Preventive measures include early ambulation or the use of anticoagulation medications and sequential compression devices in nonambulatory patients.

Malnutrition can occur after a TBI as patients may be less responsive, confused and agitated, or have impaired swallow function. In addition, energy demands after a TBI are thought to be higher than those of a noninjured individual. Appetite stimulant medications may be used in cases where the patient has an intact swallow ability but inadequate nutritional intake. If the patient is at risk for aspiration due to swallowing dysfunction, a softer consistency or thickened diet may be necessary. If the patient has swallow dysfunction that is severe enough or decreased overall function to the point where he or she is unable to engage in oral intake, a nasogastric tube or gastrostomy tube can be placed to provide access for nutritional support.

Bowel-related issues such as delayed gastric emptying, constipation, nausea, and gastroesophageal reflux are commonly encountered problems in the TBI patient with impaired mobility and more severe deficits. Stool softeners, laxatives, and motility agents are often used to try to keep the patient's bowel movements regular. Antiemetic agents and proton pump inhibitors are used to decrease symptoms of nausea and reflux. Attempts are usually made to avoid anticholinergic and antihistamine medications as they can impair cognition.

Urological dysfunction after a TBI can result in both overactivity and retention of urine. Bladder overactivity can lead to incontinent episodes as the bladder contracts uncontrollably. These patients benefit from a timed voiding program and the use of medications to increase the bladder capacity or decrease bladder contractility. Urinary retention can also develop after a TBI due to bladder hyporeflexia, where the bladder fails to contract normally, or bladder sphincter dyssynergia, where the bladder contracts against a closed urethral sphincter. This latter condition is more often associated with injury to the spinal cord and often requires intermittent catheterizations to empty the bladder and the use of medications to relax the sphincter muscle and facilitate voiding. Urodynamic studies may be beneficial in determining the mechanism of dysfunction.

Spasticity, or an involuntary velocity-dependent increase in muscle resistance to passive range of motion, can develop after a brain injury. Evaluating and managing spasticity is important to avoid such complications as pain, skin breakdown, functional compromise, and joint contractures. Physical approaches to treating spasticity include removing noxious stimuli, repositioning and stretching the affected extremity, and using pressure or vibration modalities. In more severe cases, splinting or serially casting the affected extremity in a stretched position may be necessary. If these physical approaches are ineffective, there are a range of pharmacologic and more invasive approaches that can be considered including oral antispasticity medications (often with limited efficacy), nerve blocks, neuromuscular blocks, intrathecal baclofen pumps, and surgical interventions.

Pressure ulcers in the TBI population most commonly occur in those patients with altered levels of consciousness due to their decreased spontaneous repositioning. Pressure ulcers develop as a result of prolonged pressure or friction over bony surfaces of the body, such as the sacrum, heels, and hips, leading to tissue ischemia. Moisture on the skin can decrease skin integrity making incontinent patients more at risk for pressure ulcer formation. Keys to prevention are diligent skin care and minimization of prolonged pressure on one area of the body. Repositioning every 2 hours is a common practice adopted in the nursing care for these patients because pressure ulcer formation has been seen in research studies after 1 to 4 hours of sustained pressure (Gefen, 2008). When a significant skin breakdown does occur, local infection and osteomyelitis (bone infection) must be considered. These infections can lead to extensive tissue damage and even become life-threatening if not treated promptly. Treatment involves addressing any infectious issues, either locally or systemically as needed. For clean wounds, local wound care and proper nutrition to prevent infection and promote healing are important.

Endocrine dysfunction can occur as a result of damage to select structures within the brain. Overt and subtle hormonal abnormalities can increase fatigue or exacerbate behavioral and cognitive impairments. Treatment entails management of symptoms and sequelae and/or hormone replacement, if necessary. Abnormalities may resolve spontaneously with time as well. Sodium derangement is a common acute endocrine complication after TBI. Hypernatremia can result from vasopressin deficiency, termed diabetes insipidus. Hyponatremia can result from the syndrome of inappropriate antidiuretic hormone (SIADH) or less commonly cerebral salt wasting, which is usually present in a volume-depleted patient.

Heterotopic ossification (HO) is the formation of bone in soft tissue or muscle. The risk factors for the formation of HO include prolonged coma and/or immobility, spasticity, edema, limb trauma, and pressure ulcers. The joints commonly involved are the hips, elbows, shoulders, and knees. HO can cause a low-grade fever as well as pain, decreased range of motion, swelling, redness, and warmth at the involved joint. Range of motion exercises, medications, and radiation treatment have been used to prevent the formation and slow the growth of HO. Surgical resection of calcified soft tissue or muscle is usually reserved for more severe cases of HO, and it is often best to wait until new bone formation has stopped before undergoing resection (Braddom, 2011).

Balance and coordination deficits may develop after a TBI due to injury to the vestibular system or the cerebellum. Injury to cranial nerve VIII, also known as the vestibulocochlear nerve, can result in hearing loss as well as vertigo. Treatment involves physical therapy for balance, vestibular therapy, medications to decrease dizziness and nausea, and patient education. Symptoms of dizziness and lightheadedness can also be seen in patients who are beginning to mobilize after a prolonged period of decreased mobility. This is often due to orthostatic hypotension, which is a significant decrease in blood pressure upon sitting or standing from a prone or supine position. Pressure support devices such as abdominal binders and stockings, avoidance of rapid changes in position, and physical therapy to try to acclimate the patient to changes in positioning are used to minimize the pressure change. In severe cases of orthostasis resistant to nonpharmacological treatment, medications can be used to sustain a normal blood pressure.

Cognitive and behavioral dysfunction after a TBI can range from severe debilitating impairments to milder subtle deficits only noticeable under situations of increased stress or fatigue. Cognitive issues can include decreased attention, reduced processing speed, memory and learning difficulties, and executive functioning difficulties in planning/organization and flexible problem solving. Behavioral problems can include disinhibition, personality alterations, outbursts of profanity, poor hygiene practices, hypersexuality (increased libido), and hyposexuality. Decreased awareness of deficits and behavioral disturbances often hinder progress in therapy. Inpatient and outpatient management of these challenges require interventions by rehabilitation professionals experienced and knowledgeable regarding TBI. Both cognitive and behavioral issues can be confusing, distressing, and/or difficult for a patient's family to manage. Family education and support by the treating team in both the inpatient and outpatient settings can serve to minimize family distress. These issues including interventions and treatment are addressed in later sections of this chapter.

Emotional lability, depression, and PTSD are common after TBI and can hinder progress and recovery from the injury. Treatment includes counseling, supportive therapy, and medication management. In patients with significant cognitive impairments, effective counseling may not be feasible. In these cases, a greater focus on medication management is indicated. Some patients develop inappropriate laughter or crying after their TBI (pathological laughter and crying). Treatment usually consists of selective serotonin reuptake inhibitor medications but other antidepressant and mood-stabilizing medications have been used as well.

Medications to facilitate cognitive recovery or manage behavioral issues are commonly used in the management of TBI throughout the course of recovery. Although there are few, if any, conclusive studies supporting the use of these medications in TBI management, there is significant evidence indicating that many of these medications can be beneficial (Chew & Zafonte, 2009; Warden et al., 2006). As such, a discussion between the treating team and the patient and/or family should occur when considering these medications. Furthermore, there may be some ethical concerns to consider when patients are unable to make decisions regarding medication use for themselves, especially with the use of medications that can alter mood or sexual behavior. Patients with TBI often display increased sensitivity to medications. They may experience typical side effects at lower doses, develop toxic encephalopathy, or reveal a worsening of their TBI-related neurological deficits after initiation of pharmacotherapy (Zasler et al., 2013). For this reason, nonpharmacological management options should always be considered before initiating medications as many issues may be more effectively and safely addressed without the initiation of medications at all. When medications are indicated, doses should be titrated up slowly to monitor for side effects. Medications with side effects that may impede cognitive recovery or exacerbate behavioral problems, such as sedatives or anticholinergics, should be avoided. Although there are medications that are usually better tolerated for most issues associated with TBI, at times it is necessary to use medications that may have significant detrimental effects on cognition or behavior when there are more pressing medical issues. In these cases, the risks and benefits of the medication must be considered and vigilance must be maintained to discontinue the medication as soon as it is appropriate to do so.

TBI REHABILITATION: A TEAM APPROACH

TBI-focused rehabilitation services are delivered by a team of specially trained professionals with specific knowledge of interventions for TBI-related issues. An interdisciplinary team approach facilitates communication among team members and allows for rapid sharing of goals for treatment that are tailored to each patient's unique rehabilitation needs. This communication among all team members is vital for an effective rehabilitation program. The rehabilitation team consists of different health care professionals under the leadership of a physician in addition to the patient and the patient's family and friends. The roles of the specific team members in both inpatient and outpatient settings are outlined in the following. However, there is significant overlap among team members in regard to interventions and treatment goals.

The TBI rehabilitation physician specializes in rehabilitation medicine for individuals with cognitive and physical deficits due to a brain injury. The physician is responsible for the overall coordination of care and continuous, often lifelong, medical and medication management of the patient.

Neuropsychologists address alterations in brain functioning that impact the patient's thinking processes, behavior, and emotions after a brain injury. The neuropsychologist will deliver psychological as well as neurocognitive interventions in both inpatient and outpatient settings to maximize the patient's awareness, adjustment to injury, and overall cognitive functioning.

Rehabilitation nurses and nurse's aides address a patient's needs in relation to safety, self-care, medication administration, proper nutrition, dressing, bowel and bladder functions, and mobility.

Physical therapists evaluate and intervene to enhance a patient's independence with mobility tasks including ambulation and transfers. This often involves treating weakness and range of motion restriction issues. They also often address cognitive barriers to safe mobility.

Occupational therapists evaluate and intervene to decrease difficulties identified in the performance of basic activities of daily living (ADLs) such as feeding, dressing, bathing, and personal grooming. Occupational therapists may also address sensory, perceptual, and cognitive deficits that can interfere with the completion of higher level ADLs such as preparing meals, managing household chores, managing childcare responsibilities, and handling finances.

Speech–language pathology therapists evaluate the communication and cognitive abilities of a patient after a TBI. Most speech–language pathology therapists will also evaluate a patient's swallow function and provide treatment to improve swallow safety as needed.

Recreational/art therapists identify areas of leisure and social interest for patients and design social and leisure programs to increase their independence, while providing a healthy outlet for expression. Often, with input from other team members, therapeutic activities are selected to increase awareness of cognitive and behavioral challenges, which can impact social functioning.

Vocational counselors assist a patient with transition back into the workforce or school once the patient is deemed safe and ready for return to these activities by the rehabilitation team. If necessary, the vocational counselor may assist the patient to find alternative employment options if acquired physical or cognitive deficits prohibit return to a prior profession or occupation.

Social workers/case managers work as part of both inpatient and outpatient teams. On the inpatient unit, they offer supportive counseling to patients and families, address financial and insurance issues related to the inpatient stay, and assist with plans regarding posthospital care. In the outpatient setting, they serve as liaisons between the rehabilitation program, insurance carriers, disability offices, and other community resources.

Patients and their families are key members of the rehabilitation team as well. (For the purposes required here, family refers to any person who is involved in the support or care of the patient, whether related to the patient or not.) Family members provide direct care and emotional support as well as insight into the patient's unique social history and behaviors. Although it is not always possible to engage the patient actively, especially early in the recovery course after a TBI, when the patient and family are invested in the rehabilitation program, the effectiveness of a treatment program improves greatly.

INPATIENT TBI REHABILITATION

Once an individual with moderate to severe TBI-related functional, cognitive, and behavioral problems has achieved medical stability in an acute care hospital setting, the patient is typically transferred to an inpatient TBI rehabilitation program. These TBI rehabilitation units can be embedded within a larger medical center or within a freestanding rehabilitation facility. Usually, acute inpatient TBI rehabilitation is the most appropriate setting for initial rehabilitation management following moderate to severe injury. To be eligible for acute inpatient rehabilitation, patients must be able to engage in and benefit from 3 total hours of therapy daily; this must consist of both physical and occupational therapy but may include speech therapy as well. In addition, to be eligible for rehabilitation at all, most health insurers in the United States require the patient to have residual physical impairments that would benefit from continued physical rehabilitation. These conditions for coverage do not recognize that cognitive and behavioral dysfunction alone can result in functional limitations as significant as those caused by physical impairments. They also tend to ignore the benefits that acute inpatient TBI rehabilitation offer in addressing the medical complications of TBI early on. Furthermore, most families (assuming the patient has a social support system at all), home care agencies, and subacute rehabilitation facilities are not equipped to manage the significant agitation and behavioral problems that may be present early on after a TBI.

In TBI inpatient rehabilitation units, the patient's functional, cognitive, and neurobehavioral impairments are addressed by the team. Communication among the different team members, family, and patient is emphasized because this approach has been shown to yield the most effective treatment after a TBI (Kosmidis, 2007). The Rancho Los Amigos Levels of Cognitive Functioning Scale, described earlier in this chapter (see Table 4.2), is often used by the interdisciplinary inpatient rehabilitation team to facilitate rapid identification of the patient's level of postinjury cognitive and neurobehavioral functioning (Leon-Carrion, 2006) and implement treatment programming appropriate to that level of functioning.

TABLE 4.2

RANCHO LOS AMIGOS LEVELS OF COGNITIVE FUNCTION SCALE

Level	Behaviors Exhibited
I	No response
II	Generalized response to stimulation
III	Localized response to stimulation
IV	Confused and agitated behavior
V	Confused with inappropriate behavior (nonagitated)
VI	Confused but appropriate behavior
VII	Automatic and appropriate behavior
VIII	Purposeful and appropriate behavior

Source: Adapted from Hagen, Malkmus, and Durham (1979).

Through the course of their stay, the team establishes a plan that the patients and families can eventually carry out on their own to manage the patient's medical, cognitive, and emotional issues after discharge from the unit. At the point of admission to inpatient rehabilitation, each member of the rehabilitation team completes an initial assessment of each patient's medical issues and physical and cognitive functioning to develop a plan of treatment. Collectively, the team determines each patient's functional level, motivation, and ability to engage in treatment. They then implement the treatment plan with the goal of maximizing the patient's medical stability, participation in therapy, safety awareness, and functional independence. As patients progress through their rehabilitation stay, team members discuss their progress within their programs on a regular basis and try to address any problematic issues that develop. Goals are adjusted as needed. Findings from these evaluations are shared with family members and patients if appropriate. Although each patient presents with a unique combination of challenges, some generalizations can be made, and these approaches are described in the following.

Altered Levels of Consciousness

For patients admitted to acute inpatient rehabilitation in a vegetative or minimally conscious state (Rancho Los Amigos levels II–III), enhancing arousal and responsiveness become the primary goals of rehabilitation interventions. In combination with medications prescribed by the physician, the team will initiate a stimulation program to enhance the patient's level of arousal. The JFK CRS-R is frequently used on inpatient TBI units to help guide programmatic interventions for patients at these levels (Giacino et al., 2002). Using the CRS-R, the team plans interventions utilizing all sensory modalities. In addition, the rehabilitation team will emphasize prevention of contractures and skin breakdown. Families are instructed on how best to communicate with their loved one and how to avoid overstimulating the patient. The amount and variety of stimulation provided increases as the patient improves.

Agitation and Behavioral Management

For patients with a Rancho Los Amigos IV–V level, the primary target of rehabilitation interventions is the treatment of inappropriate behaviors. During this phase of recovery, individuals typically present with psychomotor restlessness, agitation, and aggressive behaviors such as kicking and hitting. The overarching goal in treatment is to maintain patient safety while at the same time facilitate the ability to self-regulate behavior. Scales such as the Agitated Behavior Scale may be used to assess the degree of behavioral dysregulation and track the efficacy of rehabilitation treatment efforts (Bogner, 2000; Corrigan, 1989). The use of behavior modification strategies and environmental modifications, such as limiting the number of visitors a patient receives, have proven beneficial in reducing agitation in TBI patients (Herbel, Schermerhorn, & Howard, 1990). Often in this phase, pharmacological agents need to be prescribed by the physician in order to manage confusion, psychomotor restlessness, and/or aggression.

Cognitive Impairments

Patients may present with impaired orientation and significant cognitive impairments, which can limit their safety awareness and ability to complete ADLs. In TBI recovery, the GOAT is frequently used to determine when a patient is demonstrating consistent orientation to place and time. Cognitive impairments may include reduced orientation to place and time, attention, information processing speed, memory, language skills, visuospatial skills, and abstract reasoning. These problems can be further exacerbated by emerging symptoms of depression and anxiety in the patient. Family members may feel relief that their loved one has survived a brain injury, but increased confusion or sadness may result when the cognitive and behavioral impairments become more apparent. This makes ongoing supportive services for families important. Education of the family and patient now progresses to detailed discussions of cognitive and behavioral changes after a TBI. Based typically on a brief neuropsychological assessment, treatment planning by the team is directed at maximizing cognitive strengths while trying to compensate for cognitive weaknesses using compensatory strategies. A memory book involving a calendar and a to-do list is typically implemented to address memory, orientation, and planning deficits. The physician may prescribe medications to try to facilitate cognitive recovery and address depression and anxiety issues as well.

Community Reentry and Transitions of Care

Patients with higher Rancho Los Amigos levels (VI–VII) may be able to follow a structured schedule and perform routine self-care tasks with minimal assistance or supervision. These patients continue to benefit from inpatient rehabilitation to increase their awareness of how residual moderate to mild cognitive impairments will impact functioning in the community. Their time in therapy allows for practicing of compensatory techniques needed for community living. The interdisciplinary goals also focus on having patients become involved in the completion of more complex cognitive and linguistic tasks, while maximizing their physical mobility and independence in ADLs. At this phase of TBI recovery, the risk of depression and anxiety increases due to increasing self-awareness of deficits (Hibbard, Uysal, Kepler, Bogdany, & Silver, 1998; Malec, Testa, Rush, Brown, & Moessner, 2007). The physician considers medications to treat these issues to facilitate cognitive recovery. The neuropsychologist closely monitors the patient's and family's ongoing emotional adjustment.

Once a patient remains medically stable and has progressed to a level of functional independence (i.e., able to perform most ADLs independently, can live relatively independently and safely in the community, and has an adequate support network to return to the community), the patient is ready for discharge back to the community. Careful patient and family education about discharge plans and needed follow-up appointments is important as the patient may still have problems with organizational skills. If patients are not completely independent or safe on their own, the team may still plan for a discharge to home if appropriate family supervision and follow-up outpatient services can be arranged. In these cases, family education is crucial as patients may have poor awareness of their deficits and limited compliance with instructions regarding maintaining safe function. If the patient does not reach independence in a timely manner and is unsuitable for return home with family support but remains medically stable, placement in a subacute rehabilitation facility is an option with most TBI patients best suited for TBI-specific subacute rehabilitation facilities. Regardless of the discharge plan, families are provided with recommendations on how to best care for the patient going forward, with emphasis placed on the importance of a structured daily routine, safety maintenance, and appropriate environmental accommodations.

MILD TBI AND OUTPATIENT REHABILITATION

Although moderate to severe TBI patients with significant residual functional, cognitive, and behavioral deficits may return home with substantial family support and continue their rehabilitation as outpatients, patients with mild TBI or those with significant recovery of cognitive functioning after their TBI represent by far the greater proportion of the patients seen for TBI rehabilitation in the outpatient setting. Approximately 5% to 15% of individuals with documented mild TBIs remain symptomatic for their entire lives (Alexander, 1995; Cassidy et al., 2004; Iverson, 2005), with many of these individuals eventually seen by outpatient TBI services. Mild TBI has been called the "invisible injury" because the majority of individuals present without noticeable physical deficits or obvious cognitive and behavioral issues at first glance. However, upon closer examination, they often have difficulty across cognitive, behavioral, and emotional domains of functioning. Ongoing physical deficits, especially balance impairments, may also be seen. Indeed, individuals with mild TBI typically present with a growing concern about how their newly acquired cognitive and behavioral changes after TBI are impacting their former roles and their current safety in the community. Often these individuals are able to function independently in the community with minimal support from family or friends, but are unable to resume the former threads of their life as related to work and relationships. Sometimes, cognitive and physical symptoms only emerge after the person with a mild TBI has attempted to return to these former life activities and roles. In many cases, it takes rejection or failure with these former relationships and roles for the patient to seek treatment.

However, even after experiencing rejection or failure, the individual may fail to connect these new difficulties with a prior mild TBI. The variable nature of mild TBI symptoms and the time after the injury when these symptoms become problematic may result in the person never seeking treatment or seeking inappropriate treatment. Those who are able to function marginally in society may be labeled as lazy or malingering. For these reasons, the CDC has prepared an online toolkit to educate the professional community about mild TBI, improve the diagnosis of mild TBI symptoms, minimize the risk of misdiagnosis, and help physicians educate patients about mild TBI and its potential long-term sequelae.

Most patients with TBI seeking outpatient rehabilitation services present with a wide array of physical (i.e., increased fatigue, decreased motor dexterity and speed, loss of the sense of smell, dizziness, visual disturbances), cognitive (i.e., reduced attention capacity, disturbances in memory and executive functioning), and emotional problems (i.e., depression, anxiety, impulsivity, restlessness, aggression, emotional lability, decreased initiation, altered libido). A focused outpatient program is typically implemented to improve the patient's overall function and quality of life while attempting to maintain maximal involvement in work/school and family roles each step of the way. However, often a delay in return to work or school is needed so that the patient is cognitively and emotionally ready to resume these roles. The goal is for patients to incorporate compensation strategies into their lives at the same time as they are trying to improve their cognitive skills. After completing their initial treatment course, it is not unusual for an individual to return briefly for further counseling in response to a significant life change such as the birth of a child, loss of a job, new responsibilities at work, or relationship changes.

During the outpatient treatment course, sessions are scheduled with the patient and family members together at times to address interpersonal issues. These may include issues related to adjusting to new family roles, changes in relationships, including sexual interactions between the patient and significant other, and concerns over the family's involvement in the patient's life (whether it is too much or too little). At other times, group sessions may be planned with other patients to address issues with social interactions and group dynamics. As in inpatient settings, the initial treatment plan evolves out of discipline-specific assessments and team decisions regarding the appropriate approach and interventions for each patient.

Neuropsychologists initiate an in-depth neuropsychological evaluation to identify the cognitive and behavioral strengths and weaknesses of each patient. The neuropsychological evaluation includes a review of medical records, comprehensive clinical interviews with the patient and significant others, and administration of a wide array of neuropsychological tests to assess attention and concentration (simple, complex, divided, and sustained), short- and long-term memory (for both visual and verbal material), language and verbal fluency abilities, information processing, and executive functioning (planning, sequencing, organization, and abstraction). Mood, personality characteristics, and behavioral issues are evaluated as well. Test performance is interpreted within the context of each patient's prior level of functioning, which is influenced by education, occupation, and age at the time of injury. In select cases, such as for those patients showing a history of pre-TBI superior intellectual abilities, exhibiting more subtle deficits, or attempting to return to academic pursuits or a high-level job, an additional focused assessment is indicated. The results of the neuropsychological evaluation are shared with the patient, appropriate family, and treatment team. Recommendations for psychology interventions based on these findings typically include cognitive remediation, individual psychotherapy, family therapy, and/or group therapy.

Cognitive remediation is aimed at identifying cognitive issues and trying to address them through retraining exercises and compensation strategies. Overall goals of cognitive remediation include increasing awareness of strengths and weaknesses, improving attention and concentration, learning to use compensatory strategies to minimize the functional impact of deficits, improving basic problem-solving skills, and enhancing social pragmatics (i.e., giving and receiving feedback, improving social skills). Cognitive therapy can be rendered simultaneously by several disciplines including neuropsychologists, occupational therapists, speech therapists, and/or vocational rehabilitation counselors with each discipline emphasizing a different aspect of retraining to increase a patient's functional, behavioral, and emotional well-being. Through communication and teamwork, cognitive remediation by the rehabilitation team can be much more effective than by one discipline alone. Without focused cognitive interventions, the patient with a mild to moderate TBI may repeatedly reexperience failures in everyday functioning. Repeated failures in valued aspects of daily functioning, such as at work and in relationships, can lead to a downward spiral in both cognitive and emotional functioning and often results in increased depression, anxiety, or emotional dyscontrol. Medications to facilitate cognitive recovery such as neurostimulants, antianxiety, antidepressant, or mood-stabilizing medications may have a role in outpatient management as an adjunct to these nonpharmacological therapies. These medications are overseen by the treating physician.

Social workers, case managers, vocational counselors, and rehabilitation counselors all can be very helpful in facilitating patients' transition back into life roles at home, work, school, and even with leisure activities. In the most effective programs, these members of the treatment team work closely with the therapists to optimize the appropriate services, supportive counseling, and education for their patients and families.

Psychotherapy is a vital component of treatment for those with mild to moderate TBI. The neuropsychologist traditionally addresses these issues with both the patient and the family.

Many patients struggle with disparities between "how they functioned before the injury" and "how they are functioning postinjury." This discrepancy is a major focus of therapeutic treatment, and patients are helped with dealing with loss, adjusting to permanent alterations in self, and managing depression and anxiety. Individuals with mild TBI may be unaware of subtle changes in their cognitive functioning and/or behavior. Education, direct feedback, and feedback from others are often utilized to help increase their awareness. Behavioral changes are commonly experienced after a mild TBI. Patients are taught behavioral management techniques to minimize dyscontrol episodes.

Physical therapy is a common referral for the management of balance impairment, vestibular symptoms, and neck pain after mild TBI. Balance impairment, which is common after mild TBI, can remain for an extended period of time and puts patients at greater risk for falls and further brain injuries. Outpatient physical therapy can be beneficial to improve these persistent balance deficits. Vestibular symptoms, including vertigo and dizziness, are frequently reported after mild TBI and can be quite distressing to the patient. They can be addressed with a specialized physical therapy program termed vestibular therapy. Physical therapy also plays a role in the treatment of concomitant myofascial neck pain that is especially common with whiplash-type injuries.

Individuals who have survived a catastrophic accident as the cause of their TBI, such as returning military servicemen and servicewomen, may present with additional challenges after their TBI such as PTSD. Erbes, Westermeyer, Engdahl, and Johnsen (2007) found that 12% of returning soldiers from the Afghanistan and Iraq conflicts met the criteria for PTSD, whereas Hibbard et al. (1998) reported that PTSD can be observed in approximately 17% of nonmilitary individuals after a TBI. Common symptoms of PTSD, such as increased irritability, trouble sleeping, and not resuming "normal" activities, are very similar to symptoms typical of mild TBI and can significantly impede recovery after a TBI if unrecognized and unaddressed. Counseling and therapy are essential to help patients identify and cope with symptoms of PTSD.

Medical management of TBI in the outpatient setting, regardless of its severity, may be lifelong. At any point after injury, appropriate medical monitoring and interventions may be necessary to address ongoing complications of TBI (discussed in an earlier section of this chapter). In addition to nonpharmacological management, medications are often necessary both in outpatient rehabilitation and after rehabilitation services have ended.

Other therapy disciplines may be involved during outpatient rehabilitation upon referral by the physician. Referrals are based on the presenting physical and functional complaints of the patient. Physical therapists may become involved with the patient who presents with issues of decreased mobility, weakness, and poor balance after a TBI. Many specialized physical therapy programs will also provide vestibular therapy to address complaints of post-TBI dizziness. Vision or eye movement dysfunction can occur after a mild TBI as well. In these situations, the physician may refer the patient to a neuro-ophthalmologist and/or a neuro-optometrist who specializes in the treatment of TBI-related vision disorders.

CONCLUSION

TBIs can be devastating and have widespread and far-reaching effects. A TBI can affect multiple facets of a person's life, including his/her behavior, emotions, cognitive function, personality, physical appearance, and physical function. This can lead to functional failures and medical complications in the acute and long-term phases of TBI recovery and may result in long-standing and permanent disability. Treatment often necessitates addressing multiple problems over many years even after a mild TBI. The impact of a TBI often extends even further, changing family dynamics, altering social interactions, and placing a financial burden on the family and society. For these reasons, it is important to address the needs of those with a TBI and the family members who support them from the initial point of injury onward. This approach requires increased awareness regarding TBI within the medical community, society as a whole, the patient's family, and, often most challengingly, the TBI patient.

Treatment following a TBI often consists of a combination of medical management of issues that arise through the life span after TBI, as well as specialized TBI rehabilitation interventions designed to optimize functional recovery. The goal of most treatment programs is to maintain medical stability while providing therapy and treatment to maximize functional ability and independence at each stage of recovery. Although it is unclear to what extent the brain actually heals versus to what extent it creates new pathways to try to restore function, there is no doubt that early and intensive clinical interventions are important for recovery and safety.

As with most other medical conditions, the best treatment for TBI is to prevent its occurrence. Prevention of TBI is especially important given that many of these injuries are avoidable. Increasing the use of helmets and better safety equipment in sports, developing better substance and alcohol abuse prevention programs, observing proper safety practices in motor vehicles such as avoiding reckless driving and wearing seat belts, removing tripping hazards and installing safety equipment in the homes of the elderly, implementing ideas to decrease TBI risk in children, such as including softer playground surfaces and providing education programs for both parents and children, and even simply paying closer attention to traffic laws when crossing the street are all simple yet effective ways to decrease the incidence of TBIs.

REFERENCES

Alexander, M. P. (1995). Mild traumatic brain injury: Pathophysiology, natural history, and clinical management. *Neurology, 45*, 1253–1260.

Annegers, J. F., Grabow, J. D., Kurland, L. T., & Laws, E. R. (1980). The incidence, causes, and secular trends of head trauma in olmsted county, Minnesota 1935–1974. *Neurology, 30*, 912–919.

Bogner, J. (2000). *The agitated behavior scale. The center for outcome measurement in brain injury*. Retrieved from http://www.tbims.org/combi/abs

Braddom, R. L. (2011). *Physical medicine and rehabilitation* (4th ed.). Philadelphia, PA: Elsevier Saunders.

Broglio, S. P., Macciocchi, S. N., & Ferrara, M. S. (2007). Neurocognitive performance of concussed athletes when symptom free. *Journal of Athletic Training, 42*, 504–508.

Cassidy, J. D., Carroll, L. J., Peloso, P. M., Borg, J., von Holst, H., & Holm, L., . . . Task Force on Mild Traumatic Brain Injury. (2004). Incidence, risk factors and prevention of mild traumatic brain injury: Results of the WHO collaborating centre task force on mild traumatic brain injury. *Journal of Rehabilitation Medicine, 43*, 28–60.

Chew, E., & Zafonte, R. D. (2009). Pharmacologic management of neurobehavioral disorders following traumatic brain injury—A state-of-the-art review. *Journal of Rehabilitation Research & Development, 46*, 851–878.

Collins, M. W., Grindel, S. H., Lovell, M. R., Dede, D. E., Moser, D. J., Phalin, B. R., . . . McKeag, D. B. (1999). Relationship between concussion and neuropsychological performance in college football players. *Journal of the American Medical Association, 282*, 964–970.

Corrigan, J. D. (1989). Development of a scale for assessment of agitation following traumatic brain injury. *Journal of Clinical and Experimental Neurospychology, 11*, 261–277.

Courtney, A. C., & Courtney, M. W. (2009). A thoracic mechanism of mild traumatic brain injury due to blast pressure waves. *Mount Sinai Journal of Medicine: A Journal of Translational and Personalized Medicine, 76*, 111–118.

De Silva, M. J., Roberts, I., Perel, P., Edwards, P., Kenward, M. G., Fernandes, J., . . . CRASH Trial Collaborators. (2009). Patient outcome after traumatic brain injury in high-middle- and low-income countries: Analysis of data on 8927 patients in 46 countries. *International Journal of Epidemiology, 38*, 452–458.

Erbes, C., Westermeyer, J., Engdahl, B., & Johnsen, E. (2007). Post-traumatic stress disorder and service utilization in a sample of service members from Iraq and Afghanistan. *Military Medicine, 172*, 359–363.

Fazio, V. C., Lovell, M. R., Pardini, J. E., & Collins, M. W. (2007). The relation between post concussion symptoms and neurocognitive performance in concussed athletes. *Neuro Rehabilitation, 22*, 207–216.

Finkelstein, E. A., Corso, P. S., & Miller, T. R. (2006). *The incidence and economic burden of injuries in the United States*. New York, NY: Oxford University Press.

Giacino, J. T., Ashwal, S., Childs, N., Cranford, R., Jennett, B., Katz, D. I., . . . Zasler, N. D. (2002). The minimally conscious state. Definition and diagnostic criteria. *Neurology, 58*, 349–353.

Giacino, J. T., Kezmarsky, M. A., DeLuca, J., & Cicerone, K. D. (1991). Monitoring rate of recovery to predict outcome in minimally responsive patients. *Archives of Physical Medicine and Rehabilitation, 72*, 897–901.

Guskiewicz, K. M., McCrea, M., Marshall, S. W., Cantu, R. C., Randolph, C., Barr, W., . . . Kelly, J. P. (2003). Cumulative effects associated with recurrent concussion in collegiate football players: The NCAA concussion study. *Journal of the American Medical Association, 290*, 2549–2555.

Guskiewicz, K. M., Weaver, N. L., Padua, D. A., & Garrett, W. E. (2000). Epidemiology of concussion in collegiate and high school football players. *American Journal of Sports Medicine, 28*, 643–650.

Herbel, K., Schermerhorn, L., & Howard, J. (1990). Management of agitated head-injured patients: A survey of current techniques. *Rehabilitation Nursing, 15*, 66–69.

Hibbard, M. R., Uysal, S., Kepler, K., Bogdany, J., & Silver, J. (1998). Axis I psychopathology in individuals with traumatic brain injury. *Journal of Head Trauma Rehabilitation, 13*, 24–39.

Hoge, C. W., Goldberg, H. M., & Castro, C. A. (2009). Care of war veterans with mild traumatic brain injury—Flawed perspectives. *New England Journal of Medicine, 360*, 1588–1591.

Joseph, B., Khalil, M., Pandit, V., Kulvatunyou, N., Zangbar, B., O'Keeffe, T., . . . Rhee, P. (2015). Adverse effects of admission blood alcohol on long-term cognitive function in patients with traumatic brain injury. *Journal of Trauma Acute Care Surgery, 78*(2), 403–408.

Kay, T., & Lezak, M. (1990). *Nature of head injury. traumatic brain injury and vocational rehabilitation*. Menomonie, WI: University of Wisconsin-Stout Research and Training Center.

Kolakowsky-Hayner, S. A., Gourley, E. V., Kreutzer, J. S., Marwitz, J. H., Cifu., D. X., & Mckinley, W. O. (1999). Pre-injury substance abuse among persons with brain injury and persons with spinal cord injury. *Brain Injury, 13*, 571–581.

Kosmidis, M. H. (2007). Review of interdisciplinary approach to the treatment of traumatic brain injury. *Journal of the International Neuropsychological Society, 13*, 557–558.

Langlois, J. A., Rutland-Brown, W., & Thomas, K. E. (2004). *Traumatic brain injury in the United States: Emergency department visits, hospitalizations, and deaths*. Atlanta, GA: Centers for Disease Control and Prevention, National Center for Injury Prevention and Control.

Langlois, J. A., Rutland-Brown, W., & Wald, M. M. (2006). The epidemiology and impact of traumatic brain injury: A brief overview. *The Journal of Head Trauma Rehabilitation, 21*, 375–378.

Leon-Carrion, J. (2006). Methods and tools for the assessment of outcome after brain injury rehabilitation. In J. Leon-Carrion, K. V. Wild, & G. Zitney (Eds.), *Brain injury treatment: Theories and practices*. Philadelphia, PA: Taylor & Francis.

Levin, H. S., O'Donnell, V. M., & Grossman, R. G. (1979). The galveston orientation and amnesia test. A practical scale to assess cognition after head injury. *The Journal of Nervous and Mental Disease, 167*, 675–684.

Levy, D. T., Mallonee, S., Miller, T. R., Smith, G. S., Spicer, R. S., Romano, E. O., . . . Fisher, D. A. (2004). Alcohol involvement in burn, submersion, spinal cord, and brain injuries. *Medical Science Monitor, 10*, 17–24.

Malec, J. F., Testa, J. A., Rush, B. K., Brown, A. W., & Moessner, A. M. (2007). Self-assessment of impairment, impaired self-awareness, and depression after traumatic brain injury. *Journal of Head Trauma Rehabilitation, 22*, 156–166.

Marion, D. W. (1999). *Traumatic brain injury*. New York, NY: Thieme Publishing Group.

Mazzini, L., Campini, R., Angelino, E., Rognone, F., Pastore, I., & Oliveri, G. (2003). Posttraumatic hydrocephalus: A clinical, neuroradiologic, and neuropsychologic assessment of long-term outcome. *Archives of Physical Medicine and Rehabilitation, 84*, 1637–1641.

McCrea, M., Hammeke, T., Olsen, G., Leo, P., & Guskiewicz, K. (2004). Unreported concussion in high school football players: Implications for prevention. *Clinical Journal of Sport Medicine, 14*, 13–17.

Multi-Society Task Force on PVS. (1994). Medical aspects of the persistent vegetative state. *New England Journal of Medicine, 330*(21, 22), 1499–1508, 1572–1579.

Scheenen, M. E., Myrthe, E. K., Harm, J. H., Gerwin, R., Yilmaz, T., & Jouke, N., (2016). Acute alcohol intoxication in patients with mild traumatic brain injury: Characteristics, recovery, and outcome. *Journal of Neurotrauma, 33*, 339–345.

Schofield, P. W., Butler, T. G., Hollis, S. J., Smith, N. E., Lee, S. J., & Kelso, W. M. (2006). Traumatic brain injury among australian prisoners: Rates, recurrence and sequelae. *Brain Injury, 20*, 499–506.

Silver, J. M., McAllister, T. W., & Yudofsky, S. C. (2005). *Textbook of traumatic brain injury*. Arlington, VA: American Psychiatric Publishing.

Teasell, R., Bayona, N., Lippert, C., Villamere, J., & Hellings, C. (2007). Post-traumatic seizure disorder following acquired brain injury. *Brain Injury, 21*(2), 201–214.

Temkin, N. R., Dikmen, S. S., & Winn, H. R. (1991). Management of head injury. Posttraumatic seizures. *Neurosurgery Clinics of North America, 2*, 425–435.

Timble, M. R. (1987). Anticonvulsant drug and cognitive function: A review of literature. *Epilepsia, 28*, S37–S45.

Warden, D. L., Gordon, B., McAllister, T. W., Silver, J. M., Barth, J. T., Bruns, J., . . . George, Z. (2006). Guidelines for the pharmacologic treatment of neurobehavioral sequelae of traumatic brain injury. *Journal of Neurotrauma, 23*, 1468–1501.

Zaloshnja, E., Miller, T., Langlois, J. A., & Selassie, A. W. (2008). Prevalence of long-term disability from traumatic brain injury in the civilian population of the United States, 2005. *Journal of Head Trauma Rehabilitation, 23*, 394–400.

Zasler, N. D., Katz, D. I., Zafonte, R. D. (2013). *Brain Injury Medicine* (2nd ed.). New York, NY: Demos Medical Publishing.

ADDITIONAL READINGS

Asikainen, I., Kaste, M., & Sarna, S. (1999). Early and late posttraumatic seizures in traumatic brain injury rehabilitation patients: Brain injury factors causing late seizures and influence of seizures on long-term outcome. *Epilepsia, 40*, 584–589.

Baguley, I. J. (2008). Autonomic complications following central nervous system injury. *Seminars in Neurology, 28*, 716–725.

Baguley, I. J., Heriseanu, R. E., Cameron, I. D., Nott, M. T., & Slewa-Younan, S. (2008). A critical review of the pathophysiology of dysautonomia following traumatic brain injury. *Neurocritical Care, 8*, 293–300.

Baguley, I. J., Heriseanu, R. E., Gurka, J. A., Nordenbo, A., & Cameron, I. D. (2007). Gabapentin in the management of dysautonomia following severe traumatic brain injury: A case series. *Journal of Neurology, Neurosurgery, and Psychiatry, 78*, 539–541.

Baguley, I. J., Nott, M. T., Slewa-Younan, S., Heriseanu, R. E., & Perkes, I. E. (2009). Diagnosing dysautonomia after acute traumatic brain injury: Evidence for overresponsiveness to afferent stimuli. *Archives of Physical Medicine and Rehabilitation, 90*, 580–586.

Barnfield, T. V., & Leathem, J. M. (1998). Incidence and outcomes of traumatic brain injury and substance abuse in a New Zealand prison population. *Brain Injury, 12*, 455–466.

Brown, C. V., Weng, J., Oh, D., Salim, A., Kasotakis, G., Demetriades, D., . . . Rhee, P. (2004). Does routine serial computed tomography of the head influence management of traumatic brain injury? A prospective evaluation. *Journal of Trauma, 57*, 939–943.

Centers for Disease Control and Prevention. (1999). *Facts about concussion and brain injury*. Atlanta, GA: Centers for Disease Control and Prevention.

Centers for Disease Control and Prevention. (2003). *Report to Congress on mild traumatic brain injury in the United States: Steps to prevent a serious public health problem*. Atlanta, GA: National Center for Injury Prevention and Control, Centers for Disease Control and Prevention.

Christensen, A., & Caetano, C. (1999). Cognitive neurorehabilitation. In D. T. Stuss, G. Winocur, & I. H. Robertson (Eds.), *Neuropsychological rehabilitation in the interdisciplinary team: The postacute stage*. New York, NY: Cambridge University Press.

Englander, J., Bushnik, T., Duong, T. T., Cifu, D. X., Zafonte, R., Wright, J., . . . Bergman, W. (2003). Analyzing risk factors for late posttraumatic seizures: A prospective, multicenter investigation. *Archives of Physical Medicine and Rehabilitation, 84*, 365–367.

Fiser, S. M., Johnson, S. B., & Fortune, J. B. (1998). Resource utilization in traumatic brain injury: The role of magnetic resonance imaging. *The American Surgeon, 64*, 1088–1093.

Frey, L. C. (2003). Epidemiology of posttraumatic epilepsy: A critical review. *Epilepsia, 44*, 11–17.

Fugate, L. P., Spacek, B. A., Kresty, L. A., Levy, C., Johnson, J., & Mysiw, W. (1997). Measurement and treatment of agitation following traumatic brain injury-II. A survey of the brain injury special interest group of the American Academy of Physical Medicine and Rehabilitation. *Archives of Physical Medicine and Rehabilitation, 78*, 924–928.

Gefen, A. (2008). How much time does it take to get a pressure ulcer? Integrated evidence from human, animal, and in vitro studies. *Ostomy Wound Management, 54*, 26–28, 30–35.

Graham, D. P., & Cardon, A. L. (2008). An update on substance use and treatment following traumatic brain injury. *Annals of New York Academy of Sciences, 1141*, 148–162.

Hagen, C., Malkmus, D., & Durham, P. (1979). Levels of cognitive functions. In *Rehabilitation of the head-injured adult: Comprehensive physical management*. Downey, CA: Professional Staff Association, Rancho Los Amigos Hospital.

Hoge, C. W., McGurk, D., Thomas, J. L., Cox, A. L., Engel, C. C., & Castro, C. A. (2008). Mild traumatic brain injury in U.S. soldiers returning from Iraq. *New England Journal of Medicine, 358*, 453–463.

Iverson, G. L. (2005). Outcome from mild traumatic brain injury. *Current Opinions in Psychiatry, 18*, 301–317.

Ivins, B. J., Schwab, K. A., Warden, D., Harvey, L. T., Hoilien, M. A., Powell, C. O., . . . Salazar, A. M. (2003). Traumatic brain injury in the U.S. army paratroopers: Prevalence and character. *Journal of Trauma Injury, Infection and Critical Care, 55*, 617–621.

Jagoda, A. S., Bazarian, J. J., Bruns, J. J., Cantrill, S. V., Gean, A. D., Howard, P. K., . . . Whitson, R. R. (2009). Clinical policy: Neuroimaging and decision making in adult mild traumatic brain injury in the acute setting. *Journal of Emergency Nursing, 35*, e5–e40.

Jennett, B. (1979). Defining brain damage after head injury. *Journal of Royal College of Physicians of London, 4*, 197–200.

Kaups, K. L., Davis, J. W., & Parks, S. N. (2004). Routinely repeated computed tomography after blunt head trauma: Does it benefit patients? *Journal of Trauma, 56*, 475–480.

Manolakaki, D., Velmahos, G. C., Spaniolas, K., de Moya, M., & Alam, H. B. (2009). Early magnetic resonance imaging is unnecessary in patients with traumatic brain injury. *Journal of Trauma, 66*, 1008–1012.

Meythaler, J. M., Peduzzi, J. D., Eleftheriou, E., & Novack, T. A. (2001). Current concepts: Diffuse axonal injury-associated traumatic brain injury. *Archives of Physical Medicine and Rehabilitation, 82*, 1461–1471.

Murray, C. J. L., & Lopez, A. D. (1996). *Global health statistics: A compendium of incidence, prevalence, and mortality estimates for over 200 conditions.* Cambridge, MA: Harvard University Press on behalf of the World Health Organization and the World Bank.

Nampiaparampil, D. E. (2008). Prevalence of chronic pain after traumatic brain injury: A systematic review. *Journal of the American Medical Association, 300*, 711–719.

National Institute of Neurological Disorders and Stroke. (2002). *Traumatic brain injury: Hope through research* (No. 02). Bethesda, MD: National Institutes of Health.

Okie, S. (2005). Traumatic brain injury in the war zone. *New England Journal of Medicine, 352*, 2043–2047.

Owens, B. D., Kragh, J. F., Jr., Wenke, J. C., Macatis, J., Wade, C. E., & Holcomb, J. B. (2008). Combat wounds in operation Iraqi freedom and operation enduring freedom. *Journal of Trauma, 64*, 295–299.

Powell, J. M., Ferraro, J. V., Dikmen, S. S., Temkin, N. R., & Bell, K. R. (2008). Accuracy of mild traumatic brain injury diagnosis. *Archives of Physical Medicine and Rehabilitation, 89*, 1550–1555.

Roberts, I., Yates, D., Sandercock, P., Farrell, B., Wasserberg, J., Lomas, G., . . . CRASH trial collaborators. (2004). Effect of intravenous corticosteroids on death within 14 days in 10008 adults with clinically significant head injury (MRC CRASH trial): Randomised placebo-controlled trial. *Lancet, 364*, 1321–1328.

Rossitch, E. Jr., & Bullard, D. E. (1988). The autonomic dysfunction syndrome: Aetiology and treatment. *British Journal of Neurosurgery, 2*, 471–478.

Slaughter, B., Fann, J. R., & Ehde, D. (2003). Traumatic brain injury in a county jail population: Prevalence, neuropsychological functioning and psychiatric disorders. *Brain Injury, 17*, 731–741.

Sosin, D. M., Sniezek, J. E., & Thurman, D. J. (1996). Incidence of mild and moderate brain injury in the United States, 1991. *Brain Injury, 10*, 47–54.

Sosin, D. M., Sniezek, J. E., & Waxweiler, R. J. (1995). Trends in death associated with traumatic brain injury, 1979 through 1992. Success and failure. *Journal of the American Medical Association, 273*, 1778–1780.

Tagliaferri, F., Compagnone, C., Korsic, M., Servadei, F., & Kraus, J. (2006). A systematic review of brain injury epidemiology in Europe. *Acta Neurochirurgica, 148*, 255–268.

Teasdate, G., & Jennett, B. (1974). Assessment of coma and impaired consciousness. A practical scale. *The Lancet, 2*, 81–84.

Temkin, N. R. (2009). Preventing and treating posttraumatic seizures: The human experience. *Epilepsia, 50*, 10–13.

Temkin, N. R., Haglund, M. M., & Winn, H. R. (1995). Causes, prevention, and treatment of post-traumatic epilepsy. *New Horizons, 3*, 518–522.

Thurman, D. J., Alverson, C., Dunn, K. A., Guerrero, J., & Sniezek, J. E. (1999). Traumatic brain injury in the United States: A public health perspective. *Journal of Head Trauma Rehabilitation, 14*, 602–615.

Wang, M. C., Linnau, K. F., Tirschwell, D. L., & Hollingworth, W. (2006). Utility of repeat head computed tomography after blunt head trauma: A systematic review. *Journal of Trauma, 61*, 226–233.

Williams, G., Morris, M. E., Schache, A., & McCrory, P. R. (2009). Incidence of gait abnormalities after traumatic brain injury. *Archives of Physical Medicine and Rehabilitation, 90*, 587–593.

CHAPTER

Rehabilitation in Burns

Patricia A. Tufaro and Abraham P. Houng

INTRODUCTION

The skin is only a few millimeters thick, yet by far, it is the largest organ of the body. The total surface area of the average person's skin spans approximately 20 square feet and makes up 16% of the total body weight. It is the first line of defense against the environment and infection and helps the body to regulate temperature and fluid balance. There are many types of tissue embedded within its layers. It provides sensory function and interface with the environment. Because of these physiological functions, an injury to the skin such as a burn can be devastating to the body.

ANATOMY AND PHYSIOLOGY

The epidermis is the most superficial outer layer of the skin, covering almost the entire body surface. Structurally, the epidermis is only about a tenth of a millimeter thick but is made of 40 to 50 rows of stacked squamous epithelial cells. It is derived from the ectoderm during embryonic development. The epidermis's main function is that it interfaces with the environment. It is an avascular region of the body, composed of mostly sloughing nonviable skin cells. It is constantly being replaced by the underlying viable cell layers. The cells of the epidermis receive all of their nutrients via diffusion of fluids from the dermis.

Almost 90% of the epidermis is made of cells known as keratinocytes. Keratinocytes develop from stem cells at the base of the epidermis and begin to produce and store the protein keratin. Keratin makes the keratinocytes very tough, scaly, and water resistant (Herndon, 2007). Melanocytes form the second most numerous cell type in the epidermis at approximately 8%. Melanocytes produce the pigment melanin, which protects the skin from ultraviolet radiation and sunburn. Langerhans cells are the third most common cells in the epidermis and make up just over 1% of all epidermal cells. The role of Langerhans cells is to detect and fight pathogens that attempt to enter the body through the skin. Finally, Merkel cells make up less than 1% of all epidermal cells but have the important function of sensing touch.

The dermis is the deep layer of the skin found under the epidermis. It is derived from the mesoderm. It is much thicker than the epidermis and gives the skin its strength and elasticity and is responsible for the skin's tactile qualities. The dermis is composed of collagen, glycosaminoglycans, elastin, and nervous tissue (Herndon, 2007). Fibroblasts, immunological cells, and endothelial cells also reside in the dermis. The dermis is where the hair follicles, sweat glands, and most of the blood vessels reside.

Within the dermis, there are two distinct regions: the papillary layer and the reticular layer. The papillary layer is the superficial layer of the dermis that borders on the epidermis. The papillary layer contains many fingerlike extensions called dermal papillae that protrude superficially toward the epidermis. Blood flowing through the dermal papillae provide nutrients and oxygen for the cells of the epidermis. The nerves of the dermal papillae are used to feel touch, pain, and temperature through the cells of the epidermis (Herndon, 2007).

The deeper layer of the dermis, the reticular layer, is the thicker and tougher part of the dermis. The reticular layer is made of dense irregular connective tissue that contains many tough collagen and stretch elastin fibers running in all directions to provide strength and elasticity to the skin (Herndon, 2007). It also contains blood vessels to support the skin cells and nerve tissue to sense pressure and pain in the skin.

Deep in the dermis is a layer of loose connective tissues known as the hypodermis, subcutis, or subcutaneous tissue. The hypodermis serves as the flexible connection between the skin and the underlying muscles and bones as well as a fat storage area. Areolar connective tissue in the hypodermis contains elastin and collagen fibers loosely arranged to allow the skin to stretch and move independently of its underlying structures. Fatty adipose tissue in the hypodermis helps to insulate the body by trapping body heat produced by the underlying muscles.

BURN INJURY

According to the American Burn Association, there were approximately 486,000 burn injuries in 2011 that required medical treatment from hospitals. Most of the injuries were minor. However, there were 3,240 fire- and smoke-related fatalities. There were 40,000 burn admissions, with 30,000 admissions to burn centers (www.ameriburn.org/resources_factsheet.php). There are about 140 burn centers in United States and Canada. These centers provide specialized burn care, from wound care to rehabilitation treatments (American Burn Association Website, n.d.-b).

BURN ASSESSMENT

Burn injury is defined by the depth and the extent of the injury. The depth is categorized as first, second, third, or fourth degree. It is also categorized as partial or full thickness injury. The extent of the injury is calculated by the percent of total body surface area (TBSA).

A first-degree or superficial burn is a localized injury that causes pain and edema. It is confined to the epithelial layer of skin. Superficial injuries usually have some localized inflammation and erythema. Topical application of a moisturizer to the exposed surface of the burned area will reduce the pain. Reepithelialization will begin within 48 hours. No restrictive scar will result.

A second-degree or partial thickness injury can be classified further into superficial partial thickness or deep partial thickness. Partial thickness injuries occur in both the epidermis and some dermis.

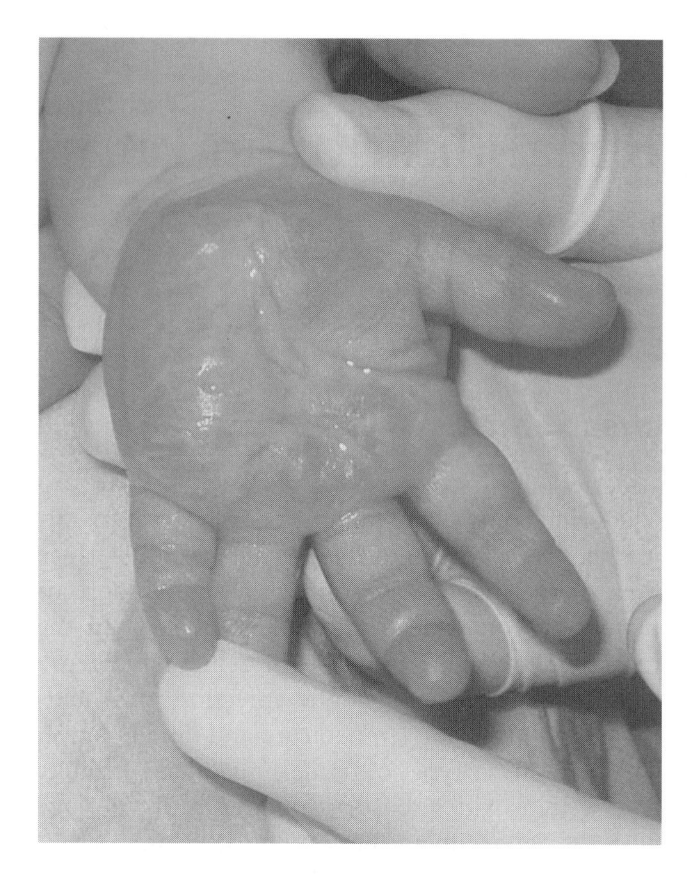

FIGURE 5.1 Superficial partial thickness injury to the palm.

Thin-walled, fluid-filled blisters can develop with a superficial partial thickness injury (Figure 5.1). The outer layer of the skin can also slough off, revealing a pink and moist wound base. A superficial partial thickness injury involves the upper level of the dermis and is expected to reepithelialize within 10 to 14 days with topical wound care.

A deep partial thickness injury usually has a more intense reddish wound base, revealing deep dermal components. It extends to the depth of the dermis, injuring a greater concentration of the adnexal hair follicles and sweat glands. This diminishes the ability for reepithelialization and results in delayed healing, taking between 14 and 21 days for completion. The appearance of this injury, in contrast to the superficial second-degree burn, shows the absence of blisters and sometimes a moderate thickness eschar. Immediate pain is less intense because the superficial nerve endings are injured by the burn at this depth. The quality of the resultant burn scar healing after these depth injuries can be poor, increasing the risk of later hypertrophy and secondary scar contracture.

A third-degree burn is also known as a full thickness injury. The entire layer of the dermis is injured. No viable dermis is left. It may reveal thrombosed vessels. The wound base may be white or have a leathery appearance. This dead tissue is called eschar (Figure 5.2). Patients typically do not experience pain in this area due to the absence of nerve endings. This injury will cause a fluid shift and protein leakage from the remaining tissue. Full thickness wounds generally trigger an immune response and require surgical intervention for final coverage.

A fourth-degree burn results from prolonged thermal contact and involves the soft tissue and underlying tendon, joint, and bones. The injured tissue at this depth is charred. Prolonged hot immersion, extended flame contact, and electrical burn injury may demonstrate this depth of tissue destruction. Extensive reconstructive procedures and, more often, amputation will result.

In order for the patient to receive proper resuscitation and care, an accurate assessment of the extent of injury is needed. The rule of 9s is a simple and quick way of estimating body surface area. It is often used by emergency medical services (EMS) and first responders. The head and the upper extremities are each 9%. The anterior torso, posterior torso, and the lower extremities are 18% each; and the genitalia makes up the remaining 1%.

Another way to estimate TBSA is by using the palm method. The patient's palm is roughly 1% TBSA. The surface area is estimated by calculating how many of the patient's palm would fit into the wound (American Burn Association, 2005).

At burn centers, a burn diagram is used to calculate the size of the burn injury. A Lund-Browder diagram is commonly utilized (Figure 5.3) to accurately assess the extent of the injury. The burn diagram subdivides the body into 30 sections, and the body proportion is adjusted for age. For instance, the head of a 0- to 1-year-old represents 19% of the TBSA and 7% in an adult. Accurate burn size is crucial because burn resuscitation is calculated based on percent body surface area burned.

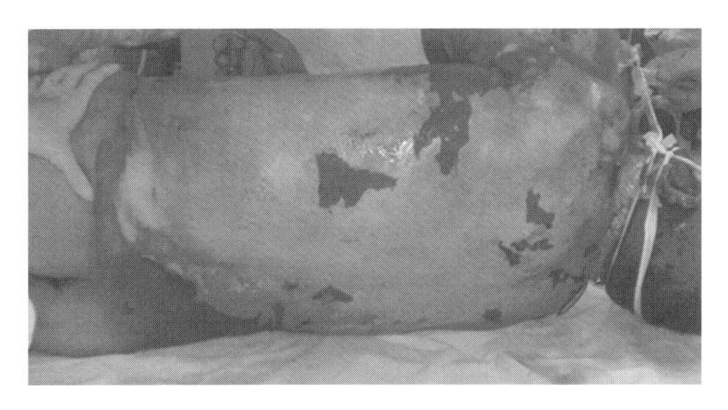

FIGURE 5.2 Full thickness burn injury to the back.

BURN MECHANISM

A scald is the most common burn injury. It is more common in the pediatric population. The mechanism is usually from a pull-down of hot liquid in the kitchen or due to bathing accidents. A scald burn from water typically results in a partial thickness injury. A scald from steam or oil leads to a much deeper burn injury (Figure 5.4).

Flame burns is the second most common burn injury. Flame burns usually present as a deep partial thickness or full thickness injury. If the patient is in an enclosed structural fire, some inhalation should be suspected. Smoke inhalation should be diagnosed with bronchoscopy.

Chemicals can cause significant injury, accounting for 30% of all burn deaths. Injury caused by liquid chemicals should be irrigated with water for at least 30 minutes. If the patient is still symptomatic after 30 minutes of irrigation, the wound should continue to be irrigated. A patient should never be placed in a tub, as it will spread the material to previously unexposed tissue. If the burn is caused by powdered chemicals, the powder should be brushed off first before irrigation, because water might activate the chemical and cause further injury. An acid or base should not be neutralized. Neutralizing an acid or base burn injury causes an exothermic reaction. Some of the chemical may be absorbed, so liver and kidney functions need to be monitored closely (Herndon, 2007).

Electrical injuries are uncommon but are the most devastating among the thermal injuries and primarily affect young, working males. Electricians, crane operators, construction workers, and power company linemen are at high risk for these injuries. They are the most frequent cause of amputations on the burn service. These injuries have many acute and chronic manifestations that are not seen in other thermal injuries.

Electrical injuries often resemble a crush injury. They involve not only the skin but deeper tissues as well. Electricity prefers lower resistance. So it

BURN DIAGRAM

Date of Burn: ______________ Admission Diagram ☐ Date: ______________

Discharge Diagram ☐ Date: ______________

Age: __________ Sex: __________ Weight: __________ Height: __________

Place of Occurance:

_____ At Home

_____ At Work

_____ Other

Type of Burn: ______________________

Inhalation Injury: Moderate ☐ Severe ☐

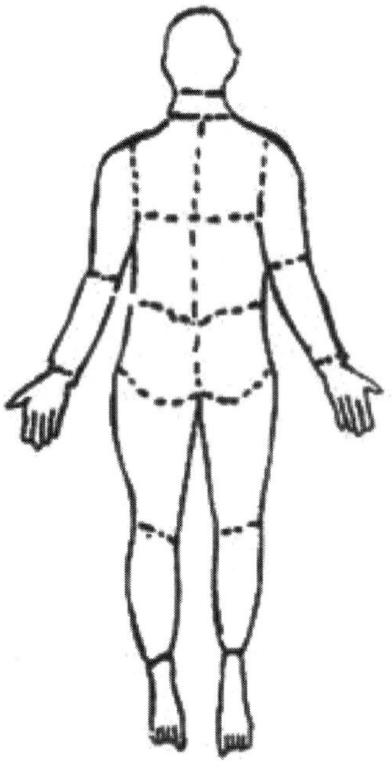

Extent of Burn: Surface Section	Age (years)				#2⁺	#3⁺
	1–4	5–9	10–15	16+		
1a. Head-front	8½	6½	5	3½		
1b. Head-back	8½	6½	5	3½		
2. Neck	2	2	2	2		
3a. Torso-R.U. ant.	3¼	3¼	3¼	3¼		
3b. Torso-L.U. ant.	3¼	3¼	3¼	3¼		
3c. Torso-R.L. ant.	3¼	3¼	3¼	3¼		
3d. Torso-L.L. ant.	3¼	3¼	3¼	3¼		
4a. Torso-R.U. post.	3¼	3¼	3¼	3¼		
4b. Torso-L.U. post.	3¼	3¼	3¼	3¼		
4c. Torso-R.L. post.	3¼	3¼	3¼	3¼		
4d. Torso-L.L. post.	3¼	3¼	3¼	3¼		
5a. Arm-R.U.	4	4	4	4		
5b. Arm-R.L.	3	3	3	3		
6a. Arm-L.U.	4	4	4	4		
6b. Arm-L.L.	3	3	3	3		
7. Hand-R.	2½	2½	2½	2½		
8. Hand-L.	2½	2½	2½	2½		
9. Buttocks-R.	2½	2½	2½	2½		
10. Buttocks-L.	2½	2½	2½	2½		
11. Genitalia	1	1	1	1		
12a. Thigh-R. ant.	3¼	4	4½	4¾		
12b. Thigh-R. post.	3¼	4	4½	4¾		
13a. Thigh-L. ant.	3¼	4	4½	4¾		
13b. Thigh-L. post.	3¼	4	4½	4¾		
14a. Leg-R. ant.	2½	2½	3	3½		
14b. Leg-R. post.	2½	2½	3	3½		
15a. Leg-L. ant.	2½	2½	3	3½		
15b. Leg-L. post.	2½	2½	3	3½		
16. Foot-R.	3½	3½	3½	3½		
17. Foot-L.	3½	3½	3½	3½		
				Total %		

% TBSA ☐

Depth code

2°=

3°=

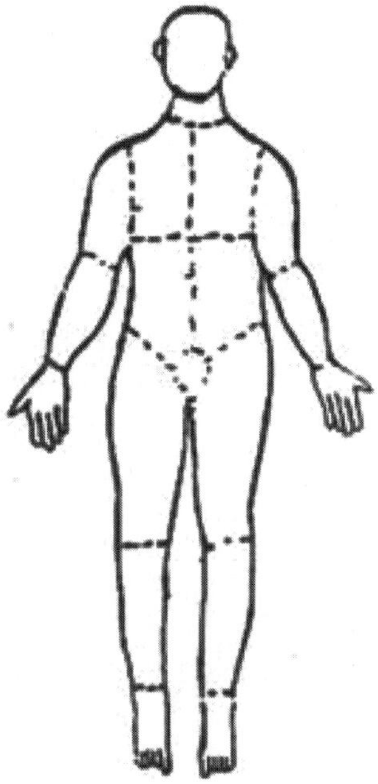

FIGURE 5.3 Lund-Browder chart for estimating total body surface area.

preferentially travels through nerve tissue. Bone has the highest resistance, so it heats up with electricity. Therefore, there can be deep thermal injury inside the muscle compartment (Figure 5.5). Rhabdomyolysis and compartment syndrome can occur (Brumback & Leech, 1995). As compartment pressures increase, an emergency escharotomy may be warranted.

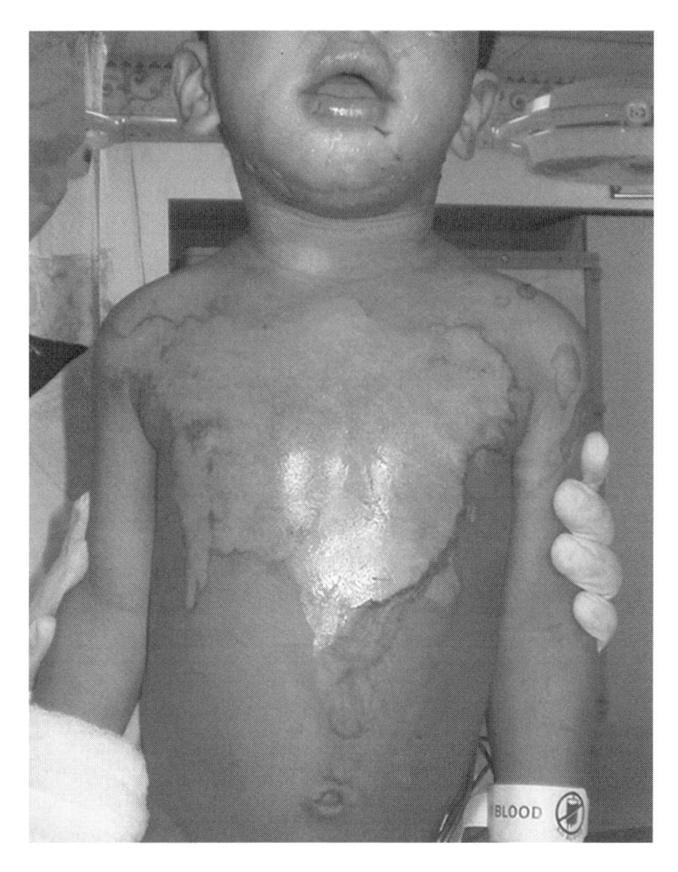

FIGURE 5.4 Typical pediatric pull-down partial thickness scald burn to the chest.

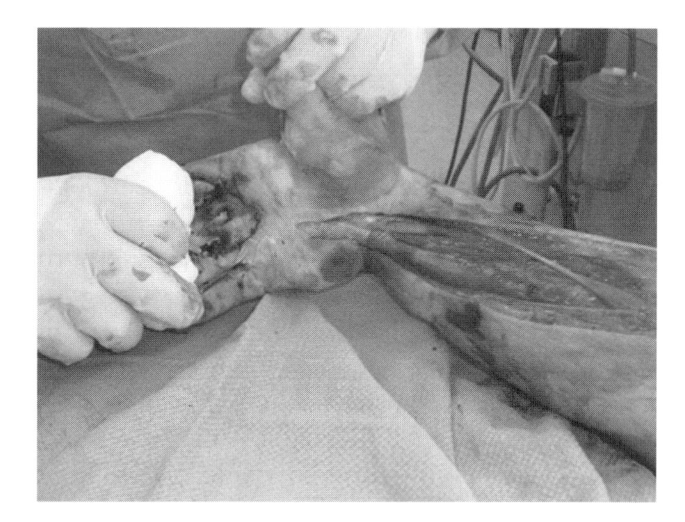

FIGURE 5.5 Electrical burn with deep muscle necrosis.

Other complications of an electrical injury include renal, septic, cardiac, neurological, and ocular. Renal failure and sepsis at times can be preventable and are treated during the acute stages of recovery. Cardiac damage is identified upon admission and treated. Neurological deficits may not present themselves until up to 2 years after injury. These may include peripheral neuropathies, generalized weakness, heterotopic ossification (HO), memory loss, and impaired attention and executive function. Cataract formation is the most frequent ocular complication. Long-term follow-up with a burn physician and/or physiatrist is imperative to ensure the most optimal outcome.

BURN CENTER TRANSFER CRITERIA

The American Burn Association defined the following as transfer criteria to specialized burn centers: any partial thickness burns that are greater than 10% TBSA; any burns that involve delicate areas: face, neck, hands, feet, or genitalia; any third-degree burns; any high-voltage electrical injuries; any chemical burns; and any inhalation injuries (American Burn Association Website, n.d.-a).

If there is a burn with concomitant trauma injury, the patient should transfer to a center, which will treat the injury that poses the greatest risk. For example, if trauma poses greater risk than the burns, the patient should be brought to a trauma center and be stabilized first before being transferred to a burn center.

BURN TREATMENT

Burn patients are trauma patients. When treating these patients initially, care should be concentrated on the patient's airway, breathing, and circulation (ABC). If the patient has significant facial burns or has smoke inhalation, he or she should have a secure airway. An oral tracheal intubation should be performed on these patients. The gold standard for diagnosing smoke inhalation is a bronchoscopy. Soot or inflammatory changes in the lower airway on bronchoscopy are diagnostic. Intravenous access should be obtained during the initial assessment. The most widely used resuscitation formula is the Parkland formula, which calculates the patient's fluid requirement in the first 24 hours. This fluid requirement is 4 mL for every percent burn for every kilogram of body weight (Baxter & Shire, 1968). Half of this fluid requirement is given in the first 8 hours. Lactated Ringer's solution is the most commonly used intravenous solution. Fluid resuscitation should be titrated to the standard end point of resuscitation, such as urine output, blood pressure, and blood lactate level.

A secondary survey is carried out after the ABC. The secondary survey consists of neurological exams and assessing the extent of burn injury. Patients with circumferential full thickness burn injuries are at a higher risk for compartment syndrome. If the patient has a circumferential burn, an escharotomy may be necessary. It is performed with an electrocautery. An escharotomy typically results in the immediate reduction of pressure; however, it is not a guarantee of tissue survival. The origin of the burn and length of exposure may be too extensive for soft tissue survival. Clinical observations of progressive distal swelling, intracompartment measurements, and pulse oximetry have been used to evaluate these conditions.

Pain is usually treated with narcotics. Intravenous morphine is given for pain relief. Anxiolytics are often used to potentiate the narcotic effect. It is common for these patients to receive large doses of narcotics for pain relief.

Once the patient is medically stabilized, attention is then turned to wound care. The wounds are first irrigated with water and cleansed with chlorhexidine soap; then loose or dead skin is derided. Nonviable skin promotes bacterial growth; therefore, it needs to be removed. Topical antibiotics are applied on the clean wound under sterile conditions. Common topical antibiotics are silver sulfadiazine and bacitracin ointment. Silver sulfadiazine is a broad-spectrum antibiotic, which does not penetrate eschar. Its side effect is a self-limiting, transient leukopenia. Bacitracin is an effective topical antibiotic against gram-positive organisms; however, it causes hypersensitivity when used for prolonged periods. Mafenide acetate is another topical antibiotic used on burns though less commonly. It penetrates eschar; however, it can be painful and causes metabolic acidosis when used on large surface areas.

Several commercially available silver-impregnated dressings are also used for wound care. Most of these dressings are designed to be used for multiple days and with wounds that will not require surgical intervention and are mostly used in the outpatient setting. Multiday dressings have played a huge role in decreasing a patient's length of stay and eliminating the need for admission altogether.

Critical care is an important part of burn care. Patients with large surface injuries will require intensive care and are often placed on mechanical ventilators. Continuous cardiac monitoring is obtained to make sure their tissue is adequately perfused. Renal insufficiency and renal failure is also common. Continuous hemodialysis is performed for patients who are unable to maintain their electrolyte or fluid balance. Infection is always a major concern in burn patients. Cultures are obtained if there are any signs of infection. Systemic antibiotics are only started when there is a high suspicion of infection or the culture is positive. Prophylactic antibiotics have no role in burn treatment.

SKIN GRAFTING

Full thickness burn injuries do not heal from underneath the wound base. They either contract in from the periphery or need excision and skin grafting for wound closure. If patients are surgical candidates, they are taken to the operating room once they are fully resuscitated.

There are two excision techniques, tangential excision and fascial excision. Tangential excision is performed by Goulian knife, hydrodissector, or ultrasonic debrider. The outer layer of nonviable skin is removed until a viable, homogeneously bleeding surface is obtained. Fascial excision is performed using a scalpel or an electrocautery. The skin and subcutaneous fat is removed, leaving the fascia intact. The goal of excision is to remove nonviable tissue and create a healthy wound bed with ample vasculature to receive skin grafts.

Once the wound has been adequately prepared, it is ready for grafting. Allograft, cadaver skin is used as a temporary wound covering if the wound bed is marginal. It is used to decrease the risk of infection and help decrease the metabolic demand on the body. However, because the skin is from another donor, the body will ultimately reject the skin. Xenograft, a product from porcine skin, is also used as a biological dressing to cover the wounds (Sood & Archauer, 2006).

An autograft is the definitive treatment for full thickness injuries. It is harvested from the patient's own body with a dermatome, a device with an oscillating blade that harvests skin (Figure 5.6). Typical donor locations include the thigh and

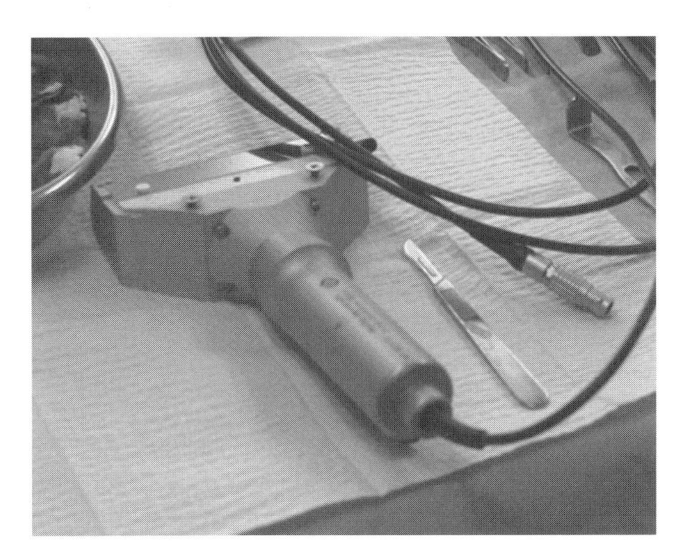

FIGURE 5.6 Dermatome used for skin harvest.

buttock region. The donor skin is usually 8 to 12 thousandth of an inch thick for a split thickness skin graft. Sheet grafts, pie crusted for drainage, generally measuring approximately 0.012 inches in thickness for the average adult, are preferred for the face, neck, hand, and fingers as they are more cosmetically appealing.

If larger wound coverage is required, it can be meshed, stretched, to cover a larger surface area. The skin can be meshed 1.5:1, 2:1, or as high as 6:1 for extremely large burns (Figure 5.7). Cosmetic outcome is worse with larger mesh. The interstices of these meshed grafts will heal by epithelialization over the scar and will be subject to somewhat greater contraction than the sheet graft. It also takes longer for the body to fill in the interstices. Conservation of donor skin will be critical when the patient has sustained greater than 50% body surface injury.

A full thickness skin graft is used in areas where contracture is a concern, such as the eyelids. Burns of the palm are also of high concern. The specialized skin of the palm and volar aspect of the fingers have a thick epidermis and a dermis rich in adnexal elements. More conservative treatment is suggested until the depth of the palmar burn is fully defined. When the palmar burn is full thickness, resurfacing via skin grafting is indicated to prevent the functional loss brought about by late palmar and digital joint contracture.

Skin substitutes have a role in some cases. Integra is one skin substitute that is a commercially available product used as temporary wound coverage (Figure 5.8). It is a bilaminar dermal regeneration template. It was initially developed to improve functional results after the acute phase of a burn injury. The dermal matrix layer is composed of bovine collagen and shark chondroitin-6-sulphate. The epidermal component is a thin layer of silicone. The deeper layer structure provides the "scaffold" for neodermis formation. The host fibroblasts migrate, proliferate, and secrete a native collagen formation within the dermal template. The endothelial cells shortly follow the fibroblasts to form a vascular network within the neodermis.

Vascularization becomes evident at approximately 2 to 4 weeks, following which the silicone layer can be removed and replaced with a thin split thickness skin graft. The product can stay on the skin for a few weeks prior to final coverage.

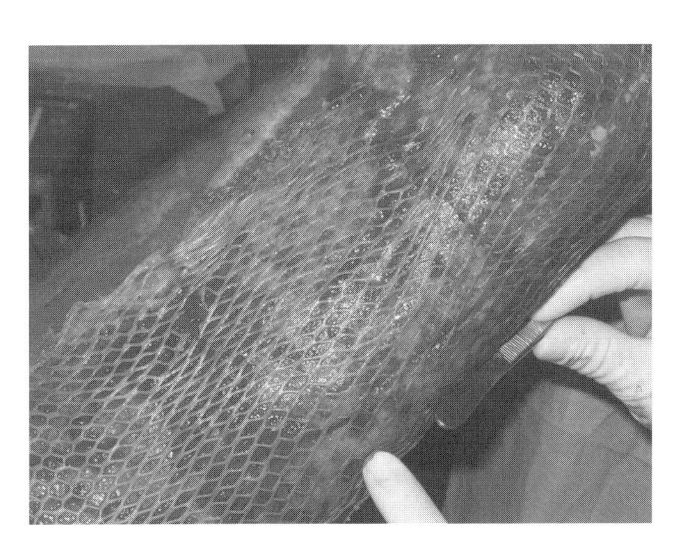

FIGURE 5.7 Meshed split thickness autograft.

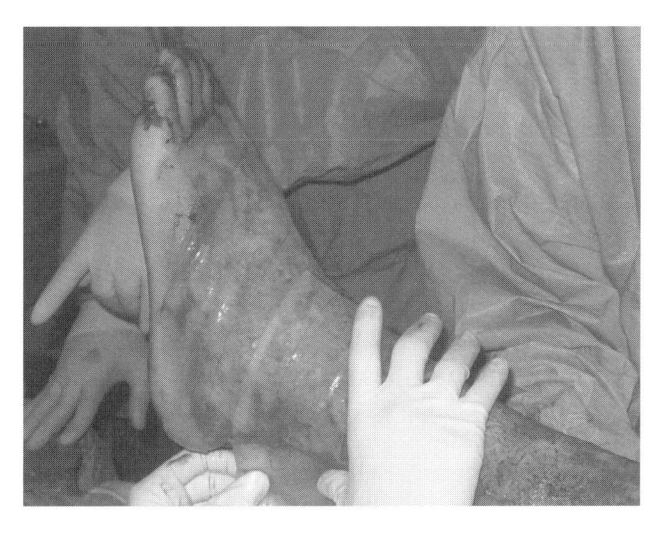

FIGURE 5.8 Integra placement over the dorsal foot and ankle.

Patients are encouraged to move 5 to 7 days after application. Active and passive range of motion (ROM) may be performed; however, friction and aggressive stretching at maximal end range should be avoided as it may cause Integra to lift up from the wound bed.

Integra is utilized in both the acute and reconstructive phases of recovery. It is most commonly placed over a joint, specifically, the axillary region; however, it can be utilized over an entire extremity. It is thought that more mobility is achieved at the joint post-Integra placement, given the thinner skin graft requirement. Donor sites also heal more quickly and, as a result, can be reharvested at a faster rate.

BURN REHABILITATION

Burn rehabilitation is a dynamic process that requires a skilled therapist. Intervention begins at the time of injury and continues until scar maturation. Both large and small burn injuries can cause lifelong deformity and disability. The leading cause of impairment following a burn injury is a hand burn (Anzarut, Chen, Shankowsky, & Tredget, 2005).

Phases of rehabilitation have been described as emergent, acute, skin grafting, and rehabilitative (Tufaro & Bondoc, 2011). A burn patient may be in one or more of these phases at any given time. He or she may even skip a phase altogether. This adds to the complexity of the treatment of the burn patient, as a therapist must have a thorough understanding of these phases to adequately tailor the treatment and progress the patient appropriately.

The ultimate goals of burn rehabilitation are to restore function and optimize the cosmetic outcome. There are many barriers to achieving this goal, specifically, scar formation, patient compliance, and lack of social supports. The scar maturation phase on average lasts 1 year; however, it can last upward of 2 years. The therapist therefore has a 1- to 2-year window to create change.

Phases of Rehabilitation

The first 24 to 72 hours after a burn injury is described as the emergent phase. The therapist's primary goals are to evaluate the patient and develop treatment goals and a plan of care. Patients are typically evaluated within the first 24 hours of admission to a burn center (Whitehead & Serghio, 2009). At this time, the treatment plan focuses on minimizing edema, obtaining optimal positioning, initiating motion, and maximizing function (Tufaro & Bondoc, 2011).

The acute phase generally extends from the emergent phase until wound closure. Wound closure is defined as surgical closure of the burn wound via skin grafting or by secondary-intention healing (Clark, 1985). Goals of therapy during the acute phase are to increase and/or preserve ROM, preserve tendon gliding and muscle activity, inhibit contraction, and promote overall function (Tufaro & Bondoc, 2011).

The skin-grafting phase begins once the surgeon deems the patient will need skin grafting. Patients who do not require surgical intervention will skip this phase. A therapist is often called at the end of surgery to apply a custom orthosis to the affected area. Typically, this orthosis is worn for approximately 5 days; however, immobilization protocols vary from facility to facility. Some prefer immobilization for 5 to 7 days, whereas others initiate motion on post-op Day 1. Graft size and location are two factors utilized in making this decision. For example, a hand graft has a higher likelihood of graft loss than the calf if early motion is initiated. The hand has many moving parts; therefore, the graft is more likely to shift or lift up from the wound bed.

The rehabilitation phase is described from the time of graft adherence or wound closure until scar maturation (Tufaro & Bondoc, 2011). The primary goals of therapy at this time are to preserve and increase joint mobility and ROM, increase strength and function, and hinder the development of scar contraction and hypertrophy. The rehabilitation phase may begin in the hospital but will continue well into the outpatient setting.

Positioning

One of the keys to the successful rehabilitation of a burn patient is proper positioning. Anti-contracture positioning and splinting must start from Day 1 and may continue for many months after injury. It applies to all patients regardless of burn depth and skin grafting and is designed to minimize edema, prevent tissue destruction, and preserve soft tissues in an elongated state to facilitate functional recovery (Apfel et al., 1994). In 2006, 95% of the surveyed burn centers reported that positioning began within 24 hours of admission as opposed to 54% in 1994 (Whitehead & Serghiou, 2009). In general, patients rest in a position of comfort; this is generally a position of flexion, which is also the position of contracture. Wounds start the healing process almost as soon as they occur and a major part of this process involves the development of contracture. Once contracture starts to develop, it can be a constant battle to achieve full movement, so preventive measures to minimize contracture development are necessary. Early compliance is essential to ensure the best possible long-term functional outcome and also to ease pain and assist with exercise regimes.

The risk of contracture is greater when the burn occurs to the flexor aspect of a joint or limb. This is due to the position of comfort being a flexed position; also, the flexor muscles are generally stronger than the extensors. If a burn was to occur on the extensor aspect of an extremity, patients can use the strength of the flexors to stretch the particular area. The flexed position is also often the position of function. Some examples include grasping, pinching, and carrying items. Students and desk workers demonstrate cervical, elbow, hip, and knee flexion. The goal of anti-contracture positioning is to counteract this natural tendency toward flexion.

It is ideal to place the joint of interest in extension and abduction to counteract the pull of the scar tissue. Patients with neck burns are advised to forego a pillow under their head. Positioning the pillow at the upper back/lower cervical region will promote cervical extension. Patients with burns in and around their axilla should be positioned at 90 to 120 degrees of shoulder abduction. Most patients find true abduction uncomfortable for long durations. It can also lead to overstretch at the brachial plexus. Positioning the shoulder in slight scaption (30–45 degrees adduction from the frontal plane) and elbow flexion has been found to be just as effective at preventing scar contracture as true abduction, while significantly improving patient compliance. This position can be maintained with a custom axillary orthosis, foam wedges, pillows, arm troughs, and bedside tables.

The upper extremity is positioned at or above heart level with the elbow in extension, forearm either supinated or neutral, wrist in neutral, and hand in an intrinsic-plus position (Apfel et al., 1994; Hildebrant, Herrmann, & Stegemann, 1993; Howell, 1994; Tilley, McMahon, & Shukalak, 2000; Villeco, Mackin, Hunter, 1992). A foam wedge is an effective and inexpensive positioning device that can be utilized with both the upper and lower extremities. It is most commonly utilized to extend the elbow and elevate the upper extremities; however, it can be utilized to abduct the extremities as well. It is easy to apply and keep in place, inexpensive, and well accepted by patients and staff. Other upper extremity elevation devices include commercial arm troughs, pillows, blankets, bedside table, and surgical netting. In the case of a palmar burn, the wrist is positioned in neutral to 30 degrees of extension, interphalangeal (IP) joints are in extension, and the first web space is in a slight stretch (Lund, 1999). This is accomplished with a custom orthosis. With circumferential hand burns, hand positioning may alternate every 12 hours to account for both a palmar and dorsal burn.

Pillows should be avoided under the knees as this can encourage hip and knee contractures. The area of most concern on the lower extremities is the ankle/heel region. When positioning the ankle, it is important to consider the heel as this is an area of high breakdown. The ankle is positioned in neutral (90 degrees) position with either a custom or a prefabricated orthosis. In many cases, the heel is suspended off the bed to prevent skin breakdown. Even if the ankle does not need specific positioning measures, the heel still needs to be addressed in the bedbound patient. A simple gel cushion can be utilized to off-load the heel or this may be applied directly under the heel. A pillow can also be utilized but is much less effective. There are many commercially available products to off-load the heel while maintaining the general position of the ankle.

Positioning does not come without risks. Patients must be monitored and frequently repositioned to ensure that complications do not arise. Devices may slip under the weight of an extremity. Patients may move when agitated or asleep, creating pressure points. Elevation beyond heart level may result in decreased arterial supply to the hand. Excessive weight-bearing stress to the olecranon of the elbow, especially with a flexed elbow, should be avoided because this may lead to breakdown and pressure on the ulnar nerve.

Orthoses

Custom orthosis fabrication is an everyday occurrence on the burn unit. Orthosis is indicated if there is total or partial restricted motion of a limb, which often occurs when a patient or a patient's body part is immobilized for any reason for a prolonged time period. Custom orthosis can be made of various materials, noting that a low-temperature thermoplastic orthosis is an ideal choice as it is lightweight, easily moldable and remoldable, and conforms extremely well to contours.

Edema, pain, and tight eschar immediately after a burn are the leading reasons why a person may demonstrate impaired ROM and therefore require an orthosis (Richard, Staley, Miller, & Warden, 1997). Whitehead and Serghiou (2009) found that 61% of the surveyed burn centers in 2006 initiated orthotic intervention within 24 hours of admission as opposed to 54% of responding centers in 1994. If the patient is alert, most facilities recommend that the orthosis only be worn when asleep. In the case of the intubated patient, orthoses are worn at all times except during burn care and therapy. Orthoses should be removed every 2 hours for cleaning to prevent patient contamination (Richard & Ward, 2005). Decisions regarding initiation of an orthosis, duration of wear, and design continue to vary significantly among burn centers.

A static orthosis is often used during the emergent and acute phases of rehabilitation. This type of orthosis has no moving parts. The goal of the orthosis is to counteract the deforming position of edema, support the extremity, and preserve joint alignment (Whitehead & Serghiou, 2009). Patients are typically immobilized when sleeping or sedated (Barillo et al., 1997; Richard, Staley, Daugherty, Miller, & Warden, 1994).

A static orthosis and/or a cast is utilized during the skin-grafting phase to immobilize the area. The therapist applies the custom orthosis and/or cast in the operating room. Wear time is variable and it can be worn upward of 5 to 7 days. The purpose of orthotic fabrication during the rehabilitation phase is to preserve ROM by opposing the force of the contracting scar, usually during periods of patient inactivity. Both static and static progressive orthoses are utilized but in some cases, dynamic orthosis may be beneficial (Lund, 1999). The term *static progressive* indicates that a static orthosis is remolded every 1to 3 days with the intent of gaining ROM at the joint. A dynamic orthosis has one or many moving parts. It has several purposes but in burn rehabilitation, it is typically fabricated to substitute for a loss of motor function or to correct a deformity by applying force to position the joint at end range with the soft tissue at a maximum length. An example of this is a dynamic proximal interphalangeal (PIP) joint flexion orthosis, which assists the PIP joint to gradually regain maximal flexion.

Hand

The hand is the body area most commonly affected by a burn injury. It is also the area most commonly splinted. To counteract the position of deforming forces and to protect the structures of the hand, an orthosis that positions the wrist in slight or neutral extension, the metacarpal phalangeal (MCP) joint in flexion, the IP joint in extension, and the thumb away from the palm is recommended. This position is commonly referred to as the *protected* or *safe* position of the hand. The position of the IP joints in extension prevents adaptive shortening of the volar plate and collateral ligaments and the development of IP joint flexion contractures.

At this time, universal dimensions for what exactly constitute the "basic" burn orthosis do not exist (Richard et al., 1994). The medical literature provides 40 different descriptions of how to position dorsal hand burns as well as a variety of names for such an orthosis. Although practitioners agree that the wrist should be in slight extension and that the MCP joints should be flexed, there is a wide range of specific joint angles cited in the literature. We recommend that the wrist be positioned in 15 to 20 degrees of extension, the MCP joints flexed 50 to 70 degrees, the IP joints extended fully, and the thumb positioned midway between radial and palmar abduction, with the thumb MCP joint flexed 10 degrees and the IP joint fully extended. In addition to maintaining thumb opposition and abduction, the orthosis must maintain the thenar web space and properly support the MCP joint of the thumb. Failure to properly support the thumb MCP joint could result in a swan neck deformity; this type of deformity mimics the shape of a swan with the PIP in hyperextension and DIP in flexion.

When applying an orthosis to a palmar hand burn, the wrist should be positioned in neutral or slight extension, the fingers in full extension and abduction, and the thumb in radial abduction and extension. This is typically called a *pan* orthosis. As healing progresses, the orthosis should be molded to maintain the palmar arches. During the rehabilitative phase, splint material lined with silicone should be utilized to further prevent palmar and digital flexion contractures. Burns involving only the thenar web space are positioned in radial abduction, but care must be taken to support the thumb MCP joint. This is typically called a *C-bar* orthosis.

Prefabricated hand orthoses can be applied; however, they are not preferred. They often are unable to accommodate the fluctuating edema of a burn patient and the bulky bandages. Prefabricated splints with cloth and/or padding should be avoided during the emergent, acute, and skin-grafting phase as they are unable to be disinfected properly.

Pediatric hand orthoses and those of an intubated patient are secured with an elastic gauze bandage. The elastic gauze promotes optimal positioning of the orthosis in patients who wear it for longer durations and is more challenging for a child to remove. In the case of an alert adult patient, hand orthoses are usually applied with strapping for easy application. If orthotic intervention is not chosen at this time, a small roll of gauze can be placed or wrapped in an intubated patient's hand to help maintain the thenar web space and the palmar arch.

A hand that is healing without complications does not have to be positioned in an orthosis unless there is a limitation of active motion. Generally, an orthosis should be applied if the finger joints lack the last 20 degrees or more in extension or less than 70 degrees of flexion and the wrist lacks 20 degrees or more of wrist flexion and/or extension. Other indicators may include guarding, significant complaints of pain, lack of use through daily activities, and noncompliance with the patient's home exercise program. A serial digit extension orthosis and/or casting fabrication should be considered during the rehabilitation phase when wounds are less of a concern (Figure 5.9).

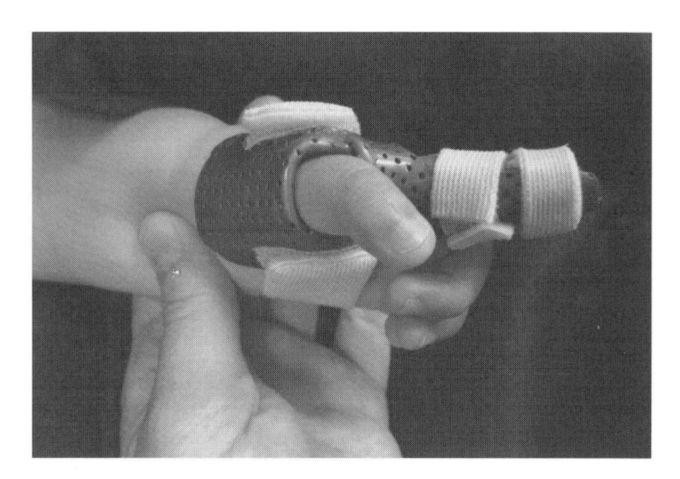

FIGURE 5.9 Static digital orthosis.

As the patient's ROM and level of arousal improves, the use of the orthosis during the day can be decreased. If the patient is unwilling or unable to cooperate, the orthosis should be worn continuously and removed only for dressing changes, self-care activities, and therapy. In these cases, casting may be considered depending on the number of open wounds. The orthosis should be worn during all hours of sleep. When an orthosis is not applied during the night, it is not unusual for the patient to experience a significant loss of motion. The therapist should be careful not to overly immobilize the patient. This can result in joint stiffness, contractures, and soft tissue adhesions. Children can tolerate immobilization longer than adults because of the elasticity of their joints and soft tissue, but they still need to be monitored (Birchenough, Gamper, & Morgan, 2008; Feldman, 2008).

Therapeutic Exercise and Function

Movement, both active and passive, is essential for an optimal outcome (Figure 5.10). A burn patient is directed to perform exercises targeting the burned area frequently throughout the day, often every awake hour (Head, 1984). If sedated, the therapists and staff perform these exercises. Self-care, instrumental activities of daily living, and play are vital to recovery and are incorporated into therapy sessions. All these activities may be performed with dressings in place. Care should be taken to avoid soiling the dressings. If a dressing is restricting movement because it is too bulky or too tight, it should be adjusted.

Although pain is often associated with movement, it will ultimately decrease over time. Initial movements are always the most painful, but each subsequent set of repetitions should be easier as the tissue stretches and the muscle-pumping action of active movement helps resolve edema, thus significantly reducing pain. The acute skin-grafting phase is the only time when motion is typically withheld. This allows for graft adherence and minimizes graft loss (Tufaro & Bondoc, 2011).

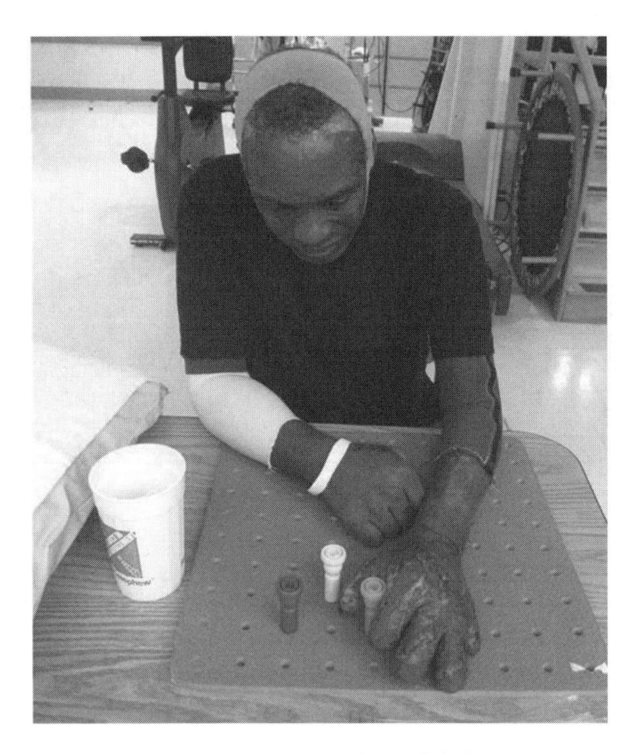

FIGURE 5.10 Fine motor activity performed during occupational therapy session.

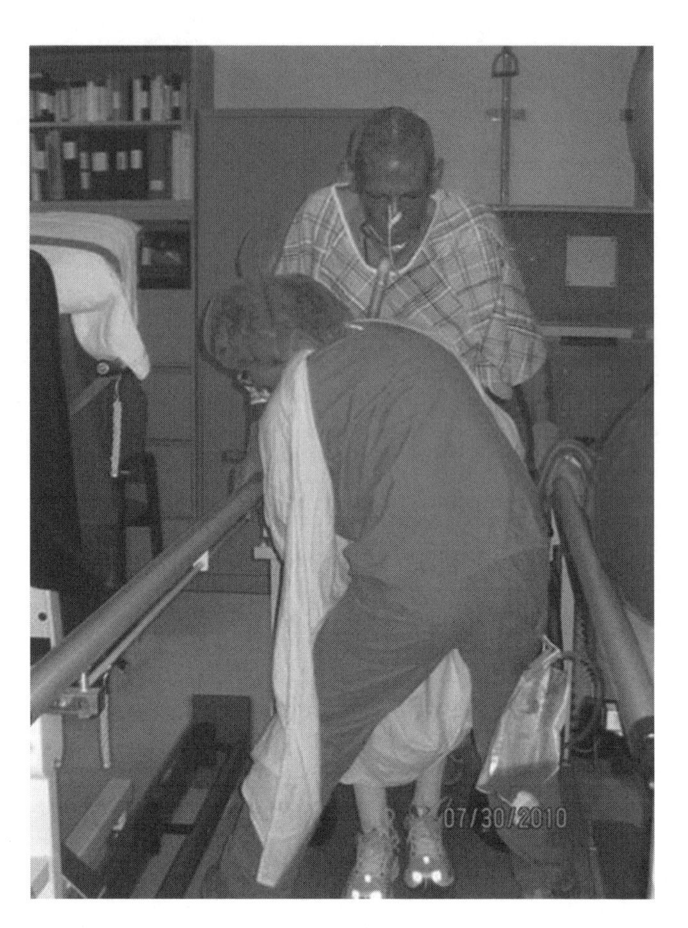

FIGURE 5.11 Early mobilization of an oxygen-dependent patient.

Patients and family members are often reluctant to engage in passive ROM due to the fear that it will cause pain. A continuous passive motion (CPM) device can be an effective modality to improve joint ROM as its movements are predictable and the patient has control over the device. The patient is able to stop at any time and adjust the parameters as tolerated. When pain and/or fear of pain is an obstacle to tolerating ROM, a CPM is an excellent alternative. It can be utilized 2 to 4 hours daily outside of therapy. Shoulder, elbow, and knee CPMs are the most common.

A significant advancement in the therapeutic intervention of the critically ill burn patient is early mobilization (Figure 5.11). Patients who are critically ill and often ventilated are being mobilized much earlier during the hospitalization. In the past, this patient population was sedated and/or activity orders were deferred until the patient was weaned off the ventilator. Now such patients are sitting on the edge of bed and in the bedside chair, standing, and ambulating despite the presence of concurrent multiple intravenous lines and mechanical ventilation. This approach to care requires that all members of the intensive care unit (ICU) team take an active role as considerable coordination among staff members is needed to achieve mobilization in this setting. Studies have shown that early mobilization decreases ICU delirium, days on mechanical ventilation, hospital-acquired paresis, and hospital length of stay, while improving overall function (Balas et al., 2013; Hilsabek, Ronnenbaum, Weir, 2015; Hopkins, Spuhler, & Thomsen, 2007; Pohlam, Pohlman, & Schwieckert, 2009).

Virtual Reality and Gaming

Pain and anxiety are complications of burn injuries that considerably influence the course of recovery, and acute pain is exacerbated by anxiety. Patients frequently experience poorly controlled procedural pain, which promotes anticipatory anxiety and, in turn, decreases pain tolerance, elevating its intensity during burn care and therapy (Byers, Bridges, Kijek, & LaBorde, 2001).

As pain medications alone tended to be insufficient in controlling these procedural symptoms, immersive virtual reality (VR) was developed to provide adjunctive nonpharmacologic analgesia through distraction. VR is a computerized technology that simulates an activity or experience. VR presence is characterized as the illusion of exploring a computer-generated virtual world (Hoffman, Patterson, Carrougher, & Sharar, 2001; Hoffman et al., 2004). Researchers propose that attention is drawn toward the virtual world, leaving less reserves of attention to focus on pain (Hoffman et al., 2004). Patients typically showed 25% to 50% reductions in pain during VR, and pain diminution in VR was correlated with the amount of enjoyment or "fun" reported by participants (Hoffman et al., 2006).

Similarly, implementation of off-the-shelf gaming systems in burn rehabilitation has been explored and has gained popularity. Studies report benefits in balance, postural control, and function (Deutsch, Borbely, Filler, Huhn, & Guarrera-Bowlby, 2008; Pigford & Andrews, 2010). It is more financially feasible than VR and has a variety of gaming options. The systems are portable and can be utilized in an individual and group setting (Saposnik et al., 2010). Off-the-shelf gaming systems promote light- to moderate-intensity activity and are enjoyable for both adolescents and adults. They have been shown to engage patients who lack the motivation and interest to complete normal exercise schedules and may be of particular advantage to burn survivors with extensive rehabilitation needs that are long-term, repetitive, and quite arduous.

Modalities

Research linking the use of physical modalities and burns is lacking. Implications for use and parameters are typically generalized from other patient populations and based on therapist experience. The most common modalities utilized are ultrasound (US), paraffin, and iontophoresis.

US has been used in the treatment of scars to increase ROM, reduce pain, and decrease scar formation (Richard, DerSarkisian, Miller, Johnson, & Staley,1999). A typical US treatment will take from 3 to 5 minutes depending on the size of the area being treated. In cases where scar tissue breakdown is the goal, this treatment time can be much longer.

Paraffin is most effective when combined with sustained stretch. This combination has been shown to cause collagen extensibility, which, in turn, makes the skin more pliable, decreases joint discomfort, and increases joint ROM. Patients with limited finger flexion can have their fingers wrapped with a self-adherent tape into a fist or their digits can be wrapped around a dowel or cone prior to applying the paraffin. Initially, the patients cannot tolerate the heat of the paraffin bath. In these cases, the paraffin can be painted on with a paintbrush or a piece of gauze (Johnson, 1984). After the paraffin has been applied, the hand is covered with plastic wrap and a towel. Later in the rehabilitation phase, a hot pack may be applied over the plastic wrap and towel layer. Paraffin should not be used on patients with wounds, fragile skin, decreased sensation, hypersensitivity to heat, or fear of hot liquids.

Iontophoresis can be effective in reducing posttraumatic scar adhesions with the use of iodine (Iodex) and methyl salicylate ointment (Langley, 1984; Tannenbaum, 1980). In the case of burn scars, saline with 0.9% to 3.0% concentration, as a means of hydrating the tough and adherent burn scars before mobilization, is more commonly utilized. Lower intensities and longer delivery time are recommended when applying iontophoresis to a burn scar because tissue resistance and permeability of a burn scar is greater than in unburned skin. To maximize tissue diffusion, the buffered pad should be left on the patient's skin for a few hours.

SCAR

Scarring is a natural part of the healing process. It is the result of the body's repair mechanism after injury (O'Brien & Pandit, 2006). In simple terms, scars are areas of fibrous tissue (fibrosis) that replace normal skin after injury. Hypertrophic or raised scarring is commonplace in grafted skin and in the case of delayed healing (wound closure >3 weeks). In hypertrophic scars, the typical process of collagen reorganization is significantly elongated and is further complicated by the excessive proliferation of dermal tissue and local chronic inflammation during the healing process (Linares, 1996; O'Brien & Pandit, 2006).

A common characteristic of a hypertrophic scar is redness. It is also raised and rigid to touch. Transient blanching is evident when gentle pressure is applied directly to the scar. As the scar matures, it becomes flatter, paler, and more pliable. The scar maturation process can last anywhere from 6 months to 2 years. Those with higher melanin pigmentation have a higher likelihood of experiencing hypertrophic scarring. Keloid scar formation is not typically seen with burn scars; however, it cannot be ruled out. A keloid is a scar that extends outside the perimeter of the original injury. Both a hypertrophic and keloid scar can be quite raised. The most common locations are earlobes, arms, pelvic region, and over the clavicle.

Other predictors of hypertrophic scar formation are the anatomical location of the burn and the timing and type of surgical intervention (McGrouther & Myer, 1991; Richard et al., 1999). Skin tension may be a factor in scar formation and contraction due to the directional variance in skin movement between the volar and dorsal skin surfaces (McGrouther & Myer, 1991). Early wound closure yields a more favorable cosmetic and functional outcome as it decreases the chance of scar formation. Despite the therapist's best efforts to minimize scarring, a contracture may be unavoidable. A loss of motion as a result of inelastic and shortened skin is deemed a burn scar contracture once the scar maturation phase is complete. Surgical intervention is required at this time. Typical scar contractures include microstomia, lip ectropion, eye ectropion, axillary, antecubital fossa flexion contractures, popliteal flexion contractures, toe extension and flexion contractures, neck contractures (lateral and flexion), abduction contracture of the thumb, and finger extension and flexion contractures (Young, Dewey, & Wolf, 2010).

Scar Evaluation

Scar rating scales have the potential to contribute to better evaluation of scar properties in both research and clinical settings, to assess the need for and efficacy of treatment, and to estimate maturation. Several methods and tools for evaluating scars have been presented. At least 18 methods of evaluation have been identified in the literature, with no reliable and consistent method. Most scar rating scales assess vascularity, pliability, height, and thickness. Some scales contain additional items such as itch. Only the Patient and Observer Scar Assessment Scale (POSAS) received a high-quality rating but only in the area of reliability for total scores and the vascularity subscale. The Vancouver Scar Scale (VSS), which is the most widely used among burn therapists, received indeterminate ratings for construct validity, reliability, and responsiveness.

Although not objective, photographs are helpful in cataloging change in a scar. They should be taken at regular intervals and in a standardized fashion. Self-healed areas, donor sites, and skin grafts should all be photographed. Currently, no published studies have evaluated the relationship between a patient's subjective scar evaluation and that of the therapist's objective measurement. Nor are there any studies that relate these two findings to function and return-to-life roles.

Scar Management

Since the 1970s, burn therapists have utilized pressure garments as the standard of care to minimize hypertrophic scarring (Abston, Larson, & Evans, 1971; Reid, 1987). This intervention is standard for anyone who has received a skin graft or experienced delayed healing (>3 weeks). Once the wound coverage has been achieved, interim pressure bandages, garments, or gloves are initiated until custom garments are received. A burn patient must be measured for custom compression garments (Figure 5.12). The goal of these garments is to provide even pressure, 25 mmHg, across the affected surfaces.

Garments are typically worn 23 hours a day. They are removed only for bathing, instances that would soil or wet the garment, and skin care. A garment requires replacement at approximately 3 months. It is difficult to achieve optimal pressure across the palm, instep, face, neck and breastplate. Foam, silicone inserts, silicone-lined splints, and enhancements

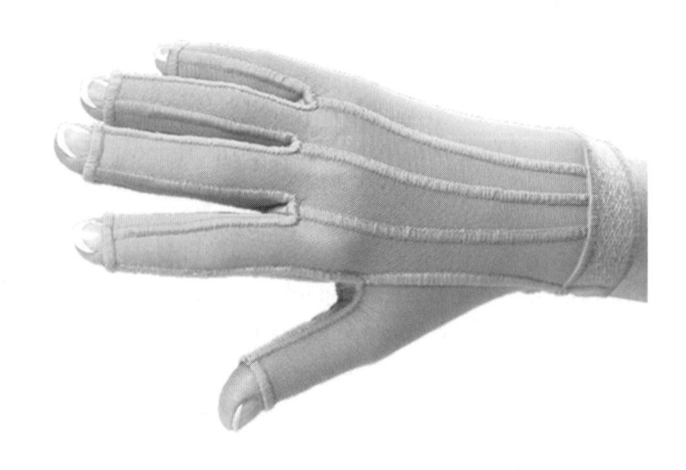

FIGURE 5.12 Custom compression glove for hypertrophic scarring.

to the custom garment are some common interventions to address this problem. Patient compliance is a concern as the garments are warm, expensive, at times may limit function, and lack long-term durability and cosmetic appeal (Bhagwanjee, Mbakaza, Stewart, & Binase, 2000; Landmann et al., 2009).

Silicone gel sheets (SGSs) are also indicated in a scar that remains raised and with decreased pliability despite the use of pressure garments (Figure 5.13). Therapists and patients report improved color and pliability of a scar following the application of SGS; however, the research in this area is weak and susceptible to bias (Fish, Musgrave, Umraw, Manuel, & Robert, 2002; Mustoe, 2008). Although the etiology is unclear, silicone gel exerts many actions on the scar. Hypotheses include the following (Puri & Ashutosh, 2009):

1. Increases hydration of stratum corneum and thereby facilitates regulation of fibroblast production and reduction in collagen production. It results in a softer and flatter scar
2. Protects the scarred tissue from bacterial invasion
3. Modulates the expression of growth factors, fibroblast growth factor β (FGF β) and tumor growth factor β (TGF β). TGF β stimulates fibroblasts to synthesize collagen and fibronectin. FGF β normalizes the collagen synthesis in an abnormal scar and increases the level of collagenases, which breaks down the excess collagen. Balance of fibrogenesis and fibrolysis is ultimately restored
4. Reduces itching and discomfort associated with scars

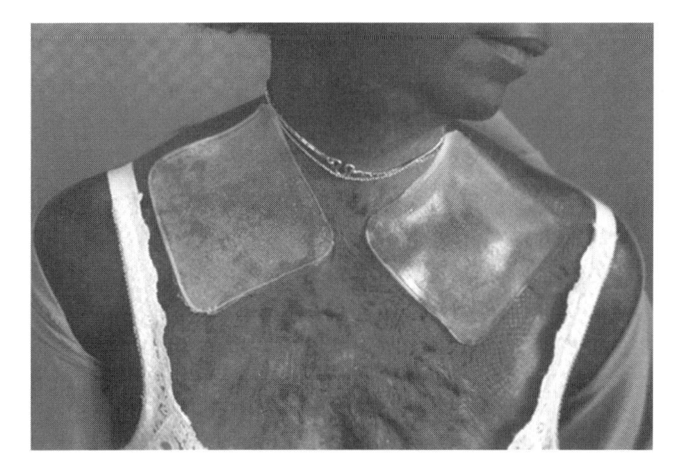

FIGURE 5.13 Adhesive silicone gel sheeting for hypertrophic scarring.

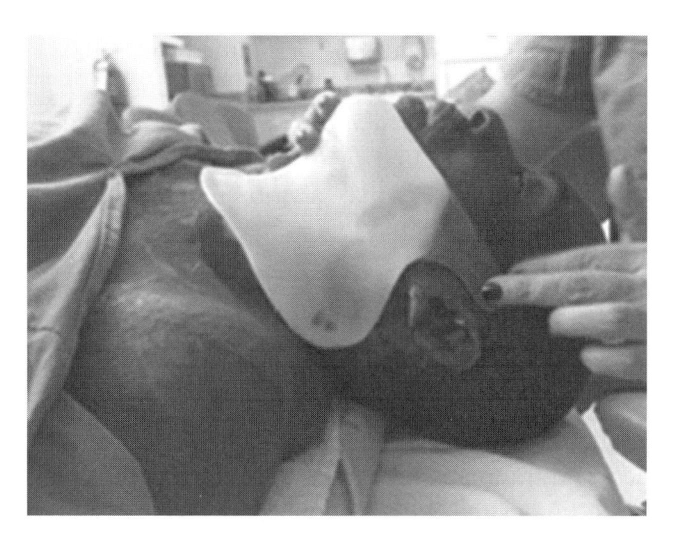

FIGURE 5.14 Static neck orthosis lined with silicone.

There are many SGS options available. The flexibility of the insert, the application site, the width, and the need for an adhesive backing are all factors to be considered (Tufaro &Bondoc, 2011). A splint lined with silicone is also an option for the face, neck, antecubital fossa, popliteal region, and hand (Figure 5.14). These areas are uneven and optimal pressure cannot be reached and/or maintained with conventional pressure garments.

Other treatment options include pulse dye laser and steroid injections. The 585 nm pulse dye laser has been shown to reduce erythema and improve the texture and elasticity of the scar (Juckette & Hartman-Adams, 2009; Young et al., 2010). Cost to the patient is often a drawback as it is frequently not covered by insurance and several treatments are required. Steroid injections have been shown to soften and shrink hardened scars (Juckette & Hartman-Adams, 2009; Young et al., 2010). This practice is often done with facial hypertrophic scars and can be quite painful. Both treatments are not yet commonplace; however, they are gaining popularity among larger burn centers.

Scar massage may be incorporated into the scar management regimen once the scar is able to withstand opposing forces. It assists in freeing adhering fibrous bands, thereby softening and remolding the scar tissue. It also has been shown to assist in alleviating itching and assisting with desensitization of the area. A lubricant may be applied. Enough pressure should be applied so that the skin blanches. Rotary, parallel, and perpendicular motions should be utilized.

The massage should be performed two to three times daily for 3 to 5 minutes (Herndon, 2007). Ideally, pressure garments are applied immediately afterward as vascularity to the area is increased. Electrical massagers may also be helpful tools for home use.

Heterotopic Ossification

HO is the creation and deposition of mature lamellar bone in muscle, tendon, and fascia. It is often seen in genetic disorders, musculoskeletal surgeries, and traumatic injuries. HO in burn patients has been associated with prolonged periods of immobilization, intubation, and time to wound closure. In addition, it has been correlated with recurring local trauma, loss of skin graft, and wound infection (Medina, Savaryn, Shankowski, Shukalak, & Edward, 2014). HO often bridges a joint causing significant pain and loss of joint motion and function.

The elbow joint has the highest occurrence, with incidence ranging from 62% to 90% in the literature (Medina et al., 2014). The hip and knee are other common areas of incidence, although with much less frequency. HO is routinely diagnosed on an x-ray. Once diagnosed, rehabilitation goals shift to preserving the available ROM. Passive ROM is acceptable within a pain-free zone. Surgical resection is preferred following skin maturation (>1 year post injury); however, the literature suggests that early removal may benefit functional outcome. Early resection (<6 months) has been shown to prevent muscle shortening, capsule contracture, and nerve entrapment (Medina et al., 2014; Young et al., 2010). Following resection, motion at the joint typically begins on postoperative day 1; however, the joint is typically protected by a static orthosis outside of therapy. Drug therapies may also be instituted to prevent bone formation and inflammation; however, these are still limited in their success. Radiation therapy is not commonplace with HO formation following a burn injury.

Common Burn Deformities

Despite improvements in care, postburn deformities are still commonplace. In general, reconstruction does not begin until after the scar maturation phase has been completed.

Surgical intervention should be performed earlier if function or safety is compromised. Understanding how the contracture developed will permit a reconstructive procedure to be successful, avoiding an early recurrence and its associated functional restriction. At the time of surgical intervention, it is assumed that all therapy has reached the maximum level of improvement. Patients are typically directed back to outpatient rehabilitation to capitalize on the gains obtained during surgery. Common postburn deformities that most often require surgical intervention include palmar, PIP joint, elbow, axillary and neck contractures, boutonniere deformities, web space contractures and syndactyly, small finger deformities, upper and lower eyelid ectropion, and perioral deformities (Figure 5.15).

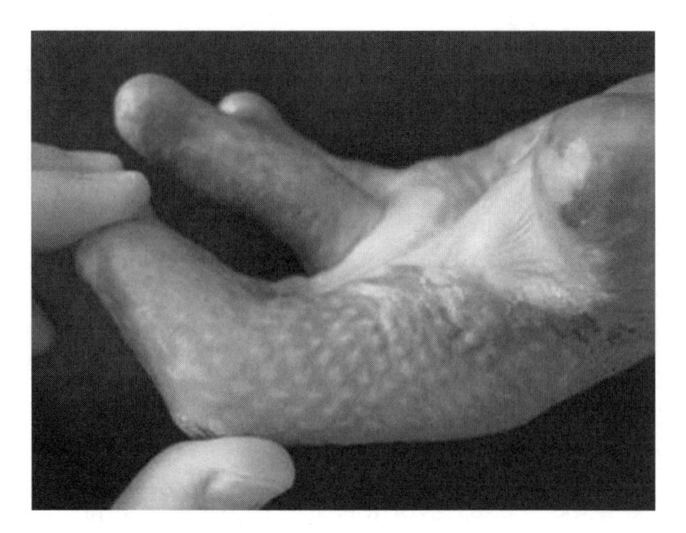

FIGURE 5.15 Second digit proximal interphalangeal joint contracture.

PSYCHOLOGICAL INTERVENTION

A burn injury is sudden and can be devastating. Burn survivors are faced with a "new" normal. They physically are forever changed, often unable to return to previous roles within their families, work, school, and community. Psychological effects are often not felt until after discharge from the hospital. As a result, burn survivors and their families must be frequently monitored for signs of emotional distress and educated on the support systems available. Functional goals should be set high and family members should be involved if possible.

Posttraumatic stress disorder (PTSD) is of high concern as it has been shown to occur in approximately 25% of all burn survivors (Fauerbach et al.,

2007; Mason, Fauerbach, & Haythornthwaite, 2010). Psychological distress after a burn injury has been shown to interfere with recovery in many ways such as making pain and itching feel worse, disrupting sleep, causing memory loss and difficulty in concentration, diminishing effort in participation in rehabilitaton programs and wound care, and reducing interest and pleasure in daily activities (Fauerbach et al., 2007; Mason et al., 2010). Burn survivors and their family members may benefit from one-on-one counseling, medications, cognitive behavioral treatment, peer support, and support groups.

Return to Work

Multiple variables affect a burn survivor's ability to return to work. Severe burn injuries often lead to cognitive impairments, contractures, weakness, psychological issues, impaired strength, and amputations. Return to work should be considered early in the course of treatment for those who were working at the time of their injury. Those injured at work often sustained hand burns and were more likely to require surgery. This negatively impacted their ability to return to work (Esselman et al., 2007).

Returning to work is affected not only by burn-related factors but also by general demographic and employment factors. Several studies have found that the mean off-work time is 17 weeks (Helm, & Walker, 1992; Helm, Walker, & Peyton, 1986). At 1 year after the burn injury, 79.7% had returned to work (Esselman et al., 2007). The topmost predictor for the time to return to work is burn severity. Patients with employment prior to the burn have an increased likelihood of returning to work. Also, a patient who is the primary wage earner in a fam ily is more likely to return to work after the injury. Physical abilities, work conditions, and wound issues were the top three return-to-work barriers reported by burn survivors.

When injured workers meet established short- and long-term goals via physical therapy and/or hand/occupational therapy but are unable to return to work due to remaining functional deficits or deconditioning, they may benefit from a higher level of therapeutic intervention designed specifically with a primary goal of returning to work. Injured workers who benefit most from these programs are usually at least 30 days out from their injury and have a job of a medium or higher physical demand category to return to. These are full-body intensive conditioning programs, called work-hardening programs. They are multidisciplinary in nature and utilize real or simulated work activities designed to restore physical, behavioral, and vocational functions. Work hardening addresses the issues of productivity, safety, physical tolerance, and worker behaviors.

Physicians may request a functional capacity evaluation (FCE) to determine safe, functional levels for an individual to either return to work or establish functional ability. It is typically completed by an occupational therapist in the outpatient setting. It provides a comprehensive evaluation that measures strength, endurance, physical demand, work level, and positional tolerance. The data gathered through this evaluation objectively define the injured employee's physical capabilities. The evaluation assists referral sources by offering information for adjudication of claims in short-long-term disability, provides return-to-work capabilities, and determines ability levels for liability cases using appropriate medical standards.

SUMMARY

Rehabilitation from a burn injury is a lengthy process, which starts on day 1 and involves a continuum of care through to scar maturation and beyond. Sustaining a burn injury, however large or small, can have a dramatic effect on the individual's physical and psychological well-being and requires teamwork and commitment to help the individual overcome the difficulties he or she may encounter. Although the path is not always easy, with the right support, therapeutic intervention, and understanding of the psychological and social challenges, the patient can reach the maximum physical, psychological, and functional outcome.

REFERENCES

Abston, S., Evans, E. B., & Larson, D. (1971). Splints and traction. In H. Polk & H. H. Stone (Eds.), *Contemporary burn management* (pp. 488–489). Boston, MA: Little, Brown.

American Burn Association. (2005). *Advanced burn life support providers manual.* Chicago, IL: American Burn Association.

American Burn Association Website. (n.d.-a). *Burn center transfer criteria*. Retrieved from http://www.ameriburn.org/BurnCenterReferralCriteria.pdf

American Burn Association Website. (n.d.-b). *Burn fact sheet*. Retrieved from http://www.ameriburn.org/resources_factsheet.php

Anzarut, A., Chen, M., Shankowsky, H., & Tredget, E. E. (2005). Quality-of-life and outcome predictors following massive burn injury. *Plastic and Reconstructive Surgery, 116*, 791–797.

Apfel, L. M., Irwin, C. P., Staley, M. J., & Richard, R. L. (1994). Approaches to positioning the burn patient. In R. L. Richard & M. J. Staley (Eds.), *Burn care and rehabilitation principles and practice* (pp. 221–241). Philadelphia, PA: F. A. Davis.

Balas, M., Burke, W., Gannon, D., Cohen, M. Z., Colburn, L., Bevil, C., . . . Vasilevskis, E. E. (2013). Implementing the awakening and breathing coordination, delirium monitoring/management, and early exercise/mobility bundle into everyday care: Opportunities, challenges, lessons learned for implementing the ICU pain, agitation, and delirium guidelines. *Critical Care Medicine, 41*, 116–127. doi:10.1097/CCM.0b013e3182a17064

Barillo, D. J., Harvey, K. D., Hobbs, C. L., Mozingo, D. W., Cioffi, W. G., & Pruitt, B. A., Jr. (1997). Prospective outcome analysis for the surgical and rehabilitative management of burns to the hands. *Plastic & Reconstructive Surgery, 100*, 1442–1451.

Baxter, C., & Shire, T. (1968). Physiological response to crystalloid resuscitation of severe burn. *Annals of the New York Academy of Sciences, 150*, 874–894.

Birchenough, S. A., Gampper, T. J., & Morgan, R. F. (2008). Special considerations in the management of pediatric upper extremity and hand burns. *Journal of Craniofacial Surgery, 19*, 933–941. doi:10.1097/SCS.0b013e318175f3f6

Brumback, R., & Leech, R. (1995). Rhabdomyolysis following electrical injury. *Seminars in Neurology, 15*, 329–334.

Byers, J. F., Bridges, S., Kijek, J., & LaBorde, P. (2001). Burn patients' pain and anxiety experiences. *Journal of Burn Care & Rehabilitation, 22*, 144–149.

Clark, R. (1985). Cutaneous tissue repair basic biologic considerations. *Journal of the American Academy of Dermatology, 13*, 701–725.

Dagum, A., & Singer, A. (2008). Current management of acute cutaneous wounds. *New England Journal of Medicine, 10*, 359. doi:10.1056/NEJMra0707253

Deutsch, J. E., Borbely, M., Filler, J., Huhn, K., & Guarrera-Bowlby, P. (2008). Use of a low-cost, commercially available gaming console (Wii) for rehabilitation of an adolescent with cerebral palsy. *Physical Therapy, 88*, 1196–1207. doi:10.2522/ptj.20080062

Esselman, P. C., Askay, S. W., Carrougher, G. J., Lezotte, D. C., Holavanahalli, R. K., Magyar-Russell, G., . . . Engrav, L. H. (2007). Barriers to return to work after burn injuries. *Archives of Physical Medicine and Rehabilitation, 88*, S50–S56.

Fauerbach, J. A., Haythornthwaite, J., & Mason, S. T. (2010). Assessment of acute pain, pain relief, and pain satisfaction. In R. Melzack & D. C. Turk (Eds.), *Handbook of pain assessment*. New York, NY: Guilford Press.

Fauerbach, J. A., McKibben, J., Bienvenu, O. J., Magyar-Russell, G., Smith. M. T., Holavanahalli, R., . . . Lezotte, D. (2007). Psychological distress following a major burn injury. *Psychosomatic Medicine, 69*, 473–482.

Feldman, M. E., & Evans, J. (2008). Early management of the burned hand. *Journal of Craniofacial Surgery, 19*, 942–950. doi:10.1097/SCS.0b013e318175f38d

Fish, J. S., Musgrave, M. A., Umraw, N., Manuel, G., & Robert, C. C. (2002). The effect of silicone gel sheets on perfusion of hypertrophic burn scars. *Journal of Burn Care & Rehabilitation, 23*, 208–214.

Head, M. D. (1984). Wound and skin care. In S. V. Fisher & P. A. Helm (Eds.), *Comprehensive rehabilitation of burns* (p. 173). Baltimore, MD: Williams & Wilkins.

Helm, P., Walker, S. C., & Peyton, S. A. (1986). Return to work following hand burns. *Archives of Physical Medicine and Rehabilitation, 67*, 297–298.

Helm, P., & Walker, S. C. (1992). Return to work after burn injury. *Journal of Burn Care & Rehabilitation, 13*, 53.

Herndon, D. (Ed.). (2007). *Total burn care*. Philadelphia, PA: Saunders Elsevier.

Hildebrant, W., Herrmann, J., & Stegemann, J. (1993). Vascular adjustment and fluid reabsorption in the human forearm during elevation. *European Journal of Applied Physiology and Occupational Physiology, 66*, 397–400.

Hilsabek, T., Ronnenbaum, J., & Weir, J. (2013). Earlier mobilization decreases length of stay in the intensive care unit. *Journal of Acute Care Physical Therapy, 2*, 204–210.

Hoffman, H. G., Patterson, D. R., Carrougher, G. J., & Sharar, S. R. (2001). Effectiveness of virtual reality based pain control with multiple treatments. *Clinical Journal of Pain, 17*, 229–235.

Hoffman, H. G., Sharar, S. R., Coda, B., Everett, J. J., Ciol, M., Richards, T., & Patterson, D. R. (2004). Manipulating presence influences the magnitude of virtual reality analgesia. *Clinical Journal of Pain, 111*, 162–168.

Hoffman, H. G., Seibel, E. J., Richards, T. L., Furness, T. A., Patterson, D. R., & Sharar, S. R. (2006). Virtual reality helmet display quality influences the magnitude of virtual reality analgesia. *Clinical Journal of Pain, 7*, 843–850.

Hopkins, R. O., Spuhler, V. J., & Thomsen, G. E. (2007). Transforming ICU culture to facilitate early mobility. *Critical Care Clinics, 23*, 81–96.

Howell, J. W. (1994). Management of the burned hand. In R. L. Richard & M. J. Staley (Eds.), *Burn care and rehabilitation principles and practice* (pp. 531–575). Philadelphia, PA: Davis.

Johnson, C. L. (1994). Physical therapists as scar modifiers. *Physical Therapy*, *64*, 1383–1387.

Juckette, G., & Hartman-Adams, H. (2009). Management of keloids and hypertrophic scars. *American Family Physician*, *80*, 253–260.

Langley, P. L. (1984). Iontophoresis to aid in releasing tendon adhesions: Suggestions from the field. *Journal of Orthopaedic & Sports Physical Therapy*, *64*, 1395.

Linares, H. A. (1996). Pathophysiology of the burn scar. In D. N. Herndon (Ed.), *Total burn care* (pp. 383–397). London, England: W.B. Saunders.

Lund, T. (1999). The Everett Idris Evans memorial lecture: edema following thermal injury—An update. *Journal of Burn Care & Rehabilitation*, *20*, 445–452.

McGrouther, D. A., & Myer, M. (1991). A study relating wound tension to scare morphology in the presternal scar using langers technique. *British Journal of Plastic Surgery*, *44*, 291.

Medina, A., Savaryn, B., Shankowski, H., Shukalak, B., & Edward, E. T. (2014). Characterization of heterotopic ossification in burn patients. *Journal of Burn Care & Researchs, 35*, 251–256. doi:10.1097/BCR.0b013e3182957768

Mustoe, T. A. (2008). Evolution of silicone therapy and mechanism of action in scar management. *Aesthetic Plastic Surgery*, *32*, 82–92.

O'Brien, L., & Pandit, A. (2006). Silicon gel sheeting for preventing and treating hypertrophic and keloid scars (Review). *Cochrane Database of Systematic Reviews, 2*, CD003826.

Pigford, T., & Andrews, A. W. (2010). Feasibility and benefit of using the Nintendo Wii Fit for balance rehabilitation in an elderly patient experiencing recurrent falls. *Journal of Student Physical Therapy Research*, *2*, 12–20.

Pohlam, A. S., Pohlman, M. C., & Schwieckert, W. D. (2009). Early physical and occupational therapy in mechanically ventilated, critically ill patients: A randomized control trial. *The Lancet*, *373*, 1874–1882.

Puri, N., & Ashutosh, T. (2009). The efficacy of silicone gel for the treatment of hypertrophic scars and keloids. *Journal of Cutaneous and Aesthetic Surgery*, *2*, 104–106. doi:10.4103/0974-2077.58527

Reid, W. H. (1987). Hypertrophic scarring and pressure therapy. *Burns*, *13*, 29–32.

Richard, R., DerSarkisian, D., Miller, S. F., Johnson, R. M., & Staley, M. (1999). Directional variance in skin movement. *Journal of Burn Care & Rehabilitation*, *20*, 259–264.

Richard, R., Staley, M., Daugherty, M. B., Miller, S. F., & Warden, G. D. (1994). The wide variety of designs for dorsal hand burn splints. *Journal of Burn Care & Rehabilitation*, *15*, 275–280.

Richard, R., Staley, M., Miller, S., & Warden, G. (1997). To splint or not to splint—Past philosophy and current practice: Part III. *Journal of Burn Care & Rehabilitation*, *18*, 251–255.

Richard, R., & Ward, R. S. (2005). Splinting strategies and controversies. *Journal of Burn Care & Rehabilitation, 226*, 392–396.

Richard, R. L., & Staley, M. J. (1994). Burn patient evaluation and treatment planning. In R. L. Richard & M. J. Staley (Eds.), *Burn care and rehabilitation principles and practice* (pp. 242–321). Philadelphia, PA: F. A. Davis.

Ripper, S., Renneber, B., Landmann, C., Weigel, G., & Germann, G. (2009). Adherence to przessure garment therapy in adult burn patients. *Burns*, *35*, 657–664. doi:10.1016/j.burns.2009.01.011

Saposnik, G., Teasell, R., Mamdani, M., Hall, J., McIlroy, W., Cheung, D., . . . Research Canada (SORCan) Working Group. (2010). Effectiveness of virtual reality using Wii gaming technology in stroke rehabilitation: A pilot randomized clinical trial and proof of principle. *Stroke, 41*, 1477–1484. doi:10.1161/STROKEAHA.110.584979

Sood, R., & Archauer, B. M. (2006). *Burn surgery-reconstruction and rehabilitation*. Philadelphia, PA: Saunders Elsevier.

Tannenbaum, M. (1980). Iodine iontophoresis in reducing scar tissue. *Physical Therapy*, *60*, 792–794.

Tilley, W., McMahon, S., & Shukalak, B. (2000). Rehabilitation of the burned upper extremity. *Hand Clinics*, *16*, 303–318.

Tufaro, P. A., & Bondoc, S. (2011). Therapist's management of the burned hand. In J. Fedorzczyk, L. Osterman, & T. Skirven (Eds.), *Rehabilitation of the hand and upper extremity* (pp. 317–341). Philadelphia, PA: Mosby.

Villeco, J., Mackin, E., & Hunter, J. (2002). Edema: Therapist's management. In J. Hunter, E. Mackin, & A. Callahan (Eds.), *Rehabilitation of the hand* (5th ed., pp. 899–913). St. Louis, MO: Mosby.

Whitehead, C., & Serghio, M. (2009). A 12-year comparison of common therapeutic interventions in the burn unit. *Journal of Burn Care & Rehabilitation, 30*, 281–287. doi:10.1097/BCR.0b013e318198a2a7

Young, A. W., Wolf, S., & Dewey, S. (2010). Rehabilitation in burns. In A. Moroz, S. Flanagan, & H. Zaretsky (Eds.), *Medical aspects of disability* (pp. 89–102). New York, NY: Springer Publishing.

6

CHAPTER

The Role of Rehabilitation in Cancer Patients

Parul Jajoo and Reema Batra

INTRODUCTION

"You have cancer" is one of the most difficult statements to say as a health care professional and to hear as a patient. It is a disease that does not discriminate among young and old, rich and poor, or healthy and sick. Unfortunately, in many cases, it is silent until it is often too late. It is these characteristics that differentiate cancer from other illnesses.

Cancer is an umbrella term for a group of diseases that are caused by the uncontrolled growth and spread of abnormal cells. The proliferation of cells is unchecked, creating an imbalance between the cancer cells and healthy cells. It is the intractability of the cancer cells, which can eventually lead to the demise of the individual. The causes of most cancers are still relatively unknown, but we do understand that it can be due to both external and internal factors. External factors, some of which can be preventable include, but are not limited to, radiation exposure, cigarette smoke, and infectious organisms, whereas internal factors include inherited mutations and abnormalities of the immune system. It is certain that the development of most cancers is a multistep process that often occurs over many years.

In 2015, there were an estimated 1,658,370 new cancer cases diagnosed and 589,430 cancer deaths in the United States (American Cancer Society, 2015). In developed countries, cancer is the second leading cause of death, whereas in poorer countries, it is the third leading cause of death. As more people are living longer and adopting unhealthy lifestyle behaviors such as smoking and high-fat diets, the rates of cancer are increasing.

In the United States, cancer is the second most common cause of death preceded by heart disease. It accounts for about one in four deaths. The lifetime risk of developing cancer in the United States is more likely in men (1 in 2) as opposed to women (slightly more than 1 in 3). Lung cancer remains the leading cause of death from cancer in both males and females. The most common cancers in men and women are prostate and breast cancer, respectively (American Cancer Society, 2015).

Because of these extremely high numbers, financial support from both public and private funding has poured into research for cancer treatment, as well as prevention and screening strategies. It is this dedication to research that has changed the landscape of cancer treatment, in many cases making it a chronic disease rather than a death sentence. Five-year survival rates increased to 68% (2004–2010), up from 49% during the period from 1975 to 1977 (American Cancer Society, 2015). These statistics vary depending on cancer type, stage, and individual patient characteristics; however, the numbers do tell us that more people are living longer with modern cancer treatment than ever before.

Treatment of cancer is specific to the type of cancer, its primary location, and the extent to which it has spread throughout the body, but general principles are applied to all cancer types. Treatments generally include surgery, radiation, and chemotherapy alone or in combination, utilizing a multidisciplinary approach with the goal of achieving the most optimal results for the patient. From the time of diagnosis to the start of treatment, most patients have encountered a surgeon, radiation oncologist, a medical oncologist, and, ideally, a rehabilitation physician. A treatment plan has likely been developed, and the patient is ready to embark on a journey that will likely be physically and emotionally draining.

The therapeutic modalities that are used in cancer management have significantly changed the way cancer is viewed by the medical field and the general population. Although patient survival has increased as a result of earlier detection and newer treatment modalities, the actual treatment process can result in other medical problems such as anemia, impaired cognition, and neuropathies that can seriously compromise patients' ability to function in their everyday lives. Many of these adverse effects of treatment are often best addressed by rehabilitation specialists who are becoming increasingly recognized as vital members of the multidisciplinary team that comprehensively cares for the cancer patient.

The origin of cancer rehabilitation can be traced back to the National Cancer Act in 1971 (Goreczny, 1995), which directed funding toward this aspect of cancer treatment. This eventually led to the National Cancer Rehabilitation Conference in 1972, sponsored by the National Cancer Institute. Four objectives were developed at this conference to improve rehabilitative support to cancer patients and include psychosocial support, optimal physical functioning, vocational counseling, and optimal social functioning (Dudas & Carlson, 1988). The increasing complexity of cancer treatment, associated prolongation of survival, and medical problems associated with treatments highlighted the issues of functionality for the patient and the need to have rehabilitation become an integral part of therapeutic planning. Multiple definitions have been proposed for cancer rehabilitation. One such example is given by Mayer and O'Connor (1989), who proposed that cancer rehabilitation is a process that assists patients in optimizing functionality in their individual environments. In that sense, rehabilitation in cancer patients uses many of the same general principles as rehabilitation for other conditions, such as stroke, traumatic brain injury, and heart disease, but applies it to the specific problems associated with cancer and its associated comorbidities. These long-term problems, often referred to as survivorship issues, are best addressed by including rehabilitation specialists in the treatment team.

The current approach to rehabilitation in cancer patients addresses the scope and course of the disease as well as the diversity of problems that may arise at unpredictable times. Dietz (1981) described four phases in the rehabilitation process: prevention, restoration, support, and palliation. Preventive strategies focus on retaining the patient's physical functioning prior to the initiation of treatment and during treatment as well. Restorative strategies are used to bring patients back to their original level of functioning after the treatment. An example of this would be upper limb range of motion exercises following mastectomy or the use of a prosthetic device in a patient who has had a limb amputation for sarcoma, permitting the patient to adapt to either temporary or permanent disabilities. If a patient reaches a phase in which the goal is palliation, there may be increasing disability as the disease progresses. These goals include, but are not limited to, pain control, psychological support, and prevention of contractures and pressure ulcers secondary to inactivity.

It has been seen in the past that the utilization of rehabilitation in cancer patients has been suboptimal. In 1978, Lehmann et al. (1978) described the problems encountered by cancer patients that required rehabilitative services. They screened more than 800 patients with various cancers and found that more than 50% of the patients had medical and functional issues that could be treated with rehabilitation. Another observation was that more than 50% of the patients who were experiencing physical problems also had psychological problems. It was concluded that this population of patients would benefit from an intervention by a rehabilitation team.

Although there have been many studies that have concluded that cancer patients can benefit from rehabilitation, there is still an underutilization of rehabilitative services. This is in part due to a lack of awareness of services offered by rehabilitation specialists and an underrecognition of the fact that patients can benefit from rehabilitation interventions. This can be improved by education of nonrehabilitation clinicians with the goal of increasing awareness of the benefits of rehabilitation, thus resulting in more patients being referred for such services. Although oncological clinicians are well aware of the disabling side effects of many cancer treatments, rehabilitation practitioners are the medical specialists with specific training in the assessment and treatment of functional impairments, such as the performance of activities of daily living, mobilization in the home and community, return to work or school, as well as how to assess and address other psychosocial needs. It is important to also assess the patient's quality of life, and this can be done using well-established scales developed by the Eastern Cooperative Oncology Group and European Organization for Research and Treatment of Cancer.

BREAST CANCER

In the United States, breast cancer is ranked as the most common cancer and the second leading cause of cancer death in women (Siegel, Miller, & Jemal, 2015). It is also the leading cause of cancer death in women between the ages of 20 and 59 years. Risk factors for developing breast cancer include older age, female gender (noting that breast cancer occurs in men, but at much lower rates than women), and personal and family history of breast cancer (Siegel et al., 2015). Although breast cancer affects women of all racial groups, in the United States, its occurrence in White women has been stable but has increased slightly in Black women (0.3% per year) from 2007 to 2011 (American Cancer Society, 2015). Although the rate is lower in Black women, the incidence is much higher at younger ages and mortality is higher than in White women. This is likely due to the cancers being more aggressive in Black women and diagnosis more frequently made at a more advanced stage. Other risk factors include, but are not limited to, weight gain after 18 years of age, hormonal replacement after menopause, physical inactivity, and alcohol consumption. Recent research has found that long-term heavy smoking may increase breast cancer risk, especially if smoking started prior to the first pregnancy. Nonmodifiable risk factors include high breast tissue density, high bone mineral density, diabetes type 2, high doses of radiation to the chest, long menstrual history (i.e., start early, end late), never having been pregnant, or having the first child after 30 years of age. An important risk factor to consider is family history and the presence of BRCA1 or BRACA2 genes, which significantly increase the risk of breast cancer in carriers as much as 65% and 47%, respectively (American Cancer Society, 2015).

Treatment options for breast cancer vary widely depending on the stage of the disease and tumor characteristics. Treatment modalities used are surgery, radiation therapy, chemotherapy, and hormonal therapy. In recent years, there has been much advancement in breast cancer therapy, resulting in improvements in survival rates.

Surgery is usually the first step in the treatment of breast cancer, unless patients have very large tumors, in which case they are offered neoadjuvant therapy, which is a medication or treatment given prior to surgery, or unless they have metastatic disease, wherein they are started on systemic chemotherapy. The type of surgery that is performed for a patient is usually a decision made by the breast surgeon, often in consultation with the medical oncologist and radiation specialist. The most common surgeries are breast conservation therapy (BCT), often referred to as lumpectomy, and mastectomy.

With BCT, the breast tumor is removed along with a small amount of the surrounding normal tissue. This is then typically followed by radiation therapy to the area. The combination of BCT and radiation therapy has been compared with mastectomy alone, with the results indicating similar outcomes with regard to patient survival (Fisher et al., 2002). For early-stage disease, sentinel lymph nodes are biopsied, meaning that only the first likely lymph nodes to which the cancer could have spread are removed. This decreases postoperative complications such as lymphedema, and survival rates are equally comparable with those of full axillary node dissection, in which all the lymph nodes in the axilla are removed (American Cancer Society, 2015). The complications that patients can experience after BCT and radiation treatment include infection, fluid collection at the incision site, rib fracture, shortness of breath, and secondary cancers. Cosmetic outcomes after BCT are usually good to excellent, using modern surgical techniques. Some factors that may influence the cosmetic outcome include the amount of breast tissue removed, patient variability such as breast size, and timing of adjuvant chemotherapy and radiation.

Although there has been a shift toward BCT, mastectomies are still performed in the United States. This procedure is usually performed if the size of the tumor is very large or if the location of the tumor makes a BCT difficult. Many times, the patient herself may opt for a mastectomy, even if a BCT is feasible; this often occurs when the patient has a fear of the cancer coming back. There are two types of mastectomies: the modified radical mastectomy (MRM) and the simple mastectomy.

MRM is removal of the tumor from the breast, the normal breast tissue surrounding the tumor, some of the chest wall tissue underlying the breast, and the nodes in the axilla. Often, an axillary lymph node dissection is performed, especially if there is concern for spread of the cancer. A simple mastectomy is the entire removal of the breast tissue without the axillary nodes, and no muscles are removed from beneath the breast. A sentinel node biopsy is performed during the procedure, and if the results are positive intraoperatively for metastatic cancer, the patient has a more extensive axillary lymph node dissection. Skin-sparing mastectomies have fallen out of favor secondary to the possibility of cancer recurrence, although nipple-sparing mastectomies are now used.

Many women opt for breast reconstruction after a mastectomy. This can be done immediately after the mastectomy or after other cancer treatments have completed. There are now many options for reconstruction, and women should consult with a plastic surgeon prior to the initial surgery to discuss which option is best for them.

Although mastectomies are relatively safe procedures, complications can occur. The more common ones are postoperative bleeding and/or hematomas, seromas, wound infection, and lymphedema. Depending on the stage of the cancer, the characteristics of the tumor found, and the type of surgery performed, chemotherapy and radiation may be used to decrease the chance of recurrence. Radiation is definitively performed if the patient has BCT, ensuring that cancer cells that may have been left behind in the breast tissue are eradicated and local control of the tumor is optimized. Radiation can also be used after mastectomy; it is usually recommended in patients who have a larger tumor or if there are more than four lymph nodes positive with cancer. Chemotherapy and hormonal therapy are also possible treatments for breast cancer. Again, the choice and duration of treatment depends largely on the tumor characteristics, such as hormone receptor positivity and the human epidermal growth factor receptor 2, or HER2/neu, status. It also depends on the stage of the tumor at diagnosis. The side effects of common chemotherapy medications are discussed elsewhere in the chapter.

Patients with primary or recurrent breast cancer can have shoulder and arm pain as well as lymphedema. The pain that is experienced includes phantom breast pain, neuroma pain, or neuralgia. Pain can extend to the neck, axilla, or chest wall. There is often a loss of shoulder function that occurs after mastectomy, lumpectomy, axillary lymph node dissection, or reconstruction. Exercise in cancer patients has numerous benefits that include decreased fatigue, increase of lean body mass, improved cardiovascular function, decreased depression, and increased range of motion.

Rehabilitation exercises for breast cancer are often prescribed with consideration of the type of surgery that was performed. If patients have a radical mastectomy or axillary lymph node dissection, they are discharged from the hospital within a day. It is necessary to instruct the patient on how to incorporate shoulder range of motion activities with a home exercise program, often accompanied by a list of illustrated exercises. This typically will include wall-walking exercises to improve flexibility in the shoulder. The patient stands about 2 feet from a wall, raises her arm to shoulder level and "climbs" her fingers up the wall, holds for a few seconds, and descends back to shoulder level. Shoulder roll exercises can also be implemented, which include standing with arms at the side of the body, moving shoulders forward and shrugging them up, and moving them backward; the patient can repeat this five times in a slow circular action. Isometric exercises can be started by using elastic bands that are differentiated by color, depending on the resistance they provide. The patient can gradually advance to isotonic exercises, which strengthen the muscle by moving the joint. Postsurgical shoulder mobilization should be gradual, with consideration of the number of days after the operation. The shoulder can be subjected to internal and external rotations as much as the patient can tolerate, starting the first postoperative day. At postoperative days 1 to 3, the patient can typically flex and abduct the shoulder up to 40° to –45°, and at postoperative days 4 to 6, the patient can advance to flex the shoulder 45° to 90° and abduct it up to 45° (Braddom, 2011). One week after surgery, the shoulder can typically be ranged based on the tolerance of the patient.

Axillary web syndrome can be seen after axillary node dissection. It is a cordlike tissue visualized within the axilla that can develop months or years after the operation. These palpable cords can extend all the way below the elbow. This can occur with a sudden increase in activity after a period of decreased range of motion. Treatment plans for axillary web syndrome should include heat, manipulation, and gradual range of motion.

Lymphedema

Lymphedema is the blockage of lymph vessels that causes increased fluid retention in the tissues. The most common cause of secondary lymphedema is surgery or radiation for breast cancer. It is also seen following treatments in cancer of the prostate, bladder, uterus, ovaries, and skin (O'Sullivan & Schmitz, 2013). The role of the lymphatic system is to transport fluid that contains proteins, large molecules, and fat. The lymphatic system reacts to cells that the body recognizes as foreign, such as the cancer cell, and produces white blood cells. Lymph nodes are a part of the immune system through which most of the lymph fluid enters the venous system.

Lymphedema occurs when the lymph load exceeds the transportation capacity of the lymph system. A dilation of lymph vessels occurs, causing valve incompetence. This fluid is filled with protein and can attract bacteria resulting in infection. These infections can cause thrombosis and clotting of the lymph vessels. Lymphedema is classified as primary and secondary. Primary lymphedema is caused by dysplasia of the lymph vessels and typically affects the extremities as a result of abnormal lymph drainage (Bellini & Hennekam, 2014). Secondary lymphedema is more common than primary, and it is due to a blockage of the lymph system that can occur after surgery or cancer treatment, such as radiation.

In the initial diagnosis of lymphedema, one can find several features such as swelling distal to the blockage of flow within the lymph system, usually not relieved by elevation, feeling of tightness, numbness and tingling, fibrotic changes of the dermis, increased chance of infection, impaired wound healing, and decreased range of motion (O'Sullivan & Schmitz, 2013). Other causes of swelling that may not be due to lymphedema are trauma, cellulitis, malignancy, complex regional pain syndrome, and deep vein thrombosis (DVT).

Lymphedema can be treated with conservative therapy. Pneumatic pumps, machines that are attached to sleeves and applied over edematous limbs, are often used. They inflate to create pressure and then deflate to promote lymph to flow in a distal-to-proximal direction, thus decreasing edema in the affected limb. Other conservative therapies, including intense physical therapy, manual lymphatic drainage, and laser therapy result in greater volume reductions in the edematous limb compared to compression garment wear, exercise, and elevation (Moseley, Carati, & Piller, 2007).

In metastatic disease, the goals for rehabilitation professionals should include attaining tolerable pain relief, allowing the patient to perform activities of daily living as independently as possible, maintaining energy levels needed for safe mobilization within their environment, and maintaining bone mineral density.

HEAD AND NECK CANCER

Head and neck cancer is not as common as some other types of cancers, but the treatment of this disease requires a prudent multidisciplinary approach, and often the patient is referred for rehabilitation because of the effects of surgery and radiation. The annual incidence of these cancers is over 40,000 persons in the United States, and it has significantly declined over the last 30 years because of the decrease in the use of tobacco (Siegel et al., 2015; Sikora, Toniolo, & DeLacure, 2004). The cancer is more frequently seen in men, but women with risk factors are susceptible to the disease.

There are many causes of head and neck cancer, but the strongest associations are tobacco, alcohol, and human papillomavirus (Smith, Rubenstein, Haugen, Hamsikova, & Turek 2010), and the risk is higher in people who combine smoking and drinking. Other risk factors include radiation exposure, occupational exposure to inhaled dust and asbestos, and genetic susceptibility.

Head and neck cancer is a general term for a variety of subtypes of cancers that are classified according to the origin of the tumor. Head and neck cancer is usually classified into six categories: oral cavity, pharynx, larynx, nasal cavity, paranasal sinuses, and salivary glands. The treatment of head and neck cancer can become quite complicated due to the number of cancer subtypes, the anatomical complexity of the head and neck region, and the need to maintain quality of life and ensure organ preservation. After treatment of the cancer, many patients find themselves working on their quality of life, undergoing rehabilitation and restoration of speech and/or swallowing.

The modalities most often used in the treatment of head and neck cancer are surgery, radiation, and systemic chemotherapy. Approximately one third of the patients present in early-stage disease, and, in general, either surgery or radiation can result in a cure. The choice between the two modalities depends largely on the patient's comorbidities, desired functional outcomes, and accessibility of the surgery. If surgery is performed, adjuvant radiation may be needed if tumor cells are identified at the margins of the resected tissue, if there is bone erosion, or if nearby lymph nodes contain cancer cells. In select cases, patients may also benefit from adjuvant chemotherapy, depending on whether they have the anticipated ability to tolerate such treatment, given the high incidence of adverse reactions to such treatment regimens.

When the cancer is more advanced but not yet metastatic, the treatment is not as straightforward. Many tumors are not resectable at this stage without first receiving chemotherapy and/or radiation that shrinks the tumor, potentially making surgical removal a viable option. When a patient is found to have metastatic disease, meaning cancer has spread to other body parts, the only modality that is used is chemotherapy. At this stage, the cancer is not curable and the goal of treatment is control of the spread of the disease and palliation.

The side effects of the treatment of head and neck cancer largely depend on the modalities used. There are several chemotherapy medications that are used, and their side effects are discussed elsewhere in the chapter. Radiation therapy can have both acute and long-term sequelae, and these occur largely because of the loss of parenchymal cells. The most common acute side effects of radiation are mucositis (inflammation of the digestive tract), odynophagia (pain with swallowing), hoarseness, xerostomia (dry mouth), dermatitis (inflammation of the skin), and weight loss. These complications typically resolve as new cells replace those that are lost following the completion of treatment. These side effects can vary and largely depend on the type of tumor being treated and patient-related factors, such as cigarette use and comorbid conditions. It is important to be aware of these potential side effects and to initiate preventive measures and/or prompt treatment when they occur, as the consequences often are so severe that they can delay treatment and ultimately affect the patient's outcome.

One of the more important preventable measures is encouraging smoking cessation once the patient begins treatment. Other than being a known cause of head and neck cancer, it can make the side effects of radiation more pronounced, even after treatment is completed. Patients should also be instructed on appropriate skin care to prevent or decrease the risk of radiation-induced dermatitis. Measures include avoidance of ultraviolet (UV) rays, wind exposure, lotions, creams, and fragrances in order to minimize irritation by chemicals.

Unfortunately, late effects can also occur in these patients after radiation. This is usually the result of injury to the stromal elements or the supportive structures of skin. Some of the more common side effects include permanent xerostomia, osteoradionecrosis of the jaw, radiation-induced fibrosis, chronic pain, airway edema requiring tracheostomy placement, and hypothyroidism.

Surgery is an integral part of the treatment of head and neck cancer, and if a patient's tumor is deemed to be completely resectable, that is often the treatment of choice if the patient is a good surgical candidate. The goal of surgical resection is to achieve a cure without compromising organ function and cosmetic outcome, both of which ultimately affect quality of life. Cancers diagnosed in their early stages can often be completely resected with low potential of organ compromise and without the need for adjuvant treatments. However, as the tumor grows and expands, surgical options become more limited and, if utilized, will often require the addition of chemotherapy and/or radiation to achieve the most beneficial outcome. There are many surgical options when it comes to head and neck cancer, and the procedure that is selected for the patient largely depends on the location and size of the tumor. Again, the more advanced cancers are usually treated with chemotherapy, radiation, or a combination of both prior to attempting a surgical resection.

Speech and Swallowing in the Head and Neck Cancer Patient

There are several phases of swallowing described according to the route the bolus of food or liquid travels after entering the mouth. These phases are not necessarily isolated from each other and may happen at the same time (Delisa & Frontera, 2010). The beginning phases are the oral preparatory and propulsive phases that occur in the oral cavity and include the preparation of the bolus prior to being swallowed. During this phase, food is chewed and moistened with saliva that helps break down food as the mouth sequentially opens and closes. At the end of this phase, when the bolus is prepared, the tongue moves up and pushes the bolus of the food into the oropharynx, initiating the pharyngeal phase. The tongue pushes the bolus and, at the same time, the epiglottis covers the trachea. The food moves from the larynx through the pharyngoesophageal sphincter and into the esophagus, beginning the last phase. The bolus travels through the esophagus and into the stomach via the gastroesophageal sphincter.

Head and neck cancer can affect any or all of these stages as well as cause speech impairments, shoulder dysfunction, neck weakness, and disfigurement, which can lead to depression. If a patient has a glossectomy (tongue removal), there is a risk of aspiration and a need for a prosthesis for the palate. A laryngectomy or radiation to the area may call for communication aids such as an electrolarynx.

Head and neck cancers can lead to impaired ability to swallow, a condition known as dysphagia. If left unaddressed, dysphagia increases the risk of food or liquid being propelled into the airways, which can cause aspiration pneumonia. A common strategy to address dysphagia is to modify diet consistency, which is often, although not always, achieved by thickening liquids and providing food consistency that easily forms into a solid bolus, thus decreasing the risk of aspiration. Specific exercises can be prescribed that strengthen oral musculature to prevent food exiting from the oral cavity. This should include techniques to exercise the tongue, such as isometric lingual exercises, which include compressing an air-filled bulb with the tip or posterior aspect of the tongue, exercising the posterior pharynx by placing the tongue on the upper teeth and pushing hard as you swallow and exercising the larynx by speaking loudly (Braddom, 2011). Patients should also learn how to eat using the chin tuck method. This involves sitting up straight and flexing the neck by placing the chin toward the chest when swallowing to prevent aspiration.

Patients who suffer from head and neck cancer must be evaluated for nutritional needs. This may include the consideration of surgically inserting a feeding tube directly into the stomach or small intestine if adequate nutrition and hydration cannot be achieved by oral intake alone. Radiation treatment may significantly reduce saliva production, thus requiring increased fluid intake and diet changes such as switching to soft consistency foods. The reduction of saliva can damage dental enamel as well; this can be prevented by the use of special toothpastes that increase saliva production.

Some head and neck cancer patients may have rehabilitation needs related to spinal accessory nerve palsy, cervical soft tissue contracture, and dysphonia, which is difficulty in speaking (Braddom, 2011). Spinal accessory nerve palsy occurs less often because radical neck dissections are falling out of favor as compared with functional dissections. Functional dissections spare the muscles, nerves, and veins of the neck. If the spinal accessory nerve is compromised, one must consider the use of rehabilitation techniques to stabilize the scapula. The spinal accessory nerve provides innervation to the trapezius muscle. If compromised by cancer treatment, spinal accessory neuropathy results in scapular winging, shoulder weakness, and restricted shoulder range of motion. In some cases, this may result in frozen shoulder, which is severely restricted range of motion that limits the use of the affected arm in addition to decreased flexibility of the chest wall. It is important to strengthen muscles that stabilize the scapula and maintain shoulder range of motion, which may include heating modalities such as ultrasound.

Cervical contractures can occur in patients who receive external beam radiation. Aggressive active and passive range of motion should be implemented during and after the radiation therapy. The patient should be given a home exercise program that includes stretching and self-massage. If left untreated, radiation-induced fibrosis can occur that results in a head-forward posture and thoracic kyphosis. Botulinum toxin can be injected in severe cases to increase cervical spine range of motion.

Head and neck cancer treatment can cause aphonia (the inability to produce voice) and dysphonia due to damaged vocal cords. This can be extremely debilitating for the patients. Patients can be taught other sources of communication such as writing, mouthing their words, or using gesturing. Following a laryngectomy, several options are available to patients such as an artificial larynx, esophageal speech, or tracheal esophageal puncture. The latter is a voice restoration procedure that involves the placement of a valve permitting air to pass into the esophagus and close off the trachea (Delisa & Frontera, 2010). Some patients do not prefer this and choose an electrolarynx. This device senses vibrations; however, the sound can be monotonous and "robotic."

MUSCULOSKELETAL CANCERS

The most common tumors afflicting the musculoskeletal system are sarcomas. These are rare tumors that can arise from any area of the mesenchymal system. However, mesenchymal cells have the capacity to mature into striated muscle, bone, cartilage, soft tissue, and adipose tissue, and the treatment of these cancers often can leave the patient with a new disability and/or a suboptimal cosmetic outcome. Therefore, even though these tumors are rare, the rehabilitation needs are high.

The biological behaviors of these tumors are varied, from indolent to aggressive, and this is largely dependent on the specific histology of the tumor cells. The tumors can affect the soft tissues, bones, and peripheral nerves. Because of the wide array of tumors that present under the sarcoma classification and the relative rarity of these tumors, there is less understanding of their biology and responsiveness to treatment. Multimodality treatment is often used, including surgery, radiation, and chemotherapy; the choice of treatment often depends on tumor location and stage. It is important to workup all patients with an unexplained deep mass of soft tissues, superficial lesions of soft tissue having a diameter of more than 5 cm, or soft tissue masses arising in childhood (Casali & Blay, 2010). In many cases, surgical resection is utilized, however, leaving patients with a functional deficit that is best addressed by rehabilitation specialists.

Rehabilitation for musculoskeletal cancers, including sarcomas, ideally begins prior to treatments and surgeries. This gives an opportunity to educate the family and patient about the goals of rehabilitation that include increasing strength and endurance as well as a means to promote safe mobility, ideally including ambulation.

Some cancers of the limb can be treated with limb-sparing surgeries. Immediate postoperative care for these patients includes rest for wound healing to decrease edema and maintain alignment of the limb and joint. Occasionally, muscles are resected and splints and orthotics can be used to compensate for lost function. Along with adaptive equipment to assist in activities of daily living, such as larger-handled utensils for eating or reachers for grabbing garments so patients can dress themselves, immediate passive range of motion is important, with particular attention paid to any restrictions imposed by the surgical technique. If a limb-sparing procedure is not feasible and an amputation is required, the length of the residual limb is dictated by the location of the tumor, which will impact rehabilitation and ultimate prosthetic prescription. If the residual limb is very short, has postoperative edema, or has a surgical wound that heals slowly, there may be a delay in fitting an upper or lower extremity prosthesis. With limb amputations, the health care professional should be watchful for the development of phantom pain, which is pain of the amputated part of the limb. Phantom sensation is a sensation that the amputated portion of the limb is still present but not perceived as painful by the patient. Residual limb pain is pain in the remaining limb. All of these conditions can be treated by the physician with various medications and other techniques.

Cancers of the trunk can result in splinting on the side of the surgery. This should be discouraged and early ambulation should be encouraged. The etiology of swelling in lower extremity cancers needs to be carefully determined, as proper treatment depends on an accurate diagnosis. Swollen limbs that appear red and tender to touch, particularly in the setting of fever and elevated white blood cell count, may be due to cellulitis and can be treated with antibiotics. A DVT or blood clot causes limb swelling but is also tender. Diagnosis is most often made with duplex ultrasound testing and may require treatment with blood-thinning medications that prevent propagation of the clot and/or insertion of a filter in the inferior vena cava that prevents the clot from traveling to the lung where it could cause a fatal pulmonary embolus. Lymphedema results in a swollen limb and at times is associated with decreased range of motion, requiring many of the treatment modalities previously described for this condition, including physical therapy.

Bone Metastases

Metastasis to the bone is a frequent complication in patients with advanced cancer. There is a focus on patients with breast and prostate cancer because of the frequency of bone metastases in these conditions. At postmortem examination, about 70% of the patients with these cancers have metastatic disease (Coleman, 2006). There are many consequences of metastasis to the bone, some common ones being severe pain, fractures, spinal cord compression, and hypercalcemia.

Bone lesions are usually classified as osteolytic or osteoblastic. Osteolytic bone lesions result from the destruction of bone, whereas osteoblastic lesions result from deposits of new bone. Patients can have one or the other type of lesion, but many patients can have characteristics of both. The common denominator of the two types of processes is that they result from an interruption of normal bone remodeling.

Patients are suspected of having bone metastasis when they present with symptoms resulting from a bone lesion. The specific diagnostic test ordered is based on the patient's symptoms. For example, a patient may experience pain in a certain area that negatively impacts the ability to perform daily activities. These symptoms would prompt the practitioner to evaluate the area with a radiological exam, usually an x-ray. Bone scans, which are nuclear medicine examinations, are helpful if bone metastases are strongly suspected even when standard x-rays fail to reveal an abnormal finding. This is because bone scans detect the lesions at earlier stages before they become apparent on standard x-rays. However, bone scans detect osteoblastic lesions better than osteolytic lesions; thus, the latter may go undetected if other diagnostic tests are not used, such as MRI and CT scans.

Spinal cord compression is another consequence of bone metastasis, but this is discussed later in the chapter. Hypercalcemia, an increase in serum calcium levels, results from an increased bone resorption and a release of calcium from the bone. This can be seen with metastasis to the bone in Stage 4 cancers. For example, when breast cancer metastasizes to the bone, the dominant lesion is osteolytic (Kim, Park, & Chung, 2015). This can result in neuropsychiatric abnormalities, gastrointestinal disturbances, renal dysfunction, and cardiac conduction abnormalities.

The treatment of bone metastasis focuses largely on the improvement of the patient's quality of life and activities of daily living. Chemotherapy and/or hormonal therapy can be used if the patient is still a candidate based on the performance status and organ function. The goals of palliative treatment in these patients are elimination of pain, preservation of skeletal integrity, and functional maintenance. One method of palliation is radiation therapy, most commonly provided by external beam radiation. This is best used when the lesions are limited to a certain number of sites, rather than in diffuse disease. External beam radiation remains the gold standard for the treatment of bone metastases and comprises the largest single component of palliative radiation therapy practice (Fairchild, 2014). Between 50% and 80% of patients gain at least partial relief of their pain following external beam radiotherapy, and complete relief may be seen in up to one third of those treated. External beam radiotherapy may be delivered to the same anatomic site of affected bone in the case of recurrent pain (Lutz & Chow, 2012).

Cancer in the bones can cause pain, fractures, and hypercalcemia and, when present in the spine, can possibly compress the spinal cord, resulting in permanent neurological damage. Bisphosphonates and the more recently approved denosumab are drugs that reduce the osteoclastic activity that reabsorb bone (Wong, Stockler, & Pavlakis, 2012).

An important issue with bony metastasis is stability and pain control. The greater the amount of cortex that is affected, the greater the risk of fractures. A risk for a fracture occurring can be a lower limb long bone lesion measuring more than 2.5 cm that involves more than 50% of the bony cortex.

A scoring system known as Mirel's encompasses four characteristics and assigns numbers to each item in the categories.

1. The site of the lesion: upper limb (1), lower limb (2), pertrochanteric (3)
2. The nature of the lesion: blastic (1), mixed (2), lytic (3)
3. The size of the lesion, a fraction of the cortical thickness: <1/3 (1), 1/3 to 2/3 (2), >2/3 (3)
4. Pain: mild (1), moderate (2), functional (3)

Based on the score, a recommendation for or against prophylactic fixation is given. A prophylactic fixation is recommended for a lesion with a score of 9 or greater; a lesion with a score of 7 or less can be managed with radiation and medication. If the lesion is an 8, the probability of a fracture is 15% and it is recommended that the physician decides what is best (Delisa & Frontera, 2010).

CENTRAL NERVOUS SYSTEM TUMORS

Central nervous system (CNS) tumors either arise from various cells within the CNS or are metastatic from another primary cancer. Because of these differing etiologies, CNS tumors can behave differently, and hence, the treatment and prognosis vary widely. The symptoms of CNS tumors are numerous. They are usually caused by local invasion into the brain and spinal cord by the tumor itself, compression of vital structures, and increased intracranial pressure caused by edema and inflammation.

CNS Metastases

Brain metastases occur in about 25% of all cancer patients (Saha, Ghosh, & Chhaya, 2013). Lung cancer accounts for approximately one half of all brain metastases, with other common cancers including renal cell carcinoma, melanoma, breast cancer, and colorectal cancer (Khuntia, 2015). The incidence of brain metastasis is increasing and is thought to be partially due to longer survival rates of patients and new imaging modalities that detect smaller cancers.

About a century ago, Paget described the "seed and soil" hypothesis, which says that brain metastases are not random but are due to certain tumor cells: "the seed" having an attraction for the environment, "the soil." The two stages of the development of metastatic disease are the migration of the tumor cells from the primary tumor to distant tissues and then the colonization of these tumor cells in their new location (Gazanfar, Toms, & Weil, 2012). Many metastatic tumors in the brain are found in watershed areas, noting that about 80% are located in the cerebral hemispheres, with the remaining in the cerebellum and brainstem.

Clinically, the symptoms vary depending on the location and the size of the tumor, as well as the surrounding edema associated with it. Because of the variability of the location of the metastases, the signs and symptoms can vary widely from patient to patient. The most common complaint is headache with or without associated nausea and vomiting, but patients can also present with focal neurological abnormalities, seizures, and cognitive dysfunction. Stroke is also a possibility, due to either hemorrhage into the tumor site or invasion or compression of a vessel from a tumor.

The management of brain metastases is usually tailored to the patient's overall prognosis. This is largely dependent on the patient's performance status, age, and extent of the primary tumor. Patients with the best prognosis have a median survival of about 7 months, whereas those with the worst prognosis have a median survival of about 2 months. If a patient has a good overall prognosis, the treatment is tailored to eradicate the brain metastases. Surgical resection is an option if the tumor location is favorable, is easy to access, there are only a limited number of lesions, and resection is not likely to result in significant functional deficits. Whole brain radiation is also recommended after the surgery to decrease the local recurrence risk. Treatment of patients with a poor prognosis is focused on the control of symptoms and maintenance of quality of life and neurological functioning. Whole brain radiation is the first line of treatment in these patients to achieve a quick relief of symptoms. Systemic chemotherapy can be used, but this is usually after radiation and surgery have not provided the desired results and the goal is for palliation only.

The treatment of the brain metastases can cause complications themselves. Current evidence supports the use of whole brain radiation when patients present with multiple metastases. However, there can be cognitive impairments and whole brain radiation should not be considered in patients who may live longer than 6 months (Lin & DeAngelis, 2015). When patients receive whole brain radiation therapy, they are at risk of both acute and long-term complications. Acute toxicities include cerebral edema, nausea, vomiting, encephalopathy, dermatitis, alopecia, and myelosuppression. More chronic problems are brain atrophy, neurocognitive dysfunction, radiation necrosis at the site of the tumor, and neuroendocrine disease. Acute toxicities are usually self-limiting, but chronic side effects can be addressed with supportive care and rehabilitative interventions. Supportive measures may include corticosteroids to control edema and anticonvulsants for seizure control.

Primary CNS Tumors

Primary brain tumors arise from different cells in the CNS, thereby creating a diverse group of tumors. Both malignant and nonmalignant tumors have an average incidence of about 7.25 per 100,000 persons (Central Brain Tumor Registry of the United States, 2014). In adults, the most common primary brain tumors are gliomas, as they make up more than 80% of these cancers. They arise from the glial cells and can be further classified as astrocytomas, anaplastic astrocytomas, and gliomas. Some other primary CNS tumors that are seen are meningiomas, pituitary tumors, lymphomas, and oligodendrogliomas. Unfortunately, even though primary CNS tumors are rare, an estimated 137,700 deaths were secondary to primary malignant brain and CNS tumors in 2015 (Central Brain Tumor Registry of the United States, 2014). The treatment for malignant gliomas and the other types of malignant brain tumors utilizes a multimodality approach to maximize the outcome of the patient. This includes, when safe, optimal surgical resection combined with adjuvant chemotherapy and/or radiation. As noted earlier, these modalities are associated with side effects, often requiring the utilization of rehabilitative efforts to positively impact the patient's quality of life.

Hydrocephalus can occur as a result of brain tumors. The classic triad of urinary incontinence, gait imbalance, and dementia seen in normal pressure hydrocephalus may be present, although in many instances, a patient may be observed to decline in function or to simply stop progressing in therapy. Tumors close to the third and fourth ventricles can obstruct the flow of cerebral spinal fluid resulting in noncommunicating hydrocephalus. Other complications include cerebral edema caused by abnormal blood vessel formation that disrupts the blood–brain barrier allowing plasma to leak into the interstitial space. Another cause of edema is cell death resulting in lost function as well as seizures. One major cause of death is uncontrolled brain edema resulting in herniation, which occurs in more than 60% of the patients with glioblastomas (Fanz, Seham, Rauh, & Eyupoglu, 2014). Depending on the type of tumor and treatments received, hemiplegia may occur, similar to what is observed following stroke. In this instance, it is important to implement aggressive rehabilitative therapies to improve the patient's ability to function as independently as possible and preserve range of motion of the weakened limbs.

Primary or metastatic brain tumors can also cause cognitive deficits. After surgical resection and subsequent relief of pressure over a particular cerebral area, cognitive function may be restored. It is important to involve speech therapy, occupational therapy, and neuropsychology in the treatment of cognitive deficits. It should be noted, however, that cognitive decline may occur if tumors cannot be surgically resected.

The goals and ultimate plan of cancer rehabilitation are guided by multiple factors, including, but not limited to, the specific physical and cognitive impairments encountered as well as the anticipated life expectancy and clinical course of the patient. Patients who have a more favorable long-term prognosis and preserved capacity to improve their functional skills should receive an aggressive course of rehabilitation. But even for patients with poorer prognoses, rehabilitation remains an important component of care in order to prevent the development of pressure ulcers, preserve joint range of motion, provide customized adaptive equipment to maintain as much independence as possible, preserve cognitive skills, and achieve relief from pain.

PERIPHERAL NERVOUS SYSTEM ONCOLOGICAL ISSUES

Patients with cancer can present with impairment related to injury of the peripheral nervous system (PNS). This can be related to the cancer, such as paraneoplastic syndromes, or to treatment, such as chemotherapy-induced peripheral neuropathy. Other factors that influence the functioning of the PNS are metabolic derangements, poor nutrition, and comorbid conditions. These neurological impairments can cause disabilities in the cancer patient that ultimately affect the quality of life.

Brachial plexopathy can occur 1 month to several years after radiation treatment directed in the proximity of the axilla. Management includes positioning the upper limb with orthoses to stabilize and improve function of joints. Range of motion exercises and physical therapy are aimed at decreasing the risk of contractures and increasing strength. Medication management must be considered for neuropathic pain, such as gabapentin or amitriptyline at night. Surgical treatments are rarely used but may include neurolysis and repairing the nerve. In severe cases, tendon or nerve grafting and transfer can be implemented (Braddom, 2011).

Paraneoplastic neurological disorders are a group of neurological disorders that rarely occur in patients with cancer. Although they do not result from metastases to the PNS, they occur from a tumor-induced autoimmune response that is directed at the nervous system. Among the most common manifestations of a paraneoplastic syndrome is myasthenia gravis that is seen in up to 40% of the patients with thymoma. Lambert-Eaton myasthenic syndrome is a similar syndrome, occurring in up to 3% of the patients with small-cell carcinoma of the lung (Sharp & Vernino, 2012).

Because most of the syndromes are immune mediated, many of the treatments focus on immune suppression and treatment of the tumor itself. For example, patients with Lambert-Eaton syndrome and myasthenia gravis are treated with intravenous immunoglobulin, which is an infusion of antibodies, or plasma exchange; both treatments can suppress the immune response and improve neurological status in the short term. If patients do not improve, it may be that the damage is irreversible at the time the treatment is instituted.

CHEMOTHERAPY

Chemotherapy is often used as the first line of treatment for advanced disease (Braddom, 2011). Although it is an effective mainstay of treatment, it is often associated with a wide array of neurological side effects that arise either directly from medication-related toxicity or indirectly from its manifestations on the metabolic system. The most common drugs to cause neurotoxicity are the platinum compounds, although many others can also be responsible.

Cisplatin, commonly used in the treatment of lung, head, and neck cancers, is known to cause peripheral neuropathy and ototoxicity. The neuropathy is largely axonal and affects myelinated sensory fibers. The patient usually begins to feel numbness, paresthesia, and sometimes pain, typically beginning distally in the toes and fingers that progresses proximally in the legs and arms as the condition worsens. This side effect is dose dependent, as most patients can tolerate doses up to 400 mg/m^2, but this varies from patient to patient. Once the patient develops neuropathy, there are some treatments to help with the symptoms. Medications such as neurontin help alleviate neuropathic pain. Patients with mild neuropathy can continue chemotherapy, but those with more disabling symptoms will need to have a discussion with their oncologist regarding the risks and benefits of continuing treatment. Discontinuing chemotherapy generally reverses the condition, although many patients may not recover fully.

Carboplatin is a drug similar to cisplatin, but the side effects of neuropathy are generally not seen when using standard doses. However, when very high doses are used for hematopoietic stem cell transplant, patients can experience a severe neuropathy. Oxaliplatin, another platinum compound used in the treatment of colorectal cancer, is associated with two types of neurotoxicity: an acute neurosensory complex, which can occur during the first few infusions of the drug, and a cumulative sensory neuropathy, which is associated with distal loss of sensation. Many preventive dosing and other treatment options for oxaliplatin induced neuropathy are available, including stopping and reintroducing the medication, prolonging the infusion time, and administering various pharmacological agents.

Other chemotherapeutic drugs that can cause neurological side effects are the vinca alkaloids, the most common being vincristine. This antineoplastic agent is widely used, and its dose-limiting toxicity is an axonal neuropathy. Patients generally have symptoms that are synonymous with diabetic neuropathy. Taxanes used as a first-lined treatment of primary breast, ovarian, and lung cancers are antimicrotubule agents that can also cause peripheral neuropathy, usually affecting the sensory fibers. The manifestations usually involve burning paresthesias of the hands and feet. Paclitaxel, a compound from the taxane family, can also cause a motor neuropathy affecting the proximal muscles. Docetaxel can also cause motor and sensory neuropathies, but these side effects are usually much less than with paclitaxel. Docetaxel can also cause fatigue in a cancer patient (Minaxi Jhawar, February 2016, personal communication).

CANCER FATIGUE

Fatigue is a common problem seen in cancer patients. It is defined by the National Comprehensive Cancer Network (NCCN) as "distressing, persistent, subjective sense of physical, emotional, and/or cognitive tiredness or exhaustion related to cancer or cancer treatment that is not proportional to recent activity and interferes with usual functioning" (NCCN, 2014). This can be associated with many causes, including a side effect of treatment, anemia, pain, emotional distress, and nutritional deficiencies. More recent studies have shown that the timing of fatigue in cancer is not related to hemoglobin levels; therefore treating low hemoglobin may not help the fatigue (Braddom, 2011). The NCCN encourages a multimodal approach that includes energy conservation, exercise, acupuncture, massage therapy, psychological intervention, and nutrition consults (2014).

Fatigue has an impact on the quality of life and cognitive tasks, which adversely affects the patient and the caregiver. Caregivers may erroneously interpret complaints of fatigue by the patient as evidence that they are giving up. Therefore, they should be instructed that it may be a symptom of their condition and treatment, rather than a manifestation of apathy or despair. Other causes of fatigue should be considered such as hypothyroidism and infection (Dy & Apostol, 2010).

Sexual dysfunction is a notable side effect of several types of cancers and their associated treatments, and this is common in musculoskeletal cancers. Chemotherapy can cause a decrease in testosterone production, which decreases libido, whereas radiation therapy can cause fibrosis of the mucus epithelium that can decrease lubrication to the vagina. In addition to specific medical intervention, counseling should be part of the treatment process with both the patient and partner, which should include encouragement to express alternative means of intimacy.

CANCER PAIN

Cancer patients experience pain that is often left untreated. The etiology of cancer-related pain is multifactorial, including, but not limited to, the tumor itself, bony metastases, or effects of the treatment, which can be due to nociceptive and/or neuropathic mechanisms (Robb, Williams, Duviver, & Newham, 2006).

Pain in spinal cord injury secondary to metastases to the spinal cord can be due to nociceptive pain and/or neuropathic pain. Nociceptive pain may arise from sprains, fractures, or other injuries. Symptoms for nociceptive pain include a localized, constant aching or throbbing pain. Nociceptive pain can also be due to instability of the spine, muscle spasms, and pain secondary to overuse. Nociceptive pain can be treated with nonsteroidal anti-inflammatory medication and spasticity treated with antispasticity medications. In neuropathic pain, trauma and neural alterations of the pain pathways can occur.

Root avulsion can also occur, creating a burning sensation to the area that is denervated. This often occurs with metastasis to the spine. Pain below the level of injury can be called central dysesthesia. This pain is constant and is described as a burning sensation with numbness and tingling. This is often treated with neuropathic pain medication and possibly epidural steroid injections. When discussing treatment options, one should consider the type of pain the patient is experiencing and the appropriate long-term goal.

Pain can also be due to neuropathic pain that is secondary to chemotherapy. Postsurgical pain can occur secondary to organ removal. It is important to know the type of pain being treated, secondary to the cancer, to develop a proper treatment plan. The goal of treatment should be to improve function and create a sense of independence so that patients can deal with their illness in a positive manner. It is important to control pain when it is acute and severe because inadequate analgesia increases the likelihood of developing chronic pain. The pain should be controlled after surgery and during chemotherapy and radiation. A balance of interventional, pharmacological, behavioral, and rehabilitation therapy is an optimal means to address pain.

Oral medications can be considered first, which can be prescribed by using the World Health Organization (WHO) guidelines. This was developed specifically for pain secondary to cancer. If a patient has bone metastasis, the best treatment is a nonsteroidal anti-inflammatory agent. This is the first suggested medication to use per the WHO pain ladder. This step also includes adjuvant medication, such as antiepileptics, for neuropathic pain that can be caused by chemotherapy or plexopathies secondary to radiation therapy. The second step includes a mild opioid, if the first step did not adequately control the patient's pain. The third step can be a strong opioid, if necessary. Prior to this, one can use interventional therapies to help with oral medications (WHO, 1990), for example, epidural injections or continuous epidural catheter infusions and neurolytic agents can also be used (phenol or alcohol) to help with thoracic pain secondary to thoracotomy or transforaminal injections into the lower thoracic foramen to help with thoracic pain (Burton, Fanciullo, Beasley, & Fisch, 2007). Radiofrequency ablation has recently been used to decrease pain caused by bone metastasis. This is a thermal destruction of the sensory nerve fibers and possibly delays tumor progression to the periosteum. Pathological fractures can be treated with vertebroplasty or balloon kyphoplasty, essentially placing cement into the compressed vertebrae to stabilize it.

Celiac plexus blocks can be used for most of the organs in the abdomen, excluding the liver. A block of the plexus can stop nociception from the visceral organs, and this eventually reduces or stops pain originating from that area. If a patient is on chronic opioids, has adverse side effects to the medication, and has a life expectancy of more than 3 months, an intrathecal pump can be inserted to deliver medications such as morphine.

SUMMARY

As cancer treatments become more advanced and patients start to live longer, the need for rehabilitation interventions becomes more apparent as patients begin to return to their daily lives and activities. It is imperative that practitioners who encounter cancer patients make assessments of their functional outcomes during and after cancer treatment. Although many survivors will eventually seek help to integrate back into the community, patients with poor prognoses can also benefit from rehabilitative services to improve their quality of life and palliation from the cancer and its treatment effects. Our goal as practitioners is ultimately to help patients feel more comfortable and provide the means to have an optimal functioning to live through cancer, from diagnosis through treatment and to recovery. Early and ongoing intervention from the rehabilitation team can make an important positive impact on function and outcomes.

REFERENCES

American Cancer Society. (2015). *Cancer facts and figures 2015*. Atlanta, Georgia: American Cancer Society. Retrieved from http://www.cancer.org

Bellini, C., & Hennekam, R. C. (2014). Clinical disorders of primary malfunctioning of the lymphatic system. In H.-W. Korf, F. Clascá, J.-P. Timmermans, P. Sutovsky, B. Singh, & T. M. Böckers (Eds.), *Advances in anatomy, embryology and cell biology* (pp. 187–188). New York, NY: Springer Publishing.

Braddom, R. L. (2011). *Physical medicine and rehabilitation*. St. Louis, MO: Elsevier Health Sciences.

Burton, A. W., Fanciullo, G. J., Beasley, R. D., & Fisch, M. J. (2007). Chronic pain in the cancer survivor: A new frontier. *Pain Medicine*, *8*, 189–198.

Casali, P. G., & Blay, J., (2010). Soft tissue sarcomas: ESMO clinical practice guidelines for diagnosis, treatment and follow up. *Annals of Oncology, 21*, 198–203.

Central Brain Tumor Registry of the United States. (2014). *CBTRUS statistical report*. Hinsdale, IL.

Coleman, R. (2006). Clinical features of metastatic bone disease and risk of skeletal morbidity. *Clinical Cancer Research*, *12*, 6243.

Delisa, J., & Frontera, W. (2010). *Delisa's physical medicine and rehabilitation: Principles and practice*. Philadelphia, PA: Lippincott Williams & Wilkins.

Dietz, J. H. (1981). *Rehabilitation oncology*. Somerset, NJ: John Wiley & Sons.

Dudas, S., & Carlson, C. E. (1988). Cancer rehabilitation. *Oncology Nursing Forum, 15*, 183–188.

Dy, S., & Apostol, C. (2010). Evidence-based approaches to other symptoms in advanced cancer. *The Cancer Journal*, *16*, 5.

Fairchild, A. (2014). Palliative radiotherapy for bone metastases from lung cancer: Evidence-based medicine? *World Journal of Clinical Oncology*, *5*(5), 845–857.

Fanz, Z., Seham, T., Rauh, M., & Eyupoglu, I. Y. (2014). Dexamethasone alleviates tumor-associated brain damage and angiogenesis. *PLOS ONE, 9*(4), e93264.

Fisher, B., Anderson, S., Bryant, J., Margolese, R. G., Deutsch, M., Fisher, E. R., . . . Wolmark, N. (2002). Twenty-year follow-up of a randomized trial comparing total mastectomy, lumpectomy, and lumpectomy plus irradiation for the treatment of breast cancer. *New England Journal of Medicine, 347*, 1233–1241.

Gazanfar, R., Toms, S., & Weil, R. (2012). The molecular biology of brain metastasis. *Journal of Oncology*, *2012*, 1–16.

Goreczny, A. J. (1995). *Handbook of health and rehabilitation psychology*. New York, NY: Springer Publishing.

Khuntia, D. (2015). Contemporart review of the management of brain metastasis with radiation. *Advances in Neuroscience, 2015*, 1–13.

Kim, H., Park, K., & Chung, W. (2015). Abstract 1543: Wogonin suppresses the production of breast cancer-derived osteolytic factors. *Cancer Research, 75*, 1543.

Lehmann, J. F., DeLisa, J. A., Warren, C. G., deLateur, B. J., Bryant, P. L., & Nicholson, C. G. (1978). Cancer rehabilitation: Assessment of need, development, and evaluation of a model of care. *Archives of Physical Medicine and Rehabilitation, 59*, 410–419.

Lin, X., & DeAngelis, L. (2015, August 17). Treatment of brain metastases. *Journal of Clinical Oncology, 33*, 3475–3484.

Lutz, S., & Chow, E. (2012). Areview of recently published radiotherapy treatment guidelines for bone metastases: Contrasts or convergence. *Journal of Bone Oncology, 1*, 18–23.

Mayer, D., & O'Connor, L. (1989). Rehabilitation of persons with cancer: An ONS position statement. *Oncology Nursing Forum, 16*, 433.

Moseley, A. L., Carati, C. J., & Piller N. B. (2007). A systemic review of common conservative therapies for arm lymphedema secondary to breast cancer treatment. *Annals of Oncology, 18*, 639–646.

National Comprehensive Cancer Network. (2014). Practice guidelines in oncology: Cancer-related fatigue. Retrieved from http://www.nccn.org

O'Sullivan, S. B., & Schmitz, T. J. (2013). *Physical rehabilitation* (pp. 588–589). Philadelphia, PA: F. A. Davis.

Robb, K. A., Williams, J. E., Duvivier, V., & Newham, D. J. (2006). A pain management program for chronic cancer-treatment-related pain. *Journal of Pain, 7*, 82–90.

Saha, A., Ghosh, S., & Chhaya, R. (2013). Demographic and clinical profile of patients with brain metastases: A retrospective study. *Asian Journal of Neurosurgery, 8*(3), 157–162.

Sharp, L., & Vernino, S. (2012). Paraneoplatic neuromuscular disorders. *Muscle and Nerve, 46*, 841–850.

Siegel, R., Miller, K., & Jemal, A. (2015). Cancer statistics, 2015. *CA: A Cancer Journal for Clinicians, 65*(1), 5–29.

Sikora, A. G., Toniolo, P., & DeLacure, M. D. (2004). The changing demographics of head and neck squamous cell carcinoma in the United States. *Laryngoscope, 114*, 1915–1923.

Smith, E. M., Rubenstein, L. M., Haugen, T. H., Hamsikova, E., & Turek, L. P. (2010). Tobacco and alcohol use increases the risk of both HPV-associated and HPV-independent head and neck cancers. *Cancer Causes & Control, 21*(9), 1369–1378.

Wong, M., Stockler, M., & Pavlakis, N. (2012). *Bisphosphonates and other bone agents for breast cancer*. Hoboken, NJ: John Wiley & Sons.

World Health Organization. (1990). *Cancer pain relief and palliative care*. Geneva, Switzerland: Author.

CHAPTER

Cardiovascular Disorders

Jonathan H. Whiteson and Gregory Sweeney

Cardiovascular disorders constituted a major health epidemic in the 20th century and will continue to do so in the 21st century also unless effective measures are taken to control or eliminate this epidemic. In the United States, and in most other industrialized countries, nearly one third of all deaths are now caused by cardiovascular diseases (CVDs)—killing one person every 40 seconds. In countries of the developing world, CVDs presently account for a quarter of all deaths, and this fraction will increase with increasing economic development and urbanization. It is estimated that CVD will be the major killer in the world by the year 2030, accounting for close to 24 million deaths annually (Mozaffarian, Benjamin, & Go, 2015). As the deaths from infectious diseases decrease, the unhealthy lifestyles of Western society will spread across the globe and will result in a greater relative mortality from cardiovascular disorders. Moreover, by the year 2050, about 70% of the world's population will be urbanized (United Nations, Department of Economic and Social Affairs, Population Division, 2014) and the prevalence of these disorders will increase not only in relative but also in absolute terms.

CVDs also represent the most common cause of disability in the United States. The American Heart Association (AHA), in 2015, estimated that there were 85.6 million people in the United States who had one or more forms of CVD. In the same year, there were an additionally estimated 73 million Americans afflicted with at least one cardiovascular risk factor for CVD. The presence of the disease, its intervention, and its determinant factors often result in physical impairments and limitations of activities of daily life. Every year in the United States, about 1 million Americans survive an acute major cardiac event or undergo a cardiac intervention. About 635,000 Americans suffer their first heart attack each year, with an additional 300,000 having a recurrent attack. In 2010, it was estimated that there were 7.6 million cardiovascular operations and procedures, an almost 30% increase over the previous 10 years. Every year, a significant percentage of individuals having either a cardiac event or a cardiac procedure will develop either physical or psychological disabilities or both.

In the United States, at present, there are about 6 million Americans who have symptoms of CVD—which can be major causes of disability by themselves. In the past decade, heart failure (HF), a condition with many symptoms, shortness of breath being the most common, became the most common diagnosis upon discharge from U.S. hospitals. The ever-growing prevalence of chronic atrial fibrillation, and its main symptom of palpitations, is on the rise as the average age of the American population increases and a greater number of individuals live beyond the age of 80 years. Such is the magnitude of the continuing cardiac disease epidemic that it is rare to find an American family that is not affected by its mortality and morbidity. Cardiovascular disorders still constitute the major health challenge to all providers of rehabilitative, physical, psychological, and vocational services. Therefore, it is imperative for all health care professionals to acquire a comprehensive understanding of the cardiovascular system and its diseases.

CARDIOVASCULAR DISORDERS

Cardiovascular disorders are those that affect the heart and the vascular system. By structural and functional criteria (or by anatomy and physiology), the heart has five components: the coronary arteries, the pericardium, the myocardium, the endocardium, and the electrical conduction system.

The Coronary Arteries

The coronary arteries are deemed to be the most important blood vessels in the body because they supply blood to the heart itself. Without normal coronary blood flow, the heart cannot carry out its function of supplying blood to the rest of the body. There are two coronary arteries: the left coronary artery and the right coronary artery. The left coronary vessel, after a short main segment, bifurcates. One of the branches is the left anterior descending coronary artery, which brings blood to the septum (the muscle between the two ventricles) and to the anterior wall of the left ventricle; the other branch is the circumflex coronary artery and is the vessel that supplies blood to the right ventricle and to the inferior wall of the left ventricle. The right coronary artery does not bifurcate and supplies blood mainly to the right ventricle. Although there are minor variations in the coronary artery network, the blood supply system is fairly similar among humans. The main variation is that in any one individual, the blood supply to the posterior wall of the left ventricle can originate from either the left circumflex artery or the right coronary artery, or from both (Figure 7.1).

Cardiovascular disorders, resulting from primary disease of the coronary arteries, are the single leading cause of death in the United States today. The cause of this coronary heart disease (CHD) can be best described as a "biopsychosocial failure"—as has already been mentioned. It is this complex constellation of biological, psychological, and social factors that has resulted in the epidemic of CHD. The risk factors for coronary atherosclerosis are abnormal blood lipids (cholesterol), high blood pressure, cigarette smoking, diabetes, obesity, and a sedentary but stressful life style. Depression has been determined to be a separate and independent risk factor. These risk factors, alone or in multiple combinations, create the initial lesion of CHD, the atherosclerotic plaque, or atheroma. Researchers have learned that the progression of atherosclerosis is a lifelong process, beginning early in life as a fatty streak in the coronary arteries and progressing to an occlusive fibrous atherosclerotic plaque. The inflammatory pathological process is one in which the endothelium, the single-cell lining of the inner surface of the coronary arteries, becomes structurally or functionally damaged. The risk factors directly or indirectly release inflammatory cytokines and other toxic enzymes that result in endothelial dysfunction. Once this endothelial barrier is altered, there is deposition of fats, calcium, and amorphous debris inside the arterial wall, which results in the development of plaques.

Eventually, the atherosclerotic plaques create rigid arterial walls and lead to progressive narrowing of the arteries, which is termed as *coronary stenosis*. Once the coronary vessel has a 70% stenosis

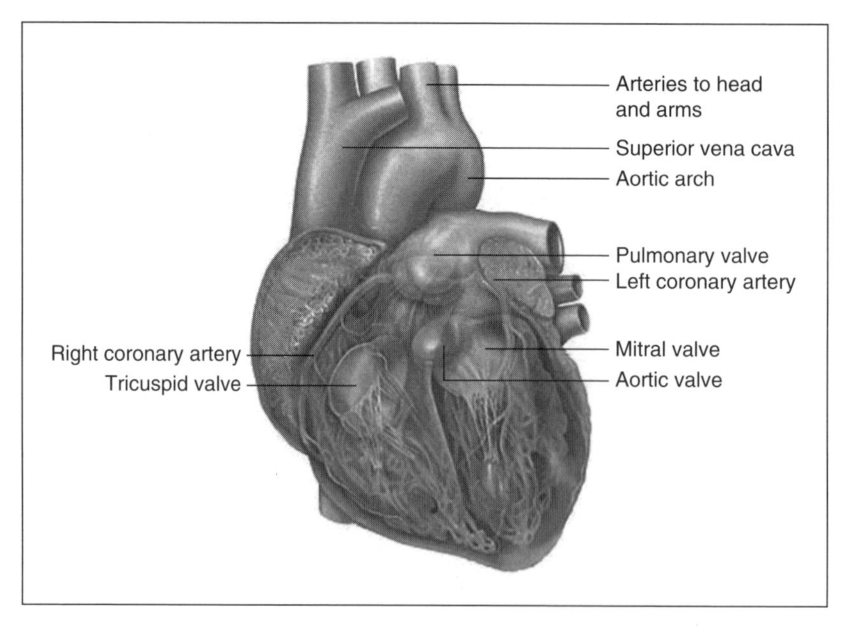

FIGURE 7.1 Interior structures of the heart.
Source: Image located at www.ynhh.org/cardiac2/heart

of the coronary artery lumen, there is reduced blood flow that may still meet the metabolic needs of the heart while that individual is in a state of rest. However, during exercise, such a narrowing can no longer allow an increase in blood flow to meet the heart tissue's increased metabolic and oxygen needs that occur with activity. Such an imbalance between oxygen demand and supply, which results in the metabolic derangement of heart cells, is called myocardial ischemia. Therefore, this type of coronary artery disease (CAD) is also known as ischemic heart disease.

Moreover, the atherosclerotic plaque is an unstable structure that can easily become damaged. At the site of an ulcerated or fissured plaque, there is a tendency to form a clot, or thrombus, and to have arterial spasm. Alone or in combination, thrombus and spasm lead to more severe stenosis and, at times, to a total or 100% occlusion of the artery. This complete cessation of all blood flow to the segment of heart muscle supplied by that artery results in the death of that muscle segment or to a heart attack or myocardial infarction (MI). An understanding of the clinical presentations of CHD must be based on this understanding of atheroma pathophysiology.

Factors that help establish the risk of this inflammatory atherosclerotic process are circulating inflammatory biomarkers that have been identified in the blood of patients with ischemic heart disease. One of the most studied inflammatory biomarkers is the high-sensitivity C-reactive protein (hs-CRP) (Rossouw et al., 2008). Numerous clinical studies have shown that measuring systemic CRP levels provides a significant clinical prognostic value in screening and identifying apparently healthy people as people with stable and unstable angina. Studies demonstrate that people with higher hs-CRP levels are on average at a higher risk of adverse cardiovascular events. This is supported with other research demonstrating that apparently healthy people who had low levels (<130 mg/dL) of the "bad" low-density lipoprotein (LDL) cholesterol but had elevated levels (>2 mg/L) of hs-CRP levels—who were treated with statin, a cholesterol-lowering agent—had a significant relative risk reduction in the incidence of unstable angina, need for coronary revascularization, and a confirmed death from cardiovascular causes (Ridker et al., 2008). Research continues into other emerging risk biomarkers of CVDs (Upadhyay, 2015). Despite this area of research, controversy remains as to whether the inflammatory biomarkers have a role in plaque formation and growth and in acute coronary artery atherosclerosis syndromes, or whether they are just predictive biomarkers of the presence of CAD and its clinical complications.

Ischemic chest pain, or angina pectoris, is one cardiac symptom in cardiac patients who have relatively slowly progressing—or "stable"—atheromas that result in coronary narrowing to more than 70% but less than a total occlusion. Other symptoms include shortness of breath—this may be the predominant or only symptom in women—nausea, sweating, and profound fatigue or weakness. Angina pectoris is described as a visceral pain because it is usually felt deeply, rather than superficially, in the chest. The angina sufferer describes the discomfort as squeezing, pressing, or crushing or as heaviness or a dull ache. Angina is usually felt in the midchest or the sternal area. It often radiates to the left arm or the jaw. It is brought on by physical exertion or by mental stress. It is relieved by the cessation of the activity that caused it. Angina usually lasts less than 5 minutes. Patients with this typical pattern are said to have the clinical syndrome of stable angina. It is estimated that at any given time, there are about 9.1 million Americans with angina pectoris (Bittner, 2008). Angina that occurs at rest, without obvious provocation, or with less effort than usual, is unstable angina. This syndrome is usually a manifestation of an unstable atheroma, which has a superimposed thrombus and spasm that has caused further acute stenosis of the coronary artery. When such unstable angina is severe in intensity or sustained in duration, it is termed preinfarction angina. It may be an indication that a 100% coronary artery occlusion is taking place. If there is total blood flow cessation for 30 minutes or more, the usual consequence is death to the segment of heart muscle supplied by the occluded artery. This muscle death is an MI, popularly known as a heart attack. The main presenting symptom of an acute MI is angina that is much more severe in intensity and that lasts for a much longer time than the typical episode of stable angina syndrome. The pain often occurs in the context of generalized symptoms such as weakness, sweating, and anxiety.

Women may be more likely to present with atypical or subtler symptoms during an acute coronary event. Although women probably experience chest pain as an acute coronary symptom as often as men, they may complain less of chest pain and be more likely than men to report neck, jaw, or back pain alone. Therefore, it can be more difficult to diagnose an MI in women than in men. Women's symptoms are not as predictable as those of men and they may appear approximately a month before the acute event occurs (Stramba-Badiale et al., 2006). In about two thirds of the cases, the initial presentation of ischemic heart disease in women may be an acute MI or a sudden cardiac death (SCD). A National Institutes of Health–sponsored research study of 515 women diagnosed with acute MI on hospitalization at five different medical centers revealed that prodromal symptoms had occurred frequently 4 to 6 months before the event. Ninety-five percent of the women reported experiencing various warning signals approximately a month before the acute event. In some of the cases, the women reported ignoring their own symptoms; in others, they sought medical assistance only to have their symptoms minimized, misdiagnosed, or ignored. The most common acute symptoms were as follows: shortness of breath, weakness, and fatigue. Notably, less than one third reported having chest pain or discomfort immediately prior to their heart attack and nearly one half reported no chest pain during any phase of the event (McSweeney et al., 2003).

During an evolving MI, many persons have a sense of impending doom and they feel they are going to die. Contrary to popular misinformation, MIs are seldom a result of physical activity. They nearly always strike at rest and often during the early morning hours, shortly after awakening. The timing of the event reflects its pathophysiology. MIs are not a consequence of myocardial demand of exercise outstripping a compromised blood supply but are caused by the sudden thrombus formation on an unstable atheroma, which then totally occludes the atherosclerotic coronary artery. In 2010, the National Center for Health Statistics reported 1,141,000 hospitalizations for primary or secondary diagnosis of an acute coronary syndrome (ACS), 322,000 for unstable angina, and 813,000 for MI. The American College of Cardiology (ACC) and the AHA have national guidelines for the clinical care of various cardiac diagnoses, and the most recent guidelines have been updated in 2015 (Mozaffarian et al., 2015). A greater emphasis has been placed on the earlier access to medical evaluation of ACSs that include unstable angina, non-ST elevation myocardial infarction (NSTEMI), and ST elevation myocardial infarction (STEMI).

Faster community emergency medical service (EMS) response time and facilitated emergency department triage of ACS have been enabled by the use of sensitive cardiac biomarkers of necrosis, such as troponins, and of emerging cardiac imaging diagnostics such as cardiac magnetic resonance imaging and coronary computed tomographic angiography. Clinical trials have further defined the best practices of initial medical or surgical interventions in patients presenting with ACS. The guidelines recommend that upon hospital discharge, patients who have been diagnosed with ACS should be prescribed the following medication regimen: aspirin (unless contraindicated), clopidogrel (Plavix), beta-blockers, angiotensin-converting enzyme inhibitors (ACEIs) or angiotensin receptor blockers if intolerant of ACEIs, and statins. In hospitalized MI patients, the use of acute thrombolytic (clot-dissolving) therapy and beta-receptor blockers has drastically reduced both the in-hospital death rate and the 1-year death rate to less than 10% for treated patients. Unfortunately, about 60% of all deaths from an acute infarction occur within 1 hour after the onset of symptoms—one half of all MI victims die before they reach the hospital and before they can receive the benefits of these new therapies. Yearly, approximately 600,000 Americans have MIs, and in spite of all these recent advances, these acute MIs still account for 15% of all deaths in the United States every year (Mozaffarian et al., 2015).

SCD is best defined as an unexpected demise with a lack of warning symptoms or prodromes. About 80% of victims of sudden death have CHD. Sudden death is usually the result of a lethal ventricular rhythm disturbance—ventricular fibrillation (VF) or ventricular tachycardia (VT)—that has its origin in the unstable electrical milieu of heart muscle cells that are affected by ischemia or that are adjacent to an area of scar caused by a prior MI. Some persons are fortunate to have the benefit of prompt cardiopulmonary resuscitation within a few minutes of being stricken. They are said to be sudden death survivors. Their long-term prognosis is poor, with a 50% chance of a subsequent fatal event within a year or 2. It is estimated that there are about 326,000 SCDs in the United States yearly (Mozaffarian et al., 2015). They account for about 50% of all the deaths from CVD. In those at significant risk for VF or VT, implantable cardioverter-defibrillators (ICDs) have been shown to decrease the frequency of sudden electrical cardiac death. An ICD is a specialized device placed in the chest wall and connected to the heart muscle like a pacemaker that detects abnormal heart rhythms and delivers an electrical shock directly to the heart to restore normal heart rhythm. The use of external defibrillators in public places such as restaurants, airports, and train and bus stations has also significantly reduced the impact of SCD in the community. In addition, the emergence of the wearable cardioverter-defibrillator (WCD) has provided a prophylactic tool for patients who are at significant risk for SCD but are not immediate candidates for ICD placement.

Silent myocardial ischemia implies that the cardiac muscle can be ischemic or infarcted without any symptoms. Silent ischemia can be detected by EKG changes in 24-hour ambulatory recordings by Holter monitors and is described in the findings of the Framingham study and other investigations that show that as many as 20% to 25% of all MIs are silent (Valensi et al., 2011). Such individuals with silent ischemia and infarction can have as their first presentation an SCD. They can also present with an ischemic cardiomyopathy where the heart muscle has suffered small multiple silent infarctions and no longer pumps efficiently. Their symptoms will be those of HF. Silent myocardial ischemia is a major component of the total ischemic burden for patients with CAD. It is estimated that approximately 2 to 3 million persons with stable CAD have evidence of silent ischemia. Approximately 40% of the patients with ischemic heart disease have acute episodes of myocardial ischemia during their lifetime, and 75% of these episodes cause no symptoms and are considered "silent." The management of silent ischemia should be directed to reduce or eliminate myocardial ischemia by risk factor modification, aggressive medical therapy, and, if deemed needed, myocardial revascularization.

Every year in the United States, over 1 million men in the total male population older than 30 years manifest symptomatic CHD for the first time. About 40% present with angina pectoris, another 40% with an acute MI, and 10% have sudden death as their first and the only symptom. In the remaining 10%, the first symptoms are those of HF, palpitations, or syncope, the sudden loss of consciousness. Coronary atherosclerosis and its clinical syndromes affect just as many women as men. Although the prevalence of CVD is not higher among women (33.9%) when compared with the total population (34.2%), more women than men die of CVD (52% of CVD deaths). The percentage of deaths caused by CVD is highest for White (39.8%) and African American (39.6%) women followed by Asian (35.8%), Hispanic or Latino (32%), and Native American (24.5%) women. CAD was the cause of half of all CVD deaths among women, and stroke was responsible for 20%. One in four women have some form of CVD and almost 6 million have a history of MI, angina pectoris, or both. Out of these, approximately 3 million have a history of MI and these women are at higher risk than men for HF. In 2008, it was estimated that 2.6 million women were living with HF. With current treatments, there is a 50% survival rate at 5 years. On average, however, women experience their clinical CHD 10 years later than men do. For example, women in their 60s have an incidence of coronary syndromes similar to that of men in their 50s. This is because of the loss of the protective effect of the female hormones, mainly estrogens, the production of which is greatly decreased at the onset of menopause (Eastwood & Doering, 2005).

There has been much interest in the use of hormone replacement therapy (HRT) to reduce the risk of CVD in postmenopausal women. Data supporting cardioprotective benefits of HRT are controversial, and other research indicates an increased risk for CHD with HRT (Grodstein, Clarkson, & Manson, 2003). Current recommendations are that HRT not be used for the primary or secondary prevention of CHD (Rossouw et al., 2007). In women felt to be at low risk for CHD with menopausal symptoms, the use of HRT can be considered for relief of those symptoms (ACOG Committee on Gynecologic Practice, 2013, June). Duration of HRT must be made on a case-by-case basis.

Function and Disability

The major determinant of impaired function and disability in CHD is angina. Coronary artery atherosclerosis is not a stable condition. For a myriad of reasons, the tonicity of the muscles in the vessel wall varies during any given time interval and so does the severity of coronary artery stenosis. Thus, an individual patient's angina pattern may have minor weekly, and even daily, variations in severity, frequency, and the level of exertion needed to provoke it. Nonetheless, a patient with a stable angina syndrome usually has a predictable functional impairment. That is, a similar number of blocks walked on a level surface or on an incline, a similar number of flights of stairs climbed, and a similar weight lifted or carried will reproducibly result in the same intensity and duration of angina pectoris. The functional impairment and disability can be best determined based on a careful history, which is unique for each individual. On the basis of this unique individual history, medical therapy can be instituted, referral to surgical intervention can be made, and rehabilitation protocols can be carried out. The estimated functional capacity and subsequent disability of an individual with angina can be confirmed by exercise stress testing. Exercise tests, whether performed on a treadmill or on a bicycle, approximate the exertion of normal activities of daily living. The goal of all stress testing is to increase the work of the heart and its muscle oxygen demand by increasing the exerciser's heart rate (HR) and systolic blood pressure. The HR should increase in proportion to how hard the heart must work to circulate blood during the exercise. The age-adjusted peak HR, 220 minus the patient's age, can be used to estimate the predicted peak HR. For example, the exercise peak HR of a 40-year-old is 180 beats per minute and that of a 60-year-old is 160 beats per minute. The actual peak HR attained during the exercise test should be used to formulate the target HR and prescribe exercise. The systolic blood pressure should rise about 60 mm from the rest level to the peak exercise level, and the diastolic blood pressure should drop slightly or remain unchanged. The increasing HRs and blood pressures are achieved by increasing the workload. On a treadmill, workload is increased by a progressively faster speed and higher incline, and on a bicycle, by gradual greater pedal resistance.

The most widely used treadmill protocol for establishing functional capacity, as well as diagnosis and prognosis, is the Bruce protocol. Typically, patients undergo an exercise stress test evaluation before and after their cardiac rehabilitation program (CRP). For those with HF, or concomitant lung disease or marked symptoms of shortness of breath, a gas-exchange metabolic evaluation (cardiopulmonary exercise testing) is performed. Other less intense exercise stress testing protocols exist, as well as testing modalities, such as a bike, and clinical judgement is used to select the protocol that will generate significant and accurate data. At least 6 minutes of exercise time is the goal of each stress test. Heart-imaging techniques used in conjunction with exercise, such as nuclear myocardial perfusion agents, nuclear ventriculograms, and echocardiography, have independent values in establishing diagnosis and prognosis and give insightful understanding of the anatomical and physiological basis for an individual's exercise tolerance and functional capacity. Whenever possible, as determined by the information gained by a medical history, a physical exam, and an exercise stress test, the functional capacity of the individual with heart disease should be described according to the classification system of the New York Heart Association (NYHA). This system establishes four functional classes, which are as follows: Class I, asymptomatic at ordinary effort level, symptoms with moderate effort; Class II, symptomatic with ordinary effort; Class III, symptomatic with minimal effort; Class IV, symptomatic at rest (no effort). This traditional functional classification is useful because it provides a common language and point of reference for all health care professionals.

■ Treatment and Prognosis

The definite and ultimate treatment of CAD is the radical correction of the biopsychosocial failure that is at its root. Primary prevention (i.e., before any clinical event has taken place) of CHD should be the main mission of all health care professionals and can be accomplished by the reduction or elimination of all of the risk factors for atherosclerosis (Mosca et al., 2007). An elevated serum cholesterol level is considered by some investigators to be the primary culprit in atherosclerosis. Some families have an autosomal dominant genetic condition called familial hypercholesterolemia. Patients who are homozygous for the gene have serum cholesterol levels as high as 1,000 mg/dL and have severe coronary and peripheral atherosclerosis during childhood and adolescence. Heterozygous individuals have a serum cholesterol level that ranges from 300 to 500 mg/dL. They also have premature and severe atherosclerosis. Homozygous individuals are only about one in a million and heterozygous only about two in a million of the U.S. population, however. Thus, the atherosclerosis epidemic is not the result of an unalterable genetic disorder but is the consequence of an atherogenic lifestyle that can be altered. It has been shown that chronic mental and emotional stress can elevate cholesterol. Numerous epidemiological and population studies, human trials of dietary intervention, and experimental animal investigations have shown the high causative correlation between an elevated serum cholesterol and atherosclerosis.

Cholesterol can be lowered below the recommended 200 mg/dL by weight loss and by reducing the consumption of saturated fats from animal sources. High-density lipoprotein (HDL) has a vascular protective effect by scooping up circulating cholesterol and bringing it to the liver for degradation. HDL cholesterol can be raised by frequent aerobic exercise. Although some research has suggested that judicious moderate alcohol consumption might benefit HDL levels, this is not recommended. Hypertension can be improved by weight loss, exercise, a diet low in salt, and stress management. When these lifestyle measures are not successful, or while they are being undertaken, if blood pressure remains significantly elevated, control of the elevated blood pressure with medication is indicated. The majority of individuals can attain target blood pressure control by a combination of interventions.

Most adult-onset diabetic patients have metabolic disease because of obesity. Weight reduction significantly lowers serum glucose levels in these patients even to normal levels. It is still controversial whether obesity by itself is an independent risk factor. There can be no argument, however, that obesity has a causative relation with all of the atherosclerotic risk factors except with smoking. The smoking of cigarettes doubles the risk of CHD. Beyond being a causative factor for atherosclerosis, it may constitute an additional separate risk for MI. The reduction of risk for infarction is 50% within 1 year after smoking cessation. Multiple studies have shown that exercise, through many mechanisms, results in reduced atherosclerosis and in a lower risk of clinical events if atherosclerosis is already present. CHD, however, is usually first treated with medication. The medical therapy of stable angina pectoris is based on an understanding of its pathophysiological basis: ischemia from an increased metabolic demand that cannot be met by a fixed supply.

Pharmaceutical intervention has as its goal the reduction or prevention of that ischemia through two main pharmacological means: an increased supply of blood to the heart muscle and a decreased demand of the heart muscle for that blood. These desired effects are accomplished by the three principal classes of cardiac pharmaceutical agents: nitrates, beta-receptor blockers, and calcium channel blockers. Nitrates are vasodilators. They exert their beneficial effects by dilating coronary arteries directly, thus increasing blood flow to the heart muscle. They also dilate peripheral veins, resulting in the peripheral pooling of blood, with a subsequent reduction in blood return to the heart, less stress on the heart wall, and finally a decreased need for oxygen. Beta-receptor blockers reduce oxygen demand by lowering the HR (or chronotropy) and are termed negative chronotropic agents. Calcium channel blockers combine the effects of nitrates and beta-blockers. Most of the available calcium channel blocker agents have both vasodilatory and chronotropic effects. Most patients with a stable angina pectoris syndrome can have their angina controlled and their functional impairment and disability eradicated with the use of one of these agents alone or with some combination or all three. Unless a contraindication exists, patients with CHD and also perhaps asymptomatic individuals with atherosclerosis risk factors should take low-dose prophylactic daily aspirin.

Patients with unstable angina pectoris require immediate hospitalization as they are at risk for an acute infarction. The treatment is based on its pathophysiologic basis: an unstable atherosclerotic plaque that creates a substrate for new thrombus and artery spasm, which, in turn, may result in total vessel occlusion and heart muscle death. Treatment with intravenous heparin is directed at the inhibition of further thrombus formation. The treatment with intravenous nitrates aims to reduce and prevent arterial spasm. Patients with an acute MI should receive immediate intravenous thrombolytic therapy with either streptokinase or tissue plasminogen activator. Promptly dissolving the occluding thrombus results in a restoration of blood flow. If this is done within the first hour or two after the onset of symptoms, there is considerable myocardial salvage. The earlier these agents are administered, the greater is the rescue of heart muscle and the patient's chance of survival. The nonmedical therapy of CHD is percutaneous coronary intervention (PCI) and coronary artery bypass graft (CABG). About an equal number of these procedures are now performed in the United States yearly. In PCI, a balloon-tipped catheter is introduced through a peripheral artery and then manipulated around the aortic arch and inserted into the coronary artery that has the occluding atheroma. The balloon inflation causes an increase of the overall vessel diameter and increased blood flow by the process of atheroma fracture and compression and by stretching of the vessel wall. The initial success rate is now more than 90%, but restenosis occurs at a rate of about 25% within 1 year of the procedure. The development of stents, cylindrical rigid metal devices that are placed within a coronary artery at the site of an angioplasty, has decreased the frequency of restenosis after percutaneous transluminal coronary angioplasty (PTCA).

PCI, developed about 30 years ago, improves the quality of life by relieving angina in patients with stable CAD and can be lifesaving in patients with extensive ischemia and ACSs. The safety of the PCI procedures has been enhanced significantly by the use of adjunctive pharmacotherapy, most importantly, antithrombotic and antiplatelet agents (Brar & Stone, 2009). PCI is best used in patients to relieve angina symptoms, to reduce medication requirements in patients with stable ischemic syndromes, and to prevent MI in patients with ACSs: unstable angina, NSTEMI, and STEMI. A meta-analysis of 17 randomized trials (Schomig et al., 2008) including the Clinical Outcomes Utilizing Revascularization and Aggressive Drug Evaluation (COURAGE) trial, with a total of 7,513 patients with stable angina treated with PCI or medical therapy, demonstrated that a 20% reduction in the odds ratio (OR) of all causes of death with PCI compared with medical treatment alone. In the nuclear substudy of COURAGE, 314 patients underwent myocardial perfusion scanning before and after PCI. The PCI group had a greater reduction in ischemia when compared with the medical therapy alone group (33%–19%). Overall, in the COURAGE trial, the aggregate data suggest that among the patients with small areas of ischemia and mild symptoms, intensive medical therapy is a viable first option, with PCI reserved for those in whom medical therapy alone is inadequate or in whom symptoms progress. In the COURAGE trial, many quality of life measures were superior in the PCI group for 3 years with the greatest benefits noted in patients with the most severe symptoms at baseline. In patients with moderate to severe ischemia or significant symptoms, an initial PCI strategy likely will lead more rapidly to an improved symptomatic state, reduce medication requirement and rehospitalization, improve quality of life, and possibly increase event-free survival (Brar & Stone, 2009).

PCI of more complex disease has become a more standard practice and has resulted in recent declines in the rates of surgical revascularization. Several randomized trials have defined the role of PCI in the management of complex CAD. For example, the Synergy between PCI with Taxus and Cardiac Surgery (SYNTAX) trial compared PCI using a drug-eluting stent (DES) with CABG among patients with triple-vessel disease or unprotected left main artery disease. Patients were randomly assigned to PCI or CABG, and at 12 months, there were no significant differences in the rates of death or MI between the two groups. However, the incidence of stroke was significantly higher in the CABG arm, whereas the repeat revascularization need was greater in the PCI arm. Moreover, in patients with unprotected left main artery disease, events were similar in the CABG and PCI groups (Serruys et al., 2009). Results similar to the SYNTAX trial were reported from the Coronary Artery Revascularization in Diabetes (CARDia) trial in which 510 patients with diabetes mellitus and multivessel disease were randomly assigned to DES, bare metal stents (BMSs), or CABG. The composite rate of death, MI, or stroke at 1 year did not significantly differ between the groups, although there were more revascularization events and fewer strokes with PCI. The results of the SYNTAX and CARDia trials suggest that patients with complex CAD can undergo PCI without an increase in the rates of death or MI. DESs have continued to evolve since the late 1990s. Pooled analyses have noted a small incremental risk in late stent thrombosis with DES compared with BMS, although the rates of death or MI are comparable with the two types of stents. The marked reduction in restenosis with DES likely offsets the excess risk of late stent thrombosis by decreasing the need for revascularization, including CABG and reducing the occurrence of ACSs after restenosis (Mauri et al., 2007). Another novel stent under investigation is the bioabsorbable stent that fully degrades in approximately 3 to 4 years. These stents may have theoretical advantages over traditional stents in that they may permit the vessel to normally remodel, minimize the frequency of late stent thrombosis, allow the vessel to respond normally to endothelial factors, and permit noninvasive stent assessments such as with multidetector CT scanning (Brar & Stone, 2009).

In CABG, saphenous veins from the legs, radial artery from the forearm, or an internal mammary artery from inside the chest wall are used as conduits to restore blood flow by bypassing the site of the atherosclerotic plaque. CABG is performed at present with an operative mortality approaching only 2%. More than 90% of operated patients achieve total or significant symptom relief. Progressive atherosclerotic occlusion of the vein grafts, through the same process that affected the native coronary arteries, is likely to occur within 10 years of surgery if the treated individuals do not change their lifestyles to reduce the risk factors for atherosclerosis. Both procedures are indicated in patients with stable angina pectoris who cannot obtain symptom relief with medical therapy. Emergency PTCA should also be performed when medical treatment alone does not appear to arrest ongoing cardiac muscle damage in unstable angina or in acute MI. Bypass surgery is indicated, regardless of symptoms, in patients who are found, by coronary angiography, to have a significant disease of the main left coronary artery segment or to have severe triple-vessel disease, especially if they have impaired left ventricular function. Several studies have shown improved survival with surgical (compared with medical) therapy in these patient subgroups with more extensive CHD. Alternative revascularization techniques include removal of the coronary atheroma by mechanical excision (coronary atherectomy) or by ablation using laser energy (laser angioplasty). Perhaps the most recent significant development in the management of CHD is the evidence that coronary atherosclerosis is reversible. It has now been convincingly shown by coronary angiography studies that coronary atherosclerosis can be reversed by lowering cholesterol with lipid-lowering agents or with changes in lifestyle.

The major determinants of prognosis in CHD are the extent and severity of the coronary atherosclerosis and of the ventricular dysfunction. CAD can be best diagnosed and evaluated by exercise stress tests and by cardiac catheterization with coronary angiography. Echocardiography and nuclear ventriculography can assess the ventricular function. The lower the left ventricular ejection fraction (the percentage of blood in the left ventricle ejected with each heartbeat, the normal being 50% or higher), the worse the prognosis. Even though the atherosclerotic epidemic still rages, there has been a significant decline in the age-adjusted mortality from all CVDs over the past 20 years. From 2001 to 2011, death rates from CVD decreased by over 30%. This reduction in mortality is partly accounted for by the creation of hospital coronary care units, development of sophisticated diagnostic tools, and advances in medical and surgical therapies. Most of the reduction is the result of changes in lifestyle.

■ Psychological and Vocational Implications

There is an undisputed relationship between CHD and psychological disorders (Khayyam-Nekouei, Neshatdoost, Yousefy, Masoumeh, & Gholamreza, 2011). Psychological disorders are definite contributors to atherosclerosis and the clinical syndromes of CAD. In turn, the diagnosis and treatment of CHD may create or worsen psychological disorders. The mechanisms whereby psychological disorders cause or accelerate coronary atherosclerosis have not been well defined. Psychosocial stresses result in increased sympathetic nervous system activity with a greater release of circulating catecholamines (epinephrine and norepinephrine) leading to elevated HRs, elevated systemic blood pressures, elevated cholesterol levels, and enhanced platelet aggregation and thrombus formation. High catecholamine levels also lower the triggering threshold for ventricular arrhythmias. Atherosclerotic vessels respond with vasoconstriction when exposed to severe psychosocial stresses. Many individuals in our society respond to mental or emotional stress by resorting to the immediate oral gratification of smoking or overeating. Poor dietary habits, with the wrong quality and quantity of foods, lead indirectly through obesity and directly through elevated saturated fat, sugar, and salt intake to a worse atherosclerosis risk profile. Stress often precedes the clinical manifestations of CHD with a positive correlation between bouts of anxiety or depression just before the onset of angina, fatal and nonfatal MI, and sudden dysrhythmic death. People with depression have a much greater mortality from CHD than the general population (Clouse et al., 2003). Social isolation also results in higher rates of sudden death.

Depression is highly prevalent after acute cardiac events, with 20% to 45% of patients having significant depression after acute MI (Mallik et al., 2005). Numerous studies indicate that depression has a prevalence from 25% to 35% in populations with CVD and is independently predictive of adverse outcomes (Rumsfeld & Ho, 2005). CABG surgery patients may have substantial perioperative depression, and the more severe the perioperative depression, the poorer the physical functional status 1 year after surgery. Depressive symptoms are a stronger predictor of poor functional improvement than previous MI, diabetes, and ventricular ejection fraction (Coulter & Campos, 2012). The relationship is more pronounced in women than in men (Moller-Leimkuhler, 2008). This may explain why women may derive less functional benefit from CABG surgery and indicates the importance of managing depression in women undergoing cardiac surgery (Mallik et al., 2005).

Patients who are depressed are significantly less likely to adhere to prescribed medications, follow lifestyle recommendations (exercise prescription and smoking cessation), and practice self-management (e.g., monitor weight and salt diet restriction in HF). Depression serves as a barrier to the delivery of optimal cardiac care. Research supports that treating depression can improve cardiovascular mortality and morbidity. Some patients treated with selective serotonin reuptake inhibitors (SSRIs) have had significantly lower overall and cardiovascular mortality. Observational data also suggest that SSRIs may be associated with a reduction in MI (Berkman et al., 2003).

Type A personality behavior—excessive drive, competitiveness, an exaggerated sense of time urgency, and free-floating hostility—is thought to be a risk factor for CHD although some studies found no correlation. A subset of patients with Type A behavior who show cynical hostility and suppressed anger may be the ones at risk for coronary disease.

Denial, a useful defense mechanism in some circumstances, may be problematic when it leads to self-destructive behavior such as a delay in getting to the hospital after the first symptoms of a MI. Denial can be maladaptive and is detrimental because it leads to noncompliance with prescribed medical therapy or risk factor modification. Anxiety is often seen during diagnostic cardiac procedures. The presentation of primary psychiatric disorders as cardiac disease when no cardiac disease exists is commonly seen in patients with chronic depression and chronic anxiety. In the United States, anxiety disorders have a prevalence of about 10%, but a higher percentage of patients with anxiety disorders and panic attacks consult cardiologists and visit emergency departments. These patients can have many of the symptoms of an acute MI, but as many as a third of all patients with chest pain syndromes referred for diagnostic coronary angiography are found to have normal coronary arteries and are diagnosed with a panic attack syndrome.

CHD has significant vocational implications. CHD causes more economic loss in the United States than any other disease or disorder. Millions of Americans are unemployed or underemployed because of the effects of CHD. The vocational counselor should consider, however, the magnitude of the problem in the context of the fact that the energy requirements of work have decreased in industrialized countries in this century. This is a result of the mechanization, automation, and computerization of labor. In 1950, 65% of all work was considered heavy labor, whereas in 1990, only 5% was deemed heavy. Therefore, through creative vocational counseling, many cardiac patients who are now unemployed could rejoin the work force. The vocational counselor should take into account the individual's cardiac diagnosis; his or her functional capacity as determined by a careful history, personal observation, and the results of the exercise stress test; and an occupational history that incorporates physical, mental, emotional, and environmental job requirements. Whenever possible, the functional status should be expressed as an NYHA class. Both the exercise tolerance on the stress test and the energy costs of work or other physical activities should be expressed in metabolic equivalents (METs). One MET is defined as the amount of oxygen consumed by an awake individual at rest. It is equivalent to 3.5 cc of oxygen per kilogram of body weight per minute. Stages of exercise and many vocational and recreational activities have been traditionally classified in terms of how many METs or multiples of the resting oxygen consumption are required by the activity. By the use of this method, results of the exercise stress test can be translated, though not precisely, to the level of exertion at work that the individual may safely perform. Rates of return to work after a cardiac event or procedure have a range of 35% to 95%.

Factors associated with a lower reemployment are severity of the cardiac condition; older age of the patient, social class, or educational level; coexisting psychological conditions; and family environment that is either not supportive or too protective. After an MI, men return to work at a rate of about 75%. Women have a lower rate of reemployment. Surprisingly, the rate for patients after coronary bypass surgery is lower at about 60%. This is paradoxical because 100% of patients have reduced myocardial function after an infarction but 90% have improved myocardial blood flow after the bypass surgery. Formal rehabilitation programs with a multidisciplinary approach that incorporates supervised exercise, education, and nutritional and psychological counseling are increasingly proving to be beneficial in many aspects. They provide an excellent environment for the effective modification of atherosclerotic risk factors, improve psychological status, and increase rates of return to work. Moreover, several recent meta-analytic studies indicate a secondary prevention benefit of increased survival and decreased cardiovascular complications.

The Pericardium

The pericardium is the sac that contains the heart. It helps to fix the heart inside the thorax, protecting it from excessive movement. It prevents direct contact with other organs in the chest, reducing friction during constant cardiac motion. It is thought to slow the spread of infection to the heart from other organs such as the lungs. The lack of a pericardium is quite compatible with life, however, and if removed, there are usually no clinical consequences.

Disease Description

The most common pericardial disease is pericarditis, or inflammation of the pericardium. This can be caused by infections from tuberculosis, bacteria, or viruses. Other causes are trauma, metabolic or autoimmune diseases, and adverse reactions to medications. Pericarditis can result in the accumulation of fluid within the two layers that make up the pericardium, termed pericardial effusion. When severe, it may result in cardiac tamponade—a choking of the heart that prevents its proper filling and emptying and may result in death. Tumors in the pericardium, either by adjacent spread or by metastasis from a distant site, can also cause pericardial effusion. Some patients, months after the acute episode of pericarditis, especially those with tuberculous pericarditis, may develop constrictive pericarditis. As the inflamed pericardium heals, it scars, contracts, and constricts the heart, resulting in a condition similar to cardiac tamponade. The pericardium can be best visualized with echocardiography.

Function and Disability

Long-term functional impairment and disability are usually not considerations in individuals with acute pericarditis because it is a short limited process without sequelae. The most common symptom in the individual with acute pericarditis is chest pain but different from that of angina pectoris. The pain is present at rest, is sharp and worsened by motion, breathing, or coughing. Cardiac tamponade's main symptoms are similar to those of HF. Chronic constrictive pericarditis presents with symptoms similar to tamponade, but its time course is more insidious. The patient may be ill for months, even years and may appear emaciated, as if suffering from terminal cancer. Functional impairment and disability in chronic constrictive pericarditis are similar to those of HF. However, in chronic pericarditis, the complete elimination of the functional impairment or disability may be possible by surgical excision of the constricting pericardium.

Treatment and Prognosis

The treatment of acute pericarditis is the direct treatment of the underlying disease causing the inflammation or infection. The threatening fluid of pericardial effusion or cardiac tamponade can be removed by inserting a small needle in the pericardial space—pericardiocentesis. A persistent or recurrent pericardial effusion can be eradicated by the definitive curative procedure of surgical resection of the pericardium. This is also the treatment for chronic constrictive pericarditis. Patients with constrictive pericarditis should not be medically managed as if HF was present. This could cause fluid depletion and dehydration and further decrease cardiac output, which will worsen symptoms and even lead to death. Prognosis for patients with pericarditis is generally excellent; individual outcomes depend on the nature of the condition causing the pericardial inflammation. Proper management of the acute condition, prompt recognition and drainage of pericardial fluid, and correct diagnosis and management of chronic constrictive pericarditis should result in a normal life span.

Psychological and Vocational Implications

The psychological and vocational implications of pericardial disease are not well studied or described. This is mainly because most pericardial disorders are neither common nor chronic. The most usual psychological manifestation is the anxiety provoked by the pain of pericarditis because it is confused by the patients, their families, and even by health care professionals, with the ischemic pain of angina or an acute MI. This situation is particularly devastating because the majority of patients with viral or traumatic pericarditis are young people. Patients with chronic constrictive pericarditis often suffer from clinical chronic depression. Their vocational evaluation should include both physiological and psychological factors.

The Myocardium

The myocardium is the heart muscle itself. It is divided into the left and the right ventricles. The left ventricle receives oxygenated blood from the lungs via the left atrium and then pumps that blood to the body via the aorta and its branches. The right ventricle receives deoxygenated blood from the body via the right atrium and then delivers that blood to the lungs for reoxygenation via the pulmonary artery.

Disease Description

Diseases of the myocardium are termed cardiomyopathy. There are three anatomical and physiological categories of cardiomyopathy, which are as follows: dilated (an enlarged heart with a thin or normal thickness muscle wall), hypertrophic (a normal size or only slightly enlarged heart with a thick muscle wall), and restrictive (a normal size heart with a thick or normal muscle wall of increased rigidity). The cardiomyopathies are best diagnosed and evaluated with echocardiography. In the United States, dilated cardiomyopathies are the most common and are most commonly caused by CHD (ischemic cardiomyopathy) as well as alcoholism, diabetes, familial/genetic, and idiopathic—unknown. Another cause of dilated cardiomyopathy is inflammation of the myocardium, or myocarditis. This is most frequently caused by a viral infection and unfortunately occurs in young individuals. In this type of cardiomyopathy, the ventricle is stretched and thinned, which can reduce the myocardial contractility. Hypertrophic cardiomyopathies are most often inherited or are the result of chronic elevated blood pressure, or hypertension. These myopathies result in a symmetrical or concentric type of hypertrophy resulting in a stiff, noncompliant left ventricle that does not relax well, and diastolic filling is limited. Hypertrophic cardiomyopathy can be nonobstructive or obstructive depending on whether the blood flow is blocked leaving the ventricle. If the thickening of the ventricle occurs in the septal wall or an area that obstructs blood flow, the condition is called hypertrophic obstructive cardiomyopathy (HOCM). Restrictive cardiomyopathies are the least common in the United States. They are caused by the infiltration or deposition of extraneous material in the heart muscle, such as iron in hemochromatosis, or amyloid. In this case, the ventricles become stiff and rigid leading to poor myocardial contraction and cardiac output.

Function and Disability

The major determinant of impaired function and disability in myocardial disease is the degree of myocardial dysfunction. All of the cardiomyopathies, by definition, entail myocardial dysfunction. In dilated cardiomyopathies, there is impaired ventricular contraction, or systole. In the hypertrophic and restrictive cardiomyopathies, the initial dysfunction is in ventricular relaxation, or diastole. In their advanced stages, the latter two myopathies may also exhibit systolic dysfunction and cardiac dilation and may progressively begin to resemble both anatomically and physiologically, a dilated cardiomyopathy. All of the cardiomyopathies may create a decreased cardiac blood output state that is insufficient to meet the metabolic needs of the peripheral tissues. This altered physiological state is called heart failure (HF). When there is a *reduced* systolic ejection fraction, HF is referred to as HF*r*EF and when there is *preserved* diastolic dysfunction, it is referred to as HF*p*EF (Yancy et al., 2013). HF is usually the pathophysiological end point of most CVDs because eventually the majority of myocardium is affected. Therefore, whether the initial disorder originated in the coronary arteries or in the cardiac valves, or whether it was the result of a systemic condition such as diabetes or hypertension, it is myocardial failure that produces the symptoms that determine functional capacity and disability.

Decreased cardiac output in HF produces low blood flow to the kidneys and activation of a neurohormonal cascade resulting in fluid retention. Fluid accumulates in the lungs resulting in the most common symptom of HF: difficulty breathing or dyspnea. In the early stages of HF, dyspnea occurs only with significant exertion and there is only mild functional impairment. As HF becomes more severe and the ventricular ejection function deteriorates, dyspnea may occur with minimal effort and even at rest. When dyspnea occurs while the patient is lying down, it is termed orthopnea; when it suddenly wakens a patient at night, it is called paroxysmal nocturnal dyspnea. The excess fluid may also cause abdominal distension, or ascites. It may cause the liver to be enlarged, a condition called hepatomegaly. The fluid deposition in the legs, which usually begins in the feet, is termed edema. The symptoms of weakness, fatigue, and lethargy indicate even more severe HF and reflect a greatly decreased cardiac blood output to all organ systems.

Functional impairment and disability are best assessed by a careful interview, with special attention given to the patient's daily activities. Treadmill exercise stress testing can be useful in determining factional capacity in patients with cardiomyopathies and is of the greatest help for those with dilated cardiomyopathies. It is not particularly useful for patients with restrictive cardiomyopathies because often their primary disease is the major contributor to their functional impairment and disability. For the assessment of functional capacity in the patient with a dilated cardiomyopathy, a gentler exercise is recommended. Before the test, it should be absolutely determined by interview and careful physical examination that the individual does not have active or decompensated HF. Particularly useful and informative for these patients are exercise tests that use imaging of ventricular function such as nuclear ventriculograms or echocardiograms. The patient's ventricular function, including global ejection fraction and segmental wall motion, at rest and with exercise, can be easily, objectively, and safely determined with both the techniques. Individuals whose ventricular function worsens with exercise are evidently more functionally limited and more likely to be disabled.

Of significance, a low left ventricular ejection fraction at rest—the best predictor of prognosis/survival in CVD—is not an accurate predictor of functional capacity. Some patients with ejection fractions below 30% can have normal exercise tolerance, whereas some patients with normal ejection fractions can have markedly reduced exercise tolerance. This paradox is accounted for by the differing peripheral adaptation between individuals. Those with a higher exercise tolerance and greater functional capacity are more physically fit individuals because of their more efficient skeletal musculature and greater oxygen extraction capability.

Treatment and Prognosis

In the medical management of the patient with myocardial failure, it is important to consider first the elimination of any conditions that might have helped to precipitate the failure. Such conditions may be internal stresses (e.g., anemia, fevers, infection, rhythm disturbances, and thyroid disorders) or they may be environmental stresses (e.g., high altitudes or excessive heat or cold). After such contributing factors are eradicated, therapy is aimed at creating the optimal hemodynamic milieu for myocardial function. This milieu can be best created by positively intervening in three components of myocardial mechanics and of HF pathophysiology. This is accomplished by increasing inotropy, or myocardial contractility; by decreasing preload, or diastolic ventricular volume; and by decreasing afterload, or the stress or tension of the heart muscle wall during the ejection of blood. By improving one of the three, the two others are also improved.

Specific treatment includes nitrates to directly decrease preload, diuretics to eliminate excess fluid and indirectly reduce preload, digitalis to directly increase inotropy, and afterload reducing agents such as vasodilators. Most patients are also advised to restrict their salt intake because high dietary salt will cause fluid retention. There is no definite cure for myocardial failure. Options in the management of advanced HF include intravenous inotrope infusions like dobutamine and milrinone (Francis, Bartos, & Adatya, 2014). Average life expectancy with advanced HF and optimum medication therapy is 1.1 years (Long, Swain, & Mangi, 2014). Device therapy in HF includes ventricular resynchronization therapy with the implantation of a biventricular pacemaker—often combined with an ICD—or implantation of a left ventricular assist device (LVAD) (European Society of Cardiology, 2010). An LVAD is a mechanical pump implanted to the left ventricle to support blood flow and cardiac output (www.nhlbi.nih.gov/health/health-topics/topics/vad). The need for this technology arose from the number of patients with advanced HF who were candidates for heart transplant vastly outstripping the number of hearts available for transplantation. Many patients who are not candidates for heart transplant are candidates for LVAD–destination therapy. Those on the heart transplant list may have an LVAD implanted as a bridge to transplant. Of significance, patients who receive heart transplant without ever getting an LVAD have an average life expectancy of 8.5 years, whereas those who get an LVAD and then heart transplant have an average life expectancy of 12.3 years. Placement of an LVAD provides time to optimize medical therapies and undergo cardiac rehabilitation so that they are in better overall health when they receive their heart transplant. Patients referred for cardiac transplantation are those who prove refractory to the best possible combination of medical therapy and are in the NYHA Class IV functional status. Without transplantation, some of these individuals may have as high as a 90% 1-year mortality. This mortality is to be compared with the survival rates of transplantation, which are currently about 85% in 1 year and about 70% in 3 years.

The prognosis of patients with cardiomyopathies depends on the kind of cardiomyopathy and the degree of myocardial dysfunction and HF present. As a general rule, the worse the ventricular function, as assessed by resting left ventricular ejection fraction, the worse the prognosis and the greater the likelihood of death from end-stage HF, cardiovascular collapse, and shock.

Psychological and Vocational Implications

The psychological and vocational implications of myocardial disease and HF are similar to those of ischemic heart disease. On average, patients with HF have a moderate to high prevalence of depression—over 20%, which is two to three times that in the general population. Some studies have reported prevalence rates as high as 60%, and higher rates of depression correlate to more advanced stages of HF (Rutledge et al., 2006). Rates of anxiety and depression are higher in patients with ICDs, approaching 25% to 35%. Anticipatory anxiety surrounding shocks delivered by the ICD after detecting an arrhythmia account for much of this.

The Endocardium

The endocardium (the heart's inner lining surface that is in contact with systemic blood) disorders are mainly those of the following four cardiac valves: the aortic, the mitral, the pulmonic, and the tricuspid. Although rare diseases may primarily involve the endocardial lining and only secondarily the valves, these are quite uncommon in the United States.

Disease Description

The principal etiologic factor of endocardial and valvular heart disease, in the developed as well as the developing countries of the world, has been rheumatic fever, a result of the body's immune response against a streptococcal infection. Rheumatic fever can result in both valvular insufficiency (or "leaky" valves) and valvular stenosis (or "tight" valves). With the introduction and widespread use of penicillin and other antibiotics to treat streptococcal infections, the incidence of rheumatic heart disease, and of valvular disease in general, has progressively and significantly decreased over the past half-century in economically developed nations. This decrease, at the same time that coronary atherosclerosis is on the increase, has limited endocardial and valvular diseases to fewer than 10% of all cases of CVD in these countries, although its prevalence remains high in underdeveloped areas of the world.

Mitral stenosis, with very few exceptions, is secondary to rheumatic heart disease. About 70% of the patients with mitral stenosis are women. Even though the left ventricle is usually normal in mitral stenosis, symptoms similar to those of HF, such as dyspnea and orthopnea, begin in these patients when they are in their 40s or 50s. The elevated pressures in the left atrium and the pulmonary vasculature that must be generated to force the blood through the stenotic mitral valve cause these symptoms. Complications of mitral stenosis such as arrhythmias can lead to symptoms of palpitations. Mitral regurgitation is caused in 50% of the cases by rheumatic fever. Pure rheumatic mitral regurgitation is more common in men than in women. Infective endocarditis, which preferentially attacks valves previously damaged by rheumatic disease, also leads to mitral regurgitation. Causative are also a variety of conditions that affect the supporting structures of the valve. There can be dilation or calcification of the mitral annulus, the ringlike orifice between the left atrium and the ventricle that the valve occupies. Also, there can be fibrosis of the papillary muscles, which, through the netlike chordae tendineae, attach the valve leaflets to the left ventricle. A unique disease entity of the mitral valve is the mitral valve prolapse syndrome. In this condition, the leaflets of the mitral valve prolapse into the left atrium during valve closure. Echocardiographic studies have suggested that the incidence of this condition may be about 5% in the female population. Aortic stenosis may be caused by rheumatic fever, by degenerative calcification of the cusps, or by a congenital condition called bicuspid aortic valve. A bicuspid aortic valve is abnormal because it has two, instead of three, cusps. This abnormality, the most common congenital cardiac abnormality, occurs in about 2% of the population. In only a small portion of that group does this congenital condition result in clinical disease. As opposed to stenosis of the mitral valve, where mainly women are affected, about 80% of adult patients with isolated aortic stenosis are men.

Aortic regurgitation is mainly rheumatic in origin, especially when found in combination with mitral valve disease. Nearly 80% of the patients with pure aortic regurgitation are men. Women are the majority of those who have concomitant mitral disease. A bicuspid aortic valve can also become insufficient. An increasing incidence of aortic regurgitation is caused by infective endocarditis. Diseases that result in the dilation of the aorta itself may also dilate the aortic valve annulus and lead to secondary aortic insufficiency. Disorders of the valves on the right side of the heart are far less common than those of the valves on the left side of the heart. Tricuspid stenosis is very uncommon and is usually secondary to rheumatic heart disease and found in association with disease of the other valves. Tricuspid insufficiency is more common than stenosis and results directly from infective endocarditis in users of intravenous drugs or indirectly from right ventricular enlargement and accompanying tricuspid annular dilation. Of all valvular disorders, those of the pulmonic valve are the rarest. The most common pulmonic valve disorder is insufficiency, secondary to pulmonary hypertension.

Function and Disability

The major determinant of impaired function and disability in endocardial disease is the severity of the valvular stenosis or insufficiency and the degree of secondary myocardial dysfunction. Valvular insufficiency and valvular stenosis both interfere with normal cardiac blood flow. Valvular insufficiency leads to a volume overload and eventual dilation of the cardiac chambers. Aortic and pulmonic stenosis may cause a pressure overload, and ventricular hypertrophy and atrial dilation. These overloads, if severe and left untreated, will invariably lead to HF. The time for the onset of symptoms is related to the severity of the valvular lesion and also to the age and physical fitness of the individual patient. Individuals with valvular disease may have the following symptoms: chest pain that has some of the features of angina pectoris, palpitations from both atrial and ventricular arrhythmias, and dyspnea most often when mitral regurgitation is present. In addition to the symptoms of HF, patients with aortic stenosis can also have chest pain indistinguishable from angina pectoris and can also have sudden death as their only clinical presentation. Disease classification by NYHA criteria is similar to that of the patient with CHD or with a cardiomyopathy. If an appropriate functional history cannot be obtained, exercise stress testing is a good objective indicator of function in these patients. It should be noted, however, that exercise testing is relatively contraindicated in patients with mild to moderate mitral stenosis and aortic stenosis and absolutely contraindicated when the stenoses are severe. With exercise testing, those with stenotic valvular disease may develop acute pulmonary edema and those with aortic stenosis may also have syncope.

Treatment and Prognosis

When possible, it is best to repair a leaking heart valve, thereby preserving as much as possible the normal structural anatomy of the valve. When the valve is not able to be repaired, a replacement valve with either a porcine (pig) valve, bovine (cow) valve, or a metal valve prosthesis may be used. Replacement with a metal prosthesis results in the need for lifelong anticoagulation.

The treatment of patients with mitral valve prolapse is mainly reassurance that they have a good prognosis. Medical treatment with beta-blockers may be necessary to treat symptoms of palpitations from their benign yet symptomatic arrhythmias. A patient with mitral valve prolapse and significant mitral regurgitation, like all other patients with valvular disease or with prosthetic valves, should have antibiotic prophylaxis before dental work or surgery to prevent acquiring endocarditis from a potential bacteremia (the introduction of bacteria into the blood), which may happen with such procedures. The prognosis of patients with valvular disease is excellent as long as replacement, repair, or valvuloplasty is performed before there is damage to the ventricles, the atria, or the pulmonary vasculature. Once the chronic volume or pressure overloads have irreversibly damaged these structures, the surgical mortality is markedly increased, from about 1% in uncomplicated cases to more than 15% in those with failing ventricles. These unfortunate individuals have a decreased life span even if the surgery is successful and the prosthetic valve has perfect function. Severely dysfunctional cardiac valves, if not repaired or replaced, usually will lead to death within 5 years.

During the past decade, there has been an increase in valve surgery through minimally invasive techniques. Reported benefits include better cosmetic outcomes and reduced surgical trauma, blood loss, incidence of atrial fibrillation, pain, and hospital stay, and a more rapid return to functional activity (Bakir et al., 2006). More recent advances include the transcatheter aortic valve replacement (TAVR), also known as transcatheter aortic valve implantation (TAVI). This procedure places a replacement valve into the old, damaged aortic valve orifice using one of two approaches: entering through the femoral artery in the groin (transfemoral approach), or via a small chest wall incision and through the tip of the left ventricle (transapical approach). The new valve is able to assume responsibility of regulating the flow of blood out of the left ventricle. This procedure is far less invasive than traditional valve replacement surgery and with fewer potential complications in high-risk, older patients with multiple comorbidities. Another minimally invasive procedure for patients with mitral regurgitation is a mitral valve clip. The clip is secured to the leaflets to reduce the amount of blood that flows back into the left atrium.

Psychological and Vocational Implications

In many respects, the psychological and vocational implications of endocardial and valvular heart disease are the same as those of the dilated cardiomyopathies, especially when secondary ventricular dysfunction exists. Unique psychological situations in valvular diseases arise because many of the patients with rheumatic valvular disease are young women of childbearing age. Often, some patients who are childless must make a decision as to whether to become pregnant even though pregnancy may worsen their cardiac condition and lead to risk of death. At times, the stress-laden decision is not whether to become pregnant but whether to terminate an advanced wanted pregnancy. Psychological intervention and support is needed before, during, and particularly after the time of decision making. Patients with mitral valve prolapse present a difficult challenge to the psychologist. These individuals, with cardiac symptoms but with a good prognosis, are often disabled for psychological, and not physiological, reasons. A team approach, with the cardiologist, psychologist, and other caregivers working together, is often more effective than an uncoordinated approach that often confuses the patient and results in further distress.

Unique vocational implications exist with patients with valvular heart disease because this is the only group of CVDs in which women constitute a majority. Patients with mitral valve prolapse and rheumatic mitral valve disease are often young women who have to care for a family and work outside the home in the context of their mitral disease. Surgical valve replacement often occurs in older women in their late 50s or early 60s who are near retirement age. Many do not return to work after the surgery. Many live alone because they have survived their husbands, who have already died from their own CHD. The rehabilitative and vocational challenges are great in this group of patients.

The Electrical Conduction System

The cardiac conduction system, made of specialized fibers, has two functions. The main cardiac pacemaker, the sinus or sinoatrial node, generates the rhythmic electrical impulse of the normal regular heart rate and rhythm. The other parts of the system include the atrioventricular (AV) node (the backup or auxiliary pacemaker), the bundle of

His, the bundle branches, and the Purkinje fibers. They all ensure the sequential and uniform propagation of the electrical current so that the cardiac cycle of ventricular systole and diastole is an organized and effective activity. As the population ages, atrial fibrillation will become more prevalent. The Framingham Heart Study showed that the lifetime risk of developing atrial fibrillation at age 40 and older is approximately one in four. The prevalence of atrial fibrillation is increasing, with predictions that the number of individuals suffering from atrial fibrillation will increase from the approximately 2.5 million at present to roughly 5.6 million over the next decades.

Disease Description

Disorders of the electrical system can result in bradycardia (slow rates of less than 60 beats per minute), tachycardia (fast rates at more than 100 beats per minute), or arrhythmias or dysrhythmias (irregular rhythms). Arrhythmias of a slow rate are bradyarrhythmias and those of a fast rate are tachyarrhythmias. Dysrhythmias can be further classified as those with an abnormal current originating from the atria or supraventricular arrhythmias, and those with an abnormal origin in the ventricles or ventricular arrhythmias. Supraventricular arrhythmias are paroxysmal atrial tachycardia (PAT), atrial flutter, atrial fibrillation, and multifocal atrial tachycardia (MAT). Although the atrial rates vary and can be as fast as 600 beats per minute, the ventricular rate in these arrhythmias, even if untreated, is generally relatively slow, because the impulses are slowed or blocked at the level of the AV node and the His bundle. MAT occurs mostly in patients with pulmonary disease. PAT can occur in normal persons without heart disease and is most commonly precipitated by anxiety or by the ingestion of excitatory agents such as alcohol and caffeine. Atrial flutter and fibrillation occur in patients with atria that are enlarged because of either ventricular dysfunction or mitral or tricuspid valvular disease. An overly active thyroid gland, or hyperthyroidism, may also cause atrial fibrillation.

Ventricular arrhythmias are of two types: VT and VF. VT and VF usually occur in patients with a dilated cardiomyopathy or a prior MI. They are rare but do occur in people with normal ventricles.

A rare congenital anomaly of the conduction system occurs in the presence of an accessory pathway, an extra bundle with conduction properties akin to those of the conduction system. Such a bundle allows the electrical activity from the atria to the ventricles to bypass the AV node and the bundle of His. Patients with these abnormalities, called preexcitation syndromes, are usually young, are prone to episodes of PAT, and can have very fast ventricular rates with atrial fibrillation. There are two types of preexcitation syndromes: Wolff–Parkinson–White syndrome and Lown–Ganong–Levine syndrome.

Cardiac electrical block is said to occur when either of the two inherent cardiac pacemakers cannot generate a normal electrical impulse or when a normal impulse is not conducted correctly through the conduction system. Fibrosis of the conduction system, which is part of the aging process, is a cause of electrical blocks in the elderly. Most blocks, however, like most arrhythmias, are the result of CHD.

Function and Disability

The functional impairments and disabilities that result from the cardiac arrhythmias fall into two major categories. One is the physiological disability from the ineffective ventricular contractions and decreased cardiac output that is secondary to a chronic arrhythmia that is too slow, too fast, or too disorganized. Atrial fibrillation is the prototype and its symptoms place the functional considerations of this arrhythmia with those of HF. The other is the psychological disability secondary to an arrhythmia that is not chronic but acute. Such an arrhythmia is unpredictable. It arrives suddenly and without any warning. VT is the prototype. The individual may have no physiological functional limitation or disability with the activities of daily life, yet may refrain from work because of fear of precipitating the arrhythmia with activity. Patients with supraventricular arrhythmias have palpitation as their most common symptom. PAT and atrial flutter are acute and not chronic arrhythmias and therefore have no functional or disability implications when they are not present. Those with atrial flutter or fibrillation may develop syncope or symptoms of HF, especially if they have the arrhythmias in the context of impaired ventricular function. Those with coexisting CAD may develop angina pectoris because the fast HRs of the arrhythmia create metabolic demands that cannot be met by the compromised blood supply through the obstructed coronary arteries. Patients whose HR in atrial fibrillation is controlled at rest can still have exertional dyspnea, as in this condition, the HR may rapidly increase with little exertion. The chaotic atrial electrical activity of atrial fibrillation creates a combination of turbulence and stasis of blood in the atria. This can lead to the complication of thrombus formation in the atria. These thrombi can dislodge and be carried by the circulation to other parts of the body. Such a traveling thrombus, or embolus, may cause obstruction of blood flow to the eyes, leading to blindness, or to the kidneys, causing renal failure. When carried to the brain, it may result in cerebral infarction, or stroke.

If VT is of a short duration (a few seconds), the patient may experience palpitation. If of a longer duration (a few minutes), syncope may occur. If sustained beyond a few minutes, degeneration to VF is likely and sudden death may ensue. Individuals with the accessory pathway syndromes will experience palpitation when PAT is their acute arrhythmia. If the arrhythmia is atrial fibrillation and of prolonged duration with a very fast ventricular rate, it may degenerate into VF and lead to SCD. The health care professional should not be deceived into complacency because the patient looks young, healthy, and vigorous. Atrial fibrillation in a patient with a preexcitation syndrome is dire. Severe bradycardia or high degrees of block, resulting in HRs of less than 30 beats per minute, can cause fatigue and dizziness because of the decreased cardiac output and the resultant diminished cerebral perfusion. When the effective rate is even slower or when the bradycardia is sudden in onset, syncope may occur.

Treatment and Prognosis

The treatment of supraventricular arrhythmias involves their prevention, quick termination, or the prompt and effective control of their fast rate. Avoiding stressful situations and the ingestion of alcohol or stimulants such as caffeine and antihistamines can prevent supraventricular arrhythmias. If the initiation of the arrhythmia is not preventable, then it may be terminated or its fast rate controlled, by medications that slow electrical conduction through the AV node such as digitalis, beta-blockers, and calcium channel blockers. Individuals whose atrial fibrillation is chronic or recurrent (paroxysmal atrial fibrillation) need to take such medications for life to control their HRs. Most of them will also require lifelong oral anticoagulation with agents such as warfarin (Coumadin), rivaroxaban (Xarelto), or apixaban (Eliquis) to prevent thrombus formation and embolization. If medication fails to abolish the arrhythmia, or if the patient is severely ill because of angina pectoris, severe HF, or shock, then prompt electrical cardioversion to try and restore normal sinus rhythm is indicated.

The treatment of sustained VT and of VF should be prompt electrical cardioversion to a normal rhythm. Younger individuals with normal ventricular function may tolerate sustained VT for short periods of time. VF is not compatible with life. Antiarrhythmic agents to prevent these ventricular arrhythmias should be prescribed only by expert cardiologists who have evaluated the arrhythmia with invasive electrophysiological studies. It is no longer acceptable to treat such patients empirically, as these agents have been found to have a high proarrhythmic potential. In up to 25% of cases, they can precipitate the very arrhythmia they are supposed to prevent or even make it worse. Patients with ventricular arrhythmias who do not respond to medical therapy may require surgical ablation of the myocardial focus from which the arrhythmia originates. Some, with recurrent episodes of VF, may require the implantation of an antiarrhythmic device, similar to a pacemaker, called an implantable automatic defibrillator, to deliver an electrical shock whenever VF occurs. The ultimate treatment of ventricular arrhythmias, however, lies in the prevention of CHD, which is present in about 80% of patients with malignant ventricular arrhythmias and sudden electrical death.

The treatment of patients with preexcitation syndromes is similar to that of those with supraventricular arrhythmias. However, great caution is needed when giving antiarrhythmic agents to these patients because a paradoxical effect may result—the arrhythmia may be made worse and faster rates may result if agents that would normally control the arrhythmia or slow down its rate are administered. In patients where arrhythmia is refractory to medical therapy or in those who have lethal atrial fibrillation with a very rapid ventricular rate, radiofrequency ablation of the accessory pathway is recommended. Cardiac electrical blocks and symptomatic bradycardia are treated with the implantation of permanent pacemakers that substitute for the heart's own pacemakers and conduction system. In recent years, technology has led to the development of even more sophisticated and smaller pacing devices that nearly duplicate the heart's electrophysiological mechanisms and allow for nearly normal ventricular hemodynamics. Cardiac resynchronization therapy (CRT), or biventricular pacing, is used in HF patients to help improve the heart's efficiency and stroke volume by restoring the normal synchrony between the right and left ventricular contractions.

The prognosis for patients with supraventricular arrhythmia under appropriate medical care is excellent. Their mortality depends on the physiological cause of the arrhythmia rather than on the arrhythmia itself. For example, those with normal hearts or with hyperthyroidism have a much better prognosis than do those whose arrhythmias are complications of structural heart disease, such as mitral stenosis or myocardial dysfunction.

The prognosis for the patient who is a survivor of sudden death and who has recurrent episodes of VF or VT is very poor. This is particularly the case for those with a dilated cardiomyopathy and a left ventricular ejection fraction of less than 20%. This poor prognosis has been ameliorated by the practice of medical therapy guided by electrophysiological testing, by newer surgical techniques, and by the use of implantable defibrillators.

The prognosis for patients with preexcitation syndrome is excellent because they usually have otherwise normal hearts. If the correct diagnosis is made and expert prompt treatment is rendered the few times it is needed, these individuals will have a normal life span. The prognosis of patients requiring pacemakers is excellent if the ventricular function is normal.

■ Psychological and Vocational Implications

The psychological implications of cardiac arrhythmias are significant. Not only is the psychologist confronted with the psychological consequences of the arrhythmias, but perhaps more importantly, psychological disorders may trigger lethal arrhythmias. As mentioned, a chronic depression or anxiety syndrome that may develop over time after repeated episodes of their sudden and unexpected tachyarrhythmia may disable patients with PAT, recurrent VT, and VF (van den Broek, Heijmans, & van Assen, 2013). They may progressively and drastically curtail their range of activities as they associate the onset of their arrhythmias with particular events, places, or times. Phobias and a repertoire of superstitious behaviors may develop in many of these individuals. Intensive psychological interventions are often necessary. Particularly difficult is the control and prevention of the psychological precipitants of the arrhythmias. It is well documented that about 1% of all patients with malignant ventricular arrhythmias have no demonstrable structural heart disease, and the only causative factor for their arrhythmia is psychological. An even greater percentage of patients with known heart disease have their potentially lethal arrhythmias triggered by psychological factors. A few medical centers have laboratories and testing protocols that elicit and identify specific thoughts, ideas, or mental images that trigger the arrhythmias in a particular individual. The judicious use of antiarrhythmic agents, in combination with beta-blockers and directed and focused psychological intervention, has proved quite successful in preventing or reducing the frequency of arrhythmias in such patients. The vocational implications of cardiac arrhythmias are also significant. The vocational counselor must undertake a careful evaluation of the work situation, with special attention given to any environmental, emotional, or mental stress that may precipitate or aggravate the arrhythmia.

DISEASES OF THE VASCULAR SYSTEM

The vascular system, also known as the peripheral vascular system, is responsible for the circulation of blood from the heart to the rest of the body and back again to the heart. Its components are the aorta, the arteries, the arterioles, the capillaries, and the veins. In this chapter, only diseases of the aorta are considered. Diseases of specific vessels and of the smaller vasculature are covered in other chapters of this book.

The Aorta

The aorta is the largest artery in the body. It receives the blood from the heart and then, through its branches, delivers that blood to the rest of the body. Because of its large size and its unique function as the receiving conduit for blood directly from the left ventricle, the walls of the aorta experience greater tension and stress than do other blood vessels. Therein lies the anatomical and physiological substrate for its diseases.

Disease Description

Arteriosclerosis develops in the aorta just as it does in the coronary arteries. Such is the extent of the process that nearly all adults in the United States are believed to have some measure of aortic arteriosclerosis. Even children and adolescents have been shown to have aortic fatty streaks, the earliest lesion of aortic arteriosclerosis. The vast majority of patients with clinical aortic disease are hypertensive men who smoke cigarettes. There are three main diseases of the aorta: aneurysms, dissections, and obstructive disease. Diseases of the aorta and its branches are best evaluated by angiography. The technique of transesophageal echocardiography is particularly useful for the evaluation of diseases of the thoracic aorta.

An aortic aneurysm is an abnormal dilation of the aorta that is susceptible to acute rupture. Aneurysms can be found in the thoracic aorta (in both its ascending and descending segments) and also in the abdominal aorta. Ascending aortic aneurysms are the ones that are least likely to be caused by arteriosclerosis. Before our age of antibiotics and organized prevention of sexually transmitted diseases, ascending aortic aneurysms were mainly caused by syphilis. At present, the most common cause of ascending aneurysms is damage of the middle layer of the aortic wall, the media. This condition is termed cystic medial necrosis and is of unknown etiology. Aneurysms of the descending thoracic aorta and of the abdominal aorta are nearly all caused by arteriosclerosis. Many patients who have thoracic aneurysms also have abdominal aneurysms, and about 10% of those with abdominal aneurysms have more than one.

Aortic dissections can occur anywhere in the aorta. A dissection takes place when the innermost of the three layers of the wall of the aorta, the intima, breaks and allows blood to flow into the wall of the aorta itself. The pressure of the blood separates the layers of the aorta. Hypertension plays a significant role in aortic dissections regardless of their location. Surgeons categorize dissections into three types: Type I dissection involves the entire aorta, from its ascending portion, around the arch, and into the abdominal aorta; Type II dissection is limited to the ascending aorta; and Type III dissection is limited to the descending aorta. Aortic obstructive disease, like coronary artery obstructive disease, impedes the adequate flow of blood. Obstruction in the aorta is most frequently noted in its terminal portion, usually at its bifurcation into the iliac and femoral arteries, the vessels that supply the lower extremities.

Function and Disability

Most patients with aortic aneurysms and dissections are free of functional impairments and disability because they are asymptomatic until the moment of the acute event. Aortic aneurysms are most often found on routine abdominal physical exam or by x-rays. Symptoms, when they do exist, may be only those of a lower back pain syndrome. Some patients may actually have been misdiagnosed as having lumbar vertebral disease.

Obstructive aortic disease does cause disability and chronic functional impairment. The most common symptom is claudication. This is pain of one or both legs, usually in the muscles of the calves, with walking. Patients may be able to walk only a few feet before disabling pain impedes further walking. They may also have pain of the thighs and buttocks with walking and at rest. They often have impotence. The functional capacity of patients with claudication and the degree of their vascular stenosis can be evaluated by Doppler ultrasound of the legs. This is performed before and after treadmill walking, using special test protocols different from those used for the evaluation of the impairment in CHD.

Treatment and Prognosis

The treatment of aortic aneurysms, dissections, and severe obstructive disease is always surgical. The acute rupture of an aortic aneurysm is nearly always a fatal event. When an abdominal aneurysm has a diameter of less than 6 cm, the probability of rupture is about 15% over a 10-year period, but if the aneurismal diameter is 6 cm or greater, there is a 50% probability of rupture in a shorter time span. The operative mortality of elective abdominal aneurysm resection is less than 10%. Resection of aneurysms of the ascending aorta or of the aortic arch carries a greater operative mortality. There is about 20% mortality in the surgical treatment of aortic dissections.

The surgical treatment of obstructive disease of the main branches of the aorta to the lower extremities is aortic–femoral bypass grafting, using synthetic conduits to restore circulation to the legs. Excellent results are achieved with little mortality and morbidity, and claudication is abolished or decreased in about 90% of patients. As in coronary disease, an alternative treatment is percutaneous balloon angioplasty, most recently with the additional placement of vascular metal stents. This procedure is particularly feasible in the dilation of discrete lesions of the iliac arteries.

The prognosis of patients with any type of arteriosclerotic disease of the aorta and its branches can be best determined in the context of their coexisting coronary artery arteriosclerosis. It is the extent and severity of the coronary disease that is the major determinant of both the operative mortality and the long-term survival of patients who undergo successful aortic or peripheral vascular surgery.

Psychological and Vocational Implications

There are usually no psychological implications in aortic disorders before the acute events of aortic aneurysm rupture and of aortic dissection because the patients are usually asymptomatic up to that time. Most of these patients had denied the potential consequences of their smoking or of their uncontrolled hypertension. The acute event has perhaps no match in all of medicine as a truly terrifying experience. Most survivors of the event, and the subsequent surgery, experience a reversal of their present psychological mind-set, become acutely aware of their mortality, and may develop chronic depression and even excessive anxiety and an overvigilant state. Such individuals can benefit from psychological intervention. A group of patients with a similar problem are those who are informed of the presence of an abdominal aortic aneurysm that is still too small to undergo surgical resection. They may spend months or even years in watchful waiting before surgery is finally indicated. Psychological implications in patients with obstructive aortic disease usually focus on their loss of self-esteem because of their inability to walk and work and principally because of impotence.

There are important vocational implications in aortic diseases. The patients who have had surgical repair of an aortic aneurysm or dissection have an even lower rate of return to work than those who have had coronary bypass surgery. This may be due to the advanced age of these patients, most of whom are in their 60s and 70s. It may also be because the surgical procedure that was performed on them is perceived as, and is in fact, more complex than coronary bypass surgery. Patients with occlusive disease have specific vocational considerations because they are unable to perform most work activity that entails walking or prolonged standing. They may be employed in jobs that require the performance of work only with the arms, and only while sitting and with infrequent walking for short distances.

CARDIAC REHABILITATION

Cardiac rehabilitation is designed to decrease the physiological and psychological effects of cardiac disease, to reduce the risk for sudden death and of reinfarction, to control cardiac symptoms, to stabilize or reverse the atherosclerotic process, and to enhance vocational status of patients. A goal of cardiac rehabilitation is also to help reduce cardiovascular risk factors by lipid control, weight loss, optimization of blood pressure and blood glucose, tobacco use cessation, stress management, and increased physical activity. Specifically, a comprehensive transdisciplinary program should improve a patient's exercise performance, promote lifestyle changes, and increase psychosocial well-being. Cardiac rehabilitation and secondary prevention programs are recognized as integral to the comprehensive care of patients with CVD and as such are recommended as useful and effective (Class I) by the AHA, ACC, American Association of Cardiovascular and Pulmonary Rehabilitation, and the Agency for Health Care Policy and Research. All conclude that CRPs should offer a multifaceted and transdisciplinary approach to the overall cardiovascular risk reduction and that programs consisting of exercise training alone are not considered cardiac rehabilitation.

Patients should be formally evaluated at the time they are enrolled in a CRP and should have a comprehensive medical history and physical examination, a review of relevant test results and treatments, and risk stratification. In order to individualize the patient's program, each clinician should design an individualized program of secondary prevention. Appropriate strategies can include nutrition counseling; weight management; blood pressure, lipid, and diabetic management; tobacco use cessation; physical activity counseling; targeted physical prescription; medication adherence; and detection and management of depression (Zellwenger, Osterwalder, Langewitz, & Pfisterer, 2004). Inherent in the patient's involvement in the CRP is the understanding that successful risk factor modification and the maintenance of a physically active lifestyle is a lifelong process.

An admission to a CRP should include a psychosocial evaluation that encompasses an identification of depression, anxiety, anger or hostility, social isolation, family distress, sexual dysfunction, and any substance abuse, using standard interview and measurement techniques. Individual or group education and counseling are warranted with referral to appropriate specialists as needed. In a study of over 500 consecutive coronary patients enrolled in cardiac rehabilitation compared with control patients not completing rehabilitation, depressive symptoms were assessed by questionnaire and mortality was evaluated at a mean follow-up of 40 months. Depressed patients had a greater than fourfold mortality than nondepressed patients (22% vs. 5%) and depressed patients who completed rehabilitation had a 73% lower mortality (8% vs. 30%; Milani & Lavie, 2007). Importantly, a reduction in depressive symptoms and the associated decrease in mortality were related to improvement in fitness. Hence, only a mild improvement in the levels of fitness was needed to produce the benefit on depressive symptoms and its associated decrease in mortality.

In terms of the safety and clinical efficacy of cardiac rehabilitation, a meta-analysis of 48 randomized clinical trials (with a total of nearly 9,000 patients out of whom only 20% were women) demonstrated that exercise-based cardiac rehabilitation had significant reductions in both all-cause mortality (odds ration [OR]: 0.80; 95% confidence interval [CI]: 0.68–0.93) and cardiac-specific mortality (OR: 0.74; 95% CI: 0.61–0.96) after a median follow-up of 15 months in both genders. In these studies, reductions in all-cause mortality ranged from 15% to 28% and reduction in cardiac mortality from 26% to 31%. Also, enrollment and participation in community-based CRPs that provide both exercise and secondary prevention education is associated with reduced mortality and fewer recurrent MIs (Witt et al., 2004).

A national study of Medicare beneficiaries to assess referral patterns for cardiac rehabilitation was conducted after individuals were hospitalized for acute MI or CABG surgery. A total of 267,427 beneficiaries who were aged 65 years and older and who survived at least 30 days after hospital discharge were enrolled in the study. Overall, cardiac rehabilitation was used for only 13.9% of patients hospitalized for acute MI and for 31% of patients who underwent CABG. Older patients, women (44% of cohort), non-Whites (8.2% of cohort), and patients with comorbidities (including HF, previous stroke, diabetes mellitus, or cancer) were significantly less likely to receive cardiac rehabilitation. CABG during index hospitalization, higher median household income, higher level of education, and shorter distance to the nearest cardiac rehabilitation facility were important indicators of higher cardiac rehabilitation utilization (Suaya, Stason, Ades, Norman, & Shepherd, 2009).

A more recent study assessed the effects of CRP on survival in a large cohort of older coronary patients. Randomized controlled trials have shown that rehabilitation improves survival, but in these trials, the participants have been predominantly middle-aged, low-, or moderate-risk, Caucasian men. This study consisted of a population of 601,099 U.S. Medicare beneficiaries who were hospitalized for coronary conditions or cardiac revascularization procedures. One- to five-year mortalities were examined in CRP users and nonusers using Medicare claims and the following three analytic techniques: propensity-based matching, regression modeling, and instrumental variables. The first method used 70,040 matched pairs and the other two used the entire cohort. Only 36% of the CRP users were women, compared to the fact that women were 50% of the nonusers. After extensive analyses to control for potential confounding variables, mortalities were 21% to 34% lower in CRP users than in CRP nonusers in this socioeconomically and clinically diverse, older population (Suaya et al., 2009).

In a study, 234 women (99 African Americans and 135 Caucasians) were surveyed 1 month after discharge from the hospital after a PCI, CABG, or MI without revascularization and they completed a 6-month follow-up survey. The findings revealed that the overall rate of referral to outpatient cardiac rehabilitation for women was only 19% and it was significantly lower for African American women compared with Caucasian women (12% vs. 24%). Only 15% of the referred women went on to enroll in the programs, with fewer African American women enrolling compared with the Caucasian women (9% vs. 19%). Controlling for age, education, angina class, and comorbidities, women with annual income less than $20,000 were 66% less likely to be referred to cardiac rehabilitation and 60% less likely to enroll when compared with women with incomes greater than $20,000. Diversity in the population of individuals referred and enrolled in CRPs and diversity of the professional caregivers of cardiac rehabilitations remains a challenge that must be addressed (Allen, Scott, Stewart, & Rohm-Young, 2004).

A recent Cochrane systematic review and meta-analysis including 63 studies and over 14,000 participants highlighted that outpatient CRPs led to a reduction in cardiovascular mortality and the risk of hospital readmission (Anderson et al., 2016). Higher levels of health-related quality of life are also reported following CRP. In our current health care environment emphasizing value-based medicine—the highest quality of care achieved at the most fiscally responsible levels of health care costs—CRP plays a key role in achieving excellence in clinical care while minimizing recurrent cardiac events and expense.

SUMMARY

The challenge of cardiovascular disorders will continue to grow as long as their prevention is not given emphasis and priority. If present trends continue, the diagnostic and therapeutic advances of the past decades may reduce cardiovascular mortality without a reduction in the prevalence of CVD and its attendant functional limitation and disability. The need of individuals with CVD for medical, psychological, rehabilitative, and vocational services may be greater than ever.

REFERENCES

ACOG Committee on Gynecologic Practice. (2013, June). ACOG committee opinion 565: Hormone therapy and heart disease. *Obstetrics & Gynecology, 121*, 1407–1410.

Allen, J. K., Scott, L. B., Stewart, K. J., & Rohm-Young, D. (2004). Disparities in women's referral to and enrollment in outpatient cardiac rehabilitation. *Journal of General Internal Medicine, 19*, 747–753.

Anderson, L., Oldridge, N., Thonpson, D., Zwisler, A. D., Rees, K., Martin, N., & Taylor, R. R. (2016). Exercise-based cardiac rehabilitation for coronary heart disease. cochrane systematic review and meta-analysis. *Journal of the American College of Cardiology, 67*, 1–12.

Bakir, I., Casselman, F. P., Wellens, F., Jeanmart, H., De Geest, R., Degrieck, I., . . . Vanermen H. (2006). Minimally invasive versus standard approach aortic valve replacement: A study in 506 patients. *The Annals of Thoracic Surgery, 81*, 1599–1604.

Berkman, L. F., Blumenthal, J., Burg, M., Carney, R. M., Catellier, D., Cowan, M. J., . . . Enhancing recovery in coronary heart disease patients' investigators (ENRICHD). (2003). Effects of treating depression and low perceived social support on clinical events after myocardial infarction: The enhancing recovery in coronary heart disease patients (ENRICHD) randomized trial. *Journal of the American Medical Association, 289*, 3106–3116.

Bittner, V. (2008). Angina pectoris: reversal of the gender gap. *Circulation, 117*, 1505–1507.

Brar, S., & Stone, G. (2009). Advances in percutaneous coronary intervention. *Current Cardiology Reports, 11*, 245–251.

Clouse, R. E., Lustman, P. J., Freedland, K. E., Griffith, L. S., McGill, J. B., & Carney, R. M. (2003). Depression and coronary heart disease in women with diabetes. *Psychosomatic Medicine, 65*, 376–383.

Coulter, S. A., & Campos, C. (2012). Identify and treat depression for reduced cardiac risk and improved outcomes. *Texas Heart Institute Journal, 39*(2), 231–234.

Eastwood, J. A., & Doering, L. V. (2005). Gender differences in coronary artery disease. *Journal of Cardiovascular Nursing, 20*, 340–351.

European Society of Cardiology. (2010). Focused update of esc guidelines on device therapy in heart failure. *European Heart Journal, 31*, 2677–2687.

Francis, G. S., Bartos, J. A., & Adatya, S. (2014). Inotropes. *Journal of the American College of Cardiology, 63*(20), 2069–2078.

Grodstein, F., Clarkson, T. B., & Manson, J. E. (2003). Understanding the divergent data on postmenopausal hormone therapy. *New England Journal of Medicine, 348*, 645–650.

Khayyam-Nekouei, Z., Neshatdoost, H., Yousefy, A., Masoumeh, S., & Gholamreza, M. (2013). Psychological factors and coronary heart disease. *ARYA Atheroscler*, *9*(1), 102–111.

Levine G. N., Bates, E. R., Blankenship, S. C., Bailey, S. R., Bittl, J. A., Cercek, B., . . . Zhao, D. X. (2015). ACC/AHA/SCAI focused update on primary PCI. *Circulation*, *67*(10), 1–50.

Long, E. F., Swain, G. W., & Mangi, A. A. (2104). Comparative Survival and Cost-effectiveness of Advanced Therapies for End-stage Heart Failure. *Circulation: Heart Failure*, *73*(3), 470–478.

Mallik, S., Krumholz, H. M., Lin, Z., Kasl, S. V., Mattera, J. A., Roumanis, S. A., . . . Vaccarino, V. (2005). Patients with depressive symptoms have lower health status benefits after coronary artery bypass surgery. *Circulation, 111*, 271–277.

Mauri, L., Hsieh, W. H., Massacre, J. M., Ho, K. K., D'Agostino, R., Cutlip, D. E. (2007). Stent thrombosis in randomized clinical trials of drug eluding stents. *New England Journal of Medicine, 356*, 1020–1029.

McSweeney, J. C., Cody, M., O'Sullivan, P., Elberson, K., Moser, D. K., & Garvin, B. J. (2003). Women's early warning symptoms of acute myocardial infarction. *Circulation*, *108*, 2619–2623.

Milani, R., & Lavie, C. J. (2007). Impact of cardiac rehabilitation on depression and its associated mortality. *American Journal of Medicine, 120*, 799–806.

Moller-Leimkuhler, A. (2008). Women with coronary artery disease and depression: A neglected risk group. *The World Journal of Biological Psychiatry, 9*, 92–101.

Mosca, L., Banka, C. L., Benjamin, E. J., Berra, K., Bushnell, C., Dolor, R. J., . . . American College of Nurse Practitioners. (2007). Evidence-based guidelines for cardiovascular disease prevention in women: 2007 update. *Circulation, 115*, 1481–1501.

Mozaffarian, D., Benjamin, E. J., & Go, A. S., (2015). AHA statistical update: Heart disease and stroke statistics—2015 update: A report from the American Heart Association. *Circulation*, *131*(4), e29–e322.

Ridker, P. M., Danielson, E., Fonseca, F. A., Genest, J., Gotto, A. M., Kastelein, J. J., . . . Koenig, W. (2008). Rosuvastatin to prevent vascular events in men and women with elevated C-reactive protein. *New England Journal of Medicine, 359*(21), 2195–2207.

Rossouw, J. E., Cushman, M., Greenland, P., Lloyd-Jones, D. M., Bray, P., Kooperberg, C., . . . Hsia, J. (2008). Inflammatory, lipid, thrombotic, and genetic markers of coronary heart disease risk in the women's health initiative trials of hormone therapy. *Archives of Internal Medicine, 168*, 2245–2253.

Rossouw, J. E., Prentice, R. L., Manson, J. E., Wu, L., Barad, D., Barnabei, V. M., . . . Stefanick, M. L. (2007). Postmenopausal hormone therapy and risk of cardiovascular disease by age and years since menopause. *Journal of the American Medical Association, 297*, 1465–1477.

Rumsfeld, J., & Ho, M. (2005). Depression and cardiovascular disease: A call for recognition. *Circulation, 111*, 250–253.

Rutledge, T., Reiss, V. A., Linke, S. E., Greenberg, B. H., & Mills, P. J. (2006). Depression in heart failure: A meta-analytic review of prevalence, intervention effects, and associations with clinical outcomes. *Journal of the American College of Cardiology*, *48*(8), 1527–1537.

Schomig, A., Mehilli, J., de Waha, A., Seyfarth, M., Pache, J., & Kastrati, A. (2008). A meta-analysis of 17 randomized trials of a percutaneous coronary intervention-based strategy in patients with stable coronary artery disease. *Journal of the American College of Cardiology, 52*, 894–904.

Serruys, P. W., Morice, M. C., Kappertein, A. P., Colombo, A., Holmes, D. R., & Mack, M. J., . . . Elisabeth, S. (2009). Percutaneous coronary intervention versus coronary-artery bypass grafting for severe artery disease. *New England Journal of Medicine, 360*, 961–972.

Stramba-Badiale, M., Fox, K. M., Priori, S. G., Collins, P., Daly, C., Graham, I., . . . Jonsson, B. (2006). Cardiovascular disease in women: A statement from the policy conference of the European Society of Cardiology. *European Heart Journal, 27*, 994–1005.

Suaya, J., Stason, W., Ades, P., Norman, S., & Shepard, S. (2009). Cardiac rehabilitation and survival in older coronary patients. *Journal of the American College of Cardiology, 54*, 25–33.

United Nations, Department of Economic and Social Affairs, Population Division. (2014). World Urbanization Prospects: The 2014 Revision, Highlights (ST/ESA/SER.A/352).

Upadhyay, R. K. (2015). Emerging risk biomarkers in cardiovascular diseases and disorders. *Journal of Lipids, 2015*, 1–50.

Valensi, P., Lorgis, L., Cottin, Y., & Lorgis, C. (2011). Prevalence, incidence, predictive factors and prognosis of silent myocardial infarction: A review of the literature. *Archives of Cardiovascular Diseases, 104*(3), 178–188.

van den Broek, K. C., Heijmans, N., & van Assen, M. A. L. M. (2013). Anxiety and depression in patients with an implantable cardioverter defibrillator and their partners. *Pacing And Clinical Electrophysiology*, *36*(3), 362–371.

Witt, B. J., Jacobsen, S. J., Weston, S. A., Killian, B. S., Meverden, R., Allison, T., . . . Roger, V. L. (2004). Cardiac rehabilitation after myocardial infarction in the community. *Journal of the American College of Cardiology, 44*, 988–996.

Yancy, C. W., Jessup, M., Bozkurt, B., Javed, B., Donald, E. C., Mark, H. D., . . . American Heart Association Task Force on Practice Guidelines. (2013). 2013 ACCF/AHA guideline for the management of heart failure. *Journal of the American College of Cardiology, 62*, e147–e239.

Zellwenger, M. J., Osterwalder, R. H., Langewitz, W., & Pfisterer, M. E. (2004). Coronary artery disease and depression. *European Heart Journal, 25*, 3–9.

CHAPTER

Chronic Pain Syndromes

Christopher Gharibo, Hersh Patel, and Steve M. Aydin

Chronic pain syndromes are composed of multifactorial relationships among biologically based neurological triggers and pathways; psychologically mediated moods, emotions, and behaviors; and socially developed responses, interactions, and consequences. The complex interplay between these factors can devastate a patient's quality of life, as well as make the diagnoses, treatment, and ongoing management of chronic pain syndromes by health care professionals exceedingly difficult, resulting in psychological and physical disability.

Chronic pain differs from acute pain in many key tenets. In acute pain, there is a gradual abatement of the signals triggered from a noxious stimulus as the cause of the perceived stimulus heals and ceases to exist as a triggering mechanism. In chronic pain, the imprinted signals and perceived pain may persist for several weeks, months, or even years after the original injury has healed. In addition, the acute pain pathway is triggered by the presence of an immediate noxious stimulus, whereas the chronic pain pathway may be spontaneously activated in the absence of an immediate physical trigger (i.e., prior traumatic injury or infection) or, in some cases, by the absence of any physiological or pathological trigger.

Treatment of chronic pain creates yet another dimension of complexity, as it requires a multimechanistic, multimodal, or multidisciplinary approach for effective management. The opioid epidemic has manifested itself with significant morbidity and mortality, as the number of overdose deaths from prescribed opioids has more than tripled in the past 20 years (Mack, 2013). For clinicians, the focus has shifted to combining nonopioid- and opioid-based pharmacological therapies that also combine interventional procedures with physiatric, psychiatric, and psychologic approaches.

PREVALENCE AND IMPACT

It is clear that the development of a chronic pain syndrome can contribute to significant morbidity in an affected individual, and when the effects are examined across a population, it is also easy to surmise that chronic pain syndromes can have significant psychosocial and medical consequences if not identified and dealt with appropriately. Previously, researchers suggested that approximately 20% to 30% of the U.S. population (Bonica, 1990) and nearly 35% of the Canadian population (Toth, Lander, & Wiebe, 2009) suffered from a chronically painful condition and that the medical resources spent annually in the diagnosis and treatment of these conditions coupled with the cost of lost productivity due to inability to work is a number that reached hundreds of billions of dollars (Gill & Frymoyer, 1997). Although controversial, the Institute of Medicine report from the Committee on Advancing Pain Research, Care, and Education in 2011 has suggested that the United States with its current population of 318,000,000 has approximately 95,000,000 chronic pain sufferers with a total societal cost ranging from $560 billion to $635 billion.

Although chronic pain syndromes can affect a significant portion of a population, their prevalence and impact is not equal across gender lines, age, and/or socioeconomic status (Wenig, Schmidt, Kohlmann, & Schweikert, 2009). In addition, coexisting psychopathology (i.e., major depressive disorder, anxiety, attention deficit disorder) is another major component of this cohort, which not only predisposes individuals to developing a chronic pain syndrome but may also exacerbate the symptoms of a newly acquired syndrome.

The complexity of the various syndromes that are discussed in this chapter has made it difficult to address chronic pain syndromes within the traditional medical model of care. Thus, the fact that these conditions require a multidisciplinary approach and a thorough understanding and commitment to addressing their respective biological, psychological, and social aspects is no surprise and has been convincingly proved as effective in numerous studies.

PATHOPHYSIOLOGY OF CHRONIC PAIN

Although an extensive discussion of the physiology of acute pain and the pathophysiology of chronic pain is beyond the scope of this chapter, an understanding of what exactly is occurring neurologically is necessary. Chronic pain is more than just "low back pain." Several questions emerge with this topic: Why is chronic pain spontaneous? Why does it persist longer than expected after an injury has healed? Why is it physically and emotionally disabling? How does it reduce a person's quality of life? To begin to address these questions, we need to discuss how this pain is initiated.

To understand the progression of acute pain to chronic pain pathophysiology, we need to understand that the process of neurological change in the peripheral and central nervous systems is a continuum. It starts with the basic mechanisms of nociception, or the ability to detect harmful stimuli, and eventually includes the structural and chemical changes in the peripheral and central nervous system, which are ultimately responsible for the more complex mechanisms of chronic pain. The process of neurological peripheral and central sensitization starts from "time zero" with the initiation of peripheral tissue injury; it is peripherally and centrally imprinted in the chronic pain population rather than initiated but reversed in the rest of the population.

The International Association for the Study of Pain (IASP) categorizes pain into two distinct classes, which may present together in the same patient: Nociceptive pain includes acute, subacute, and inflammatory pain and results from noxious stimuli and inflammation, which is largely considered protective, adaptive, and "normal." Neuropathic pain often implies chronic pain and has peripheral and central nervous system components.

Chronic pain often is mixed nociceptive and neuropathic (e.g., failed back surgery syndrome and osteoarthritis) or primarily neuropathic and is associated with imprinted neuroanatomical (e.g., neuroplastic rewiring, sodium channel, and alpha-receptor upregulation) and chemical changes (e.g., glutamate and aspartate release) in the peripheral and central nervous systems, which result in abnormal processing.

Such changes often result in clinical symptoms and signs of spontaneous and paresthetic pain that is associated with dysesthesias (unpleasant sensations evoked by various stimuli), allodynia (pain evoked by a normally nonpainful stimulus), and hyperalgesia (disproportionate pain due to a stimulus considered to be already painful).

Peripheral "nociceptors" are free nerve endings that exist throughout the body and respond to potential tissue-damaging stimuli (Bonica, 1990). In the chronic pain patient, often in the absence of a noxious stimulus, a lowered activation threshold of peripheral nociceptors or aberrant spontaneous firing by, for example, a peripheral neuroma, maintains the sensitivity of the central nervous system to afferent input. These peripheral signals are transmitted by myelinated A-delta and A-beta fibers, as well as unmyelinated C fibers, which can respond to a variety of chemical, mechanical, and thermal stimuli in the periphery.

The large-diameter A-beta fibers are myelinated and respond primarily to light touch and moving stimuli, such as vibration, whereas A-delta fibers, which are myelinated, small-diameter fibers, and unmyelinated C fibers respond to noxious stimuli. A-delta and C fibers are known as nociceptors, or pain fibers, because they respond maximally to noxious stimulation. These nociceptors respond to noxious mechanical, thermal, and chemical stimuli (Fields, Basbaum, & Heinricher, 2005).

The first-order nociceptive afferents, which are nerves along the pathway that communicate up to the central nervous system, terminate in the Rexed lamina of the dorsal horn of the spinal cord. For example, the unmyelinated C fibers terminate primarily in the Rexed lamina 1 and the myelinated pain fibers terminate in laminae 1, 3, 4, and 5. The second-order neurons that project from the dorsal horn to the thalamus and cortex, some of which are known as wide dynamic range (WDR) neurons, expand to receive a wider range of impulses. In essence, WDR neurons are activated by both noxious and non-noxious stimuli and are thought to be responsible for central mechanisms of allodynia. These second-order neurons project to the higher centers primarily via the spinothalamic tracts and project to the medial and posterior nuclei of the thalamus, which, in turn, project to the sensory cortex (Raj, 1996).

The Gate Control Theory of Pain published by Wall and Melzack introduced the concept of spinal pain modulation. The pain modulation concept has since been broadened to encompass the pain-processing parts of the peripheral and central nervous systems, including the descending pathways that are all thought to be responsible for chronic pain pathophysiology and individual differences of pain perception (Figure 8.1).

The descending cerebrospinal pathways can be inhibitory or excitatory. These tracts involve connections from periaqueductal gray in the midbrain to the nucleus raphe magnus, reticular formation, and lower dorsal horn centers that receive the primary afferents. These pathways are modulated primarily by noradrenergic and serotonergic neurotransmitters, which help explain why certain antidepressants are effective treatments for chronic pain. Antidepressants can also address the patient's coexisting anxiety and depression, which are inextricably linked to the chronic pain population.

Immediately following an injurious stimulus, the barrage of stimuli that are generated in the primary afferents in the periphery travel toward the second-order neurons and higher centers in the central nervous system. This process induces peripheral and central sensitization, also known as "windup," where the primary afferents, dorsal horn, and higher centers become progressively hypersensitized to repetitive afferent stimulation. In the chronic pain patient, this is often coupled with diminished descending inhibition on the afferent impulses. The end result is exaggerated afferent impulse activity that reaches the higher centers that are ultimately processed as chronic pain.

In essence, there are neuroanatomic, neuroplastic, and neurochemical changes as well as associated sensitization in the progression from acute to chronic pain pathophysiology. The neurological sensitization process starts immediately upon tissue injury, which typically reverses, resulting in the resolution of the pain. However, when this neurological process does not reverse, chronic pain results. The interactions between the ascending and descending pathways play an important role in chronic pain development, perception, and modulation.

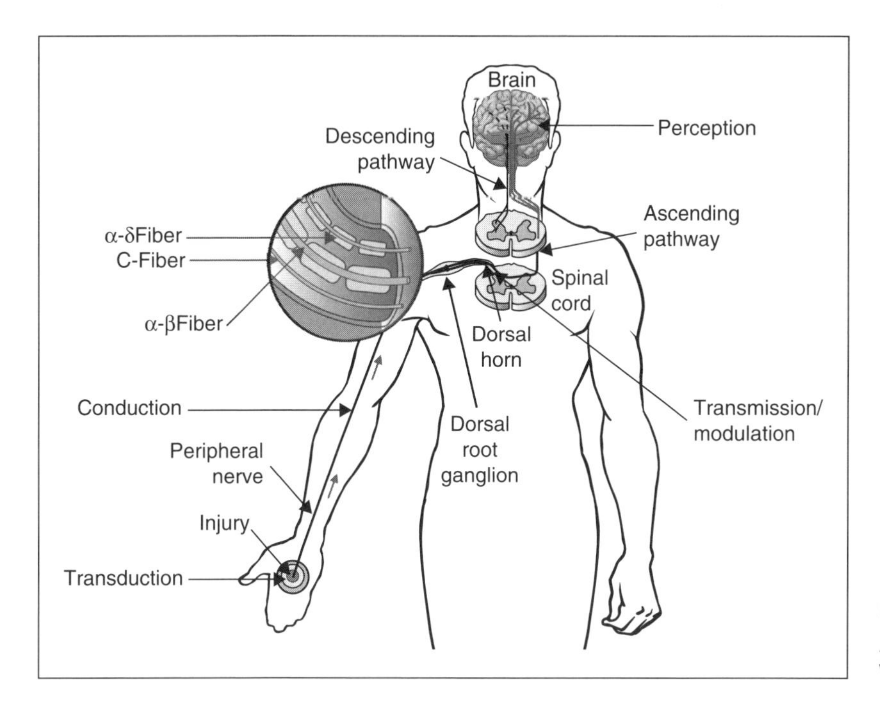

FIGURE 8.1 Physiology of pain perception.
Source: Galer and Dworkin (2000); Irving and Wallace (1997); Woolf (2004).

COMPONENTS OF DISABLING CHRONIC PAIN SYNDROMES

Biopsychosocial Component

In addition to the biological and physiological basis for chronic pain, there are strong correlations with psychological and social factors that contribute to the etiology, onset, and progression of chronic pain syndromes. Major psychological contributors to chronic pain may include problems such as a lack of self-control, poor coping, emotional turmoil, low self-esteem, and negative thinking. Social factors that affect chronic pain syndromes are numerous and, among other factors, include gender, culture, family dynamics, employment issues, socioeconomic status, religion, and income.

The importance of understanding and addressing psychosocial contributors to chronic pain syndromes is underscored by the fact that these nonbiological factors can have both a direct and indirect effect on the patient's mind and body. For instance, patients' persistence of negative thinking may preclude them from allowing themselves to believe that treatment modalities will relieve their pain. Furthermore, patients' cultural beliefs may limit them from being able to effectively communicate all aspects of their pain to a practitioner. In light of these factors, it is clear that a multidisciplinary approach to the chronic pain patient, including physicians, nurses, psychologists, social workers, and other allied health care professionals, is essential in the care of many chronic pain patients.

Neuropathic Component

In addition to the nociceptive components that can contribute to acute pain and eventually lead to chronic pain, more subtle neuropathic pain conditions need to be identified early to direct targeted treatment. Neuropathic components are prevalent in scenarios where direct injury to nerve components is obvious (i.e., mechanical nerve trauma) and in settings where obvious pathology to nerves is less explicit (i.e., diffuse back pain). Commonly, the neuropathic component may manifest as numbness, paresthesias (abnormal sensation), allodynia (pain from a stimulus that does not normally cause pain), hyperalgesia (increased response to stimulus), motor weakness, anhidrosis (inability to perspire), and/or dysautonomia (improperly functioning autonomic system). In addition to chronic pain and the aforementioned symptoms, systemic neuropathies due to conditions such as diabetes or chronic alcoholism may produce bowel and bladder dysfunction, heat and cold intolerance, and sexual dysfunction. Therefore, the importance of identifying the neuropathic component is essential for the effective management of any chronic pain syndrome.

Depression and Anxiety Components

An undiagnosed mental illness, especially a depressive or anxious mood disorder, can interfere with the effective treatment of a chronic pain syndrome. Given the high prevalence of depression, anxiety, and other psychiatric conditions in chronic pain patients, it is important to screen patients for the presence of such conditions and refer them for appropriate treatment (Alschuler, Theisen-Goodvich, Haig, & Geisser, 2008). Mental health issues may manifest themselves as lack of motivation, lack of general physical activity, and/or feelings of hopelessness or worthlessness and are often best elucidated by a mental health care professional such as a pain psychologist or psychiatrist. Without addressing the depressive components of chronic pain, patients will continue not only to experience significant impairment in their ability to participate in treatment modalities, but to also exhibit low energy and be markedly limited in the performance of their basic activities of daily living.

Quality of Life

Given the high incidence of physical and psychosocial impairment in chronic pain patients, the negative effect on a patient's quality of life can be enormous. Detailed functional and psychological assessments of the chronic pain patient can identify areas to address to improve the patient's quality of life. One aspect of coping with chronic pain that has been shown to have a positive association with quality of life is a patient's willingness to accept his or her pain (Mason, Mathias, & Skevington, 2008). The assessment of improvements in the quality of life of a patient suffering from a chronic pain syndrome over time is a useful outcome measure that can be applied to determine the effectiveness of the overall management of a single patient or to assess the advantages of a specific chronic pain therapy.

HEADACHES

Migraine and chronic headache accounts for a large number of lost workdays, billions of dollars annually in health care costs, and loss of productivity in the United States. Migraineurs cost American employers about $13 billion per year because of missed workdays and impaired work function. Direct medical costs for migraine care are about $1 billion per year (Hu, Markson, Lipton, Stewart, & Berger, 1999). Data from the National Ambulatory Medical Care Survey and National Hospital Ambulatory Medical Care Survey indicate that headache is among the top 20 reasons for outpatient medical visits and among the top five for emergency department (ED) visits.

Migraine is a prevalent episodic chronic disease that affects sufferers during their most productive years. Individuals with severe migraine are typically incapacitated by a throbbing headache, nausea and/or vomiting, and sensitivity to light and/or sound (Levin, 2008). A migraine headache is debilitating due to the fact that it interferes with family obligations and social plans, impairs work responsibilities, produces emotional stress, and challenges a health-related quality of life (Levin, 2008). It also increases the risk for other physical and psychiatric comorbidities.

As opposed to the vast majority of medical syndromes, the diagnosis and development of a treatment plan for headaches relies almost solely on a patient's historical description of his or her symptomatology. The value of laboratory analysis and radiological testing is not in the confirmation of a primary diagnosis of a headache syndrome, but instead in ruling out a secondary cause of pain related to entities such as tumors, neurodegenerative disease, increased intracranial pressure, or vascular pathology.

It is important to assess the extent of impairment and disability in headache sufferers. Reliable, validated self-administered questionnaires can be clinically helpful. A number of these have been developed to quantify disability such as the Subjective Symptoms Assessment Profile, the Headache Disability Inventory, and the Migraine Disability Assessment Questionnaire.

Migraine and chronic daily headache are serious afflictions and are recognized as potentially serious and disabling chronic pain syndromes. Many patients require a combination of pharmacological therapy and avoidance of common triggers to manage their symptoms. Most of these therapies, especially the acute abortive and acute analgesic therapies, are accompanied by significant side effects. Therefore, differentiating between migraines and other common types of headaches has become more important with the advent of manual and cognitive therapies in the management of headaches. Efficacy of manual therapy in primary tension-type headaches (Chiabi & Russel, 2014) and cognitive behavioral therapy (CBT) in chronic headaches (Harris, Loveman, Clegg, Easton, & Berry, 2015) creates new alternatives for patients struggling with limited pharmaceutical options.

Traditionally, the etiology of these headaches has been described as a central phenomenon, but more recently, extracranial trigger sites have been identified with decompression leading to improved symptomatology (Janis, Dhanik, & Howard, 2011). Botulinum toxin-A injections at these trigger sites can be used as an effective preventive therapy for chronic migraines, whereas surgical decompression or neurectomy of select sites may provide long-term improvements after compression is confirmed (Guyuron et al., 2009).

Although there are numerous pharmacological, interventional, and behavioral modalities aimed at treating headache syndromes, there is a need for further research into the etiologies and innovative therapies (Kernick, 2005), which can result in improved management of these chronic pain syndromes.

LOW BACK AND LEG PAIN

Low back pain is one of the most common experiences of humankind. Although studies reveal that back pain affects 60% to 80% of the adult population in the United States, it is probably experienced by nearly everyone at some point in his or her life. The point prevalence of low back pain is estimated to be approximately 30%. The diagnosis and treatment of refractory chronic low back pain represents one of the greatest challenges to medicine.

The Quebec Task Force on Spinal Disorders found that more than 90% of low back pain episodes improve spontaneously within 3 weeks of onset. The Task Force recommended against diagnostic tests, including imaging studies, for low back pain within the first 4 to 6 weeks. In 1994, the Agency for Health Care Policy and Research published guidelines for the treatment of acute low back pain (Bigos et al., 1994). The consensus was that more than 90% of acute low back pain patients recover spontaneously within 1 month, regardless of treatment.

Surveys conducted in the United States reveal that low back pain accounts for approximately 15 million office visits annually, with total associated health care–related and productivity losses exceeding $100 billion annually. Because of the limitations of currently available medical therapies for low back pain and other conditions, up to 40% of the population resorts to alternative therapeutic modalities (Bigos et al., 1994; Derby, Bogduk, Anat, & Schwarzer, 1993). The portion that continues with conventional medical treatment will often undergo progressively more invasive and expensive therapeutic modalities that may end in one or more surgeries in an attempt to obtain pain relief.

Low back pain is a leading cause of disability in people younger than 45 years and accounts for roughly 40% of all disability claims. The cost of medical treatments, days off from work, and worker's compensation payments results in an annual cost to society of tens of billions of dollars.

The vast majority of low back pain is acute and muscular in origin, although other etiologies should be considered. The differential diagnosis of low back pain is vast and, as noted in Table 8.1, includes visceral and nonmusculoskeletal processes as well. However, the vast majority of low back pain is caused by biomechanical processes that develop with years of poor posture and age-related degenerative changes. The spine and its attached elements degenerate simultaneously, resulting in pain that may originate from multiple sources.

The most common examples include muscle sprains and strains, osteoarthritis of the lumbosacral spine, and other anatomical abnormalities such as herniated nucleus pulposus, degenerative disc disease, and spinal stenosis. The structures that can be major contributors to low back pain are muscles, intervertebral discs, zygapophyseal joints, the posterior longitudinal ligament, nerve roots, dura, and ligamentum flavum.

The typical low back pain patient often suffers from more than one musculoskeletal diagnosis and presents with multiple pain generators. A thorough history and physical examination with particular attention to the musculoskeletal and nervous systems is essential while ruling out more serious conditions such as the low back pain of cancer, infection, or vascular etiology. Although commonly performed, the use of MRI and CT of the lumbar spine has been criticized because of their sensitivity, causing the physician to focus on anatomic abnormalities that are unrelated to the patient's pain. The results of MRI or CT scan of the lumbar spine and electromyography (EMG) are not diagnostic and are mainly useful to corroborate clinical suspicions identified during the history and physical examination, or plan for invasive therapeutic interventions.

TABLE 8.1

CAUSES OF LOW BACK PAIN
• Muscle sprain/strain
• Herniated nucleus pulposus
• Degenerative disc disease
• Annular fissure/tear
• Zygapophyseal (facet) joint arthropathy
• Spinal central canal or foraminal stenosis
• Osteoarthritis of the hip
• Spondylolisthesis
• Ankylosing spondylitis
• Epidural abscess/hematoma
• Discitis
• Osteomyelitis
• Primary or metastatic cancer
• Referred: abdominal aortic aneurysm, pancreatitis, renal colic, etc.

One common generator of low back pain is a lumbosacral radiculopathy (spinal nerve root pathology) caused by degeneration of or injury to an intervertebral disc in the spinal column. Disc disease is accompanied by the triggering of an inflammatory cascade, the chemical mediators of which in turn exert a noxious effect on the nearby spinal nerves (Mchaourab & Knight, 2009). As these spinal nerves, which exit the spinal cord in the lower back and link the back and the lower extremities to the central nervous system, are irritated, they can transmit inflammatory pain that travels from the lower back to the legs. This is typically manifested in patients describing pain that starts in their back and characteristically "shoots" down one or both of their legs toward their feet.

Another prevalent cause of low back pain is spinal arthropathy and the accompanying inflammation of a key joint of the spinal column known as the zygapophyseal or facet joint. The facet joints of the spine run from the cervical region all the way down to the lumbosacral area, are in almost constant motion, and play a significant role in allowing twisting, bending, and rotation of the human body. Over time, facet joints, similar to any other joint in the body, can become arthritic, destabilize, or lose their cartilage, which causes the synovium to inflame and the bony components of the joint to hypertrophy, causing arthritic pain and compressive radiculopathy (Czervionke & Fenton, 2008).

Routine clinical evaluations of low back pain patients fail to provide a specific diagnosis in up to 85% of cases (Bigos et al., 1994). Diagnostic spinal injections can provide additional information, which in conjunction with the history, physical examination, and results of imaging studies, may aid in identifying the most probable anatomic basis for the pain. Subsequently, a precisely directed therapeutic spinal injection can provide significant relief with minimal risk to the patient when compared with surgery. The challenge presented to the physician is to identify the major pain generator(s) and to decide which to treat first, while avoiding the structures that appear abnormal on the MRI but do not contribute to the patient's symptoms.

Although some references recommend bedrest for the treatment of low back pain, it has been shown to impede recovery. Prolonged inactivity and deconditioning propagate the conditions responsible for low back pain, making recovery more difficult. Currently, maintenance of the patient's activity and work status, participation in a physical rehabilitation program, and pain management have become the cornerstones of treating low back pain patients.

Because of the dire statistics on persistent low back pain, a patient with low back pain that has persisted beyond a 4-week period should be referred to a specialist. This level of care is necessary to provide the patient with sufficient pain control to allow physical therapy and reverse the physical deconditioning that insidiously develops. For example, Katz (2006) published that 80% of workers who report an episode of low back pain will usually return to work within 1 month. By 3 months, about 90% of those with the episode of lower back pain return to work. However, less than 5% will never return to work. The subset of individuals who do not return to work account for 75% of the cost for the treatment of low back pain. Furthermore, if a patient is out of work due to low back pain for greater than 6 months, he or she has a 50% likelihood of returning to work. At 1 year, the likelihood of the individual returning to work drops to 25%. The longer an individual remains out of work due to low back pain, the lesser the likelihood of him or her returning to work (Katz, 2006).

Low back pain affects costs related to work loss, disability, and worker's compensation. According to published data, there are approximately 150 million workdays lost as a result of low back pain every year, and low back pain has been reported to be responsible for 40% of absences from work, the second leading source of work absences after the common cold (Shaw, Linton, & Pransky, 2006).

Furthermore, back pain is the most common cause for filing worker's compensation claims and the most common cause of work-related disability in people younger than 45 years. Economically, the average cost of a worker's compensation claim for low back pain was $8,300, more than twice the average cost of $4,075 for other compensable claims.

Katz also noted that the 5% of patients who have low back pain and do not return to work by 3 months account for 75% of health care costs incurred by those with low back pain (Katz, 2006). These costs include medications, outpatient visits, physical therapy, peripheral and spinal injections, ED visits, hospitalizations, and surgery. As the volume of low back pain–related health care utilization increases without evidence of corresponding clinical improvement, more scientifically validated therapies are demanded by insurers, employers, and other stakeholders.

COMPLEX REGIONAL PAIN SYNDROME

Complex regional pain syndrome (CRPS) is predominantly a neuropathic and partly musculoskeletal pain syndrome associated with autonomic disturbance. At least 50,000 new cases of CRPS are diagnosed in the United States annually, with women being three times more likely to be affected (Bruehl, 2010). What used to be referred to as "reflex sympathetic dystrophy" and "causalgia" have been reclassified by the IASP as "CRPS Type I" and "CRPS Type II," respectively. The syndromes are similar in that they are both characterized by a spectrum of sensory, motor, autonomic, trophic, and dystrophic changes. The differentiating factor between them is the evidence of obvious nerve damage in CRPS Type II, which is lacking in CRPS Type I.

Although the pain and characteristic symptoms of CRPS are usually localized over an initial injured location, it is not uncommon for the symptoms to spread to both adjacent and remote unaffected areas. Typically, the most bothersome symptoms for patients can be "electrical" shooting and "burning" pains, but additional complaints may include allodynia, dysesthesia, and hyperalgesia. Autonomic dysfunction (hyperhidrosis and color or temperature changes of the skin) and altered motor function (tremors, inability to use muscles secondary to pain, and painful range of motion leading to atrophy and motion-limiting contractures) may also be present.

A distinguishing factor between CRPS and other forms of neuropathic pain is the regional distribution of pain compared to a pattern more consistent with the territory of a single peripheral nerve. The pain itself may not be proportionate to the inciting injury as well. To make the diagnosis of CRPS, the symptoms cannot be attributable to another pathology or condition.

A complex interplay of various pathophysiologic mechanisms within the peripheral and central nervous systems contribute to the development of CRPS. Alterations of sympathetic and catecholaminergic function, peripheral and central sensitization and neurogenic inflammation, and altered somatosensory representation in the brain, genetics, and psychology influence the presentation and chronicity of the disease process. The multifactorial nature of CRPS allows for a spectrum of symptoms, which not only makes diagnosing difficult, but the management even more complex.

Early recognition and referral of the CRPS patient to a multidisciplinary pain treatment clinic is essential so that the diagnosis can be made and appropriate therapy initiated. A delay in diagnosis and treatment can be a source of devastating impairment as it can result in irreversible physical, neurological, and psychological damage. Clinical diagnosis relies on patient history, physical examination, and the findings of musculoskeletal degeneration and secondary pain from the chronic processes of the syndrome. The symptoms and signs must be consistent with time-dependent effects of CRPS, such as atrophy, dystrophy, contractions, and secondary pain. Hypoesthesia and hyperalgesia are common in the earlier months, which progresses to anesthesia dolorosa with ongoing disease (Veldman, Reynen, Arntz, & Goris, 1993). The chronic pain that follows the acute phase is often present at rest and resistant to treatment. No difference in pathophysiologic mechanisms or treatment responsiveness exists between the two types of CRPS other than that Type II may require direct surgical management of the underlying nerve injury.

Various diagnostic criteria have been developed for appropriately identifying CRPS pathology. Patients with CRPS endure derangement of normal physiologic responses, which makes it difficult to identify when these changes become pathologic CRPS and not another diagnosis from an acute injury. The original diagnostic criteria were developed by the IASP in 1994 and were modified in 2003 to improve specificity (Table 8.2).

The mainstay of treatment for CRPS is based on physical and occupational therapy aimed to return and preserve function, prevent loss of range of motion, and prevent contractures and atrophy. Most symptoms of CRPS resolve within the first 12 months, but an estimated 25% fulfill the IASP diagnostic criteria at 12 months from chronicity and require further management. Common therapies include rehabilitation, pharmacological treatment, psychological counseling, and interventional approaches. Therapy may be tailored to the predominant pathophysiology at play (Figure 8.2).

Pharmacologic treatments used by clinicians are largely empirical and influenced by personal experiences and preferences. The most convincing evidence exists with intravenous bisphosphonates in patients with disease duration of less than 6 months. Neuropathic and antinociceptive medications such as gabapentin, opioids, and antidepressants are commonly used with support inferred from the benefits demonstrated through other neuropathic conditions.

Interventional techniques enable patients to participate in effective physical and occupational

TABLE 8.2

HARDEN/BRUEHL CRPS DIAGNOSTIC CRITERIA
CRPS TYPE I
1. Continuing pain, which is disproportionate to any inciting event
2. Must report at least one symptom in three of the following four categories: • **Sensory:** Reports of hyperesthesia and/or allodynia • **Vasomotor:** Reports of temperature asymmetry and/or skin color changes and/or skin color asymmetry • **Sudomotor/edema:** Reports of edema and/or sweating changes and/or sweating asymmetry • **Motor/trophic:** Reports of decreased range of motion and/or motor dysfunction (weakness, tremor, dystonia) and/or trophic changes (hair, nails, skin)
3. Must display at least one sign at time of evaluation in two or more of the following categories: • **Sensory:** Evidence of hyperalgesia (to pinprick) and/or allodynia (to light touch and/or temperature sensation and/or deep somatic pressure and/or joint movement) • **Vasomotor:** Evidence of temperature asymmetry (>1°C) and/or skin color changes and/or asymmetry • **Sudomotor/edema:** Evidence of edema and/or sweating changes and/or sweating asymmetry • **Motor/trophic:** Evidence of decreased range of motion and/or motor dysfunction (weakness, tremor, dystonia) and/or trophic changes (hair, nails, skin)
4. There is no other diagnosis that better explains the signs and symptoms
CRPS TYPE II Type II of CRPS Is similar to Type I but with evidence of a peripheral or central nerve injury
CRPS NOS Patients who do not fully meet the clinical criteria, but whose signs and symptoms cannot be better explained by another diagnosis

CRPS, complex regional pain syndrome; NOS, not otherwise specified.

Source: Harden, Bruehl, and Stanton-Hicks (2007).

therapy by breaking the cycle of pain. Implantation of spinal cord stimulators has been shown to provide significant improvements in function in CRPS Type I with more cost-effectiveness than physical therapy and pharmaceutical management (Taylor, Van Buyten, & Buchser, 2006). Other procedures include sympathetic blockade, which has moderate evidence for effectiveness, nerve decompression or denervation procedures, neuroma resection, and neurolysis after identifying a source through nerve blocks. Surgical intervention may be effective in noxious stimuli maintained by anything that entraps, compresses, or distorts the nerve. Ultimately, diagnosis and effective management of CRPS requires a keen understanding of the multimechanistic pathophysiology of the syndrome.

PELVIC PAIN

Chronic pelvic pain has been defined as pain causing functional disability that has lasted for at least 6 months and is otherwise not solely attributable to pathologies such as malignancy, inflammatory bowel disease, prostatitis, pelvic inflammatory disease, endometriosis, or dysmenorrhea. It is an ailment that negatively affects a significant number of men and women around the world. In some family practice cohorts, it has been estimated that upward of 20% to 25% of women suffer from this chronic pain syndrome, a number that rivals that of migraine headaches, back pain, and asthma (Grace & Zondervan, 2004). Although the overall prevalence of the condition is likely much less than that, chronic pelvic pain is a problem that leads to increasing morbidity, health care utilization, and economic impact every year. The appropriate diagnosis and subsequent treatment of pelvic pain can help prevent the deleterious consequences this syndrome can have on the patient's personal and occupational well-being.

To date, the etiologies of chronic pelvic pain have yet to be thoroughly elucidated. According to published results, more than 60% of chronic pelvic pain sufferers stated that the cause of their pain had no single identifiable causative factor (Latthe, Latthe, Say, Gülmezoglu, & Khan, 2006). Several immunohistochemically based hypotheses have led to the identification of specific upregulated molecules in the human tissues of chronic pelvic pain sufferers. Transient receptor potential vanilloid Type-1 has been shown to inhabit

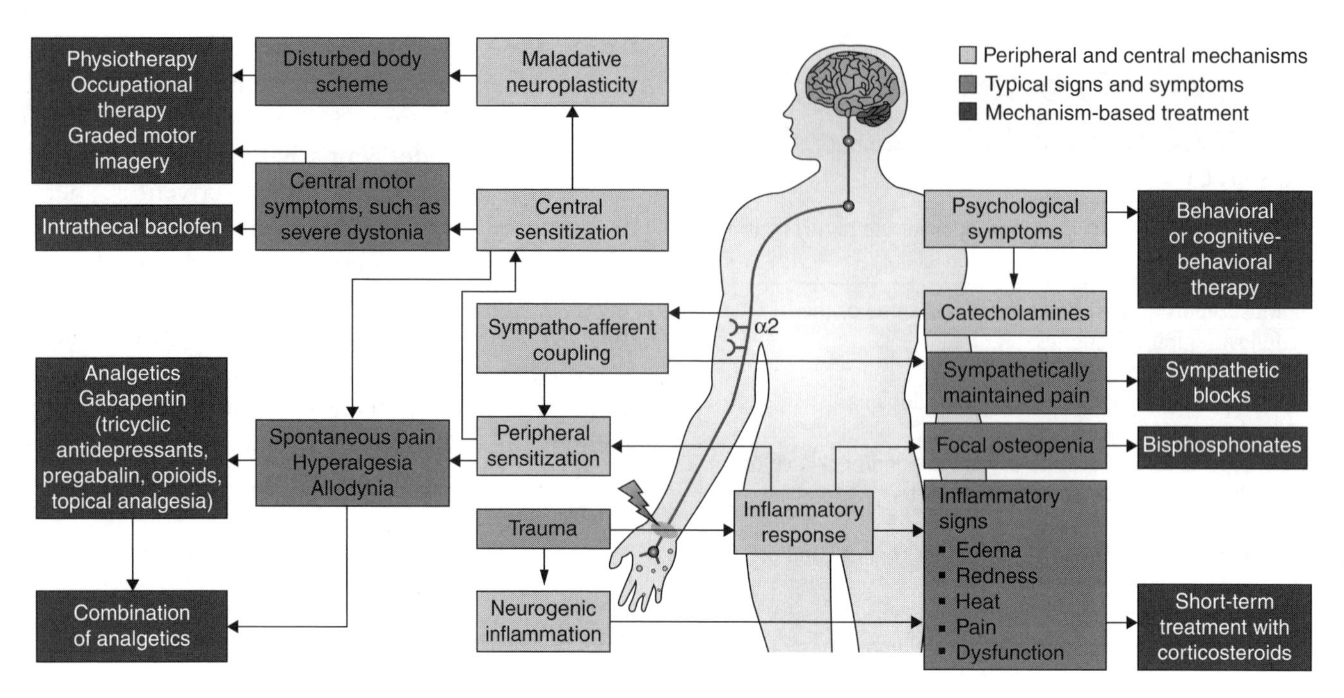

FIGURE 8.2 Pathophysiology and mechanism-based treatment options in complex regional pain syndrome (CRPS).
Source: Gierthmühlen, Binder, and Baron (2014).

a greater percentage of biopsied endometriotic lesions in women with chronic pelvic pain in comparison with their unaffected cohorts (Poli-Neto et al., 2009). In addition, it has been proven that the vascular endothelial growth factor manifests a significantly higher expression in association with subsequent immature vascularization in chronic pelvic pain patients (Kiuchi et al., 2009). These exciting new discoveries have not only expanded on previous hypotheses relating the etiology of chronic pelvic pain to vascular and neuropathic causes, but have also laid the groundwork for potential drug therapies that will target the cause of this syndrome, as opposed to the symptomatic treatment that is the current mainstay of treatment.

Despite the myriad of modalities that have been commonly prescribed by physicians for the treatment of chronic pelvic pain, there is no consensus regarding the choice of treatment because of a lack of scientifically proven data regarding various interventions. The spectrum of therapeutic options ranges from the noninvasive to surgery, as depicted in Table 8.3.

A recent Cochrane Library review outlined the documented efficacy and ineffectiveness of several commonly used treatment regimens for chronic pelvic pain (Stones, Cheong, & Howard, 2005). On the basis of data garnered from several randomized controlled trials, the review supported the use of ultrasound scanning in conjunction with reassurance and counseling, the prescription of progesterone or goserelin (a synthetic hormonal analog) for pelvic congestion, and the utilization of a multidisciplinary approach to assessment and treatment as proven effective treatment modalities. Although adhesiolysis, laparoscopic uterine nerve ablation, extracorporeal shock wave therapy, and the prescription of selective serotonin reuptake inhibitor antidepressants have yet to show a statistically significant benefit in the chronic pelvic pain population in appropriately powered and replicated randomized controlled trials, positive outcomes using these modalities have been described in the literature and thus continue to be used as part of treatment regimens.

With the significant burden that chronic pelvic pain places on both individuals and our society as a whole, further research in the field elucidating the etiology and best practices in diagnosis is needed. In addition, as this chronic pain syndrome continues to cause significant disability and economic hardship related to its multifaceted treatment options, outcomes-based research focusing on the efficacy of both expensive and affordable invasive and noninvasive therapies is warranted.

TABLE 8.3

INTERVENTIONS AIMED AT RELIEF OF CHRONIC PELVIC PAIN

Noninvasive	Medical	Surgical
Exercise	NSAIDs	Laparoscopy
Diet modification	Oral contraceptives	Adhesiolysis
Acupuncture	Progesterone	Ventral suspension
Cognitive behavioral therapy	Danazol	Presacral neurectomy
Psychotherapy	GnRH analogs	Laparoscopic uterine nerve ablation
Biofeedback	Intrauterine contraceptive devices	Ovarian vein ligation
Meditation	Antidepressants	Hysterectomy/ oophorectomy
Hypnosis	Anticonvulsants	Ovarian drilling
Ultrasound scanning	Analgesics	Endometrial ablation

GnRH, gonadotropin-releasing hormone; NSAID, nonsteroidal anti-inflammatory drug.

Source: Stones et al. (2005).

MULTIDISCIPLINARY PAIN TREATMENT

Over the years, a multidisciplinary approach to the treatment of chronic pain has been proven to be superior to single-discipline treatments such as medication management or rehabilitation alone. As evaluation methods and treatment modalities have evolved, the development of multidisciplinary pain centers has led to the consolidation of a patient's overall chronic pain management. The growth of multidisciplinary centers has also allowed for more effective management of chronic pain patients by not only identifying and alleviating physical and emotional pain but also implementing effective strategies to help cope with chronic pain. To provide a comprehensive slew of services, a multidisciplinary approach often includes physicians (i.e., anesthesiologists, neurologists, physiatrists, surgeons, radiologists, and psychiatrists), physical therapists, occupational therapists, nurses, psychologists, and providers of complementary medicine.

In addition to its multipronged therapeutic approach to the chronic pain condition, the success of a multidisciplinary approach is rooted in the effective sharing of information and data between members of the multidisciplinary team. Communication and knowledge sharing among team members can help to elucidate the true etiology of a patient's pain and, in turn, better direct specific therapeutic interventions.

Pharmaceutical Approach

Various medications can be used for the treatment of chronic pain. The strategy is to provide balanced, multimechanistic analgesia that maximizes the antinociceptive effect while reducing the overall side effects and end-organ effects of each individual medication. More recently, the opioid epidemic has driven clinicians toward eliminating or reducing opioids from their practice. The National Institutes of Health Office of Disease Prevention recently conducted a review of research regarding opioid therapy for chronic pain and found that most clinical studies lasted 6 weeks or less although there are studies that extend as long as 6 months (Reuben et al., 2015). Therefore, the long-term use of opioids has no proven efficacy and may increase the risk of tolerance and addiction. Most moderate-severe subchronic or chronic pain can be controlled with nonopioids such as nonsteroidal anti-inflammatory drugs (NSAIDs), muscle relaxants, anticonvulsants, antidepressants, and nonpharmacological approaches.

Interventional Approach

Interventional techniques, as described by the Medicare Payment Advisory Commission, are minimally invasive procedures that include needle placement of drugs in targeted areas, ablation of targeted nerves, and some surgical techniques, including discectomies and the implantation of intrathecal infusion pumps or spinal cord stimulators. These interventions can be divided into diagnostic and therapeutic strategies for the management of chronic pain. Some common procedures are described here.

Diagnostic Interventional Techniques

When symptomatology or noninvasive imaging fails to provide an appropriate diagnosis in difficult cases of chronic pain, procedures such as selective nerve root blocks, sympathetic nerve blocks, facet joint injections, or provocation lumbar discography may be utilized. Diagnostic spinal root nerve blocks are performed based on the theory that if a particular nerve is responsible for mediating the patient's symptoms, then anesthetizing the nerve will provide temporary relief (Datta et al., 2013). This technique focuses on radicular pain, where the single symptom of pain arises from specific spinal nerve roots.

A sympathetic nerve block may be used for the evaluation of chronic pain associated with sympathetic undertones. The most common blocks include stellate, superior hypogastric, ganglion impar, and celiac plexus. The concept of the block is to disrupt sympathetic signaling to increase blood flow to the areas of pain. A test block establishes sympatholysis as an effective treatment, followed by radiofrequency ablation at the ganglionic site for chronic relief.

Facet, or zygapophyseal, joint degeneration modulates spinal pain through capsular stretch, nerve impingement, and inflammation. The joint itself has an abundant supply of nerves that produce spinal and referred pain, creating susceptibility for arthritic changes that lead to instability and injury. Diagnosing facet joint degeneration also involves a test block where a local anesthetic is administered to the medial branches of the dorsal rami supplying these joints. Radiofrequency ablation of the medial branches may be considered for long-term relief.

Percutaneous discography involves injection of contrast into the suspected disc to evaluate its pathoanatomy and illicit pain when imaging reveals multiple levels of abnormal discs. This information about the structure and sensitivity of the intervertebral discs may guide patients to make informed decisions about treatment and modifications of activity (Manchikanti et al., 2013). Potential therapeutic treatments following diagnosis are described in the following.

Therapeutic Interventional Techniques

Therapeutic interventions may involve simple techniques, such as needling for trigger points, or more complex surgeries like kyphoplasty that require fluoroscopic guidance and involve percutaneous access to the spinal column. These are generally same-day procedures that rarely require fasting unless sedation is involved.

Epidural Steroid Injections

Epidural steroid injections attempt to reduce inflammation surrounding spinal nerves via the injection of glucocorticoids and local anesthetics into the epidural space. Patients with disabling neck, arm, low back, or leg pain from spinal stenosis, spondylolysis, herniated disc, degenerative disc, or sciatica may experience pain relief from these injections. The goal of this therapy is to reduce pain and facilitate rehabilitation with physical therapy and exercise.

Interlaminar and transforaminal approaches are two common techniques used during these procedures. With interlaminar epidural injections, the medication is introduced into a space between the lamina of adjacent vertebra using either a paramedian or midline approach with the needle. Transforaminal epidural injections involve an oblique approach in order to access the opening, or foramina, between the vertebrae where the nerve roots exit. Limited data exist comparing the two techniques; however, evidence exists for both techniques being more efficacious than caudal injections (Wilkinson & Cohen, 2012). The review article by Wilkinson and Cohen (2012) notes three studies asserting some efficacy of transforaminal injections over interlaminar, but with limited data.

The effects of epidural steroid injections tend to be temporary, lasting from a week up to a year, but provide substantial benefits to patients experiencing back pain. With proper placement, more than 50% of patients experience pain relief, leading to improvements in mental health and quality of life while avoiding the adverse effects of pharmaceutical and surgical interventions. Overall, data strongly suggest that epidural steroid injections provide short-term relief for radicular symptoms but less compelling evidence for long-term relief.

Intrathecal Pump

Intrathecal delivery of analgesics through pumps offers direct administration of medications to the spinal cord via an intrathecal catheter attached to a pump that is implanted into a pocket created within the anterior abdominal wall. The pumps are utilized primarily for cancer pain and intractable pain of non-cancer origin where the patient is not a candidate for surgical intervention, but can also be used in failed back surgery syndrome, reflex sympathetic dystrophy, causalgia, arachnoiditis, or chronic pancreatitis. The direct delivery of analgesics to the spinal column reduces the oral medication requirements for pain control and thereby reduces overall side effects. Antispasmodics may also be administered via the pump to reduce spasticity in cerebral palsy, multiple sclerosis, stroke, brain injury, or spinal cord injury.

Spinal Cord Stimulator

Spinal cord stimulators consist of a battery-powered pulse generator that sends mild electric current to the spinal cord via electrodes placed into the posterior epidural space. The electrical activity alters the neurochemistry of the local dorsal horn and thereby suppresses the hyperexcitability of the neurons creating a warm sensation that replaces the painful response. There is some evidence showing positive, long-term effects on refractory angina pain, severe ischemic limb pain secondary to peripheral vascular disease, CRPS Type I and Type II, peripheral neuropathic pain, and failed back surgery syndrome (Cameron, 2004).

Vertebral Augmentation—Vertebroplasty and Kyphoplasty

Vertebral body augmentation techniques are commonly used for compression fractures secondary to malignancies or osteoporosis. Kyphoplasty involves the use of a balloon to form a cavity within the collapsed vertebral body followed by injection of cement into the cavity to stabilize the damaged bone and reduce or eliminate the pain. Alternatively, vertebroplasty accomplishes the same without the creation of a cavity, but rather through direct injection of cement into the vertebral body.

Physiatric Approach

The physiatric, or physical medicine and rehabilitation, approach to chronic pain syndromes emphasizes the performance of a comprehensive musculoskeletal and appropriate neuromuscular history and examination with an emphasis on both structure and function as it applies to diagnosing chronic pain problems and developing rehabilitation programs. The approach includes assessments of static and dynamic flexibility, strength, coordination, and agility of the peripheral joint, spine, and soft tissue in patients with pain conditions. The examination also commonly entails a thorough neurological assessment. The physiatric approaches discussed elsewhere in the book are integrated and utilized concomitantly with the pharmacological, interventional, and, sometimes, surgical treatments that a patient may also be prescribed to achieve functional restoration by treating multiple problems multidimensionally.

Neurological Approach

The neurological approach entails a detailed neurological history and physical, which includes a neurological examination that assesses mental status, cranial nerves, motor function, sensory function, reflexes, cerebellar function, and gait. Obtaining and interpreting neuroimaging of the brain and/or spine as well as radiographs of bony structures and joints will not only aid in the diagnosis of a chronic pain pathology but also help direct appropriate therapy.

Psychiatric Approach

The full psychiatric evaluation of a chronic pain patient to elucidate psychiatric and pain comorbidities can be helpful in the management of chronic pain syndromes. Unrecognized conditions such as substance abuse, and mood, anxiety, somatoform, factitious, and personality disorders can hinder the treatment of chronic pain if not simultaneously and appropriately addressed. In addition to counseling patients regarding the potential effects of pain and psychotropic medications on mental status, this arm of the multidisciplinary pain treatment program can be effective at tackling psychosocial contributors to chronic pain pathologies by referring patients for psychological or psychiatric treatments as well as by teaching patients coping and stress-relieving strategies.

Psychological Approach

CBT is a treatment strategy that is commonly used as part of a comprehensive approach to managing chronic pain syndromes. Through CBT, a patient is able to reconceptualize beliefs that pain is uncontrollable and unavoidable into beliefs that it is manageable and does not have to control his or her life. The success of CBT lies in its ability to distract a patient from his or her pain, which will reduce autonomic activity and, in turn, provide an enhanced sense of self-control. Four commonly used techniques of this approach are explained in the following.

Guided Imagery

This technique has the patient focus on a multisensory imaginary scene. Typically, the image is elicited from the patient, and the therapist guides the patient through the image, substituting sensations such as warmth or numbness for pain.

Progressive Muscular Relaxation

By being taught to alternately tense and relax individual muscle groups throughout the body, the patient is able to learn the difference between feelings of tension and relaxation.

Biofeedback

Through the use of modalities such as EMG or nerve stimulation, a chronic pain patient can learn relaxation techniques and the ability to self-regulate physiological pain processes.

Hypnosis

This technique teaches relaxation strategies and enables the patient to experience an analgesic reinterpretation of the pain, experiencing numbness, for example, instead of pain.

CONCLUSION

In summary, it is important to note that successful chronic pain management is best achieved via a coordinated multimodal, multidisciplinary approach. The complex and sometimes cryptic nature of chronic pain syndromes often lends them to being best approached in both diagnosis and treatment by providers and modalities from differing specialty backgrounds. In addition, recent literature has shown outcomes supporting the fact that a multidisciplinary approach to chronic pain may actually result in a reduction in overall health care costs (Cunningham, Rome, Kerkvliet, & Townsend, 2009). This fact is important to keep in mind, as the prevalence of and costs associated with chronic pain syndromes are continuing to rise as mentioned throughout this chapter. Therefore, a successful and efficient approach to chronic pain involves a number of different practitioners specializing in multiple disciplines, concurrently applying various interventions in a coordinated, multidisciplinary fashion.

REFERENCES

Alschuler, K. N., Theisen-Goodvich, M. E., Haig, A. J., & Geisser, M. E. (2008). A comparison of the relationship between depression, perceived disability, and physical performance in persons with chronic pain. *European Journal of Pain, 12,* 757–764.

Bigos, S., Bowyer, O., Braen, G., Brown, K., Deyo, R., Haldeman, S., et al. (1994). *Acute low back problems in adults.* Clinical practice guidelines No. 14. (AHCPR Publication No. 95–0642). Rockville, MD: Agency for Health Care Policy and Research, Public Health Service, U.S. Department of Health and Human Services.

Bonica, J. J. (1990). Anatomic and physical basis of nociceptive and pain. In J. J. Bonica (Ed.), *The management of pain* (2nd ed., pp. 28–94). Philadelphia, PA: Lea & Febiger.

Bruehl, S. (2010). An update on the pathophysiology of complex regional pain syndrome. *Anesthesiology, 113*(3), 713–725.

Cameron, T. (2004). Safety and efficacy of spinal cord stimulation for the treatment of chronic pain: A 20-year literature review. *Journal of Neurosurgery Spine, 3*(100), 254–267.

Chaibi, A., & Russel, M. B. (2014). Manual therapies for primary chronic headaches: A systematic review of randomized controlled trials. *Journal of Headache and Pain, 15,* 67.

Cunningham, J., Rome, J., Kerkvliet, J., & Townsend, C. (2009). Reduction in medication costs for patients with chronic nonmalignant pain completing a pain rehabilitation program: A prospective analysis of admission, discharge, and 6-month follow-up medication costs. *Pain Medicine, 10,* 787–796.

Czervionke, L., & Fenton, D. (2008). Fat-saturated MR Imaging in the detection of inflammatory facet arthropathy (facet synovitis) in the lumbar spine. *Pain Medicine, 9,* 400–406.

Datta, S., Manchikanti, L., Falco, F. J. E., Calodney, A. K., Atluri, S., Benyamin, R. M., . . . Cohen, S. P. (2013). Diagnostic utility of selective nerve root blocks in the diagnosis of lumbosacral radicular pain: Systematic review and update of current evidence. *Pain Physician, 16*, Se145–Se172.

Derby, R. D., Bogduk, N., Anat, D., & Schwarzer, A. (1993). Precision percutaneous blocking procedures for localizing spinal pain. *Pain Digest, 3,* 89–100.

Fields, H. L., Basbaum, A. I., & Heinricher, M. M. (2005). Central nervous system mechanisms of pain modulation. In S. McMahon & M. Koltzenburg (Eds.), *Textbook of Pain* (5th ed., pp. 125–142). Burlington, MA: Elsevier Health Sciences.

Galer, B. S., & Dworkin, R. H. (2000). *A clinical guide to neuropathic pain.* Minneapolis, MN: McGraw-Hill.

Gierthmühlen, J., Binder, A., & Baron, R. (2014). Mechanism-based treatment in complex regional pain syndromes. *Nature Reviews Neurology, 10*(9), 518–528.

Gill, K., & Frymoyer, J. W. (1997). Management of treatment failures after decompressive surgery. In J. W. Frymoyer (Ed.), *The adult spine: Principles and practice* (2nd ed., pp. 2111–2133). Philadelphia, PA: Lippincott-Raven.

Grace, V. M., & Zondervan, K. T. (2004). Chronic pelvic pain in New Zealand: Prevalence, pain severity, diagnoses and use of the health services. *Australia and New Zealand Journal of Public Health, 28,* 369–375.

Guyuron, B., Reed, D., Kriegler, J. S., Davis, J., Pashmini, N., & Amini, S. (2009). A placebo-controlled surgical trial of the treatment of migraine headaches. *Plastic Reconstructive Surgery, 124*, 461–468.

Harden, R. N., Bruehl, S., Stanton-Hicks, M., & Wilson, P. R. (2007). Proposed new diagnostic criteria for complex regional pain syndrome. *Pain Medicine, 8*(4), 326–331.

Harris, P., Loveman, E., Clegg, A., Easton, S., & Berry, N. (2015). Systematic review of cognitive behavioural therapy for the management of headaches and migraines in adults. *British Journal of Pain, 9*, 1–12.

Hu, H., Markson, L. E., Lipton, R. B., Stewart, W. F., & Berger, M. L. (1999). Burden of migraine in the United States: Disability and economic costs. *Archives of Internal Medicine, 1,* 813–818.

Irving, G. A., & Wallace, M. S. (1997). *Pain management for the practicing physician.* New York, NY: Churchill Livingstone.

Janis, J. E., Dhanik, A., & Howard, J. H. (2011). Validation of the peripheral trigger point theory of migraine headaches: Single-surgeon experience using botulinum toxin and surgical decompression. *Plastic Reconstructive Surgery, 128*, 123–131.

Katz, J. N. (2006). Lumbar disc disorders and low-back pain: Socioeconomic factors and consequences. *The Journal of Bone and Joint Surgery, 88*, 21.

Kernick, D. (2005). An introduction to the basic principles of health economics for those involved in the development and delivery of headache care. *Cephalalgia, 25,* 709–714.

Kiuchi, H., Tsujimura, A., Takao, T., Yamamoto, K., Nakayama, J., Miyagawa, Y., . . . Okuyama, A. (2009). Increased vascular endothelial growth factor expression in patients with bladder pain syndrome/interstitial cystitis: Its association with pain severity and glomerulations. *British Journal of Urology International, 104,* 826–831.

Latthe, P., Latthe, M., Say, L., Gülmezoglu, M., & Khan, K. S. (2006). WHO systematic review of preva-lence of chronic pelvic pain: A neglected reproductive health morbidity. *BMC Public Health, 6,* 177.

Levin, M. (2008). The international classification of headache disorders and classification and diagnosis of migraine. In M. Levin (Ed.), *Comprehensive review of headache medicine* (pp. 59–72). New York, NY: Oxford University Press.

Mack, K. A. (2013). Drug-induced deaths - United States, 1999–2010. *Morbidity and Mortality Weekly Report Surveillance Summary, 62*(Suppl. 3), 161–163.

Manchikanti, L., Abdi, S., Atluri, S., Benyamin, R. M., Boswell, M. V., Buenaventura, R. M., . . . Hirsch, J. A. (2013). An update of comprehensive evidence-based guidelines for interventional techniques in chronic spinal pain: Guidance and recommendations. *Pain Physician, 16*, S49–S283.

Mason, V. L., Mathias, B., & Skevington, S. M. (2008). Accepting low back pain: Is it related to a good quality of life? *Clinical Journal of Pain, 24*, 22–29.

Mchaourab, A., & Knight, K. (2009). Management of axial back pain: A critical view. *Techniques in Regional Anesthesia and Pain Management, 13,* 65–66.

Medicare Payment Advisory Commission Report to the Congress. (2001, December). *Paying for Interventional Pain Services in Ambulatory Settings.*

Poli-Neto, O. B., Filho, A. A., Rosa e Silva, J. C., Barbosa, H. F., Candido Dos Reis, F. J., & Nogueira, A. A. (2009). Increased capsaicin receptor TRPV1 in the peritoneum of women with chronic pelvic pain. *Clinical Journal of Pain, 25,* 218–222.

Raj, P. P. (1996). Pain mechanisms. In P. P. Raj (Ed.), *Pain medicine: A comprehensive review* (pp. 12–23). St. Louis, MO: Mosby.

Reuben, D. B., Alvanzo, A. A., Ashikaga, T., Bogat, G. A., Callahan, C. M., Ruffing, V., . . . Steffens, D. C. (2015). National institutes of health pathways to prevention workshop: The role of opioids in the treatment of chronic pain. *Annals of Internal Medicine, 162*(4), 295–300.

Shaw, W., Linton, S., & Pransky, G. (2006). Reducing sickness absence from work due to low back pain: How well do intervention strategies match modifiable risk factors? *Journal of Occupational Rehabilitation, 16,* 591–605.

Stones, W., Cheong, Y. C., & Howard, F. M. (2005). Interventions for treating chronic pelvic pain in women. *Cochrane Database of Systematic Reviews*, CD000387. doi:10.1002/14651858

Taylor, R. S., Van Buyten, J. P., & Buchser, E. (2006). Spinal cord stimulation for complex regional pain syndrome: A systematic review of the clinical and cost-effectiveness literature and assessment of prognostic factors. *European Journal of Pain, 10*(2), 91–101.

Toth, C., Lander, J., & Wiebe, S. (2009). The prevalence and impact of chronic pain with neuropathic pain symptoms in the general population. *Pain Medicine, 10*, 918–929.

Veldman, P. H., Reynen, H. M., Arntz, I. E., & Goris, R. J. (1993). Signs and symptoms of reflex sympathetic dystrophy: prospective study of 829 patients. *The Lancet, 342*(8879), 1012–1016.

Wenig, C. M., Schmidt, C. O., Kohlmann, T., & Schweikert, B. (2009). Costs of back pain in Germany. *European Journal of Pain, 13*, 280–286.

Wilkinson, I. M., & Cohen, S. P. (2012). Epidural Steroid Injections. *Current Pain and Headache Reports, 16*, 50–59.

Woolf, C. J. (2004). Pain: Moving from symptom control toward mechanism-specific pharmacologic management. *Annals of Internal Medicine, 140*, 441–451.

CHAPTER

Diabetes Mellitus

Antonia M. Carbone, Joseph Tribuna, Elfie Wegner, Stuart Green, and Amy Miano

INTRODUCTION

Diabetes mellitus is a pandemic affecting more than 380 million people worldwide, posing significant public health challenges (Hu, Satija, & Manson, 2015; Nathan, 2015). In the United States, over 29.1 million people have diabetes, of which 8.1 million people are undiagnosed (Centers for Disease Control and Prevention [CDC], 2014).

Additionally, it is estimated that 86 million adults in the United States have prediabetes, a condition characterized by elevated glucose levels that often precedes a diagnosis of type 2 diabetes. Those with prediabetes are 10 times more likely to develop type 2 diabetes if lifestyle modifications are not implemented (CDC, 2014; Knowler et al., 2009; Popp Switzer, Elhanafi, & San Juan, 2015).

Diabetes costs an estimated $245 billion and is the seventh leading cause of death (American Diabetes Association [ADA], 2013b, 2014b). It is a disease of dysfunctional glucose metabolism characterized by insufficient insulin secretion, or resistance to insulin, resulting in hyperglycemia (Triplitt, Repas, & Alvarez, 2014). If chronically uncontrolled, diabetes is associated with significant long-term health consequences. The rate of hospitalization and death from stroke are greater in those diagnosed with diabetes compared to those without diabetes (CDC, 2014). Other potential complications from uncontrolled diabetes include heart disease, retinopathy, nephropathy, foot ulcers, and amputations, often resulting in decreased quality of life, functional limitations, and disability (Kalyani, Saudek, Brancati, & Selvin, 2010; Kalyani et al., 2012; Yekta, Pourali, & Ghasemi-Rad, 2011).

CLASSIFICATION OF PREDIABETES AND DIABETES

The ADA 2015 position statement defines prediabetes as fasting blood glucose greater than or equal to 100–125 mg/dL (also referred to as impaired fasting glucose) and a 2-hour oral 75-g glucose tolerance test with a plasma glucose of greater than or equal to 140 to 199 mg/dL (also referred to as impaired glucose tolerance). The hemoglobin A1C (HbA1C) test can also be utilized to define those who are at increased risk of diabetes. Based on its position paper, the ADA considers those individuals with HbA1Cs between 5.7% and 6.4% prediabetic. It should be noted that the World Health Organization (WHO) defines impaired fasting glucose as 110 to 125 mg/dL (WHO, 2015).

Diabetes can be classified into many categories and subtypes. Type 1 diabetes is due to beta cell destruction in the pancreas and an ultimate deficiency of insulin. Type 2 diabetes is a result of a progressive defect in the secretion of insulin and insulin resistance. Gestational diabetes mellitus (GDM) is generally diagnosed in the second and third trimester of pregnancy. The last category is characterized by specific types of diabetes, which are due to other medical causes. These include individuals with genetic defects in beta cell function, genetic defects in insulin action, exocrine pancreatic diseases such as cystic fibrosis, and drug- or chemical-induced diabetes caused by medications used for HIV/AIDS and after organ transplantation.

DIAGNOSTIC CRITERIA

ADA guidelines recommend diagnosing diabetes utilizing any of the following testing modalities: a fasting blood glucose of greater than or equal to 126 mg/dL obtained after an 8-hour fast, a 2-hour plasma glucose greater than or equal to 200 mg/dL obtained after ingestion of a 75-g glucose load dissolved in water, a random plasma glucose greater than or equal to 200 mg/dL obtained from a symptomatic individual, or an HbA1C value greater than or equal to 6.5% performed at a laboratory using a method that is certified by the National Glycohemoglobin Standardization Program (NGSP; standardized to the Diabetes Control and Complications Trial [DCCT] reference assay). The guidelines further recommend repeat testing of patients in the absence of unequivocal hyperglycemic symptoms (Inzucchi et al., 2015).

PREVALENCE AND INCIDENCE

Prediabetes

In 2012, 86 million adults had prediabetes, an increase from 79 million in 2010 (ADA, 2014b). A study evaluating the prevalence of prediabetes found an increase from 1999 to 2005 (38.5%–45.9%) in adults 50 to 64 years old. Moreover, an increase was seen from 2006 to 2010 (41.3%–47.9%) in adults 65 to 74 years old (Caspersen, Thomas, Beckles, & Bullard, 2015). A study by Nichols et al. showed that those with fasting blood glucose levels of 100 to 125 mg/dL progressed to diabetes at an annual rate of 1.34% (Nichols, Hillier, & Brown, 2007). More recent literature states that 5% to 10% of those with prediabetes will convert to a diagnosis of diabetes annually (Tabak, Herder, Rathmann, Brunner, & Kivimaki, 2012).

Diabetes

Worldwide, the prevalence of diabetes mellitus is estimated to be 400 million (Hu et al., 2015; Nathan, 2015). Approximately 9.3% of the population in the United States had diabetes in 2012 (ADA, 2014b). An analysis evaluating trends in the incidence and prevalence of type 2 diabetes from 1980 to 2012 found that incidence and prevalence doubled in the United States from 1990 to 2008 and plateaued from 2008 to 2012 (Geiss et al., 2014). The incidence per 1,000 persons was 3.2, 8.8, and 7.1 in 1990, 2008, and 2012, respectively. The prevalence per 100 persons was 3.5, 7.9, and 8.3 in 1990, 2008, and 2012, respectively. Potential explanations for the doubling of incidence and prevalence from 1990 to 2008 include improved survival rates, aging populations, and sedentary lifestyles. The plateau occurring from 2008 to 2012 may have occurred as a result of the use of HbA1C in diagnosing diabetes. The HbA1C reflects glucose levels over a 3-month period and is less sensitive but more specific when compared to fasting blood glucose, which may have impacted trends related to incidence and prevalence (ADA, 2010).

An estimate of 1.25 million children and adults in the United States have type 1 diabetes (ADA, 2014b). Global prevalence estimates were 1.93 per 1,000 in 2009 (Dabelea et al., 2014). There were 18,436 young people with type 1 diabetes in the United States in 2009, increase in incidence of 2.72% per year for males and 2.57% per year for females (Chiang, Kirkman, Laffel, & Peters, 2014; Lawrence et al., 2014). Type 1 diabetes accounts for only 5% of all cases of diabetes, whereas type 2 diabetes accounts for 90% to 95% (ADA, 2014b; CDC, 2014). A study conducted by Gregg et al. evaluated the lifetime risk of developing diabetes and life years lost due to diabetes using data from the National Health Interview Survey. Lifetime risk for developing diabetes was 40.2% for men and 39.6% for women between 2000 and 2011. Life years lost due to diabetes was 5.8 and 6.8 for men and women diagnosed at age 40 (Gregg et al., 2014).

GDM occurs in up to 9.2% of the pregnancies (DeSisto, Kim, & Sharma, 2014). Mothers with gestational diabetes and their children are more likely to develop type 2 diabetes in the future (Kitzmiller, Dang-Kilduff, & Taslimi, 2007). Therefore, testing for GDM during the third trimester of pregnancy is important for reducing potential complications for both the mother and the newborn.

RISK FACTORS FOR THE DEVELOPMENT OF DIABETES

Type 1 Risk Factors

Sex, Age, Race/Ethnicity

There is no difference between the sexes in the risk for type 1 diabetes. Although type 1 diabetes is usually diagnosed in children or young adults, it can occur at any age. The disease is most often diagnosed in those between 14 and 17 years of age. Non-Hispanic White children have higher rates of type 1 diabetes (CDC, 2014). Ethnicity is thought to play a role because of differences in genetic variations that occur in human leukocyte antigen alleles in different geographic locations. For example, Scandinavia has the highest incidence, whereas northern Europe and the United States have an intermediate rate (Powers, 2015a).

Genetic

Genetics plays an important role in the risk for type 1 diabetes. Those with family members with type 1 diabetes have a 15-fold increased risk for the disease (Chiang et al., 2014). Variations in HLA alleles play a role and differ based on ethnicity and geographic location (Powers, 2015a).

Environmental/Lifestyle

Cold weather is considered a risk factor for type 1 diabetes because the diagnosis is more common during winter months or in areas with cold climates (Waernbaum & Dahlquist, 2015). Viruses may also have the potential to increase the risk (Bergamin & Dib, 2015). Early diet may impact the risk of acquiring type 1 diabetes. Those who are breastfed are less likely to develop the disease. In addition, those who are introduced to solid foods later may also be at greater risk.

Physiological

Autoantibodies are said to be present in those with type 1 diabetes years prior to diagnosis. Screening for autoantibodies often present in those with type 1 diabetes may delay the progression of type 1 diabetes (Simmons & Michels, 2015).

Type 2 Risk Factors

Sex, Age, Race/Ethnicity

The risk of type 2 diabetes is the same in men and women. However, the odds of developing diabetes are projected to increase by 30% in women by the year 2020 (Ibe & Smith, 2014). Increasing age is a risk factor for type 2 diabetes, likely a result of weight gain and decreased muscle mass as people age. Type 2 diabetes most often occurs in those 30 years of age or older.

African Americans, Hispanics, American Indians, Asian Americans, and Pacific Islanders have the greatest risk of type 2 diabetes (ADA, 2013a). Asian Indians have one of the highest conversion rates from normoglycemia to hyperglycemia (Anjana et al., 2015).

Genetic

Evidence supports that diabetes is a genetic disease affecting beta cell mass and function. Those with two parents with diabetes have a 40% increased risk of type 2 diabetes (Powers, 2015a).

Environmental/Lifestyle

The majority of type 2 diabetes cases is thought to occur as a result of environmental and lifestyle factors in individuals with a genetic predisposition. Obesity is a major determinant of insulin resistance, causing the accumulation of fatty acids contributing to impaired insulin signaling and insulin resistance. Western diets consisting of highly processed foods as well as fast foods that are high in fat contribute to the development of type 2 diabetes.

Physiological

The degree of insulin resistance and impaired insulin secretion differ among those with diabetes. Both play a role in the development of diabetes in addition to excessive hepatic glucose production and abnormal metabolism of muscle and fat (Powers, 2015a).

FUNCTIONAL PRESENTATION OF DIABETES

Type 1 and Type 2 at Onset

Classifying patients as either type 1 or type 2 diabetes is often not clearly defined. Clinical presentations and the disease progression can vary widely in both type 1 and type 2 diabetes, often overlapping and therefore making either diagnosis difficult.

Type 1 diabetes is due to beta cell destruction, which leads to absolute insulin deficiency. Type 2 diabetes is associated with a progressive insulin secretory defect in the background of insulin resistance (Inzucchi et al., 2015). The hallmark symptoms of polyuria and polydipsia accompanied with weight loss can be the presenting complaints in both type 1 and type 2 diabetes. The initial symptoms of hyperglycemia in type 2 diabetes are related to an insidious increase in hyperglycemia therefore delaying diagnosis. Patients with type 1 diabetes require treatment with insulin at the onset.

Type 1 and 2: Acute Complications

Diabetic ketoacidosis (DKA) is an acute event resulting from insulin deficiency. DKA is often associated with type 1 diabetes and may possibly be due to undiagnosed type 1 diabetes, infection, serious illness, or insulin omission (MacArthur, 2015). It is characterized by elevated glucose, ketone levels along with a low metabolic pH due to acidosis, potentiating altered consciousness, and coma (MacArthur, 2015). Mortality is reported to be 0.2% to 2% in developed countries (Thuzar, Malabu, Tisdell, & Sangla, 2014).

Hyperosmolar hyperglycemic state (HHS) is the acute hyperglycemic event occurring in patients with type 2 diabetes, characterized by severe hyperglycemia, hyperosmolarity, and dehydration in the absence of ketoacidosis and more frequently seen in the elderly with infection as the precipitating cause (Pasquel & Umpierrez, 2014). The key difference between DKA and HHS is that with HHS, insulin is present. The overall estimated mortality rate is as high as 20%, which is 10 times higher than the mortality in patients with DKA (Pasquel & Umpierrez, 2014).

PREDIABETES, TYPE 1, AND TYPE 2: LONG-TERM COMPLICATIONS

Chronically uncontrolled blood glucose contributes to a number of long-term complications including microvascular and macrovascular complications and increased mortality.

Microvascular Complications

Approximately 28.5% or 4.2 million people in the United States have had diabetic retinopathy between 2005 and 2008 (CDC, 2014). Proliferative retinopathy and nephropathy are more likely to occur in those with chronically elevated HbA1C (Nordwall et al., 2015). Retinopathy is said to take 5 years to develop after the onset of hyperglycemia. However, once progression has occurred, it can be permanent and can cause blindness. The use of telemedicine in screening for retinopathy has been used to reduce the progression of retinopathy (Zimmer-Galler, Kimura, & Gupta, 2015). Diabetes is the leading cause of kidney failure, responsible for 44% of the diagnoses in 2011. Additionally, 228,924 people were on dialysis or had a kidney transplant as a result of diabetic nephropathy (CDC, 2014). Adequate blood glucose and blood pressure control will decrease the risk or slow the progression of both retinopathy and nephropathy (Inzucchi et al., 2015).

Macrovascular Complications

Diabetes accelerates macrovascular disease, affecting arteries that supply the brain and heart. Elderly adults with impaired fasting blood glucose have higher baseline rates of heart disease when compared to elderly adults with normal fasting blood glucose (Samaras et al., 2015). Prediabetes is an important modifiable risk factor for stroke prevention (Fonville, Zandbergen, Koudstaal, & den Hertog, 2014). Many patients with diabetes will likely receive statin therapy and antihypertensive medications to decrease cardiovascular risks associated with high low-density lipoprotein (LDL) cholesterol and increased blood pressure. Aspirin is often recommended for those with diabetes to reduce cardiovascular events. Metformin has also been shown to have cardiovascular benefits (Inzucchi et al., 2015).

Mortality

Cardiovascular disease is a major cause of morbidity and mortality in patients with diabetes. A review of prospective cohort studies showed that those with prediabetes had an increased risk of all-cause and cardiovascular mortality (Huang et al., 2014). Approximately 65% of those with diabetes die from heart disease or stroke (American Heart Association, 2012). The overall risk of death is said to be double that of those without a diagnosis of diabetes. Newer medications used to treat diabetes such as empagliflozin may decrease cardiovascular death when added to standard glucose-lowering regimens (Zinman et al., 2015).

ECONOMIC COSTS OF PREDIABETES AND DIABETES

Global expenditures associated with diabetes were $548 billion in 2013 (Hu et al., 2015). National costs associated with prediabetes, diabetes, and gestational diabetes are $44 billion, $277 billion (diagnosed and undiagnosed), and $1.3 billion, respectively (ADA, 2013b; Dall et al., 2014). Between 2007 and 2012, the cost of prediabetes increased by 74% (Cefalu, Petersen, & Ratner, 2014). Costs associated with diagnosed diabetes increased by 41% between 2007 and 2012 (ADA, 2013b), whereas the costs of undiagnosed diabetes increased by 82% (Cefalu et al., 2014). The approximate cost per case is $10,970, $5,800, $4,030, and $510 for diagnosed diabetes, gestational diabetes, undiagnosed diabetes, and prediabetes, respectively (Dall et al., 2014).

REDUCING OR PREVENTING THE INCIDENCE OF DIABETES

Lifestyle modifications may delay or prevent progression to type 2 diabetes for a period of up to 10 years (Knowler et al., 2009). Consequently, policy changes are being encouraged, which consist of promoting walking, bicycling, and reduction of junk foods (Hu et al., 2015).

The Diabetes Prevention Research Group evaluated the effect of lifestyle modifications such as 5% weight loss in patients with prediabetes and found that the incidence of diabetes was decreased by 58% (Knowler et al., 2002). The Diabetes Prevention Program is being piloted in some primary care settings to reduce the incidence of diabetes (Ackermann, Finch, Brizendine, Zhou, & Marrero, 2008).

Unique measures have been evaluated to prevent type 2 diabetes including social marketing campaigns, the use of lifestyle reminders via text messaging, and prediabetes risk assessment tools. Social marketing campaigns are being explored to prevent type 2 diabetes in low-income and minority youth by changing perspectives using a public health literacy framework (Rogers et al., 2014). A study by Ram et al. evaluated the impact of sending healthy lifestyle reminders via text message to patients at a risk of diabetes. Improved lifestyle scores associated with a decreased risk of developing diabetes was seen in those receiving text message reminders (Ram et al., 2014). Several risk assessment tools are available to detect those with prediabetes (Barber, Davies, Khunti, & Gray, 2014).

Prevention of diabetes is critical, as many of the complications of hyperglycemia occur prior to the diagnosis of type 2 diabetes (Nichols, Arondekar, & Herman, 2008).

TREATMENT OF PREDIABETES AND DIABETES

Prediabetes

Weight loss, dietary modifications, increased physical activity, and pharmacotherapy agents can be used to treat prediabetes and reduce or prevent the incidence of diabetes (Daniele, Abdul-Ghani, & DeFronzo, 2014; Palermo, Maggi, Maurizi, Pozzilli, & Buzzetti, 2014; Popp Switzer et al., 2015; Rattay & Rosenthal, 2014). Weight loss decreases progression from prediabetes to diabetes (Gillies et al., 2007; Knowler et al., 2002). A goal of 7% weight loss for those with prediabetes is recommended (Inzucchi et al., 2015). Medications indicated for type 2 diabetes have been studied at higher doses for weight loss. Liraglutide 3.0 mg received an indication approved by the U.S. Food and Drug Administration (FDA) for weight loss and it may be considered for those with prediabetes (Pi-Sunyer et al., 2015). A healthy diet is associated with a 20% reduction in the incidence of type 2 diabetes (Esposito et al., 2014).

Exercise can oppose the mechanisms that promote insulin resistance and promote glucose uptake independent of insulin (Buresh, 2014). A study by Rejeski et al. showed that those with diabetes without preexisting cardiovascular disease who underwent intensive lifestyle intervention for weight loss had a slower decline in physical functioning compared to those who received diabetes support and education alone (Rejeski et al., 2015).

Pharmacotherapy agents shown to reduce the incidence of diabetes include metformin, pioglitazone, and acarbose (Choudhary, Kalra, Unnikrishnan, & Ajish, 2012; Daniele et al., 2014).

Diabetes

Treatment goals for type 2 diabetes are often individualized based on the patient's age, comorbid conditions, cardiovascular risk, and propensity for hypoglycemia. In general, goals include lowering HbA1C to less than 7% to reduce microvascular complications. Macrovascular complications may also be reduced if treatment for blood glucose control is obtained soon after diagnosis (Inzucchi et al., 2015). The goal for HbA1C may vary depending on patient-specific factors. For example, a goal HbA1C of less than 8% may be recommended for elderly patients with an increased risk of hypoglycemia. Pharmacotherapy for the treatment of type 2 diabetes is selected based on patients' initial HbA1C and other factors including cost and side effect profiles. Treatment goals for those with type 1 diabetes include an A1C goal of less than 7.5%. Patients should be monitored for hypertension, hyperlipidemia, nephropathy, neuropathy, and retinopathy. Treatment consists of injections of basal insulin, which targets blood glucose at night and between meals and prandial insulin, which targets blood glucose after meals, or continuous subcutaneous insulin infusion via insulin pumps. Education is needed regarding the various factors affecting insulin requirements such as anticipated activity and carbohydrate intake.

Components of the treatment of diabetes include medication, medical nutrition therapy, exercise, and self-monitoring of blood glucose (SMBG). Self-management education and support is an integral component of the treatment of diabetes because it may improve outcomes and result in cost savings (Inzucchi et al., 2015).

■ Medication[1]

Type 2 diabetes is a progressive disease and therefore several medications may be required to obtain adequate glucose control, and eventually insulin therapy is indicated for many. Oral metformin is considered an optimal first-line treatment due to its efficacy, low cost, and lack of propensity to cause hypoglycemia and weight gain. Additional agents may be prescribed with metformin or another first-line agent if the patient presents with diabetes that has progressed (HbA1C ≥7.5%) or if the patient does not obtain adequate glucose control with metformin alone. Additional agents are selected by taking into account patient-specific factors, as there are advantages and disadvantages for each medication. Insulin is selected as initial therapy in patients presenting with severe type 2 diabetes such as those with an HbA1C greater than 9% or patients who are unable to maintain adequate glucose control with other medications (Tamez-Perez, Proskauer-Pena, Hernrndez-Coria, & Garber, 2013). Insulin is required for the treatment of type 1 diabetes in order to survive because those with type 1 diabetes are insulin deficient.

There are many factors that may make it difficult for patients to adhere to their medication regimens. Medication adherence may be affected by medication side effects or the required frequency of dosing. Table 9.1 describes various medication-related side effects that may occur in patients who are being treated for diabetes. Some strategies that may be used to improve adherence include hypoglycemia awareness, the use of insulin pen devices, reducing the financial burden of insulin to the patient, and providing additional support from nurses, pharmacists, psychiatrists, and other mental health professionals (Davies et al., 2013).

[1]Portions of this text were previously published in Burg and Oyama (2015). Copyright 2015, reproduced with permission of Springer Publishing Company, LLC.

TABLE 9.1

MEDICATION-RELATED FACTORS THAT MAY IMPACT PATIENTS WITH DIABETES

Medication-Related Factors	Specific Causes and/or Medications
Hypoglycemia (low blood sugar)	Hypoglycemia may occur with certain medications used to treat diabetes, especially in elderly patients. Symptoms of hypoglycemia may include sweating, hunger, confusion, and fatigue. When severe and prolonged, hypoglycemia may cause altered levels of consciousness, seizure, and even death (Cryer, Davis, & Shamoon 2003). Examples of medications used for the treatment of diabetes that may cause hypoglycemia are sulfonylureas, which include glyburide (DiaBeta, Micronase), glipizide (Glucotrol, Glucotrol XL), and glimepiride (Amaryl). Insulin may also cause hypoglycemia. Repaglinide (Prandin) and nateglinide (Starlix) can cause hypoglycemia, although the incidence is less than with sulfonylureas, and is worse if the medication is taken without a meal. Pramlintide (Symlin) may cause hypoglycemia with insulin. Medications used for the treatment of diabetes, which do not cause hypoglycemia include metformin, miglitol, acarbose, sitagliptin, saxagliptin, linagliptin, alogliptin, and canagliflozin. Rosiglitazone and pioglitazone do not cause hypoglycemia but have several more serious potential adverse effects, which may preclude their use.
Weight gain	Weight gain may occur in patients taking sulfonylureas such as glyburide (DiaBeta, Micronase), glipizide (Glucotrol, Glucotrol XL), and glimepiride (Amaryl). Weight gain may also occur in those taking repaglinide (Prandin), or nateglinide (Starlix) or those taking insulin. Pioglitazone (Actos) and rosiglitazone (Avandia) may also cause weight gain. Medications used for the treatment of diabetes that do not cause weight gain include metformin, miglitol, acarbose, sitagliptin, saxagliptin, linagliptin, alogliptin, canagliflozin, pramlintide, exenatide (Byetta), liraglutide (Victoza), and exenatide XR (Bydureon).
Diarrhea, flatulence, abdominal discomfort	Diarrhea is a common side effect of metformin and may occur in up to 50% of patients. Some methods to diminish gastrointestinal side effects of metformin include using an extended-release formulation of the medication and starting the medication at a low dose and increasing the dose in 500-mg increments on a weekly basis until the target dose is reached. Diarrhea, flatulence, and abdominal discomfort may occur in a large percentage of patients taking acarbose (Precose) or miglitol (Glyset), but these side effects usually lessen after 4–8 weeks of treatment. Doses of miglitol and acarbose should be titrated to reduce potential gastrointestinal side effects. Sulfonylureas such as glyburide (DiaBeta, Micronase), glipizide (Glucotrol, Glucotrol XL), and glimepiride (Amaryl) may cause indigestion although it is a less common side effect of sulfonylureas. Exenatide (Byetta), liraglutide (Victoza), and exenatide XR (Bydureon) may cause diarrhea. The incidence of diarrhea is highest with exenatide (Byetta).
Nausea	Sulfonylureas such as glyburide (DiaBeta, Micronase), glipizide (Glucotrol, Glucotrol XL), and glimepiride (Amaryl) may cause nausea. Metformin can cause nausea, especially upon initiation of treatment. Pramlintide (Symlin) may cause nausea and vomiting Exenatide (Byetta), liraglutide (Victoza), and exenatide XR (Bydureon) may cause nausea and vomiting.
Headache	Sulfonylureas such as glyburide (DiaBeta, Micronase), glipizide (Glucotrol, Glucotrol XL), and glimepiride (Amaryl) may cause headache. Exenatide (Byetta), liraglutide (Victoza), and exenatide XR (Bydureon) may cause headache.
Frequent dosing	Repaglinide (Prandin) and nateglinide (Starlix) are dosed three times daily. Acarbose (Precose) and miglitol (Glyset) are dosed three times daily. Pramlintide (Symlin) requires three additional injections each day because it cannot be mixed with insulin.

Source: Burg and Oyama (2015).

Medical Nutrition Therapy

Medical nutrition therapy is recommended for those with type 1 and type 2 diabetes as well as those with prediabetes (Parker, Byham-Gray, Denmark, & Winkle, 2014). A pilot trial showed that a low-carbohydrate diet, in addition to behavioral changes, may decrease HbA1C and reduce the need for medications (Saslow et al., 2014). Because medical nutrition therapy can improve outcomes such as HbA1C and result in cost savings, it should be part of the overall treatment plan in those with diabetes (Inzucchi et al., 2015).

Exercise

Exercise delays progression of diabetes, reduces morbidity and mortality, and improves quality of life (Pozzo et al., 2014). Benefits include reduction of cardiovascular risk, decreased blood pressure, improved high-density lipoprotein (HDL) cholesterol, increased muscle mass, and weight loss (Powers, 2015b). Aerobic and resistance training reduce coronary heart disease risk scores independent of weight loss (Balducci et al., 2012). Additionally, a "spillover effect" may occur in those who participate in resistance training and also improve dietary habits (Halliday et al., 2014). Exercise should be individualized to avoid potential complications that may occur during exercise, including hypoglycemia, hyperglycemia, or musculoskeletal problems. Those with retinopathy should not perform vigorous exercises due to risk of retinal detachment (Powers, 2015b). Although there is evidence to support exercise in improving blood glucose, many are not meeting exercise targets recommended by the ADA of 150 minutes/week. Behavioral goal setting, feedback, and self-monitoring should be used to promote change (Bushman, 2014).

Self-Monitoring of Blood Glucose

SMBG allows patients to test their blood glucose at any time and provides guidance regarding whether adjustments in diet, exercise, or dosages of medications are needed. Although the effects of SMBG on HbA1C are controversial, patients are often motivated to alter their behaviors based on the results (Inzucchi et al., 2015). A 2015 study showed that more frequent SMBG of more than 3.5 times per day was associated with achieving target HbA1C levels in type 1 diabetics using continuous insulin infusion pumps (Murata et al., 2015).

PSYCHOSOCIAL AND VOCATIONAL IMPLICATIONS[2]

Psychosocial Factors in Diabetes

The two major behavioral factors in diabetes care are the numerous tasks required to manage the condition and the psychosocial factors that impact each patient's ability to perform these tasks (Meichenbaum & Turk, 1987). See Table 9.2 for psychosocial factors affecting patients with diabetes.

Diabetes self-management involves a complicated, demanding, and relentless treatment routine that impacts virtually all aspects of a patient's life (work, school, family, and friends). A typical day in the life of a person living with diabetes will vary according to the type of diabetes (1 or 2), disease status, comorbidities, and treatment regimen. Especially significant is whether the treatment plan includes oral medication, a combination of oral and injectable medication, or insulin alone. Examples of ideal daily self-care tasks include checking glucose at least two times daily, reading food labels, keeping a food diary, keeping a glucose level log, meal planning, counting carbohydrates/portion sizes, eating timely meals, exercising daily and self-treatment of potential hypoglycemia, taking medications as prescribed and as variably necessary based on continuous assessments of glucose levels, and arranging and keeping multiple medical appointments.

In an essay, which illustrates not only the demanding nature of diabetes but also the disease's emotional impact, one particularly diligent man with insulin-dependent diabetes described his days as follows:

> Every morning the first thing I do is search my apartment for my blue case. In it is my . . . glucometer, lancet, syringes, and other blood

[2]Portions of this text were previously published in Burg and Oyama (2015). Copyright 2015, reproduced with permission of Springer Publishing Company, LLC.

TABLE 9.2

PSYCHOSOCIAL-RELATED FACTORS THAT MAY IMPACT PATIENTS WITH DIABETES	
Psychosocial-Related Factors	**Specific Considerations**
History/stage of diabetes	Emotional response to diabetes and coping mechanisms. Consider using Problem Areas in Diabetes (PAID) Questionnaire for assessment. Experience with multigenerational family diabetes.
Concurrent medical conditions	Nondiabetic experiences with loss, medical expenses, and physical limitations can lower patient's threshold for diabetes-related stresses. Diabetes-related conditions such as renal failure, visual impairment, obesity, pain, and neuropathy further complicate capacity for self-care.
Physical limitations	Effects of neuropathy: • Reduced manual dexterity (difficulty with insulin injections) • Ambulation difficulties Visual impairment (difficulty with glucose testing and injections) Shortness of breath Amputations
Use of durable medical equipment	Assess need and availability. May benefit from physical therapy/occupational therapy evaluation.
Medications	Is the person with diabetes: • Able to describe medications and purpose? • Able to describe medication regimen accurately? • Able to describe a plausible method for adherence to prescribed regimen? Is there evidence of medication nonadherence? Is the patient experiencing side effects of the medication? Are there competing medication costs? Assess complexity of medication routine. Who sets up, reminds, administers, renews, and picks up diabetes supplies and medications if patient is not independent in medication routine?
Financial status	Does the individual have health insurance? Can the individual afford medications and supplies? (Glucose test strips range in cost from $.50 to $1.50 or more per strip. Free glucometers, which may be distributed to physician offices by manufacturers' representatives frequently require use of the more costly test strips.)
Cognitive status	Forgetfulness, confusion, impaired decision making, and other factors can diminish ability to manage diabetes routine without support. Consider using the VA-SLUMS (Veterans Administration-St. Louis University Mental Status) cognitive screening tool available online (familymed.uthscsa.edu/geriatrics/tools/SLUMS.pdf).
Education/literacy level	Does the patient need help understanding self-care techniques, routines, nutrition, etc.? Avoid medical jargon. Explore options for adapting instructions and routines as needed, including creating visual prompts if necessary. Use language translation services whenever necessary.
Behavioral health concerns—past and current	Depression, anxiety, eating disorders, trauma, loss history, personality disorders, other major psychiatric disorders, and substance use may all impact the patient's ability to self-manage diabetes care.
Use/misuse of alcohol and other substances, past and current	Both alcohol use and smoking raise blood sugar level and increase the likelihood of medical complications in persons with diabetes (www.cdc.gov). How does use of alcohol and other substances interrelate with patient's family/friend network?
Diabetes-specific emotional distress	See PAID questionnaire available at www.dawnstudy.com

(*continued*)

TABLE 9.2 (*continued*)

PSYCHOSOCIAL-RELATED FACTORS THAT MAY IMPACT PATIENTS WITH DIABETES	
Psychosocial-Related Factors	**Specific Considerations**
Change history and readiness to change	Explore prior experience with making changes in daily behaviors (quitting smoking, exercising, losing weight, changing diet, etc.). Assess stage of change, decisional balance regarding improving diabetes self-care behaviors.
Current self-care behaviors/ barriers to self-care	Quality of patient's current diabetes self-care, facilitators, barriers. Self-Care Inventory Revised (SCI-R; Weinger, Butler, Welch, & La Greca, 2005).
Family responsibilities/stresses	Does the patient need assistance coping with caregiving for others family members (i.e., childcare, elder care, care of disabled family member)? Are there adequate, stable finances or competing financial demands that interfere with purchasing supplies or needed equipment?
Work responsibilities/stresses	Does the patient have the ability (time, privacy, hygienic conditions) during the workday for blood glucose testing, medications, and other needs? Is the patient experiencing any diabetes-related discrimination? What are the patient's coping techniques? Assess organizational and time management skills.

Source: Burg and Oyama (2015).

glucose testing paraphernalia. . . . I test my blood at least four times a day: in the morning, before lunch, before dinner, and before bedtime. On days when I exercise, I may test two times before vigorous activity to ensure my blood sugar is high enough and one time after I exercise to ensure that I have not gone too low. If I feel strange sometime during the day, I will test again . . . I write the data in my log book, in which I keep a tally of my glucose levels. . . . I project where I want [my glucose level] to be throughout the remainder of the day, whether I can eat, how much I can eat, how much insulin I should inject, and whether I can exercise or must wait to get my sugars higher. Usually [for the first reading of the day], I come in at . . . the [glucose level] goal I have set for myself. If I meet this goal, give or take ten points, I feel a sense of accomplishment, a willingness to meet the day. If the read-out is much above . . . my mood changes abruptly. "A poor beginning," I say to myself, "What did I do? What on earth did I eat yesterday?" The next few minutes are spent reconstructing my last night's meals and insulin injections, adjusting my dose for the day, and thinking about what I can eat for breakfast. I do not expect to be perfect, and I know there are times when things get out of control either because I ate too much or injected too little. . . . There have been many times when I have thought I was low—when I even felt low—and my meter has told me the opposite and vice versa. . . . Many times I can think of no good reason for the discrepancy. When my mental image of my physical self conflicts with my meter, I have a problem. Do I doubt myself, or do I doubt my meter? . . . The discrepancy between the reading and my expectation makes me redouble my efforts to remember what I could have forgotten, what I might have done wrong. Only when I remember do I feel in control once again. (Cevetello, 2011)

Psychological factors impacting self-care may be emotional or other than emotional. Emotional distress (most commonly depression, anxiety, and the psychological impact of stressors) will negatively impact the ability of patients to engage in optimal self-care (Anderson, Freedland, Clouse, & Lustman, 2001; Jacobson, de Groot, & Samson, 1994; Rubin & Peyrot, 1992). Psychological factors other than depression and anxiety may also directly impact self-care. These factors include cognitive capacity, self-efficacy, and readiness to change, among others. The clarity and organization of the patient's thinking and such key factors as the patient's intelligence, attention skill, working memory, and social acuity will inevitably determine the patient's ability to understand and implement self-management strategies. These qualities will also impact motivation by enhancing or limiting the patient's understanding of the consequences of poor self-management. Patients with limited cognitive skills, limited literacy, or impaired auditory processing will also struggle to use helpful informational resources and supports. Similarly, social skills deficits will tend to limit the social support on which chronic disease self-management critically relies. Self-efficacy is fundamental to a patient's motivation and ability to self-manage chronic disease and lifestyle changes. Both of these factors, as well as others, will determine whether the patient moves along the change continuum from precontemplation to action (Prochaska & DiClemente, 1983). Motivation to change is the crux on which all of the desired behavioral changes depend. Given the proper motivation, a patient will use tools and supports already at hand to produce desired change, or he or she can easily be helped to acquire additional tools and support as and if needed (Prochaska, Norcross, & DiClemente, 2007). For all of these reasons, and for addressing the psychological issues described in the following text, the presence of a behavioral health specialist (BHS) in medical settings and as part of the health care team is critical.

Children and Adolescents With Diabetes

It is often acknowledged that diabetes is the entire family's disease, as the care needs of the patient with diabetes touch and overlap virtually all aspects of the family's routine. At no time is this more evident than when the patient is a child or teen. For the BHS in primary care settings, the focus of support can be the parent as much as the child or teen. Stress related to caring for a child with diabetes affects both the child and the parent in (a) increased risk for poor mental health outcomes for parents, (b) potential impairment of parents' ability to manage the child's illness, (c) increased stress experienced by the child, and (d) negative influence on the child's diabetes self-management (Streisand, Swift, Wickmark, Chen, & Holmes, 2005). Furthermore, diabetes-related parenting stress is associated with parents' level of confidence in their ability to manage the child's diabetes, owning much of the responsibility for the child's diabetes management, and high levels of worry about a possible episode of severe low blood glucose level (Streisand et al., 2005). All of these are areas of potential intervention and support. Finding the balance between age-appropriate independence and safety in managing the child's or teen's diabetes is a complex and constantly shifting process.

As a child with diabetes grows, care and parenting challenges shift. In the infant and toddler years, key challenges involve keeping up with the complex and rapidly changing insulin demands of the growing child. This complexity can make finding reliable and safe childcare difficult and can have negative consequences on the family's income. School-age children are faced with stigma and "feeling different" from peers and adults along with increasing responsibility for their own diabetes care (Ayala & Murphy, 2011).

In children with diabetes, the major family challenge is to maintain normal developmental expectations for the child's behavior and relations with others. The temptation to overfocus on the child's illness and to lessen expectations for the child's functioning is significant. A common pathological family dynamic is for the child's diabetic episodes to arise as a mechanism for shifting attention away from other problematic family relationships, especially those concerning the parents (Minuchin et al., 1975; Minuchin & Fishman, 1979).

The shift in responsibility for self-care continues through adolescence. Parents may prematurely hand over responsibility to adolescents out of weariness of conflicts and intense management demands, but many teens do not have the problem-solving skills and maturity to manage their diabetes independently. Shared responsibility for diabetes management tasks has been associated with less depression, less anger, higher diabetes self-efficacy, and better metabolic control (Helgeson, Reynolds, Siminerio, Escobar, & Becker, 2008). By ages 10 to 12 years, many children may be able to self-manage some aspects of their diabetes care. Parents may undermine the expected shift to self-care by encouraging dependency, reflecting parental fears and anxiety. The health care team can support parents and teens by facilitating trust and positive communication that is supportive and nonblaming (Ivey, Wright, & Dashiff, 2009).

Although many adolescents are confronted with the decisions and risks related to driving and choosing whether to smoke or use alcohol or be sexually active, diabetic teens face greater health risks associated with these activities than do nondiabetic teens. Health care providers can offer supportive conversation and education to assist teens in thoughtful decision making and can assist in developing problem-solving skills (Ayala & Murphy, 2011).

From the child's or teen's perspective, diabetes requires the integration of a complicated routine requiring heightened awareness while also working through the usual developmental tasks of forming social relationships, becoming autonomous, and separating from family. Health care providers must therefore be alert for signs of stress and childhood depression. The rate of depression among youth with diabetes is almost twice that of the highest estimate of depression in youth in general. Symptoms include increased irritability, moodiness, loss of interest and pleasure, change in sleep pattern and appetite, drop in school performance, poor diabetes control, and a sense of being overwhelmed. Childhood depression has been associated with poor metabolic control and episodes of DKA (Ayala & Murphy, 2011; Delamater, 2009).

Disordered Eating and Diabetes

Eating disorders and diabetes share common ground. The near-constant attention to diabetes-specific self-care behaviors such as detailed meal planning, precision in food portions, and careful monitoring of exercise and blood glucose parallel the rigid thinking about food and body image found in nondiabetic women with eating disorders (Goebel-Fabbri, Fikkan, Connell, Vangsness, & Anderson, 2002). Although the prevalence of eating disorders among youth and adults with diabetes is reportedly inconclusive, estimates are that adolescents with diabetes may have a risk between two and three times greater of developing an eating disorder than their peers without diabetes (Pereira & Alvarenga, 2007). Estimates of the prevalence of disturbed eating behavior (DEB) among individuals with type 1 diabetes range from 10% to 49%, with approximately 28% of girls and 9% of boys with type 1 diabetes scoring above the cutoff for DEB (Wisting, Froisland, Skrivarhaug, Dahl-Jorgensen, & Ro, 2013). The prevalence of DEB has been shown to increase dramatically with age, from about 33% for females between ages 14 and 16 to nearly 50% for females between ages 17 and 19, as well as with weight (highest rates with obese patients; Wisting et al., 2013). DEBs place patients with diabetes at risk for serious complications such as visual impairment, kidney failure, and cardiovascular disease (Pereira & Alvarenga, 2007).

Insulin Manipulation

Insulin manipulation is a weight control measure uniquely available to adolescents with diabetes. A 2008 study of disordered eating and body dissatisfaction among adolescents with type 1 diabetes found that 10.3% of girls and 1.4% of boys with type 1 diabetes reported skipping insulin in the past year as a weight control measure. The study showed that 7.4% of girls and 1.4% of boys reduced their insulin dosages (Ackard et al., 2008). In Wisting et al., one third of the study participants reported skipping their insulin dose entirely at least occasionally after overeating (Wisting et al., 2013).

Health care providers who are attuned to DEBs can help identify concerns about weight, body image, and self-esteem by incorporating these topics into their routine discussions with patients with diabetes. Routine and annual screenings for disturbed eating and increased psychosocial focus are recommended for young patients with type 1 diabetes especially among females, older adolescents, and individuals with higher body mass index (BMI; Wisting et al., 2013).

Stress, Anxiety, and Diabetes

Stressors are believed to impact diabetes, either causing or impacting care and outcomes. Although stress can directly impact blood glucose levels, stress most directly impacts diabetes when stressful events weaken the resources and supports essential for diabetes self-management and care. Lack of health insurance, for example, will limit access to medical care and health system supports. Unemployment will increase food insecurity and nutritional deficits. Interpersonal losses, such as death or illness in the family or divorce, will decrease social support (Walker, Gebregziabher, Martin-Harris, & Egede, 2014). The stress associated with poor social conditions (e.g., job strain) can impact development of diabetes (Baumert et al., 2014). The stressors that trigger posttraumatic stress disorder (PTSD) have also been associated with the development of diabetes (Roberts et al., 2015). Those with prediabetes, at high risk for development of diabetes, may be especially impacted by stress, with increased weight as a mediating factor (Virtanen et al., 2014). Diabetes appears more prevalent in patients with anxiety (as well as depression) at baseline (Engum, 2007). Additionally, there may be a higher rate of anxiety disorders in those with diabetes (Huang, Chiu, Lee, & Wang, 2011). The essential presumed relationship between diabetes and anxiety is the heightened state of vigilance—the core feature of anxiety—that is demanded by the attention required for the condition of diabetes, especially its active self-care. There are specific aspects of diabetes self-management that are anxiety inducing, such as fear of hypoglycemic episodes and fear of injections. But there are mixed reports about an independent relationship between anxiety disorders and diabetes, other than etiologically (Grigsby, Anderson, Freedland, Clouse, & Lustman, 2002; Scott, 2014).

Fear of Hypoglycemia

Managing the risk of developing hypoglycemia is part of the daily routine of a person with diabetes. Persons with type 1 diabetes average 43 symptomatic episodes of hypoglycemia a year, whereas persons with type 2 diabetes who are treated with insulin experience an average of 16 symptomatic episodes a year (Perlmuter, Flanagan, Shah, & Singh, 2008). Patients with type 1 diabetes also typically experience up to two severe hypoglycemic episodes a year, whereas those with type 2 diabetes experience about one severe episode every 5 years. The risk of severe hypoglycemic episodes increases with the number of years of insulin treatment. Although the symptoms of hypoglycemia can warn of an impending hypoglycemic episode, they can also create anxiety and fear of future episodes. Severe hypoglycemic episodes often occur during sleep, leaving individuals unable to recognize symptoms and take action to counter them. Nocturnal hypoglycemia is estimated to affect 50% of adults with diabetes and 78% of children and is suspected to contribute to the 6% mortality rate of persons with type 1 diabetes below the age of 40 (Perlmuter et al., 2008).

It is no wonder that fear of hypoglycemia is a well-known emotional occurrence. The fear can motivate some individuals to purposely keep their blood glucose levels above recommended levels as a precaution against a hypoglycemic episode, despite knowing the long-term consequences of high blood sugar levels. Further complicating matters, individuals with anxiety can confuse symptoms of anxiety (sweating, dizziness) with warning signs of a hypoglycemic episode, leading to unnecessary overeating (Sabourin & Pursley, 2013).

Sexual Dysfunction

Both women and men with diabetes are at increased risk for sexual dysfunction (decreased desire, arousal dysfunction, and orgasmic dysfunction). In a 2003 study, a total of 27% of women and 22% of men with diabetes reported sexual dysfunction. More women with diabetes reported sexual dysfunction than their peers who did not have diabetes (15%), citing decreased lubrication. Men with diabetes are at increased risk for erectile dysfunction occurring at an earlier age than their counterparts without diabetes. Both women and men who reported sexual dysfunction also reported more depressive symptoms than their peers without sexual dysfunction. Both women and men with more diabetes complications were more likely to report more sexual dysfunction. Predictors of sexual dysfunction differed between men and women. For men, significant predictors included the presence of diabetes complications and high age. For women, the significant predictor was depression (Enzlin, Mathieu, Van Den Bruel, Vanderschueren, & Demyttenaere, 2003).

Needle Phobia in Persons With Diabetes

The repeated exposure to needle sticks, especially for those who begin as children, as in type 1 diabetes, can exacerbate anxiety even to pathologic levels (Cemeroglu et al., 2014). Expected or "normal" anxiety will fluctuate as coping skills and social supports are acquired, are strengthened, or degrade. But a phobia, once established, is less likely to moderate and should be identified and treated. Effective treatment of phobias—needle phobias or otherwise—is a well-established therapeutic intervention of short duration (typically 10 sessions or less) and can even be done effectively on a self-help, bibliotherapy-guided basis. Where such treatment services are integrated and available in the primary care setting, they are more likely to be accessed and used. This is especially needed in primary care settings, because more than 90% of patients with diabetes receive most of their care in primary care practices (Hiss, 1996; Rothman & Wagner, 2003).

Depression and Diabetes

The prevalence of depression among people with diabetes is approximately twice as high as for those without diabetes, affecting more than 40% of all persons with diabetes (Anderson et al., 2001; Gonzalez, Peyrot et al., 2008; Peyrot & Rubin, 1997). The relationship between diabetes and depression is symbiotic: Diabetes invites depression, and depression seems to worsen the severity of diabetes and its complications. Depression has been found to be associated with a wide variety of diabetes complications, including neuropathy, retinopathy, and sexual dysfunction (Lin et al., 2006; Lin et al., 2010; Naranjo, Fisher, Arean, Hessler, & Mullan, 2011). Compared to individuals with diabetes alone, those with both depression and diabetes have more symptoms, increased work disability, and increased use of medical services. Diabetes-specific emotional distress such as depression, anxiety, and stress are negatively correlated with self-care in type 1 and type 2 diabetics (Weinger et al., 2005).

The relationship between depression and diabetes involves both biological and behavioral factors. The physiological aspects of depression seem to contribute to poor glycemic control, thereby increasing diabetes complications; the behavioral effects of depression seem to negatively impact self-care behaviors (adherence to diet, checking blood glucose, taking medications as prescribed, exercising).

Once depression exists in the person with diabetes, characteristic features of depression may negatively impact diabetes self-care. Depression-related withdrawal from social interaction may lessen social support. Negative thinking about the self may lessen self-efficacy and motivation. Depression-related fatigue, low energy, and sleep of poorer quality are threats to the energy and activity levels required to manage diabetes. Cognitive changes associated with depression, including difficulties in concentration, may also make self-care more difficult. Neuropathic pain may exacerbate depression. The anxiety already associated with diabetes (fears of hypoglycemia, anxiety about needles) is likely to intensify.

Routine psychosocial screening and assessment of depression is recommended by the U.S. Preventive Services Task Force but is especially indicated in patients with chronic conditions including diabetes ("Screening for depression in adults: U.S. Preventive Services Task Force Recommendation Statement," 2009). Strategies such as reminder prompts for behavioral health providers to screen for diabetes in patients with depression have been shown to be useful (Gote & Bruce, 2014). When depression is diagnosed, treatment should be provided. The current standard of care is the combination of antidepressant medication and counseling (ADA, 2014a).

Although treatment of depression alone has not been shown to improve self-care behaviors, comprehensive interventions that address both depression and self-care can have positive effects on both emotional status and self-care behaviors (Gonzalez, Peyrot, et al., 2008; Gonzalez, Safren et al., 2008).

Substance Use and Diabetes

Problematic substance use is associated with poor self-care and lack of attention to health (Minugh, Rice, & Young, 1998; Zhu et al., 2015). Although problematic for all those with substance use problems, such inattention to health can be disastrous for those with diabetes. Health care providers should routinely screen diabetic patients for substance use problems and encourage strong, ongoing collaborative communication between primary care and specialized substance use treatment settings (Walter & Petry, 2014).

Family Dynamics and Social Support

For most adults, including adults with diabetes, the family represents the most important source of social support. Health care providers should therefore be actively interested in the patient's family relations, assessing the availability of supportive family, identifying family problems from the patient's perspective, and offering active assistance to improve the patient's relationship with family, whether through counseling directly, or by taking steps to help the patient engage family members in aspects of the patient's care.

However, there are many patients who have no significant social support in their lives. This is especially problematic for people with a complex, chronic condition such as diabetes (Reeves et al., 2014). People with more social support do better with self-care behaviors (Gleeson-Kreig, Bernal, & Woolley, 2002; Lloyd, Wing, Orchard, & Becker, 1993; Wen, Shepherd, & Parchman, 2004). Friends and community organizations may also be important sources of support. People with diabetes may be much more likely to initiate and maintain exercise routines if the routines are done with supportive others.

Peer illness support groups or organizations can offer strong support. In most states, the ADA offers peer support groups. These are often hospital based and can be identified through local or online self-help clearinghouses. Health care providers should create or use an existing database of support organizations for patients and create mechanisms for disseminating such information to patients and encouraging them to use them. Offering group visits for patients with diabetes can also provide significant peer support.

Cognitive and Functional Capacity

Strong cognitive capacities and skills are required for the ideal self-management of diabetes. As described earlier, diabetes self-care is complex. Cognitive limitations or impairments from concomitant depression, other psychiatric conditions, developmental condition, or age- or disease-related changes can negatively impact the management of diabetes. Additionally, those patients in midlife with diabetes may have a greater incidence of cognitive decline than those who do not have diabetes (Rawlings et al., 2014). To address cognitive limits, the health care team must identify the underlying condition(s) and institute appropriate treatments. Identifying and mobilizing social and structural supports for the cognitively impaired patient will be the critical intervention. This might include family support and support from day care or residential programs.

Variability in patients' physical status will impact diabetes care and self-care. A patient who is not ambulatory will need home-based and remote services and may not be able to visit the office easily or at all. A variety of physical limitations may need accommodation. Sensory impairments will require hearing and vision adaptations. Administering medication, especially insulin injections, can be dangerous for unsupervised patients with visual impairment. Alternative means for diabetic patients to access good nutrition and exercise may need to be arranged. Screening should identify such conditions and proactively offer or arrange whatever adjustment and services are needed. The physical environment is another variable. Ideal environments for diabetes care would offer easy access to exercise-friendly areas, including safe, readily available roadways and sidewalks for bicycling and walking. Similarly, an ideal diabetes care environment would have supermarkets and other venues that make nutritious food choices easily available. Many patients do not live in such areas.

Finances

The affordability of diabetes medication and supplies (e.g., glucometer, needles, test strips) is a care barrier for many patients. Health care providers can help patients apply for medicines through drug company patient assistance programs. An interdisciplinary team of providers should have access, through social work support, to available resources, including insurance and benefit options, and relevant community services. Whenever possible, generic medicines at lower cost should be prescribed. Other financial issues, which may impact those with diabetes, include food insecurity, funds for transportation to medical appointments, costs for gym and exercise equipment access, housing instability, and even affordability of co-payments for medical care.

Stress Management

Stress management is a term commonly used (and understood by patients) for how people deal with life's challenges and the problematic human responses, which commonly arise. In terms of clinical outcomes, studies suggest a relationship between stress and blood glucose levels and diabetes-related problems. Stress can directly affect glucose levels' response to medication and can impact self-care (Faulenbach et al., 2012). There are a variety of stress management approaches (Sobol-Pacyniak, Szymczak, Kwarta, Loba, & Pietras, 2014). Relaxation techniques (e.g., progressive muscle relaxation, diaphragmatic breathing, meditation, yoga, tai chi, chi gong) are often taught as stress management skills. Such techniques are ideally used preventively to lower baseline levels of arousal from routine, daily stressors and as preparation for responding to stress exacerbations. Simply learning to pay more attention to bodily tension, such as that commonly experienced in the shoulders, face, or belly, and then employing such simple measures as regularizing and deepening breathing, sighing, stretching, or repeating a self-soothing statement (silent or verbalized) can be effective in reducing dysfunctional arousal in stressful situations (Koloverou, Tentolouris, Bakoula, Darviri, & Chrousos, 2014).

Disability and Employment

People with diabetes face significant employment barriers. The primary cause of this problem is employer and societal bias against those with observable diseases and a related lack of accommodation and support. There is nothing inherently disabling in diabetes: Every element of the condition, including its required care and its medical outcomes, either causes no work-limiting consequences or could be easily accommodated. The secondary cause is the association between diabetes and depression, because people with depression are also less likely to obtain and sustain employment. In part, this is because depression can be disabling, negatively impacting motivation and function. But employer and societal bias, including limited access to adequate care, also plays a role in that relationship (Anderson et al., 2014; Ervasti et al., 2014; Herquelot, Gueguen, Bonenfant, & Dray-Spira, 2011).

SUMMARY/FUTURE DIRECTIONS

Prevalence of both diabetes and prediabetes is on the rise and projected to affect more than 483 million and 470 million people by 2030, respectively (CDC, 2010; Tabak et al., 2012). Lifestyle modification is the key to the prevention of type 2 diabetes, with a relative risk reduction of 40% to 70% (Bergamin & Dib, 2015). Consistently elevated blood glucose results in increased morbidity and mortality and is associated with functional disabilities including limited joint mobility and decreased quality of life (American Heart Association, 2012; Larkin et al., 2014; Vanstone, Rewegan, Brundisini, Dejean, & Giacomini, 2015). Diabetes self-management support and education is critical to optimizing glycemic control. There have been significant advances in diabetes management including improved technology, increased understanding, and stepwise treatment guidelines (Chatterjee & Davies, 2015). New emerging technologies determine the association between lifestyle behaviors and clinical outcomes related to type 2 diabetes, which will provide feedback to patients, potentially affecting their behavior (Spruijt-Metz, O'Reilly, Cook, Page, & Quinn, 2014). Multidisciplinary intervention is an effective strategy for managing patients with diabetes; educating patients and team care may prevent complications associated with disability and reduced quality of life (Inzucchi et al., 2015; Jiao et al., 2014; Morey-Vargas & Smith, 2015).

REFERENCES

Ackard, D. M., Vik, N., Neumark-Sztainer, D., Schmitz, K. H., Hannan, P., & Jacobs, D. R., Jr. (2008). Disordered eating and body dissatisfaction in adolescents with type 1 diabetes and a population-based comparison sample: Comparative prevalence and clinical implications. *Pediatric Diabetes, 9*(4 Pt 1), 312–319. doi:10.1111/j.1399-5448.2008.00392.x

Ackermann, R. T., Finch, E. A., Brizendine, E., Zhou, H., & Marrero, D. G. (2008). Translating the diabetes prevention program into the community. The DEPLOY pilot study. *American Journal of Preventive Medicine, 35*(4), 357–363. doi:10.1016/j.amepre.2008.06.035

American Diabetes Association. (2010). Diagnosis and classification of diabetes mellitus. *Diabetes Care, 33*(Suppl. 1), S62–S69. doi:10.2337/dc10-S062

American Diabetes Association. (2013a). Age, race, gender, and family history. Retrieved from http://www.diabetes.org/are-you-at-risk/lower-your-risk/nonmodifiables.html?referrer=https://www.google.com

American Diabetes Association. (2013b). Economic costs of diabetes in the U.S. in 2012. *Diabetes Care, 36*(4), 1033–1046. doi:10.2337/dc12-2625

American Diabetes Association. (2014a). Executive summary: Standards of medical care in diabetes–2014. *Diabetes Care, 37*(Suppl. 1), S5–S13. doi:10.2337/dc14-S005

American Diabetes Association. (2014b). Statistics about diabetes. Retrieved from http://www.diabetes.org/diabetes-basics/statistics/?referrer=https://www.google.com

American Heart Association. (2012). Cardiovascular diseases and diabetes. Retrieved from http://www.heart.org/HEARTORG/Conditions/Diabetes/WhyDiabetesMatters/Cardiovascular-Disease-Diabetes_UCM_313865_Article.jsp/#.WAACDVeMD-Y

Anderson, J. E., Greene, M. A., Griffin, J. W., Jr., Kohrman, D. B., Lorber, D., Saudek, C. D., . . . Siminerio, L. (2014). Diabetes and employment. *Diabetes Care, 37*(Suppl. 1), S112–S117. doi:10.2337/dc14-S112

Anderson, R. J., Freedland, K. E., Clouse, R. E., & Lustman, P. J. (2001). The prevalence of comorbid depression in adults with diabetes: A meta-analysis. *Diabetes Care, 24*(6), 1069–1078.

Anjana, R. M., Shanthi Rani, C. S., Deepa, M., Pradeepa, R., Sudha, V., Divya Nair, H., . . . Mohan, V. (2015). Incidence of diabetes and prediabetes and predictors of progression among Asian Indians: 10-year follow-up of the Chennai Urban Rural Epidemiology Study (CURES). *Diabetes Care, 38*(8), 1441–1448. doi:10.2337/dc14-2814

Ayala, J. M., & Murphy, K. (2011). Managing psychosocial issues in a family with diabetes. *MCN, The American Journal of Maternal/Child Nursing, 36*(1), 49–55. doi:10.1097/NMC.0b013e3181fc5e94

Balducci, S., Zanuso, S., Cardelli, P., Salvi, L., Mazzitelli, G., Bazuro, A., . . . Pugliese, G. (2012). Changes in physical fitness predict improvements in modifiable cardiovascular risk factors independently of body weight loss in subjects with type 2 diabetes participating in the Italian Diabetes and Exercise Study (IDES). *Diabetes Care, 35*(6), 1347–1354. doi:10.2337/dc11-1859

Barber, S. R., Davies, M. J., Khunti, K., & Gray, L. J. (2014). Risk assessment tools for detecting those with pre-diabetes: A systematic review. *Diabetes Research and Clinical Practice, 105*(1), 1–13. doi:10.1016/j.diabres.2014.03.007

Baumert, J., Meisinger, C., Lukaschek, K., Emeny, R T., Rückert, I.-M., Kruse, J., & Ladwig, K.-H. (2014). A pattern of unspecific somatic symptoms as long-term premonitory signs of type 2 diabetes: Findings from the population-based MONICA/KORA cohort study, 1984–2009. *BMC Endocrine Disorders, 14*(1), 87. doi:10.1186/1472-6823-14-87

Bergamin, C. S., & Dib, S. A. (2015). Enterovirus and type 1 diabetes: What is the matter? *World Journal of Diabetes, 6*(6), 828–839. doi:10.4239/wjd.v6.i6.828

Buresh, R. (2014). Exercise and glucose control. *Journal of Sports Medicine and Physical Finess, 54*(4), 373–382.

Burg, M. A., & Oyama, O. (Eds.). (2015). *The behavioral health specialist in primary care: Skills for integrated practice*. New York, NY: Springer Publishing.

Bushman, B. (2014). Promoting exercise as medicine for prediabetes and prehypertension. *Current Sports Medicine Reports, 13*(4), 233–239. doi:10.1249/jsr.0000000000000066

Caspersen, C. J., Thomas, G. D., Beckles, G. L., & Bullard, K. M. (2015). Secular changes in prediabetes indicators among older-adult Americans, 1999–2010. *American Journal of Preventive Medicine, 48*(3), 253–263. doi:10.1016/j.amepre.2014.10.004

Cefalu, W. T., Petersen, M. P., & Ratner, R. E. (2014). The alarming and rising costs of diabetes and prediabetes: A call for action! *Diabetes Care, 37*(12), 3137–3138. doi:10.2337/dc14-2329

Cemeroglu, A. P., Can, A., Davis, A. T., Cemeroglu, O., Kleis, L., Daniel, M. S., . . . Koehler, T. J. (2014). Fear of needles in children with type 1 diabetes mellitus on multiple daily injections (MDI) and continuous subcutaneous insulin infusion (CSII). *Endocrine Practice*, 1–25. doi:10.4158/ep14252.or

Centers for Disease Control and Prevention. (2010). Number of Americans with diabetes projected to double or triple by 2050. Retrieved from http://www.cdc.gov/media/pressrel/2010/r101022.html

Centers for Disease Control and Prevention. (2014). *National diabetes statistics report: Estimates of diabetes and its burden in the United States*. Retrieved from http://www.cdc.gov/diabetes/pubs/statsreport14/national-diabetes-report-web.pdf

Cevetello, J. (2011). *Evocative objects: Things we think with*. Cambridge, MA: MIT Press.

Chatterjee, S., & Davies, M. J. (2015). Current management of diabetes mellitus and future directions in care. *Postgraduate Medical Journal, 91*(1081), 612–621 doi:10.1136/postgradmedj-2014-133200

Chiang, J. L., Kirkman, M. S., Laffel, L. M., & Peters, A. L. (2014). Type 1 diabetes through the life span: A position statement of the American Diabetes Association. *Diabetes Care, 37*(7), 2034–2054. doi:10.2337/dc14-1140

Choudhary, N., Kalra, S., Unnikrishnan, A. G., & Ajish, T. P. (2012). Preventive pharmacotherapy in type 2 diabetes mellitus. *Indian Journal of Endocrinology and Metabolism, 16*(1), 33–43. doi:10.4103/2230-8210.91183

Cryer, P. E., Davis, S. N., & Shamoon, H. (2003). Hypoglycemia in diabetes. *Diabetes Care*, *26*(6), 1902–1912.

Dabelea, D., Mayer-Davis, E. J., Saydah, S., Imperatore, G., Linder, B., Divers, J., . . . Hamman, R. F. (2014). Prevalence of type 1 and type 2 diabetes among children and adolescents from 2001 to 2009. *Journal of the American Medical Association, 311*(17), 1778–1786. doi:10.1001/jama.2014.3201

Dall, T. M., Yang, W., Halder, P., Pang, B., Massoudi, M., Wintfeld, N., . . . Hogan, P. F. (2014). The economic burden of elevated blood glucose levels in 2012: Diagnosed and undiagnosed diabetes, gestational diabetes mellitus, and prediabetes. *Diabetes Care, 37*(12), 3172–3179. doi:10.2337/dc14-1036

Daniele, G., Abdul-Ghani, M., & DeFronzo, R. A. (2014). What are the pharmacotherapy options for treating prediabetes? *Expert Opinion on Pharmacotherapy, 15*(14), 2003–2018. doi:10.1517/14656566.2014.944160

Davies, M. J., Gagliardino, J. J., Gray, L. J., Khunti, K., Mohan, V., & Hughes, R. (2013). Real-world factors affecting adherence to insulin therapy in patients with type 1 or type 2 diabetes mellitus: A systematic review. *Diabetes Medicine, 30*(5), 512–524. doi:10.1111/dme.12128

Delamater, A. M. (2009). Psychological care of children and adolescents with diabetes. *Pediatric Diabetes, 10*(Suppl. 12), 175–184. doi:10.1111/j.1399-5448.2009.00580.x

DeSisto, C. L., Kim, S. Y., & Sharma, A. J. (2014). Prevalence estimates of gestational diabetes mellitus in the United States, Pregnancy Risk Assessment Monitoring System (PRAMS), 2007–2010. *Preventing Chronic Disease, 11*, E104. doi:10.5888/pcd11.130415

Engum, A. (2007). The role of depression and anxiety in onset of diabetes in a large population-based study. *Journal of Psychosomatic Research, 62*(1), 31–38. doi:10.1016/j.jpsychores.2006.07.009

Enzlin, P., Mathieu, C., Van Den Bruel, A., Vanderschueren, D., & Demyttenaere, K. (2003). Prevalence and predictors of sexual dysfunction in patients with type 1 diabetes. *Diabetes Care, 26*(2), 409–414.

Ervasti, J., Vahtera, J., Pentti, J., Oksanen, T., Ahola, K., Kivekas, T., . . . Virtanen, M. (2014). The role of psychiatric, cardiometabolic, and musculoskeletal comorbidity in the recurrence of depression-related work disability. *Depression and Anxiety, 31*(9), 796–803. doi:10.1002/da.22286

Esposito, K., Chiodini, P., Maiorino, M. I., Bellastella, G., Panagiotakos, D., & Giugliano, D. (2014). Which diet for prevention of type 2 diabetes? A meta-analysis of prospective studies. *Endocrine, 47*(1), 107–116. doi:10.1007/s12020-014-0264-4

Faulenbach, M., Uthoff, H., Schwegler, K., Spinas, G. A., Schmid, C., & Wiesli, P. (2012). Effect of psychological stress on glucose control in patients with type 2 diabetes. *Diabetic Medicine: A Journal of the British Diabetic Association, 29*(1), 128–131. doi:10.1111/j.1464-5491.2011.03431.x

Fonville, S., Zandbergen, A. A., Koudstaal, P. J., & den Hertog, H. M. (2014). Prediabetes in patients with stroke or transient ischemic attack: prevalence, risk and clinical management. *Cerebrovascular Diseases, 37*(6), 393–400. doi:10.1159/000360810

Geiss, L. S., Wang, J., Cheng, Y. J., Thompson, T. J., Barker, L., Li, Y., . . . Gregg, E. W. (2014). Prevalence and incidence trends for diagnosed diabetes among adults aged 20 to 79 years, United States, 1980–2012. *Journal of the American Medical Association, 312*(12), 1218–1226. doi:10.1001/jama.2014.11494

Gillies, C. L., Abrams, K. R., Lambert, P. C., Cooper, N. J., Sutton, A. J., Hsu, R. T., & Khunti, K. (2007). Pharmacological and lifestyle interventions to prevent or delay type 2 diabetes in people with impaired glucose tolerance: Systematic review and meta-analysis. *BMJ: British Medical Journal, 334*(7588), 299. doi:10.1136/bmj.39063.689375.55

Gleeson-Kreig, J., Bernal, H., & Woolley, S. (2002). The role of social support in the self-management of diabetes mellitus among a Hispanic population. *Public Health Nursing, 19*(3), 215–222.

Goebel-Fabbri, A. E., Fikkan, J., Connell, A., Vangsness, L., & Anderson, B. J. (2002). Identification and treatment of eating disorders in women with type 1 diabetes mellitus. *Treatments in Endocrinology, 1*(3), 155–162.

Gonzalez, J. S., Peyrot, M., McCarl, L. A., Collins, E. M., Serpa, L., Mimiaga, M. J., & Safren, S. A. (2008). Depression and diabetes treatment nonadherence: A meta-analysis. *Diabetes Care, 31*(12), 2398–2403. doi:10.2337/dc08-1341

Gonzalez, J. S., Safren, S. A., Delahanty, L. M., Cagliero, E., Wexler, D. J., Meigs, J. B., & Grant, R. W. (2008). Symptoms of depression prospectively predict poorer self-care in patients with Type 2 diabetes. *Diabet Medicine, 25*(9), 1102–1107. doi:10.1111/j.1464-5491.2008.02535.x

Gote, C., & Bruce, R. D. (2014). Effectiveness of a reminder prompt to screen for diabetes in individuals with depression. *The Journal for Nurse Practitioners, 10*(7), 456–464. doi:10.1016/j.nurpra.2014.04.021

Gregg, E. W., Zhuo, X., Cheng, Y. J., Albright, A. L., Narayan, K. M., & Thompson, T. J. (2014). Trends in lifetime risk and years of life lost due to diabetes in the USA, 1985–2011: A modelling study. *Lancet Diabetes Endocrinol, 2*(11), 867–874. doi:10.1016/s2213-8587(14)70161-5

Grigsby, A. B., Anderson, R. J., Freedland, K. E., Clouse, R. E., & Lustman, P. J. (2002). Prevalence of anxiety in adults with diabetes: A systematic review. *Journal of Psychosomatic Research, 53*(6), 1053–1060.

Halliday, T. M., Davy, B. M., Clark, A. G., Baugh, M. E., Hedrick, V. E., Marinik, E. L., . . . Winett, R. A. (2014). Dietary intake modification in response to a participation in a resistance training program for sedentary older adults with prediabetes: Findings from the resist diabetes study. *Eating Behaviors, 15*(3), 379–382. doi:10.1016/j.eatbeh.2014.04.004

Helgeson, V. S., Reynolds, K. A., Siminerio, L., Escobar, O., & Becker, D. (2008). Parent and adolescent distribution of responsibility for diabetes self-care: Links to health outcomes. *Journal of Pediatric Psychology, 33*(5), 497–508. doi:10.1093/jpepsy/jsm081

Herquelot, E., Gueguen, A., Bonenfant, S., & Dray-Spira, R. (2011). Impact of diabetes on work cessation: Data from the GAZEL cohort study. *Diabetes Care, 34*(6), 1344–1349. doi:10.2337/dc10-2225

Hiss, R. G. (1996). Barriers to care in non-insulin-dependent diabetes mellitus. The Michigan experience. *Annals of Internal Medicine, 124*(1, Pt. 2), 146–148.

Hu, F. B., Satija, A., & Manson, J. E. (2015). Curbing the diabetes pandemic: The need for global policy solutions. *Journal of the American Medical Association, 313*(23), 2319–2320. doi:10.1001/jama.2015.5287

Huang, C. J., Chiu, H. C., Lee, M. H., & Wang, S. Y. (2011). Prevalence and incidence of anxiety disorders in diabetic patients: A national population-based cohort study. *General Hospital Psychiatry, 33*(1), 8–15. doi:10.1016/j.genhosppsych.2010.10.008

Huang, Y., Cai, X., Chen, P., Mai, W., Tang, H., Huang, Y., & Hu, Y. (2014). Associations of prediabetes with all-cause and cardiovascular mortality: A meta-analysis. *Annals of Medicine, 46*(8), 684–692. doi:10.3109/07853890.2014.955051

Ibe, A., & Smith, T. C. (2014). Diabetes in U.S. women on the rise independent of increasing BMI and other risk factors; a trend investigation of serial cross-sections. *BMC Public Health, 14*, 954. doi:10.1186/1471-2458-14-954

Inzucchi, S. E., Bergenstal, R. M., Buse, J. B., Diamant, M., Ferrannini, E., Nauck, M., . . . Matthews, D. R. (2015). Management of hyperglycemia in type 2 diabetes, 2015: A patient-centered approach: Update to a position statement of the American Diabetes Association and the European Association for the Study of Diabetes. *Diabetes Care, 38*(1), 140–149. doi:10.2337/dc14-2441

Ivey, J. B., Wright, A., & Dashiff, C. J. (2009). Finding the balance: Adolescents with type 1 diabetes and their parents. *Journal of Pediatric Health Care, 23*(1), 10–18. doi:10.1016/j.pedhc.2007.12.008

Jacobson, A. M., de Groot, M., & Samson, J. A. (1994). The evaluation of two measures of quality of life in patients with type I and type II diabetes. *Diabetes Care, 17*(4), 267–274.

Jiao, F. F., Fung, C. S., Wong, C. K., Wan, Y. F., Dai, D., Kwok, R., & Lam, C. L. (2014). Effects of the multidisciplinary risk assessment and management program for patients with diabetes mellitus (RAMP-DM) on biomedical outcomes, observed cardiovascular events and cardiovascular risks in primary care: A longitudinal comparative study. *Cardiovasc Diabetol, 13*(1), 127. doi:10.1186/s12933-014-0127-6

Kalyani, R. R., Saudek, C. D., Brancati, F. L., & Selvin, E. (2010). Association of diabetes, comorbidities, and A1C with functional disability in older adults: results from the national health and nutrition examination survey (NHANES), 1999–2006. *Diabetes Care, 33*(5), 1055–1060. doi:10.2337/dc09-1597

Kalyani, R. R., Tian, J., Xue, Q. L., Walston, J., Cappola, A. R., Fried, L. P., . . . Blaum, C. S. (2012). Hyperglycemia and incidence of frailty and lower extremity mobility limitations in older women. *Journal of the American Geriatrics Society, 60*(9), 1701–1707. doi:10.1111/j.1532-5415.2012.04099.x

Kitzmiller, J. L., Dang-Kilduff, L., & Taslimi, M. M. (2007). Gestational diabetes after delivery. Short-term management and long-term risks. *Diabetes Care, 30*(Suppl. 2), S225–S235. doi:10.2337/dc07-s221

Knowler, W. C., Barrett-Connor, E., Fowler, S. E., Hamman, R. F., Lachin, J. M., Walker, E. A., & Nathan, D. M. (2002). Reduction in the incidence of type 2 diabetes with lifestyle intervention or metformin. *New England Journal of Medicine, 346*(6), 393–403. doi:10.1056/NEJMoa012512

Knowler, W. C., Fowler, S. E., Hamman, R. F., Christophi, C. A., Hoffman, H. J., Brenneman, A. T., . . . Nathan, D. M. (2009). 10-year follow-up of diabetes incidence and weight loss in the diabetes prevention program outcomes study. *The Lancet, 374*(9702), 1677–1686. doi:10.1016/s0140-6736(09)61457-4

Koloverou, E., Tentolouris, N., Bakoula, C., Darviri, C., & Chrousos, G. (2014). Implementation of a stress management program in outpatients with type 2 diabetes mellitus: A randomized controlled trial. *Hormones (Athens), 13*(4), 509–518. doi:10.14310/horm.2002.1492

Larkin, M. E., Barnie, A., Braffett, B. H., Cleary, P. A., Diminick, L., Harth, J., . . . Nathan, D. M. (2014). Musculoskeletal complications in type 1 diabetes. *Diabetes Care, 37*(7), 1863–1869. doi:10.2337/dc13-2361

Lawrence, J. M., Imperatore, G., Dabelea, D., Mayer-Davis, E. J., Linder, B., Saydah, S., . . . D'Agostino, R. B., Jr. (2014). Trends in incidence of type 1 diabetes among non-Hispanic white youth in the U.S., 2002–2009. *Diabetes, 63*(11), 3938–3945. doi:10.2337/db13-1891

Lin, E. H., Katon, W., Rutter, C., Simon, G. E., Ludman, E. J., Von Korff, M., . . . Walker, E. (2006). Effects of enhanced depression treatment on diabetes self-care. *The Annals of Family Medicine, 4*(1), 46–53. doi:10.1370/afm.423

Lin, E. H., Rutter, C. M., Katon, W., Heckbert, S. R., Ciechanowski, P., Oliver, M. M., . . . Von Korff, M. (2010). Depression and advanced complications of diabetes: A prospective cohort study. *Diabetes Care, 33*(2), 264–269. doi:10.2337/dc09-1068

Lloyd, C. E., Wing, R. R., Orchard, T. J., & Becker, D. J. (1993). Psychosocial correlates of glycemic control: The pittsburgh epidemiology of diabetes complications (EDC) Study. *Diabetes Research and Clinical Practice, 21*(2–3), 187–195.

MacArthur, C. (2015). Ketoacidosis in diabetes: Recognition and avoidance. *Practice Nursing, 26*(8), 393–399. doi:10.12968/pnur.2015.26.8.393

Meichenbaum, D., & Turk, D. C. (1987). *Facilitating treatment adherence: A practitioner's guidebook*. New York, NY: Plenum Press.

Minuchin, S., Baker, L., Rosman, B. L., Liebman, R., Milman, L., & Todd, T. C. (1975). A conceptual model of psychosomatic illness in children. Family organization and family therapy. *Archives of General Psychiatry, 32*(8), 1031–1038.

Minuchin, S., & Fishman, H. C. (1979). The psychosomatic family in child psychiatry. *Journal of the American Academy of Child Psychiatry, 18*(1), 76–90.

Minugh, P. A., Rice, C., & Young, L. (1998). Gender, health beliefs, health behaviors, and alcohol consumption. *The American Journal of Drug and Alcohol Abuse, 24*(3), 483–497.

Morey-Vargas, O. L., & Smith, S. A. (2015). BE SMART: Strategies for foot care and prevention of foot complications in patients with diabetes. *Prosthetics and Orthotics International, 39*(1), 48–60. doi:10.1177/0309364614535622

Murata, T., Tsuzaki, K., Yoshioka, F., Okada, H., Kishi, J., Yamada, K., & Sakane, N. (2015). The relationship between the frequency of self-monitoring of blood glucose and glycemic control in patients with type 1 diabetes mellitus on continuous subcutaneous insulin infusion or on multiple daily injections. *Journal of Diabetes Investigation, 6*(6), 687–691. doi:10.1111/jdi.12362

Naranjo, D. M., Fisher, L., Arean, P. A., Hessler, D., & Mullan, J. (2011). Patients with type 2 diabetes at risk for major depressive disorder over time. *The Annals of Family Medicine, 9*(2), 115–120. doi:10.1370/afm.1212

Nathan, D. M. (2015). Diabetes: Advances in diagnosis and treatment. *Journal of the American Medical Association, 314*(10), 1052–1062. doi:10.1001/jama.2015.9536

Nichols, G. A., Arondekar, B., & Herman, W. H. (2008). Complications of dysglycemia and medical costs associated with nondiabetic hyperglycemia. *American Journal of Managed Care, 14*(12), 791–798.

Nichols, G. A., Hillier, T. A., & Brown, J. B. (2007). Progression from newly acquired impaired fasting glusose to type 2 diabetes. *Diabetes Care, 30*(2), 228–233. doi:10.2337/dc06-1392

Nordwall, M., Abrahamsson, M., Dhir, M., Fredrikson, M., Ludvigsson, J., & Arnqvist, H. J. (2015). Impact of HbA1c, followed from onset of type 1 diabetes, on the development of severe retinopathy and nephropathy: The VISS Study (Vascular Diabetic Complications in Southeast Sweden). *Diabetes Care, 38*(2), 308–315. doi:10.2337/dc14-1203

Palermo, A., Maggi, D., Maurizi, A. R., Pozzilli, P., & Buzzetti, R. (2014). Prevention of type 2 diabetes mellitus: Is it feasible? *Diabetes/Metabolism Research and Reviews, 30*(Suppl. 2), 4–12. doi:10.1002/dmrr.2513

Parker, A. R., Byham-Gray, L., Denmark, R., & Winkle, P. J. (2014). The effect of medical nutrition therapy by a registered dietitian nutritionist in patients with prediabetes participating in a randomized controlled clinical research trial. *Journal of the Academy of Nutrition and Dietetics, 114*(11), 1739–1748. doi:10.1016/j.jand.2014.07.020

Pasquel, F. J., & Umpierrez, G. E. (2014). Hyperosmolar hyperglycemic state: A historic review of the clinical presentation, diagnosis, and treatment. *Diabetes Care, 37*(11), 3124–3131. doi:10.2337/dc14-0984

Pereira, R. F., & Alvarenga, M. (2007). Disordered eating: Identifying, treating, preventing, and differentiating it from eating disorders. *Diabetes Spectrum, 20*(3), 141–148. doi:10.2337/diaspect.20.3.141

Perlmuter, L. C., Flanagan, B. P., Shah, P. H., & Singh, S. P. (2008). Glycemic control and hypoglycemia: Is the loser the winner? *Diabetes Care, 31*(10), 2072–2076. doi:10.2337/dc08-1441

Peyrot, M., & Rubin, R. R. (1997). Levels and risks of depression and anxiety symptomatology among diabetic adults. *Diabetes Care, 20*(4), 585–590.

Pi-Sunyer, X., Astrup, A., Fujioka, K., Greenway, F., Halpern, A., Krempf, M., . . . Wilding, J. P. (2015). A randomized, controlled trial of 3.0 mg of liraglutide in weight management. *New England Journal of Medicine, 373*(1), 11–22. doi:10.1056/NEJMoa1411892

Popp Switzer, M., Elhanafi, S., & San Juan, Z. T. (2015). Change in daily ambulatory activity and cardiovascular events in people with impaired glucose tolerance. *Current Cardiology Reports, 17*(3), 562. doi:10.1007/s11886-015-0562-3

Powers, A. C. (2015a). Diabetes mellitus: Diagnosis, classification, and pathophysiology. In D. Kasper, A. Fauci, S. Hauser, D. Longo, J. L. Jameson, & J. Loscalzo (Eds.), *Harrison's principles of internal medicine* (19th ed.). Retrieved from http://accesspharmacy.mhmedical.com/content.aspx?bookid=1130&Sectionid=79752868

Powers, A. C. (2015b). Diabetes mellitus: Management and therapies. In D. Kasper, A. Fauci, S. Hauser, D. Longo, J. L. Jameson, & J. Loscalzo (Eds.), *Harrison's principles of internal medicine* (19th ed.). Retrieved from http://accesspharmacy.mhmedical.com/content.aspx?bookid=1130&Sectionid=79752952

Pozzo, M. J., Mociulsky, J., Martinez, E. T., Senatore, G., Farias, J. M., Sapetti, A., . . . Lemme, L. (2014). Diabetes and quality of life: initial approach to depression, physical activity, and sexual dysfunction. *American Journal of Therapeutics*, *23*(1), e159–e171. doi:10.1097/01.mjt.0000433949.24277.19

Prochaska, J. O., & DiClemente, C. C. (1983). Stages and processes of self-change of smoking: Toward an integrative model of change. *Journal of Consulting and Clinical Psychology, 51*(3), 390–395.

Prochaska, J. O., Norcross, J. C., & DiClemente, C. C. (2007). *Changing for good: A revolutionary six-stage program for overcoming bad habits and moving your life positively forward.* New York, NY: Harper Collins.

Ram, J., Selvam, S., Snehalatha, C., Nanditha, A., Simon, M., Shetty, A. S., . . . Ramachandran, A. (2014). Improvement in diet habits, independent of physical activity helps to reduce incident diabetes among prediabetic Asian Indian men. *Diabetes Research and Clinical Practice, 106*(3), 491–495. doi:10.1016/j.diabres.2014.09.043

Rattay, K. T., & Rosenthal, M. (2014). Reversing the diabetes epidemic: A role for primary care in identifying pre-diabetes and referral to an evidence-based program. *Delaware Medical Journal, 86*(10), 307–313; quiz 317.

Rawlings, A. M., Sharrett, A. R., Schneider, A. L., Coresh, J., Albert, M., Couper, D., . . . Selvin, E. (2014). Diabetes in midlife and cognitive change over 20 years: A cohort study. *Annals of Internal Medicine, 161*(11), 785–793. doi:10.7326/M14-0737

Reeves, D., Blickem, C., Vassilev, I., Brooks, H., Kennedy, A., Richardson, G., & Rogers, A. (2014). The contribution of social networks to the health and self-management of patients with long-term conditions: A longitudinal study. *PLOS ONE, 9*(6), e98340. doi:10.1371/journal.pone.0098340

Rejeski, W. J., Bray, G. A., Chen, S. H., Clark, J. M., Evans, M., Hill, J. O., . . . Ip, E. H. (2015). Aging and physical function in type 2 diabetes: 8 years of an intensive lifestyle intervention. *Journals of Gerontology. Series A: Biological Sciences and Medical Sciences, 70*(3), 345–353. doi:10.1093/gerona/glu083

Roberts, A. L., Agnew-Blais, J. C., Spiegelman, D., Kubzansky, L. D., Mason, S. M., Galea, S., . . . Koenen, K. C. (2015). Posttraumatic stress disorder and incidence of type 2 diabetes mellitus in a sample of women: A 22-year longitudinal study. *JAMA Psychiatry*, 72, 203. doi:10.1001/jamapsychiatry.2014.2632

Rogers, E. A., Fine, S., Handley, M. A., Davis, H., Kass, J., & Schillinger, D. (2014). Development and early implementation of the bigger picture, a youth-targeted public health literacy campaign to prevent type 2 diabetes. *Journal of Health Communication, 19*(Suppl. 2), 144–160. doi:10.1080/10810730.2014.940476

Rothman, A. A., & Wagner, E. H. (2003). Chronic illness management: What is the role of primary care? *Annals of Internal Medicine, 138*(3), 256–261. doi:10.7326/0003-4819-138-3-200302040-00034

Rubin, R. R., & Peyrot, M. (1992). Psychosocial problems and interventions in diabetes. A review of the literature. *Diabetes Care, 15*(11), 1640–1657.

Sabourin, B. C., & Pursley, S. (2013). Psychosocial issues in diabetes self-management: Strategies for healthcare providers. *Canadian Journal of Diabetes, 37*(1), 36–40. doi:10.1016/j.jcjd.2013.01.002

Samaras, K., Crawford, J., Lutgers, H. L., Campbell, L. V., Baune, B. T., Lux, O., . . . Sachdev, P. (2015). Metabolic burden and disease and mortality risk associated with impaired fasting glucose in elderly adults. *Journal of the American Geriatrics Society, 63*(7), 1435–1442. doi:10.1111/jgs.13482

Saslow, L. R., Kim, S., Daubenmier, J. J., Moskowitz, J. T., Phinney, S. D., Goldman, V., . . . Hecht, F. M. (2014). A randomized pilot trial of a moderate carbohydrate diet compared to a very low carbohydrate diet in overweight or obese individuals with type 2 diabetes mellitus or prediabetes. *PLOS ONE, 9*(4), e91027. doi:10.1371/journal.pone.0091027

Scott, K. M. (2014). Depression, anxiety and incident cardiometabolic diseases. *Current Opinion in Psychiatry, 27*(4), 289–293. doi:10.1097/yco.0000000000000067

Simmons, K. M., & Michels, A. W. (2015). Type 1 diabetes: A predictable disease. *World Journal of Diabetes, 6*(3), 380–390. doi:10.4239/wjd.v6.i3.380

Sobol-Pacyniak, A. B., Szymczak, W., Kwarta, P., Loba, J., & Pietras, T. (2014). Selected factors determining a way of coping with stress in type 2 diabetic patients. *BioMed Research International, 2014*, 1–7. doi:10.1155/2014/587823

Spruijt-Metz, D., O'Reilly, G. A., Cook, L., Page, K. A., & Quinn, C. (2014). Behavioral contributions to the pathogenesis of type 2 diabetes. *Current Diabetes Reports, 14*(4), 475. doi:10.1007/s11892-014-0475-3

Streisand, R., Swift, E., Wickmark, T., Chen, R., & Holmes, C. S. (2005). Pediatric parenting stress among parents of children with type 1 diabetes: the role of self-efficacy, responsibility, and fear. *Journal of Pediatric Psychology, 30*(6), 513–521. doi:10.1093/jpepsy/jsi076

Tabak, A. G., Herder, C., Rathmann, W., Brunner, E. J., & Kivimaki, M. (2012). Prediabetes: A high-risk state for diabetes development. *The Lancet, 379*(9833), 2279–2290. doi:10.1016/s0140-6736(12)60283-9

Tamez-Perez, H. E., Proskauer-Pena, S. L., Hernrndez-Coria, M. I., & Garber, A. J. (2013). AACE comprehensive diabetes management algorithm 2013. Endocrine practice. *Endocrine Practice, 19*(4), 736–737. doi:10.4158/ep13210.lt

Thuzar, M., Malabu, U. H., Tisdell, B., & Sangla, K. S. (2014). Use of a standardised diabetic ketoacidosis management protocol improved clinical outcomes. *Diabetes Research and Clinical Practice, 104*(1), e8–e11. doi:10.1016/j.diabres.2014.01.016

Triplitt, C. L., Repas, T., & Alvarez, C. (2014). Diabetes mellitus. In J. T. DiPiro, R. L. Talbert, G. C. Yee, G. R. Matzke, B. G. Wells, & L. Posey (Eds.), *Pharmacotherapy: A pathophysiologic approach* (9th ed.). Retrieved from http://accesspharmacy.mhmedical.com/content.aspx?bookid=689&Sectionid=45310509

U.S. Preventive Services Task Force. (2009). Screening for depression in adults: U.S. preventive services task force recommendation statement. *Annals of Internal Medicine, 151*(11), 784–792. doi:10.7326/0003-4819-151-11-200912010-00006

Vanstone, M., Rewegan, A., Brundisini, F., Dejean, D., & Giacomini, M. (2015). Patient perspectives on quality of life with uncontrolled type 1 diabetes mellitus: A systematic review and qualitative meta-synthesis. *Ontario Health Technology Assessment Series, 15*(17), 1–29.

Virtanen, M., Ferrie, J. E., Tabak, A. G., Akbaraly, T. N., Vahtera, J., Singh-Manoux, A., & Kivimaki, M. (2014). Psychological distress and incidence of type 2 diabetes in high-risk and low-risk populations: The whitehall II cohort study. *Diabetes Care, 37*(8), 2091–2097. doi:10.2337/dc13-2725

Waernbaum, I., & Dahlquist, G. (2015). Low mean temperature rather than few sunshine hours are associated with an increased incidence of type 1 diabetes in children. *European Journal of Epidemiology, 31*, 61–65. doi:10.1007/s10654-015-0023-8

Walker, R. J., Mulugeta. G., Bonnie, M.-H., & Leonard, E. E. (2014). Relationship between social determinants of health and processes and outcomes in adults with type 2 diabetes: Validation of a conceptual framework. *BMC Endocrine Disorders, 14*(1), 82. doi:10.1186/1472-6823-14-82

Walter, K. N., & Petry, N. M. (2014). Patients with diabetes respond well to contingency management treatment targeting alcohol and substance use. *Psychology, Health & Medicine*, 1–11. doi:10.1080/13548506.2014.991334

Weinger, K., Butler, H. A., Welch, G. W., & La Greca, A. M. (2005). Measuring diabetes self-care: A psychometric analysis of the self-care inventory-revised with adults. *Diabetes Care, 28*(6), 1346–1352.

Wen, L. K., Shepherd, M. D., & Parchman, M. L. (2004). Family support, diet, and exercise among older Mexican Americans with type 2 diabetes. *Diabetes Education, 30*(6), 980–993.

World Health Organization. (2015). WHO Diabetes fact sheet no. 312. Retrieved from http://www.who.int/mediacentre/factsheets/fs312/en

Wisting, L., Froisland, D. H., Skrivarhaug, T., Dahl-Jorgensen, K., & Ro, O. (2013). Disturbed eating behavior and omission of insulin in adolescents receiving intensified insulin treatment: A nationwide population-based study. *Diabetes Care, 36*(11), 3382–3387. doi:10.2337/dc13-0431

Yekta, Z., Pourali, R., & Ghasemi-Rad, M. (2011). Comparison of demographic and clinical characteristics influencing health-related quality of life in patients with diabetic foot ulcers and those without foot ulcers. *Diabetes, Metabolic Syndrome and Obesity, 4*, 393–399. doi:10.2147/dmso.s27050

Zhu, Q., Lou, C., Gao, E., Cheng, Y., Zabin, L. S., & Emerson, M. R. (2015). Drunkenness and its association with health risk behaviors among adolescents and young adults in three Asian cities: Hanoi, Shanghai, Taipei. *Drug and Alcohol Dependence, 147*, 251–256. doi:10.1016/j.drugalcdep.2014.10.029

Zimmer-Galler, I. E., Kimura, A. E., & Gupta, S. (2015). Diabetic retinopathy screening and the use of telemedicine. *Current Opinion in Ophthalmology, 26*(3), 167–172. doi:10.1097/icu.0000000000000142

Zinman, B., Wanner, C., Lachin, J. M., Fitchett, D., Bluhmki, E., Hantel, S., . . . Inzucchi, S. E. (2015). Empagliflozin, cardiovascular outcomes, and mortality in type 2 diabetes. *New England Journal of Medicine, 373*(22), 2117–2128. doi:10.1056/NEJMoa1504720

CHAPTER 10

Epilepsy

Anuradha Singh and Stephen Trevick

Epilepsy is the fourth most common neurological condition in the United States (Hirtz et al., 2007). A seizure is defined as a change in the clinical state of a patient due to excessive synchronous neuronal depolarization. This change can have a myriad of presentations, but the most commonly observed clinical changes are motor, sensory, psychic, and autonomic. About 1% to 2% of the general population suffers from seizures, and every one in 26 people experiences at least one seizure in his or her lifetime (Institute of Medicine, 2012). In general, seizures may be provoked or unprovoked and can be broadly classified into two types: focal or generalized. A single seizure does not necessarily mean that a person has epilepsy; epilepsy is defined as more than two unprovoked seizures. The common risk factors for developing epilepsy include febrile seizures during childhood, brain lesions, head trauma with loss of consciousness, meningitis, encephalitis, and a family history of seizures. The cause of epilepsy in an individual may often go completely unknown. Several chromosomal derangements, genetic mutations (de novo or familial), inborn errors of metabolism, and neurophakomatoses are commonly associated with epilepsy. Epilepsy is also common in patients with developmental delays, cerebral palsy, autism, and learning disabilities. About 50% of patients with intellectual disabilities with an IQ less than 50 have epilepsy (Lhatoo & Sander, 2001).

"Everything that shakes is not epilepsy." Other transient, paroxysmal disorders, such as migraines or transient ischemic attacks (TIAs), can be confused with seizures. However, seizures typically represent "positive" symptoms such as marching, tingling, or motor activity versus TIAs that produce more "negative" symptoms, like numbness or weakness.

CLASSIFICATION AND ETIOLOGY

The International League Against Epilepsy (ILAE) has revised the classification of epilepsy and epilepsy syndromes multiple times (Trinka et al., 2015). In the new classification, simple partial seizures are now referred to as focal seizures, and complex partial seizures are referred to as "focal dyscognitive seizures with alteration of consciousness" (see Table 10.1). The grand mal, or tonic–clonic, seizures are now referred to as "convulsions" in the new classification. Petit mal is also an obsolete term and is replaced by "absence seizures" (Figure 10.1). There are revised guidelines for the classification of seizures based on pathogenesis (genetic, structural-metabolic, unknown) and age of onset. The classification of epilepsy syndromes did not change significantly in the new classification. These syndromes are still classified based on seizure types, age of onset, diurnal pattern, family history, response to treatment, prognosis, etiology, and severity. The idiopathic epilepsies are now considered "genetic" in origin. The genetic defect may arise at a chromosomal or molecular level. The word "genetic" does not mean the same as "inherited," as de novo mutations may arise. Having a genetic etiology does not preclude environmental contribution to the epilepsy. Some common examples of idiopathic generalized syndromes include childhood absence, juvenile absence, and juvenile myoclonic epilepsy. The common childhood epileptic encephalopathies include Lennox–Gestaut syndrome, West syndrome, Dravet syndrome, progressive myoclonic epilepsies, and so forth, all of which are associated with progressive cognitive and motor delays.

Epilepsy with seizures originating in the temporal lobe is more common than frontal lobe epilepsy

TABLE 10.1

BASIC CLASSIFICATION OF EPILEPSY	
Focal	**Generalized**
Focal Dyscognitive Secondarily generalized tonic–clonic	Absence (typical and atypical) Myoclonic Primarily generalized tonic–clonic Tonic Atonic Clonic–tonic–clonic

(Figures 10.2 and 10.3). Parietal and occipital lobe epilepsies represent a very small percentage of epilepsy syndromes (Manford, Hart, Sander & Shorvon, 1992). People with epilepsy may or may not have a preceding aura (warning), but the presence of an aura favors possible focal epilepsy. Patents with generalized epilepsy may rarely experience auras as well. Common auras experienced by people with epilepsy include unpleasant smell or odor, difficulty speaking, dizziness, nausea, headache, unusual stomach sensations, déjà vu (feelings of familiarity) and jamais vu (feelings of unfamiliarity), depersonalization, derealization, visual changes, extreme fear, anxiety, goose bumps, and sweating. Common motor activity during dyscognitive seizures coming from the temporal regions include repetitive movements such as fumbling with hands or clothing (automatisms), lip smacking (oromasticatory automatisms), and pacing or wandering. Motor activity during frontal lobe seizures can be complex bilateral bizarre movements with or without vocalizations. A marching sensory aura seems to originate from the sensory cortices and is referred to as the "Jacksonian march." Repetitive clonic movements involving one side of the body may result from excitability in the motor areas of the contralateral hemisphere. Visual auras are encountered in focal seizures arising from the posterior temporal or occipital regions and can be elementary or more complex.

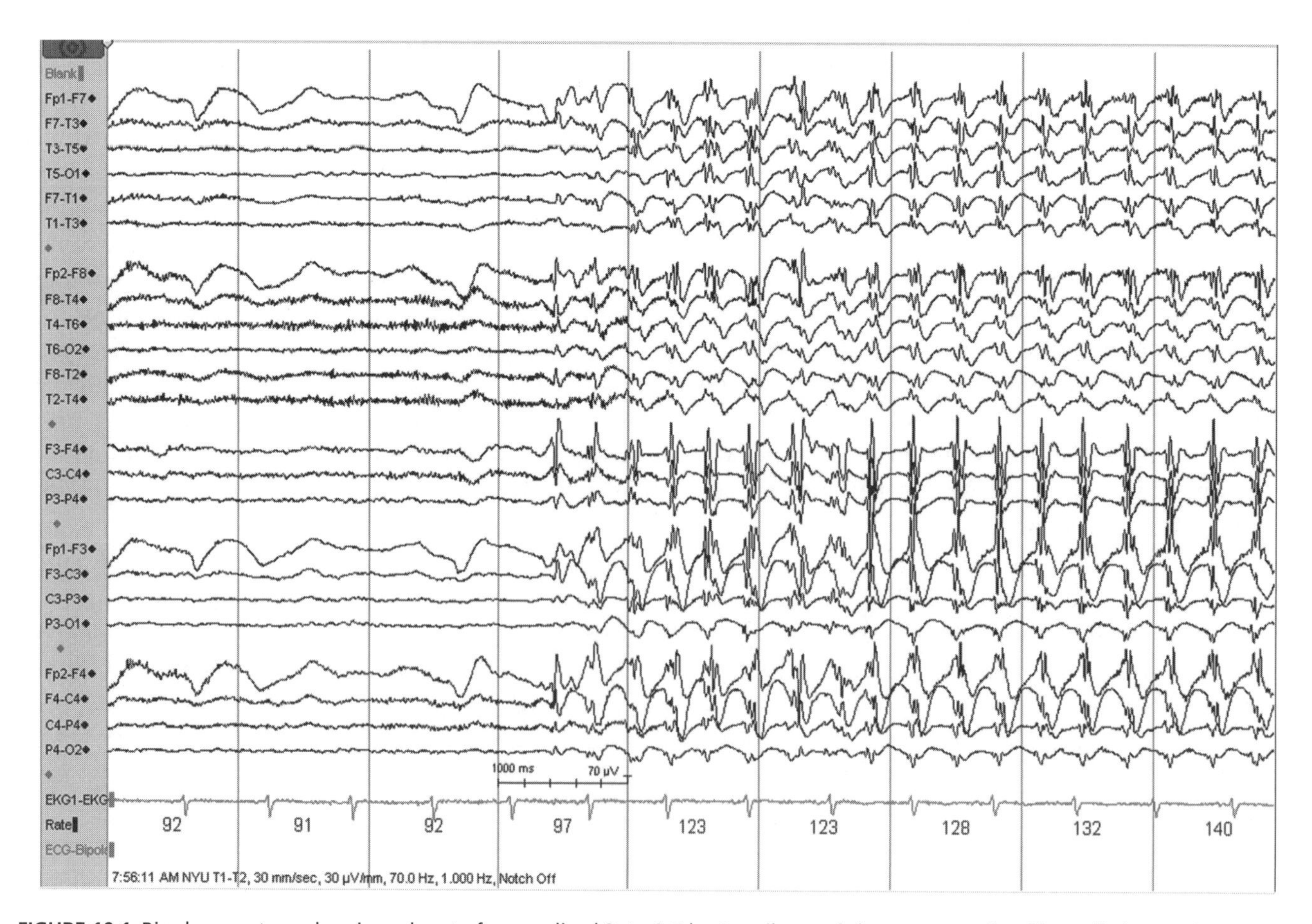

FIGURE 10.1 Bipolar montage showing a burst of generalized 3- to 3.5-hertz spikes and slow waves epileptiform discharges in a patient during a brief absence seizure.

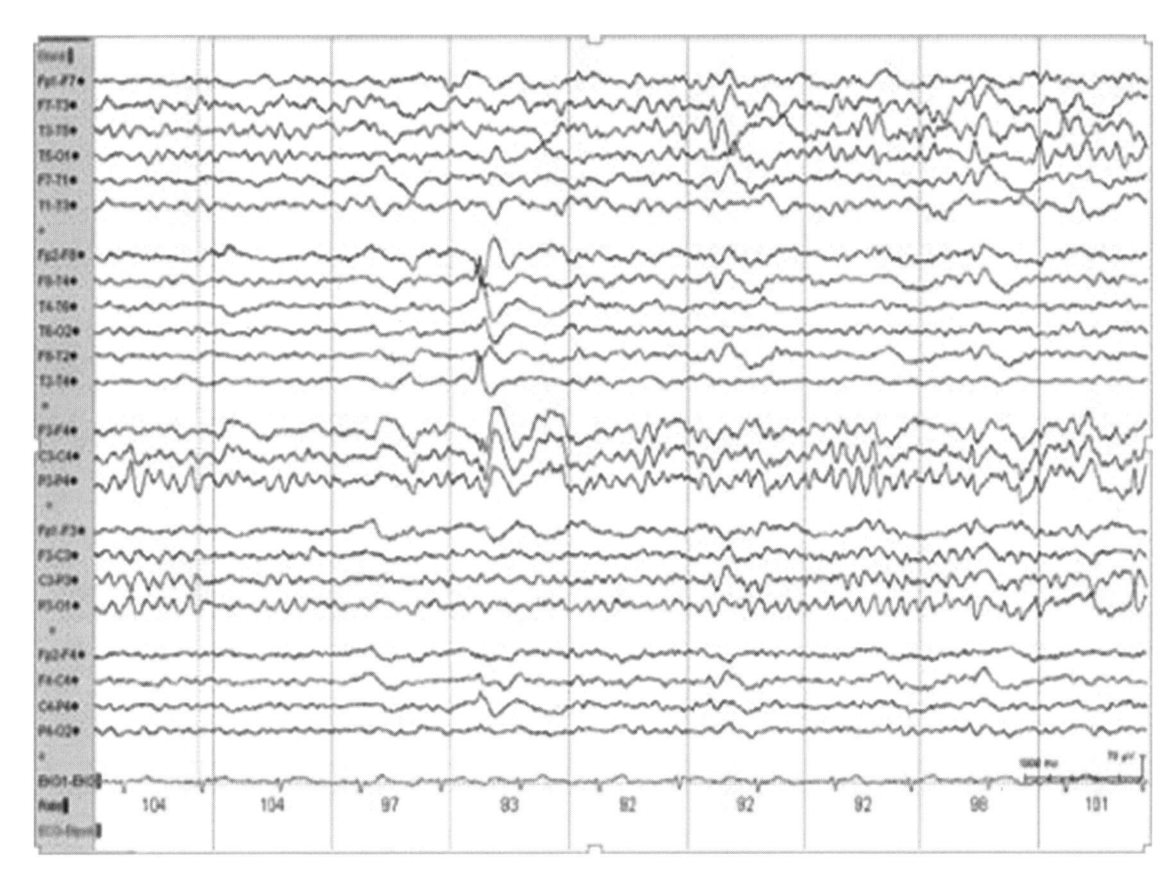

FIGURE 10.2 Bipolar montage EEG tracing showing right focal epileptiform discharge in a patient with right temporal lobe epilepsy. Note that right hemispheric leads are represented in even numbers (e.g., FP2, F4, F8, T4, P4, O2) and left hemispheric leads as odd numbers (e.g., FP1, F3, F7, T3, P3, O1) conventionally.

The common etiopathogenesis associated with epilepsy include:

- **Mesial temporal sclerosis** (MTS; Figure 10.4a)
- **Congenital:** neuronal migrational disorders such as focal cortical dysplasia, periventricular nodular heterotopia (PVH), subcortical heterotopia (SBH), lissencephaly (smooth brain with lack of gyri), pachygyria (thickened and cobblestone cortex), polymicrogyria, hemimegalencephaly (unilateral diffuse hypertrophy of one cerebral hemisphere), schizencephaly
- **Low-grade tumors**: gangliogliomas, dysembryoplastic neuroepithelial tumors (DNETs), hypothalamic hamartomas
- **High-grade tumors:** anaplastic astrocytomas, glioblastoma multiforme (GBM)
- **Vascular**: stroke (ischemic or hemorrhagic; Figures 10.4c and d)
- **Neurocutaneous syndromes:** tuberous sclerosis, neurofibromatosis Type 1 and 2, Sturge–Weber syndrome
- **Infectious:** bacterial, fungal, parasitic (neurocysticercosis), meningitis and encephalitis, TORCH infections (toxoplasmosis, other [syphilis, varicella-zoster, parvovirus B19], rubella, cytomegalovirus [CMV], and herpes infections)
- **Inflammation/autoimmune:** lupus (8% of patients); other autoimmune disease (Sjögren's and Hashimoto's encephalopathy), multiple sclerosis (approximately 5%–10%), neurosarcoidosis, limbic encephalitis, Morvan's syndrome, paraneoplastic syndromes, acute disseminated encephalomyelitis (ADEM)
- **Vascular malformations:** cavernomas (Figure 10.4b), arteriovenous malformations (AVMs)
- **Trauma:** subdural, epidural, intraparenchymal, subarachnoid
- **Degenerative:** progressive myoclonic epilepsies, Alzheimer's disease, frontotemporal dementia, neuronal ceroid lipofuscinosis (dementia, ataxia, seizures—myoclonic and convulsions and blindness); Rett syndrome

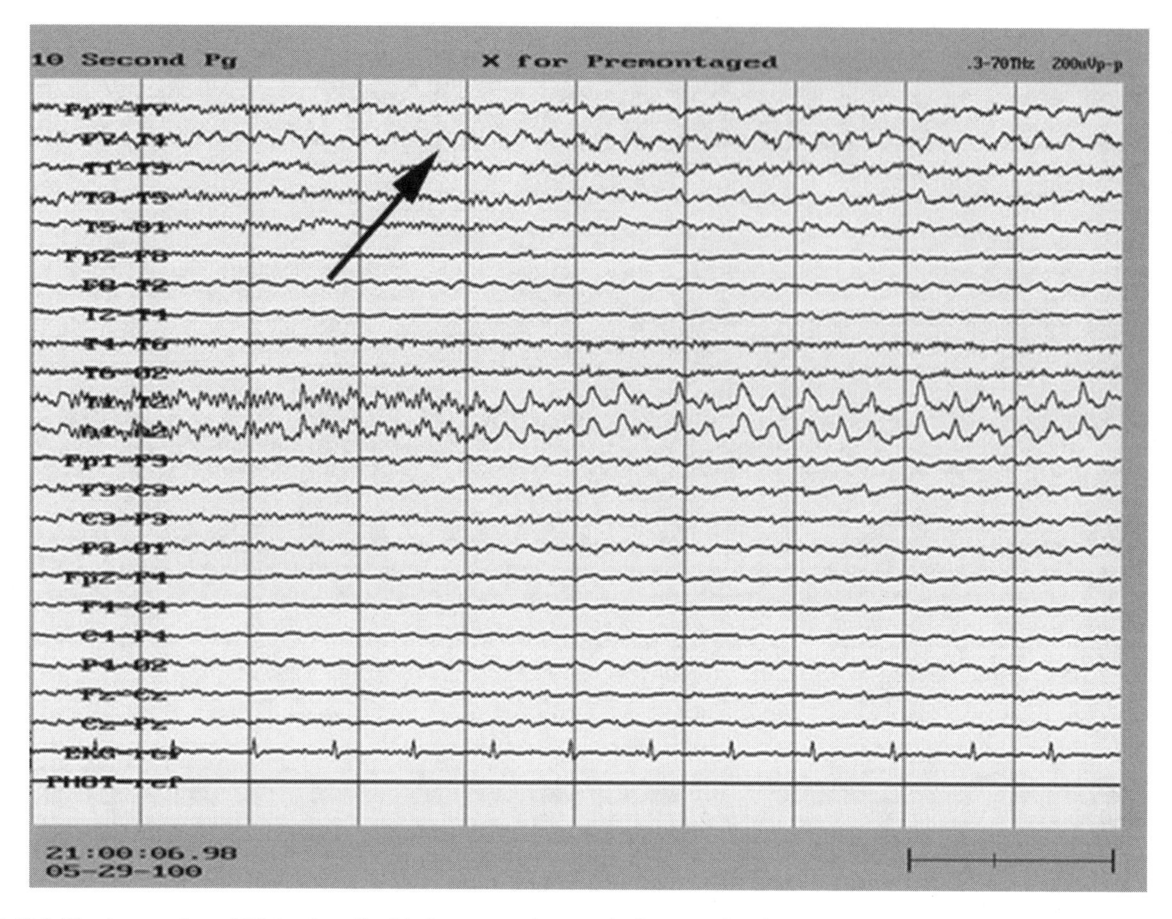

FIGURE 10.3 Bipolar montage EEG tracing; the black arrow points to the low amplitude 3- to 4-hertz rhythmic ictal activity during a temporal lobe seizure.

- **Chromosomal abnormalities:** Angelman syndrome, Prader–Willi syndrome
- **Hypoxic–ischemic insults:** birth injuries, cardiopulmonary arrest
- **Hypertensive encephalopathies:** posterior reversible encephalopathy syndrome (PRES)
- **Toxic:** ethanol, ephedrine, brupropion, amitryptiline, chemotherapeutic agents, tramadol, cefepime, tacrolimus, imipenem, metronidazole, penicillin, lithium
- **Endocrine disorders:** hyperthyroidism
- **Psychiatric disorders:** nonepileptic seizures (NESs)

Common provoking factors for seizures are sleep deprivation, alcohol withdrawal, stress, nonadherence to medication, different phases of menstruation in female patients, and photic stimulation. Provoked seizures do not require administration of antiseizure medications. Acute symptomatic seizures, for example, seizures arising from acute head trauma, acute stroke, or acute infection/inflammation of the brain, may only need a short course of treatment, although long-term administration of antiseizure medications may be necessary if there is residual epilepsy. In general, focal epilepsy is more resistant to medical treatment than generalized epilepsy. Medically refractory epilepsy (MRE) is defined as a failure of adequate trials of two tolerated and appropriately chosen and used antiepileptic drug (AED) schedules (whether as monotherapies or in combination) to achieve sustained seizure freedom. It is important to note that no specific seizure frequency is necessary to meet the definition. Thus, an individual with one seizure per year can be regarded as treatment resistant.

Forty-seven percent of the patients respond to the first antiepileptic medication tried and 13% are seizure-free on the second, but only 1% respond to the third monotherapy choice. About 32% of focal epilepsy patients continue to be medically intractable (Brodie & Kwan, 2002). The best prognosis for seizure control is response to the first anticonvulsant. The risk factors for continued intractability include frequent multiple seizures, simple partial seizures, autism, cognitive impairment,

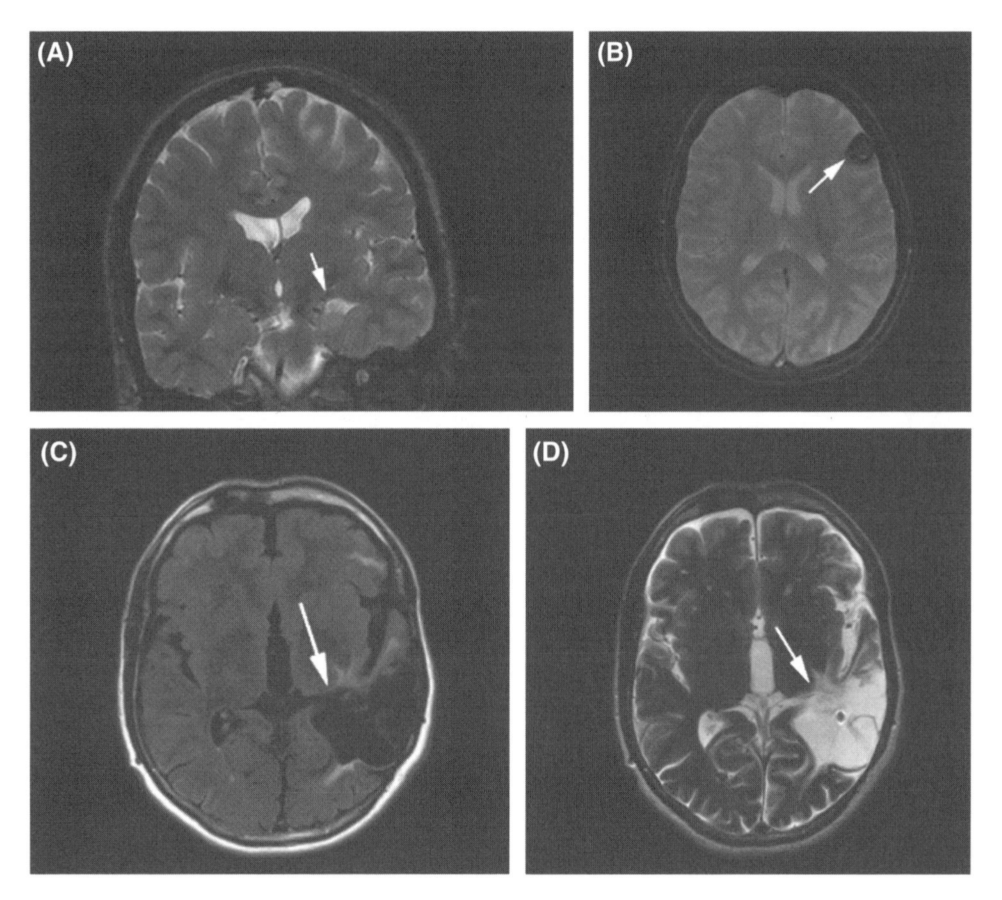

FIGURE 10.4 Some pathologies that can cause epilepsy. MRI brain T2-weighted coronal images showing left hippocampal atrophy and dilatation of the left temporal horn of the lateral ventricle **(A)**. MRI axial images of the brain HemoFLASH sequence showing left frontal cavernoma **(B)**. MRI brain axial fluid attenuated inversion recovery (FLAIR) image **(C)** and T2-weighted image **(D)** show an old hemorrhagic stroke in the left temporoparietal region; patient had medically refractory seizures.

history of status epilepticus, symptomatic lesional epilepsy, and onset of epilepsy less than 2 years of age or more than 12 years of age. Surgical resection of epileptogenic zone in patients with MTS, malformations of cortical development, low-grade gliomas (ganglioglioma, dysembryoplastic neuroepithelial tumor, neurocytoma, etc.), cavernoma, or encephalomalacia have proved to reduce the seizure burden in patients with MRE.

Mortality in epilepsy is two to three times greater than in the general population. Polytherapy, frequent seizures (especially nocturnal and tonic–clonic seizures), female sex, frequent changes in AEDs, lack of supervision, and symptomatic epilepsy (epilepsy related to developmental syndromes) confer higher risks of sudden unexplained death in epilepsy (SUDEP). SUDEP is fortunately uncommon but does exist and is defined as sudden, unexpected, witnessed or unwitnessed, nontraumatic and nondrowning death in epilepsy, excluding status epilepticus (Annegers & Coan, 1999). Autopsy should not show any anatomical or toxicological cause for death.

Seizures have significant economic impact on our health care system related to missed days from work, loss of job opportunities, or even total dependence on caretakers. Some patients with severe childhood epileptic encephalopathies (static or neurodegenerative), cerebral palsy, or postencephalitis or posttraumatic epilepsy have to be institutionalized. It is not uncommon for their caregivers to give up their careers to take care of people with epilepsy. Patients should be screened for any coexisting depression, anxiety, or memory problems and should be counseled about driving restrictions, safety and injury prevention, diagnosis, treatment options, and other lifestyle factors that may affect seizure control (e.g., sleep deprivation, alcohol/drug use). Women of child bearing age with epilepsy should be counseled about the teratogenic effects of antiepileptic drugs and the role of folic acid supplementation.

Nonepileptic events (psychogenic or nonpsychogenic) show profound delays in diagnosis despite the emergence of growing epilepsy centers nationwide. Patients with NESs can often have coexisting epileptic seizures. About 41% of patients with NESs continue to remain on at least one or multiple medications (Reuber et al., 2003). This demonstrates hesitancy on the part of physicians to wean off all antiseizure medications despite the diagnosis.

DIAGNOSTIC TESTS

Neurological consultation includes a history and a physical examination and routine labs (complete blood count, basic metabolic panel, liver function test, magnesium, phosphorus). Further diagnostic workup includes routine EEG and MRI. Initial imaging includes an MRI brain with epilepsy protocol, which includes volumetric T1-weighted sequence, proton density, gradient echo sequences, T2-weighted sequences, and fluid attenuated inversion recovery (FLAIR) sequences in oblique coronal and axial images. Various imaging modalities such as MRI, functional MRI (f-MRI), PET, single-photon emission computed tomography (SPECT), magnetoencephalography (MEG), and diffusion tensor imaging (DTI) are used for presurgical evaluation.

The awake and sleep EEGs are screened for epileptiform discharges, which is a sign of cortical hyperexcitability. A normal EEG does not support or refute the diagnosis of epilepsy. A sleep-deprived EEG increases the yield of finding abnormalities on the EEG, and signs of cortical hyperexcitability are more frequent during drowsiness. Neuroimaging cannot confirm a diagnosis of epilepsy; rather, its purpose is to find the cause. MRI of the brain is generally superior to CT, also known as a CAT scan, because it is better able to detect small lesions such as MTS or cortical dysplasias. Single-photon emission CT and positive emission tomography (PET) are not used in the initial evaluation of seizures and are only used when patients are evaluated for possible neurosurgical treatment for uncontrolled epilepsy.

Since the early 1990s, many new antiepileptic medications (gabapentin, oxcarbazepine, felbamate, lamotrigine, tiagabine, topiramate, levetiracetam, pregabalin, lacosamide, rufinamide, eslicarbazepine, and perampanel) have been approved by the U.S. Food and Drug Administration (FDA; Table 10.2). The so-called third generation of antiseizure medications, such as eslicarbazepine, are not necessarily more effective but are better tolerated than older versions such as carbamazepine and oxcarbazepine.

TABLE 10.2

FIRST- AND SECOND-GENERATION ANTIEPILEPTIC DRUGS	
First Generation	**Second Generation**
phenobarbital (Luminal)	gabapentin (Neurontin)
phenytoin (Dilantin)	levetiracetam (Keppra)
ethosuximide (Zarontin)	lamotrigine (Lamictal)
primidone (Mysoline)	oxcarbazepine (Trileptal)
carbamazepine (Tegretol)	tiagabine (Gabitril)
valproate (Depakote)	topiramate (Topamax)
methsuximide (Celontin)	felbamate (Felbatol)
	lacosamide (Vimpat)
	vigabatrin (Sabril)
	rufinamide (Banzel)
	eslicarbazepine (Aptiom)
	perampanel (Fycompa)

Functional hemispherectomies are indicated in conditions such as Rasmussen's encephalitis, porencephalic or large hemispheric infarcts, and hemimegalencephaly. Corpus callosotomy, severing of the connection between the two sides of the brain, is done in patients with drop attacks and patients with frequent partial seizures with secondary generalization. Incomplete or almost complete corpus callosotomy prevents secondary generalization, decreasing the morbidity and mortality associated with primarily or secondarily generalized seizures (Table 10.3).

The ketogenic diet (KD) is another option for children who have MRE, as a recent meta-analysis indicated greater than 50% seizure reduction for 60% of the children treated (Henderson, Filloux, Alder, Lyon, & Caplin, 2006). Table 10.4 enlists various options from a stringent diet (classical KD) to more plausible options.

Vagus nerve stimulation (VNS) was approved by the FDA in 1997 and more than 100,000

TABLE 10.3

TYPES OF CORPUS CALLOSOTOMY		
% Corpus Callosotomy	**Rationale**	**Adverse Effects**
Anterior two thirds to four fifths	Spares splenium of the corpus callosum, which relays visual information	Disconnection syndrome, alien hand syndrome
Total (90%)	Further reduction of epileptic spread	Disconnection syndrome, alien hand syndrome, language impairment, memory loss

devices have been implanted. In VNS, a pacemakerlike device is implanted in the chest with leads, which the surgeon wraps around the left vagus nerve. Because vagal innervation of the sinoatrial node is preferentially from the right vagus, the left vagus is used to avoid any cardiac consequences. It is FDA approved for refractory focal epilepsy but is often used for refractory generalized epilepsy as well. The device is typically set to stimulate every few minutes but may be triggered by the patient by waving a magnet over the stimulator if a seizure is felt to be imminent. The precise antiepileptic mechanism of VNS is not known, but it is thought to work via multiple pathways, including neurotransmitter modulation, changes in cerebral blood flow, and suppression of interictal epileptiform discharges. The vagus nerve synapses bilaterally on the nucleus of the solitary tract (NTS), which projects to brainstem nuclei (the dorsal raphe magnus and locus coeruleus) that modulate norepinephrine and serotonin diffusely in the brain. The NTS has widespread connections to limbic, reticular, and autonomic cerebral structures.

Responsive neurostimulation (RNS): Whereas VNS stimulation is delivered chronically, regardless of whether a seizure is occurring or not, in RNS, stimulation is delivered only if brain rhythms indicate that a seizure is underway or imminent. To do this, EEG leads and a small computer that which monitor the intracranial EEG continuously are implanted intracranially. The patient is able to upload the recordings to an external computer for inspection by an epileptologist. The epileptologist will choose settings on the stimulator that determine what EEG patterns should trigger stimulation. RNS is also FDA approved for refractory partial epilepsy. Studies to date show that its efficacy is comparable to that of VNS (Bergey et al., 2015).

TABLE 10.4

VARIOUS DIETARY OPTIONS FOR PERSONS WITH EPILEPSY				
Diet Type	**Ratios**	**What Is Restricted**	**Starting the Diet**	**Adverse Effects and Downfalls***
Classic ketogenic diet	Fat-to-protein ratio 3:1 or 4:1	Calories/protein	Inpatient monitoring of glucose/ketones and family teaching	Hyperlipidemia, kidney stones, poor growth, osteopenia, requires blood monitoring
Modified Atkins Diet (MAD)	10–15 g/day carbs; 20 g/day in older patients	Carbohydrates	Outpatient	Some need to advance to classic KD for better seizure control
Medium-chain triglyceride (MCT) diet	MCT substituted for long-chain triglycerides used in classic KD	Calories/protein	Outpatient, start slow to decrease gastrointestinal upset	Gastrointestinal upset
Low glycemic index treatment (LGIT)	40–60 g/day	Carbohydrates, specifically glycemic index of carbs <50	Outpatient	Does not produce ketone bodies

*Similar side effects for all diets, but decreased in MAD/LGIT/MCT.

Deep brain stimulation (DBS) is used for many complaints, including symptoms of Parkinson's, essential tremor, obsessive-compulsive disorders, depression, and Tourette's syndrome. Unlike RNS, in DBS, the same area of the brain is stimulated for a specific indication. Like in VNS, a stimulator is implanted in the chest; unlike VNS, the stimulation is done intracranially via electrodes implanted through the skull and targeted to deep structures. For epilepsy, the main target in current practice is the anterior nucleus of the thalamus (ANT). The ANT is an important component of the limbic system and has been shown to be involved in many kinds of epilepsy. The Stimulation of the Anterior Nucleus of Thalamus for Epilepsy (SANTE) trial published in 2010 demonstrated the efficacy of ANT stimulation for seizure reduction (Fisher et al., 2010). Table 10.5 lists the advantages and disadvantages of various neurostimulation devices and Table 10.6 compares the existing neurostimulation devices.

Neuropsychological Assessment

Brain injury and epilepsy have an intimate and complex connection. Only 4% of epilepsy overall is attributed to trauma (Annegers, 2001). However, approximately 40% of those applying to the University of Washington's Regional Epilepsy Center Vocational Services indicated on their program application form that they had had a head injury. This discrepancy is likely related to the severity of epilepsy after traumatic brain injury (TBI), the cognitive effects of the initial trauma itself, and the increased risk of trauma and repeat injury in those with generalized seizures. In 582 falls admitted at the University of British Columbia, 90.9% of those due to seizures had intracranial hematomas, whereas the rate of hematomas was only 39.8% of those due to other causes (Zwimpfer, Brown, Sullivan, & Moulton, 1997).

Research has shown significantly decreased cognitive performance in individuals with many generalized tonic–clonic seizures or prolonged seizures characterized as status epilepticus (Dodrill, 1986). Although all seizures have the potential to affect cognition, the very changes in the brain that lead to epilepsy may induce measurable impairment. One study found a rate of attentional, executive, or memory deficits of 75% in patients with newly diagnosed epilepsy (Witt & Helmstaedter, 2012).

Seizures can be associated with many regions of the brain involved in a wide variety of cognitive tasks. Similarly, diffuse spreading of ictal activity in generalized seizures can affect many different cognitive systems. Research by Hermann, Filloux, Alder, Lyon, and Caplin (2006), Hermann et al. (2008), Oyegbile et al. (2004), and Rausch, Le, and Langfitt (1997) indicates that common cognitive concerns for individuals with epilepsy include attention, speed of mental processing, memory, learning, executive function, and cognitive

TABLE 10.5

ADVANTAGES AND DISADVANTAGES OF NEUROSTIMULATION	
Advantages	**Disadvantages**
No allergies (rash), no systemic side effects	Expensive
No drug-to-drug interactions	Infection 1.7% with VNS 5% with DBS
No cognitive side effects	Recurrent laryngeal nerve injury or vocal cord paralysis (rare)
Different mechanism of action from antiseizure medications	Requires general anesthesia
Reversible	More follow-up MD appointments needed to set parameters
Sense of control (magnet empowerment)	Intracerebral hemorrhage (5%–7% risk with DBS)
Improved quality of life	

DBS, deep brain stimulation; VNS, vagus nerve stimulation.

TABLE 10.6

COMPARISON OF NEUROSTIMULATION DEVICES			
	VNS	**DBS**	**RNS**
Target	Left vagus	Bilateral: anterior nucleus of thalamus	Specific epileptogenic zone
Type	Scheduled Intermittent	Scheduled Intermittent	As needed
Surgery	Minimally invasive	Invasive	Invasive
Stimulation	Bipolar, biphasic peripheral	Bipolar or unipolar Biphasic direct brain stimulation	Highly variable direct brain stimulation
Sensing	N/A	N/A	Multiple detection methods
Programming	Transcutaneous	Transcutaneous	Transcutaneous

DBS, deep brain stimulation; RNS, responsive neurostimulation; VNS, vagus nerve stimulation.

flexibility. Neuropsychological testing, that is, detailed evaluation of multiple domains of cognitive function by a psychologist specifically trained in this procedure, can help elucidate specific deficits in these varied domains.

Commonly used neuropsychological batteries include the Halstead–Reitan Neuropsychological Battery (Reitan & Wolfson, 1985) and the Luria-Nebraska Neuropsychological Battery (Goldin, Hammeke, & Parisch, 1980). Dodrill (1978) has established a comprehensive battery of 16 discriminative measures more sensitive to brain impairment and epilepsy. This battery includes Halstead's Neuropsychological Battery for Adults, the Aphasia Screening Test, the Trail Making Test, the Logical Memory and Visual Reproduction parts of the Wechsler Memory Scale-Form I, the Sensory-Perceptual Examination, the Stroop Test, and the Seashore Tonal Memory Test. In recent years, other neuropsychological batteries have been adapted incorporating some of the original with newer instruments to include measures of "malingering." Neuropsychological testing is important both before and after surgery for epilepsy, particularly to assess the surgical impact on memory and language functioning. The testing can also be helpful in clarifying epileptic foci.

It is important to emphasize that among studies conducted at the University of Washington (Fraser, Clemmons, Dodrill, Trejo, & Freelove, 1986) with clients actively engaged in vocational rehabilitation services, aspects of cognitive impairment consistently discriminated between those who were able to go to work and maintain a job for 1 year and those who could not secure a job through our program (i.e., they tried to secure work through the program but were unsuccessful). Specific predictive impairments were visual/spatial problem-solving and motor deficits. Most of these clients had job experience that was characterized as unskilled or semiskilled work, and the brain impairments were affecting their employability. Clients with cognitive impairments affecting job stability typically require longer training or coached work experience to secure and maintain competitive job placement. They also benefit from learning compensatory strategies to cope with their difficulties. For clients with a long history of generalized tonic–clonic seizures, neuropsychological test results can be facilitative relative to rehabilitation planning.

Psychosocial Assessment

Epilepsy is strongly associated with a variety of psychiatric problems and diagnoses. There are many causes of this, some of which are still being elucidated. What is known is that rates of depression and anxiety in particular are much higher in persons with epilepsy than the general public. The rates of a major depressive episode (by the *Diagnostic and Statistical Manual of Mental Disorders* criteria) in people with epilepsy is approximately 30% (Hermann, Seidenberg, & Bell, 2000) compared to the estimated 16% in the general population

(Johnson et al., 2004; Kessler et al., 2003). This increases to 50% in those with refractory or uncontrolled epilepsy (Gilliam & Kanner, 2002). Anxiety is less well studied; however, clinically significant disorders of anxiety have been measured at a point prevalence of 11% versus 5.6% in the general populace (Gaitatzis, Carroll, Majeed, & Sander, 2004). Psychosis, usually around the time of seizures (also known as peri-ictal psychosis) is a particular entity discussed elsewhere but affects approximately 7% of persons with epilepsy (Adams et al., 2008). Of particular concern, people with epilepsy are at a 25-fold higher risk of completing suicide than others (Gaitatzis, Trimble, & Sander, 2004). An increase in suicide is maintained even when controlled for identified psychiatric disorders (Kwon et al., 2011).

There are many factors leading to the association between psychiatric diagnoses and epilepsy. These include, but are not limited to, the stress of living with a potentially disabling and highly unpredictable illness, social stigma of this diagnosis, medication effects, surgical morbidity, and direct neurobiological effects of seizures. Furthermore, there is some evidence that the underlying biochemical nature of the brains of people with epilepsy can lead to some of these diagnoses. Higher rates of depression, anxiety, bipolar disorder, psychosis, and suicide attempts have been found even prior to the onset of the first seizure (Adelöw, Andersson, & Tomson, 2012; Hesdorffer et al., 2012). The contributing factors are discussed individually in the following. Identification of the activity of each of these factors in individuals with epilepsy and psychosocial maladjustment or complaints can provide multiple inroads for treatment and support.

The same measures used in the clinical environments for the quantification of psychosocial function may be utilized in clients with epilepsy. These measures include the Minnesota Multiphasic Personality Inventory-2 (MMPI-2), the Personality Assessment Inventory (PAI), the Millon Clinical Multiaxial Inventory III, the Beck Depression Inventory-II, the Symptom Checklist-90-Revised, computerized psychiatric diagnostic interviews (Diagnostic Interview Schedule), and structured clinical interviews (the Mini-International Neuropsychiatric Interview, Structured Clinical Interview for *DSM-5* [SCID-5]).

A psychosocial assessment tool specifically for clients with epilepsy was developed in 1980 by the name of the Washington Psychosocial Seizure Inventory (WPSI). This inventory, developed by Dodrill, Batzel, Queisser, and Temkin, is still in wide use and has been well characterized and demonstrated to identify specific areas of concern to the client (Chang & Gehlert, 2003). This empirically derived measure has 132 items, which clients can typically complete in approximately 20 to 30 minutes. Other quality-of-life instruments have also been developed more recently (e.g., Liverpool Quality of Life Battery, Quality of Life in Epilepsy Inventory [QOLIE]-89 item, QOLIE-31 item). The QOLIE-89 is used particularly widely across neurological illnesses and takes into account a variety of functional measures, thereby discerning the effects of many of the difficulties discussed earlier facing clients with epilepsy. Recently, a brief, 25-item patient report instrument was developed, the Personal Impact of Epilepsy Scale (PIES), which correlated well with the QOLIE-31 and other seizure impact inventories (Fisher, Nune, Roberts, & Cramer, 2015).

PSYCHOLOGICAL AND VOCATIONAL IMPLICATIONS

Incidence of Psychosocial Maladjustment

An early review of WPSI findings showed that 50% of the respondents had moderate to severe psychosocial maladjustment in the majority of measured scales (Trostle, 1988). The same group found a rate of severe maladjustment of 50% to 60% in those sent for evaluation at a special epilepsy center, in comparison with only 19% in a general sample (Trostle, Hauser, & Sharbrough, 1986), indicating a higher rate of maladjustment in those requiring a higher level of specialized care. For those clients in whom a high level of maladjustment is indicated by one of the inventories mentioned in the preceding discussion, a referral for more comprehensive psychological or neuropsychiatric evaluation would be indicated

Factors Influencing Psychosocial Adjustment

Given the wide range of factors affecting psychosocial function in people with epilepsy, a cognitive framework is helpful to approach these patients. One may organize these effects into neurological, treatment related, psychosocial (or modifiable), and demographic (or not modifiable). These factors were explored by Fraser and Clemmons (1989).

In the neurological category, items such as early age of onset, additional disabilities, associated neuropsychological impairment, and type of seizure activity have been found to be important variables. Those with generalized seizures reported a greater level of limitations in social activities and associated hopelessness (Pompili et al., 2014). Refractory (drug-resistant) seizures significantly lowered QOLIE, as did elevated overall seizure frequency (Elsharkawy, Thorbecke, Ebner, & May, 2012).

AEDs have a variety of side effects, which can directly and indirectly affect psychological states both positively and negatively. For example, levetiracetam (Keppra) is known to cause irritability and valproate (Depakote) can cause depression, whereas lamotrigine (Lamictal) has mood-stabilizing and elevating properties. Many are associated with sedation and weight gain and can require frequent monitoring. Surgery for epilepsy has become an increasingly widely used option for people with refractory epilepsy and has been demonstrated to have an overall positive effect on QOLIE in these patients (Elsharkawy et al., 2012), although persistent deficits in neurological or cognitive function from surgery can be disabling.

Under the psychosocial category, a number of variables are identified, including perceived stigma and limitations, adjustment to seizures, vocational status, financial status, parental fears, limited socialization and recreation, divisive or dysfunctional parenting styles, and poor relationships with parents, siblings, and intrusive grandparents. Other more immediate issues, such as considerable life event changes, availability of social support, and perceived locus of control or self-efficacy, seem to affect adjustment (Bautista, Shapovalov, & Shoraka, 2015).

Basic demographic issues such as age, sex, education, and intelligence can be important. Age seems to positively correlate with adaptation to seizures, whereas younger clients can be more unsettled or find their lives more disrupted by a new, severe illness. Young men tend to have the most difficulty adjusting (Fraser, Trejo, Temkin, Clemmons, & Dodrill, 1985). There was no significant association of race with WPSI ratings in people with epilepsy (Gehlert, Difrancesco, & Chang, 2000).

Vocational Implications

In discussing vocational evaluation and planning, many issues arise. These may be thought of in relationship to the seizure condition itself, associated disabilities, medication concerns, and seizure disclosure. These categories are discussed in the following text.

■ Clarification of Seizure Status

First and foremost, it is important to clarify the current status of the patient's seizures and the level of control. If further neurological evaluation is required, a client may be directed to a clinical center (a directory of these may be found via the National Epilepsy Foundation; www.epilepsyfoundation.org) so that more sophisticated assessment and/or 24-hour EEG-video monitoring can be conducted. NESs are events mimicking seizure activity that may be either organic or psychological in origin. Organic causes include other forms of loss of consciousness (or syncope) or other medical problems causing alterations of awareness or movement. Psychogenic nonepileptic seizures (PNESs; previously known as pseudoseizures or hysterical seizures) may arise from a variety of psychological mechanisms. However, these are generally unconsciously produced though a mechanism more generally known as a conversion disorder. Although they are not related to measurable, pathologic discharges in the brain, they do primarily occur in people with a coexisting, verified seizure disorder, making advanced and specialized care even more vital.

Epileptic seizures generally fall into generalized or partial seizure, depending on whether the whole brain or only part of the brain is involved. Partial seizures may generalize to the whole brain (secondary generalization), where loss of consciousness is inevitable. Seizures that remain partial may impair consciousness in which case they are known as "focal seizures with impairment of consciousness or awareness," or they may not, in which case they are described as "focal seizures without impairment of consciousness or awareness." In order to clarify the status of this incredibly varied diagnosis, some of the following points should be answered.

1. The specific type of seizure the client currently has, with a clear description of what occurs during a seizure. Of particular importance is establishing whether there is a loss of consciousness.
2. What type of seizure control has the client achieved? If the seizures are not controlled, it is important to understand whether there is any pattern to their occurrence. Seizures may follow a daily or, in women, a menstrual, cycle. Factors such as alcohol or drug use/withdrawal, lack of sleep, illness (particularly fever), missed medication doses, and flashing lights may bring on seizures. Other, less common exacerbations do exist rarely and can be idiosyncratic.
3. Does the client have a specific warning or aura (actually the initial part of the seizure) before the occurrence of a full seizure? A warning can be a feeling of lightheadedness, a rising sensation in the abdomen, other strange sensations, or déjà vu experiences. A consistent aura is helpful in that it allows an individual to take safety precautions (e.g., sitting down, lying down, or otherwise removing oneself to a safe area before the seizure is in full progress).
4. What is involved in the recovery period? Some individuals can go directly back to work, others will require a brief nap, and, often with generalized seizures, a whole day may be required to return to function and work.
5. Has the client ever been otherwise injured as a result of a seizure? A lack of injury may be reassuring to employers.
6. Does the client have any other disabilities? One study at a tertiary care facility (Fraser, Clemmons, Andrechak, Dodrill, & Temkin, 1991) showed that 89% of the clients served had one or more additional disabilities. It is particularly important to note whether there has been an additional head injury that precipitated the seizures or whether a head injury came about as a result of seizure activity. Other disabilities or medical concerns will require specific assessment.
7. What type of medication is the client taking, is it appropriate, and is he or she complying with the recommended medication and dosages? Is the neurological follow-up recent? If there have been recent changes in the seizure frequency, does the client require reassessment for medications or even surgery?

Answering these questions can aid in appropriate placement. If a client has minimized or miscommunicated symptoms, he or she may be placed in a work situation where problems such as quick loss of consciousness may lead to injury. However, if seizures are more controlled, or if a reliable aura can alert to any danger, certain types of physical work may be safer than otherwise assumed. It is important to remember that many types of seizures impair awareness and the clients may not themselves be able to recall or describe what happens during a seizure. A report (Bryant-Comstock, Hogan, Shumaker, & Tennis, 1997) indicates that a client's own perception of seizure severity, using the Liverpool Seizure Severity Scale, may be a better discriminator of employability than other seizure variables (e.g., seizure frequency).

■ Additional Disabilities

As discussed, a majority of clients with epilepsy coming for vocational rehabilitation services will have additional disability or concerns. Most commonly, cognitive or psychological impairment will require clarification. Vocational rehabilitation staff should be alert to factors that may have caused seizures, including head injury or other neurological assaults, as well as the myriad of effects of seizures as described in the preceding text. All these may lead to specific problems, such as memory deficits or spatial reasoning difficulty, which may point away from specific job placements. However, compensatory mechanisms may be available depending on the specific demands of the job. Awareness of the clients' specific needs will help improve their comfort with the rehabilitation program and their likelihood of success. Again, review of any available neuropsychological assessments will be of vital aid in this process.

Appropriate psychological support is similarly vital to the client's success. The path back to job success and independence is fraught with challenges. Unidentified or undertreated anxiety and depression will hamper this process. Although the rehabilitation staff must be specifically sensitive to cognitive and emotional concerns, other injuries or disabilities may be present and should also be addressed.

Medication Issues

The area of medication management deserves significant attention. There are several medications used in the management of seizures and unfortunately many have unpredictable or severe side effects. It is of utmost importance that the client's medical providers are aware of these effects and that their regimen is tailored to that client's specific needs. Medications such as Phenytoin, Phenobarbital, or Topiramate (Topamax), often causes mild cognitive clouding. This is generally not troubling in day-to-day life; however, it can be a significant problem for someone who needs to work with numbers or is involved in tasks taxing working memory. Where this may have been an appropriate medication before job placement, another medication may need to be used thereafter.

Other medications, such as lamotrigine (Lamictal), may actually help with concentration and depression. Valproic acid (Depakote) can cause weight gain and sedation, but can also decrease impulsivity and stabilize moods. It is the job of the treating physician to know the specific benefits and risks of each medication. Often, collaboration between a patient's neurologist and psychiatrist can help lead to the optimal regimen, given the overlap in medications used by both professions. An awareness of the common effects of AEDs on the part of the vocational rehabilitation staff can, however, help to identify needs for medication adjustment. A chart of commonly used medications and their effects is provided in Table 10.7. It is important to note that these side effects are not universal and often improve or remit over time.

These medications can be complicated and can require a long period of consistent use to both stabilize the amount of medication in the blood and have their beneficial effect on seizure prevention. Some medications such as lamotrigine require long, slow titrations to achieve a therapeutic dose.

TABLE 10.7

MEDICAL AND NEUROPSYCHOLOGICAL EFFECTS OF ANTIEPILEPTIC MEDICATIONS

Generic Name	Brand Name	General Side Effects	Neurological/Psychological Side Effects	Possible Benefits
Carbamazepine	Tegretol	Nausea, drug–drug interactions, electrolyte abnormalities	Drowsiness (mild), double vision	Mood stabilization
Felbamate	Felbatol	Nausea, weight loss	Insomnia, imbalance	Arousal, weight loss
Gabapentin	Neurontin	Infrequent	Drowsiness (moderate)	Decreased anxiety. Can treat insomnia
Lamotrigine	Lamictal	Rash (can be severe)	Infrequent	Treats depression and can be stabilizing and improve cognition
Levetiracetam	Keppra	Infrequent	Irritability, rarely depression	
Phenobarbital	Luminal	Drug–drug interactions	Sedation, dependence, imbalance	
Phenytoin	Dilantin	Thickened gums, drug–drug interactions	Imbalance, double vision	
Topiramate	Topamax	Weight loss, sensory complaints	Cognitive "clouding," depression	Weight loss
Valproic acid	Depakote	Weight gain, nausea, hair loss	Tremor, drowsiness (moderate)	Mood stabilization, improved impulse control, stimulates appetite

Sudden cessation of medications can actually bring on seizures through withdrawal. Inconsistent usage of medications can therefore be dangerous through a variety of medications. When switching medications, the second medication is often introduced slowly in order to avoid side effects, and the first is then slowly removed to ensure continued seizure control. It is therefore not uncommon that clients with inconsistent medical follow-up can end up taking more medications than any one provider had intended. It is therefore important to encourage consistent medication usage through reminders and medication boxes, as well as good follow-up with the provider.

Disclosure of Seizure Status

Disclosure of a seizure condition is a very individual decision. For most people, we recommend that seizures be clearly discussed if they could affect work performance, preferably at the end of the interview, after they have had the opportunity to discuss their work-related background and skills. Although it is not necessary to mention on a job application, it can still be discussed with the interviewer, allowing any concerns to be addressed. There can be a number of different approaches to disclosing. If seizures are well controlled, only occur at night, or are mild without loss of consciousness, disclosure may not be necessary. A client may decide then only to share this information after some time at a job or only to closer friends and coworkers. The Americans with Disabilities Act, which was implemented in 1992, and amended in 2008, requires reasonable accommodation of employees. Many jobs may need only minor modifications to the worksite (such as layer of padding on a concrete floor or reassignment of minimal work tasks [e.g., having a coworker do some minimal driving that is required on the job if the client lacks a driver's license because of epilepsy]). Although people with controlled or uncontrolled epilepsy are covered under the 2008 amendments to the Americans with Disabilities Act, litigation is slow, and it is better to negotiate these problems directly with employers when able.

Studies show that the attendance and performance records for people with epilepsy are equal to or better than those of the general working population (McLellan, 1987). Average time lost due to seizures was approximately 1 hour for every 1,000 hours worked by individuals with active seizure conditions (Risch, 1968), and over a 13-year period in the state of New York, there were more accidents in the workplace caused by sneezing or coughing on the job than accidents related to seizures (Sands, 1961). Hiring people with epilepsy does not increase industrial insurance and most states have second injury funds protecting an employer from bearing responsibility for total disability if the client has a seizure on the job that results in inability to work again. Relatively few jobs at this time require working directly with heavy machinery, and many machines have "kill switches" or plastic guards to prevent injury in the setting of sudden loss of consciousness, even if a client is not warned by a preceding aura. Often seizures can be controlled to the extent where such concerns are no longer active.

A commonly used working guideline is that those who are seizure-free for 6 months are considered in good control and may be exposed to the same basic activities as the general population. Rules regarding drivers licenses vary by state, but driving is often allowed with this level of seizure control. Jobs involving direct interaction with heights or boiling/molten materials do present active concerns, although harnesses and fire-retardant clothing may minimize these risks sufficiently to allow participation. Obviously, these must be assessed on a case-by-case basis. The Job Accommodation Network in West Virginia (www.jan.wvu.edu) or university departments and their vocational rehabilitation, occupational therapy, or assistive technology units can be contacted for accommodation or ideas specific to individual seizure-related concerns. The Epilepsy Foundation in Washington, DC, has extensive online resources and a variety of local affiliates with employment programs (www.epilepsy.com). The American Epilepsy Society has a resource site for physicians and employers on Epilepsy and Employment within the Practice Tools link (www.aesnet.org).

CONCLUSION

This chapter reviewed medical, psychosocial, and vocational implications of epilepsy as a disability. With greater understanding of third-generation anticonvulsants' benefits, people with epilepsy should be more employable. Seizures can take on a wide variety of forms and are associated with many different issues. However, all of the service professionals supporting a client with epilepsy may benefit from sensitivity to the types of needs that may arise. In our experience, with good medical and psychosocial/vocational assessment and targeted intervention, the seizure condition itself and associated disabilities can be worked with, and successful job placement and community integration can be achieved.

REFERENCES

Adams, S. J., O'Brien, T. J., Lloyd, J., Kilpatrick, C. J., Salzberg, M. R., & Velakoulis, D. (2008). Neuropsychiatric morbidity in focal epilepsy. *The British Journal of Psychiatry, 192*(6), 464–469.

Adelöw, C., Andersson, T., Ahlbom, A., & Tomson, T. (2012). Hospitalization for psychiatric disorders before and after onset of unprovoked seizures/epilepsy. *Neurology, 78*(6), 396–401.

Annegers, J. F. (2001). The epidemiology of epilepsy. In E. Wyllie (Ed.), *The treatment of epilepsy: Principles and practice* (3rd ed., p. 135). Philadelphia, PA: Lippincott Williams & Wilkins.

Annegers, J. F., & Coan, S. P. (1999). SUDEP: Overview of definitions and review of incidence data. *Seizure, 8*(6), 347–352.

Bautista, R. E., Shapovalov, D., & Shoraka, A. R. (2015). Factors associated with increased felt stigma among individuals with epilepsy. *Seizure, 30*, 106–112.

Bergey, G. K., Morrell, M. J., Mizrahi, E. M., Nair, D., Goldman, A., King-Stephens, D., . . . Seale, C. G. (2015). Long-term treatment with responsive brain stimulation in adults with refractory partial seizures. *Neurology, 84*(8), 810–817.

Brodie, M. J., & Kwan, P. (2002). Staged approach to epilepsy management. *Neurology, 58*(Suppl. 5), 52–58.

Bryant-Comstock, I., Hogan, P., Shumaker, S., & Tennis, P. (1997). Relation of seizure severity to employment status and education [Abstract]. *Epilepsia, 38*(Suppl.), 135.

Chang, C. H., & Gehlert, S. (2003). The washington psychosocial seizure inventory (WPSI): Psychometric evaluation and future applications. *Seizure, 12*, 261–267.

Dodrill, C. B. (1978). A neuropsychological battery for epilepsy. *Epilepsia, 19*, 611–623.

Dodrill, C. B. (1986). Correlates of tonic-clonic seizures with intellectual, neuropsychological, emotional, and social functions in patients with epilepsy. *Epilepsia, 27*, 399–411.

Elsharkawy, A. E., Thorbecke, R., Ebner, A., & May, T. W. (2012). Determinants of quality of life in patients with refractory focal epilepsy who were not eligible for surgery or who rejected surgery. *Epilepsy & Behavior, 24*(2), 249–255.

Fisher, R., Salanova, V., Witt, T., Worth, R., Henry, T., & Gross, R., . . . SANTE Study Group. (2010). Electrical stimulation of the anterior nucleus of thalamus for treatment of refractory epilepsy. *Epilepsia, 51*(5), 899–908.

Fisher, R. S., Nune, G., Roberts, S. E., & Cramer, J. A. (2015). The personal impact of epilepsy scale (PIES). *Epilepsy & Behavior, 42*, 140–146.

Fraser, R. T., & Clemmons, D. C. (1989). Vocational and psychosocial interventions for youth with seizure disorders. In B. Hermann & N. I. Siedenberg (Eds.), *Childhood epilepsies: Neuropsychological, psychosocial, and intervention aspects* (pp. 201–220). Chichester, England: John Wiley & Sons.

Fraser, R. T., Clemmons, D. C., Andrechak, N., Dodrill, C. B., & Temkin, N. (1991). *Prevocational intervention in epilepsy rehabilitation: Outcome and pre/postintervention employability correlates.* Seattle, WA: American Epilepsy Society.

Fraser, R. T., Clemmons, D. C., Dodrill, C. B., Trejo, W., & Freelove, C. (1986). The difficult to employ in epilepsy rehabilitation: Predictors of response to an intensive intervention. *Eplepsia, 27*, 220–224.

Gaitatzis, A., Carroll, K., Majeed, A. W., & Sander, J. (2004). The epidemiology of the comorbidity of epilepsy in the general population. *Epilepsia, 45*(12), 1613–1622.

Gaitatzis, A., Trimble, M. R., & Sander, J. W. (2004). The psychiatric comorbidity of epilepsy. *Acta Neurologica Scandinavica, 110*(4), 207–220.

Gehlert, S., Difrancesco, A., & Chang, C. H. (2000). Black-white differences in the psychosocial outcomes of epilepsy. *Epilepsy Research, 42*(1), 63–73.

Gilliam, F., & Kanner, A. M. (2002). Treatment of depressive disorders in epilepsy patients. *Epilepsy & Behavior, 3*(5S), 2–9.

Goldin, C. J., Hammeke, T. A., & Parisch, A. D. (1980). *The Luria-Nebraska neuropsychological battery: Manual.* Los Angeles, CA: Western Psychological Services.

Henderson, C. B., Filloux, F. M., Alder, S. C., Lyon, J. L., & Caplin, D. A. (2006). Efficacy of the ketogenic diet as a treatment option for epilepsy: Meta-analysis. *Journal of Clinical Neurology, 21*(3), 193–198.

Hermann, B. P., Jones, J. E., Sheth, R., Koehn, M., Becker, T., Fine, J., . . . Seidenberg, M. (2008). Growing up with epilepsy: A two-year investigation of cognitive development in children with new onset epilepsy. *Epilepsia, 49*, 1847–1858.

Hermann, B. P., Seidenberg, M., & Bell, B. (2000). Psychiatric co-morbidity in chronic epilepsy: Identification, consequences, and treatment of major depression. *Epilepsia, 41*(Suppl. 2), S31–S41.

Hermann, B. P., Seidenberg, M., Dow, C., Jones, J., Rutecki, P., Bhattacharya, A., & Bell, B. (2006). Cognitive prognosis in chronic temporal lobe epilepsy. *Annals of Neurology, 60*, 80–87.

Hesdorffer, D. C., Ishihara, L., Mynepalli, L., Webb, D. J., Weil, J., Hauser, W. A. (2012). Epilepsy, suicidality, and psychiatric disorders: A bidirectional association. *Annals of Neurology, 72*(2), 184–191.

Hirtz, D., Thurman, D. J., Gwinn-hardy, K., Mohamed, M., Chaudhuri, A. R., & Zalutsky, R. (2007). How common are the common, neurologic disorders? *Neurology, 68*(5), 326–337.

Institute of Medicine. (2012). *Epilepsy across the spectrum: Promoting health and understanding*, Washington, DC: National Academies Press.

Kwon, C., Liu, M., Quan, H., Thoo, V., Wiebe, S., & Jetté, N. (2011). Motor vehicle accidents, suicides, and assaults in epilepsy: A population-based study. *Neurology, 76*(9), 801–806.

Lhatoo, S. D., & Sander, J. W. (2001). The epidemiology of epilepsy and learning disability. *Epilepsia, 42*(Suppl. 1), 6–9.

Manford, M., Hart, Y. M., Sander, J. W., & Shorvon, S. D. (1992). The national general practice study of epilepsy. The syndromic classification of the international league against epilepsy applied to epilepsy in a general population. *Archives of Neurology, 49*(8), 801–808.

McLellan, D. L. (1987). Epilepsy and employment. *Journal of Social and Occupational Medicine, 3*, 94–99.

Oyegbile, T. O., Dow, C., Jones, J., Bell, B., Rutecki, P., Sheth, R., . . . Hermann, B. P. (2004). The nature and course of neuropsychological morbidity in chronic temporal lobe epilepsy. *Neurology, 62*, 1736–1742.

Pompili, M., Serafini, G., Innamorati, M., Montebovi, F., Lamis, D. A., Milelli, M., . . . Buttinelli, C. (2014). Factors associated with hopelessness in epileptic patients. *World Journal of Psychiatry, 4*(4), 141–149.

Rausch, R., Le, M. T., & Langfitt, J. L. (1997). Neuropsychological evaluation: Adults. In J. Engel & T. A. Pedley (Eds.), *Epilepsy*. Philadelphia, PA: Lippincott-Raven.

Reitan, R. M., & Wolfson, D. (1985). *The halstead-reitan test battery: Theory and clinical interpretations.* Tucson, AZ: Neuropsychology Press.

Reuber, M., Pukrop, R., Bauer, J., Helmstaedter, C., Tessendorf, N., & Elger, C. E. (2003). Outcome in psychogenic nonepileptic seizures: 1 to 10-year follow-up in 164 patients. *Annals of Neurology, 53*, 305–311.

Risch, F. (1968). We lost every game . . . but. *Rehabilitation Record, 9*, 16–18.

Sands, H. (1961). Report of a study undertaken for the committee on neurological disorders in industry. *Epilepsy News, 7*, 1.

Trinka, E., Cock, H., Hesdorffer, D., Rossetti, A. O., Scheffer, I. E., Shinnar, S., . . . Lowenstein, D. H. (2015). A definition and classification of status epilepticus - Report of the ILAE task force on classification of status epilepticus. *Epilepsia, 56*(10), 1515–1523.

Trostle, J. A. (1988). Social aspects of epilepsy. In W. A. Hauser (Ed.), *Current trends in epilepsy: A self-study course for physicians (Unit 1)*. Landover, MD: Epilepsy Foundation of America.

Trostle, J. A., Hauser, W. A., & Sharbrough, F. (1986). Self-regulation of medical regimens among adults with epilepsy in Rochester. *Epilepsia, 27*, 640.

Witt, J. A., & Helmstaedter, C. (2012). Should cognition be screened in new-onset epilepsies? A study in 247 untreated patients. *Journal of Neurology, 259*(8), 1727–1731.

Zwimpfer, T. J., Brown, J., Sullivan, I., & Moulton, R. J. (1997). Head injuries due to falls caused by seizures: A group at high risk for traumatic intracranial hematomas. *Journal of Neurosurgery, 86*(3), 433–437.

CHAPTER

Hematological Disorders

Bruce G. Raphael and Richard J. Lin

Blood contains a variety of mature differentiated cells that have specialized functions. The different kinds of cell include the red blood cells that carry oxygen to the tissues, the white blood cells that help fight infection, and the platelets, which are the blood-clotting cells. The white blood cells are further divided into a variety of cell types. The two most important white blood cell types are the granulocytes, which fight bacterial infection, and the lymphocytes, which make the antibodies, control the immune reactions, and help with viral infections. New cells are required constantly to replace the old, and hence, there is a need for a stem cell, which is defined as the self-renewing progenitor cell that, under appropriate stimulus, divides and matures into various blood cells. The majority of these stem cells are in a resting state in the bone marrow in humans. The process of division and maturation is a complex operation; mistakes in the control and programmed cell death lead to abnormal accumulation of precursor cells at various stages of maturation. Cancers that develop because of abnormal proliferation of the white blood cells in the blood are known as leukemia, and in the lymph nodes are called lymphoma. The final stage of maturation of B-lymphocytes is plasma cells that produce immunoglobulins to fight infection, and malignant transformation of plasma cells in the bone marrow is known as multiple myeloma (Williams, Butler, Ersley, & Lichtman, 1990).

LYMPHOMA

Disease Description

Lymphomas are a malignant proliferation of one of the white blood cell types—lymphocytes—which are divided into B-lymphocytes and T-lymphocytes. B-lymphocytes are cells that go through a complicated maturation process in which only a portion of the genetic material that codes for antibody production is activated, so each B-cell produces a single antibody against a specific foreign protein. T-lymphocytes go through similar maturation, with activation of other portions of the genetic material. These cells then specialize in helping (helper cells) or suppressing (suppressor cells) the immune reaction. Once formed, these cells migrate to the lymph nodes, and when exposed to a foreign protein or an infectious agent, those lymphocytes programmed to make the specific antibody against the abnormal antigen will divide, enlarge, and multiply, producing a large number of cells that ultimately mature into plasma cells in the bone marrow, which in turn produce antibodies to neutralize the invading organism. The T-helper cells aid this reaction; when the organism is cleared, T-suppressor cells inhibit the immune reaction and the swollen lymph gland shrinks back to the quiescent state (Skarin, 1989).

When one of the maturing and dividing lymphocytes undergoes malignant change and divides uncontrollably, an accumulation of these cells occurs as a tumor, called a lymphoma. The cause of this malignant change is chromosomal breaks or gene mutations that occur during the division and maturation of each individual lymphocyte, which leads to activation of genes involved in differentiation, proliferation, and cell death. The result is either uncontrolled growth (Williams et al., 1990) or lack of programmed cell death, both of which lead to an accumulation of clonal malignant cells. Although certain viruses (the Epstein–Barr virus and T-cell lymphotrophic virus) have been implicated in a small number of B- and T-cell lymphomas, respectively, most of these genetic changes occur as a consequence of mistakes in the complex act of gene replication and division, generating chromosomal translocations, deletions, and amplifications (Shankland, Armitage, & Hancock, 2012). Five percent of all cancers in the United States are lymphomas, with 70% to 80% of B-cell origin and the rest derived from T-cells (Skarin, 1989). There is a rising incidence of aggressive lymphoma in patients with AIDS and in patients on chronic immunosuppressive drugs (i.e., posttransplant state). The speculative cause of these lymphomas is excessive immune stimulation of B-lymphocytes with chromosomal breaks and poor immune surveillance by the reduced number of T-lymphocytes, which are destroyed by the AIDS virus (Raphael & Knowles, 1990).

Pathology

The lymphomas are all classified by the appearance of malignant lymphocytes on the biopsy slides of the tumor. As stated earlier, normal lymphocytes go through various stages of maturation. A lymphoma is an accumulation of clonal, malignant lymphocytes that are arrested at one stage of maturation. Clinical behavior of the tumor is often correlated with the level of maturation of the abnormal lymphocyte. Hence, classification of lymphomas is divided into three categories: (a) low, (b) intermediate, and (c) high grade (Rosenberg, 1982). Low-grade lymphomas contain cells that are smaller, slower growing, and often asymptomatic. Intermediate-grade lymphomas have cells that are larger and faster growing. High-grade lymphomas are very fast growing, immature lymphocytes, which often present in extranodal as well as nodal tissues. In addition, the tumor can present in a nodular (follicular) pattern or diffusely, replacing the architecture of the lymph node. Slower growth is associated with the former pattern, and more aggressive behavior is related to the latter (Table 11.1; Rosenberg, 1982). Subsequently, the realization based on immunologic staining of cells, molecular studies, and the understanding of genetic translocations and mutation have led to further classifications called the Revised European American Lymphoma (REAL) classification in 1994 and the World Health Organization (WHO) classification in 2008 (Swerdlow et al., 2008). Classification based on cytogenetic abnormalities is not shown in Table 11.1, and is beyond the scope of this chapter. However, it is important to note that tumors that look the same but have different genetic mutations have led to the understanding of why some patients are cured whereas others with the same disease do not respond to the same treatment. Hence, this new information is being used to develop new protocols targeting the molecular defects resulting from these changes (Schouten, 2007; Shankland et al., 2012).

Functional Presentation

Patients usually present with swollen, growing lymph glands (nodal disease) or tumors in other organs, such as spleen and liver (extranodal disease). Patients can be asymptomatic (A) or have one or more of the B symptoms, which include fever, drenching night sweats, loss of 10% of body weight, and itching. An evaluation, called "staging," is done to determine the extent of disease. This includes a proper physical examination to determine any lymph node group that is enlarged, or any abnormal organ enlargement. In addition, CT scans of chest, abdomen, and pelvis are done to determine internal organ and nodal involvement. A bone marrow biopsy is used to examine whether it is involved by lymphoma. In addition, cerebrospinal fluid is analyzed to determine central nervous system involvement in higher grade lymphomas because of a higher chance of spread with these aggressive tumors. PET scans have recently been added to the evaluation methods of lymphomas. Radioactive sugar is given intravenously which rapidly accumulates in tumor cells because tumor cells use more sugar to fuel their increased metabolic activity compared with normal cells. The amount of radioactivity in the tumor cells can be followed both during and after chemotherapy to determine

TABLE 11.1

CLASSIFICATIONS OF LYMPHOMA
Low grade Malignant lymphoma, small lymphocytic Malignant lymphoma, follicular, predominantly small cleaved cell Malignant lymphoma, follicular, mixed small and large cell
Intermediate grade Malignant lymphoma, follicular, predominantly large cell Malignant lymphoma, diffuse, mixed small and large cell Malignant lymphoma, diffuse large cell cleaved
High grade Diffuse large cell, immunoblastic Malignant lymphoma, lymphoblastic Malignant lymphoma, small noncleaved cell

TABLE 11.2

STAGING OF LYMPHOMA	
Stage	Characteristics
I	Involvement of a single lymph node region or single extra modal organ or site
II	Involvement limited to one side of the diaphragm with two or more lymph node regions
III	Involvement of lymph node regions on both sides of the diaphragm
IV	Diffuse or disseminated involvement of one or more extra lymphatic organs

completeness of response to therapy (Friedberg & Chengazi, 2003). The stage of disease is then determined by the number of lymph nodes involved and the presence of disease in other organs (Table 11.2). Prognosis is dependent on the type of lymphoma, as well as age, functional status, stage, and clinical presentation (Matasar & Zelenetz, 2008). This has led to a commonly used international prognostic index and risk stratification (Table 11.3). When applied to 2,031 patients with aggressive lymphomas, these risk groups had 5-year survival rates of 73%, 51%, 43%, and 26%, respectively (The International Non-Hodgkin's Lymphoma Prognostic Factors Project, 1993).

TABLE 11.3

PROGNOSTIC FACTORS AND RISK STRATIFICATION
Prognostic factors Age < or > 60 years ECOG performance status Advanced stage (III or IV) >1 extranodal sites of involvement
Presence of symptoms Serum lactate dehydrogenase level increased
Risk group stratification according to the International Prognostic Index (total number of above-listed features) 0–1: Low risk 2: Low intermediate risk 3: High intermediate risk 4–5: High risk

ECOG, Eastern Cooperative Oncology Group.

Treatment

The vast majority of lymphomas present in multiple areas of the body, as abnormal lymphocytes, are free to travel to other areas of the body through the blood. Hence, localized treatment with surgery or radiation is rarely curative unless for early stages (Ruthoven, 1987; Skarin, 1989). Treatment is, therefore, primarily chemoimmunotherapy, in which chemicals are used to poison the growing malignant cells. Combinations of drugs have resulted in more remissions and cures, although the number of poor prognostic factors, as noted in Table 11.3, influence response rates. In addition to chemotherapy and external irradiation to shrink the disease, in the last decade, biologic agents have been added to treatment regimens. These include manufactured monoclonal antibodies directed at proteins on the cancer cell that attack the tumor cells directly, antibodies that are conjugated with a radioactive substance or toxin allowing preferential targeting of the tumor, and a vaccine produced from the tumor cells that stimulate an immune reaction in the patient against the cancer cell (Fanale & Younes, 2007; Hsu et al., 1997). Low-grade lymphomas can be controlled for many years, with median survival of 7 to 10 years, but are rarely curable (Shankland et al., 2012; Skarin, 1989). Recently, there has been a large number of newer agents, in particular, monoclonal antibodies, that are manufactured in large quantities that target the lymphocytes. When these new agents were added to existing chemotherapeutic protocols, responses improved and it was hoped that it would result in either cure or long-term control of the lymphoma growth (Berdeja, 2003). A recent study comparing survival in modern combination chemotherapy and monoclonal antibody treatment with historical controls from the 1980s and 1990s appears to suggest that complete remission and duration of remission is longer, and overall survival is also improved (Fisher et al., 2005). That said, cures in low-grade lymphomas remain rare and frequent relapses is the rule rather than the exception. For example, patients with high-risk follicular lymphoma typically have a 2-year relapse rate of close to 60% (Freedman, 2015).

The intermediate lymphomas now have a 50% to 70% cure rate, depending on stage and prognostic factors, using combinations of multiple chemotherapy agents (Shankland et al., 2012; Skarin,

1989). The addition of monoclonal antibodies has also influenced these lymphomas, and cure rates increased in all prognostic risk categories by 10% to 15% (Michallet & Coiffier, 2009). High-grade lymphomas are treated with intensive doses of chemotherapy, leading to 80% to 90% cures in children and 30% to 50% cure rate in adults, but individuals who relapse often die within a year (Magrath et al., 1996) unless they are able to be salvaged with bone marrow transplantation (Philip et al., 1995).

Lymphomas are very sensitive to chemotherapy, but no drug is specific for only the tumor cell. This leads to the side effects of chemotherapy: Normal-growing cells are affected, as well as specific organs that are sensitive to the toxic effects of these agents. The disability that patients experience may be—in part, due to the presence of the tumor in a disease site—shortness of breath with lung involvement and debilitation from fevers and weight loss. Alternatively, they may be related to the side effects of the chemotherapy. These drugs are toxins that poison the tumor cells but may also injure normal cells. Examples are Adriamycin, which can damage the heart and cause mucositis, or Oncovin, which causes peripheral neuropathy. It should be noted that specialized and expensive treatments might add further barriers to care in lower socioeconomic groups. A disparity in survival figures between Whites and Blacks has already been demonstrated in lymphoma treatment (Han et al., 2008).

Bone marrow transplantation is increasingly used in patients who do not respond to primary treatment. High-dose chemotherapy is used to kill the lymphoma that was resistant to conventional treatment. Stem cells harvested from the patient (autologous transplant) or from a tissue-matched relative (allogeneic transplant) are stored before the high-dose chemotherapy and given back to rescue the patient from the lethal effects of high-dose chemotherapy on the bone marrow. Other organs are damaged during the intensive therapy, infections are frequent, and immunosuppressive drugs are needed in the case of allogeneic transplant to prevent the donor's immune cells from infecting the recipient's cells (graft vs. host). The result is a prolonged, complicated hospital stay with multiple manifestations of organ damage. As patients recover, they typically have been bedridden, unable to eat owing to chemotherapy-induced gastric damage, and debilitated from previous infection. Hence, a lengthy recovery period is the norm with active rehabilitation by physiotherapy, psychology, and dietary services (Steinberg, Asher, Bailey, & Fu, 2015).

MYELOMA

Disease Description

Multiple myeloma is the type of hematological cancer derived from a single plasma cell that has undergone malignant transformation. The plasma cell is an immunoglobulin-secreting cell that helps fight off foreign "invaders." As each plasma cell produces only one antibody, a clone of malignant cells derived from the original transformed cell produces increased amounts of that one immunoglobulin called a paraprotein or M-protein. The accumulation of the increased monoclonal serum protein and the malignant plasma cells in the bone marrow that produces them causes the kidney problems, bone lesions, anemia, and hypercalcemia that is seen in myeloma. Normal bone marrow contains less than 5% plasma cells. In multiple myeloma there is usually more than 30% plasma cells where they interfere with the production of normal blood cells (Raab et al., 2009).

Multiple myeloma is the second most common hematological malignancy in the United States (after non-Hodgkin lymphoma). There are over 25,000 new cases of myeloma in the United States each year, representing 15% of all blood cancers and 1% of all types of cancer. The average age of onset is 70 years. It is more common in men and, for unknown reasons, is twice as common in African Americans as in White Americans (Raab et al., 2009).

Pathology

B-lymphocytes accumulate in the lymph nodes and mature under appropriate stimulation, leave the node and become either long-lived memory cells or travel to the bone marrow where they further differentiate into a plasma cell. Plasma cells then secrete one type of antibody, each leading the normal mixture of gammaglobulins in our body that provide defense against microbes. A malignant transformation of one of the precursor plasma cells leads to an accumulation of malignant plasma cells, as seen on a biopsy of the bone marrow in a patient with myeloma. The malignant transformation is caused by chromosomal breaks and gene mutations often through rearrangement or amplification; the control is lost and cells proliferate to form a malignant clone (or clones; Corre, Munshi, & Avet-Loiseau, 2015).

The malignant myeloma cells have an affinity for the bone marrow environment where they establish a destructive relationship with other stromal (bone matrix) cells, which promotes growth of the plasma cells. The myeloma cells secrete substances called osteoclastic activating factor that cause bone destruction and lead to a further proliferation of the myeloma cells. They also produce a large excess of antibodies that are deposited in various organs leading to kidney failure, polyneuropathy, and various other myeloma-associated symptoms (Raab et al., 2009).

Functional Presentation

The extra plasma cells in the bone marrow crowd out the normal bone marrow cells and cause bone destruction as well as inhibit normal immunoglobulin production from the normal plasma cells, leading to the diverse clinical presentations and variable clinical signs. A mnemonic commonly used for the common symptoms of multiple myeloma is CRAB: C = calcium (elevated), R = renal failure, A = anemia, B = bone lesions (Raab et al., 2009). The bone destruction leads to pain and bone fractures, which affect rehabilitation even after the disease is under control. Other possible symptoms include opportunistic infections (e.g., pneumonia) due to low normal-functioning immunoglobulins and the abnormal antibodies that attach to nerves and cause peripheral neuropathy. Multiple myeloma can produce all classes of immunoglobulin with IgG paraproteins as the most common, followed by IgA, and IgM. IgD and IgE myeloma are very rare. In addition, an antibody is made up of heavy and light chains which are separately produced and combined to form a full immunoglobulin molecule. The cell may produce excess of the light chains, called kappa (κ) or lambda (λ), which are smaller in size and tend to be filtered by the kidney and lead to kidney damage. True "nonsecretory" myeloma (not producing immunoglobulins) is very rare and accounts for approximately 1% to 3% of all multiple myeloma patients. In 2014, the International Myeloma Working Group updated the diagnostic criteria for symptomatic myeloma, asymptomatic myeloma, and monoclonal gammopathy of undetermined significance (MGUS), which are listed in Table 11.4 (Rajkumar et al., 2015).

TABLE 11.4

DIAGNOSTIC CRITERIA FOR MULTIPLE MYELOMA AND RELATED DISORDERS
Myeloma Clonal plasma cells >10% on bone marrow biopsy or (in any quantity) in a biopsy from other tissues (plasmacytoma), and any one of the following: Evidence of end-organ damage as defined by *CRAB* symptoms Clonal bone marrow plasma cell percentage >60% Involved:uninvolved serum free light chain ratios ≥100 >1 focal lesions on MRI studies
Smoldering myeloma Serum monoclonal protein ≥30 g/L or urinary protein >500 mg per 24 hours and/or clonal bone marrow plasma cells 10%–60% Absence of myeloma-defining events or amyloidosis
Monoclonal gammopathy of undetermined significance (MGUS) Serum paraprotein <30 g/L and/or clonal plasma cells <10% on bone marrow biopsy Absence of myeloma-defining events or amyloidosis

Source: Rajkumar et al. (2015).

Treatment

The International Staging System can help to predict survival, with a median survival of 62 months for Stage I disease, 45 months for Stage II disease, and 29 months for Stage III disease (Greipp et al., 2005).

- Stage I: β_2 microglobulin (β2M) <3.5 mg/L, albumin ≥3.5 g/dL
- Stage II: β2M < 3.5 mg/L and albumin <3.5 g/dL; or β2M 3.5 mg/L to 5.5 mg/L irrespective of the serum albumin
- Stage III: β2M ≥5.5 mg/L

Treatment for multiple myeloma is focused on control of the clonal plasma cell population and consequently decrease the signs and symptoms of disease. Initial treatment depends on the patient's age and medical comorbidities. In recent years, the focus of treatment is on novel agents that inhibit the machinery of plasma cells, or affect the bone marrow matrix cells to prevent the signals of growth that were mentioned earlier as critical to plasma cell survival. The use of proteosome inhibitors such as bortizomib (Velcade) and immune modulators such as lenalidomide (Revlimid) have dramatically increased response rates over standard chemotherapy but have side effects such as peripheral neuropathy and diarrhea that contribute to disability. Once in partial remission from these agents, the use of high-dose chemotherapy with autologous hematopoietic stem-cell transplantation has become the preferred treatment for fit patients under the age of 65 to 70. Autologous stem cell transplantation is not curative, but does prolong overall survival and result in deeper reduction in tumor cells at the expense of more toxic side effects and deconditioning. The natural history of myeloma is of relapse following treatment, which may be caused by intratumor heterogeneity. Depending on the patient's condition, the prior treatment modalities used, and the duration of remission, options for relapsed disease include retreatment with the original regimen, use of other novel regimens, and a second autologous stem cell transplant. In addition to direct treatment of the plasma cell proliferation, bisphosphonates (e.g., pamidronate or zoledronic acid) are routinely administered to prevent fractures. This preventive approach has led to less bone pain, fractures, and long-term disability (Moreau, Attal, & Facon, 2015).

LEUKEMIA

Disease Description

Acute leukemia is characterized by an abnormal proliferation of immature white blood cells. As stated earlier, lymphoma represents an accumulation of lymphocytes arrested at one stage of maturation leading to the different lymphomas based on the level of maturation of the malignant cell. Leukemia is the accumulation of the earliest white blood cells, called blasts or progenitor cells. These cells normally divide and mature into the white cells that help fight infections, but eventually die. Hence, stem cells also must self-renew so that they can be called upon again and again to repopulate the constant turnover of bone marrow cells. Hence, the effect of lack of maturation is the presence of large numbers of these young cells in the bone marrow and lack of normal bone marrow cells. Patients then present with signs and symptoms of low red blood cell count (anemia), such as weakness and shortness of breath with activity, decreased white blood cells (granulocytopenia) with infection and fever, and a low platelet count (thrombocytopenia) with bleeding. In addition, infiltration of various organs by these tumor cells can lead to enlargement of liver, spleen, and lymph nodes, as well as to gum hypertrophy and skin nodules (Williams et al., 1990).

The incidence of acute leukemia is 9 cases per 100,000 individuals, and the incidence rises with age (DeVita, Hellman, & Rosenberg, 1989). Unlike some other tumors, however, acute leukemia is the most common childhood malignancy. There are two main forms of acute leukemia: acute lymphoblastic leukemia (ALL) is a cancer of the earliest stages of lymphocyte maturation, and acute nonlymphoblastic leukemia (ANLL) usually is a malignancy of the progenitor of the granulocyte series called the myeloblast. ALL occurs more often in the young; ANLL is more common with adults. Cytogenetic studies show a variety of chromosomal breaks and mutations associated with different types of leukemia. The proteins encoded by these mutated genes cause dysregulation of division and maturation, and hence accumulation of myeloblasts or lymphoblasts (Berman, 1997). Recent studies also reveal molecular evidence of progressive cytogenetic evolution of multiple clone of leukemia stem cells from preleukemia state to acute leukemia and disease relapse (Shlush & Mitchell, 2015).

Pathology

Patients' routine blood tests show low levels of all blood cells (pancytopenia) and/or the presence of early white cell forms (blasts). Bone marrow analysis shows a hypercellular specimen with almost complete replacement by early white cell forms. Only a few remaining normally maturing blood cells can be found. Morphology, staining characteristics, biochemistry, and immunologic typing can help differentiate between ANLL and ALL. In addition, cytogenetic and molecular analysis is done to characterize the type of leukemia as well as to indicate prognosis (Frankfurt, Licht, & Tallman, 2007). The realization that response to treatment is affected by the genetic mutations led

TABLE 11.5

CLASSIFICATION OF MYELOID LEUKEMIA
Acute myeloid leukemia with recurrent genetic abnormalities
Acute myeloid leukemia with myelodysplasia-related changes
Therapy-related myeloid neoplasms
Acute myeloid leukemia, not otherwise specified
Myeloid sarcoma
Myeloid proliferations related to Down syndrome
Blastic plasmacytoid dendritic cell neoplasm

Source: Vardiman et al. (2009).

to the WHO recently classifying myeloid leukemia using genetic, morphologic, and previous exposure to DNA-damaging agents (Vardiman et al., 2009; Table 11.5). Long-term survival with standard chemotherapy would range from 70% to 80% for patients with good-risk cytogenetics and/or molecular mutations to 10% or less for patients with poor-risk features and/or advanced age and suboptimal performance status (Kadia, Ravandi, O'Brien, Cortes, & Kantarjian, 2015).

Functional Presentation and Treatment

Patients with lymphoma and myeloma present with tumor and related symptoms, but they generally have adequate normal blood cells and can tolerate chemotherapy as outpatients. Patients with acute leukemia usually present as critically ill, with signs and symptoms of lack of normal blood elements. If they present late in the course of the disease, the white blood cell counts are elevated because the leukemic cells have multiplied in the bone marrow and spilled into the blood, or there is organ dysfunction due to infiltration by the tumor cells. Hence, patients are admitted immediately and stabilized by correcting the anemia with red blood cell transfusions, treated for any uncontrolled infection resulting from lack of mature white blood cells, transfused platelets to control bleeding, and started on chemotherapy to kill the leukemia cells. Although treatment for ANLL differs from treatment for ALL, the principle is the same. Induction therapy involves large doses of chemotherapy to poison the tumor cells (Gale & Foon, 1987; Hoelzer & Gale, 1987). However, these drugs are toxic to all blood cells, resulting in the death of the few remaining normal bone marrow cells and the development of aplasia in the bone marrow. Once chemotherapy stops and the tumor cells die, the normal stem cells in the marrow that are resistant to chemotherapy divide and their progeny cells mature and repopulate the marrow over the next 3 weeks. Until sufficient cells grow to produce the necessary mature, functioning peripheral blood cells, the patient remains sick and must receive antibiotics, fluids, and transfusions on a daily basis. Remissions occur in up to 80% of cases, but relapses are common. Additional consolidation chemotherapy is given after recovery to prevent recurrence (Gale & Foon, 1987; Hoelzer & Gale, 1987) but with variable success depending on the cytogenetic abnormality (Kadia et al., 2015; King & Rowe, 2007). The repetitive chemotherapy injury further slows bone marrow recovery, adding days of admissions to the hospital, and resulting in more disability.

Furthermore, the chemotherapy drugs are toxic to other organs as well as bone marrow. Myopathy (disorders of the muscle) caused by steroids and neurotoxicity from the drug vincristine is common in the treatment of ALL. Heart damage from anthracycline chemotherapy drugs and fluid overload due to multiple intravenous fluids and transfusions are common to all patients. Finally, nausea, mouth sores, and gastric irritation are typical with this type of chemotherapy, making adequate nutritional intake difficult and further adding to the general level of poor nutrition and debilitation. In cases of relapse, as well as in some experimental protocols for patients in remission, allogeneic bone marrow transplantation is offered as a way of using very high doses of chemotherapy to rid the body of any remaining leukemia cells, using the normal stems from a donor infused back into the patient after chemotherapy is completed to replenish the stem cells and subsequent normal blood production, and prevent any further relapses (Brissot & Mohty, 2015). The physical problems secondary to this intensive therapy are multiplied, compared with conventional therapy. Hence, patients with leukemia face months of treatment and weeks of hospitalization with each treatment. The resulting physical, psychological, and financial toll is substantial.

Psychological and Vocational Implications

A further discussion of the relationship of cancer and psychosocial adaptation can be found in

Chapter 6. However, several points that are unique to lymphoma, myeloma, and leukemia are discussed here.

As stated earlier, lymphoma and leukemia affect a wider age range than do most cancers, and the psychosocial implications vary with age. Daiter, Larson, Weddington, and Ultmann (1988) surveyed younger adults, aged 18 to 36, with leukemia and lymphoma. As might be expected, patients with less favorable prognoses experienced more stress but also significant personal growth and maturation. In addition, family and friends who provided social support reported not only more stress when dealing with the sicker patient with poor prognosis but also sometimes expressed more prolonged anxiety after treatment was completed than did the patient. Psychological stress has been reported to be lower for leukemia than for breast cancer. Treatment with chemotherapy and radiation to younger patients with acute leukemia, particularly ALL, may add developmental disability to the list of long-term deficits. There is up to a 30% risk of school-related problems, especially in those patients treated for central nervous system involvement (Mulhern, Friedman, & Stone, 1988). Adolescents require different types of support, and negotiating treatment is more demanding (Penson et al., 2002).

Older patients have additional concerns about financial matters, how their spouses and children are coping and functioning, and interpersonal relationships at work. Depression, sleep disorder, and anxiety over personal appearance are common. Long-term survivors also have persistent problems; one study reported 73% of patients with Hodgkin's disease having at least one of five problems, including decreased energy level, negative body image, depression, employment problems, and marital problems (Fobair et al., 1986). In addition, the rising incidence of leukemia with age, and secondary leukemia owing to previous chemotherapy, results in many difficult decisions concerning therapy and quality-of-life issues (Sekeres et al., 2004). However, a recent review looking at quality-of-life parameters 6 months after chemotherapy in older patients in remission from acute myeloid leukemia demonstrated that those patients who remained in remission had a gradual improvement of all parameters (Alibhai et al., 2009). Hence, while the chance of long-term remission in patients older than 60 years is smaller, those who do have a remission can a relatively normal quality of life.

Finally, because bone marrow transplantation has become a common therapy for refractory lymphoma and leukemia, studies of the psychosocial morbidity of these procedures have been completed. Jenkins, Linington, and Whittaker (1991) report a 40% prevalence of depression with impaired function, but most cases were temporary and resolved with resumption of normal activities and return to work. Wolcott, Wellisch, Fawzy, and Landsverk (1986) also reported that 15% to 20% of bone marrow transplant recipients have a degree of psychological distress that would benefit from intervention. Somerfield, Curbow, Wingard, Baker, and Fogarty (1996) noted a list of most frequently endorsed fears of transplant patients, which included increased vulnerability to illness, uncertain future, reduced energy, and inability to have children. In addition, heightened concern over somatic symptoms led to panic attacks that the cancer is returning. In particular, patients with continuing medical problems were more likely to need help. In addition to routine physical therapy, aerobic training has been tested on patients after high-dose chemotherapy and shown to reduce fatigue and enhanced physical performance (Dimeo et al., 1997).

In summary, patients with leukemia, lymphoma, and myeloma require intensive chemotherapy and, in some cases, repeated hospitalizations, which can lead to a host of psychological and vocational difficulties. Remarkably, most patients adapt well, but significant numbers may benefit from at least temporary counseling and rehabilitation services. The psychological aspects of survivorship need attention as well as physical rehabilitation. Two recent studies show that both physical and emotional recovery after bone marrow transplantation is delayed with psychological symptoms persisting longer. Three to five years are required before most patients have fully recovered and rehabilitative interventions, such as physical, occupational, and psychological therapies, are beneficial to reduce fatigue and improve quality of life (Broers, Kaptein, Le Cessie, Fibbe, & Hengeveld, 2000; Syrjala et al., 2004). Finally, a comprehensive, holistic approach to rehabilitation must be utilized when available, given the profound psychological and behavioral implications of the transplantation process (Steinberg et al., 2015).

DISORDERS OF HEMOSTASIS

Hemostasis is the process by which blood clots in response to injury to the vessels. When a vessel is cut, it may constrict, reducing blood flow and bleeding. Platelets, the blood-clotting cells, then adhere to the open wound and clump together to form a plug. In a highly orchestrated and sequential manner, coagulation factors are activated from an inactive proenzyme form one after another, ultimately resulting in the last coagulation factor fibrinogen (Factor I) converting to fibrin. Fibrin strands mesh with platelets forming a stable clot that will not break down until the vessel repairs itself. Abnormal bleeding may occur when there is a defect in the number or function of the platelets or any of the 13 coagulation factors (Johari & Loke, 2012). Hemophilia A and B are the most common congenital deficiencies of these plasma coagulation proteins. We discuss them in more detail as prototypes of a chronic bleeding disorder.

HEMOPHILIA

Disease Description

As stated previously, there are 13 coagulation factors. Factor XII is activated first, and then a series of factors are converted to their active form. This cascade of activation is stopped or slowed if there is a deficiency of any one factor required to convert the next factor. Mutations of the genes responsible for the proper levels of the coagulation proteins result in their decreased production and impairment of clot formation. Factor VIII is the most common congenital factor deficiency, accounting for 75% of hemophilia. It is a rare disease, however, with an incidence of 1 in 10,000 male births (Williams et al., 1990). A gene on the X chromosome encodes the protein. Hence, males need inherit only one defective gene from the mother to be affected. Females, who have two X chromosomes, are rarely affected.

Hemophilia B, a deficiency of Factor IX, is also an X-linked recessive hemorrhagic disease. It occurs in 1 of 75,000 male births and is clinically indistinguishable from hemophilia A (Williams et al., 1990). The diagnosis of both of these disorders is made by functionally assaying the plasma for the level of either protein compared with normal plasma.

Functional Presentation

The genes controlling production of either Factor VIII or IX on the X-chromosome may have one of many mutations. This can lead to either no production, decreased production, or production of a defective protein. Hence, the patient can present with mild, moderate, or severe hemorrhagic disease, depending on the amount of active protein produced. Activity of the protein is measured in a timed clotting assay and compared with normal plasma. Mothers of hemophilia patients are obligate carriers and have 50% or greater activity. Individuals with mild hemophilia have 6% to 25% activity, rarely bleed spontaneously, and usually are discovered after excessive bleeding secondary to trauma or surgery. Moderately affected individuals have 1% to 5% levels of the active protein and have rare episodes of spontaneous bleeding but can hemorrhage with any trauma. Finally, patients with less than a 1% level have severe disease, with frequent spontaneous hemorrhage from early childhood (Williams et al., 1990). Patients can bleed anywhere, but bleeding into joints (hemarthrosis), soft tissue (such as muscle), urine (hematuria), and the brain are common. Chronic bleeding into joints results in inflammation, scarring, and restriction of movement. Bleeding into the brain or spinal canal can lead to nerve damage with both functional and psychological disabilities.

Treatment and Prognosis

The general principle of treatment of hemophilia is, first, to avoid drugs that can interfere with clotting, particularly aspirin and other nonsteroidal anti-inflammatory agents that inhibit platelet function (Williams et al., 1990). Second, early recognition of bleeding episodes or potential trauma and treatment with replacement Factor VIII or IX is imperative (Oldenburg, 2015). Concentrates of these factors from normal plasma are commercially available. The number of units of coagulation protein infused depends on the initial level of the factor in the patient's plasma and the level of factor desired. Minor trauma or bleeding may require factor levels of only 20% of normal to stop bleeding, whereas major hemorrhage, especially intracranial, will require larger doses to raise levels of the factor to more than 50% of normal (Kasper & Dietrich, 1985; Williams et al., 1990). If surgery is required, Factors VIII and IX must be raised before the operation. Because Factor VIII is degraded in the plasma, half the dose is gone in 8 to 12 hours; treatment is given every 12 hours for several days to allow healing and prevent late hemorrhage. Factor IX has a longer half-life, 18 to 24 hours, and reinfusion can take place less often. In fact, prophylactic replacement for the patient severely affected by hemophilia has become the rule rather than treating only after a bleeding episode.

Prognosis improved with the advent of factor concentrate treatment in the 1960s, with fewer severe bleeds, less crippling arthritis from hemarthrosis, and less intracranial bleeding. Complications of multiple transfusions, such as hepatitis and AIDS, have greatly influenced the prognosis. New preparation techniques have eliminated hepatitis and HIV from Factor VIII concentrates and the risks of infection now is very small. However, many older patients with hemophilia, particularly those who were severely affected and hence needed many transfusions, were infected by HIV in the 1980s and ultimately died of AIDS. Younger patients appear safe from transmission of these viruses because of the new concentrates, and a long-acting Factor VIII and IX are now available allowing for less frequent and hence more convenient administration (Mahlangu et al., 2015; Powell et al., 2013).

Psychological and Vocational Implications

The medical advancement of efficient factor replacement led to a great improvement in the psychosocial aspect of caring for patients with hemophilia. A study from the Netherlands (Rosendaal et al., 1990) showed that most patients consider their health and quality of life no different from that of the general population. In addition, those who were employed had positions consistent with their education. In the older patient, however, joint damage correlated with increased disability and decrease in successful marriage and having children. Twenty-two percent of patients were unemployed and receiving some disability compensation. Vocational training should stress jobs that limit potentially hazardous situations. Patients who are on effective replacement therapy can compete equally for most jobs. It is clear that programs like home therapy slow the rate of progression of arthropathy, and most young patients with hemophilia who are under appropriate medical care can and should be fully employed and lead normal lives (David & Feldman, 2015).

However, the patients who were infected with the AIDS virus during therapy from 1980 to 1985 will require special psychological help and will experience greater disability. Social counseling for sexual partners is imperative. The impact of this tragic complication should be temporary as future patients are protected by the newer generation of coagulation factor replacement products.

SICKLE CELL DISEASE AND THALASSEMIAS

Disease Description

Normal red blood cells have a biconcave shape with a pliable cell membrane and cytoplasm in the center filled with a protein called hemoglobin. This protein is a combination of two alpha-globin chains and two beta-globin chains forming a complex molecule that binds an iron-containing heme molecule in the center, which allows the protein to bind oxygen. Hemoglobin is soluble in the cytoplasm, so the red cell shape can change and thereby squeeze through small vessels to deliver the oxygen to the tissues. Sickle cell disease occurs when both beta chains have one amino acid changed from a glutamic acid to valine in the sixth position of a 146-amino acid chain that makes up the beta-globin protein molecule (Williams et al., 1990). This substitution of one amino acid for another causes lining up of the hemoglobin molecules producing stacking, forming a tubular insoluble structure, and causing the red cell to assume a nonpliable sickle shape. This process occurs only when the hemoglobin molecule has lost the oxygen molecule at the level of the tissue, and it can be reversed by reoxygenating the hemoglobin in the lungs as the blood returns to the left side of the heart. However, permanent membrane change occurs after several cycles of sickling and unsickling, resulting in an irreversibly sickled cell. The resultant cellular defect leads to the main manifestations of disease, which include (a) premature destruction of the cells, called hemolytic anemia, (b) vascular occlusion of vessels (due to plugging of vessels by sickle cells that cannot pass through the small capillaries) and subsequent tissue infarction, and (c) increased susceptibility to infection.

Patients with sickle cell disease are homozygous for the abnormal gene controlling beta-chain production. Hence, both parents must be at least heterozygous for the abnormal gene. The frequency of one abnormal gene in the African America population is 1 in 12, and the incidence of sickle cell anemia is 1 in 650 in African Americans (Williams et al., 1990). Milder forms of this disease can be seen with one sickle beta-gene and either deletion of the other beta-gene (thalassemia) or occurrence of a second type of sickle gene, called sickle C. The latter results from replacement of the glutamic acid by lysine at the sixth position on the beta chain (Rees, Williams, & Gladwin, 2010; Williams et al., 1990).

In contrast to sickle cell anemia where there is a qualitative defect of hemoglobin, thalassemias are a group of genetically inherited hemoglobinopathies characterized by quantitatively reduced or absent synthesis of normal hemoglobin. This is due to a decreased production of alpha chain production in alpha (α) thalassemia or beta chains in beta (β) thalassemia. Beta thalassemia is relatively asymptomatic with one of two beta genes being defective resulting in mild anemia. However, if both genes are inherited missing, the patient cannot produce enough hemoglobin to live, with severe anemia developing at 6 months of age and requiring transfusions for the rest of the patient's life. As the alpha gene is a duplicated gene, everyone has four genes, and even three missing leads to mild-to-moderate anemia called Hb H disease; but four missing is incompatible with life and the child dies in utero owing to lack of hemoglobin (hydrops fetalis). Depending on the defective globin gene involved, patients with defected beta-globin genes have beta-thalassemia, and those with defected alpha-globin genes have alpha-thalassemia (Martin & Thompson, 2013).

Functional Presentation

Patients usually present in the first decade of life with complications of the three main characteristics of sickle cell disorder. As stated earlier, anemia results from hemolysis secondary to irreversible shape change and the quick breakdown of blood cells, with large amounts of hemoglobin being released into the blood, converted into bilirubin, and secreted into the bile. Bile stones develop early, and the clinical picture is that of a patient with anemia, jaundice, and recurrent gallstone attacks. Also, the bone marrow expands, producing extra red blood cells to make up for the anemia, causing bone deformity. This hypercellular marrow is susceptible to vitamin deficiency and viral infection, leading to an abrupt decrease in production, a condition called aplastic crisis (Rees et al., 2010).

The second set of clinical symptoms results from the plugging of small blood vessels by the nonpliable sickle cells termed vaso-occlusive crisis. Infarction of any organ and, in particular, bone, results in a painful crisis. In addition, strokes and cardiac and pulmonary infarction are major complications of the vaso-occlusive crisis. Leg ulcers develop for the same reason, heal poorly because of poor tissue perfusion, and can cause physical disability. In a recent study, children with more severe sickle cell disease and more vascular episodes had language-processing deficits (Schatz, Puffer, Sanchez, Stancil, & Roberts, 2009).

Finally, the spleen, an organ that helps clear certain infectious agents from the blood, shrinks, and is nonfunctional as a result of many infarctions in early childhood. The result is a susceptibility to infections, particularly pneumococcal pneumonia. Another infectious complication results from the combination of devitalized bone and a propensity for *salmonella* to lodge in the diseased gallbladder, leading to seeding of the bone and salmonella osteomyelitis (Rees et al., 2010).

Patients with thalassemia have widely variable clinical presentations, ranging from nearly asymptomatic to severe anemia (beta-thalassemia major) requiring lifelong blood transfusions with complications in multiple organ systems. Patients may present with severe anemia as early as the first 6 months of life when fetal hemoglobin F production declines, as well as abdominal distention from hepatosplenomegaly of extramedullary hematopoiesis. The severity of beta-thalassemia in adults can be described based on blood transfusion requirements. Beta-thalassemia major describes patients who require regular blood transfusions, usually more than 8 to 12 times per year. The consequence of ineffective red cell production is marked erythroid expansion that can cause significant bony abnormalities in long bones and skulls, such as cortical thinning with expansion of the medullary space, which then become prone to pathologic fractures.

To prevent this, the ineffective red cell production is inhibited by chronic transfusions, but this leads to iron overload with damage to the heart and liver resulting in early death. Iron chelators can delay this accumulation but are not entirely effective (Martin & Thompson, 2013).

Treatment and Prognosis

There is no specific treatment for acute manifestations of sickle cell disease; hence, most therapy is supportive in treatment of the complications. Painful crises are treated with fluids, pain medication, and careful search for causes, such as an infection (Charache, 1974). Pain control usually requires narcotics in the acute crisis and doctors have been reluctant to prescribe enough medication because of the manifestation of vaso-occlusive disease, the sociocultural factors in pain assessment, and fears of potential addiction (Lin, Evans, Wakeman, & Unterbrink, 2015; Wright & Adeosum, 2009). This appears to be worse for the patients with more or longer crisis following a hospital admission. A recent study demonstrated that post-discharge pain control and functional limitation outcomes were worse for the group of 2- to 18-year-old patients with sickle cell (Brandow, Brousseau, & Panepinto, 2009) who had more severe crisis. Early recognition of infection, administration of prophylactic antibiotics, and vaccination may forestall or prevent other complications (Scott, 1985). If painful crisis persists or there is infarction of a major organ (brain, lung, or heart), exchange transfusion is performed to remove some of the sickle red cells. Normal red cells are transfused to lower the concentration of sickle hemoglobin to 50% (Charache, 1974). At this level, no significant sludging, further thrombosis, or complications will occur. This effect is temporary; however, as the transfused red cells die and are replaced by patient's own cells with hemoglobin S (Hb S), then symptoms recur. In addition, transfusion carries risks of infection, allergy, and sensitization to donor blood. Hence, this mode of treatment is used only for severe cases.

New approaches to therapy are centered on the reduction of intracellular Hb S concentration and pharmacologic induction of hemoglobin F (Hb F) as a substitute for Hb S (Bunn, 1997). This has resulted in the use of hydroxyurea, an oral chemotherapeutic agent, which can cause an increase in Hb F and reciprocal decrease in Hb S. The decreased concentration of Hb S then leads to reduced sickling and reduction in symptoms. The exposure to chemotherapy and potential complications has limited its use to patients with more frequent and severe attacks. However, the efficacy, safety, and cost-effectiveness of hydroxyurea have been well established (Moore, Charache, Terrin, Barton, & Ballas, 2000). Unfortunately, hydroxyurea is used in less than 25% of patients with sickle cell disease who could benefit from it, according to results from a large-scale epidemiologic study (Stettler, McKierman, Melin, Adejoro, & Walczak, 2015).

The mainstay of therapy for thalassemia remains red blood cell transfusion, which then necessitates iron chelation. The timing of transfusion therapy is largely based on clinical assessment and the impact of anemia on the patient's symptoms, such as impaired growth, bony deformities, and fatigue. Specific transfusion regimens should target pretransfusion hemoglobin of 9 to 10 g/dL. Maintaining this hemoglobin level suppresses endogenous erythropoietin levels and reduces marrow expansion and extramedullary hematopoiesis. Most patients will require 10 to 20 mL/kg of packed red blood cells every 2 to 4 weeks to maintain this goal (Martin & Thompson, 2013).

Bone marrow transplantation and possible gene therapy, in which the normal beta-globin gene is placed in the patient's stem cell, remain the only curative treatment for sickle cell disease and thalassemia, but many technical hurdles still remain and the potential for transplantation-related mortality, graft rejection, and graft-versus-host disease is high (King & Shenoy, 2014). Prognosis has improved with good supportive care, particularly in pediatric mortality although the reduction in the last 20 years is less for older children (Yanni, Grosse, Yang, & Olney, 2009). However, frequent admissions for painful crisis, the complication of sickle cell disease, narcotic use and abuse due to chronic pain, and absence from school and work lead to significant psychological and vocational problems.

Psychological and Vocational Implications

Several authors have documented the psychological impact on a patient with chronic painful disease (Barrett et al., 1988; Damlouji, Kevess-Cohen,

Charache, Georgopoulos, & Folstein, 1982). In one study, the findings suggested that a relationship between the chronicity and dependence on the medical care system was the best predictor of psychosocial functioning (Damlouji et al., 1982). Others have shown links between medical complications and psychopathology (Barrett et al., 1988). The psychological impact can include drug addiction, hysterical conversion reaction, and malingering, as well as low self-esteem, dependency, and depression (Barrett et al., 1988). Likewise, depression, anxiety, and somatic comorbidities have been shown to be associated with poor physical and mental health–related quality of life among patients with beta-thalassemia (Azarkeivan et al., 2009).

Adolescents with sickle cell disease and thalassemia must deal with defining their personal identity along with their chronic illness. Delays in sexual maturation and adolescent growth spurt contribute to poor self-image. Physical limitations, particularly in sports, also lead to low self-esteem. Fifteen percent of patients between the ages of 13 and 40 have been reported to be depressed (Kinney & Ware, 1996). Osteoporosis, fracture, and bone pain occur in 46%, 36%, and 34%, respectively, of patients with thalassemia (Vogiatzi et al., 2009).

Physical limitations stemming from stroke in childhood, along with decreased IQ (Hariman, Griffith, Hartig, & Keehn, 1991) and medical complications, may contribute to both psychosocial and vocational limitations. The greatest dysfunction was found in areas of employment, finances, sleep habits, and performance of daily activities (Barrett et al., 1988). Hence, the implications of these findings suggest a strong need for vocational rehabilitation services, training in areas of communication and self-esteem (Barrett et al., 1988), medical treatment, and psychological help for depression and drug dependence. The prevalence of this disease in the Black population, who are chronically underserved by the health care system and the difficulty of obtaining affordable insurance, as well as maintaining a job with insurance benefits, has necessitated development of a national policy to pay for the costs and develop treatments for these patients (Nietert, Silverstein, & Abboud, 2002).

A national sickle cell disease program with regional centers has been established to provide the comprehensive care required (Scott, 1985). The centers provide cost-effective day treatment to handle the majority of patient complaints that are neither emergent nor life-threatening. The physical and psychological damage from repeated painful crises require continued care as an outpatient, and the mission of these centers is also to provide psychological, rehabilitative, and vocational services for the patient and family (Koshy & Dorn, 1996). However, not all patients, especially adult and young adolescent patients, receive state-of-the-art care, and the National Heart, Lung, and Blood Institute and the U.S. Department of Health and Human Services announced a sickle cell disease initiative in 2011 to increase access to health care systems and providers and to improve coordination of care in a "medical home" (www.nhlbi.nih.gov/about/directorscorner/messages/hhs-announces-sickle-cell-disease-initiative). A comprehensive overview and management guideline has been developed as a result (Yawn et al., 2014).

REFERENCES

Alibhai, S. M. H., Leach, M., Gupta, V., Tomlinson, G. A., Brandwein, J. M., Saiz, F. S., & Minden, M. D. (2009). Quality of Life beyond 6 months after diagnosis in older adults with acute myeloid leukemia. *Critical Reviews in Oncology-Hematology, 69*, 168–174.

Azarkeivan, A., Hajibeigi, B., Alavian, S. M., Lankarani, M. M., & Assari, S. (2009). Associates of poor physical and mental health-related quality of life in beta thalassemia-major/intermedia. *Research Journal of Medical Sciences, 14*, 349–355.

Barrett, D. H., Wisotzek, I. E., Abel, G. G., Rouleau, J. L., Platt, A. F., Pollard, W. E., & Eckman, J. R. (1988). Assessment of psychosocial functioning of patients with sickle cell disease. *Southern Medical Journal, 81*, 745–750.

Berdeja, J. G. (2003). Immunotherapy of lymphoma: Update and review of the literature [Review]. *Current Opinion in Oncology, 15*, 363–370.

Berman, E. (1997). Recent advances in the treatment of acute leukemia. *Current Opinion in Hematology, 4*, 256–260.

Brandow, A. M., Brousseau, D. C., & Panepinto, J. A. (2009). Post discharge pain, functional limitations and impact on caregivers of children with sickle cell disease treated for painful events. *British Journal of Haematology, 144*, 782–788.

Brissot, E., & Mohty, M. (2015). Which acute myeloid leukemia patients should be offered transplantation? *Seminar Hematology, 52*, 223–231.

Broers, S., Kaptein, A. A., Le Cessie, S., Fibbe, W., & Hengeveld, M. W. (2000). Psychological functioning and quality of life following bone marrow transplantation: A 3-year follow-up study. *Journal of Psychosomatic Research, 48*, 11–21.

Bunn, H. F. (1997). Pathogenesis and treatment of sickle cell disease. *New England Journal of Medicine, 337*, 762–769.

Charache, S. (1974). The treatment of sickle cell anemia. *Archives of Internal Medicine, 133*, 698–705.

Corre, J., Munshi, N., & Avet-Loiseau, H. (2015). Genetics of multiple myeloma: Another heterogeneity level? *Blood, 125*, 1870–1876.

Daiter, S., Larson, R. A., Weddington, W. W., & Ultmann, J. E. (1988). Psychosocial symptomatology, personal growth and development among young adult patients following the diagnosis of leukemia or lymphoma. *Journal of Clinical Oncology, 6*, 613–617.

Damlouji, N. F., Kevess-Cohen, R., Charache, S., Georgopoulos, A., & Folstein, M. F. (1982). Social disability and psychiatric morbidity in sickle cell anemia and diabetes patients. *Psychosomatics, 23*, 925–931.

David, J. A., & Feldman, B. M. (2015). Assessing activities, participation, and quality of life in hemophilia: Relevance, current limitations, and possible options. *Seminars in Thrombosis and Hemostasis, 41*, 894–900.

DeVita, V. T., Hellman, S., & Rosenberg, S. A. (Eds.). (1989). *Cancer: Principles and practice of oncology* (3rd ed.). Philadelphia, PA: J. B. Lippincott.

Dimeo, F. C., Tilmann, M. H., Bertz, H., Kanz, L., Mertelsmann, R., & Keul, J. (1997). Aerobic exercise in the rehabilitation of cancer patients after high dose chemotherapy and autologous peripheral stem cell transplantation. *Cancer, 79*, 1717–1722.

Fanale, M. A., & Younes, A. (2007). Monoclonal antibodies in the treatment of non-Hodgkin's lymphoma. *Drugs, 67*, 333–350.

Fisher, R., Leblanc, M., Press, O. W., Maloney, D. G., Unger, J. M., & Miller, T. P. (2005). New treatment options have changed the survival of patients with follicular lymphoma. *Journal of Clinical Oncology, 23*, 8447–8452.

Fobair, P., Hoppe, R. T., Bloom, J. R., Cox, R., Varghese, A., & Spiegle, D. (1986). Psychosocial problems among survivors of Hodgkin's Disease. *Journal of Clinical Oncology, 4*, 805–814.

Frankfurt, O., Licht, J. D., & Tallman, M. S. (2007). Molecular characterization of acute myeloid leukemia and its impact on treatment. *Current Opinion in Oncology, 19*, 635–649.

Freedman, A. (2015). Follicular lymphoma: 2015 updates on diagnosis and management. *American Journal of Hematology, 90*, 1171–1178.

Friedberg, J. W., & Chengazi, V. (2003). PET scans in the staging of lymphoma: Current status. *Oncologist, 8*, 438–447.

Gale, R. P., & Foon, K. A. (1987). Therapy of acute myologenous leukemia. *Seminars in Hematology, 24*, 40–54.

Greipp, P. R., San Miguel, J., Durie, B. G., Crowley, J. J., Barlogie, B., Bladé, J., . . . Westin, J. (2005). International staging system for multiple myeloma. *Journal of Clinical Oncology, 23*, 3412–3420.

Han, X., Kilfoy, B., Zheng, T., Holford, T. R., Zhu, C., Zhu, Y., & Zhang, Y. (2008). Lymphoma survival patterns by WHO subtype in the United States, 1973–2003. *Cancer Causes & Control, 19*, 841–858.

Hariman, L. M. P., Griffith, E. R., Hartig, A. L., & Keehn, M. T. (1991). Functional outcomes of children with sickle-cell disease affected by stroke. *Archives of Physical Medicine and Rehabilitation, 12*, 498–502.

Hoelzer, D., & Gale, R. P. (1987). Acute lymphoblastic leukemia in adults: Recent progress, future directions. *Seminars in Hematology, 24*, 27–39.

Hsu, F. J., Caspor, C. B., Czerwinski, D., Kwak, L. W., Liles, T. M., Syrengelas, A., . . . Levy, R. (1997). Tumor-specific idiotype vaccines in the treatment of patients with B-cell lymphoma: Long term results of a clinical trial. *Blood, 89*, 3129–3135.

The International Non-Hodgkin's Lymphoma Prognostic Factors Project. (1993). A predictive model for aggressive Non-Hodgkin's Lymphoma. *The New England Journal of Medicine, 329*, 987–994.

Jenkins, P. L., Linington, A., & Whittaker, J. A. (1991). A retrospective study of psychosocial morbidity in bone marrow transplant recipients. *Psychosomatics, 32*, 65–71.

Johari, V., & Loke, C. (2012). Brief overview of the coagulation cascade. *Disease Month, 58*, 421–423.

Kadia, T. M., Ravandi, F., O'Brien, S., Cortes, J., & Kantarjian, H. M. (2015). Progress in acute myeloid leukemia. *Clinical Lymphoma, Myeloma & Leukemia, 15*, 139–151.

Kasper, C. K., & Dietrich, S. L. (1985). Comprehensive management of hemophilia. *Clinics in Haematology, 14*, 489–512.

King, A., & Shenoy, S. (2014). Evidence-based focused review of the status of hematopoietic stem cell transplantation as treatment of sickle cell disease and thalassemia. *Blood, 123*, 3089–3094.

King, M. E., & Rowe, J. M. (2007). Recent developments in acute myelogenous leukemia therapy. *The Oncologist, 12*, 14–21.

Kinney, T. R., & Ware, R. E. (1996). The adolescent with sickle cell anemia. *Hematology-Oncology Clinics of North America, 10*, 1255–1264.

Koshy, M., & Dorn, L. (1996). Continuing care for adult patients with sickle cell disease [Review]. *Hematology-Oncology Clinics of North America, 10*, 1265–1273.

Lin, R. J., Evans, A. T., Wakeman, K., & Unterbrink, M. (2015). A mixed-methods study of pain-related quality of life in sickle cell vaso-occlusive crises. *Hemoglobin, 39*, 305–309.

Magrath, I., Adde, M., Shad, A., Venzon, D., Seibel, N., Gootenberg, J., . . . Horak, I. D. (1996). Adults and children with small non-cleaved-cell lymphoma have a similar excellent outcome when treated with the same chemotherapy regimen. *Journal of Oncology, 14*, 925–934.

Mahlangu, J., Powell, J. S., Ragni, M. V., Chowdary, P., Josephson, N. C., Pabinger, I., . . . Pierce, G. F. (2015). Phase 3 study of recombinant factor VIII Fc fusion protein in severe hemophilia A. *Blood, 123*, 317–325.

Martin, A., & Thompson A. A. (2013). Thalassemias. *Pediatric Clinics of North America, 60*, 1383–1391.

Matasar, M. J., & Zelenetz, A. D. (2008). Overview of lymphoma diagnosis and management. *Radiologic Clinics of North America, 46*, 175–198.

Michallet, A. S., & Coiffier, B. (2009). Recent developments on the treatment of aggressive non-Hodgkin Lymphoma. *Blood Reviews, 23*, 11–23.

Moore, R. D., Charache, S., Terrin, M. L., Barton, F. B., & Ballas, S. K. (2000). Cost-effectiveness of hydroxyurea in sickle cell anemia. Investigators of the multicenter study of hydroxyurea in sickle cell anemia. *American Journal of Hematology, 64*, 26–31.

Moreau, P., Attal, M., & Facon, T. (2015). Frontline therapy of multiple myeloma. *Blood, 125*, 3076–3084.

Mulhern, R. K., Friedman, A. G., & Stone, P. A. (1988). Acute lymphoblastic leukemia: Long-term psychological outcome [Review]. *Biomedicine & Pharmacotherapy, 42*, 243–246.

Nietert, P. J., Silverstein, M. D., & Abboud, M. R. (2002). Sickle cell anaemia: Epidemiology and cost of illness. *Pharmacoeconomics, 20*(6), 357–366.

Oldenburg, J. (2015). Optimal treatment strategies for hemophilia: Achievements and limitations of current prophylactic regimens. *Blood, 125*, 2038–2044.

Penson, R. T., Rauch, P. K., McAfee, S. L., Cashavelly, B. J., Clair-Hayes, K., Dahlin, C., . . . Lynch, T. J., Jr. (2002). Between parent and child: Negotiating cancer treatment in adolescents. *The Oncologist, 7*, 154–162.

Philip, T., Guglielmi, C., Hagenbeek, A., Somers, R., Van Der Lelie, H., Bron, D., . . . Chauvin, F. (1995). Autologous bone marrow transplantation as compared with salvage chemotherapy in relapses of chemo-sensitive non-Hodgkin's lymphoma. *The New England Journal of Medicine, 330*, 1540–1545.

Powell, J. S., Pasi, K. J., Ragni, M. V., Ozelo, M. C., Valentino, L. A., Mahlangu, J. N., . . . B-LONG Investigators. (2013). Phase 3 study of recombinant factor IX Fc fusion protein in hemophilia B. *The New England Journal of Medicine, 369*, 2313–2323.

Raab, M., Podar, K., Breitkreutz, I., Richardson, P. G., & Anderson, K. C. (2009). Multiple myeloma. *The Lancet, 374*, 324–339.

Rajkumar, S. V., Dimopoulos, M. A., Palumbo, A., Blade, J., Merlini, G., Mateos, M., . . . San Miguel, J. F. (2015). International myeloma working group updated criteria for the diagnosis of multiple myeloma. *The Lancet Oncology, 15*, e538–e548.

Raphael, B. G., & Knowles, D. M. (1990). Acquired immunodeficiency syndrome-associated non-Hodgkin's lymphoma. *Seminars in Oncology, 17*, 361–366.

Rees, D. C., Williams, T. N., & Gladwin, M. T. (2010). Sickle-cell disease. *The Lancet, 376*, 2018–2031.

Rosenberg, S. A. (Chairman). (1982). National cancer institute sponsored study of classifications of non-Hodgkin's lymphomas: Summary and description of a working formulation for clinical usage. *Cancer, 49*, 2112–2135.

Rosendaal, F. R., Smit, C., Varekamp, L., Bröcker-Vriends, A. H., Van Dijck, H., Saurmeijer, T. P., . . . Briët, E. (1990). Modern hemophilia treatment: Medical improvements and quality of life. *Journal of Internal Medicine, 228*, 633–640.

Ruthoven, J. J. (1987). Current approaches to the treatment of advanced-stage non-Hodgkin's lymphoma. *Canadian Medical Association Journal, 136*, 29–36.

Schatz, J., Puffer, E. S., Sanchez, C., Stancil, M., & Roberts, C. W. (2009). Language processing deficits in sickle cell disease in young school-age children. *Developmental Neuropsychology, 34*, 122–136.

Schouten, H. C. (2007). Diagnosis, staging and prognostic factors. *Annals of Oncology, 18*(Suppl. 1), i22–i28.

Scott, R. B. (1985). Advances in the treatment of sickle cell disease in children. *American Journal of Diseases of Children, 139*, 1219–1222.

Sekeres, M. A., Stone, R. M., Zahrieh, D., Neuberg, D., Morrison, V., De Angelo, D. J., . . . Lee, S. J. (2004). Decision-making and quality of life in older adults with acute myeloid leukemia or advanced myelodysplastic syndrome. *Leukemia, 18*, 809–816.

Shankland, K. R., Armitage, J. O., & Hancock, B. W. (2012). Non-Hodgkin lymphoma. *The Lancet, 380*, 848–857.

Shlush, L., & Michell, A. (2015). AML evolution from preleukemia to leukemia and relapse. *Best Practice & Research Clinical Haematology, 28*, 81–89.

Skarin, A. T. (1989). Non-Hodgkin's lymphoma. *Archives of Internal Medicine, 34*, 209–242.

Somerfield, M. R., Curbow, B., Wingard, J. R., Baker, F., & Fogarty, L. A. (1996). Coping with the physical and psychosocial sequelae of bone marrow transplantation among long-term survivors. *Journal of Behavioral Medicine, 19*, 163–184.

Stettler, N., McKierman, C. M., Melin, C. Q., Adejoro, O. O., & Walczak, N. B. (2015). Proportions of adults with sickle cell anemia and pain crises receiving hydroxyurea. *Journal of the American Medical Association, 313*, 1671–1672.

Steinberg, A., Asher, A., Bailey, C., & Fu, J. B. (2015). The role of physical rehabilitation in stem cell transplantation patients. *Support Care Cancer, 23*, 2447–2460.

Syrjala, K. L., Langer, S. L., Abrams, J. R., Storer, B., Sanders, J. E., Flowers, M. E., & Martin, P. J. (2004). Recovery and long-term function after hematopoietic cell transplantation for leukemia or lymphoma. *Journal of the American Medical Association, 291*, 2335–2343.

Swerdlow, S. H., Campo, E., Harris, N. L., Jaffe, E. S., Pileri, S. A., Stein, H., . . . Vardiman, J. W. (2008). *WHO classification of tumors of haematopoietic and lymphoid tissues* (4th ed.). Lyon, France: IARC Press.

Vardiman, J. W., Thiele, J., Arber, D. A., Brunning, R. D., Borowitz, M. J., Porwit, A., . . . Bloomfield, C. D. (2009). The 2008 revision of the World Health Organization (WHO) classification of myeloid neoplasms and acute leukemia: rationale and important changes. *Blood, 114*, 937–951.

Vogiatzi, M. G., Macklin, E. A., Fung, E. B., Cheung, A. M., Vichinsky, E., Olivieri, N., . . . Giardina, P. J. (2009). Bone disease in thalassemia: A frequent and still unresolved problem. *Journal of Bone and Mineral Research, 24*, 543–557.

Williams, W. J., Butler, E., Ersley, A. J., & Lichtman, M. A. (Eds.). (1990). *Hematology* (4th ed.). New York, NY: McGraw-Hill.

Wolcott, D. L., Wellisch, D. K., Fawzy, F. I., & Landsverk, J. (1986). Adaptation of adult bone marrow transplant recipient long-term survivors. *Transplantation, 41*, 478–484.

Wright, K., & Adeosum, O. (2009). Barriers to effective pain management in sickle cell disease. *British Journal of Nursing, 18*, 158–161.

Yanni, E., Grosse, S. D., Yang, Q., & Olney, R. S. (2009). Trends in pediatric sickle cell disease-related mortality in the United States 1983–2000. *Journal of Pediatrics, 154*, 541–545.

Yawn, B. P., Buchanan, G. R., Afenyi-Annan, A. N., Ballas, S. K., Hassell, K. L., James, A. H., . . . John-Sowah, J. (2014). Management of sickle cell disease: Summary of the 2014 evidence-based report by expert panel members. *Journal of the American Medical Association, 312*, 1033–1048.

CHAPTER

Developmental Disabilities

Kristin C. Thompson, Richard J. Morris, and Yvonne P. Morris

Research related to developmental disabilities can be traced back to the 1820s and the work of Jean Itard, a French physician, and his attempts to educate Victor, the Wild Boy of Aveyron (Humphrey, 1962). Victor was a child who had been found living in the woods, and having little language or other developmentally appropriate skills. Although it was unknown how long Victor was living in the woods, it was thought that he was between 9 and 12 years old and had lived in the woods for the majority of his life (Harlan, 1976). According to Humphrey (1962), Itard believed that Victor's condition could be cured, as Itard felt that the cause of Victor's "apparent subnormality" was his lack of experience and social interactions that form an integral part of development. He placed Victor under his care for 5 years at the Paris institution where he worked. Although Victor improved over this period, he did not achieve Itard's initial expectations and predictions of becoming "normal." Nevertheless, Itard's work with Victor was fundamental to further work and research in developmental delays and disabilities.

Itard's work influenced the writings, research, and treatment practices of a number of early practitioners and researchers in the field of developmental disabilities, notably Edouard Seguin. Their writings, in turn, led directly to the building of residential schools and facilities in the United States for individuals having intellectual or other developmental disabilities. The first facility was established in Watertown, Massachusetts, in 1848, as part of the Perkins Institution for the Blind (Macmillan, 1982), and the second was built in Syracuse, New York, in 1851, as an independent facility for people with intellectual and other developmental disabilities. Although the primary residents of these facilities were children, adults and adolescents were also placed in these institutions. These persons, as well as those across the country who manifested similar characteristics, were over the next 100 years, formally referred to as "feebleminded" or, in later years, as "mentally defective." In addition to these general diagnostic labels, more specific levels of "feebleminded" and "mentally defective" were given depending on an individual's level of intellectual functioning. Specifically, "idiot" was a category of feeblemindedness for those with the very lowest level of intellectual functioning, "imbeciles" were in the middle range of intellectual impairment, and "morons" were those who were in the mild range of intellectual impairment (Kanner, 1948).

Seguin and others (e.g., Samuel Howe) intended for residential schools and facilities to be established on an experimental basis as educational institutions (versus being custodial asylums), their thought being that this type of intervention could allow for intensive training and education in skills to function adequately in society, and then these individuals would return to their original homes within the community (Morris & Kratochwill, 2008). Unfortunately, few individuals who entered these institutions were ever returned to their community, and by the beginning of the 20th century, the educational schools became instead state custodial institutions (Baumeister, 1970; Blatt, 1984; Kanner, 1964; Morris & Kratochwill, 2008; Wolfensberger, 1972). This custodial emphasis began to change in the late 1960s and early 1970s with positive developments in the deinstitutionalization and normalization movements (e.g., Blatt, 1968; Blatt & Kaplan, 1966; Nirje, 1969; Wolfensberger, 1969, 1972), legal advocacy for individuals having an intellectual disability (e.g., Friedman, 1975; *Halderman v. Pennhurst*, 1977; *New York State Association for Retarded Children v. Rockefeller*, 1973; *Pennsylvania Association for Retarded Children v. Commonwealth of*

Pennsylvania, 1971; *Wyatt v. Stickney*, 1971), and the introduction of behavior modification and applied behavior analysis treatment procedures (e.g., Ayllon & Azrin, 1968; Baer, Wolf, & Risley, 1968; Gardner, 1971; Kazdin, 1975; Lovaas & Bucher, 1974; Morris, 1976; Schaefer & Martin, 1969; Thompson & Grabowski, 1972; Watson, 1973).

The deinstitutionalization movement was successful in reducing the number of individuals with disabilities living in custodial institutions, with there being a nearly 95% decline of people being cared for in state psychiatric facilities since the 1950s (Torrey, Fuller, Geller, Jacobs, & Rogasta, 2012). However, some writers maintain that this decline was not the result of adequate interventions being provided but, rather, to a type of "transinstitutionalization" in which the care of these individuals had merely been transferred to short-term institutions, such as medical hospitals, nursing homes and long-term care facilities, or even correctional facilities (Sisti, Segal, & Emanuel, 2015).

DESCRIPTION OF DISABILITY

As described by the American Psychiatric Association (APA), developmental disabilities encompass a wide range of diagnostic conditions, each of which is manifested in individuals before 22 years of age (APA, 2013). Behaviors and impairments are typically observed early in the individual's life, often during infancy or early childhood, with the presence of a developmental disability typically reflecting differences in the way a child develops intellectual, language, mobility, and/or social and emotional skills. Hallmark symptoms associated with a developmental disability typically involve a child not meeting early developmental milestones, such as walking or talking within the typical age range. Major forms of developmental disabilities include intellectual disability, autism spectrum disorder, cerebral palsy, and spina bifida (Boyle et al., 2011).

While some symptoms may decrease over an individual's life span, the impairments related to a developmental disability are considered to be chronic or lifelong, requiring services and interventions over extended periods of time or even the lifetime (APA, 2013). Some of the common characteristics that are often found in persons with developmental disabilities are functional limitations in some or most of the following areas: self-care and self-help skills, receptive and/or expressive language, cognition and learning ability, mobility, self-direction, economic independence, and the ability to live independently without assistance (APA, 2013; Developmental Disabilities Act, 1984; Developmental Disabilities Assistance and Bill of Rights Act, 2000). In addition, many individuals with a developmental disability are characterized as scoring in the significantly below average range on standardized intelligence tests. This chapter focuses on two broad types of developmental disabilities, namely, intellectual disability and autism spectrum disorder.

FUNCTIONAL PRESENTATION

Intellectual Disability

In 1959, the American Association of Mental Deficiency—now called the American Association on Intellectual and Developmental Disabilities (AAIDD)—defined an intellectual disability in terms of a person's level of intelligence and level of adaptive behavior. This definition has been modified and revised over the years, with the AAIDD currently defining an intellectual disability as follows: "Intellectual disability is characterized by significant limitations in both intellectual functioning and in adaptive behavior as expressed in conceptual, social, and practical adaptive skills. This disability originates before age 18" (Schalock et al., 2010, p. 1). The APA's *Diagnostic and Statistical Manual for Mental Disorders, Fifth Edition* (*DSM-5*; 2013), provides a similar definition of intellectual disability, although it does not provide a specific age requirement but rather specifies that the symptoms/impairments must have begun during the developmental period. The definition of intellectual disability reflects the multidimensional underpinnings of the disability, including the need for deficits in both intellectual and adaptive functioning. Consistent with good testing practice, the evaluation of intellectual and adaptive functioning should be assessed within the context of environmental and personal factors, including culture, race and ethnicity, linguistic diversity, and sensory, motor, and behavioral factors.

Intelligence refers to overall mental ability, including capacity to solve and learn. Limitations in intellectual functioning are generally assessed through the use of individually administered, standardized IQ tests. In general, scores that are two or more standard deviations below the mean are typically viewed as falling into the intellectual disability range (Schalock et al., 2010). As most IQ tests have a mean of 100 and a standard deviation of 15, the requisite IQ score for a diagnosis of intellectual disability is generally accepted to be 70 or lower. Given that IQ assessment instruments have a degree of error of measurement associated with them (typically, plus or minus five points), the ceiling IQ score for intellectual disability is generally considered to be 75, with IQ being reported as a confidence band (e.g., scores between 65 and 75) rather than as a finite score (Schalock et al., 2010). It is important to note, however, the while the AAIDD provides a range of IQ scores to guide the diagnosis of intellectual disability, the *DSM-5* (APA, 2013) no longer provides this same guideline. For example, the *DSM-5* generically states in its diagnostic criteria for intellectual disability that intellectual impairment must be present, while in a later discussion it indicates that the intellectual impairment is typically considered to be an IQ that is around or lower than 70. Specifically, the *DSM-5* states that "Individuals with intellectual disability have scores of approximately two standard deviations or more below the population mean, including a margin for measurement error . . ." (APA, 2013, p. 37).

Adaptive behavior is defined by the AAIDD (Schalock et al., 2010) as the conceptual, social, and practical skills people use in order to function in their everyday lives. Conceptual skills include communication skills, money and calculation skills, and self-direction. Social skills include interpersonal skills and the ability to understand and follow rules and laws. Practical skills include skills in personal and instrumental activities of daily living (e.g., meal preparation, travel, health care, safety), as well as job-related skills (Schalock et al., 2010). Measurement of adaptive behavior typically occurs through direct observation of the individual in situations where these skills are required, by interviewing those who know the individual well (e.g., parent or other caregiver), or through a combination of these procedures.

Adaptive behavior is also commonly assessed through the use of standardized tests of adaptive behavior that have been normed on the general population, subsequently providing an estimate of the individual's adaptive skills in comparison to the individual's same-age peer group. Limitation in adaptive functioning is typically conceptualized as scores on standardized tests that are two or more standard deviations below the mean for overall adaptive skills, or for at least one of the three types of adaptive functioning (i.e., conceptual, social, or practical skills; APA, 2013; Schalock et al., 2010). Two instruments that are commonly used to assess adaptive behavior in persons who may have an intellectual disability are the Vineland Adaptive Behavior Scales, Second Edition (VABS; Sparrow, Cicchetti, & Balla, 2005) and Adaptive Behavior Assessment System, Third Edition (ABAS; Harrison & Oakland, 2015).

■ Severity Levels

Intellectual disability has traditionally been divided into levels of severity, with these levels linked to the individual's level of intellectual functioning or IQ score. In the early 1900s, Henry Goddard, a psychologist who strongly advocated for standardized intellectual assessments, first proposed a classification system for intellectual disability based on the Binet–Simon concept of mental age (Binet & Simon, 1916). With this classification system, individuals having an intellectual disability with the lowest mental age level (less than 3 years of age) were classified as idiots. Imbeciles had a mental age of 3 to 7 years, and morons had a mental age between 7 and 10 years (Binet & Simon, 1916).

In the 1950s, Heber (1959) developed a classification system based on deficits in measured intelligence and adaptive behavior (personal-social and sensory-motor). This system, however, proved unworkable, and in 1961 Heber revised the intellectual disability classification manual, linking severity classification to an IQ score on the Stanford Binet Intelligence Scale (Heber, 1961). Specific categories included borderline (IQ range of 68–83), mild (IQ range of 52–67), moderate (IQ range of 36–51), severe (IQ range of 20–35), and profound (IQ below 20). A subsequent revision in the categories reduced the categories to four levels of intellectual disability: mild, moderate, severe, and profound (Grossman, 1983). In 1968, the APA's *Diagnostic and Statistical Manual of Mental*

Disorders, Second Edition (*DSM-II*; APA, 1968) also linked IQ scores to level of severity of the intellectual disability and had similar classification categories as reported by Heber.

The *DSM-5* (APA, 2013) defines intellectual disability similar to more recent *DSM* editions in that it requires both impairments in intellectual and adaptive functioning; however, guidelines have changed so that the level of severity is *not* determined based on IQ score but rather on the deficits in one's adaptive functioning and subsequent level of support required (see Table 12.1). This change has served to deemphasize the impact of a person's specific IQ score, which is important as it is more difficult to obtain a reliable IQ score for significantly impaired individuals, and IQ has not been found to be perfectly correlated with the level of support an individual may need. Categorizing severity based on level of support needed is also more in line with current recommendations from the AAIDD. In this regard, beginning in 1992, the AAIDD proposed a reconceptualization of the levels of severity of intellectual disability based on intensities of support a person required in order to function successfully in society (Luckasson et al., 2002). These recommendations were not widely accepted for several years, as they were not in line with many state and federal policies regarding how severity was defined and support services subsequently provided. The AAIDD categories for level of support are listed and described in Table 12.2.

There has long been some level of disagreement in the literature regarding the most appropriate method of diagnosing the severity level of an intellectual disability, particularly given the impact that the designated level of severity may have on the individual qualifying for local, state, and federal services (e.g., Conyers, Martin, Martin, & Yu, 2002; Luckasson et al., 2002). The extent of disagreement has been mediated, in part, with the *DSM-5* eliminating IQ score as the primary identifying factor, and both the *DSM-5* and AAIDD focusing on the level of impairment in an individual's skills rather than on a specific IQ score representing the individual's level of need. Nevertheless, some professionals maintain that the categorical approach of *DSM-5* to classifying the severity of intellectual disability remains flawed because it fails to view a person's need on a continuum (Schalock et al., 2010).

Etiology and Prevalence

It is estimated that the prevalence of intellectual disabilities in the general population of the United States is approximately 1% (APA, 2013). Prevalence rates for students in U.S. public schools who receive special education services have dropped significantly over the past 25 years to less than 1% of the student population (U.S. Department of Education, 2014). This decline may reflect increased differentiation of these students from others who have overlapping disabilities (e.g., autism), a reluctance on the part of school administrators to diagnose a mild intellectual disability, and/or an increased use of nondiagnostic multicategorical classrooms (Harris, 2005). Globally, prevalence rates for intellectual disability range from 1%

TABLE 12.1

INTELLECTUAL DISABILITY SEVERITY LEVEL AND ASSOCIATED DESCRIPTION OF LEVEL OF ADAPTIVE FUNCTIONING

Severity Level	Description of Adaptive Functioning Impairment
Mild	Difficulty learning, poor higher-level thinking skills, difficulty with abstract thinking; weak money management; difficulty reading social cues and understanding social situations; vocational training needed
Moderate	Limited academic skills; limited language skills, enough to impact the development of relationships; difficulty working without support; needs prompts for daily life activities
Severe	Little understanding of math; inability or very limited ability to read; speech in single words or short phrases; requires support for all daily activities (e.g., eating, dressing, personal hygiene); cannot work
Profound	No academic skills; typically nonverbal; requires continuous support for all daily activities

Source: Adapted from APA (2013).

TABLE 12.2

DEFINITION AND EXAMPLES OF AMERICAN ASSOCIATION ON INTELLECTUAL AND DEVELOPMENTAL DISABILITIES (AAIDD) INTENSITIES OF SUPPORTS

Level of Support	Description
Intermittent	Provided on an "as needed" basis. Characterized by the individual needing additional support during times of transition, crisis, or other times of uncertainty (e.g., job loss or acute medical crisis).
Limited	This level of support is for individuals with intellectual disabilities who have the ability to improve their adaptive functioning skills if provided appropriate education and training (e.g., vocational training). The type of support may change, but the intensity is consistent over time.
Extensive	This level provides ongoing, daily support in at least some environments (e.g., work, school, and/or home), and it is long term.
Pervasive	This level of support is characterized by its high level of intensity and constancy. This is the most intense level of support and would entail providing daily interventions to help the individual function and survive, and applies to nearly every aspect of the individual's routine (e.g., feeding, dressing, personal hygiene).

Source: Adapted from Schalock et al. (2010).

to 5%, with it being suggested that prevalence rates vary across the globe based on socioeconomic status and age (Maulik, Mascarenhas, Mathers, Dua, & Saxena, 2011). Interestingly, although there is a lack of consensus regarding how to define the level of severity of an intellectual disability (i.e., defining severity via IQ score, level of adaptive functioning, or a combination of IQ and adaptive functioning), research has shown that the use of IQ score alone can be appropriately used for determining the prevalence of intellectual disability in a population (Obi, Van Naarden Braun, Drews-Botsch, Devine, & Yeargin-Allsopp, 2011).

In regard to classification of intellectual disability, mild intellectual disability is the most commonly diagnosed category, with it being suggested that as many as 85% of those people diagnosed as having an intellectual disability fall within this category. Approximately 10% of individuals with intellectual disability are classified as being in the moderate range, 3% to 4% are in the severe range, and 1% to 2% are classified as being in the profound range (APA, 2013).

An appreciable amount of research has been devoted to determining the causes of intellectual disabilities, with several causes of intellectual disability being identified. The three major known causes of intellectual disability are Down syndrome, fetal alcohol syndrome, and fragile X syndrome (Boyle et al., 2011); however, there are hundreds of other factors that have been identified as contributing to intellectual disability. For example, the Online Mendelian Inheritance in Man (OMIM) database lists over 1,000 genetic conditions that are associated with intellectual disabilities (OMIM, 2016). In addition to these latter genetic conditions, other causal factors that have been identified include problems during pregnancy that interfere with brain development in utero (e.g., preeclampsia, infections, malnutrition, fetal alcohol syndrome, drug use), problems during childbirth (e.g., being deprived of oxygen for an extended period of time), and early childhood infections (e.g., meningitis). It has been estimated that approximately 50% of the cases involving intellectual disability are due to genetic causes and the rest are due to environmental impacts (Winnepenninckx, Rooms, & Kooy, 2003).

As a general rule, the more severe the intellectual disability, the more likely it is that the intellectual disability can be attributable to an identifiable medical or physical condition; however, the actual cause is often identified in less than half of all reported cases (McDermott, Durkin, Schupf, & Stein, 2007). For known cases, prenatal factors (e.g., Down syndrome, maternal alcohol consumption) are implicated as causal factors more often than are perinatal (e.g., hypoxia, fetal malnutrition, various infections) or postnatal (e.g., head injury, malnutrition, seizure disorder) factors (Handen, 2007; Matson, Terlonge, & Minshawi, 2008; Whitaker, 2013). For individuals whose intellectual disability is not accounted for by medical or physical conditions, social deprivation, neglect, abuse, and inadequate levels of environmental stimulation are considered to be primary contributing factors to the etiology of intellectual disability (Handen, 2007; Matson et al., 2008; Whitaker, 2013).

Autism Spectrum Disorder

In the past, the APA (1980, 2000) categorized the group of neurodevelopmental disorders characterized by impaired social interaction, deficits in verbal and nonverbal communication, and restrictive and/or stereotyped patterns of behavior, activities, and/or interests under a general classification called pervasive developmental disorders (PDD). This umbrella term included such mental disorders as autism spectrum disorder, Asperger's disorder, Rett's disorder, and childhood disintegrative disorder (APA, 2000). The disorders had overlapping diagnostic criteria and were commonly viewed as related disorders. For example, Rett's disorder was a disorder that was primarily found in females and was characterized by regression in motor skills during early childhood, hand-wringing movements, and regression of cognitive skills (APA, 2000; Mount, Hastings, Reilly, Cass, & Charman, 2003). Childhood disintegrative disorder, which was first added in 1994 to the APA's *Diagnostic and Statistical Manual for Mental Disorder, Fourth Edition* (*DSM-IV*), described children having this disorder as demonstrating a significant loss of skills in communication, social relationships, play, and adaptive behavior after a period of at least 2 years of typical development (APA, 2000). Asperger's disorder, which was also added to the *DSM-IV* in 1994, was considered as a more mild form of autism in which there were symptoms of atypical behaviors and impaired social interactions, but no communication difficulties (APA, 2000).

Given the similar descriptions and overlapping diagnostic criteria for the various pervasive developmental disorders, this general classification was eliminated in the *DSM-5* (APA, 2013), and many of the previously specific disorders (i.e., Rett's disorder, Asperger's disorder, and childhood disintegrative disorder) were grouped together under a new broader category, called autism spectrum disorder (ASD). According to the APA (2013), a primary reason for combining these disorders into one category was that research had found that it was often difficult to differentiate one of the more specific disorders from the others, which resulted in the inconsistent application of the specific diagnoses across different clinics. While this change in diagnostic classification and related terminology impacts reported incidence and prevalence rates to some degree, initial research has reported that approximately 91% of children who had previously been given a diagnosis of a PDD based on the criteria listed in the *DSM-IV* continued to qualify under the diagnostic criteria for ASD in the *DSM-5* (Huerta, Bishop, Duncan, Hus, & Lord, 2012).

■ Definition

More than 70 years ago, Leo Kanner (1943) described a group of 11 children who displayed a similar pattern of behaviors that he indicated were appreciably different from those of other childhood behavior disorders. Hans Asperger also described a group of children in 1944 who manifested similar behaviors to those described by Kanner (Wing, 1976). Kanner called this form of childhood psychopathology "early infantile autism" and noted that among its characteristics were marked withdrawal; dislike of being held; unresponsiveness to people as well as to the environment; manipulation of objects in a rigid, stereotyped manner; lack of appropriate play; failure to acquire normal speech; echolalia and difficulties with pronoun use; anxious insistence on sameness in the environment; excellent rote memories; normal physical appearance; and good cognitive potential.

These characteristics observed by Kanner still largely characterize current models of ASD, as symptoms include impairments in social functioning, communication, and behavior. While previous editions of the *Diagnostic and Statistical Manual for Mental Disorders* required symptoms to be present prior to age 3 (e.g., APA, 1994; 2000), the *DSM-5* states only that the impairments must be present starting in the early developmental period (APA, 2013). In addition, although the *DSM-IV* previously included three categories in which deficits must be present (i.e., reciprocal social interaction; communication; and, restricted, repetitive behaviors, interests or activities), the *DSM-5* includes only two major categories: (a) ". . . deficits in social communication and social interaction across settings," and (b) "restricted, repetitive patterns of behavior, interests, or activities" (APA, 2013, p. 50).

"Deficits in social communication and social interaction across settings" may be observed in several ways. It may include the child having delays in language or limited language skills, with studies suggesting that 30% to 50% of individuals diagnosed with autism never develop meaningful speech (e.g., Tanguay, 2000; Wodka, Mathy, & Kalb, 2013). Social communication deficits may also be observed by the child or adolescent having difficulty participating in back-and-forth conversation and being relatively unable to engage in "social chitchat" or "small talk." Communication deficits may also include the individual having difficulty using or understanding nonverbal communication such as gestures, head nods, or appropriate facial expressions (e.g., smiling to show happiness). Other symptoms of poor social communication and social interaction may include difficulty forming friendships or other social relationships, or having very limited interest in forming relationships. Social impairments may also be observed in the individual having difficulty understanding the feelings and perspective of others (APA, 2013).

"Restricted, repetitive patterns of behavior, interests, or activities" typically includes atypical behaviors such as repetitive motor movements (e.g., hand flapping or rocking), echolalia, inflexibility and unreasonable insistence on sameness in daily routines, attachment to or preoccupations with unusual objects or topics (e.g., a historical event, rocks, car tires), and narrow interests that are extremely intense and/or unusual (APA, 2013). More recent research has suggested that restricted and repetitive behaviors can better serve individuals by subdividing the behaviors into two different subcategories, including "repetitive sensory motor" and "insistence on sameness," as this could direct research regarding etiology and intervention (e.g., Bishop et al., 2012).

Similar to intellectual disabilities, the diagnosis of ASD is classified in regard to the individual's level of severity (i.e., Levels 1–3), with the specific level assigned to a person based on the extent of his or her impairment and, subsequently, the level of support required for him or her. For example, a "high functioning" person having ASD is one whose symptoms cause only mild impairments and, therefore, may only need limited support to function independently in society. Conversely, an individual with ASD who has "severe impairments" is likely to require intensive, lifelong support. Table 12.3 provides a description of impairment and related severity levels of ASD.

TABLE 12.3

EXAMPLES OF IMPAIRMENT AND RELATED SEVERITY LEVEL OF AUTISM SPECTRUM DISORDER

Severity Level	Examples of Impairment
Level 1	*Requires support* Noticeable deficits in social communication skills when supports are not in place; difficulty making friends; rigidity is to a degree that it causes interference in functioning; poor planning and organization may impair independence.
Level 2	*Requires substantial support* Marked deficits in social communication even with supports in place; limited social relationships; limited language and communication skills; rigidity to a degree that it is obvious to the casual observer and interferes with functioning across contexts.
Level 3	*Requires very substantial support* Very limited social communication skills; minimal social interaction; rigidity to a degree that transition and change causes significant distress.

Source: Adapted from APA (2013).

It should be noted that many individuals with ASD have comorbid psychiatric diagnoses, including attention deficit/hyperactivity disorder and bipolar disorder (e.g., Giovinazzo, Marciano, Giana, Curatolo, & Porfiroio, 2013; Joshi, Biederman, Petty, Goldin, Furtak, & Wozniak, 2013; Vannucchi, Masi, Toni, Dell'Osso, Marazziti, & Perugi, 2014). Additional comorbid disorders include intellectual disability, sleep problems, and gastrointestinal problems (Liu, Hubbard, Faber, & Adams, 2006; Tsai, 2006). In this regard, it has been reported that about 70% of children with ASD who are older than 8 years of age receive some form of psychoactive medication in a given year (Oswald & Sonenklar, 2007). In contrast, research has also suggested that pharmacological treatment has limited success (Charlop-Christy, Malmberg, Rocha, & Schreibman, 2008; Ozonoff, Goodlin-Jones, & Solomon, 2007; Tsai, 2006) and, if used, is more effective when it targets specific impairments like inattention or irritability (Dove et al., 2012).

Etiology

The specific cause(s) of ASD are currently unknown, but it is largely thought that genetic factors are the primary contributing factors to this developmental disability (e.g., Gupta & State, 2007; Pennington, McGrath, & Peterson, 2009b; Schaefer & Mendelsohn, 2013). The Autism Genetic Resource Exchange (AGRE) has provided for a DNA repository and family registry of genotypic and phenotypic information since 1997, with hundreds of studies utilizing these data for identifying loci on several genes that are significantly associated with autism (AGRE, 2016). The popular assumption is that these genetic factors lead to abnormalities in the development of brain structures which, in turn, may influence cognitive, social, and behavioral functioning.

As the use of neuroimaging procedures has grown in research centering on ASD (e.g., Brambilla et al., 2003; Haar, Berman, Behrmann, & Dinstein, 2014), it has consistently been demonstrated that there are abnormalities and differences at the most basic level of the brain for individuals with ASD (e.g., reduced neuronal structures, reduced neuronal activity, and more cerebral volume). Related to this, the Autism Brain Imaging Data Exchange (ABIDE) was created to provide for a registry of R-fMRI, MRI, and phenotypic information of individuals with ASD in order to promote research and knowledge in this area (Di Martino et al., 2014).

In addition to structural differences, research has found functional differences in the brains of individuals with versus without ASD. Abnormalities have included reduced responsiveness to novel stimuli, lower activation of mirror neurons on certain tasks, increased variability in regional metabolic rates, and altered serotonergic function (e.g., Amaral, Schumann, & Nordahl, 2008; Anderson et al., 2002; Pennington et al., 2009b; Rane et al., 2015). Related to this, researchers have also suggested that there may be poor synchronization between various regions of the brain, so that each area of the brain is functioning independently (e.g., Just, Cherkassky, Keller, & Minshew, 2004; Peters et al., 2013). This atypical activity can then have direct implications on cognitive, social, and behavioral functioning. For example, researchers from Cambridge, England, were the first to discover that when trying to decipher facial expressions and related emotions, the amygdala (i.e., the emotional control center of the brain) was underactive in individuals with ASD (Baron-Cohen, 1995), which may lead to more difficulty in accurately interpreting facial expressions.

Prevalence

Estimates of the prevalence of ASD have varied over the years, ranging between 4.5 and 147 per 10,000 individuals (e.g., Chakrabarti & Fombonne, 2005; CDC, 2014; Fombonne, 2002, 2003b; Rice et al., 2007; Yeargin-Allsopp et al., 2003), with a general trend showing rates increasing over time. For example, research from the 1960s estimated that ASD occurred in approximately 4.5 out of 10,000 people (Lotter, 1966), whereas by the 1980s it was estimated that the ratio was approximately 10 per 10,000 people (Burd, Fisher, & Kerbesbian, 1987). According to the Centers for Disease Control and Prevention (CDC, 2014), at the present time it is estimated that 1 in every 68 children is diagnosed with autism (equivalent to 147 per 10,000). This latter estimate suggests that ASD is more common than the total combined prevalence of childhood cancer, juvenile diabetes, and pediatric AIDS, in that it is estimated that 1.5 million individuals in the United States and tens of millions of persons worldwide have an autism diagnosis (CDC, 2014).

There has been increasing debate over the factors that may be contributing to the increase in ASD diagnoses. For example, there has been a fair amount of attention paid in recent years in the print and news media, as well as over the Internet, regarding the belief that childhood vaccinations—usually the combined measles, mumps, and rubella (MMR) vaccine—lead to ASD. In this regard, a study by Andrew Wakefield and colleagues (Wakefield et al., 1998) was published that described eight children whose first symptoms of autism appeared within 1 month after they received the MMR vaccine. Although this study was retracted by the scientific journal, *The Lancet*, where it was first published because it was found that Dr. Wakefield's data were inaccurately collected, interpreted, and reported (Wakefield et al., 2010), many people continue to believe that there is a link between autism and vaccines or between autism and other environmental factors. However, to date, there have been no empirically based studies published in refereed scientific journals that link environmentally based casual factors to autism (e.g., Newschaffer et al., 2007; Taylor, Swerdfeger, & Eslick, 2014).

Given the lack of evidence indicating that environmental influences contribute to the increase in ASD across the globe, one might speculate that the change in prevalence rates is due to a variety of indirect factors, such as a broader understanding by health professionals of this disorder and its related symptoms, more accurate diagnostic practices, and better assessment methods available to identify prevalence. In this regard, funding for ASD research grew nearly 45% from 2008 to 2012, with over $1.2 billion being awarded for autism-related research during this time (Government Accountability Office, 2015) which, in turn, could contribute to increased public knowledge and the identification of individuals with ASD. In regard to methodology for assessing prevalence, Frombonne (2003a) speculated that prevalence appeared to have increased because older survey research underestimated the true prevalence of ASD. He noted that (a) children with milder or high-functioning types of ASD were often missed in surveys, (b) younger children were underrepresented because assessment techniques used in the diagnosis of infants and preschool-aged children were less sensitive than techniques used for older children, (c) older children were underidentified because the newer diagnostic criteria for ASD were not in place when they were diagnosed, and (d) with the increasing availability in the 1990s of developmental disability services for children with ASD, schools and other educational service agencies became more likely to identify and provide programs for children with ASD. In addition, Williams, Higgins, and Brayne (2006) conducted a meta-analysis of 60 studies that estimated the prevalence of autism, and found that 61% of the variation in prevalence estimates could be attributed to differences in diagnostic criteria, age of children screened, and/or study location. Moreover, in a study conducted in California, Croen, Grether, Hoogstrate, and Selvin (2002) found that while the prevalence rate for ASD increased over time, the prevalence rate for intellectual disability had gone down. They, therefore, speculated that some children who would have previously been diagnosed with intellectual disability were now being diagnosed with ASD.

Finally, increases in the prevalence of ASD are also likely related to the changes in the diagnostic criteria over time. The recent change in the *DSM-5* eliminated subcategories of PDD (e.g., Rett's disorder, Asperger's disorder, child disintegrative disorder) and reclassified these individuals into the general category of ASD. This change is likely to have an impact on current prevalence rates versus those from, for example, a decade ago, as current ASD diagnostic criteria now include some individuals who had been previously categorized under a different diagnostic category.

TREATMENT AND PROGNOSIS

Historically, treatment programs for individuals with developmental disabilities were quite limited and did not typically include counseling and psychotherapy services (see e.g., Cowen, 1963; Stacey & DeMartino, 1957). Moreover, individuals who were severely impaired often lived in institutional settings where they received custodial care (Morris & Kratochwill, 2008). Although people who were higher functioning also often lived in institutional settings, they were more likely to participate in educational programs within these institutions, as publically funded educational programs within local community settings were scarce. When such community-based educational programs were available, they were more likely to be found in private and parochial schools. In addition, when individuals functioning in the moderate-to-mild range of intellectual disability were able to live and be educated outside of the institutional setting, they were typically educated in segregated classroom settings or school settings (i.e., segregated classroom or school settings for "trainable" and "educable" students).

More contemporary approaches to treatment for individuals with developmental disabilities can be traced to the behavior modification treatment research of the 1960s and 1970s (see e.g., Ayllon & Azrin, 1968; Gardner, 1971; Kazdin, 1975; Lovaas, 1977; Matson & McCartney, 1981; Morris, 1976; Tharp & Wetzel, 1969; Thompson & Grabowski, 1972; Ullmann & Krasner, 1965; Ulrich, Stachnik, & Mabry, 1966). Many contemporary behavioral treatment programs use an applied behavior analysis approach and are based on the assumption that the antecedents of a behavior, as well as the consequences of a behavior, can be manipulated so that the likelihood that a behavior will be repeated is either increased or reduced depending on the nature of the consequences that are applied. Behavioral treatment programs have been widely used in helping individuals with developmental disabilities develop and strengthen their positive behavioral skills, including adaptive behavior and coping skills, functional language skills, and social skills. Behavioral programs are frequently used for children with intellectual disabilities, as well as those with ASDs. Over the past decade, however, social thinking programs have also become more popular in helping to improve the language and social skills for children with ASD, with these programs utilizing social learning theory (e.g., Bandura, 1969) to directly teach skills such as perspective taking and reciprocal social interaction (Winner & Crooke, 2009).

Intellectual Disability

So much has been written about the effectiveness of behavior modification programs for individuals with intellectual disabilities that few professionals today would question its utility and role in assisting people to live more comfortable and humane lives, independent of their level of intellectual disability (see e.g., Alberto, Heflin, & Andrews, 2002; Carr, Turnbull, & Horner, 1999; Cole & Gardner, 1993; Handen, 2007; Lakhan, 2014; Matson et al., 2008; Matson, Laud, & Matson, 2004; Medeiros, 2015; Pennington et al., 2009a; Sturmey & Didden, 2014; Wacker & Berg, 1988). Behavior modification programs are highly effective because they can successfully be used both to develop and strengthen positive behaviors and skills (e.g., independent living skills, assertiveness, communication, social, job skills), as well as reduce and eliminate problem behaviors (e.g., self-injurious behavior, physical aggression; Sturmey & Didden, 2014). While various curricula have been created over the past few decades, the basic behavioral principles and procedures underlying these curricula have remained the same over time since they were first introduced by B.F Skinner (e.g., Skinner, 1938, 1953) and later applied directly to work with children and adults in the 1950s and 1960s (see e.g., Ayllon & Azrin, 1968; Ayllon & Michael, 1959; Baer, Wolf, & Risley, 1968; Bandura, 1969; Graziano, 1971; Tharp & Wetzel, 1969; Ullmann & Krasner, 1965; Ulrich, Stachnik, & Mabry, 1966).

Reinforcement Procedures

Reinforcement is typically defined as an event that immediately follows a specific behavior that has been designated for change (called the target behavior), and that results in an increase in the frequency in which the target behavior occurs (e.g., Skinner, 1938, 1953). Because reinforcement is defined, for our purposes, in terms of its effects on the person, something that might be reinforcing to one individual may not be reinforcing to another person. Therefore, it is very important when using reinforcement procedures to make sure that the clinician, teacher, counselor, parent, or other care provider knows what a reinforcer is for the person with whom he or she is working.

There are typically five categories of positive reinforcement: social praise ("Very good," "Great job," You're terrific," etc.), nonverbal messages (smiling, tickling, hugging, etc.), edibles (small amounts of the person's favorite foods, snacks, or drinks), objects (toys, tokens, ink markers, etc.), and activities (watching a video, playing games on a computer/tablet, going to the park, etc.; Miltenberger, 2011; Morris, 1985). The positive reinforcers used by the clinician, teacher, counselor, parent, or other care provider should be appropriate for the individual's age. The most commonly used method for distributing positive reinforcers is through the use of a token economy program (see e.g., Ayllon & Azrin, 1968; Kazdin, 1975; Miltenberger, 2011; Morris, 1985). Another procedure that relies on positive reinforcement to increase a behavior is "shaping." This reinforcement procedure is used to teach a complex target behavior to the individual in successive steps, with each step gradually leading to the desired behavior. For example, instead of teaching the individual a whole complex behavior pattern at once, such as cooking dinner, the behavior of cooking dinner would be broken into small parts (e.g., locating the recipe on food package, finding a pot, boiling water, adding ingredients listed on the package, setting a timer, etc.). Each part is then taught in succession, being rewarded individually until all parts are learned and the complex behavior pattern can be learned and rewarded (Morris, 1985).

Reinforcement is a highly supported behavioral intervention for individuals with an intellectual disability, and it has been used successfully to teach a variety of target behaviors to individuals with intellectual disabilities, including academic skills (e.g., Adibsereshki, Abkenar, Ashoori, & Mirzamani, 2015; Burton, Anderson, Prater, & Dyches, 2013; Lovaas, 2003; Morris & McReynolds, 1986), adaptive skills (e.g., Sturmey & Didden, 2014), communication skills, and social skills (e.g., Matson et al., 2004, 2008; Matson & McCartney, 1981).

Behavior-Reduction Procedures

Behavior-reduction procedures involve the introduction of a dissatisfying or unpleasant event immediately following a person's performance of the target behavior, with this resulting in a decrease in the probability that the target behavior will occur again the next time the same antecedent or situational stimuli are present (Skinner, 1938, 1953). While research has found these methods to be effective in reducing maladaptive behaviors, it has also been recommended that these procedures be used in conjunction with positive reinforcement (Morris, 1985; Sturmey & Didden, 2014). The most commonly used behavior-reduction procedures are extinction, time-out from positive reinforcement, response cost, and overcorrection (Miltenberger, 2011; Morris, 1985).

Extinction refers to the removal of the reinforcing consequences that normally follow a particular target behavior (Skinner, 1953). For example, if it is determined that attention from a caregiver (albeit negative) is a reinforcer for a child having a behavioral outburst, then the attention would be removed by the caregiver going into a different room or not responding to the outburst. To use this procedure, the clinician or caregiver must be able to (a) identify those consequences that are reinforcing or maintaining the person's undesirable behavior, (b) determine whether those consequences will follow the person's behavior each time the behavior is performed, (c) control the occurrence of those consequences, and (d) be consistent in the use of the procedure each time the target behavior is performed (Martin & Pear, 2015; Miltenberger, 2011; Morris, 1985). If these conditions cannot be met, then another behavior-reduction procedure should be used.

Time-out from positive reinforcement involves removing the person from an attractive and positively reinforcing situation (or withdrawing a positive reinforcing activity) for a particular period of time immediately following the individual's performance of the undesirable target behavior. The type of time-out setting in which the individual is placed is very important and should contain fewer positive aspects than the positive reinforcing area. Three types of time-out procedures have consistently been applied for individuals having an intellectual disability, including contingent observation, exclusion time-out, and seclusion time-out (Iwata, Rolider, & Dozier, 2009).

Contingent observation involves having the person who performs the undesirable target behavior step away from the reinforcing setting (e.g., small group discussion, athletic event, group vocational activity) for a specified period of time and watch the other people in the setting perform the appropriate behaviors and receive positive reinforcement from the clinician or caregiver. The person then rejoins the group after the specific time has elapsed. Exclusion time-out, on the other hand, removes the person from the setting for a specific time but also places him or her in a position in which he or she cannot view the setting. Typically, the individual is not moved to another room or environment with this procedure; rather, he or she is placed in an isolated area in the same room with his or her back to the group activity. A third procedure, known as seclusion time-out, involves removing the individual from the reinforcing situation for a specific period of time and placing him or her in a safe, supervised, and isolated area that is separate from the reinforcing setting. The isolated area must be well ventilated, well lit, and unlocked, and the person must be monitored closely (Miltenberger, 2011; Morris, 1985).

Another behavior-reduction procedure is response cost. This procedure is typically combined with a token-economy positive reinforcement method, and it involves placing a cost on a person's performance of a specific undesirable target behavior. Thus, this procedure consists of the removal or withdrawal of a particular quantity of reinforcers (tokens) from the person each time he or she performs the target behavior (Miltenberger, 2011; Morris, 1985).

As noted, these behavior-reduction procedures have been used effectively to decrease the frequency of or eliminate the occurrence of a wide variety of target behaviors, including physical aggression, verbal aggression, disruptive behaviors, property destruction, stealing, noncompliance, self-injurious behavior, and self-stimulation (Sturmey & Didden, 2014). However, if used, these procedures *should only be used* in conjunction with positive reinforcement procedures where the clinician or caregiver is also teaching the individual alternative, desirable behaviors (Morris, 1985). In contrast to the use of behavior reduction procedures, Matson et al. (2008) have commented that a number of writers in the field of intellectual disability have objected to the use of these methods, maintaining that they are not necessary. In this regard, Matson et al. are promoting the use of positive behavior support (PBS) in interventions with people having an intellectual disability and challenging behaviors, citing both ethical and clinical considerations for why PBS is more appropriate (see e.g., Carr et al., 1999; LaVigna & Willis, 2012). The AAIDD (2010) has also submitted position statements promoting the use of PBS over behavior-reduction procedures.

The foundation of the PBS approach is in applied behavior analysis, and it involves the replacement of undesirable or challenging behaviors with more desirable prosocial behaviors and skills. The assumption underlying PBS is that it reduces the need for behavior-reduction methods such as time-out procedures while also promoting positive changes in the person's behavior(s). PBS makes use of "functional behavior assessment" to determine the frequency, antecedents, and consequences of the challenging behavior(s), as well as the situations and settings under which the behavior(s) occurs. Once this assessment is completed, an intervention plan can be implemented that focuses on preventing the undesirable or challenging behavior(s) from occurring and/or providing the individual with PBS for engaging in more desirable behaviors (e.g., Crone & Hawken, 2015; Storey & Post, 2014). It is notable that while PBS has become a more widely used and supported intervention, research supporting the effectiveness of it for reducing maladaptive behaviors has been variable (e.g., Matson et al., 2008; Sturmey & Didden, 2014) for individuals with developmental disabilities.

Modeling/Imitation Learning Procedures

Behavior change that results from the observation of another person has typically been referred to as modeling (Bandura, 1969; Bandura & Walters, 1963). The modeling procedure consists of an individual, called the model (e.g., therapist, parent, teacher), and a person, called the observer (e.g., the child). The observer typically observes the model performing the desirable target behavior in a familiar setting, where the model experiences reinforcement for engaging in the behavior. Another approach to modeling follows Skinner's (1938, 1953) position, in which the clinician, teacher, counselor, parent, or other care provider first demonstrates the target behavior and then reinforces the person for successfully imitating the target behavior of the therapist. Modeling or imitation learning often reduces the amount of time that a person needs to learn a particular target behavior.

Modeling and imitation learning have been found to be effective in teaching individuals with intellectual disabilities such prosocial behaviors as social skills, communication skills, and recreational activities (e.g., Mason, Davis, Boles, & Goodwyn, 2013; Mason, Ganz, Parker, Burkey, & Cmargo, 2012). Video modeling has become more common, with this being a modeling technique that allows the person to either model himself or herself on video, observe himself or herself on video during the completion of a task, or observe videos of others completing activities (Sturmey & Didden, 2014). Although this has been a useful behavioral intervention, there are certain preconditions that must be met for it to be effective. First, the person should have the ability to attend to the various aspects of the modeling situation. Second, the individual should have the motor skills and coordination needed to reproduce the modeled behavior. Finally, the individual should be motivated to perform the target behavior that he or she has observed (Bandura, 1969; Rimm & Masters, 1979). If any of these factors are absent, the clinician, counselor, teacher, or other care provider should consider using another behavior modification procedure to teach the target behavior.

Autism Spectrum Disorder

Although Kanner (1943) postulated that autism was innate or genetic in origin, it was commonly assumed until the mid-1960s that a central contributor to autism was a pathological parent–infant relationship (e.g., Bettelheim, 1950, 1967, 1974; Kanner, 1948). As a result, the most widely used therapeutic approach was psychoanalytically based treatment. An alternative approach to this was presented by Rimland (1964), in which he reviewed literature on ASD and concluded that it had a biological basis and should be treated accordingly. His book stimulated a great deal of interest in the biological bases of autism, and subsequently more treatment programs were developed that were based on Rimland's assumption that ASD had a neurological or biochemical origin.

Behavior Modification Procedures

Most contemporary intervention programs for the treatment of ASD are based on the use of behavior modification procedures to improve social skills, communication, and functional behaviors. As described earlier, behavior modification focuses on a prescribed and structured method of teaching objectively defined behaviors and skills. Presently, behavioral approaches are the only evidence-based interventions for children with ASD (e.g., Charlop-Christy et al., 2008; Ozonoff et al., 2007; Pennington, 2009; Smith & Iadarola, 2015; Sturmey & Didden, 2014). However, while research is limited, social learning theory approaches (e.g., Bandura, 1969; Bandura & Walters, 1963) are also increasingly being used (Sturmey & Didden, 2014; Wang et al., 2013).

One of the earliest behavior modification programs for the treatment of autism was proposed by Lovaas and his associates (e.g., Lovaas, 1977). They used behavior modification techniques to treat many of the behaviors associated with autism, including increasing the frequency of eye contact, developing functional speech and social skills, and reducing self-injurious and stereotypic behaviors. Lovaas and his associates used an approach called discrete trial training (DTT) in which each task given to a child consisted of a request to perform a specific action, followed by a response from the child, and a direct and immediate reaction from the therapist. Lovaas (1987) reported on the results of a treatment study in which preschool children with autism received intensive behavioral treatment (i.e., more than 40 hours per week of intensive one-to-one behavioral intervention), while similar children in a control group received less intensive treatment (i.e., 10 hours per week of behavioral treatment). Results indicated that 47% of the children in the intensive treatment group, compared with 2% of the children in the control group, achieved normal intellectual functioning and were placed in their regular first-grade educational program. Lovaas further reported that these latter findings were maintained over time (McEachin, Smith, & Lovaas, 1993). Consistent with Lovaas's structured approach using behavior modification procedures, more contemporary research reviews have concluded that the most successful intervention programs for preschool children with autism are those that use a structured, functional approach to problem behaviors; focus on teaching attention, imitation, communication, social, and play skills; have a low student-to-staff ratio; and have a high level of family involvement with family members involved in the treatment program (e.g., Dawson & Osterling, 1997; National Research Council, 2001; Sturmey & Didden, 2014).

Behavioral interventions have been found to be effective for a variety of adaptive behavior skills, including social and communication skills. In terms of social skills, behavioral methods such as modeling and imitation learning have commonly been used to teach primary social skills such as eye contact, attention, and response to the immediate environment, as well as more complex social skills such as play, social behavior, and perspective taking (e.g., theory of mind). Interventions may be implemented on a 1:1 basis, as well as in small group and classroom settings; peer modeling, video modeling, and direct instruction have all been found to be beneficial in improving skills (e.g., Mason et al., 2013; Reichow & Volkmar, 2009; Sturmey & Didden, 2014; Wang et al., 2013).

In regard to using behavioral strategies to teach communication skills, most programs focus primarily on the development of functional language, using positive reinforcement and shaping procedures for imitating the clinician's vocalizations. When vocalizations are combined with visual strategies (e.g., picture icons, drawings, objects, and/or written words), these methods have been found to be even more effective (Charlop-Christy et al., 2008). Augmentative and alternative communication (AAC) models rely strongly on reinforcement for teaching communication skills and have strong evidence of effectiveness (e.g., Ganz et al., 2011, 2012). The picture exchange communication system (PECS; Bondy & Frost, 2002) is a specific AAC model using behavioral methods to teach functional communication skills. Nonverbal individuals are reinforced for exchanging a picture of something they want (such as a glass of water or swinging on a swing) for the actual item or activity. The program initially teaches requesting and then moves into teaching more complex communication skills, with researchers finding that this is highly effective in helping individuals with ASD acquire functional communication skills (Ganz et al., 2012). There have also been some attempts in using AAC to help decrease challenging behaviors (presumably, by reducing frustration in helping the individual communicate needs and desires); however, evidence supporting its effectiveness for this has been minimal (Walker & Snell, 2013).

The Treatment and Education of Autistic and related Communication-Handicapped Children (TEACCH) model relies heavily on charting behaviors and reinforcement to help improve communication and other skills in children (Schopler, Mesibov, & Hearsey, 1995). Studies have found this comprehensive intervention model to be applicable across the life span (Van Bourgondien & Coonrod, 2013) and have long-term positive effects (D'Elia et al., 2014).

In addition to developing social and communication skills, behavioral strategies have been found to be effective in reducing maladaptive behaviors. Many programs for treating problem or challenging behaviors incorporate a functional behavior assessment prior to the start of treatment in order to determine the frequency, antecedents, and consequences of variables in the environment that are maintaining the behavior, with antecedents commonly being thought to fall into one of three groups: attention-motivated behavior, escape-motivated behavior, and sensory reinforcement–motivated behavior (e.g., Charlop-Christy et al., 2008; Dunlap & Fox, 1999). Programs have traditionally used extinction and positive reinforcement techniques to treat such problematic or challenging behaviors (e.g., Odon et al., 2003; Sturmey & Didden, 2014). Applied behavior analysis has also been found effective in reducing repetitive behaviors (Boyd, McDonough, & Bodfish, 2012), and other positive reinforcement techniques have been found to be successful in reducing self-injurious behaviors (e.g., Sturmey, Maffei-Almodovar, Madzharova, & Cooper, 2012) and disruptive behaviors (e.g., Carr, Severtson, & Lepper, 2009; Chen & Ma, 2007).

As intervention research has continued to advance in this area, professionals have also identified some difficulties with using behavioral approaches. For example, some have noted that difficulties may arise when primarily using positive reinforcement programs with children having ASD, as these children may not be motivated to learn the actual behavior or skills being taught (Charlop-Christy et al., 2008). In addition, it may be difficult to identify any salient or age-appropriate reinforcers. Along with reinforcement procedures, generalization of skills learned has also been an area of concern in using behavior modification strategies for individuals with ASD. For example, while the Lovaas method was found to be an effective program for teaching communication and social skills, problems have been noted in how the treatment results were generalized to other behaviors, people, and environments. In addition, the robotic responding to stimulus cues on the part of children were sometimes reported, as well as a dependency on the stimulus prompt from the adult (Charlop-Christy et al., 2008). To address these problems, behavioral treatment programs that focused on teaching behaviors in the natural environment using natural contingencies were developed. Early programs established using this approach included pivotal response training (e.g., Koegel et al., 1989; Koegel & Koegel, 2012), incidental teaching (McGee, Krantz, & McClannahan, 1985), milieu training (Christensen-Sandfort & Whinnery, 2013; Kaiser, Yoder, & Keetz, 1992), and modified incidental teaching sessions (Charlop-Christy, Carpenter, Le, LeBlanc, & Kellet, 2002). Integrating these approaches into the various behavioral programs has been reported to have good generalization of treatment effects, and they are described as more likely to be used by parents and others in naturally occurring situations (e.g., Charlop-Christy et al., 2008; Lane, Lieberman-Betz, & Gast, 2015; Suhrleinrich et al., 2013).

Other Interventions

A relatively new method of intervention for ASD is that which relies on social learning theory and cognitive skills, with this approach typically being reserved for those individuals having at least average verbal skills (Winner & Crooke, 2009, 2014). These approaches are based on the presumption that the traditional behavior modification method of teaching social skills is not as effective for higher functioning individuals as it does not help them understand *why* they need to engage in certain social skills, such as making eye contact with someone who is speaking to you. Social Thinking (Winner, 2008), for example, is an approach that utilizes social stories to help teach and model social problem-solving skills, social perception and interpretation, and reciprocal interaction. This method strives to teach social skills and more nuanced social responses that a person can then use to navigate a variety of social situations. While this approach is still in a relatively early phase of investigation, research has suggested that it can be an effective method of improving social-communication skills in individuals with ASD (Lee et al., 2015).

Finally, given the frequency of hyper- and hyporeactivity to sensory stimulation that is common in individuals having ASD, professionals have attempted to identify interventions that can effectively treat such reactivity. Perhaps, the most widely known and used of these procedures is sensory integration therapy (Ayers, 1972, 1979). This treatment focuses primarily on three senses: tactile (i.e., touch), vestibular (i.e., motion and balance), and proprioception (i.e., joints and ligaments). Although numerous anecdotal reports emphasize the beneficial effects of sensory integration therapy, empirical reviews have consistently not reported any efficacy of this procedure (e.g., Shaw, 2002; Smith, Mruzek, & Mozingo, 2005; Sturmey & Didden, 2014).

PSYCHOLOGICAL AND VOCATIONAL IMPLICATIONS

As a result of the deinstitutionalization and normalization movements that began in the late 1960s and early 1970s, as well as the research advances in behavior modification treatment, many individuals with developmental disabilities are living in group homes, semi-independent apartments/homes, or independent living residences rather than in institutional settings. Although this situation certainly reflects the advances that have taken place over the past 35 to 40 years in implementing intervention methods that address various social, emotional, academic, and behavioral problems found in some individuals having developmental disabilities, certain issues continue to be present in the field. Specific issues include the living conditions of these individuals, their activity level, and their perceptions of the quality of life and level of productivity (e.g., Brown & Faragher, 2014; Migliore & Butterworth 2008; Morisse, Vandemaele, Claes, Claes, & Vandevelde, 2013).

In addition, issues remain involving the maximization of treatment gains through the generalization of behaviors that have been modified or successfully developed in these individuals. Such generalization involves transferring the acquired behaviors to a variety of settings in the person's natural environments, and in the maintenance of the person's treatment gains over time (e.g., Cole & Gardner, 1993; Hammel, Lai, & Heller, 2002; Luftig & Muthert, 2005; Matson et al., 2008; Smith, Parker, Taubman, & Lovaas, 1992). These issues have significant implications when assessing the long-term success of both the psychological and vocational aspects of a person's intervention and habilitation plans (see e.g., Handen, 2007; Matson et al., 2008). Future research needs to continue to address these areas to further assist people having a developmental disability in moving forward socially, educationally, emotionally, and vocationally in order for them to be able to lead meaningful, fulfilling, and productive adult lives with as much independence and personal satisfaction as possible.

REFERENCES

Adibsereshki, N., Abkenar, S. J., Ashoori, M., & Mirzamani, M. (2015). The effectiveness of using reinforcements in the classroom on the academic achievement of students with intellectual disabilities. *Journal of Intellectual Disabilities, 19*, 83–93.

Alberto, P., Heflin, L. J., & Andrews, D. (2002). Use of the timeout ribbon procedure during community-based instruction. *Behavior Modification, 26*, 297–312.

Amaral, D. S., Schumann, C. M., & Nordahl, C. W. (2008). Neuroanatomy of autism. *Trends in Neuroscience, 31*, 137–145.

American Association on Intellectual and Developmental Disabilities. (2010). *Behavioral supports: Joint position statement of AAIDD and the ARC*. Washington, DC: Author.

American Psychiatric Association. (1968). *Diagnostic and statistical manual of mental disorders* (2nd ed.). Washington, DC: Author.

American Psychiatric Association. (1980). *Diagnostic and statistical manual of mental disorders* (3rd ed.). Washington, DC: Author.

American Psychiatric Association. (1994). *Diagnostic and statistical manual of mental disorders* (4th ed.). Washington, DC: Author.

American Psychiatric Association. (2000). *Diagnostic and statistical manual of mental disorders* (4th ed., Text Revision). Washington, DC: Author.

American Psychiatric Association. (2013). *Diagnostic and statistical manual for mental disorders* (5th ed.). Arlington, VA: American Psychiatric Publishing.

Anderson, G. M., Gutkecht, L., Cohen, D. J., Brailly-Tabard, S., Cohen, J. H. M., Ferrari., P., . . . Tordjman, S. (2002). Serotonin transporter and promoter variants in autism: Functional effects and relationship to platelet hyperserotonemia. *Molecular Psychiatry, 7,* 831–836.

Autism Genetic Resource Exchange. (2016). Retrieved from http://research.agre.org/program/descr.cfm

Ayers, A. J. (1972). *Sensory integration and learning disorders.* Los Angeles, CA: Western Psychological Associates.

Ayers, A. J. (1979). *Sensory integration and the child.* Los Angeles, CA: Western Psychological Associates.

Ayllon, T., & Azrin, N. H. (1968). *The token economy: A motivational system for therapy and rehabilitation.* New York, NY: Appleton-Century-Crofts.

Ayllon, T., & Michael, J. (1959). The psychiatric nurse as a behavioral engineer. *Journal of the Experimental Analysis of Behavior*, 2, 323–334.

Baer, D., Wolf, M., & Risley, T. (1968). Some current dimensions of applied behavior analysis. *Journal of Experimental Analysis of Behavior, 1,* 91–97.

Bandura, A. (1969). *Principles of behavior modification.* New York, NY: Holt.

Bandura, A., & Walters, R. H. (1963). *Social learning and personality development.* New York, NY: Holt.

Baron-Cohen, S. (1995). *Mindblindness. An essay on autism and theory of mind.* Cambridge, MA: MIT Press.

Baumeister, A. A. (1970). The American residential institution: Its history and character. In A. A. Baumeister & E. Butterfield (Eds.), *Residential facilities for the mentally retarded* (pp. 1–28). Chicago, IL: Aldine.

Bettelheim, B. (1950). *Love is not enough.* Glencoe, IL: Free Press.

Bettelheim, B. (1967). *The empty fortress.* New York, NY: Free Press.

Bettelheim, B. (1974). *A home for the heart.* New York, NY: Knopf.

Binet. A., & Simon, T. (1916). *The development of intelligence in children*. Baltimore, MD: Lippincott Williams & Wilkins.

Bishop, S. L., Hus, V., Dunca, A., Huerta, M., Gotham, K., Pickles, A., . . . Lord, C. (2013). Subcategories of restricted and repetitive behaviors in children with autism spectrum disorders. *Journal of Autism and Developmental Disorders, 43,* 1287–1297.

Blatt, B. (1968). The dark side of the mirror. *Mental Retardation, 6,* 42–44.

Blatt, B., & Kaplan, F. (1966). *Christmas in purgatory: A photographic essay on mental retardation.* Boston, MA: Allyn & Bacon.

Bondy, A., & Frost, L. (2002). *A picture's worth: PECS and other visual communication strategies in autism.* Bethesda, MD: Woodbine House.

Boyd, B. A., McDonough, S. G., & Bodfish, J. W. (2012). Evidence-based behavioral interventions for repetitive behaviors in autism. *Journal of Autism and Developmental Disorders*, *42*, 1236–1248.

Boyle, C. A., Boulet, S., Schieve, L., Cohen, R. A., Blumberg, S. I., Yeargin, A. M., . . . Korgan, M. D. (2011). Trends in the prevalence of developmental disabilities in US children, 1997–2008. *Pediatrics, 127,* 1034–1042.

Brambilla, P., Harden, A., di Nemi, S. U., Perez, J., Soares, J. C., & Barale, F. (2003). Brain anatomy and development in autism: Review of structural MRI studies. *Brain Research Bulletin, 61*(6), 557–569. doi:10.1016/j.brainresbull.2003.06.001

Brown, R. J., & Faragher, R. M. (2014). *Quality of life and intellectual disability: Knowledge application to other social and educational challenges.* Hauppauge, NY: Nova Science Publishers.

Burd, L., Fisher, W., & Kerbesbian, J. (1987). A prevalence study of pervasive developmental disorders in North Dakota. *Journal of the American Academy of Child and Adolescent Psychiatry, 26,* 700–703.

Burton, C. E., Anderson, D. H., Prater, M., & Dyches, T. (2013). Video self-modeling on an iPad to teach functional math skills to adolescents with autism and intellectual disability. *Focus on Autism and Other Developmental Disabilities, 28*, 67–77.

Carr, J. E., Severtson, J. M., & Lepper, T. L. (2009). Noncontingent reinforcement is an empirically supported treatment for problem behavior exhibited by individuals with developmental disabilities. *Research in Developmental Disabilities, 30,* 44–57.

Carr, E. G., Turnbull, A. P., & Horner, R. H. (1999). *Positive behavior support in people with developmental disabilities: A research synthesis.* Washington, DC: AAMR.

Centers for Disease Control and Prevention. (2014). *Identified prevalence of autism spectrum disorder.* Retrieved from http://www.cdc.gov/ncbddd/autism/data.html

Chakrabarti, S., & Fombonne, E. (2005). Pervasive developmental disorders in preschool children: Confirmation of high prevalence. *American Journal of Psychiatry, 162,* 1133–1141.

Charlop-Christy, M. H., Carpenter, M., Le, L., LeBlanc, L. A., & Kellet, K. (2002). Using the picture exchange communication system (PECS) with children with autism: Assessment of PECS acquisition, speech, social-communicative behavior, and problem behavior. *Journal of Applied Behavioral Analysis, 35,* 213–231.

Charlop-Christy, M. H., Malmberg, D. B., Rocha, M. L., & Schreibman, L. (2008). Treating autistic spectrum disorder. In R. J. Morris & T. R. Kratochwill (Eds.), *The practice of child therapy* (3rd ed., pp. 299–335). New York, NY: Lawrence Erlbaum & Associates.

Chen, C. W., & Ma, H. H. (2007). Effects of treatment on disruptive behaviors: A quantitative synthesis of single-subject researches using the PEM approach. *The Behavior Analyst Today, 8,* 380–396.

Christensen-Sandfort, R. J., & Whinnery, S. B. (2013). Impact of milieu teaching on communication skills of young children with autism spectrum disorder. *Topics in Early Childhood Special Education, 32,* 211–222.

Cole, C. L., & Gardner, W. I. (1993). Psychotherapy with developmentally delayed children. In T. R. Kratochwill & R. J. Morris (Eds.), *Handbook of psychotherapy with children and adolescents* (pp. 426–471). Boston, MA: Allyn & Bacon.

Conyers, C., Martin, T. L., Martin, G. L., & Yu, D. (2002). The 1983 AAMR Manual, the 1992 Manual, or the Developmental Disabilities Act: Which do researchers use? *Education and Training in Mental Retardation and Developmental Disabilities, 37,* 310–316.

Cowen, E. (1963). Psychotherapy and play techniques with the exceptional child and youth. In W. M. Criuckshank (Ed.), *Psychology of exceptional children and youth* (2nd ed., pp. 526–592). Englewood Cliffs, NJ: Prentice-Hall.

Croen, L. A., Grether, J. K., Hoogstrate, J., & Selvin, S. (2002). The changing prevalence of autism in California. *Journal of Autism and Developmental Disorders, 32,* 207–215.

Crone, D. A., & Hawken, L. S. (2015). *Building positive behavior support systems in schools: Functional behavior assessment* (2nd ed.). New York, NY: Guilford Press.

Dawson, G., & Osterling, J. (1997). Early intervention in autism: Effectiveness and common elements of current approaches. In M. J. Guralnick (Eds.), *The effectiveness of early intervention* (pp. 307–325). Baltimore, MD: Brookes.

Developmental Disabilities Act. (1984). Washington, DC: U.S. Governemet Printing Office.

Developmental Disabilities Assistance and Bill of Rights Act (PL 106-402). (2000). Washington, DC: U.S. Government Printing Office.

D'Elia, L., Valeri, G., Sonnino, F., Fontana, I., Mammone, A., & Vicari, S. (2014). A longitudinal study of the TEACCH program in different settings: The potential benefits of low intensity intervention in preschool children with autism spectrum disorder. *Journal of Autism and Developmental Disorders, 44,* 615–626.

Di Martino, A., Yan, C. G., Denio, E., Castellanos, F. X., Alaerts, K., Anderson, J. S., . . . Milhan, M. P. (2014). The autism brain imaging data exchange: Towards a large-scale evaluation of the intrinsic brain architecture in autism. *Molecular Psychiatry, 19,* 659–667. doi:10.1038/mp.2013.78

Dove, D., Warren, Z., McPheeters, M. L., Taylor, J. L., Sathe, N. A., & Veenstra-VanderWeele, J. (2012). Medications for adolescents and young adults with autism spectrum disorders: A systematic review. *Pediatrics, 130,* 717–726.

Dunlap, G., & Fox, L. (1999). A demonstration of behavioral support for young children with autism. *Journal of Positive Behavior Interventions, 1,* 77–87.

Fombonne, E. (2002). Prevlalence of childhood disintegrative disorder. *Autism, 6,* 149–157.

Fombonne, E. (2003a). Editorial. *Journal of the American Medical Association, 289,* 49.

Fombonne, E. (2003b). Epidemiological surveys of autism and other pervasive developmental disorders: An update. *Journal of Autism and Developmental Disorders, 33,* 365–382.

Friedman, P. (1975). *The rights of the mentally retarded.* New York, NY: Avon.

Ganz, J. B., Earles-Vollrath, T. L., Mason, R. A., Rispoli, M. J., Heath, A. K., & Parker, R. I. (2011). An aggregate study of single-case research involving aided AAC: Participant characteristics of individuals with autism spectrum disorders. *Research in Autism Spectrum Disorders, 5,* 1500–1509.

Ganz, J. B., Earles-Vollrath, T. L., Mason, R. A., Rispoli, M. J., Heath, A. K., & Parker, R. I. (2012). A meta-analysis of single case research on aided augmentative communication systems with individuals with autism spectrum disorders. *Journal of Autism and Developmental Disorders, 42,* 60–74.

Gardner, W. I. (1971). *Behavior modification: Applications in mental retardation.* Chicago, IL: Aldine.

Giovinazzo, S., Marciano, S., Giana, G., Curatolo, P., & Porfirio, M. C. (2013). Clinical and therapeutic implications of psychiatric comorbidity in high functioning autism/Asperger comorbidity in high functioning autism/Asperger syndrome: An Italian study. *Open Journal of Psychiatry, 3,* 329–334.

Government Accountability Office. (2015). *Federal autism research: Updated information on funding from fiscal years 2008 through 2012.* Washington, DC: Author.

Graziano, A. M. (1971). *Behavior therapy with children.* Chicago, IL: Aldine-Atherton.

Grossman, H. J. (Ed.). (1983). *Classification in mental retardation.* Washington, DC: American Association on Mental Deficiency.

Gupta, A., & State, M. (2007). Recent advances in the genetics of autism. *Biological Psychiatry, 61,* 429–437.

Haar, S., Berman, S., Behrmann, M., & Dinstein, I. (2014). Anatomical abnormalities in autism? *Cerebral Cortex, 35*(14). doi:10.1093/cercor/bhu242

Halderman v. Pennhurst, 446 F. Supp. 1295 (1977).

Hammel, J., Lai, J. S., & Heller, T. (2002). The impact of assistive technology and environmental interventions on function and living situation status with people who are ageing with developmental disabilities. *Disability and Rehabilitation, 24*, 93–105.

Handen, B. L. (2007). Intellectual disability (mental retardation). In E. J. Mash & R. A. Barkley (Eds.), *Assessment of childhood disorders* (4th ed., pp. 551–597). New York, NY: Guilford Press.

Harlan, L. (1976). *The wild boy of Aveyron*. Cambridge, MA: Harvard University Press.

Harris, J. C. (2005). *Intellectual disability: Understanding its development, causes, classification, evaluation, and treatment*. New York, NY: Oxford University Press.

Harrison, P., & Oakland, T. (2015). *ABAS-3: Adaptive behavior assessment system* (3rd ed.). Torrance, CA: Western Psychological Services.

Heber, R. F. (1959). A manual on terminology and classification in mental retardation. *American Journal on Mental Deficiency, 64*(Monograph Supp), 1–111.

Heber, R. F. (1961). Modifications in the manual on terminology and classification in mental retardation. *American Journal on Mental Deficiency, 65*, 499–500.

Huerta, M., Bishop, S. L., Duncan, A., Hus, V., & Lord, C. (2012). Application of DSM-5 criteria for autism spectrum disorder to three samples of children with DSM-IV diagnoses of pervasive developmental disorders. *American Journal of Psychiatry, 169*, 1056–1064.

Humphrey, G. (1962). Introduction. In J. M. C Itard (Ed.), *The wild boy of Aveyron* (G. Humphrey & H. Humphrey, Trans.). New York, NY: Appleton-Century-Crofts.

Iwata, B. A, Rolider, N. U., & Dozier, C. L. (2009). Evaluation of time-out programs through phased withdrawal. *Journal of Applied Research in Intellectual Disabilities, 22*, 203–209.

Joshi, G., Biederman, J., Petty, C., Goldin, R. L., Furtak, S. L., & Wozniak, J. (2013). Examining the comorbidity of bipolar disorder and autism spectrum disorders: A large controlled analysis of phenotypic and familial correlates in a referred population of youth with bipolar I disorder with and without autism spectrum disorders. *The Journal of Clinical Psychiatry, 74*, 578–586. doi:10.4088/JCP.12m07392

Just, M. A., Cherkassky, V. L., Keller, T. A., & Minshew, N. J. (2004). Cortical activation and synchronization during sentence comprehension in high-functioning autism: Evidence of underconnectivity. *Brain, 127*(8), 1811–1821. doi:10.1093/brain/awh199

Kaiser, A. P., Yoder, P. J., & Keetz, A. (1992). Evaluation milieu training. In S. F. Warren & J. Reichle (Eds.), *Causes and effects in communication and language intervention* (pp. 9–47). Baltimore, MD: Brookes.

Kanner, L. (1943). Autistic disturbances of affective contact. *Nervous Child, 2*, 217–250.

Kanner, L. (1948). *Child psychiatry*. Springfield, IL: Charles C. Thomas.

Kanner, L. (1964). *A history of the care and study of the mentally retarded*. Springfield, IL: Charles C. Thomas.

Kazdin, A. E. (1975). *Behavior modification in applied settings*. Homewood, IL: Dorsey.

Kazdin, A. E. (2001). *Behavior modification in applied settings* (6th ed.). New York, NY: Wadsworth.

Koegel, R. L., & Koegel, L. K. (2012). *The PRT pocket guide: Pivotal response treatment for autism spectrum disorders*. Baltimore, MD: Brookes Publishing Company.

Koegel, R. L., Schreibman, L., Good, A., Cerniglia, L., Murphy, C., & Koegel, L. K. (1989). *How to teach pivotal behavior to children with autism: A training manual*. Santa Barbara: University of California.

Lakhan, R. (2014). Behavioral management in children with intellectual disabilities in a resource-poor setting in Barwani, India. *Indian Journal of Psychiatry, 56*, 39–45.

Lane, J. D., Lieberman-Betz, R., & Gast, D. L. (2015). An analysis of naturalistic interventions for increasing spontaneous expressive language in children with autism spectrum disorder. *Journal of Special Education, 50*(1), 49–61. doi: 10.1177/0022466915614837

LaVigna, G. W., & Willis, T. J. (2012). The efficacy of positive behavioral support with the most challenging behavior: The evidence and its implications. *Journal of Intellectual and Developmental Disability, 37*, 185–195.

Lee, K. Y. S., Crooke, P. J., Lui, A. L. Y., Kan, P. P. K., Luke, K. L., Mak, Y. M., . . . Wong, I. (2015). The outcome of a social cognitive training for mainstream adolescents with social communication deficits in a Chinese community. *International Journal of Disability, Development and Education, 63*(2), 201–223. doi:10.1080/1034912X.2015.1065960

Liu, X., Hubbard, J. A., Faber, R. A., & Adams, J. B. (2006). Sleep disturbances and correlates of children with autism spectrum disorder. *Child Psychiatry and Human Development, 27*, 179–191.

Lotter, V. (1966). Epidemiology of autistic conditions in young children. *Social Psychiatry, 1*(3), 124–137. doi:10.1007/bf00584048

Lovaas, O. I. (1977). *The autistic child*. New York, NY: Irvington.

Lovaas, O. I. (1987). Behavioral treatment and normal education and intellectual functioning in young autistic children. *Journal of Consulting and Clinical Psychology, 55*, 3–9.

Lovaas, O. I. (2003). *Teaching individuals with developmental delays*. Austin, TX: Pro-Ed.

Lovaas, O. I., & Bucher, B. D. (Eds.). (1974). *Perspectives in behavior modification with deviant children*. Englewood Cliffs, NJ: Prentice-Hall.

Luckasson, R., Borthwick-Duffy, S., Buntinx, W. H. E., Coulter, D. L., Craig, E. M., Reeve, A., . . . Tasse, M. J. (2002). *Mental retardation: Definition, classification, and systems of supports* (10th ed.). Washington, DC: AAMR.

Luftig, R. L., & Muthert, D. (2005). Patterns of employment and independent living of adult graduates with learning disabilities and mental retardation of an inclusionary high school vocational program. *Research in Developmental Disabilities, 26*, 317–325.

MacMillan, D. L. (1982). *Mental retardation in school and society*. Boston, IL: Little, Brown.

Martin, G., & Pear, J. J. (2015). *Behavior modification: What is it and how to do it* (10th ed.). United Kingdom: Psychology Press.

Mason, R. A., Davis, H. S., Boles, M. B., & Goodwyn, F. (2013). Efficacy of point-of-view video modeling: A meta-analysis. *Remedial and Special Education, 34*, 333–345. doi:10.1177/0741932513486298

Mason, R. A., Ganz, J. B., Parker, R. I., Burke, M. B., & Camargo, S. P. (2012). Moderating factors of video-modeling with other as model: A meta-analysis of single-case studies. *Research in Developmental Disabilities, 33*, 1076–1086.

Matson, J. L., Laud, R. B., & Matson, M. L. (Eds.). (2004). *Behavior modification for persons with developmental disabilities: Treatments and supports*. Kingston, NY: NADD Press.

Matson, J. L., & McCartney, J. R. (Eds.). (1981). *Handbook of behavior modification with the mental retarded*. New York, NY: Plenum.

Matson, J. L., Terlonge, C., & Minshawi, N. F. (2008). Children with intellectual disabilities. In R. J. Morris & T. R. Kratochwill (Eds.), *The practice of child therapy* (4th ed., pp. 337–361). New York, NY: Lawrence Erlbaum & Associates.

Maulik, P. K., Mascarenhas, M. N., Mathers, C. D., Dua, T., & Saxena, S. (2011). Prevalence of intellectual disability: A meta-analysis of population-based studies. *American Journal of Intellectual and Developmental Disabilities, 116*, 360–370. doi:10.1352/1944-7558-116.5.360

McDermott, S., Durkin, M. S., Schupt, N., & Stein, Z. A. (2007). Epidemiology and etiology of mental retardation. In J. W. Jacobson, J. A. Mulikc, & J. Rojann (Eds.), *Handbook of intellectual and developmental disabilities* (pp. 3–40). New York, NY: Springer Publishing.

McEachin, J. J., Smith, T., & Lovaas, I. O. (1993). Long-term outcome for children with autism who received early intensive behavioral treatment. *American Journal of Mental Retardation, 97*, 359–372.

McGee, G. G., Krantz, P. J., & McClannahan, L. E. (1985). The facilitative effects of incidental teaching on preposition use by autistic children. *Journal of Applied Behavioral Analysis, 18*, 17–31.

Medeiros, K. (2015). Behavioral interventions for individuals with intellectual disabilities exhibiting automatically-reinforced challenging behavior: Stereotypy and self-injury. *Journal of Psychological Abnormalities in Children, 4*, 1–8. doi:10.4172/2329-9525.1000141

Migliore, A., & Butterworth, J. (2008). Trends in outcomes of the vocational rehabilitation program for adults with developmental disabilities. *Rehabilitation Counseling Bulletin, 52*, 35–44.

Miltenberger, R. G. (2011). *Behavior modification: Principles and procedures* (6th ed.). Belmont, CA: Wadsworth Publishing.

Morisse, F., Vandemaele, E., Claes, C., Claes, L., & Vandevelde, S. (2013). Quality of life in persons with intellectual disabilities and mental health problems: An explorative study. *The Scientific World Journal, 2013*, 1–6. doi:10.1155/2013/491918

Morris, R. J. (1976). *Behavior modification with children: A systematic guide*. Cambridge, MA: Winthrop.

Morris, R. J. (1985). *Behavior modification with exceptional children: Principles and practices*. Glenview, IL: Scott-Foresman.

Morris, R. J., & Kratochwill, T. R. (2008). Historical context of child therapy. In R. J. Morris & T. R. Kratochwill (Eds.), *The practice of child therapy* (4th ed., pp. 1–5). New York, NY: Lawrence Erlbaum & Associates.

Morris, R. J., & McReynolds, R. A. (1986). Behavior modification with special needs children: A review. In R. J. Morris & B. Blatt (Eds.), *Special education: Research and trends* (pp. 66–130). New York, NY: Pergamon Press.

Mount, R. H., Hastings, R. P., Reilly, S., Cass, H., & Chjarman, T. (2003). Toward a behavioral phenotype for Rett syndrome. *American Journal on Mental Retardation, 108*, 1–12.

National Research Council. (2001). *Educating children with autism*. Washington, DC: National Academies Press.

New York State Association for Retarded Children v. Rockefeller, 357 F. Supp. 752 (1973).

Newschaffer, C. J., Croen, L. A., Reaven, J., Reynolds, A. M., Rice, C. E., Schendel, D., . . . Windham, G. C. (2007). The epidemiology of autism spectrum disorders. *Annual Review of Public Health, 28*, 235–258.

Nirje, B. (1969). The normalization principle and its human management implications. In R. B. Kugel & W. Wolfensberaer (Eds.), *Changing patterns in residential services for the mentally retarded* (pp. 179–195). Washington, DC: President's Commission on Mental Retardation.

Obi, O., Van Naarden, B. K., Baio, J., Drews-Botsch, C., Devine, O., & Yeargin-Allsopp, M. (2011). Effect of incorporating adaptive functioning scores on the prevalence of intellectual disability. *American Journal of Intellectual and Developmental Disabilities, 116*, 360–370. doi:10.1352/1944-7558-116.5.360

Odom, S. L., Brown, W. H., Frey, T., Karasu, N., Smith-Canter, L. L., & Strain, P. S. (2003). Evidence-based practices for young children with autism: Contributions for single-subject design research. *Focus on Autism and Other Developmental Disabilities, 18*, 166–175.

Online Mendelian Inheritance in Man. (2016). Intellectual disability [Data file]. Retrieved from http://omim.org

Oswald, D. P., & Sonenklar, N. A. (2007). Medication use among children with autism spectrum disorders. *Journal of Child and Adolescent Psychopharmacology, 17*, 348–355.

Ozonoff, S., Goodlin-Jones, B. L., & Solomon, M. (2007). Autism spectrum disorders. In E. J. Mash & R. A. Barkley (Eds.), *Assessment of childhood disorders* (4th ed., pp. 487–525). New York, NY: Guilford.

Pennington, B. F. (2009). *Diagnosing learning disorders* (2nd ed.). New York, NY: Guilford.

Pennington, B. F., McGrath, L. M., & Peterson, R. L. (2009a). Intellectual disability. In B. F. Pennington (Ed.), *Diagnosing learning disorders* (2nd ed., pp. 181–226). New York, NY: Guilford.

Pennington, B. F., McGrath, L. M., & Peterson, R. L. (2009b). Autism spectrum disorder. In B. F. Pennington (Ed.), *Diagnosing learning disorders* (2nd ed., pp. 108–151). New York, NY: Guilford.

Pennsylvania Association for Retarded Children v. Commonwealth of Pennsylvania, 334 F. Supp. 1257 (1971).

Peters, J. M., Taquet, M., Vega, C., Jeste, S. S., Fernandez, I. S., Tan, J., . . . Warfield, S. K. (2013). Brain functional networds in syndromic and non-syndromic autism: A graph theoretical study of EEG connectivity. *BMC Medicine, 11*(54). doi:10.1186/1741-7015-11-54

Rane, P., Cochran, D., Hodge, S. M., Haselgrove, C., Kennedy, D. N., & Frazier, J. A. (2015). Connectivity in autism: A review of MRI connectivity studies. *Harvard Review of Psychiatry, 23*, 223–244.

Reichow, B., & Volkmar, F. (2009). Social skills interventions for individuals with autism: Evaluation for evidence-based practices within a best evidence synthesis framework. *Journal of Autism and Developmental Disorders, 40*, 149–166.

Rice, C. E., Baio, J., Van Naarden Braun, K., Doernberg, N., Meaney, F. J., & Kirby, R. S. (2007). A public health collaboration for the surveillance of autism spectrum disorders. *Pediatric and Perinatal Epidemiology, 21*(2), 179–190. doi:10.1111/j.1365-3016.2007.00801.x

Rimland, B. (1964). *Infantile autism.* New York, NY: Appleton-Century-Crofts.

Rimm, D. C., & Masters, J. C. (1979). *Behavior therapy: Techniques and empirical findings.* New York, NY: Academic Press.

Schaefer, H. H., & Martin, P. L. (1969). *Behavior therapy.* New York, NY: McGraw-Hill.

Schaefer, G. B., & Mendelsohn, N. J. (2013). Clinical genetics evaluation in identifying the etiology of autism spectrum disorders: 2013 guideline revisions. *Genetics in Medicine, 15*, 399–407. doi:10.1038/gim.2013.32

Schalock, R. L., Borthwick-Duffy, S. A., Bradley, V. J., . . . Yeager, M. H. (2010). *Intellectual disability: Definition, classification, and systems of supports* (11th ed.). Washington, DC: AAIDD.

Schopler, E., Mesibov, G. B., & Hearsey, K. (1995). Structured teaching in the TEACCH system. In E. Schopler & G. B. Mesibov (Eds.), *Learning and cognition in autism* (pp. 243–268). New York, NY: Plenum.

Shaw, S. R. (2002). A school psychologist investigates sensory integration therapies: Promise, possibility, and the art of placebo. *Communique, 31*, 5–6.

Sisti, D. A., Segal, A. G., & Emanuel, E. J. (2015). Improving long-term psychiatric care: Bring back the asylum. *Journal of the American Medical Association, 313*, 243–244. doi:10.1001/jama.2014.16088

Skinner, B. F. (1938). *The behavior of organisms.* New York, NY: Appleton-Century-Crofts.

Skinner, B. F. (1953). *Science and human behavior.* New York, NY: Macmillan.

Smith, T., & Iadarola, S. (2015). Evidence base update for autism spectrum disorder. *Journal of Clinical Child & Adolescent Psychology, 44*, 897–922.

Smith, T., Mruzek, K. W., & Mozingo, D. (2005). Sensory integrative therapy. In J. W. Jacobson, R. M. Foxx, & J. A. Mulick (Eds.), *Controversial therapies for developmental disabilities* (pp. 331–350). Mahwah, NJ: Erlbaum.

Smith, T., Parker, T., Taubman, M., & Lovaas, O. I. (1992). Transfer of staff retraining from workshops to group homes: A failure to generalize across settings. *Research in Developmental Disabilities, 13*, 57–71.

Sparrow, S. S., Cicchetti, D. V., & Balla, D. A. (2005). *Vineland-II: Vineland adaptive behavior scales* (2nd ed.). Circle Pines, MN: AGS.

Stacey, C. L., & DeMartino, M. F. (Eds.). (1957). *Counseling and psychotherapy with the mentally retarded.* Glencoe, IL: Free Press.

Storey, K., & Post, M. (2014). *Positive behavior supports for adults with disabilities in employment, community, and residential settings.* Springfield, IL: Charles C. Thomas.

Sturmey, P., & Didden, R. (2014). *Evidence-based practice and intellectual disabilities.* Hoboken, NJ: John Wiley & Sons.

Sturmey, P., Maffei-Almodovar, L., Madzharova, M., & Cooper, J. (2012). Self-injurious behavior. In P. Sturmey & M. Hersen (Eds.), *The handbook of evidence-based practice in clinical psychology: Children and adolescents* (Vol. 1, pp. 477–492). Hoboken, NJ: Wiley.

Suhrleinrich, J., Stahmer, A. C., Reed, S., Schreibman, L., Reisinger, E., & Mandell, D. (2013). Implementation challenges in translating pivotal response training into community settings. *Journal of Autism and Developmental Disorders, 43*, 2970–2976.

Tanguay, P. M. (2000). Pervasive developmental disorders: A ten year review. *Journal of the American Academy of Child and Adolescent Psychiatry, 39*, 1079–1095.

Taylor, L. E., Swerdfeger, A. L., & Eslick, G. D. (2014). Vaccines are not associated with autism: An evidence-based meta-analysis of case-control and cohort studies. *Vaccine, 32*, 3623–3629.

Tharp, R. G., & Wetzel, R. J. (1969). *Behavior modification in the natural environment*. New York, NY: Academic Press.

Thompson, T., & Grabowski, J. (Eds.). (1972). *Behavior modification of the mentally retarded*. New York, NY: Oxford University Press.

Torrey, E., Fuller, D., Geller, J., Jacobs, C., & Rogasta, K. (2012). *No room at the inn: Trends and consequences of closing public psychiatric hospitals*. Arlington, VA: Treatment Advocacy Center.

Tsai, L. Y. (2006). Autistic disorders. In M. Dulcaan & J. Weiner (Eds.), *Essentials of child and adolescent psychiatry*. Arlington, VA: American Psychiatric Publishing.

Ullmann, L., & Krasner, L. (Eds). (1965). *Case studies in behavior modification*. New York, NY: Holt.

Ulrich, R., Stachnik, T., & Mabry, J. (1966). *Control of human behavior*. Glenview, IL: Scott Foresman and Company.

U.S. Department of Education. (2014). *Thirty-sixth annual report to congress on the implementation of the Individuals with Disabilities Education Act*. Washington, DC: Author.

Van Bourgondien, M. E., & Coonrod, E. (2013). TEACCH: An intervention approach for children and adults with autism spectrum disorders and their families. In S. Goldstein & J. A. Naglieri (Eds.), *Interventions for autism spectrum disorders* (pp. 75–105). New York, NY: Springer Publishing.

Vannucchi, G., Masi, G., Toni, C., Dell'Osso, L., Marazziti, D., & Perugi, G. (2014). Clinical features, developmental course, and psychiatric comorbidity of adult autism spectrum disorders. *CNS Spectrums, 19*, 157–164.

Wacker, D. P., & Berg, W. K. (1988). Behavioral habilitation of students with severe handicaps. In J. C. Witt, S. N. Elliot, & F. M. Greshman (Eds.), *Handbook of behavior therapy in education* (pp. 719–737). New York, NY: Plenum.

Wakefield, A. J., Anthony, A., Murch, S. H., Thomson, M., Montgomery, S. M., Davies, S., . . . Walker-Smith, J. A. (2010). Retraction: Enterocolitis in children with developmental disorders. *American Journal of Gastroenterology, 105*, 1214. doi:10.1038/ajg.2010.149

Wakefield, A. J., Murch, S. H., Anthony, A., Linnell, J., Casson, D. M., Malik, M., . . . Walker-Smith, J. A. (1998). Ileal-lymphoid-nodular hyperplasia, non-specific colitis, and pervasive developmental disorder in children. *The Lancet, 351*, 637–641.

Walker, V. L., & Snell, M. E. (2013). Effects of augmentative and alternative communication on challenging behavior: A meta-analysis. *Augmentative and Alternative Communication, 29*, 117–131.

Wang, S. Y., & Parilla, R. (2013). Meta-analysis of social skills intervention of single-base research for individuals with autism spectrum disorders: Results from three-level HLM. *Journal of Autism and Developmental Disorders, 43*, 1701–1716. doi:10.1007/s10803-012-1726–1722

Watson, L. (1973). *Child behavior modification*. New York, NY: Pergamon Press.

Whitaker, S. (2013). *Intellectual disability: An inability to cope with an intellectually demanding world*. London, England: Palgrave Macmillian.

Williams, J. G., Higgins, J. P. T., & Brayne, C. E. G. (2006). Systematic review of prevalence studies of autism spectrum disorders. *Archives of Disease in Childhood, 91*, 8–15.

Wing, L. (1976). *Early childhood autism* (2nd ed.). Elmsford, NY: Pergamon Press.

Winnepenninckx, B., Rooms, L., & Kooy, R. F. (2003). Mental retardation: A review of the genetic causes. *The British Journal of Developmental Disabilities, 49*(96), 29–44. doi:10.1179/096979503799104138

Winner, M. G. (2008). Social thinking: Cognition to enhance communication and learning. In K. D. Buron & P. Wolfburg (Eds.), *Learners on the autism spectrum* (pp. 209–231). Shawnee Mission, KS: Autism Asperger Publishing Company.

Winner, M. G., & Crooke, P. J. (2009). Social thinking: A training paradigm for professionals and treatment approach for individuals with social learning/social pragmatic challenges. *Perspectives on Language Learning and Education, 16*, 62–69.

Winner, M. G., & Crooke, P. J. (2014). Executive functioning and social pragmatic communication skills: Exploring the threads in our social fabric. *Perspectives on Language Learning and Education, 21*, 42–50.

Wodka, E. L., Mathy, P., & Kalb, L. (2013). Predictors of phrase and fluent speech in children with autism and severe language delay. *Pediatrics, 131*, 2012–2221.

Wolfensberger, W. (1969). The origin and nature of our institutional models. In R. B. Kugel & W. Wolfensberger (Eds.), *Changing patterns in residential services for the mentally retarded* (pp. 59–171). Washington, DC: President's Commission on Mental Retardation.

Wolfensberger, W. (1972). *The principle of normalization in human services*. Washington, DC: National Institute on Mental Retardation.
Wyatt v. Stickney, 325 F. Supp. 781 (1971).
Yeargin-Allsopp, M., Rice, C., Karapurkar, T., Doernberg, N., Boyle, C., & Murphy, C. (2003). Prevalence of autism in a US metropolitan area. *Journal of the American Medical Association, 289*, 49–55.

13

CHAPTER

Neuromuscular Disorders

Anna Shor, Athena M. Lolis, and Aleksandar Beric

INTRODUCTION

Neuromuscular disorders are a complex and heterogeneous group of disorders that ultimately impair the general function of the skeletal muscles. These disorders can affect all ages from newborns to the elderly, and vary in severity, ranging from mild to very severe, and sometimes are fatal. The vast majority of these disorders are relentlessly progressive and disabling. Despite considerable recent advances in many aspects of medicine, particularly genetics and molecular biology, there are no curative treatments for most of the neuromuscular disorders. Many other organ systems are frequently involved in these disorders in addition to the musculoskeletal dysfunction. Management of these disorders requires an interdisciplinary team approach that focuses on anticipatory and preventive measures as well as active interventions to address the primary and secondary aspects of the disorder. The team should ideally consist of neuromuscular specialists, as well as physical, occupational, and speech therapists. Other services that need to be involved in the care of these patients are orthopedic surgeons, pulmonologists, cardiovascular specialists, otolaryngologists, gastrointestinal physicians, pain specialists, and social workers, and they should address different aspects of the disorder and its impact on the patient. This approach greatly improves quality of life, longevity, and patient's independence. The cornerstone of management for a patient with neuromuscular disorders is rehabilitation. An effective rehabilitation program is critical not only for maintaining a patient's quality of life but also for optimizing physical and psychosocial function.

Electrodiagnostic testing, which consists of nerve conduction (NC) studies and electromyography (EMG), is a common tool used to help establish a diagnosis. NC testing includes electroneurography, which records and assesses sensory nerve function—sensory nerve action potentials (SNAP) and motor nerve testing with recording of compound muscle action potential (CMAP). In the process, three main parameters are assessed: latency and amplitude of the response and conduction velocity of the nerve. In addition, duration of the response is assessed in some conditions. NC studies are usually done with surface electrodes both for stimulation of the nerves and for recordings of sensory nerve and muscle responses. EMG records events from different muscles during three main states: relaxation-rest, graded voluntary contraction, and maximal voluntary contraction. Parameters that are assessed during relaxation include so-called spontaneous activity in a form of fibrillation potentials and positive sharp waves that indicate denervation of the muscle as a result of an innervating nerve lesion. During voluntary activation of the muscle, different parameters of motor units are assessed that can differentiate muscle from nerve diseases, and furthermore indicate if there are signs of either early or remote reinnervation. Activity during maximal voluntary effort assesses if there is any loss of motor units indicating either injury or disease of motor nerve axons or alpha motoneurons. NC studies/EMG are used to confirm the presence and extent of nerve and/or muscle damage and further delineate the nature of the nerve damage differentiating between demyelination and axonal damage. Segmental demyelination, also known as simple demyelination, implies injury of either myelin sheaths or Schwann cells that produce myelin, resulting in the breakdown of myelin with sparing of the axons (see Figure 13.1). It can occur by different mechanisms: mechanically by acute or chronic nerve compression, immune-mediated lesions, or genetic coding abnormalities as in hereditary disorders of Schwann cell/myelin metabolism. Axonal degeneration, also known

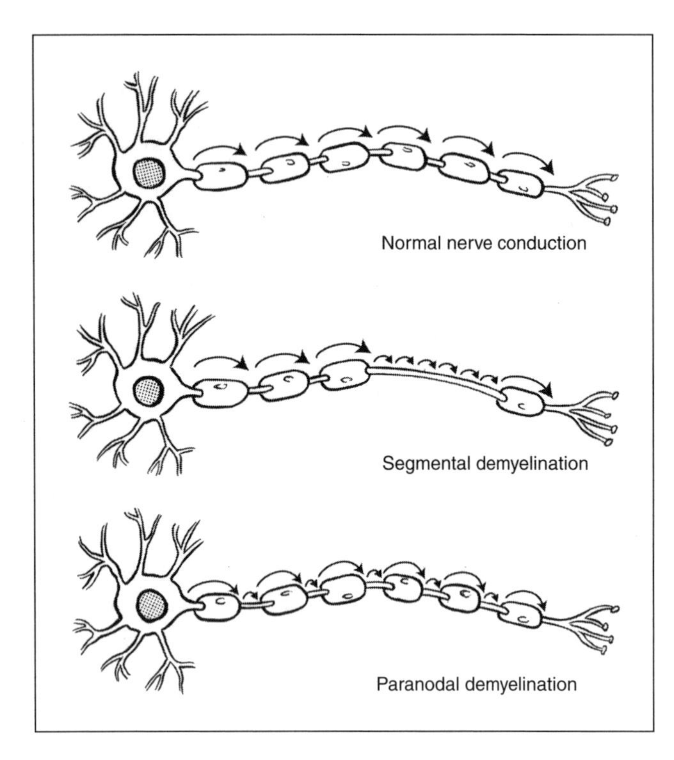

FIGURE 13.1 Nerve conductions.

as axonopathy, is the most common pathological reaction of the peripheral nerve. Axonopathy occurs in conjunction with breakdown of the myelin sheath that usually clinically presents at the most distal part of the nerve cell body: a process known as dying back neuropathy.

PERIPHERAL NERVE DISORDERS

Peripheral nerve disorders can be classified into mononeuropathy, multiple mononeuropathies, polyneuropathy, plexopathy, radiculopathy, and polyradiculopathy. The pattern of sensory loss and/or concomitant weakness helps to localize the lesion and its etiology. For example, symmetric proximal and distal weakness with sensory loss should bring acute immune-mediated polyneuropathy to mind, whereas symmetric sensory loss without significant weakness is suggestive of a slowly progressive axonal polyneuropathy. We explore these disorders in this section.

Mononeuropathy

Entrapment/and or compression neuropathies of the upper and lower extremities have the potential to cause significant disability. They are commonly a result of either occupational or recreational activities due to ischemia or mechanical pressure. They typically present with pain, numbness, paresthesias, and if severe enough, weakness in the distribution of the injured nerve.

Upper Limb Mononeuropathies

Suprascapular Neuropathy

This nerve is commonly entrapped at the level of the suprascapular notch. This lesion is most often seen in repetitive overhead loading activities, such as those done by certain athletes (swimmers and volleyball players). The nerve is derived from the upper trunk of the brachial plexus (C5, C6 roots) and innervates the supraspinatus and infraspinatus muscles, as seen in Figure 13.2. Clinical presentation is shoulder pain and weakness. If the site of compression is at the suprascapular notch, then shoulder external rotation and abduction will be weak as both the supraspinatus and infraspinatus muscles are affected. If it is at a more distal site, then just the infraspinatus will be affected. The diagnosis is confirmed with electrodiagnostic testing and abnormalities found only in infraspinatus and/or supraspinatus muscles without involvement of muscles innervated by the C5 root, nerves derived from the upper trunk of the brachial plexus and/or paraspinal muscles. It is imperative to rule out a brachial plexopathy and cervical radiculopathy. Imaging of the scapula is often needed to rule out any space-occupying lesions that may compress the suprascapular nerve. Once the diagnosis is made, physical therapy can be targeted to strengthen the shoulder. If there is a structural lesion, such as a cyst compressing the nerve, surgical intervention is warranted, followed by physical therapy.

Median Nerve Neuropathies

This is the most frequently encountered compressive neuropathy. While the most common site of compression is at the wrist, it is important to note that other less common sites of compression need to be considered in the differential diagnosis and include entrapment of the nerve between the heads of the pronator teres muscle and in the forearm where it may affect the anterior interosseous nerve. The median nerve arises from the lateral and medial cords of the brachial plexus with nerves originating from C5–T1 roots. It provides sensation to the

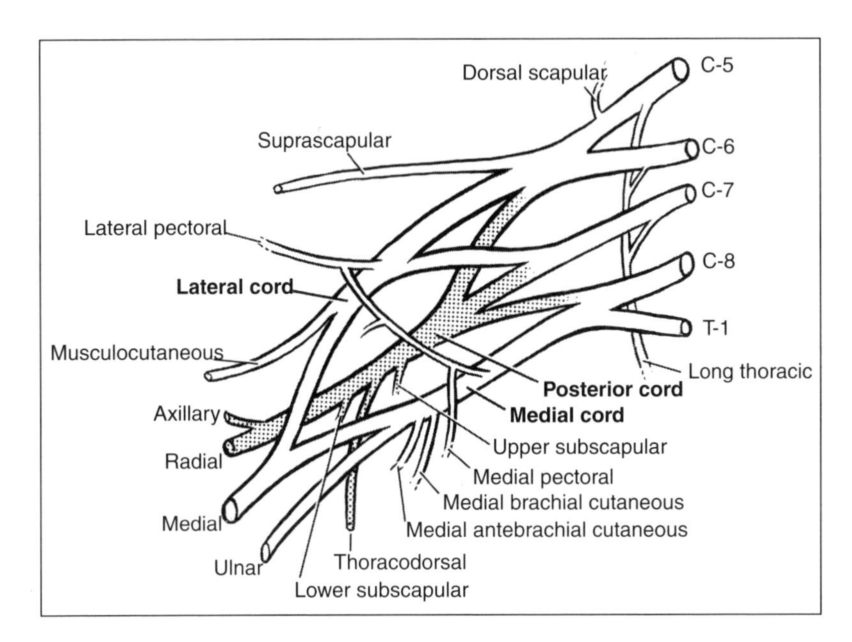

FIGURE 13.2 Brachial plexus.

lateral aspect of the palm, dorsal terminal phalanges, and volar surfaces of the thumb, index, and middle finger, as well as the radial aspect of the fourth digit. Its motor component innervates the thenar eminence muscles (except for the adductor pollicis brevis) and the flexor muscles of the forearm (with the exception of the flexor digitorum profundus to the ring and little finger). Figure 13.3 is a diagram of the median nerve.

Pronator Teres Syndrome. This condition is caused by the median nerve becoming entrapped in the forearm by the heads of the pronator teres muscle. There is usually no detectable weakness, but patients present with pain in the elbow, forearm, and wrist that is worsened by forearm pronation and supination. Electrodiagnostic testing is performed to rule out brachial plexopathy, or entrapment at the wrist, that can mimic this disorder.

Anterior Interosseous Syndrome. Clinical presentation is weakness of the thumb and index finger flexion. There is no sensory loss as this is a pure motor nerve, but there might be a poorly defined forearm pain. Electrodiagnostic testing will show evidence of denervation with variable chronicity in the flexor pollicis longus and pronator quadrates muscles, depending on the length of time the injury has been present.

Carpal Tunnel Syndrome. Carpal tunnel syndrome (CTS) is characterized by numbness, tingling, and pain, which worsens at night, in the median nerve distribution. In severe cases, there may be hand weakness and thenar atrophy. It commonly results from median nerve compression at the wrist

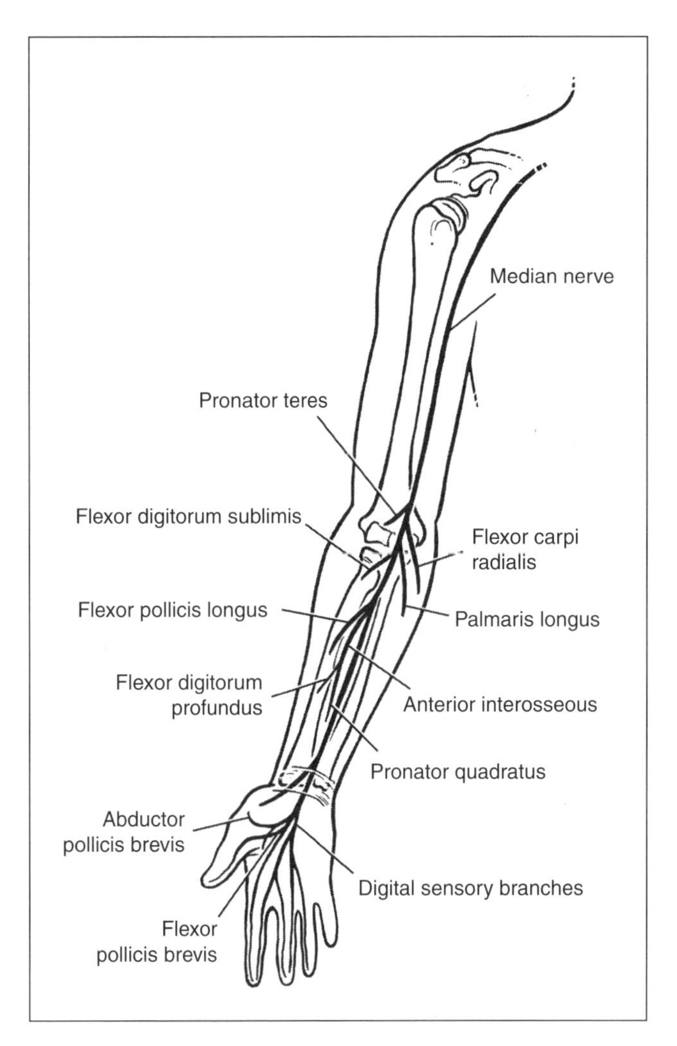

FIGURE 13.3 Median nerve.

where it crosses the carpal tunnel. There are both regional and systemic predispositions to developing this syndrome. Trauma, inflammation, tumors, and any anatomic anomalies can predispose one to developing CTS. Systemic causes include diabetes, renal disease, and amyloidosis. The incidence and prevalence are higher among working groups exposed to repetitive manual labor. CTS usually has a unilateral presentation, but is frequently a bilateral disease. NC studies revealing delay of electrical activity along the motor and sensory fibers of the medial nerve as it crosses the carpal tunnel is both diagnostic and useful in differentiating axonal versus compressive-demyelinating process. Therapies include wearing wrist splints to limit the longitudinal and transverse movements of the wrist (mainly wrist flexion). Additionally, there can be symptomatic relief from steroid injections into the carpal tunnel. Surgery is a last resort when nonoperative treatment has been exhausted or when there is electrodiagnostic evidence of severe involvement of the nerve.

Ulnar Neuropathy

This nerve is the terminal branch of the medial cord of the plexus and contains the fibers from C8–T1 roots. It provides motor innervation to the flexor carpi ulnaris, part of the flexor digitorum profundus (4th and 5th digit), and the majority of the intrinsic hand muscles (besides the thenar eminence). Common sites of entrapment are at the elbow (vast majority) and in Guyon's canal. The clinical presentation is that of paresthesias and/or sensory loss in the ulnar side of the fourth digit and the entire fifth digit. As the condition progresses, weakness will develop in the hand with progressive atrophy of hand intrinsic muscles.

Cubital Tunnel Syndrome. This is entrapment of the ulnar nerve in the ulnar groove or the cubital tunnel. The cubital tunnel is a space in which the ulnar nerve passes through as it makes its way to the hand. The space is created by the medial epicondyle of the humerus, the olecranon process of the ulna, and the arch between the humeral and ulnar heads of the flexor carpi ulnaris muscle.

It is the second overall most common entrapment neuropathy. It commonly occurs as the nerve runs very superficial at this level and is susceptible to repeated trauma. Additionally, constant flexion and extension at the elbow can also raise the intraneural pressure or lead to nerve subluxation out of sulcus, which may lead to nerve injury. Both NC studies and EMG are useful in confirming the site of a lesion as well as determining the degree of axonal and demyelinating components. Elbow splints and protection from further injury to the elbow area are the first choice in treatment, while surgical decompression and ulnar nerve transposition is reserved for more advanced situations, as the surgical outcome is not as successful as with carpal tunnel decompressions.

Guyon's Canal Compression. The most common causes of compression at this site are space-occupying lesions, such as ganglions, or occupational activities involving manual labor that put pressure and high force on the hand. The clinical presentation differs from cubital tunnel syndrome because the nerve is compressed at the canal or distally, resulting in loss of only palmar sensation, as the dorsal cutaneous branch is spared. There are four different areas of compression in the canal; hence there are slightly different clinical presentations depending on degree of involvement of motor and/or sensory branches. Figure 13.4 is a diagram of Guyon's canal. Consequently there are different NC studies/EMG patterns corresponding to different clinical presentations.

Radial Nerve Neuropathy. This nerve is predisposed to being entrapped and/or to a compression injury at the axilla, spiral groove of the humerus, or the elbow. The nerve is a continuation of the posterior

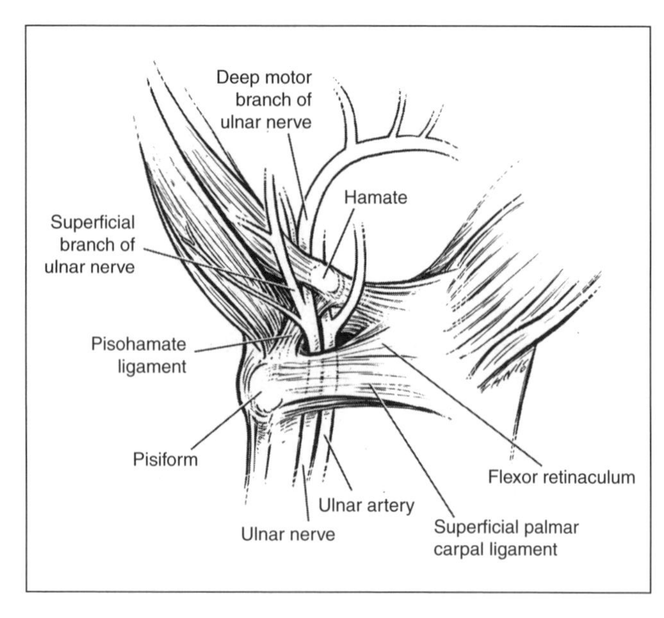

FIGURE 13.4 Guyon's canal.

cord of the brachial plexus with root derivation from C5–T1 levels. Figure 13.5 is a diagram of the radial nerve. In the upper arm, it innervates the triceps brachii muscle, and after entering the spiral groove it innervates the brachioradialis and extensor carpi radialis longus muscles. After that it divides into a superficial branch and a deep branch. The superficial branch provides sensation, whereas the deep branch is the motor branch called the posterior interosseous nerve. Radial nerve lesions at the level of axilla are usually due to a humeral fracture. Compression at the spiral groove is related to arm positioning during sleep, the so-called Saturday night palsy. There is often sensory loss in the anterolateral forearm, as well as dorsoradial aspect of the hand. Wrist drop is also seen, but a compression at the level of the spiral groove will spare triceps function as noted by normal elbow extension strength. All incomplete lesions are treated conservatively with expectation for a full recovery. Only complete transection is treated surgically with primary repair or grafts at a later time.

Posterior interosseous syndrome presents usually as painless finger and thumb extension weakness without marked wrist drop as the branch innervating the extensor carpi radialis muscle is proximal to the posterior interosseous nerve. It is purely a motor syndrome usually caused by nerve entrapment at the Arcade of Frohse, which is part of the supinator muscle.

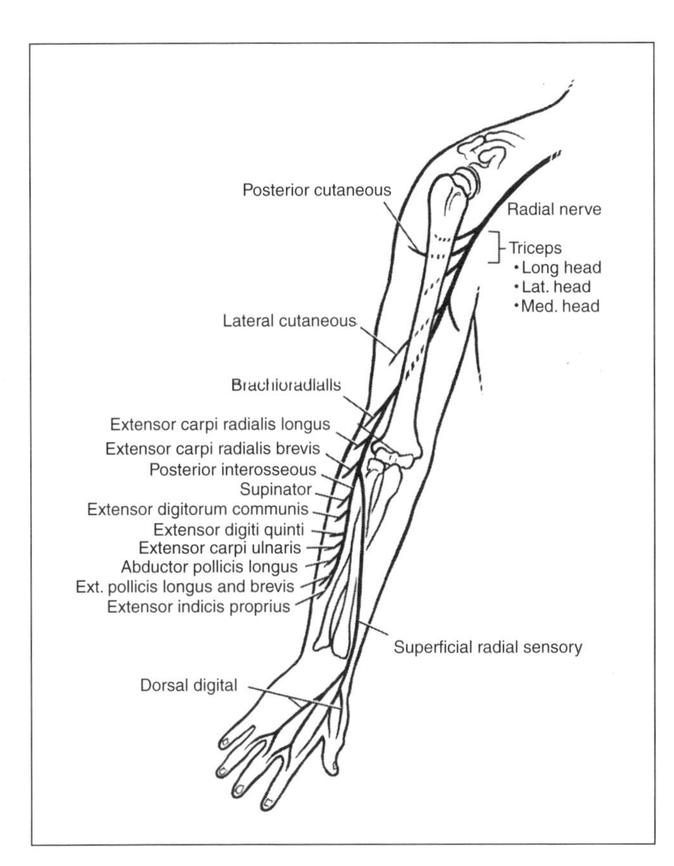

FIGURE 13.5 Radial nerve.

Lower Limb Entrapment Neuropathies

Lower limb entrapment neuropathies can lead to significant disabilities, but they are not as common as upper extremity mononeuropathies.

Lateral Femoral Cutaneous Nerve

This nerve provides sensation to the lateral thigh. It arises from the dorsal divisions of the lumbar plexus and emerges over the lateral border of the psoas muscle, crossing over the iliacus muscle toward the anterior superior iliac spine. It then passes under the inguinal ligament, through the lacuna musculorum, and then over the sartorius muscle into the thigh, where it divides into an anterior and a posterior branch. Figure 13.6 is a diagram of the lateral

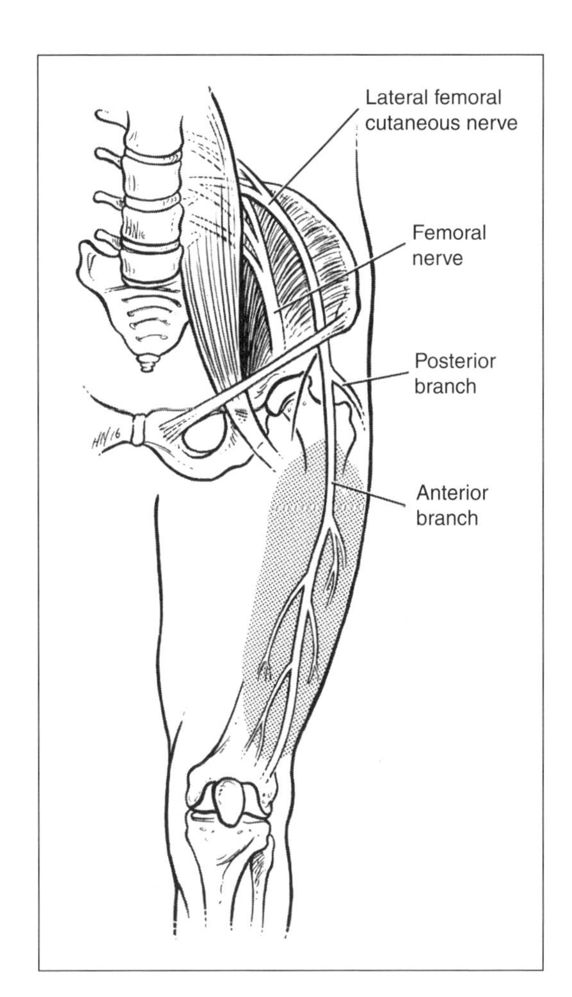

FIGURE 13.6 Lateral femoral cutaneous nerve.

femoral cutaneous nerve. Compression of this nerve is called meralgia paresthetica. The most common site of compression is at the inguinal ligament. There is sensory loss and pain usually in the form of tingling-burning in the upper lateral thigh. Common conditions that can be associated with this are obesity, pregnancy, sudden extreme changes in weight, or wearing tight clothing. Rarely, it can arise as a side effect from a pelvic surgery. Diagnosis is usually clinical based on characteristic presentation and objective findings. Electrodiagnostic testing is useful to rule out other conditions that can mimic meralgia paresthetica, such as lumbar radiculopathy, and to prompt further investigation of other causes when the study is either normal or there are bilaterally symmetric findings. NC studies have limited utility if the SNAP are bilaterally small or not present, as it is often technically difficult to elicit them. Similar issues are encountered when lateral femoral cutaneous nerve cortical somatosensory evoked potentials (SEP) are used for diagnosing this condition. Treatment of meralgia paresthetica is conservative. Oral therapeutics, such as nonsteroidal anti-inflammatory medications, and neuropathic agents, such as gabapentin, are usually prescribed. Refractory cases may be amenable to selective blocks or radiofrequency ablation. There is no role for active physical therapy in this condition, though if weight gain is suspected to be a causing factor, weight loss can be recommended.

Common Peroneal Neuropathy at the Fibular Neck

The common peroneal nerve is derived from the dorsal branches of the fourth and fifth lumbar nerves and from the first sacral nerve. It descends along the lateral side of the popliteal fossa and then winds around the fibular head. After that, it divides into the deep peroneal nerve and superficial peroneal nerve. The most common site of entrapment is around the fibular head, where it is very superficial and often palpable through the skin. Symptoms of entrapment include impaired foot dorsiflexion, and eversion and sensory loss or burning pain in the lateral lower leg and dorsum of the foot. The interweb space between the first and second digit is spared if only the superficial peroneal nerve is entrapped. Compression can result from tumors, habitual leg crossing, sudden weight loss, trauma, and positioning from anesthesia. There are hereditary causes such as hereditary neuropathy with liability to pressure palsies, which is inherited in an autosomal dominant pattern and is caused by dysfunction of the *PMP22* gene causing the myelin to become unstable and extremely sensitive to compression, such as that from leg crossing in the case of the peroneal nerve. Electrodiagnostic testing will show demyelination and conduction block in the peroneal nerve CMAP as it traverses the fibular head. It is imperative to perform NC studies and EMG to rule out a sciatic neuropathy and L5 radiculopathy, which can have a similar clinical presentation. Surgery is indicated only if there is a focal compression from a tumor or cyst seen on neuroimaging. Otherwise, the mainstay of treatment involves aggressive physical therapy for gait training, strengthening, and stretching. Orthoses such as an ankle foot orthotic (AFO) is commonly prescribed to keep the ankle in a neutral position and prevent the foot drop from interfering with the gait.

Tarsal Tunnel Syndrome

This syndrome is also known as posterior tibial neuralgia. It occurs when the tibial nerve is compressed in the tarsal tunnel, which is a canal formed between the medial malleolus and the flexor retinaculum. Symptoms consist of shooting pain, numbness, or burning in the bottom of the foot and toes. Proposed causes of tarsal tunnel include orthopedic deformities such as flat feet or fallen arches. Additionally, bone spurs, swelling, and ganglion cysts within the tunnel can cause compression. Systemic disease such as diabetes and arthritis can also increase the pressure within the tunnel. Electrodiagnostic testing is imperative in establishing a diagnosis. On NC studies, the sural SNAP will be normal, while the medial and/or lateral plantar nerves will either be absent or with significantly decreased amplitude. Depending on the chronicity of the compression, EMG may show membrane instability in the abductor hallucis, flexor digitorum brevis, and/or abductor digiti quinti muscles. Therapy is targeted to symptom control with nonsteroidal anti-inflammatory medications and neuropathic pain agents. Orthosis such as splints and braces can be tried to keep the foot in a neutral position and limit the amount of movement and pressure on the foot. Injections can be attempted if conservative treatment fails. Surgery for tarsal tunnel release for refractory cases can also be pursued. Any space-occupying lesion can be removed surgically and neurolysis can be performed, or any adhesions can be carefully dissected and the nerve can be released from flexor retinaculum.

Polyneuropathy

Polyneuropathy can result from axonal degeneration, segmental demyelination, or a combination of both. Axonal degeneration is a pathologic reaction of the peripheral nerve in which the myelin sheath breaks down concomitantly with the axon in the process that usually starts at the most distal part of the nerve. This produces the dying back or length-dependent neuropathy. In segmental demyelination, there is injury of either myelin sheaths or Schwann cells resulting in the breakdown of myelin with sparing of the axons. This can occur mechanically by acute or chronic nerve compression, through immune-mediated demyelinating neuropathies, or via hereditary disorders of Schwann cell/myelin metabolism.

Sensory symptoms of neuropathy are decreased light touch, pinprick, vibration, proprioception, temperature, paresthesias, allodynia, neuropathic pain, and hyperalgesia. Motor nerve dysfunction manifests as weakness, atrophy, gait abnormalities, muscle cramps, and tremors. In certain neuropathies, there can also be autonomic dysfunction such as hypotension, anhydrosis, xerostomia, gastroparesis, diarrhea, urinary dysfunction, sexual dysfunction, and pupillary abnormalities.

■ Acquired Polyneuropathy

Acquired polyneuropathies can be divided into dysmetabolic, immune-mediated, infectious, carcinomatous, drug-induced/toxic and, lastly, cryptogenic.

Dysmetabolic Polyneuropathies

In this subgroup, symptoms and signs are typical of a length-dependent neuropathy. Sensory loss usually begins distally in the toes, and then gradually progresses over time up the legs. If the neuropathy is severe enough, it can also be present in the fingers and rarely can extend all the way up the arms. On examination, there is initially pain and temperature sensation loss due to preferential involvement of the small nerve fibers. As the disease progresses, the larger fibers are impacted resulting in light touch and vibratory sensory loss and suppression of muscle stretch reflexes. Usually, motor function is preserved earlier in the disease with only some mild atrophy or weakness of foot intrinsic muscles. Later in the disease, motor nerves are also affected. Diabetes is the most common cause of peripheral neuropathy in the developed world. Other causes include vitamin deficiencies such as B1, B6, niacin, and B12, renal disease, and systemic illnesses such as amyloidosis. Electrodiagnostic testing may be completely normal early on in the disease, or can have values in the lower end of normative data. These findings are due to the fact that the small myelinated and unmyelinated nerve fibers, which are affected early in the disease course, do not contribute to the SNAP. Eventually, with progression of the disease, SNAP amplitudes decrease and slowing of conduction velocities (CV) ensue involving the sural and superficial nerves first. With further progression, motor responses amplitudes become lower with prolonged distal latencies. However, there should be no evidence of conduction slowing to suggest demyelination, presence of conduction block, and/or temporal dispersion. Although EMG is typically normal, there can be evidence of denervation with membrane instability (fibrillation and positive sharp waves) if the neuropathy is severe. EMG may also reveal chronic neurogenic changes (larger amplitudes and/or polyphasic motor unit action potentials [MUAP]) with decreased recruitment pattern if the condition has been present for a long period of time.

There is no cure for neuropathy; however, the symptoms can be managed to provide an adequate quality of daily living. The treatment of most polyneuropathies often depends on identifying the causative agent and attempting to correct or control it. Pharmacologic therapy is targeted at relieving the neuropathic pain. There are many neuropathic agents, such as gabapentin, pregabalin, nortriptyline, topical lidocaine, and capsaicin. Physical therapy is often indicated for balance and gait training. If the neuropathy is severe enough to cause muscle weakness, strengthening and stretching exercises as well as orthoses and assistive gait devices should be utilized to improve patient function. Another important aspect of physical therapy is the home safety evaluation. Often, the gait dysfunction is worse at night, when the visual input for maintaining balance is lacking, which can result in falls. A home evaluation is important to ensure that there are proper rails and other safety measures in place.

Immune-Meditated Polyneuropathies

The two most common immune-mediated polyneuropathies seen are acute immune-mediated polyneuropathy (AIDP) and chronic immune-mediated polyneuropathy (CIDP).

AIDP is a rare, but important, disease that can lead to life-threatening respiratory failure. It is an immune-mediated response that causes myelin damage. A majority of patients have an antecedent viral or gastrointestinal illness. The clinical presentation is one of a rapidly progressing weakness of an ascending paralysis. It usually starts with distal weakness, but cranial nerves can also be affected early on. On examination, one can see symmetric weakness, sensory loss, hyporeflexia, and dysautonomia. On electrodiagnostic testing, there is characteristic slowing of conduction velocities in the demyelinating range with or without temporal dispersion and conduction block. The F-waves are preferentially affected by the disease and are often absent at the very onset of symptoms. F-waves are usually used to evaluate motor conduction problems in the proximal part of nerves. The F-waves essentially are CMAPs that are elicited by supramaximal antidromic stimulation of a nerve. The axons that are stimulated have depolarization waves travel back to the spinal cord (antidromic), depolarize some anterior horn cells that are excitable enough to fire back depolarization waves toward the muscle fibers (orthodromic) and generate the F-wave. Roughly 5% of anterior horn cells have that capacity and those belong to small intrinsic hand and foot muscles only.

Management is usually in an intensive care unit setting owing to the respiratory and autonomic complications, and consists of treatment with immune globulin and in some more rapidly progressing cases, with plasma exchange.

AIDP can be a significant cause of long-term disability. Overall, the mortality associated with AIDP is low: 3% of patients die of complications. The progressive phase is limited to 4 weeks and most patients generally have a favorable outcome. According to Khan (2012), 30% of patients with rapid progression require ventilator support and 20% may have residual permanent severe disability with deficits in ambulation or the need for ventilator assistance. More than one third of patients require inpatient rehabilitation with a multidisciplinary approach. Inpatient rehabilitation programs and postdischarge individualized home-based therapy programs are required. They include a range of motion exercise for the limbs, breathing exercises with patients who have respiratory difficulties, home modifications for access, gait training with or without splints, assistive devices, and activities of daily living training. Those patients who have AIDP-related residual motor and sensory deficits at 1 year usually have neuropathic pain, foot drop necessitating ankle–foot orthoses and locomotion difficulty requiring other assistive devices.

CIDP is a symmetric polyradiculoneuropathy or polyneuropathy, affecting motor and sensory fibers, proximal and distal limbs, and infrequently cranial nerves and the central nervous system (CNS) occurring in a progressive or stepwise progressive or relapsing course. The characteristic symptoms are weakness and altered sensation and paresthesias. Fifteen percent to 20% of patients present with Guillain–Barre syndrome (AIDP) initially. The male to female ratio is 2:1 and the incidence increases until the age of 60. On electrodiagnostic testing, there is slowing of motor and sensory conduction velocities where the proximal nerve segments may have a greater degree of reduction of conduction velocity than distal segments. There are many illnesses that can be associated with CIDP, such as HIV, chronic active hepatitis, lymphoma, connective tissue disorders, and disorders of the bone marrow, to name a few. A therapeutic trial of plasma exchange, course of steroids, and nowadays, intravenous immunoglobulin (IVIG) usually results in unequivocal improvement of the neurologic disability score and/or in neurophysiological parameters. This therapy may need to be chronic.

Other Causes of Neuropathy

Infections with either bacteria or viruses such as herpes zoster, leprosy, Lyme, and HIV often can be associated with neuropathy. There are a number of cancer-related neuropathies, such as with lymphoma, myeloma, or carcinomatosis. There are many drugs and toxins that can cause neuropathy. Toxins include mercury, lead, ethylene oxide, and dimethylaminopropionitrile to name a few. Chemotherapeutic agents are notorious for causing neuropathy such as vinca alkaloids (vincristine), cisplatin, paclitaxel, and the podophyllotoxins (etoposide and teniposide). Some other drugs used to treat cancers and infections such as thalidomide and interferon also can cause peripheral neuropathy.

Critical Illness Neuropathy

This disease of the peripheral nerves often occurs as a complication from a prolonged hospitalization for a severe injury or illness. Typically the patient will present with predominantly distal weakness and/or difficulty with extubation. The diagnostic criteria for this entity include the onset of weakness following critical illness such as sepsis, multiorgan failure, respiratory failure, or septic inflammatory response syndrome (SIRS). Electrodiagnostic testing is performed to rule out any other illnesses, such as AIDP. The typical findings on NC studies are loss of amplitudes or absence of SNAPs and CMAPs. On EMG, there is evidence of acute membrane instability with active widespread denervation. More severe underlying illness is associated with a more severe neuropathy. There is no treatment for critical illness neuropathy. The treatment is supportive with physical therapy, occupational therapy, and respiratory therapy, as well as correction of the underlying metabolic and systemic illness. In the past, therapies such as administration of testosterone derivatives, immunoglobulins, growth hormone, and antioxidant therapy were tried without any benefit. Hermans and DeJonghe (2008) reported that several trials showed that intensive insulin therapy reduced the critical illness neuropathy electrophysiologic markers and shortened the need for supportive ventilation for at least 1 week. Recovery usually occurs within weeks in mild cases, and within months in severe cases. About 50% of patients have a full recovery, although the more severe neuropathy can be associated with a poor prognosis.

Hereditary Polyneuropathy

This group of diseases presents with slowly progressive weakness, muscle atrophy, and sensory loss.

Charcot–Marie–Tooth (CMT) is the most common hereditary polyneuropathy. It is classically associated with an insidious onset of distally predominant motor and sensory loss, muscle wasting, and pes cavus. The majority of patients with CMT will have onset of symptoms in the first to second decade of life, although there is significant variability ranging from severe deficits in early childhood to only mild features in very late life. CMT1 is a dominantly inherited, hypertrophic, predominantly demyelinating form. CMT2 is a dominantly inherited predominantly axonal form. Dejerine–Sottas disease is a severe form of demyelinating neuropathy clinically present in infancy with hypotonia and delayed motor development. CMTX is inherited in an X-linked manner. CMT4 includes the various demyelinating autosomal recessive forms of CMT disease. While there is no cure, the symptoms should be addressed with a multidisciplinary approach; neuropathic pain should be treated, physical therapy with emphasis on stretching to prevent contractures and improve or restore function, orthoses and other assistive devices such as walkers and wheelchairs as needed.

Mononeuritis Multiplex

This is a type of polyneuropathy that consists of painful, asymmetrical, asynchronous sensory and motor peripheral neuropathy involving nerves in different distributions. It can occur secondary to systemic diseases such as vasculitis, sarcoid, amyloid, diabetes, polyarteritis nodosa, or lupus. It can also be related to a paraneoplastic syndrome or lymphoma. Recovery is often seen, with a repeated flare up of the same nerves or new ones can get involved a few years later. Symptoms include pain, numbness, paresthesias, and weakness in different nerve distributions. Electrodiagnostic testing is imperative in establishing a diagnosis. NC studies reveal SNAPs with decreased amplitudes and conduction velocities of nerves in different distributions. CMAPs will often show axonal loss manifested primarily in decreased amplitude with or without mild slowing of conduction velocities. EMG will have a wide array of manifestations depending on the chronicity of the symptoms. There are common signs of denervation and membrane instability, neurogenic motor units, and loss of recruitment. Treatment usually depends on the etiology underlying the neuropathy. Physical therapy is recommended; however, the specific treatment plan should be determined based on the affected nerves and the clinical presentation of the patient. Therapy should aim to prevent contractures and maintain strength through the use of range of motion and strengthening exercises. Braces or splints to help improve independence are recommended. Safety training is also imperative. Occupational therapies address the need for adaptive techniques to assist with the safe completion of activities of daily living and are paramount for patient well-being. Pharmacologic therapy can be divided into symptom control and disease modification. Symptom control should include neuropathic pain management with agents such as gabapentin, tricyclics, and anticonvulsants. Treatment should target the underlying process, but corticosteroids as well as immunosuppresants, such as IVIG, are usually helpful as the underlying process is presumably immune mediated.

Plexopathy

Plexopathies involving the brachial plexus and lumbar and sacral plexus are exceedingly rare. The fibers that travel through the plexus can be affected by compression, traction, stretch, radiation, and laceration.

The brachial plexus is more commonly affected than the lumbar and sacral plexus. In the upper extremity, they can occur as a result of birth injuries, falls, penetrating injuries, or vehicle trauma. They often lead to physical disability, stress, and socioeconomic hardship (Ko, 2011). The roots and trunks are frequently more affected than the division, cords, and terminal branches. The dorsal root ganglia hold the cell bodies of the sensory nerve and lie outside the spinal canal. When the spinal roots are avulsed from the cord, a preganglionic injury will occur. In this setting, electrodiagnostic testing of the sensory nerve action potential will be normal, whereas in a postganglionic lesion they will be affected. This distinction is important to make as in preganglionic lesions, prognosis for recovery is poor with little to no role for surgical intervention. In brachial plexus lesions, if the nerves are not avulsed by surgical repair, nerve grafting or neurolysis may be indicated. The type of repair utilized is typically dependent on the underlying mechanism of the injury.

Lesions of the lumbar and sacral plexus are exceedingly rare. When they do occur, they most often are related to trauma with many nerves being affected at multiple sites. Other etiologies include inflammation, infections, neoplasms, and paraneoplastic processes. Diabetes can also present as a neuralgic amyotrophy or even as amyotrophy affecting the femoral nerve predominantly.

Electrodiagnostic testing is imperative in delineating the extent of the lesion and is also helpful in prognostication (partial lesions with lesser nerve distribution involvement have excellent reinnervation and outcome).

Radiculopathy

One of the most common complaints in the population today is neck and back pain. Often, this pain will have a radicular component (pain and/or sensorimotor deficit due to compression of a nerve root). Most common causes of radiculopathy are degenerative disc disease, disc herniations, spondylosis, spinal instability, spinal stenosis, and rarely, tumors. Patients with radiculopathy may complain of pain, weakness, or numbness in the distribution of the nerve that is being compressed. History alone is often the most important component in establishing a working clinical diagnosis.

■ Cervical Radiculopathy

Radiculopathies are described by the nerve root that is being compressed: C2 radicular pain can manifest itself as eye and/or ear pain and headache; C3 and C4 symptoms tend to be vague neck pain and trapezius area pain; C5 pain occurs in the shoulder and radiates down the ventral arm to elbow or even below the elbow; C6 radiculopathy is associated with pain down the superior lateral aspect of the arm into the first two digits; C7 pain radiates down the dorsal aspect of the arm, through the elbow, and into the third digit; C8 symptoms move down the inferior medial aspect of the arm into the fourth and fifth digits, while T1 radiculopathy involves the medial forearm; C5 radiculopathy may show weakness in the deltoid muscle; C6 radiculopathy presents with weakness in the biceps brachii and extensor carpi radialis muscles (evaluated by testing of elbow flexion and wrist extension); C7 weakness is typically seen in the triceps brachii muscle, as well as in the wrist flexion/extension; C8 and/or T1 root pathology causes weakness in the intrinsic muscles of the hand, as evaluated by finger spread (adduction/abduction) and grip. Muscle stretch reflexes also tend to be decreased (asymmetric) in the setting of radiculopathy (Caridi, Pumberger, & Hughes, 2011).

■ Lumbar Radiculopathy

Tarulli and Raynor (2007) reported that the prevalence of lumbosacral radiculopathy is approximately 3% to 5%, distributed equally in men and women. L1 radiculopathy is extremely uncommon. Typical presentation is one of pain, paresthesias, and sensory loss in the inguinal region, without significant weakness. Infrequently, subtle involvement of hip flexion is noted. L2 radiculopathy produces pain, paresthesias, and sensory loss in the anterolateral thigh. Weakness of hip flexion may occur. Disc herniation is an uncommon cause of L3 radiculopathy, although is more common than with higher lumbar roots. Pain and paresthesias involve the medial thigh and knee, with weakness of hip flexors, hip adductors, and knee extensors; the knee jerk may be depressed or absent. L4 radiculopathy is produced most commonly by disc herniation. Sensory symptoms involve the medial lower leg in the distribution of the saphenous nerve. L3 radiculopathy presents with the knee extension and hip adduction weakness; additionally, foot dorsiflexion weakness may be sometimes observed (due to variable L4 innervation of the tibialis anterior muscle). The knee jerk may be depressed or absent. The most common cause of L5 radiculopathy is disc herniation. Foot drop is the salient clinical feature, with associated sensory symptoms involving the anterolateral leg and dorsum of the foot. In addition to weakness of ankle dorsiflexion, L5 radiculopathy commonly produces weakness of toe extension and flexion, foot inversion and eversion, and hip abduction. S1 radiculopathy also is caused commonly by intervertebral disc herniation, with associated weakness of foot plantar flexion, knee flexion, and hip extension. Subtle weakness of foot plantar flexion may be demonstrated by having patients stand or walk on their toes. Sensory symptoms typically involve the lateral foot and sole. The ankle jerk is depressed or absent (Tarulli & Raynor, 2007).

Electrodiagnostic testing is imperative in establishing the diagnosis, especially as other underlying diseases need to be evaluated for. The symptoms of a C6 radiculopathy can often present very similar to carpal tunnel median nerve lesions, and a C8 radiculopathy can be confused for an ulnar neuropathy. Neurophysiologic testing is necessary to differentiate between these entities. In radiculopathies, the SNAPs and CMAPs should show no abnormalities in latency, amplitude, and conduction velocity. EMG may show mild findings of abnormal spontaneous activity to widespread denervation with neurogenic motor units and a pattern of decreased interference if there is profound weakness in the appropriate muscle groups.

Treatment options depend on the severity of the symptoms. Physical therapy for stretching and strengthening is often recommended. Oral therapeutics including the use of nonsteroidal anti-inflammatory medications and steroids can also be given in combination with the trial of physical therapy. Pain management is geared toward targeted injections to the proposed pain generators, including facet injections, foraminal injections, and epidural injections. Epidural injections are commonly used to treat pain caused by radiculopathy that can be caused by conditions such as disc herniations and spinal stenosis, whereas facet injections target pain caused by inflamed facet joints, and foraminal injections target the side of the spine where a specific nerve root exits.

MOTOR NEURON DISEASES

Motor neuron diseases can be divided into heritable and sporadic, as well as classified based on the degree of upper motor neuron or lower motor neuron involvement.

Lower Motor Neuron Diseases

This includes heritable diseases such as spinal muscular atrophy (SMA) and spinobulbar muscle atrophy (SBMA). SMA can present at birth, in childhood, or in early adulthood, while SBMA typically presents in later adulthood. SMA presents with progressive proximal weakness that ultimately leads to problems with ambulation. There is no sensory loss or other upper motor neuron signs. The mode of inheritance is autosomal dominant. In SBMA, there is a bulbar weakness in addition to lower motor neuron findings in the lower extremities. This disease is X-linked owing to a CAG repeat expansion in the androgen receptor gene.

Upper Motor Neuron Disease

Primary lateral sclerosis (PLS) is a disorder of progressive upper motor neuron dysfunction. It is extremely rare, and represents 1% to 4% of all patients with motor neuron disease (Stratland & Barohn, 2015a). Symptoms typically present in the fifth or sixth decade of life, with stiffness, clumsiness, dysarthria, dysphagia, and emotional lability. Weakness, spasticity, and hyperreflexia often begin in the legs. The progression is slow. PLS is a diagnosis of exclusion. Workup should include B12, HIV, Human T-Lymphotropic Virus type I (HTLV) and paraneoplastic tests, MRI of neuroaxis, cerebrospinal fluid analysis, and electrodiagnostic testing. There is no cure, and therapies are geared toward helping to alleviate symptoms and to improve function. Physical therapy and occupation therapy for range of motion, gait and balance training, and assistive devices are the mainstays of treatment (Stratland & Barohn, 2015a). Oral therapeutics that are usually used to relieve spasticity include baclofen, tizanidine, or Valium. The placement of an intrathecal baclofen pump may ultimately be beneficial. For management of secretions, oral anticholinergics are the first-line drugs of choice with Botox injections indicated only when oral medications are ineffective. Lastly, combination dextromethorphan and quinidine is the only U.S. Food and Drug Administration (FDA)–approved agent for pseudobulbar affect.

Amyotrophic Lateral Sclerosis

Amyotrophic lateral sclerosis (ALS), also known as Lou Gehrig's disease, should be strongly considered when there is a combination of upper and lower motor neuron findings. The annual incidence rate is 1.52 per 100,000 person years. There is a higher prevalence in men compared to woman with a male-to-female ratio of 1:56. Overall, ALS is twice as common in Caucasians compared to African Americans (Stratland & Barohn, 2015a). The clinical features suggestive of ALS include insidious onset of painless weakness and muscle wasting, typically starting in one limb before spreading to others. There is muscle stiffness, spasticity, cramps, and fasciculations. There can be head drop, as well as bulbar symptoms, and unexplained restrictive airway disease. The median time from diagnosis to death is 2.5 to 3 years. Several factors are associated with a faster progression including bulbar symptoms at onset, older age at symptom onset, shorter duration of symptoms, and reduced vital capacity. There are regional ALS variants. Patients who have either the lower motor neuron variant or the upper motor neuron variant have a slower disease progression.

The diagnosis is based on clinical history and physical examination findings. Electrodiagnostic testing is very useful for diagnosis confirmation with evidence of both widespread denervation (fibrillation, fasciculations, and positive sharp waves) and reinnervation (large, frequently unstable motor units of increased duration with reduced interference pattern). Additional investigations should always be obtained to rule out any other disorders that can present with both upper and lower motor neuron dysfunction (such as coexistence of both cervical and lumbar spinal stenosis with multilevel radiculopathies). These tests include MRI of the brain and spine and screening for infection (HIV, Lyme), toxins (heavy metals), malignancy (lymphoma, paraneoplastic syndromes), and autoimmune diseases (GM1 antibodies).

The clinical diagnosis of ALS is broken down by probabilities according to the revised El Escorial Criteria. "Clinically definite" demonstrates the presence of upper and lower motor neuron signs in the bulbar region and in two to three spinal cord levels. "Clinically probable" is considered when there are upper and lower motor neuron signs in two spinal cord levels with the upper motor neuron signs, rostral to the lower motor neuron signs. "Clinically probable-laboratory supported" is considered when there are upper and lower motor neuron signs in one spinal cord level, and lower motor neuron signs in two levels. "Clinically possible" is defined as displaying upper and lower motor neuron signs in one region, upper motor neuron signs found alone in two regions, or lower motor neuron signs found rostral to the upper motor neuron findings (Stratland & Barohn, 2015a).

All patients diagnosed with ALS should be followed in a specialized multidisciplinary clinic. Respiratory function needs to be carefully monitored. Noninvasive ventilation should be considered to treat respiratory insufficiency, both to lengthen survival time and to slow the rate of forced vital capacity decline. Speech and swallowing functions need to be closely monitored. If swallowing problems are present, diet adjustment and ultimately feeding tube placement might be needed. Assistive communication devices are frequently necessary to allow effective communication. Physical and occupational therapy are needed to maintain as much independent function for as long as possible and to provide braces and wheelchairs as needed in conjunction with a physician familiar with the needs of these patients. Excessive salivation can be treated with Botox or anticholinergics. Currently there is only one FDA-approved therapeutic drug for ALS, riluzole, which can only prolong life expectancy by 3 months and improve respiratory outcome. The mechanism of action is thought to be decreasing glutamate toxicity on the motor neurons. Dextromethorphan and quinidine combination is an FDA-approved treatment for pseudobulbar affect (involuntary uncontrollable episodes of crying or laughing) frequently present in patients with ALS. Lastly, end of life discussions and advanced directives should be addressed to optimize a peaceful and dignified death (Jackson, McVey, & Rudnicki, 2015).

■ Polio (Post-Poliomyelitis Syndrome)

Laffont and Julia (2010) reported that there is an estimate of 20 million individuals affected by poliomyelitis worldwide. It is an infectious disease of the neurologic system, and over the years has been the cause of most motor disabilities in the world (Boyer, Tiffreau, & Rapin, 2010). Polio is caused by an enterovirus and most commonly affects children and young adults. The virus attacks the anterior horn cells of the spinal cord and brainstem, which leads to asymmetric limb muscle weakness, and in some cases respiratory and bulbar weakness as well. This is followed by the recovery phase in which there is a nerve terminal sprouting leading to reinnervation of previously denervated muscle fibers. Electrodiagnostic testing of affected muscles often show neurogenic enlarged motor units in the absence of any acute denervation. There are many complications that are seen in polio survivors. There is a high incidence of tendon disease, especially at the rotator cuff and elbow. There is arthritis, commonly affecting the lower limbs. Osteoporosis is more common in polio survivors than in the general population. There is back pain often present with a radicular component. Secondary scoliosis can aggravate symptoms as well. Fatigue is the most common sequela reported by patients, as well as decreased attention, concentration, and memory difficulties, thought to be due to involvement of brain structures, especially in the reticular activating system (Laffont & Julia, 2010).

Post-polio syndrome is a clinical entity affecting polio survivors with the new onset of symptoms, several years or decades after the initial polio attack, which was followed by a period of stability (Boyer, Tiffreau, & Rapin, 2010). These symptoms include new onset muscle weakness, atrophy, fatigue, muscle or joint pain, sleep disorders, dysphonia/dysphagia, or respiratory insufficiency. The prevalence has been reported from 15% to 80% (Tiffrenau & Rapin, 2010). Halstead and Rossi (1985) suggested one of the first cohesive criteria for diagnosis of post-polio syndrome. Currently, according to Farbu and Gilhus (2006), the consensus from the European Federation of Neurologic Societies suggests that the criteria for this diagnosis should include: Halstead criteria of confirmed history of polio, partial recovery after the acute episode, and period of functional stability of at least 15 years with new onset of symptoms such as fatigue, joint pain, weakness, or atrophy that cannot be otherwise explained.

Clinical neurophysiological studies are essential in establishing this diagnosis. The diagnosis of a lower motor neuron syndrome, showing an ongoing denervation–reinnervation process supports the diagnosis (Farbu & Gilhus, 2006). Additionally, any other muscle or nerve disorders such as radiculopathy, entrapment neuropathies, or polymyositis should also be excluded.

There is no effective treatment for the post-polio syndrome. Different therapeutic agents were tried in the past. Based on Class I studies, acetylcholinesterase inhibitors, steroids, as well as amantadine had no significant effect on muscular strength or fatigue in post-polio syndrome patients (Farbu & Gilhus, 2006). Gonzalez, Olsson, and Borg (2010) reported similar results were found in studying the effect of IVIG. Restless legs syndrome, which is a common complaint in patients with post-polio syndrome, can be successfully treated with dopamine agonists (Gonzalez & Olsson, 2006).

In the past, there have been claims that muscular overuse and training can worsen the symptoms of post-polio syndrome and even provoke further muscle loss. However, there are no prospective studies that show that increased muscle activity or training will lead to loss of strength when compared to the absence of training and therapy. On the contrary, patients who exercise regularly report fewer symptoms and are at a higher functional level than those who are inactive (Gonzalez & Olsson, 2006). Aquatic physical therapy is the treatment of choice for post-polio syndrome, as it is possible to do muscular training in a controlled resistance environment and also to perform an assisted active autonomous workout on deficient muscles in an antigravity setting. This also helps to create proper conditions for relieving musculoskeletal pain (Tiffrenau & Rapin, 2010). Patients with post-polio syndrome should also be supplied with appropriate orthoses and braces based on individual needs. Braces can restrict unwanted movements and support joints and muscles while helping to improve mobility and reduce pain. Besides orthoses, assistive devices to increase functional activity, including crutches, manual and electric wheelchairs, and motorized scooters, can also be considered (Gonzalez, Olsson, & Borg, 2010). Lastly, early recognition of respiratory impairment and timely introduction of noninvasive ventilator aids prevents or delays further respiratory decline and the need for invasive respiratory aids. Group training, regular follow-ups, and patient education and support groups are important for the patient's well-being and mental status (Gonzalez & Olsson, 2006).

DISEASES OF THE NEUROMUSCULAR JUNCTION

The neuromuscular junction (NMJ) is a synaptic structure composed of the nerve terminal, with acetylcholine vesicles, the junctional cleft, and the muscle endplate on the postsynaptic membrane containing acetylcholine receptors (AChR). The NMJ is depicted in Figure 13.7. At the nerve terminal, there are small numbers of vesicles available for immediate release; a mobilization store serves as backup to this immediately available store and a larger pool of vesicles serves as a reserve supply. Normally, an action potential travels along the motor axon to the motor nerve terminus where it causes depolarization, resulting in opening of voltage-gated calcium channels. The calcium enters the presynaptic membrane and initiates release of acetylcholine (ACh) into the synaptic cleft. ACh diffuses across the synaptic cleft and binds to ACh receptors (AChR) causing sodium and potassium flux across the membrane and resulting in a depolarizing endplate potential (EPP). When the EPP reaches the threshold (10–15 mV), a muscle fiber action potential is initiated, causing a muscle contraction.

The NMJ disorders are divided into presynaptic and postsynaptic conditions, depending on where there is the pathology in relationship to the synaptic cleft.

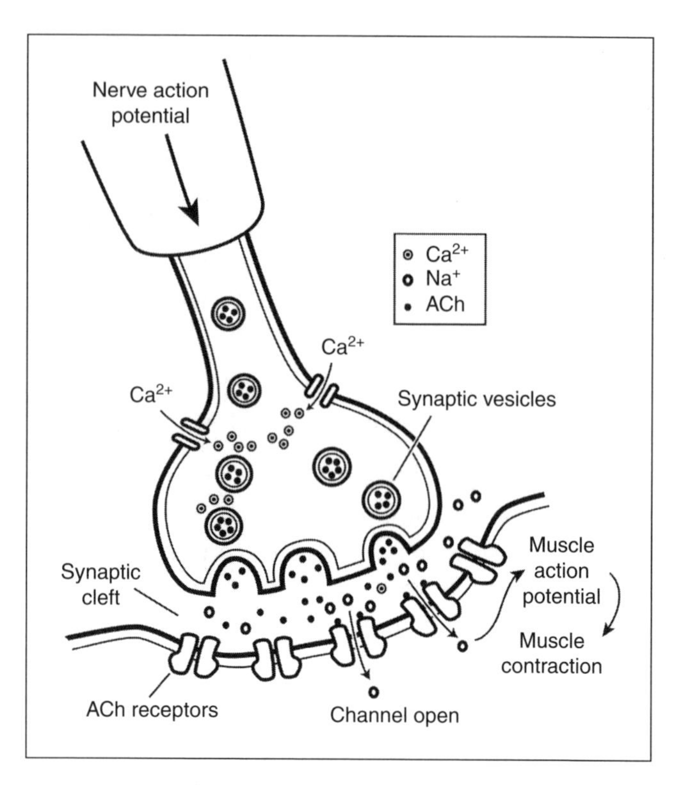

FIGURE 13.7 Neuromuscular junction.

Two main presynaptic entities are Lambert–Eaton myasthenic syndrome and botulism.

Lambert–Eaton Myasthenic Syndrome

In Lambert–Eaton myasthenic syndrome (LEMS), antibodies against the P/Q type of the voltage-gated calcium channel block the ability of calcium to flow into the nerve terminal during the depolarization, thus disrupting the release of ACh. This disruption of ACh release ultimately leads to a reduced number of fibers contracting, and causes the clinical manifestation of weakness, decreased reflexes, and autonomic symptoms. There are two types of LEMS: paraneoplastic and sporadic autoimmune. Paraneoplastic LEMS is most often associated with small-cell lung cancer.

Age of onset is typically over 40 years. The most common presenting symptom is leg weakness, followed by more generalized weakness, muscle pain or stiffness, dry mouth, arm weakness, diplopia, and dysarthria (2%). Autonomic dysfunction, including dry mouth, blurred vision, hypohidrosis, constipation, and orthostatic hypotension, occurs in up to 75% to 80% of patients with LEMS. Hypoactive tendon reflexes are typically seen with frequent transient postexercise facilitation of diminished reflexes.

Diagnosis is confirmed by positive serologic testing and electrophysiological studies, which display characteristic features of low compound muscle action potentials, a decrement at 3Hz repetitive nerve stimulation, and facilitation with exercise or high-frequency repetitive stimulation. Treatment involves cancer monitoring and treatment. Usually, treating the cancer improves the symptoms significantly. The drug of choice for LEMS is 3,4-diaminopyridine, which inhibits presynaptic voltage-gated potassium channels, thereby prolonging the nerve action potential and increasing release of ACh into the synaptic cleft. The alternative therapies are immunosuppressive medications, with prednisone and azathioprine, and ACh esterase inhibitors.

Botulism

Botulism is another presynaptic disorder of neuromuscular transmission. Botulinum toxin is a neurotoxin with a mechanism of action that disrupts peripheral nervous system cholinergic transmission presynaptically, by impairment of the fusion and release of the vesicles containing ACh, thereby causing skeletal muscle weakness and autonomic dysfunction. There are four modes of transmission: food-borne, wound, infant, and "other" (in which the patient is not an infant, there is no wound, and no history of suspicious food ingestion). Clinical features classically involve cranial and bulbar palsies followed by descending weakness of the limbs, respiratory failure, and autonomic dysfunction. Electrodiagnostic testing is important in the evaluation and diagnosis. Treatment is supportive, and administration of antitoxin is beneficial in selected cases.

There is a variety of therapeutic and cosmetic uses of botulinum toxin. In neuromuscular disorders it is frequently used to treat spasticity and sialorrhea.

Myasthenia Gravis

Myasthenia gravis (MG) is the most common autoimmune disease affecting the NMJ, and is considered a postsynaptic disorder. Most frequently, it is caused by antibodies against NMJ proteins, either the nicotinic acetylcholine receptor (nAChR) or the muscle-specific tyrosine kinase (MuSK). Approximately 80% to 85% of generalized MG and 50% of ocular MG have antibodies against nAChRs. There are three nAChR-Ab types: binding, blocking, and modulating. MuSK-antibody positive MG usually presents with predominantly ocular, facial, and bulbar symptoms. Even in "seronegative" cases of MG, there are low affinity antibodies against clustered AchRs detected in near 50% to 60% cases (Jacob, Viegas, Lashley, & Hilton-Jones, 2009). Alternatively, in a much rarer form, muscle weakness is caused by a genetic defect in some portion of the NMJ that is inherited at birth.

Prevalence of myasthenia is 1 to 2 per 10,000 and it is increasing owing to better diagnosing tools and survival. There is a bimodal age of onset: early (usually women less than 40 years) and late (males after age of 60 years).

Clinically, MG presents as fluctuating painless muscle weakness and fatigue of the extraocular muscles, facial muscles, bulbar muscles, neck musculature, and extremities. Patients may present with nasal or slurred speech with upper eyelid weakness with double vision or with difficulty swallowing. When the extremities are affected, the proximal muscles are usually more severely involved than the distal ones. The weakness is often worse with activity, but improved by rest. The disease does not involve cardiac or smooth muscle, nor is there an alteration of cognitive skills, coordination, sensation, or autonomic function.

Several physiological, pathological, and iatrogenic factors exacerbate myasthenia and can lead to myasthenic crisis with respiratory failure. The most common are infection, trauma, surgery, toxic–metabolic disturbances, as well as certain medications. The most common offending agents are aminoglycosides, sulfonamide, quinidine, clindamycin, tetracyclines, chloroquine, muscle relaxants, sedatives, narcotics, anticonvulsants, Dilantin, and ethosuximide. Myasthenic crisis affects approximately 10% to 15% of patients. MuSK antibody myasthenia patients are more likely to develop myasthenic crisis. Predictors of a crisis include a poor vital capacity due to respiratory muscle weakness and an inability to keep the airway patent.

The diagnosis of MG is suspected based on the fluctuating nature of weakness, and confirmed by administration of the rapidly acting ACh inhibitor, edrophonium, also known as the Tensilon test. A positive test is manifested by dramatic clinical improvement. The nAChR antibodies should be checked and are positive in 80% to 85% of generalized MG. If they are negative, the MuSK antibodies should be tested. Other antibodies, such as anti–striated muscle antibodies and anti-titin antibodies are also associated with MG with thymoma (Yamamoto, 2001). Electrodiagnostic testing is very helpful to confirm the diagnosis and rule out other neurological conditions. Repetitive nerve stimulation shows decremental response (more than 10% decline in amplitude). Single fiber EMG is the most sensitive test, revealing increased jitter and blocking, indicating NMJ transmission defect.

The use of radiographic studies (chest x-ray and chest CT scans) is important in the evaluation and identification of those patients with thymoma.

Myasthenia is treated with medications such as ACh esterase inhibitors or immunosupressants, and, in selected cases, thymectomy (surgical removal of the thymus). Pyridostigmine (Mestinon) is the most common first line treatment. It inhibits the action of ACh esterase, allowing acetylcholine to remain longer at the NMJ. This increases the ability to generate a muscle action potential. Prednisone is the first-line immunosuppressant treatment for MG and is the most consistently effective therapy for MG. The vast majority of patients do not achieve adequate symptomatic improvement with cholinesterase inhibitor therapy alone and require prednisone.

To avoid steroid-induced side effects, the "steroid-sparing" immunosuppressive agents are used to allow reductions of corticosteroid dose. Among these agents, the most commonly used are azathioprine, cyclosporine, methotrexate, and cyclophosphamide.

For the acute exacerbation of myasthenic symptoms in patients with myasthenic crisis, or when rapid correction of symptoms is necessary (e.g., prior to surgery), there are rapidly acting immunotherapies that include IVIG therapy, the mechanism of action of which is to bind and neutralize the antibodies and plasmapheresis, which works by removing antibodies. They have quick onsets of action compared with the therapies described earlier, but shorter effect, usually between 4 and 6 weeks.

Thymectomy has been a mainstay of treatment for MG; however, a more recent rigorous evidence-based evaluation concluded that thymectomy might only improve the chance of remission (Gronseth & Barohn, 2000).

Even though there are not enough studies to prove the benefit of exercise in MG, it was established that there are no harmful effects. Furthermore, it was proposed that MG patients may benefit from exercise by reversing their baseline deconditioning. Regular mild–moderate level of exertion of aerobic exercises and respiratory training have been shown to improve MG functional status, respiratory endurance, self-perception of physical fitness, and decrease fatigue. Based on these studies, current recommendations for the patients with MG are exercising during cooler times of the day, avoiding prolonged endurance-type exercises, and working out only after adequate rest (Anziska & Sternberg, 2013).

MUSCLE DISEASES

Myopathy refers to a clinical disorder of the skeletal muscles. Myopathies present as pure motor syndromes without any disturbance of sensory or autonomic function. Symptoms are usually symmetric and affect preferentially proximal muscles, but there are certain types with predominant involvement of the distal muscles.

Myopathies can be divided into two main groups: inherited and acquired.

Hereditary Myopathies

Hereditary myopathies are progressive muscle disorders caused by mutations in the genes needed for normal muscle structure and function. They share some common features; however, the severity varies significantly among the different disorders.

Hereditary myopathies can be subdivided into four main categories:

1. Muscular dystrophies
2. Congenital myopathies
3. Metabolic myopathies
4. Mitochondrial myopathies

■ Muscular Dystrophies

Muscular dystrophies are a group of inherited muscle disorders characterized by variable degrees and distribution of muscle wasting and weakness. In several dystrophies the heart can be seriously affected, sometimes in the absence of clinically significant weakness. Most of the diseases have their corresponding genes and their protein products identified, which is essential in establishing the diagnosis; however, there are no proven cures for any of the disorders as of yet. Stem cell and gene therapy are currently being investigated as potential for cure.

Dystrophinopathies include Duchenne muscular dystrophy (DMD) and Becker muscular dystrophy (BMD).

Duchenne Muscular Dystrophy

DMD is the most common and severe form of muscular dystrophy. The prevalence of DMD is 1.7 per 10,000 individuals. DMD is transmitted by an X-linked recessive inheritance. DMD is caused by the mutation of the *Xp21* gene loci, which codes for the sarcolemmal protein, dystrophin, an important cytoskeletal protein localized to the inner surface of the sarcolemma membrane. The mutation causes absence (or severe reduction) of dystrophin. The disease primarily affects boys, but in rare cases it can affect girls. Clinical severity depends on the amount or remaining functioning dystrophin (the lesser, the more severe).

Clinical features of DMD includes muscle weakness, usually beginning at age 2 to 4. Muscles affected initially include those of the hips, pelvic area, and thighs, resulting in delay in walking, waddling type gait, frequent falls, and difficulty climbing stairs. Weakness of the knee and hip extensors results in difficulty arising from the floor with a child climbing up the thighs, pushing down on them to extend the hips and trunk (Gower's sign). There is progressive lordotic posture (due to hip extensor weakness). The calves often are enlarged (pseudohypertrophy of calf muscles). Later, muscles of the shoulders, arms, and trunk are also involved. Fractures of the arms and legs are frequent. Children also frequently have mild cognitive impairment or global developmental delay (Banihani et al., 2015; Mirski & Crawford, 2014). Patients are usually wheelchair bound by 10 years of age. They later develop contractures of the hip and knee flexors, ankle plantar flexors, as well as the elbow and wrist flexors and scoliosis. Scoliosis in DMD typically occurs in the second decade. Scoliosis, in combination with progressive weakness, results in impaired pulmonary function, which in turn can cause acute respiratory failure. Bracing is known to be ineffective to stop the progression of scoliosis in these children. Spinal stabilization is recommended to correct significant spinal deformity. DMD also affects cardiac muscles and causes primary dilated cardiomyopathy. It is clinically apparent in about one third of patients by age 14 years, one half by 18 years, and all patients older than 18 years (Nigro, Comi, Bain, & Politano, 1990). There are also frequent conduction abnormalities with different types of arrhythmias.

Becker Muscular Dystrophy

BMD is closely related and allelic with DMD, with the same X-linked recessive pattern of inheritance; however, dystrophin is present, either in decreased amount or decreased function, at 20% to 80% of normal level, as opposed to completely or nearly absent dystrophin in DMD. Subsequently, BMD is characterized by later onset and milder symptoms. It is a slowly progressive muscle weakness of the legs and pelvis. Patients usually remain ambulatory until at least age 15 and commonly into adulthood, and even into old age. Intellectual disability and contractures are also not common. Although skeletal muscle involvement is less severe than in DMD, cardiac involvement in BMD is often more evident (Yazawa et al., 1987). Also, conduction abnormalities are more frequent and can result in fascicular and bundle branch block and can progress to complete heart block.

Emery–Dreifuss Muscular Dystrophy

Emery–Dreifuss muscular dystrophy (also known as humeroperoneal muscular dystrophy) can be inherited as an X-linked, autosomal dominant, or autosomal recessive, disorder, and is caused by mutations in the emerin (*Xq28*) or lamin A/C genes (*1q21*). It can present in childhood or in adults. It presents with early contractures, before any clinically significant weakness of the Achilles tendons, resulting in an equinus positioning of the feet and toe walking; elbow flexors, which restricts elbow extension; and posterior cervical muscles, limiting neck flexion. This can later result in extensive contractures of the cervical and lumbar extensor muscles, restricting spine forward flexion. The progression is usually slow with muscle weakness and wasting in humeroperoneal distribution first, and proximal limb-girdle musculature later in the disease. Cardiomyopathy with conduction defects and arrhythmias are frequent and cardiac disease presents by age 30 years.

Limb-Girdle Muscular Dystrophy

Limb-girdle muscular dystrophy (LGMD) is a muscular dystrophy with predominantly proximal limb-girdle distribution of weakness. So far, 15 genetically different types have been described, with significant clinical and genetic heterogeneity (seven with autosomal dominant and 12 with autosomal recessive inheritance). Most childhood-onset LGMDs are associated with predominantly lower extremity weakness, whereas most adult onsets present with shoulder and pelvic girdle weakness. Several types are associated with significant cardiac involvement.

Facioscapulohumeral Muscular Dystrophy

Facioscapulohumeral muscular dystrophy is the third most common type of muscular dystrophy. It is an autosomal dominant disorder with defect in the *DUX4* gene on chromosome 4. The age of onset is variable, from early childhood to adult life. The severity of this disorder ranges from mild to very severe (infantile form). The disease derives its name from the muscle groups that are mainly affected, first those of the face and shoulder girdle, followed by foot extensors, and later pelvic muscles. The heart is not usually affected, although arrhythmias and conduction defects have been described (Laforêt, 2001). There is a characteristic "Popeye" appearance due to wasting and weakness of the biceps and triceps, with relative prominence of the forearm. Mild restrictive lung disease occurs in approximately 50% of patients.

Oculopharyngeal Muscular Dystrophy

Oculopharyngeal muscular dystrophy (OPMD) is a rare autosomal dominant myopathy linked to chromosome 14. As its name implies, it is characterized by ocular and pharyngeal muscle involvement. Onset is around the third decade of life, affecting the extraocular muscles and upper facial muscles causing ptosis, dysarthria, and dysphagia. It can also be associated with proximal and distal upper (and sometimes lower) extremity weakness. It is a slowly progressive myopathy; however, ptosis can occlude vision, and severe dysphagia may lead to weight loss and death if not treated.

Myotonic Dystrophy

Myotonic dystrophy (DM) is a clinically and genetically heterogeneous disorder with both muscle weakness and myotonia (slowed relaxation following a normal muscle contraction), as well as other organ and system involvement. There are two major forms: DM1 (also known as Steinert's disease), caused by a mutation of the dystrophia myotonica protein kinase gene (*DMPK* gene) on chromosome *19q13*, and DM2, which is a milder form caused by mutation of zinc finger protein 9 gene located on chromosome *3q 21.3*. They are usually inherited in an autosomal dominant fashion.

DM is more than just a muscle disorder, as in addition to muscle weakness and myotonia, it is also characterized by involvement of many other organs and systems, including cardiac conduction abnormalities, cataracts, testicular failure, hypogammaglobulinemia, insulin resistance, cognitive disorders, and others. The weakness most frequently involves facial muscles, sternocleidomastoids, distal muscles of the forearm, and hand intrinsic muscles, which leads to compromised finger dexterity, and ankle dorsiflexor weakness causing bilateral foot drop. Less commonly, weakness can occur in the quadriceps, respiratory muscles, palatal and pharyngeal muscles, tongue, and extraocular muscles. There is common characteristic facial appearance in DM1 with long and narrow face and high arched palate. In DM2, neck flexors and finger flexors muscles are affected in the earliest stages. The hip girdle weakness is often the presenting feature of DM2 with difficulties arising from a squat position or from a chair, or climbing stairs. Myotonia is usually more prominent in the early stages of the disease and usually more pronounced in facial, jaw, tongue, and hand intrinsic muscles (Machuca-Tzili, Brook, & Hilton-Jones, 2005). It is aggravated by cold and stress and is universally present in DM1, and in 75% of patients with DM2. DM1, and possibly DM2, are associated with a significantly increased risk of cardiomyopathy, heart failure, conduction disorders, and arrhythmias (Lund et al., 2014).

Congenital Myopathies

The congenital myopathies (or muscular dystrophies) are genetically determined conditions in which muscular dystrophy is evident at birth or in infancy. They are characterized by hypotonia (in severe cases, the presentation is that of the floppy infant with a frog-leg posture), weakness (including facial), feeding difficulties, hypoactive deep tendon reflexes, delayed motor milestones, with normal cognitive development. Some disorders are associated with dysmorphic features such as dolichocephaly, a long, narrow face, high-arched palate, pectus excavatum, kyphoscoliosis, and dislocated hips. Muscle weakness tends to be stable or slowly progressive over time. Rarely, these disorders present in late childhood or adolescence, and typically have mild symptoms and minimal progression.

Metabolic Myopathies

Metabolic myopathies encompass a group of rare, inherited disorders arising from defects in glycogen breakdown (glycogenolysis), glucose utilization (glycolysis), fatty acid transport and oxidation, and energy production along the mitochondrial respiratory chain (Adler & Shieh, 2015).

Most patients with a metabolic myopathy have exercise intolerance ranging from myalgias or cramps to rhabdomyolysis. Usually, metabolic myopathies present during periods of increased need for energy such as physiologic stress/exertion, illness, or surgery/anesthesia. The presentation with progressive muscular weakness, usually proximal, mimicking inflammatory myopathy or muscular dystrophy, is less common.

Metabolic myopathies can be subclassified into groups according to the type of specific metabolic pathway affected.

Disorders of Glycogen Metabolism

Disorders of glycogen metabolism are disorders that result from abnormal storage, breakdown, or utilization of glycogen. The main symptoms and signs for all the disorders in this group are muscle cramps, exercise intolerance and easy fatigability, progressive weakness, and recurrent myoglobinuria. Many other systems and organs can be preferentially affected in different disorders of glycogenolysis leading to liver dysfunction, hepatomegaly, failure to thrive, hypoglycemia (sometimes with seizures), gross motor delay, peripheral neuropathy, cardiac involvement, and hemolytic anemia with jaundice, splenomegaly, and others.

Fifteen types of glycogen storage disease (GSD) have been identified and two disorders of glycogen metabolism (glucose transporter 2 [GLUT2] deficiencies and aldolase A deficiency) with established genetic mutations are known, causing their corresponding enzyme deficiencies. They all have characteristic clinical features with a wide range of severity from very mild to life-threatening, and fatal.

Disorders of Lipid Metabolism

Disorders of lipid metabolism can cause metabolic myopathies by disruption of triglyceride degradation, carnitine uptake, long-chain fatty acids mitochondrial transport, or b-oxidation.

Frequently these disorders present in infancy or early childhood with failure to thrive, or hypotonia. In adult onset, these disorders usually have milder forms, presenting as proximal muscle weakness, exercise intolerance, myalgias, neck weakness, myoglobinuria, hepatomegaly, and ophthalmoplegia. Additional manifestations may include cardiomyopathy or transient hepatic dysfunction, and encephalopathy.

Mitochondrial Myopathies

The mitochondria are cellular organelles responsible for oxidative phosphorylation, the final common pathway for aerobic energy production. Mitochondrial myopathies include a broad range of clinical phenotypes, making the diagnosis frequently challenging. Mitochondrial disease should be suspected when there is a history of possible maternal inheritance. There are, however, sporadic mutations as well. Another clue to mitochondrial disease is involvement of other organs with high energy requirements (i.e., brain, heart, skeletal muscle). Mitochondrial myopathies usually present with moderate aerobic activities like walking or jogging. They can range from mild exercise intolerance and exertional myalgias (with or without myoglobinuria), to exercise-induced dyspnea or rhabdomyolysis. The pattern of muscle involvement is highly variable with proximal limb muscle weakness being the most common presentation (DiMauro, Schon, Carelli, & Hirano, 2013). There are some syndromes with distinct clinical features (Kearns–Sayre syndrome, lactic acidosis and stroke-like episodes [MELAS], and others) which allow clinicians to go directly to targeted gene testing.

Diagnostic Approach to Inherited Myopathies

The diagnostic approach is similar for most of the inherited muscular disorders. When such a disorder is suspected, a careful family history should always be obtained. The characteristic clinical findings and clinical suspicion should guide more tailored investigation and specific tests (such as slit lamp examination for cataracts; cardiac workup for cardiomyopathy and arrhythmias, etc.).

Routine blood test should include creatine kinase (CK), and other muscle enzymes, such as lactate dehydrogenase (LDH), aspartate aminotransferase (AST), alanine aminotransferase (ALT), and aldolase. They are markers of muscle breakdown that can be elevated, with levels varying depending on the specific disorder and its severity. If metabolic myopathy is suspected, levels of specific compounds in the blood and/or urine (lactate, pyruvate, uric acid, carnitine, ketones, glucose, ammonia, myoglobin, liver transaminases, potassium, calcium, phosphate, creatinine, urinary ketones, myoglobin, etc.) should be checked. There are additional disorder-specific tests available (forearm ischemic exercise test for disorders of glycogen metabolism, etc.).

EMGs/NC studies are helpful, but usually are not obligatory, except in certain disorders with characteristic EMG findings, such as myotonic dystrophy, as it can rule out other neuromuscular disorders and demonstrate a characteristic myopathic EMG pattern.

A muscle biopsy can be nonspecific in some disorders, but can also be diagnostic, for example, in DMD where it reveals absent dystrophin, glycogen accumulation, and PAS+ vacuoles in glycogen storage disorders, or classic ragged red fibers in mitochondrial disorders.

The confirmatory tests for nearly all these disorders are genetic testing and mutation analysis.

Management and Treatment of Inherited Myopathies

Despite considerable advances in the realms of genetics and molecular biology that have identified most of the genetic mutations and their corresponding protein deficiencies, there are no curative treatments for any inherited myopathies or muscular dystrophies. Many clinical trials are currently assessing the potential efficacy of gene therapy and myoblast transplantation in several muscular dystrophies, and they look promising. Meanwhile, current management of these disorders should concentrate on an interdisciplinary approach. The emphasis should be on organs and systems involved in each particular case (respiratory, cardiac, ophthalmologic, ears–nose–throat [ENT], speech, physical therapy, occupational therapy, and cognitive therapy), with an aim to improve quality of life, longevity, and independence.

The ultimate goal of therapy is to slow disease progression. The cornerstone of management is physical therapy with a focus on strength, maintenance of range of motion, and avoidance of prolonged immobility. It is important to emphasize that the old dogma, that patients with muscle disease should refrain from exercise owing to potential physical stress–induced muscle tearing and potential disease exacerbation, should no longer be practiced. There is growing evidence that exercise, both aerobic and strength training, seems not to be harmful and may even be beneficial for most of the muscle diseases (Anziska & Sternberg, 2013; Kierkegaard, Harms-Ringdahl, Edström, Holmqvist, & Tollbäck, 2011; Lindeman et al., 1995). Most patients with muscle diseases require stretching to prevent contractures, splints or orthotics to preserve independent ambulation. In more advanced stages of the disease, assistive devices might be useful to maintain function. In cases of contractures limiting muscle functions, surgical release is indicated. Surgery is also indicated in cases of progressive scoliosis, as it corrects and prevents the progression of spinal deformity with subsequent improvement of lung function and overall improves posture and comfort.

Neuromuscular electrical stimulation (NMES) is widely used in rehabilitation to prevent disuse atrophy and recover muscle mass and function in immobilized patients. There is growing evidence of safety and benefit of NMES use in many of the inherited myopathies (Chisari, Bertolucci, Dalise, & Rossi, 2013; Colson et al., 2010).

There are new and exciting developments in the world of physiatry, with new devices in the armamentarium proving to be beneficial in neuromuscular disorders. These include body weight–supported (BWS) treadmill ambulation, and robotic-assisted training, which uses an active extra exoskeleton (Anziska & Sternberg, 2013).

In addition to physical therapy focusing on the muscle functions, functions of other systems and organs involved in each disorder should be closely monitored. In many of the myopathies, progressive weakness may lead to dysphagia and increased risk of aspiration pneumonia. To prevent it, dysphagia should always be assessed and diets changed to the appropriate consistency, considering the possibility of a feeding tube if nutrition and hydration needs cannot be met with oral intake alone.

Many of the inherited myopathies present with varying degrees of cardiac involvement and patients should be closely monitored for evidence of cardiomyopathy and arrhythmias (with electrocardiography and echocardiography) with early medical management and, if needed, use of cardiac devices including pacemakers, defibrillators, and ventricular assist devices.

In addition to a general interdisciplinary approach, certain types of specific therapy may be beneficial for different inherited myopathies. In DMD and BMD, glucocorticoids and some other immunosuppressive drug therapies are the mainstays of treatment; however, there is no strong evidence for long-term effectiveness of these agents on the course of the disease. In oculopharyngeal muscular dystrophy, special glasses with eyelid crutches can be useful and blepharoplasty can improve ptosis. In metabolic myopathies many enzyme-replacement therapies (ERT) are currently being investigated and have very reassuring results. Other therapeutic measures, such as special diets and supplements (creatine, carnitine, succinate, coenzyme Q10, CoQ10 with riboflavin combination, medium-chain triglycerides and triheptanoin diet, etc.) can be beneficial and are mainstay interventions for some disorders (Chan, Reichmann, Kögel, Beck, & Gold, 1998). Liver transplantation and bone marrow transplantation are helpful in specific disorders in this group. Also, patients with these disorders should avoid prolonged aerobic exercises, prolonged fasting, and exposure to cold to reduce the risk of muscle pain and rhabdomyolysis.

Acquired Myopathies

Acquired myopathies is a group of muscle disorders that are not inherited and not caused by genetic abnormalities, but rather caused by a wide spectrum of environmental factors. These factors include nutritional issues and deficiencies, drugs and toxins, infections, acquired metabolic dysfunctions, and others.

Acquired myopathies can be subdivided into five main categories:

- Idiopathic inflammatory myopathies (IIM)
- Infectious myopathies
- Myopathies associated with systemic illness
- Drug induced/toxic myopathies
- Endocrine myopathies

Idiopathic Inflammatory Myopathies

IIM are a group of chronic, autoimmune conditions affecting primarily the proximal muscles. There are four major entities: dermatomyositis, polymyositis, immune-mediated necrotizing myopathy, and inclusion body myositis, which are clinically, histologically, and pathogenically distinct. All these disorders share the common feature of immune-mediated muscle injury; however, different histopathological characteristics among these conditions suggest that different pathogenic processes underlie each of the inflammatory myopathies. These disorders may occur in isolation or in association with cancers, or with connective tissue diseases.

Dermatomyositis

Dermatomyositis is more common in women, and can present at any age. Onset can be acute, over a couple of weeks, or more insidious. Weakness characteristically involves proximal leg muscles and, to a lesser degree, arm muscles. Weakness either is accompanied or is preceded by a characteristic skin rash (erythematous, photosensitive rash on the neck, back, and shoulders referred to as the shawl sign); heliotrope rash that is often associated with periorbital edema; and erythematous scaly rash over the knuckles (Gottron's papules); however, it can develop years later, and can be very mild. Patients typically present with difficulty rising from a chair, climbing stairs, lifting objects, and combing their hair. Interstitial lung disease occurs in 10% to 20% of patients with dermatomyositis, and presents as dyspnea and nonproductive cough. Incidence of cancer is increased, ranging from 6% to 45%, in adult dermatomyositis patients (Amato & Greenberg, 2013; Bohan, Peter, Bowman, & Pearson 1977).

Polymyositis

Polymyositis is a heterogeneous group of disorders rather than one distinct entity. It is frequently difficult to make a diagnosis owing to lack of strict diagnostic criteria. Generally, it is similar to dermatomyositis but without skin involvement. It usually manifests in adults, more commonly in women, over the age of 20 years. It presents typically with progressive neck flexor and symmetric proximal limb muscle weakness, which develops over weeks to months. Myalgias and tenderness are common complaints, as well as difficulty swallowing. Heart and lungs are frequently affected. There is also high incidence of polyarthritis (up to 45%). The risk of malignancy in polymyositis is also high, but lower than in dermatomyositis.

Necrotizing Autoimmune Myopathy

Necrotizing autoimmune myopathy is more recently identified as a separate entity. It usually presents with proximal weakness and often myalgia that may begin acutely or more insidiously. Some drugs are implicated as triggers of the immune response. Necrotizing autoimmune myopathy can be associated with connective tissue disease (usually scleroderma or mixed connective tissue disease) or cancer (paraneoplastic-necrotizing myopathy, which is usually severe and rapidly progressive).

Sporadic Inclusion Body Myositis

Sporadic inclusion body myositis is the most common myopathy and presents in patients over the age of 40 years, with a male-to-female ratio of 3:1. It presents as a slowly progressive proximal and distal weakness in the arms and legs that usually develops after the age of 50 years. It is unique from other inflammatory myopathies in that it involves both the proximal and distal muscles, and is frequently asymmetrical. The weakness and atrophy starts in flexor forearm muscles (i.e., wrist and finger flexors), and in the quadriceps muscles, leading to tripping and falling. Dysphagia is very common in inclusion body myositis and may be the presenting feature; it can be severe enough to require esophageal dilation or cricopharyngeal myotomy. Facial weakness may also be present. It is also different from other inflammatory myopathies in that it is not associated with myocarditis, lung disease, or malignancies, and is notoriously resistant to immunotherapies.

Diagnostic Evaluations and Laboratory Studies for IIM

Serum CK level is the most sensitive measure but does not correlate with the severity of the symptoms; it might normalize with treatment. In DM, 70% to 80% will have up to 50 folds levels, while in inclusion body myositis, serum CK is normal or only mildly elevated. Other muscle enzymes and connective tissue disease autoantibodies (ANA, antiSS-A, antiSS-B, anti-Smith, anti-RNP, anti-Scl70, anticentromere antibodies) should also be checked. Myositis-specific antibodies (MSA) can offer a prognosis for a subset of patients, usually predicting poor treatment response. EMG/NC studies are usually nonspecific, revealing myopathic features (usually with evidence of significant denervation). There can also be a mild axonal sensory neuropathy (particularly in inclusion body myositis). The EMG/NC study also helps to exclude other neuromuscular disorders, and can also guide the biopsy. Moderately weak muscle should be chosen for biopsy to increase the yield. Muscle biopsy with specific findings, characteristic for each disorder, is the gold standard to make the diagnosis and to differentiate inflammatory myopathy from some muscular dystrophies.

Management and Treatment of IIM

The main goals of IIM therapy are to restore muscle strength, decrease inflammation, and prevent damage to other organs. Treatment should involve a multidisciplinary approach: neurology, rheumatology, dermatology, pulmonology, and physical, occupational, and speech therapies. It is also essential to evaluate for potential underlying malignancies and treat them. Corticosteroids are the first-line treatment for adult onset dermatomyositis, polymyositis, and necrotizing autoimmune myopathy. These disorders usually respond well to immunotherapy, while inclusion body myositis usually does not. It is important to differentiate between relapse and steroid-induced myopathy in case of initial improvement with subsequent symptomatic worsening. The EMG can be helpful in differentiating between the two, revealing irritability of muscle membrane in case of the former. Second-line agents include methotrexate, azathioprine, mycophenolate, and immunoglobulin. These agents are usually added to corticosteroids in patients with severe weakness or other organ system involvement, but can be used alone (as steroid-sparing strategy) in case there are serious steroid-induced side effects.

Physical and occupation therapy along with orthotic devices if needed, are essential to retain and improve motor function, range of motion (ROM), and prevent contractures. They also help prevent steroids side effects such as weight gain, osteoporosis, and Type 2 fiber atrophy. There is growing evidence for safety and benefits of physiotherapy and home exercise programs in inflammatory myopathies (Alexanderson & Lundberg, 2012; Varjú, Pethö, Kutas, & Czirják, 2003). Strengthening programs twice weekly can be started as early as 2 to 3 weeks from the acute phase. With severe cases, passive ROM exercises can be done for 3 months, until strength improves, at which point strengthening exercises are initiated. In addition, combining physical exercise programs with oral creatine supplementation in the first 6 months following the acute phase of dermatomyositis/polymyositis can lead to superior outcomes (Chung et al., 2007).

Infectious Myopathies

Infectious myopathies are considered rare; however, many that are currently classified as IIMs might have an underlying infectious etiology. Many infectious agents, including viruses, bacteria, fungi, and parasites, can infect muscle. Viral etiologies typically cause diffuse myalgias and/or myositis, whereas bacteria and fungi usually lead to a local myositis, especially at sites compromised by prior trauma, vascular problems, or surgery. The parasitic etiologies (toxoplasma, amoeba, trichinella, cysticercus, etc.) are also rare causes of muscle invasion and inflammation. Different diagnostic tools are used depending on the presentation and suspected cause, including muscle enzymes, laboratory testing for specific microorganism, imaging, EMGs, and biopsy. Management is based on appropriate antibiotic therapy or surgery. Disorders of this group usually have a good prognosis if the causative agent is eliminated; however, the prognosis is less favorable in chronic infections (HIV, HTLV, etc.).

Myopathy Associated With Systemic Diseases

Endocrine diseases are generally associated with hormonally mediated systemic alterations in metabolism. At any time during the course of many endocrinopathies, muscle may become affected. These disorders usually have other characteristic multiorgan features, but when myopathy is a presenting manifestation the diagnosis can be very challenging. The weakness is typically symmetric or rapidly becomes symmetric with muscle pain, cramps, spasms, and at times muscle atrophy may be present. The most common endocrine myopathy is steroid myopathy from endogenous hypercortisolism due to Cushing's disease. Other common endocrine abnormalities leading to myopathies are due to abnormalities of the thyroid, parathyroid, adrenal, pituitary glands, ovaries/testes, and the pancreas. The diagnosis is usually based on identifying the specific endocrinologic disease. The CK concentration in endocrine myopathies often does not correlate with muscle weakness. Therapy usually focuses on correcting the endocrinopathy, typically followed by improvement or resolution of myopathy.

Amyloid myopathy is rare, but may also be underdiagnosed (Spuler, Emslie-Smith, & Engel, 1998). Amyloid myopathy usually presents with symmetric proximal weakness predominantly afflicting the elderly (in sporadic forms), but there is a wide range with genetic forms of familial amyloidosis (with mutations in gelsolin and transthyretin) presenting at a young age. Transthyretin gene mutations are typically associated with distal weakness and polyneuropathy. In cases of sporadic amyloidosis, a diagnosis of monoclonal gammopathy of undetermined significance (MGUS) or multiple myeloma should be considered. Pathology underlying this myopathy is amyloid deposition around small blood vessels causing muscle fiber necrosis and regeneration. Almost one half of the patients have enlarged muscles and frequent involvement of many other systems and organs (gastrointestinal, peripheral nerve, renal and cardiac systems). The diagnostic tools helping to establish the diagnosis are laboratory studies as well as electrodiagnostic testing. Typically, an elevated CK is present. On NC study/EMG, there is evidence of myopathy with or without denervation, and at times also polyneuropathy; MRI shows characteristic reticulation of the subcutaneous fat; serum and urine protein immunoelectrophoresis show dysproteinemia with monoclonal peak. The gold standard for the diagnosis is a muscle biopsy with special fluorescent Congo red stain. There is no specific therapy. The prognosis is poor and different immunotherapies are currently being investigated.

Myopathies of Systemic Inflammatory Diseases

Myopathies of systemic inflammatory diseases—disorders such as systemic lupus erythematosus, rheumatoid arthritis, scleroderma, and Sjögren's syndrome—can be associated with skeletal muscle vasculitis. More than one half of patients with systemic inflammatory diseases have various degrees of skeletal muscle involvement. The presentation can be of substantial myalgias and some degree of weakness with systemic signs of weight loss and fever, arthralgias, and involvement of other organ systems.

The condition is usually suspected by the presence of signs and symptoms of the primary disease and supported by lab studies and characteristic biopsy (evidence of vasculitis by presence of fibrinoid necrosis and inflammation). Usually these disorders respond well to immunosuppressive therapies.

Critical Illness Myopathy

Critical illness myopathy (CIM) is an acute process causing muscle dysfunction and disruption of the normal muscle fiber structure in critically ill patients. It is a frequent finding in the ICU setting and occurs in up to 50% of severe ICU patients (Stevens et al., 2007), and up to 100% in patients with septic shock or multiorgan failure. Sepsis, multiple organ failure, drugs (particularly intravenous corticosteroids and NMJ blocking agents) hyperglycemia, and inflammation (with inflammatory cytokines promoting muscle protein degradation) all play roles in the pathophysiology of CIM. Immobility is another independent and important contributing factor in disuse atrophy and wasting. Patients may lose half their muscle mass, resulting in severe physical disability. CIM usually presents with generalized muscle weakness of the limb and respiratory muscles, with facial muscle sparing.

CIM is usually suspected clinically based on acute onset of generalized weakness after the onset of critical illness. The main disorder that CIM should be differentiated from is critical illness neuropathy (clinically differentiated based on abnormal sensory examination). Electrophysiological investigation plays a critical role in establishing the diagnosis (particularly differentiating between neuropathy and myopathy), and muscle biopsy should be done if EMG is limited and cannot reliably confirm the diagnosis. The biopsy characteristically reveals myofiber atrophy (especially of Type 2 fibers) and variable degree of necrosis and regeneration. There are no specific treatments for CIM and therapy should target the underlying critical illness. Almost one third of people discharged from the ICU with diagnosis of CIM will have a variable degree of permanent weakness, and in severe cases, persistent tetraparesis and ventilator dependency. It was recently shown in a randomized controlled trial that minimizing sedation together with early rehabilitation in ICU patients resulted in better functional outcomes compared with patients receiving standard treatment (Schweickert, 2009).

Toxic Myopathies

Multiple drugs and toxins can cause myopathy. The clinical and pathological features depend on the causative agent and on individual susceptibility to a given compound, ranging from mild to severe (at times with massive rhabdomyolysis and acute renal failure) and from transient symptoms to chronic myopathy. Drug-induced myopathy is among the most common causes of muscle disease.

There are different categories of toxic myopathy brought on by multiple causes or agents. These include necrotizing myopathy that occur primarily from lipid-lowering drugs, steroid myopathy, hypokalemic myopathy induced by diuretics or other compounds that lower serum potassium levels, inflammatory myopathies, vacuolar myopathies, and others. Several different mechanisms result in muscle damage depending on the causative agent—alcohol, cocaine, glucocorticoids, lipid-lowering drugs—and cause direct toxicity to the muscle. Immunologically induced inflammation may result from treatment with D-penicillamine or interferon alpha. Muscle damage may be indirect as a result of a drug-induced coma with subsequent ischemic muscle compression, drug-induced hypokalemia (e.g., diuretics), drug-induced hyperkinetic states, hyperthermia related to cocaine use, or neuroleptic malignant syndrome.

It is important to consider toxic/drug-induced myopathy in patients with new onset muscle pain and weakness in patients on different drug therapies, as these myopathies can be potentially very severe and fatal. Diagnostic tools helping in establishing the diagnosis include CK, and other muscle enzymes, EMG, and muscle biopsy. Most of these myopathies are reversible with discontinuation of offending agents.

Neuromuscular disorders include disorders of the peripheral nerves, plexuses, spinal roots, motor neurons, NMJs, and muscles. Despite significant variations in etiologies, genetic factors, ages of onset, clinical presentations, and organs involved, the main feature common to all these disorders is weakness. The weakness from these disorders cannot only be attributed to muscle degeneration caused by the disease itself, but also from disuse atrophy and contractures. In addition to disease-specific treatments when available, there is a significant impact on overall health by the reduced physical activity, making early and effective rehabilitation programs the cornerstone of the management for patients with neuromuscular disorders.

REFERENCES

Adler, M., & Shieh, P. B. (2015). Metabolic myopathies. In W. S. David & D. A. Chad (Eds.), *Seminars in neurology* (Vol. 35, No. 4, pp. 385–397). New York, NY: Thieme Medical Publishers.

Alexanderson, H., & Lundberg, I. E. (2012). Exercise as a therapeutic modality in patients with idiopathic inflammatory myopathies. *Current Opinion in Rheumatology*, *24*(2), 201–207.

Amato, A. A., & Greenberg, S. A. (2013). Inflammatory myopathies. *CONTINUUM: Lifelong Learning in Neurology*, *19*(6, Muscle Disease), 1615–1633.

Anziska, Y., & Sternberg, A. (2013). Exercise in neuromuscular disease. *Muscle & Nerve*, *48*(1), 3–20.

Banihani, R., Smile, S., Yoon, G., Dupuis, A., Mosleh, M., Snider, A., & McAdam, L. (2015). Cognitive and neurobehavioral profile in boys with duchenne muscular dystrophy. *Journal of Child Neurology*, *30*(11), 1472–1482.

Bohan, A., Peter, J. B., Bowman, R. L., & Pearson, C. M. (1977). A computer-assisted analysis of 153 patients with polymyositis and dermatomyositis. *Medicine*, *56*(4), 255–286.

Boyer, F. C., Tiffreau, V., & Rapin, A. (2010). Post polio syndrome: Pathophysiology hypotheses, diagnosis criteria, medication therapeutics. *Annals of Physical and Rehabilitation Medicine*, *53*, 34–41.

Caridi, J., Pumberger, M., & Hughes, A. (2011). Cervical radiculopathy: A review. *HSS Journal, 7*(3), 265–272.

Chan, A., Reichmann, H., Kögel, A., Beck, A., & Gold, R. (1998). Metabolic changes in patients with mitochondrial myopathies and effects of coenzyme Q10 therapy. *Journal of Neurology*, *245*(10), 681–685.

Chisari, C., Bertolucci, F., Dalise, S., & Rossi, B. (2013). Chronic muscle stimulation improves muscle function and reverts the abnormal surface EMG pattern in Myotonic Dystrophy: A pilot study. *Journal of Neuroengineering and Rehabilitation*, *10*(1), 1.

Chung, Y. L., Alexanderson, H., Pipitone, N., Morrison, C., Dastmalchi, M., Ståhl-Hallengren, C., . . . Lundberg, I. E. (2007). Creatine supplements in patients with idiopathic inflammatory myopathies who are clinically weak after conventional pharmacologic treatment: Six-month, double-blind, randomized, placebo-controlled trial. *Arthritis Care & Research*, *57*(4), 694–702.

Colson, S. S., Benchortane, M., Tanant, V., Faghan, J. P., Fournier-Mehouas, M., Benaïm, C., . . . Sacconi, S. (2010). Neuromuscular electrical stimulation training: A safe and effective treatment for facioscapulohumeral muscular dystrophy patients. *Archives of Physical Medicine and Rehabilitation*, *91*(5), 697–702.

DiMauro, S., Schon, E. A., Carelli, V., & Hirano, M. (2013). The clinical maze of mitochondrial neurology. *Nature Reviews Neurology*, *9*(8), 429–444.

Farbu, E., & Gilhus, N. E. (2006). EFNS guideline on diagnosis and management of post polio syndrome. Report of an EFNS task force. *European Journal of Neurology, 13*, 795–801.

Gonzalez, H., Olsson, T., & Borg, K. (2010). Management of post polio syndrome. *The Lancet (Neurology)*, *9*, 634–642.

Gronseth, G. S., & Barohn, R. J. (2000). Practice parameter: Thymectomy for autoimmune myasthenia gravis (an evidence-based review) report of the quality standards subcommittee of the American Academy of Neurology. *Neurology*, *55*(1), 7–15.

Halstead, L. S., & Rossi, C. D. (1985). New problems in old polio patients: Results of a survey of 539 polio survivors. *Orthopaedics, 8*, 845–850.

Hermans, G., & DeJonghe, D. (2008). Clinical review: Critical illness neuropathy and myopathy. *Critical Care, 12*, 238.

Jackson, C., McVey, A., & Rudnicki, S. (2015). Symptom management and end of life care in amyotrophic lateral sclerosis. *Neurology Clinics, 33*, 889–908.

Jacob, S., Viegas, S., Lashley, D., & Hilton-Jones, D. (2009). Myasthenia gravis and other neuromuscular junction disorders. *Practical Neurology*, *9*(6), 364–371.

Khan, F., & Amatya, B. (2012). Rehabilitation interventions in patients with acute demyelinating inflammatory polyneuropathy: A systemic review. *European Journal of Physical Rehabilitation Medicine*, *48*, 507–522.

Kierkegaard, M., Harms-Ringdahl, K., Edström, L., Holmqvist, L. W., & Tollbäck, A. (2011). Feasibility and effects of a physical exercise programme in adults with myotonic dystrophy type 1: A randomized controlled pilot study. *Journal of Rehabilitation Medicine*, *43*(8), 695–702.

Ko, I. (2011). Clinical, electrophysiologic findings in adult patients with non traumatic plexopathies. *Annals of Rehabilitation Medicine, 35*, 807–815.

Laffont, I., & Julia, M. (2010). Aging and sequelae of poliomyelitis. *Annals of Physical and Rehabilitation Medicine, 53*, 24–33.

Laforêt, P., Eymard, B., Becane, H. M., Ounnoughene, Z., Varin, J., Lazarus, A., . . . Jeanpierre, M. (2001). Cardiac involvement in facioscapulohumeral muscular dystrophy: The experience of salpetriere hospital in 2001. *Neuromuscular Disorders, 11*, 616–617.

Lindeman, E., Leffers, P., Spaans, F., Drukker, J., Reulen, J., Kerckhoffs, M., & Köke, A. (1995). Strength training in patients with myotonic dystrophy and hereditary motor and sensory neuropathy: A randomized clinical trial. *Archives of Physical Medicine and Rehabilitation*, *76*(7), 612–620.

Lund, M., Diaz, L. J., Ranthe, M. F., Petri, H., Duno, M., Juncker, I., . . . Melbye, M. (2014). Cardiac involvement in myotonic dystrophy: A nationwide cohort study. *European Heart Journal*, *35*(32), 2158–2164.

Machuca-Tzili, L., Brook, D., & Hilton-Jones, D. (2005). Clinical and molecular aspects of the myotonic dystrophies: A review. *Muscle & Nerve*, 32(1), 1–18.

Mirski, K. T., & Crawford, T. O. (2014). Motor and cognitive delay in Duchenne muscular dystrophy: Implication for early diagnosis. *The Journal of Pediatrics*, *165*(5), 1008–1010.

Nigro, G., Comi, L. I., Politano, L., & Bain, R. J. I. (1990). The incidence and evolution of cardiomyopathy in Duchenne muscular dystrophy. *International Journal of Cardiology*, 26(3), 271–277.

Schweickert, W. D., Pohlman, M. C., Pohlman, A. S., Nigos, C., Pawlik, A. J., Esbrook, C. L., . . . Schmidt, G. A. (2009). Early physical and occupational therapy in mechanically ventilated, critically ill patients: A randomised controlled trial. *The Lancet*, *373*(9678), 1874–1882.

Spuler, S., Emslie-Smith, A., & Engel, A. G. (1998). Amyloid myopathy: An underdiagnosed entity. *Annals of Neurology*, *43*(6), 719–728.

Stevens, R. D., Dowdy, D. W., Michaels, R. K., Mendez-Tellez, P. A., Pronovost, P. J., & Needham, D. M. (2007). Neuromuscular dysfunction acquired in critical illness: A systematic review. *Intensive Care Medicine*, *33*(11), 1876–1891.

Stratland, J., & Barohn, R. (2015a). Patterns of weakness, classification of motor neuron disease, and clinical diagnostics of sporadic amyotrophic lateral scelerosis. *Neurology Clinics, 33*, 735–748.

Stratland, J., & Barohn, R. (2015b). Primary lateral sclerosis. *Neurology Clinics, 33*, 749–760.

Tarulli, A., & Raynor E. (2007). Lumbosacral radiculopathy. *Neurologic Clinics, 25*, 387–405

Tiffrenau, V., & Rapin, A. (2010). Post polio syndrome and rehabilitation. *Annals of Physical and Rehabilitation Medicine, 53*, 42–50.

Varjú, C., Pethö, E., Kutas, R., & Czirják, L. (2003). The effect of physical exercise following acute disease exacerbation in patients with dermato/polymyositis. *Clinical Rehabilitation*, *17*(1), 83–87.

Yamamoto, A. M., Gajdos, P., Eymard, B., Tranchant, C., Warter, J. M., Gomez, L., . . . Garchon, H. J. (2001). Anti-titin antibodies in myasthenia gravis: Tight association with thymoma and heterogeneity of nonthymoma patients. *Archives of Neurology*, *58*(6), 885–890.

Yazawa, M., Ikeda, S., Owa, M., Haruta, S., Yanagisawa, N., Tanaka, E., & Watanabe, M. (1987). A family of Becker's progressive muscular dystrophy with severe cardiomyopathy. *European Neurology*, *27*(1), 13–19.

Musculoskeletal Disorders

Efren Caballes

14

CHAPTER

INTRODUCTION

Musculoskeletal disorders (MSDs) are among the most common causes of disability in the community. Disorders of the musculoskeletal system may result from hereditary, congenital, or acquired pathologic processes. Risk for developing a disorder varies by age, occupation, activity level, and lifestyle. For example, the Bureau of Labor Statistics indicates that professions such as home health aides who assist with care for the elderly, delivery truck drivers, freight handlers, laborers, nursing aides, and orderlies experience more musculoskeletal problems than the general population.

In 2011, about 3 million workplace injuries were reported in private industries, more than half of which involved an injury severe enough that work restrictions, job transfer, or time off from work was required (Bureau of Labor Statistics, U.S. Department of Labor). The back (36%), shoulder (12%), and knee (12%) were most often injured (Bureau of Labor Statistics, U.S. Department of Labor, 2012). In 2007, the cost for workers' compensation care in the United States was approximately $50 billion (Leigh & Marcin, 2012).

An understanding of a patient's work and occupational history is critical for clarifying how related the injury is to work, preventing future injuries, and maximizing the return-to-work process. Symptoms that may impact return to work may include recurring pain, stiff/painful joints, swelling, or dull aches. Additionally, psychosocial risk factors may be associated with work-related injuries and can affect recovery. Psychiatric comorbidities and maladaptive pain coping behaviors are associated with delayed recovery from low back pain.

Regardless of the cause of impairment, functional loss is defined as the inability to ambulate effectively on a sustained basis for any reason, including pain associated with underlying musculoskeletal impairment or inability to perform fine and gross movements effectively on a sustained basis.

Although there is a wide range of conditions that may result in work-related disability, the goal of this chapter is to provide the clinician with an overview of the most commonly occurring MSDs affecting the working population, including low back pain, rotator cuff (RTC) tendinopathy, acromioclavicular (AC) joint arthritis, and carpal tunnel syndrome (CTS). This discussion offers insight into the physical and psychosocial considerations used to develop a patient-centered approach to MSDs aimed at improving functional outcomes and effective return-to-work strategies.

LOW BACK PAIN

Etiology and Role of the Workplace and Physical Activities

Low back pain is a highly prevalent cause of disability (Centers for Disease Control and Prevention [CDC], 2001) and one of the most expensive heath conditions, costing Americans approximately $50 billion annually (National Institute of Neurological Disorders and Stroke, 2015). As much as 70% to 90% of the population experience at least one episode of low back pain in their lifetime (Rubin, 2007). Low back pain can result in decreased productivity and absenteeism (Waddell, 2004). Furthermore, it is one of the leading causes of lost work time (Stewart, Ricci, Chee, Morganstein, & Lipton, 2003). According to the U.S. Bureau of Labor Statistics, among work-related musculoskeletal injuries and illnesses resulting in lost time from work, 42%

were back-related conditions that resulted in a median of 7 days of lost work time annually (Bureau of Labor Statistics. U.S. Department of Labor, 2012).

Pathophysiology/Clinical Presentation

The evaluation of patients with complaints of low back pain should begin with a thorough history and physical examination. The medical history should elicit details of pain, including location, character, onset, duration, exacerbating and relieving factors, radiating pain, constitutional symptoms, and past medical history. Details of any recent trauma should also be investigated. It is crucial to first identify the possibility of any serious cause of the patient's low back pain by detailing the presence of any "red flags." Saddle anesthesia (loss of sensation in the buttocks, perineum, and inner surfaces of the thighs), recent bowel or bladder dysfunction, or severe or progressive neurologic deficit suggests cauda equina syndrome, which refers to a characteristic pattern of neuromuscular and urogenital symptoms resulting from compression of the lumbosacral nerve roots below the conus medullaris and requires urgent intervention.

Often in patients presenting with low back pain, the definitive pain generator is not identified. The differential diagnosis is broad and may include lumbar strain, myalgia, lumbar radiculopathy, lumbar degenerative disc disease, sacroiliac joint dysfunction, lumbar spondylosis, and facet arthropathy. Physical examination should begin with inspection to identify a gross deformity or loss of normal lumbar lordosis and palpation to elicit areas of tenderness over the spinous process, paraspinal muscles, or sacroiliac joints. Range of motion (ROM) should be assessed to determine the presence of any limitations as well as exacerbation and alleviation of pain during specific movements. Increased pain with spine flexion is characteristic of disc herniation, whereas pain with extension suggests spinal stenosis. A complete neurologic examination is performed, including sensory and motor testing, and deep tendon reflexes (Eck & Riley, 2004). Nerve root tension signs should also be evaluated, including the straight-leg raise test and femoral nerve tension sign. Straight-leg raise testing is performed with the patient lying supine while the physician elevates the straight lower extremity so as to place tension on the nerve roots. A positive sign is elicited if radicular symptoms—reproducible radiating pain into the lower extremity along the course of a spinal nerve root—are reproduced at greater than 30° of elevation. With the femoral nerve tension sign, the patient is prone, and the clinician flexes the knee to 90°, and then extends the hip while supporting the pelvis against the table. This places tension on the femoral nerve and can reproduce radicular pain in the anterior thigh.

Acute pain that is localized to the low back without radiating symptoms is most often caused by lumbar strain. The lumbar disc is composed of a gel substance (nucleus pulposus) surrounded by outer collagen fibers, which are arranged in a crossed pattern (annulus fibrosus). These discs are further supported by the anterior and posterior longitudinal ligaments. Together, the vertebral disc complex resists spinal compression. During axial rotation and flexion of the spine, the annular fibers are placed at a mechanical disadvantage. A common mechanism for herniation is combined flexion, rotation, and compression of the spine (Borg-Stein, Elson, & Brand, 2012). The clinical presentation of disc-related low back pain is primarily divided into three subtypes: axial pain, radicular pain, or combined. Axial discogenic low back pain often presents as severe episodes of acute pain, muscle spasm, and time lost from work. The symptoms are exacerbated by prolonged sitting, standing, or axial loading. There are no neurologic deficits. Patients may also present with radicular pain without back pain, most often in the L5 or S1 nerve root distribution. Sitting puts more pressure on the spine than standing, as the muscles that are normally engaged to support the spine turn off and cause strain. An inflexible spine may be more susceptible to damage in routine activities. There is greater risk for herniated discs in the lumbar spine.

Persistent axial low back pain lasting more than a few weeks requires further investigation to determine its cause. Facet joints, also known as zygapophyseal joints, are small joints connecting consecutive vertebral bodies. They are synovial-lined joints with hyaline cartilage. Increased loading conditions of the spine involving extension and rotation has been presumed to increase the risk for facet arthropathy. Repetitive hyperextension and rotation can lead to inflammation and synovitis. Additionally, in older patients with other degenerative changes, such as loss of disc height, a greater load is placed through the facet. Patients with facet-mediated pain often have reproduction of pain with combined extension and rotation. Avoidance of this motion leads to axial pain, stiffness, and impaired motion. On examination, there may be point tenderness to palpation in the paraspinal region over the corresponding facet joint. Associated radicular pain may also occur from the proximity of the inflammatory mediators to the exiting nerve root. Facet referral patterns are nonspecific and levels may overlap (Borg-Stein et al., 2012).

Pain radiating into the buttocks or lower extremities indicate nerve root impingement, which may occur in the setting of compromised discs, ligamentous hypertrophy, facet arthrosis, and spondylolisthesis. The lumbar spinal canal is surrounded anteriorly by the vertebral bodies, the disc, and the posterior longitudinal ligament. The lateral margin is comprised of the pedicles and the lateral extension of the ligmentum flavum. Posteriorly, the border is lined by the ligmentum flavum, facet joints, and laminae. As the spinal nerves exit at each level, the neuroforamina are surrounded by the discs and vertebral bodies anteriorly, by the facets posteriorly, and by the pedicles superior and inferiorly (Figure 14.1). Degenerative changes of any of these components can lead to compression of the neural elements.

Many individuals may have evidence of mechanical compression of the nerve roots without pain. Symptoms develop in the lower extremities when there is inflammation and irritation of the nerve root. An inflammatory reaction may occur if the normal motion is obstructed, leading to tension and disruptions of the neural architecture (Garfin, Herkowitz, & Mirkovic, 1999). Initially, lumbar stenosis presents as vague low back pain and stiffness relieved with rest and exacerbated with activity. Depending on the location, the pain typically begins in the low back and radiates toward the buttocks or lower extremities. Symptoms include numbness, tingling, and pain that present in a dermatomal or myotomal distribution related to the level of neuroforaminal stenosis. Often, patients will complain of a feeling of weakness, cramping, diffuse paresthesias, and a dull, aching pain. Classically, these symptoms are described as a neurogenic claudication, which are exacerbated with spinal extension and are rapidly improved with flexion. On physical examination, specific motor deficits are uncommon. Diminished or absent reflexes corresponding to the suspected nerve root may be present.

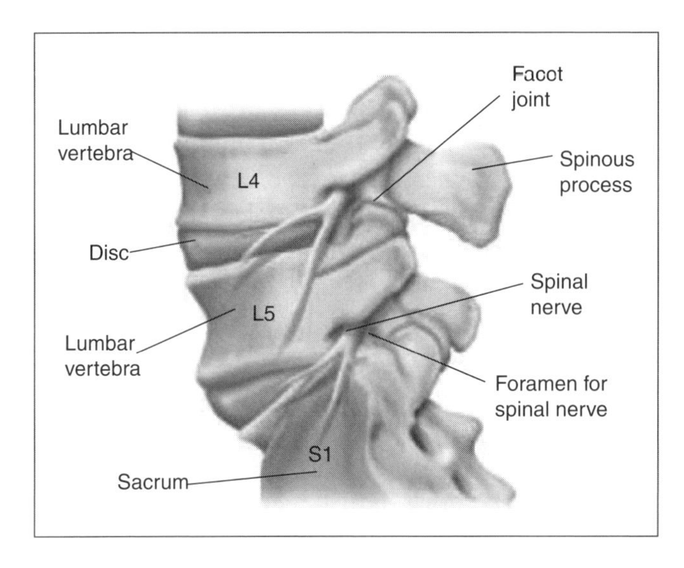

FIGURE 14.1 Lumbar spine anatomy.

Diagnostic Studies

Diagnostic tests range from plain radiographs, MRI, electromyography and nerve conduction studies (EMG/NCS), and interventional procedures such as facet blocks or medial branch blocks. X-rays and MRIs should complement a carefully obtained history and physical as several studies have shown that asymptomatic patients may have abnormal findings on both imaging modalities (Jensen et al., 1994). MRI is most useful when imaging correlates with the patient's symptoms and clinical findings. EMG/NCS is a sensitive test that detects functional abnormalities in the nerves and muscles such as in the setting of peripheral nerve injuries, neuropathies, radiculopathies, and plexopathies. Injuries to nerves due to pathology in the spine may also be confirmed on EMG/NCS, especially if symptoms and physical examination findings correspond to results.

Differentiating between low back pain originating from facet-mediated pain and discogenic pain is difficult. Interventional procedures such as medial branch blocks are useful to help confirm diagnosis. Medial branches are the nerve fibers that innervate each individual facet joint. Each joint is innervated by two separate medial branches. For example, the L4–L5 facet joint is innervated by the L3 and L4 medial branches. Low-volume intra-articular anesthetic injection and medial branch blocks under fluoroscopic guidance are the most accepted methods for diagnosing facet-mediated pain (Cohen & Raja, 2007). If the patient experiences pain relief after the block, the facet joint that was targeted is believed to be the source of pain, and is used to help guide further treatment plans.

Treatment, Return to Work, Prevention

Returning to work after an episode of low back pain is a complex process involving many interrelated factors including fear avoidance, pain catastrophizing, and confidence issues (Besen, Young, & Shaw, 2015). Initial management emphasizes pain reduction with short-term use of nonsteroidal anti-inflammatory drugs (NSAIDs) or opioid medications to reduce acute symptoms. Corsets and braces do not produce any long-term improvements and may lead to deconditioning of core muscles. Physical therapy may include manual treatments, lumbar and core stabilization, modalities, and a graded exercise program. A neutral-based isometric trunk-strengthening program is progressed as tolerated to resistive strengthening, motion, and aerobic conditioning. In the setting of lumbar degenerative disc disease, lumbar epidural steroid injections are indicated for radicular pain that does not respond to these measures. However, the technical difficulty of the procedure increases in patients who have severe degenerative changes in the spine (Garfin et al., 1999). In the case of intractable radicular pain or progressive neurologic deficit, lumbar discectomy is offered. Diagnostic medial branch blocks are predictive of the efficacy of radiofrequency ablation—a procedure that uses radio waves to stop the lumbar medial branch nerve from transmitting pain signals from the injured facet to the brain—for the treatment of facet arthropathy. Additionally, aspiration and corticosteroid injection is helpful in the treatment of synovial cysts in the facet.

Return to work after completion of treatment can be difficult. An essential element of developing a successful treatment plan requires having realistic expectations for outcomes. Educating the patient that return to work with residual symptoms is acceptable. For example, it is not unusual for patients to return to work with restrictions and while continuing treatment. Restrictions may range from limited lifting, pushing, and pulling. However, return to work is impacted by job-specific activities. Therefore, a detailed history of job-specific responsibilities is important. A functional capacity evaluation (FCE) may be needed to evaluate other work options that patients may have if their current job responsibilities do not allow them to return. The FCE is performed by a licensed physical therapist and is a standardized way to collect information regarding the patient's physical abilities to determine whether or not they can return to their job.

Although an accurate diagnosis and thoughtful treatment plan is important, the best option is injury prevention. Prevention usually occurs with education of proper lifting and ergonometric evaluation. Ergonometric evaluations ensure the proper position of equipment to minimize any work-related injuries. Correct computer monitor height and appropriate seating are examples of changes that may result from an ergonometric evaluation. Worksite physical activity programs are a feasible way of conducting primary prevention. Both strength training and all-round physical exercise have proven effective for relief from musculoskeletal pain symptoms (Burton et al., 2005).

SHOULDER PAIN

RTC Tendinopathy

Epidemiology

The prevalence of asymptomatic RTC tears is high, particularly with increasing age (Yamaguchi et al., 2001). RTC tears are extremely common, affecting at least 10% of persons aged older than 60 years in the United States (Reilly, Macleod, Macfarlane, Windley, & Emery, 2006). An estimated 75,000 to 250,000 patients per year undergo RTC surgery in the United States (Vitale et al., 2006). Interestingly, in patients who do have surgical repair of RTC tears, the failure rate is between 25% and 90% (Bishop et al., 2006), yet patients whose repairs fail report satisfaction levels and outcome scores that are nearly indistinguishable from those whose repairs are intact (Slabaugh et al., 2010).

Pathophysiology and Clinical Features

RTC disorders can be divided into primary and secondary causes. Primary causes can be attributed to the patient's underlying anatomy, such as outlet impingement, compromised microvascular supply, and age-related degeneration. Outlet impingement refers to changes that have occurred to the AC joint. The AC joint is the bony roof that sits above the RTC muscles. Arthritic changes to the AC joint can cause injury to the muscle. Age-related degeneration is associated with intrinsic tendinopathy. As one ages, there is an increased frequency of partial-thickness and full-thickness tears of the cuff muscles. These degenerative changes are commonly observed in workers who execute overhead activity, such as seen with painters and plumbers. The superficial side of the supraspinatus tendon, also known as the bursal side, maintains a higher blood supply compared with the side of the muscle that is above the glenohumeral articular surface (Figure 14.2). RTC muscles may be susceptible to a decrease in blood circulation due to increased intramuscular pressures along the articular surface. Secondary sources include glenohumeral instability.

The patient presenting with a full-thickness RTC tear can have a variety of complaints including pain, weakness, functional loss, and decreased ROM (Ianotti, 1994). In the setting of a known acute, traumatic, full-thickness RTC tear, repair within 3 weeks of injury has been suggested as optimal (Bassett & Cofield, 1983). Anatomically, an increased duration of a full-thickness RTC tear may contribute to increased tear size or fat atrophy of the RTC muscle (Goutallier, Postel, Bernageau, Lavau, & Voisin, 1994). With regard to traumatic RTC tears, the duration of symptoms has been related to muscular atrophy, tendon retraction, tear size, and operative outcomes (Feng, Guo, Nobuhara, Hashimoto, & Mimori, 2003). However, duration of symptoms may not be the best historical feature to use when one is deciding a treatment approach for patients with symptomatic, atraumatic, full-thickness RTC tears (Unruh et al., 2014).

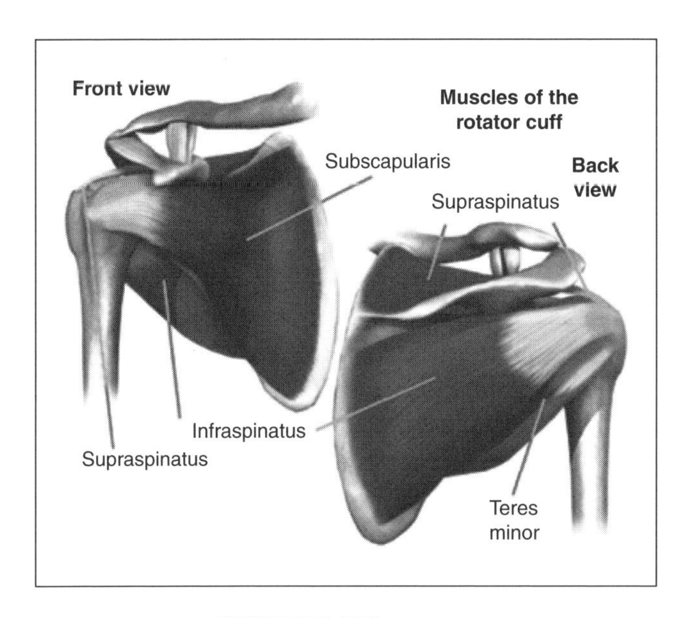

FIGURE 14.2 RTC anatomy.

Diagnostic Studies

Obtaining a proper and detailed history is vital in diagnosing RTC injuries. The practitioner has to rule out other pathologies including referred neck pain or cardiac pain. One has to identify the patient's chief complaint and acquire more detailed information: handedness, onset, location, duration, exacerbating/alleviating symptoms, and radiation of pain. In addition, one should inquire about weakness, numbness, catching/popping of shoulder, instability, night pain, pain when lying on affected arm, and ROM. It is important to gather both social and occupational information. Some patients may have tried alternative treatment options prior to seeking medical evaluation so it is beneficial to identify these sources of treatment modalities such as ice or heat; medications such as acetaminophen, NSAIDs, aspirin; physical therapies; injections; or surgical interventions. One should follow a systematic approach when performing the physical examination: inspection, palpation, ROM, manual muscle strength testing, sensation, reflexes, and special testing.

Radiologic studies can be invaluable in diagnosing RTC disorders. The initial workup should entail x-rays of the shoulder. MRI is highly sensitive and specific in identifying RTC injuries. Disadvantages of MRI include cost and the necessity of the patient to remain absolutely still during the study. Ultrasound (US) is an alternate study that may be considered. It is of low cost and extremely precise in identifying RTC.

Treatment

Current rehabilitation programs for the painful shoulder conditions focus on restoration of functional ability rather than focusing solely on resolution of symptoms. The shoulder works as a link in the kinetic chain of joint motions and muscle activations to produce optimum athletic function. Functional shoulder rehabilitation should start with establishment of a stable base of support and muscle facilitation in the trunk and legs, and then proceed to the scapula and shoulder as healing is achieved and proximal control is gained. The pace of this "flow" of exercises is determined by achievement of the functional goals of each segment in the kinetic chain. In the early rehabilitation stages, the incompletely healed shoulder structures are protected by exercises that are directed toward the proximal segments. As healing proceeds, the weak scapular and shoulder muscles are facilitated in their reactivation by the use of the proximal leg and trunk muscles to reestablish normal coupled activations. Closed chain axial loading exercises form the basis for scapular and glenohumeral functional rehabilitation, as they more closely simulate normal scapula and shoulder positions, proprioceptive input, and muscle activation patterns. In the later rehabilitation stages, glenohumeral control and power production complete the return of function to the shoulder and the kinetic chain. In this integrated approach, glenohumeral emphasis is part of the entire program and is toward the end of rehabilitation, rather than being the entire program and being at the beginning of the program (Kibler, McMullen, & Uhl, 2012).

One large multicenter, prospective, cohort study demonstrated that physical therapy is effective in the nonoperative treatment of atraumatic full-thickness RTC tears. Physical therapy is not ideal for all patients, and some will elect to undergo surgery early. Others may be at risk for symptom or RTC tear progression. Decisions regarding surgery should be made individually with each patient but should include information that a physical therapy program is highly effective in alleviating symptoms (Kuhn et al., 2013).

It is helpful to know whether the patient's primary concern is pain, weakness, and/or functional loss. The relationship between pain and RTC integrity is not clear (Dunn et al., 2014). However, RTC repairs that remain intact do have better strength. One of the clinical methods used to assess shoulder function is the Constant Score, which consists of four variables including pain, activities of daily living (ADLs), ROM, and strength. One study demonstrated that the Constant Score is no different for patients undergoing RTC repair and patients treated nonoperatively at 6 months, but a difference does develop after that time favoring the RTC repair group. It is conceivable that this difference is related to strength gains, suggesting that patients who present with weakness or functional loss may be better served with RTC repair compared with patients who present with pain, who might be successfully managed nonoperatively (Dunn et al., 2013).

Return to work following treatment depends on the severity of the injury, handedness of the individual, and job requirements. If the dominant limb is affected, this will increase days away from work. It is also important to note that return to work will be postponed for months if surgery is performed. On average, when surgery is not required, the return to work following a shoulder injury typically ranges from 5 to 9 days (Bureau of Labor Statistics, 2008).

AC Joint Arthritis

Epidemiology

Osteoarthritis of the AC joint is a common and potentially debilitating condition of the shoulder, resulting in pain and physical limitations with overhead and cross-body movements. Clinically, osteoarthritis is the most common disorder of the AC joint, and it has numerous causes. As such, the ability to recognize, diagnose, and treat osteoarthritis of the AC joint is important when patients present with shoulder pain (Mall et al., 2013).

Pathophysiology

The AC joint plays a role in overall shoulder girdle motion and scapular positioning (Cadet, Ahmad, & Levine, 2008). Joint motion at the AC joint is critical for scapular kinesis, coupling clavicular and scapular motion, and thus scapular dyskinesis has been associated with AC joint injury (Kibler, Sciascia, & Wilkes, 2012). The small articular surface area and high loads experienced with everyday activity result in very high contact stresses within the AC joint (Colegate-Stone et al., 2010). Oblique orientation of the articular surfaces, incongruences of the articular surfaces, and degeneration of the disc can exacerbate these stresses, subjecting local areas of articular cartilage to very high stresses and accelerating osteoarthritic changes (Docimo, Kornitsky, Futterman, & Elkowitz, 2008).

Degenerative joint disease of the AC joint can occur owing to age-related degeneration of the intra-articular disc, posttraumatic arthropathy, distal clavicle osteolysis, inflammatory arthropathy, joint instability, and impingement. Similar to the meniscus of the knee, the intra-articular disc degenerates by fraying, tearing, and forming holes, macerated by defects in the chondral surface. This in turn leads to osteoarthritis (Petersson, 1983).

Clinical Presentation

Clinical diagnosis of AC joint osteoarthritis can be challenging. Common symptoms include pain with passive and active motion of the shoulder joint, most notable with overhead and cross-body occupational activities (Simovitch, Sanders, Ozbaydar, Lavery, & Warner, 2009). Pain is predominantly referred to the anterolateral aspect of the shoulder and sometimes to the neck, deltoid, and trapezius muscles as well. Similar symptoms can be observed with cervical spine disorders, RTC injury, and subacromial impingement. Thus, the examiner must be meticulous in the physical examination and imaging review to eliminate other probable causes. Mechanical symptoms such as popping, catching, or grinding within the joint can be present as well (Shaffer, 1999). Because of commonly concomitant RTC tears, labral injury, and biceps tendonitis, determining the contribution of the AC joint to the patient's pain requires careful examination. A careful examination of the entire shoulder girdle, including scapular movement, is essential and should be combined with a cervical spine examination to rule out contribution from cervical lesions (Brown, Roberts, Hayes, & Sales, 2000). On visual inspection, swelling, deformity, or prominence of the lateral clavicle may suggest AC joint instability (Chronopoulos, Kim, Park, Ashenbrenner, & McFarland, 2004). Palpation frequently yields tenderness, which is sensitive but nonspecific (Hegedus et al., 2008). Specific provocative tests include the cross-body adduction test and the AC resisted extension test. In the cross-body adduction test, the shoulder is brought to 90° of forward flexion and maximal adduction. Pain at the AC joint with this maneuver is considered a positive test (Chronopoulos et al., 2004).

Diagnostic Studies

Radiographic findings suggestive of degenerative osteoarthritis include joint space narrowing, subchondral cysts, osteophytes, and subchondral sclerosis (Ernberg & Potter, 2003). These findings must be interpreted in light of the history and physical examination, given the frequency of asymptomatic AC joint osteoarthritis (Mall et al., 2013). Although plain films are sufficient to diagnose AC joint degenerative joint disease, patients often undergo advanced imaging as part of the evaluation for concomitant injuries. MRI provides superior visualization of soft tissue, and may reveal capsular hypertrophy, effusion, and subchondral edema (Ernberg & Potter, 2003). Three-dimensional imaging of the AC joint is best visualized in the coronal oblique plane. Caudal osteophytes and capsular hypertrophy seen on MRI are predictive of increased pain relief with intra-articular injection (Strobel, Pfirrmann, Zanetti, Nagy, & Holder, 2003). MRI can also be useful when there is an acute injury, because edema can help localize the zone of injury and involved structure. US can also be used to assess joint space and detect osteophytes, cortical irregularities, or changes in echogenicity suggestive of capsular disruption (Figure 14.3) (Ernberg & Potter, 2003). Joint injection can be used both diagnostically and therapeutically using a mixture of short- and long-active anesthetic and corticosteroid (Mall et al., 2013). After palpating the bony landmarks, the clinician can advance the needle perpendicular to the articulation and into the joint capsule. Accuracy of the injection is improved with the use of US guidance, which yields an increased frequency of reaching the intra-articular space (Daley, Bajaj, Bisson, & Cole, 2011).

Treatment

The most common modes of nonoperative treatment include physical therapy, activity modification, immobilization, NSAIDs, and intra-articular injections (Rabalais & McCarty, 2007). Physical therapy can increase ROM, flexibility, and strength

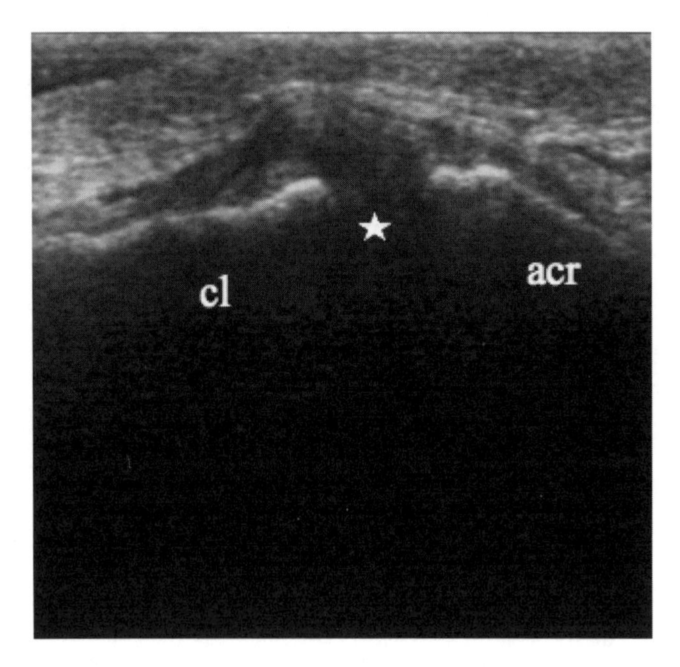

FIGURE 14.3 Ultrasound image of acromioclavicular (AC) joint arthritis. Cortical irregularity noted in the acromion (acr) and clavicle (cl). Asterisk represents joint space narrowing with a characteristic "geyser sign" suggestive of AC joint capsule disruption.

particularly within the periscapular musculature and RTC (Shaffer, 1999). Avoidance of repetitive, aggravating overhead and cross-body activity can also relieve pain. Patients who fail a trial of other nonoperative measures can be considered for intra-articular injection.

CARPAL TUNNEL SYNDROME

Etiology and Role of the Workplace and Physical Activities

CTS is the most common and best studied of all focal neuropathies. CTS is an entrapment median neuropathy, which is commonly seen in workers who are engaged in heavy manual occupations or light, repetitive tasks involving the wrist and hand. CTS cases related to occupational exposures result in a substantial burden of worker's compensation claims, lost work time and productivity, and disability. It is estimated that one in five patients presenting with upper limb pain, numbness, tingling, and weakness have CTS. In the United States, the prevalence of CTS in working populations ranges from 1.7% to 21% and is generally higher than the rates of 1% to 4.9% observed in the general population (Fan et al., 2015).

An understanding of biomechanics is an essential basis for accurately assessing, diagnosing, and treating CTS associated with computer use. CTS may develop due to repetitive microtrauma, often related to sustained or frequently repeated tasks in the setting of suboptimal ergonomics. The median nerve is subjected to increased pressure within the carpal tunnel during excessive wrist flexion or extension, which can occur when typing on a keyboard that is too high or too low. However, not all wrist or hand symptoms are related to CTS. Therefore, the entire kinetic chain within the upper extremity should be evaluated including the neck, shoulder, elbow, and forearm. Biomechanical evaluation includes a detailed understanding of the posture and positions the worker, and physical layout of the workstation. Also, it is important to understand the potential role of underlying degenerative changes as preexisting pathology may predispose to work-related exacerbations (Foye, Cianca, Prather, & John, 2002).

Pathophysiology and Clinical Presentation

The median nerve is derived from the lateral and medial cord of the brachial plexus and follows a path at the elbow close to the brachial artery. Within the carpal tunnel, which lies at the level of the wrist, the median nerve is accompanied by nine flexor tendons, including the four tendons of the flexor digitorum superficialis, the four tendons of the flexor digitorum profundus, and the flexor pollicis longus tendon. The walls of the carpal tunnel are made of fibro-osseous tissue, which is inelastic and unyielding to pressure. Fluid dynamics in CTS subjects demonstrate that intracarpal pressure is elevated and dissipation of this pressure is abnormally slow relative to controls (Cobb, Cooney, & An, 1995). Large myelinated fibers in the carpal tunnel are most susceptible to mechanical and ischemic damage. In CTS, microscopic studies have shown that disruption of myelin and the nodes of Ranvier results in conduction abnormalities, and when severe enough, axonal death (Sunderland, 1978). Damage to the median nerve from CTS can result in sensory changes and muscle weakness of the hand.

A directed history and physical examination is essential for the diagnosis of CTS. Patients with CTS generally experience numbness, tingling, or burning sensations in the thumb, index, middle, and radial half of the ring fingers and palm. Additionally, Phalen's maneuver (patient is asked to hold the wrists in forced flexion by pushing the dorsal surfaces of both hands together for 30–60 seconds causing increased pressure in the carpal tunnel) and reverse Phalen's maneuver (similar to Phalen's but with the wrists maintained in full extension by pressing the palms against each other) may elicit reproducible symptoms in the hand. For those patients with long-standing CTS, muscular atrophy and corresponding weakness of the thenar eminence may be observed, and this consequently results in the loss of grip and pinch strength as well as deficits in fine motor control. In more severe cases of CTS, atrophy of the thenar eminence and thumb abduction and opposition weakness can be appreciated. Sensory deficits in the hand are generally associated with poor manual performance for patients with peripheral nerve injuries, and impairments in the tactile sensation of patients with chronic CTS have adverse impacts on grasp force and dexterity. In addition, patients with CTS have reported problems generating sufficient grip force to use hand tools.

Diagnostic Studies

Electrodiagnostic studies are valuable because they can identify nerve pathology, localize the site of the lesion, and provide information regarding the severity of the nerve involvement. These studies offer the distinct advantage of providing objective data, which may quantify the degree of impairment in a manner independent of the patient's pain behaviors. The key finding for CTS is slowed conduction velocity localized to the segment of the median nerve passing through the carpal tunnel. In early and mild CTS, mild sensory nerve conduction slowing across the carpal tunnel is often the only abnormal finding. As CTS progresses, sensory peak latency, which represents how much signal reaches the recording electrode, is progressively delayed and the amplitude becomes smaller, suggesting significant demyelination or injury to the axons. Needle EMG can provide further evidence of denervation. With severe CTS, electrodiagnostic evidence of axonal loss of motor nerves can be seen in intrinsic hand muscles innervated by the median nerve, including the abductor pollicis brevis (Werner & Andary, 2011).

Treatment, Return to Work, Prevention

Oral NSAIDs are often used. Protected immobilization using a nighttime wrist brace that reduces nocturnal wrist flexion and extension is often of benefit. A recent prospective study showed that local steroid injections into the carpal tunnel can be effective in treating CTS and may be considered as an option. Educating the patient about avoiding overuse and activity modification is essential to prevent recurrence.

Occupational therapy or physical therapy may provide short-term modalities, such as ice or electric stimulation, to decrease pain and thus facilitate active stretching or strengthening. Patient education regarding proper body mechanics is also important. Some therapists are trained to perform worksite analysis, which can provide information critical for decisions about return to work.

A wide variety of ergonomic factors are relevant to the employee who uses a computer. Although there is some debate regarding the strength of the published research to confirm the usefulness of ergonomic interventions in video display terminal users, it seems probable that such interventions are a worthwhile component of a comprehensive rehabilitation plan. With CTS, ergonomic intervention should focus on hand and wrist positioning. Also, a modified job description that permits the employee to alternate work duties with less repetitive activities should be implemented, if available and feasible (Foye et al., 2002).

Because increased pressure on the median nerve within the carpal tunnel has been associated with excessive wrist flexion or extension, these positions should be avoided. If the keyboard is too low or too high (relative to the forearms), the computer user will excessively extend or flex the wrists while typing. Thus, interventions in this case require coordination between the chair height, forearm supports, forearms, wrists, hands, and keyboard. The forearms should be relatively horizontal to the floor and the wrist should be in a neutral position. The volar aspect of the wrist can be supported during typing by a wrist support placed on the desktop or support tray in front of the keyboard. The wrist support should be padded and without sharp or square edges. The mouse position also needs consideration to ensure that it meets the same criteria outlined for the keyboard (i.e., located at a height that fosters a neutral wrist position [no excessive extension or flexion] and perhaps with a padded wrist support on the desktop or support tray just in front of the mouse).

CTS is one of the most common occupational MSDs and considered the leader in the amount of lost work time among major disabling injuries. In order to reduce disability and economic burden associated with this condition, it is important to make an accurate diagnosis and to initiate appropriate treatment promptly. Furthermore, more research will be necessary to identify personal and workplace factors that can be incorporated into the primary prevention of CTS.

CONCLUSION

MSDs are a major problem that affects the employee, employer, and the economy. The difficulty of treating MSDs, whether it is back pain, shoulder pain, or CTS, is the multifactorial issues that surround each condition. Although effective treatment options may be in place for the physical disorder, the overall treatment of each condition is complicated by non-occupational, emotional, and psychosocial factors. The ideal treatment includes a multidisciplinary approach coupled with effective communication regarding treatment goals and outcomes. Prevention through education and ergonometric evaluation of workstations is ideal. Unfortunately, the ideal is rarely achieved. Overall, the incidence and prevalence of MSDs in the United States continue and deserves continued diligent medical attention.

REFERENCES

Bassett, R. W., & Cofield, R. H. (1983). Acute tears of the rotator cuff. The timing of surgical repair. *Clinical Orthopaedics and Related Research*, *175*, 18–24.

Besen, E., Young, A., & Shaw, W. (2015). Returning to work following low back pain: Towards a model of individual psychosocial factors. *Journal of Occupational Rehabilitation*, *25*, 25–37.

Bishop, J., Klepps, S., Lo, I. K., Brd, J., Gladstone, J. N., & Flatow, E. L. (2006). Cuff integrity after arthroscopic versus open rotator cuff repair: A prospective study. *Journal of Shoulder and Elbow Surgery, 15*, 290–299.

Bjelle, A., Hagberg, M., & Michaelson, G. (1981). Occupational and individual factors in acute shoulder-neck disorders among industrial workers. *British Journal of Industrial Medicine, 38*(4), 356–363.

Borg-Stein, J., Elson, L., & Brand, E. (2012). The aging spine in sports. *Clinics in Sports Medicine*, *31*, 473–486.

Brown, J. N., Roberts, S. N., Hayes, M. G., & Sales, A. D. (2000). Shoulder pathology associated with symptomatic acromioclavicular joint degeneration. *Journal of Shoulder and Elbow Surgery, 9*(3), 173–176.

Bureau of Labor Statistics. (2008). Nonfatal occupational injuries and illnesses requiring days away from work, 2011. *United States Department of Labor, 2012*. Retrieved from http://www.bls.gov/news.release/pdf/osh2.pdf

Burton, A. K., Balagué, F., & Cardon, G. (2005). How to prevent low back pain. *Best Practice & Research: Clinical Rheumatology, 19*(4), 541–555.

Cadet, E., Ahmad, C. S., & Levine, W. N. (2008). The management of acromioclavicular joint osteoarthrosis: Debride, resect, or leave it alone. *Instructional Course Lectures*, *55*, 75–83.

Centers for Disease Control and Prevention. (2001). Prevalence of disabilities and associated health conditions among adults—United States. *Journal of the American Medical Association*, *285*(12), 1571–1572.

Chronopoulos, E., Kim, T. K., Park, H. B., Ashenbrenner, D., & McFarland, E. G. (2004). Diagnostic value of physical tests for isolated chronic acromioclavicular lesions. *American Journal of Sports Medicine, 32*(3), 655–661.

Cobb, T. K., Cooney, W. P., & An, K. (1995). Pressure dynamics of the carpal tunnel and flexor compartment of the forearm. *The Journal of Hand Surgery*, *20*, 193–198.

Cohen, S. P., & Raja, S. N. (2007). Pathogenesis, diagnosis, and treatment of lumbar zygapophysial (facet) joint pain. *Anesthesiology*, *106*(3), 591–614.

Colegate-Stone, T., Allom, R., Singh, R., Elias, D. A., Standring, S., & Sinha, J. (2010). Classification of the morphology of the acromioclaviular joint using cadaveric and radiologic analysis. *Journal of Bone and Joint Surgery*, *92*(5), 743–756.

Daley, E. L., Bajaj, S., Bisson, L. J., & Cole, B. J. (2011). Improving injection accuracy of the elbow, knee, and shoulder: Does injection site and imaging make a difference? A systematic review. *American Journal of Sports Medicine*, *39*(3), 656–662.

Docimo, S. Jr., Kornitsky, D., Futterman, B., & Elkowitz, D. E. (2008). Surgical treatment for acromioclavicular joint osteoarthritis: patient selection, surgical options, complications, and outcome. *Current Reviews in Musculoskeletal Medicine*, *1*(2), 154–160.

Dunn, W. R., Kuhn, J. E., Keith, M. B., Julie, Y. B., Robert H. B., & James L. C., . . . Rick, W. W. (2013). Defining indications for rotator cuff repair: predictors of failure of non-operative treatment of chronic, symptomatic, full-thickness rotator cuff tears. *Journal of Shoulder and Elbow Surgery, 22*(4), e28.

Dunn, W. R., Kuhn, J. E., Sanders. R., An, Q., Baumgarten, K. M., Bishop, J. Y., . . . Wright, R. W. (2014). Symptoms of pain do not correlate with rotator cuff tear severity: A cross sectional study of 393 patients with symptomatic atraumatic full thickness rotator cuff tears. *The Journal of Bone and Joint Surgery, 96*(10), 793–800.

Eck, J. C., & Riley, L. H. (2004). Return to play after lumbar spine conditions and surgeries. *Clinics in Sports Medicine, 23*, 367–379.

Ernberg, L. A., & Potter, H. G. (2003). Radiographic evaluation of the acromioclavicular and sternoclavicular joints. *Clinics in Sports Medicine, 22*(2), 255–275.

Fan, Z. J., Harris-Adamson, C., Gerr, F., Eisen, E. A., Hegmann, K. T., & Bao, S., . . . Rempel, D. (2015). Associations between workplace factors and carpal tunnel syndrome: A multi-site cross sectional study. *American Journal of Industrial Medicine, 58*, 509–518.

Feng, S., Guo, S., Nobuhara, K., Hashimoto, J., & Mimori, K. (2003). Prognostic indicators for outcome following rotator cuff repair. *Journal of Orthopaedic Surgery, 11*, 110–116.

Foye, P., Cianca, J., Prather, H., & John, C. C. (2002). Cumulative trauma disorders of the upper limb in computer users. *Archives of Physical Medicine and Rehabilitation, 83*, S12–S15.

Garfin, S. R., Herkowitz, H. N., & Mirkovic, S. (1999). Spinal stenosis. *The Journal of Bone and Joint Surgery, 81*(4), 572–586.

Goutallier, D., Postel, J. M., Bernageau, J., Lavau, L., & Voisin, M. C. (1994). Fatty muscle degeneration in cuff ruptures. Pre- and postoperative evaluation by CT scan. *Clinical Orthopaedics and Related Research, 304*, 78–83.

Hegedus, E. J., Goode, A., Campbell, S., Morin, A., Tamaddoni, M., & Moorman, C. T., . . . Cook, C. (2008). Physical examination tests of the shoulder: A systematic review with meta-analysos of individual tests. *British Journal of Sports Medicine, 42*(2), 80–92.

Ianotti, J. P. (1994). Full-thickness rotator cuff tears: factors affecting surgical outcome. *Journal of the American Academy of Orthopaedic Surgeons, 2*, 87–95.

Jensen, M. C., Brant-Zawadzki, M. N., Obuchowski, N., Modic, M. T., Malkasian, D., & Ross, J. S. (1994). Magnetic resonance imaging of the lumbar spine in people without back pain. *The New England Journal of Medicine, 331*, 69–73.

Kibler, B., Sciascia, A., & Wilkes, T. (2012). Scapular dyskinesis and its relation to shoulder injury. *Journal of the American Academy of Orthopaedic Surgeons, 35*(2), 316–329.

Kibler, W. B., McMullen, J., & Uhl, T. (2012). Shoulder rehabilitation strategies, guidelines, and practice. *Operative Techniques in Sports Medicine, 20*, 103–112.

Kuhn, J., Dunn, W. R., Sanders, R., An, Q., Baumgarten, K. M., & Bishop, J. Y., . . . MOON Shoulder Group. (2013). Effectiveness of physical therapy in treating atraumatic full-thickness rotator cuff tears: A multicenter prospective cohort study. *Journal of Shoulder and Elbow Surgery, 22*, 1371–1379.

Leigh, J. P., & Marcin, J. P. (2012). Workers compensation benefits and shifting costs for occupational injury and illness. *Journal of Occupational and Environmental Medicine, 54*(4), 445–450.

Mall, N., Foley, E., Chalmers, P. N., Cole, B. J., Romeo, A. A., & Bach, B. R. (2013). Degenerative joint disease of the acromioclavicular joint. *The American Journal of Sports Medicine, 41*, 2684–2692.

National Institute of Neurological Disorders and Stroke. (2015). Low back pain fact sheet. Retrieved from http://www.ninds.nih.gov/disorders/backpain/detail_backpain.htm

Nonfatal occupational injuries and illnesses requiring days away from work, 2011 [news release]. (2012). Washington, DC: Bureau of Labor and Statistics, U.S. Department of Labor. Retrieved from http://www.bls.gov/news.release/osh2.nr0.htm

Petersson, C. J. (1983). Degeneration of the acromioclavicular joint: A morphological study. *Acta Orthopaedica Scandinavica, 54*(3), 434–438.

Rabalais, R. D., & McCarty, E. (2007). Surgical trwatment of symptomatic acromioclavicular joint problems: A systematic review. *Clinical Orthopaedics and Related Research, 455*, 30–37.

Reilly, P., Macleod, I., Macfarlane, R., Windley, J., & Emery, R. J. H. (2006). Dead men and radiologists don't lie: A review of cadaver and radiologic studies of rotator cuff tear prevalence. *The Annals of The Royal College of Surgeons of England, 88*, 116–121.

Rubin, D. I. (2007). Epidemiology and risk factors for spine pain. *Neurologic Clinics, 25*(2), 353–371.

Simovitch, R., Sanders, B., Ozbaydar, M., Lavery, K., & Warner, J. J. (2009). Acromioclavicular joint injuries: diagnosis and management. *Journal of the American Academy of Orthopaedic Surgeons, 25*(9), 968–974.

Shaffer, B. S. (1999). Painful conditions of the acromioclavicular joint. *Journal of the American Academy of Orthopaedic Surgeons, 7*(3), 176–188.

Slabaugh, M. A., Nho, S. J., Grumet, R. C., Wilson, J. B., Seroyer, S. T., & Frank, R. M., . . . Verma, N. N. (2010). Does the literature confirm superior clinical results in radiographically healed rotator cuffs after rotator cuff repair? *Arthroscopy, 26*, 393–403.

Stewart, W. F., Ricci, J. A., Chee, E., Morganstein, D., & Lipton, R. (2003). Lost productive time and cost due to common pain conditions in the us workforce. *Journal of the American Medical Association, 290*(18), 2443–2454.

Strobel, K., Pfirrmann, C. W., Zanetti, M., Nagy, L., & Holder, J. (2003). MRI features of the acromioclavicular joint that predict pain relief from intraarticular injection. *American Journal of Roentgenology, 181*(3), 755–760.

Sunderland, S. (1978). *Nerve and nerve injuries*. Edinburgh, Scotland: Churchill Livingston.

Svendsen, S. W., Gelineck, J., Mathiassen, S. E., Bonde, J. P., Frich, L. H., Stengaard-Pedersen, K., & Egund N. (2004). Work above shoulder level and degenerative alterations of the rotator cuff tendons: A magnetic resonance imaging study. *Arthritis & Rheumatism, 50*(10), 3314–3322.

Unruh, K. P., Kuhn, J. E., Sanders, R., An, Q., Baumgarten, K. M., & Bishop, J., . . . Dunn, W. R. (2014). The duration of symptoms does not correlate with rotator cuff tear severity or other patient-related feature: a cross-sectional study of patients with atraumatic, full-thickness rotator cuff tears. *Journal of Shoulder and Elbow Surgery, 23*, 1052–1058.

Vitale, M. A., Vitale, M. G., Zivin, J. G., Braman, J. P., Bigliani, L. U., & Flatow, E. L. (2006). Rotator cuff repair: An analysis of utility scores and cost-effectiveness. *Journal of Shoulder and Elbow Surgery, 16*, 181–187.

Waddell, G. (2004). *The back pain revolution* (2nd ed.). Edinburgh, Scotland: Churchill Livingstone.

Werner, R. A., & Andary, M. (2011). Electrodiagnostic evaluation of carpal tunnel syndrome. *Muscle & Nerve, 44*, 597–607.

Workplace injuries and illnesses–2011 [news release]. (2012, October 25). Washington, DC: Bureau of Labor and Statistics, U.S. Department of Labor. Retrieved from http://www.bls.gov/news.release/osh.nr0.htm

Yamaguchi, K., Tetro, A. M., Blam, O., Evanoff, B. A., Teefy, S. A., & Middleton, W. D. (2001). Natural history of asymptomatic rotator cuff tears: A longitudinal analysis of asymptomatic tears detected sonographically. *Journal of Shoulder and Elbow Surgery, 10*, 199–203.

CHAPTER

Pediatric Disorders: Cerebral Palsy and Spina Bifida

Joan T. Gold and David H. Salsberg

INTRODUCTION

Physically challenged children present with a variety of developmental and neuromuscular disabilities that are often difficult to diagnose, hard to remediate, and impossible to cure. Approximately one in six children in the United States have such special needs (Boyle et al., 2011). There is a disproportionate demand on the supportive services that these patients require with an approximate threefold demand on emergency department care; finding a "medical home" for such patients and establishing effective coordination of multidisciplinary care are extremely challenging (Lin, Margolis, Yu, & Adirim, 2014). These demands are accompanied by psychological and neuropsychological issues that also require major ongoing interventions to maximize functional potentials.

The restrictions imposed by such disabilities may not permit the patient the motoric control or the experiences to acquire skills at the same rate as the typically developing child. Accordingly, secondary developmental delays may occur (Missuna & Pollack, 1991). Medical complications unique to the underlying diagnosis, with frequent hospitalizations and surgeries, social isolation, parental dependency, and financial burdens, are stressors for patients, parents, and siblings (Worley, Rosenfeld, & Liscomb, 1991a, 1991b).

It is the purpose of this chapter to discuss cerebral palsy and spina bifida, two of the more common handicapping conditions of childhood, and the strategies that allow for appropriate medical treatment and rehabilitation. This information permits the health professional to serve as an advocate for optimization of care, prevention of complications, referral to early intervention programs, and placement of the child in the least restrictive school setting. Additionally, potentially abusive and neglectful behaviors of parents and caretakers may be circumvented (Benedict, White, Wulff, & Hall, 1990).

This chapter addresses the wide range of emotional challenges that face children diagnosed with chronic medical disorders and disabilities. Children with spina bifida and cerebral palsy require attention to their psychological issues and neuropsychological challenges to facilitate both rehabilitation courses and general functioning within a community setting (Gerring et al., 2008; Max et al., 2002; Pellock, 2004). Significant family stressors and multicultural factors have an impact on the child's developmental growth (Morison, Bromfield, & Cameron, 2003). The holistic care of children with disabilities requires a multidisciplinary approach that fully integrates the child's developmental, cognitive, and psychological issues, as well as family and cultural dynamics, in addition to the medical presentation (Spates, Samaraweera, Plaiser, Souza, & Otsui, 2007).

CEREBRAL PALSY

Cerebral palsy is a descriptive clinical term that denotes a group of static encephalopathies of diverse etiologies resulting from nonprogressive lesions of the brain sustained in the prenatal, perinatal, or postnatal periods. The disorder is characterized by abnormalities in muscle tone, muscle control and movement, and postures, of which spasticity is the most common type of presentation, occurring in 65% to 80% of cases. Secondary dysfunction and deformities occur, but there is not the frank regression in function seen with neurodegenerative disorders, such as the leukodystrophies. Other symptoms of cerebral dysfunction, such as learning disabilities, mental retardation, and seizures, may be seen, but it is the motoric dysfunction that is essential to the diagnosis of the condition (Ingram, 1955).

Incidence

The incidence of cerebral palsy in the past 20 years has remained at 2 cases per 1,000 births in the United States (Nelson & Ellenberg, 1986), with approximately 400,000 patients currently being affected. There was a concern that with survival of more medically fragile, lower birth weight infants, the incidence may have increased, despite advances in intrapartum monitoring that can herald fetal distress (albeit with a false-positive rate approaching 99.8%; Grant, O'Brien, Joy, Henessy, & MacDonald, 1989; Stanley & Blair, 1991; Vohr & Msall, 1997). However, more recent studies do not support this and greater proportion of lower birth weight infants are surviving unscathed, with better management of their brain injury, chronic lung disease, and sepsis (Hack & Costello, 2008). The cases that do occur may also be less severe with a reduction in the number of cases of quadriplegia, a relative increase in the numbers of spastic diplegia, and an overall reduction in the incidence of later seizure disorders (Sigurdardottir, Halldorsdottir, Thorkelsson, Thorarensen, & Vik, 2009). A further reduction in incidence may not be easily forthcoming as prenatal etiologies in a majority of cases (Ford, Kitchen, Doyle, Richards, & Kelly, 1990) cannot be clinically identified. Intervention may be required in a greater percentage of the population as more than 40% of the group may require special education services, although they are not specifically diagnosed with cerebral palsy.

Etiology and Risk Factors

Cerebral palsy was first described by Little in 1843 in infants born prematurely; they developed increased tone and incoordination primarily affecting the lower extremities, or what is now termed as spastic diplegia. With changes in medical treatment, a reduced association with dystocia (difficult labor), erythroblastosis (Rh-negative blood incompatibility), and encephalitis, and an increased association with multiple births, prematurity, acquired hydrocephalus (following intracranial hemorrhage and antenatal infection), and trauma have been noted (Capute, Shapiro, & Palmer, 1981; O'Callaghan et al., 2011).

Accordingly, fewer patients are affected with the writhing movement disorder of athetosis, seen with erythroblastosis and subsequent deposition of abnormal hemoglobin pigments into the basal ganglia, and a greater number of patients have diffuse cerebral dysfunction, with spasticity and cognitive dysfunction.

Etiology can be identified in up to 71% of quadriplegics (those patients with equal involvement of all four extremities) and 40% of nonquadriplegics (Naeye & Peters, 1989). A gestational age of less than 32 of 40 weeks is the greatest predictor for the development of cerebral palsy, although children born at 34 to 36 weeks gestation still have a threefold risk of incurring cerebral palsy (Petrini et al., 2009). Other risk factors, such as maternal mental retardation, birth weight of less than 2,001 g, presence of congenital malformations, and symptomatic intoxications, such as fetal alcohol syndrome, support a largely prenatal etiology (Coorsen, Msall, & Duffy, 1991; Ellenberg & Nelson, 1981). Factors that result in chronic antenatal hypoxia with brain injury include maternal anemia, preeclampsia/gestational hypertension, a drop in third-trimester blood pressure, postterm delivery, and multiple births (Nelson, 1989). These events have a high association with the presence of congenital malformations.

A prenatal etiology for cerebral palsy has been identified in up to 50% to 60% of patients (Holm, 1982; Naeye & Peters, 1989), most presenting with hypotonia, ataxia, or hemiplegia (unilateral limb involvement). In utero infections, in association with maternal fever during labor (Nelson, 1998), have been demonstrated as one of the predisposing factors in the etiology of cerebral palsy. Inflammatory markers such as cytokines and interferon levels of cord blood are frequently elevated in the population of patients who progress to have spastic diplegia (Nelson, 1998; Rousset et al., 2008).

Thrombotic events in utero, which are really early onset ischemic strokes, may also explain many cases of cerebral palsy. Analysis of cord blood levels for Protein S and Protein C deficiencies, conditions that predispose to hypercoagulability, and in utero stroke may be of value in patients who are subsequently diagnosed as having the hemiplegic variety of cerebral palsy (Gibson, Mac Lennan, Goldwater, & Dekker, 2003). Identification of a parental coagulopathy or other serological markers could potentially provide for early designation of a population at risk, with more prompt and effective initiation of early intervention therapeutic services and for the development of a preventive protocol (Kraus, 1997).

A perinatal etiology has been identified in only about 10% to 15% of cases although placental abruption, cord prolapse, and uterine rupture, when they do occur, can be significant (Nelson, 2008). Factors thought to be characteristic of birth asphyxia, such as meconium staining and fetal distress, are more often the result of nonasphyxial disorders that have been present as chronic stressors in the pregnancy and clinically may not have a way of being identified, tracked, or ameliorated (Nelson, 1989). True perinatal asphyxia may be related to obstetrical complications, such as placental abruption, nuchal cord, or meconium aspiration. Such an etiology is often accompanied by seizures in the newborn period and evidence of other organ system dysfunction due to anoxia such as cardiac, renal, and/or hepatic dysfunction. Other perinatal etiologies include central nervous system bleeding (Williams, Lewandowski, Coplan, & D'Eugenio, 1987) and meningeal infections. Patients in this group are most likely to be spastic. When the diagnosis of a hypoxic ischemic encephalopathy is made, it is most often associated with central gray matter damage especially of the palladium. This finding has been strongly associated with severe motor impairment (Krageloh-Mann, 2015; Martinez-Biarge et al., 2011).

A postnatal etiology occurs in about 10% of patients (Holm, 1982). Factors include head trauma, of an accidental or inflicted (abusive) nature, central nervous system infections, and cerebrovascular accidents. Such patients are likely to be hemiparetic. A mixed etiology occurs in about 7% of cases (Holm, 1982). In some cases, there may be multifactorial factors that result in cumulative risk.

Neonatal indicators for the development of static encephalopathy include intracranial hemorrhage, seizures, microcephaly (small head size), hypertonia or hypotonia, abnormal suck/cry/grasp reflexes, jitteriness, temperature instability, and feeding difficulties (Nelson & Ellenberg, 1979). Apgar scores that reflect immediate neonatal status are not as predictive as once thought (Nelson & Ellenberg, 1981). Periventricular hemorrhage in association with attenuation of the white matter about the ventricles (periventricular leukomalacia [PVL]) with formation of cysts, which can be demonstrated on head ultrasound or other neuroimaging studies, correlates with the development of cerebral palsy (Graham, Levene, & Trounce, 1987). PVL is associated with birth trauma, asphyxia and respiratory failure, cardiopulmonary defects, premature birth/low birth weight with associated immature cerebrovascular development, and lack of appropriate autoregulation of cerebral blood flow in response to hypoxic–ischemia insult. Other pertinent findings on neuroimaging may include lesions of the basal ganglia, cortical and subcortical lesions, malformations, and focal infarcts (Bax, Tydeman, & Flodmark, 2006).

Brain cells known as oliogodendrocytes are vulnerable to the exposure of free-radical chemicals that are liberated during these events. They are further compromised by poor circulation and the presence of cytokines that are seen with inflammation and infection. There is not currently a "dosage" factor related to the risk of the development of cerebral palsy that can be calculated. While there are many single genes that may influence the effects of inflammation in a positive or negative way, no statiscally significant association has been made (Wu, Croen, Vanderwerf, Geifand, & Torres, 2011). If this process is identified earlier and better delineated by newer imaging studies, such as diffusion imaging and other studies, which are not yet routinely available or demonstrated as the standard of care, it might possible to develop treatment that would have more direct efficacy on treating the brain injury. Such options could potentially include use of drugs that reverse the effects of free radicals and other inflammatory chemicals such as the use of interleukin-10 (Bell & Hallenback, 2002; Mesples, Plaisant, & Gressens, 2003; Rezaie & Dean, 2002).

Delineation of an etiology may imply a specific clinical presentation and prognosis that permits parents to be supplied with an overview of the child's potential outcome. Counseling of parents that actions during the time of conception and pregnancy are most likely unrelated to the development of the cerebral palsy permits feelings of guilt to be assuaged and promotes better acceptance of the child.

Functional Presentation

Cerebral palsy is classified on the basis of etiology, muscle tone, and the anatomical distribution of neurological abnormalities. Pyramidal or spastic (clasp-knife) cerebral palsy is the most common. Resistance is noted when muscles are stretched rapidly beyond a critical point. Associated hyperreflexia, up-going plantar responses (toes move upward in response to stimulation of the plantar surface of the foot), prolonged contraction of muscles, inability to isolate fine motor movements, co-contractions of agonist and antagonist muscles, and misfiring of muscles during ambulation resulting in gait abnormalities are found. Quadriplegia occurs in about 20% of these cases, with diffuse cortical involvement, and, in the most disabled, widespread atrophy occurs with cavity formation and decreased white matter density. Hemiplegia occurs in about 30% and is associated with atrophy/gliosis of the cerebral hemisphere opposite the side of muscle weakness, likely caused by a vascular disturbance. Liquifaction necrosis may occur, resulting in a porencephalic cyst (Mannino & Traunor, 1983).

Diplegics, who comprise more than 50% to 65% of this population, are generally, but not exclusively, premature infants who have undergone significant intraventricular hemorrhages (Blair & Stanley, 1990; Hagberg & Hagberg, 1989). The periventricular areas have cortical radiations to the lower extremities, which are more involved with spasticity than the upper extremities; this differentiates these patients from quadriplegics, in whom all extremities are involved to the same degree. Diplegia, and cerebral palsy, in general, in premature infants is most correlated with PVL as discussed earlier, and is demonstrable on head ultrasound, CT scan, and MRI studies. The severity of these findings seems to correlate with the degree of the child's sensorimotor involvement. Infants in this group, who also demonstrate thalamic lesions, are more likely to have severe motor and cognitive dysfunction (Yokochi, 1997). Monoplegia and triplegia (affecting one and three limbs, respectively) are rare. Bilateral involvement is the most common presentation, occurring in 75% of preterm and 45% of term patients (Hagberg & Hagberg, 1996).

Extrapyramidal or nonspastic types of cerebral palsy are responsible for about 20% of cases. Patients who have athetosis or rigidity have basal ganglia dysfunction that accounts for their movement disorders. Patients with ataxia have difficulties with balance and position sense, resulting from cerebellar pathology. Diagnostic workup is most important with ataxias, as posterior fossa brain tumors and degenerative inherited diseases, such as ataxia telangiectasia and Friedreich's ataxia, may have similar presentations.

Patients with hypotonia have widespread damage to cortical and subcortical areas, so spasticity cannot be mounted as a response, and they have the poorest prognosis for cognitive and motor function. Some patients with hypotonia may become athetoid with time. The remaining cases have mixed features (i.e., diffuse cerebral involvement and impaired motor function). Cerebral palsy can also be classified on the basis of functional performance. This is not only helpful for clinical clarity but can serve as a way of delineating response to a specific clinical intervention.

In recent years, the Gross Motor Function Classification System (GMFCS) has been introduced with acceptable validity and reliability (Palisano et al., 1997; Palisano, Rosenbaum, & Bartlett, 2008; Rosenbaum et al., 2007; Rutz, Tirosh, Thomason, Barg, & Graham, 2012). It is based on a five-point grading system ranging from those children who are nonambulant (V) to children who ambulate in the community without orthotics or other devices (I). Alternatively, for ambulatory patients, the 6-minute walk test coupled with measurement of oxygen consumption can also be utilized to reflect functional changes (Maltais, Robitaille, Dumas, Boucher, & Richarsd, 2012).

Differential Diagnosis

Up to 40% of patients with an initial diagnosis of cerebral palsy have been incorrectly diagnosed. Other disorders that present with gross motor delays, aberrant tone, and abnormal movement patterns include mental retardation, neurodegenerative disorders, hydrocephalus, subdural effusions, slowly growing brain tumors, spinal cord lesions, muscular dystrophy, spinal muscular atrophy, and congenital cerebellar ataxias. Obviously, prognosis, inheritance patterns, and treatment vary widely in these disorders.

Investigations that may be helpful in substantiating or excluding the diagnosis of cerebral palsy include the following: CT or MRI scans to assess structural lesions, ultrasound of the head to exclude the possibility of intraventricular hemorrhage, lumbar puncture to exclude elevated protein in the cerebrospinal fluid that is seen in association with neurodegenerative disorders, serum uric acid and blood and urine assays for amino and organic acids to exclude congenital metabolic disorders, viral and parasitic titers (TORCH) to exclude the possibility of an intrauterine-acquired infection, and chromosomal studies to exclude such abnormalities, especially in children with dysmorphia. Recent studies have begun to investigate the usefulness of diffusion tensor imaging (DTI) and fiber tracking in delineating the primary and secondary degenerative changes in cerebral white matter and deep gray matter in patients with cerebral palsy and to explore any possible reorganization of the axonal architecture.

Associated Medical Problems

Mental retardation coexists in 50% to 60% of patients with cerebral palsy, communication and learning disorders in 40% to 50%, visual problems including strabismus and myopia in 50%, deafness in 6% to 16%, seizure disorders in 33% to 38%, and orthopedic deformities in 50% (Robinson, 1973). Visual problems are not only important in terms of learning and school-related tasks, but also affect head and hand movements that influence gross motor coordination, including ambulation and self-care skills.

Generalized seizures are most common in patients with quadriplegia, and partial seizures are most common in those patients with hemiplegia (Carlson, Hagberg, & Olssom, 2003). Electroencephalograms and visual- and auditory-evoked potentials are helpful in delineation of such problems. The superimposed seizures and medication effects also increase the risk of behavioral problems and need for counseling in this population (Carlsson, Olsson, Hagberg, & Beckung, 2008).

The parietal lobe syndrome is characterized by hemiplegia, limb length discrepancies (the upper extremity being more affected), and sensory deficits as manifested by reduced two-point discrimination, stereognosis, and graphesthesia (Staheli, Duncan, & Schafer, 1960). A less common triad, seen with erythroblastosis-related disease, includes kernicterus (bilirubin deposition from red blood cell breakdown in the basal ganglia) with resultant athetosis, hearing loss, and paralysis of upward gaze. This is less commonly seen owing to a reduction in the incidence of athetoid cerebral palsy but can still be demonstrated in the older population with cerebral palsy.

Oropharyngeal incoordination may result in poor oral intake, with failure to thrive, occasionally necessitating placement of a gastrostomy tube for caloric supplementation. Misdirected swallowing and gastroesophageal reflux may result in aspiration pneumonias. Poor hand function, pooling of saliva, and abnormal muscle tone can result in poor dental hygiene and malocclusion (Rosenstein, 1982). Restrictive pulmonary disease may result from hypertonicity, and scoliosis may further limit endurance (Rothman, 1978). Bladder spasticity and sphincteric incoordination, rather than cognitive limitations, may result in urinary incontinence and may be responsive to uropharmacological and behavioral management (Keating, McCarron, James, Gruenberg, & Lonczak, 1985; McNeal, Hawtrey, Wolraich, & Mapel, 1983).

Owing to these comorbidities, patients undergo multiple procedures including botulinum toxin injections, feeding gastrostomies, ventriculoperitoneal shunts, and ophthalmologic surgery often depending on their GMFCS level, with more dependent patients requiring more interventions (Erkin, Colha, Ozel, & Kirbiyik, 2010; McLellan, Cipparone, Giancola, Armstrong, & Bartlett, 2012).

Orthopedic complications include the development of limb contractures and deformities, dislocations, especially at the hips, and scoliosis due to prolonged muscle imbalance. All of these conditions may require medical and therapeutic attempts at normalization of tone and/or surgical interventions as described subsequently. Fractures may occur in these patients as a result of osteopenia concomitant with spasm and secondary effects of anticonvulsant administration. In nonambulatory children with quadriplegis, lumbar spine bone mineral density may be decreased by as much as 58%, and up to 39% of the patients may suffer nontraumatic hip fractures (King, Levin, Schmidt,

Oestreich, & Heubi, 2003). Prolonged periods of immobilization following orthopedic procedures may exacerbate this tendency with up to a 34% loss in bone mineral density occurring over a 4- to 6-week period (Szalay, Harriman, Eastlund, & Mercer, 2008). Initial studies suggest that the use of bisphosphonate infusions (Pamidronate) may be helpful in treatment of this complication (Henderson, Lark, & Kecskemethy, 2002). Oral agents need to be considered carefully, as they usually require the patient to sit upright for at least 1 hour, which is potentially difficult in this population. Dietary deficiencies may also require supplementation with calcium and vitamin D.

The long-term effects of sedentary lifestyle not of their choosing may have an effect not only on bony fragility of patients with cerebral palsy, but on overall health, sense of well-being, and cardiovascular fitness as well (Morris, 2008), although specific studies in this area are lacking.

Clinical Findings and Prognostic Indicators

Cerebral palsy may be difficult to identify in a patient who is younger than 1 year of age. Although gross motor milestones may be delayed, hypertonicity, movement disorders, and early hand dominance may have not yet occurred (Levine, 1980). Although the brain lesion that results in the encephalopathy is static, the child's neurological appearance may vary with growth and maturation of the brain. The infant with spastic quadriparesis is generally identified by 5 months of age; diplegics are not identified until 12 months of age, on average, and hemiplegics at 21 months (Harris, 1989). Difficulty in diagnosis is compounded by the plasticity of the immature nervous system, with compensatory branching of the corticospinal tract fibers (Farmer, Harrison, Ingram, & Stephens, 1991), allowing cerebral palsy to "disappear" in up to 55% of cases (Tardorf, 1986). There is also recent evidence to indicate potential neuronal repair in white matter in association with PVL (Haynes et al., 2011). Labeling an infant as "high risk" may result in overinterpretation of normal physical findings (Ashton, Piper, Warren, Stewin, & Byrne, 1991).

Motor development in the subtypes of cerebral palsy varies, but common denominators exist (Bobath & Bobath, 1975). Abnormal positioning of the hands, hypertonicity of the neck extensors, inability to isolate lower extremity movements (i.e., an all-flexor or all-extensor pattern), difficulty in bringing the elbows across midline suggestive of increased tone, poor head control, microcephaly, abnormal deep tendon reflexes, persistence of grasp reflexes, and up-going plantar responses beyond 12 months of age are all suspect findings. Lack of symmetrical movement and early onset of hand dominance are suggestive of a hemiparesis. Not only may gross motor activities be delayed, but when performed, they may be carried out in an abnormal way, often with utilization of abnormal, stereotypical primitive reflexes to initiate the movement (see subsequent discussion). The use of head arching to initiate rolling and crawling on the abdomen with both legs being flexed simultaneously rather than on all fours in a reciprocal manner are two examples of these behaviors. In the absence of frankly abnormal gross motor movements or reflex abnormalities, the lack of variation of limb movements may also be a finding indicative of a static encephalopathy (Bruggink et al., 2008).

Major support for the diagnosis of cerebral palsy is given by the persistence of primitive reflexes. These subcortical reflexes are normally suppressed by 6 months of age. They can always be summoned but are modulated by more advanced learned motor activities. When these reflexes occur each time a child is placed in a position, they interfere with that child's ability to change position, and to assume and maintain an antigravity position. These reflexes include the symmetric and asymmetric (fencer) tonic neck reflexes, the tonic labyrinthine response, positive support reaction, and the Moro (startle) response. Postural reactions such as head and neck righting responses may be delayed or absent. The persistence of more than one reflex beyond 2 years of age, in association with the child's inability to sit, is negatively associated with future ambulation (Capute, 1978; Sala & Grant, 1995). Conversely, the ability of the child to sit by 2 years correlates with a good prognosis for ambulation. More recently, identification of certain patterns of antigravity movements, such as head lifting, sitting with upper extremity support, and ambulating 10 steps, may stratify the population with cerebral palsy into five different types of patients where motor development can be more definitely assessed (Palisano, Rosenbaum, Walter, & Hanna, 1997). However, these studies are preliminary and should not be utilized as a way of limiting therapeutic services or other medical interventions at this time.

Children who do not ambulate by 7 to 8 years of age are usually unable to do so, unless limited therapeutic services have not been provided prior to this time. Ninety-eight percent of hemiplegics, 75% of diplegics, and 50% of quadriplegics will ambulate according to studies performed in the past (Molnar & Gordon, 1976). Of those patients with quadriplegia, 25% will be independent, 50% will require assistance, and 25% will utilize wheelchairs as their means of community ambulation. Most patients with the ataxia variant of cerebral palsy will ambulate. Hypotonic and rigid patients have the poorest prognosis for ambulation (Molnar, 1979). These studies were performed prior to newer interventions such as selective dorsal rhizotomy and placement of intrathecal baclofen pumps (ITBP); it is yet to be determined if such interventions will result in significant alterations of these prognostic parameters. Children ambulate abnormally because of static and dynamic muscle dysfunction (Sutherland, 1984). Gaits are energy inefficient, resulting in fatigability and limited endurance (Mossberg, Linton, & Friske, 1990).

Fine motor, personal–social, and language skills may also be impaired to a variable degree. The Amiel-Tison Scale, Milani-Comparetti Scale, Denver Developmental Screening Test, and the Bayley Scale of Infant Development III are some of the tools that have been developed for documentation and tracking of these dysfunctions. Periodic neuropsychological evaluations to include nonverbal measures as appropriate and the assessment of social, personality, and educational functioning are recommended.

Therapeutic Interventions

Direct treatment for cerebral palsy is for the most part unavailable. However, use of certain physical supports and medications has recently indicated that potential for change and effective treatment is possible. Treatment trials of total body and head cooling for the reduction of effects of hypoxic ischemic encephalopathy have suggested potential reduction in both death and disability (Eicher, Wagner, & Katikaneni, 2004; Shah, Ohlsson, & Perlman, 2007). The use of extracorporeal membrane oxygenation in patients with severe respiratory distress syndrome has been demonstrated as having additional efficacy over traditional ventilatory support, and although these infants are at risk, they have improved survival and need further assessments as to later neuropsychological outcomes (Wagner et al., 2007).

Certain pharmacological agents have been demonstrated to modulate the stressors that may result in a static encephalopathy and appear to be of statistical benefit. The use of prenatal glucocorticoids (dexathamethasone) treatment administered to mothers of preterm infants may reduce the risk of intraventricular hemorrhage and PVL. The protective effect may occur owing to direct stabilization of the vasculature of the fetal brain and a reduction of the acid–base fluctuations that ensue with reduced/aborted respiratory distress syndrome for which these steroids are administered. The risk of the development of cerebral palsy in such a group may be reduced from 22% to 10% (Salakor et al., 1997; Sotriadis et al., 2015). Research has also suggested that the use of free-radical scavengers and blockers of receptors of excitatory amino acids could limit the tissue damage that is sustained by neonates with perinatal asphyxia (Vannucci, 1990). Magnesium sulfate, which is used to protect mothers from the hypertension associated with preeclampsia, may also offer a protective effect by acting as a vasodilator to the fetal brain (Hirtz & Nelson, 1998; Rouse et al., 2008) although results of some of these studies are somewhat equivocal (Galvin, 1998). Indomethacin, a nonsteroidal antiinflammatory agent used in the treatment of infants to close a patent ductus arteriosus, has also been recently utilized as a neuroprotective agent to decrease the risk of intraventricular hemorrhage in premature neonates. Other secondary treatments include therapy, tone-altering medications, provision of adaptive equipment to enhance patients' level of function, and orthopedic and neurosurgical procedures that correct deformities and normalize tone, as discussed subsequently (Diamond, 1986; Lord, 1984; Ronan & Gold, 2007).

Therapeutic systems share the goals of maintenance of joint range, prevention of contractures, normalization of tone, improvement in interaction with the environment, postural control, assumption of antigravity postures, development of muscular control and coordination, and education of the family (Deaver, 1956; Kottke, Halpern, Easton, Ozel, & Burrill, 1978). Many systems are axiomatic, being based on the concept of neuroplasticity in the child, avoidance of abnormal movement patterns, and the importance of sensorimotor learning in cognitive development (Matthews, 1988). Controlled studies are difficult to design, as parents are unwilling to assign their child to a nontreatment group (Guyatt et al., 1986; Martin & Epstein, 1976; Tirosh & Rabino, 1989). It has also been problematic to document the clinical effectiveness of early intervention programs, but there is a strong sense of the clinical effectiveness of such treatment (Palmer et al., 1990; Resnick, Eyler, Nelson, Eitman, & Bucciarelli, 1987; Spittle, Orton, Anderson, Boyd, & Doyle, 2015). Meta-analyses of such interventions have revealed that when services were initiated in at-risk infants prior to 6 months of age, an improvement of 9 to 13 points in IQ testing results. The developmental stimulation, rather than physical therapy alone, may be responsible for enhancement of gross motor and cognitive skills (Palmer, Shapiro, & Wachtel, 1988). This is a rationale offered by proponents of the system of conductive education (Hill, 1990). Systems have been proposed by Rood, Knott and Voss, Brunstrom, Temple Fay, and Dolman-Delacato (patterning; Halpern, 1984), but the Bobath type of treatment generally prevailed in this setting, although motor learning theory may recently be preempting this type of intervention. According to Bobath principles, by placing the affected child in a position in which the effects of abnormal tone and postures are deemphasized, voluntary muscular control may develop, in a proximal-to-distal fashion, paving the way for more functional activities, and the use of the upper extremities for something other than support (Finnie, 1974). Secondary reductions in tone may result in improvement in oromotor control, feeding, speech, and respiration (Nwaobi & Smith, 1986). Motor learning treatment is a more task-directed application where the child learns by limb placement and repetition of the motor tasks required (Tscharnuter, 2002; Valvano, 2004).

Other systems have been developed to deal with the visual–manual and spatial learning difficulties that may coexist (Bachrach & Greenspun, 1990). Additional options include training the patient in age-appropriate self-care skills and behavior modifications.

The weakness noted in the muscles of patients with cerebral palsy is a recently described entity. It is felt to be multifactorial in its etiology possibly due to sarcopenia or decreased muscle mass in premature infants, abnormal neural maturation, disorganized neuronal recruitment patterns, impaired reciprocal inhibition, and reduced elasticity among other factors (Mockford & Caulton, 2010). This may also have an implication for the development of cardiorespiratory fitness rather than being attributed to disuse alone (Butler, Scianni, & Ada, 2010). Traditionally, strengthening programs were felt to be contraindicated in spastic conditions such as cerebral palsy, as such efforts were thought to reenforce the patterns of spasticity that already existed. However, newer studies do not support this notion. Strengthening has been documented as resulting in improvement of hip and knee strength, gait pattern marked by a reduction in crouching and better control of walking speed, and in Gross Motor Functional Measurement (GMFM) ratings (Andersson, Grooten, Hellsten, Kaping, & Mattson, 2003). Similar efficacy has also been recently demonstrated for upper extremity function with use of an arm cranking device (Unnithan et al., 2007).

Efficacy not only exists for younger patients, but teenagers and even patients in the fifth decade of age have shown demonstrable improvements without negative effects or increases in Ashworth scores (a spasticity measurement scale; Damiano, Kelly, & Vaughn, 1995; Damiano, Vaughn, & Abel, 1995). Therefore, neurological maturation or cessation of growth is not a contraindication to efficacy of services. However, most adults with cerebral palsy need to be educated on maintaining their own physical regimen to maintain both endurance and range of motion while preventing pain (Gorter, Holty, Rameckers, Hans, & Rob, 2009), with more formal therapeutic interventions indicated in response to a more generalized change in their physical status, injury, or surgical intervention.

Abstracted from the experience with adult patients with hemiplegia who have had strokes, constraint-induced movement therapy has been used in children with hemiplegia, with documented improvement (Pierce, Daly, Gallaghger, Gershkoff, & Schaumburg, 2002). However, it is advisable that children selected for such treatment be able to perceive that these efforts are not punative. Recently, more efficacy has been ascribed to bimanual upper extremity training in patients with hemiplegia (Facchin et al., 2011).

Although there are clinical proponents, the efficacy of other treatments, such as hyperbaric oxygenation, use of the Adeli suit for proximal stabilization (Bar-Haim et al., 2006), craniosacral therapy, massage, acupuncture and acupressure, hippotherapy, and aquatherapy, has not been scientifically substantiated (Fragala-Pinkham, Dumas, Barlow, & Pasternak, 2009; Hurvitz, Leonard, Ayyangar, & Nelson, 2003). Parental perceptions of improvement may not be in accordance with more objectifying measures (Duncan, Barton, Edmonds, & Blashill, 2004).

Although considered a type of passive exercise, pediatric supported standing programs have been utilized with positive results when used in a 5-day-per-week program; benefits have been documented for bone mineral density, hip stability, range at hips, knees, ankles, and modulation of abnormal tone (spasticity; Paleg, Smith, & Glickman, 2013).

Body weight–supported treadmill training is more recently utilized. This intervention has been demonstrated as improving patients' walking speed and gait kinematics without a negative effect on baseline spasticity (Chrysagis, Skorilis, Stavrov, Grammatopoulou, & Kootsouki, 2012). It may work centrally by reducing corucal processing demands of children with cerebral palsy (Kurz, Wilson, Corr, & Volkman, 2012).

Despite multiple studies, the optimal frequency and intensity of therapy to be provided to the child with cerebral palsy has not been determined. However, studies suggest that intensive therapy provided three times or more per week may have a modest effect in improving gross motor performances, especially in children of about 2 years of age (Arpino, Vescio, DeLuca, & Curatolo, 2010).

A variety of modalities, including shaking and cold, are believed to exert effects at the level of the vestibular receptors, muscle spindles, and the Golgi tendon apparatus. Heat is relatively contraindicated, especially in a nonverbal population who cannot express discomfort. Nerve and motor point blocks and biofeedback have also been used (Halpern, 1982; Kassover, Tauber, Au, & Pugh, 1986). Nerve blocks in contrast to motor point blocks not only resulted in weakness, but concurrent and undesirable sensory deficits/dysesthesias and are therefore used less frequently.

Botulinum A toxin, derived from denatured clostridium, injected into the muscles of patients with cerebral palsy has been shown to transiently reduce spasticity for a period of about 4 months by decreasing acetylcholine release at motor nerve endings, thereby blocking neuromuscular transmission in a controlled fashion. This temporary reduction in tone may permit reduction of dynamic deformities, such as talipes equinus by reducing tone in spastic gastrocnemius muscles, knee flexion contractures by injection into the hamstrings, and reduction in scissoring following injection into hip adductors. Strengthening of agonist muscle groups also assists in improvement of gait and function. Improvement in gait and posture, reduction in oxygen consumption (Balaban, Tok, Tan, & Mathews, 2012), pain management, and facilitation of care have also been documented (Strobi et al., 2015). Three different types of preparations are available, each with different dosage recommendations. Experience in the use of botulinum toxin in patients less than 2 years of age is limited (Bakheit, 2010) and is not yet approved (Druschel, Althuizes, Funk, & Placezek, 2013).

Both upper and lower extremity muscles may be treated. The treatment has the advantage of specifically targeting certain areas, rather than globally reducing tone so that loss of trunk and proximal control are much less of a concern. Tendon-lengthening procedures may be deferred on this basis until the patient is older, but it is uncertain if such interventions will reduce the total number of surgical interventions that the patient will eventually require (Korman, Mooney, Smith, Goodman, & Mulvaney, 1993). However, studies in animal models suggest that when given early in development, it may promote growth of muscles, altering the development of contractures (Cosgrove & Graham, 1994). Other studies suggest that injection of botulinum toxin in conjunction with serial casting of lower extremity deformities may approach the results obtained from percutaneous tendon lengthenings (Glantzman, Kim, Swaminathan, & Beck, 2004; Hayek, Gershon Weintroub, & Yizhar, 2010) or selective dorsal rhizotomy (see subsequently), although the number of injection sites (Satila et al., 2008) and protocols vary widely, making analysis of results difficult (Kelly, MacKay-Lyons, Berryman, Hyndman, & Wood, 2008; Molenaers, Desloovere, & DeCat, 2001). The advantages of this treatment are the relative ease of administration, although younger children may require sedation when deeper muscles are injected, and development of usually only mild side effects, which include local soreness to muscles and generalized transient myalgias. More serious, but infrequent, side effects include an association with aspiration pneumonia in patients with pseudobulbar palsy and spastic quadriparesis, global muscle weakness and atrophy (Ansved, Odergren, & Borg, 1997), urinary and fecal incontinence, development of antibodies not associated with clinical disease (Goschel, Wohlfarth, Frevert, Dengler, & Bigalke, 1997), possible potentiation of weakness seen with aminoglycoside antibiotics and depolarizing agents, and acute allergic reactions (Preiss, Condie, Rowley, & Graham, 2003).

Botulinum toxin injections have also been utilized to control drooling in pediatric patients by injecting into the salivary glands.

Oral medications, including diazepam, dantrolene sodium, baclofen, and tizanidine, can be tried to reduce tone. Although these may be effective, diazepam has central, sedative effects, is habit forming, and is relatively undesirable in patients who may already have cognitive limitations. It has, however, been reported to decrease tone and improve lower extremity range and spontaneous movements without daytime drowsiness in children with cerebral palsy (Mathew, Mathew, Thomas, & Antonisamy, 2005). Dantrolene, which reduces tone by modulating calcium regulation into muscles, is metabolized by the liver, and thus is not a good option for children who may be concurrently prescribed anticonvulsant medications, which are also metabolized by the same route, potentially placing a child at risk for hepatic dysfunction (Zarfonte, Lornard, & Elovic, 2004). Baclofen may also have a sedative effect when used orally and can result in constipation in a population already predisposed to this problem. Tizanidine is a newer drug that works on alpha-adrenergic nerve endings; it is similar to an antihypertensive medication from which it is derived, and therefore, blood pressure needs to be monitored carefully with its introduction. Reduction of nocturnal spasms in children with spastic quadriparesis has been reported with its use (Tanaka et al., 2004).

Appropriate prescription of seating devices for nonambulatory patients permits positioning in an upright manner, improved eye contact, enhanced interaction with the environment, decreased effect of hypertonicity (which pushes the patient out of the chair and adducts the hips), and enhanced feeding, respiration, and ability to use communication devices (Bergen & Colangelo, 1982). Power wheelchairs have been prescribed as early as 14 months of age. Despite concerns that mobility would decrease and the child would become more dependent, the reverse had been demonstrated. Patients' communication scores and their Pediatric Evaluation of Disability Inventory (PEDI) functional skills improved significantly (Jones, McEwen, & Neas, 2012).

Orthotics are prescribed to prevent progression of deformities, provide stability, and enhance function. Traditional leather and metal braces have given way to custom-molded plastic orthoses that are lighter and that more easily control angular (varus/valgus) deformities. Full control, hip-knee-ankle-foot orthoses are generally used for positioning, but are too heavy for functional ambulation. Variations of these devices exclude the medial metal uprights and thigh cuffs and may be helpful for children with toe walking and dynamic internal rotation at the hips. Ankle-foot orthoses are indicated to improve ankle dorsiflexion and control equinus deformities. Spring-assisted devices are generally contraindicated as rapid stretch may exacerbate spasticity. Orthoses used to maintain muscle length must be worn for at least 6 hours per day to achieve a physiological effect (Tardieu & Lespargot, 1988). The use of tone-reducing orthoses with full footplates and the toes maintained in extension (Bronkhorst & Lamb, 1987; Hinderer & Harris, 1988) may have a direct effect on muscle ultrastructure with resultant increase in sarcomere (muscle unit) length (Tardieu, de la Tour, Bret, & Tardieu, 1982). It is important to discuss these findings with parents/guardians, so that compliance with the recommended wearing schedule is achieved. Ankle-foot orthoses may have hinges incorporated at the ankles to allow for active ankle dorsiflexion and to facilitate movements from sitting to standing (Wilson, Haideri, Song, & Telford, 1997). Orthoses that extend to just above the ankles (supramalleolar orthoses) can control foot alignment, but do not control the ankle joints (Carlson, Vaughan, Damiano, & Abel, 1997). The long-term effect of orthoses in reducing deformity and need for subsequent surgical intervention is controversial (Crenshaw et al., 2000; Sankey, Anderson, & Young, 1989).

Night splints may also be utilized to prevent progression of equinus deformities but do not have the functional advantage in gait that day splints demonstrate with improvement of GMFM scores (Zhao, Xiao, Li & Du, 2013).

Total contact splinting and use of serial casting are other orthotic options that can be considered for tone reduction and improvement in range. Neoprene garments to improve sensory feedback and proximal stability have also recently been used. There have been some preliminary reports of reduction of peripheral tone and improved quality of gait pattern with their use (Siracusa, Taylor, Geletka, & Overby, 2005).

For maximally involved children, the use of a walking frame with casters provides trunk alignment and support, in conjunction with hip-knee-ankle orthoses. Although functional ambulation is not possible with such devices, their utilization permits tolerance of the upright posture, increased weight bearing, and a sense of movement for the child, which may be psychologically rewarding (Stallard, Major, & Farmer, 1996). Similarly, body weight–supported treadmill training has been explored as a means of enhancing reciprocal stepping patterns as a preliminary activity to prepare for ambulation (Dieruf et al., 2009; Eisenberg, Zuk, Carmeli, & Katz-Leuer, 2009).

Recently, treadmill treatment combined with transcranial stimulation had demonstrated better stability, increased cadence step length, step width, and gait velocity with support (Grecco, Mendonca, Duarte, Zsinon, & Olivelra, 2014).

Threshold electrical stimulation can be utilized as an adjunct to traditional therapeutic interventions. Low-intensity transcutaneous stimulation can be applied to a variety of weak, superficial muscles, nocturnally. Theoretically, the resultant increase in blood flow to these muscles at a time when growth hormone levels are highest encourages their growth. This permits the traditional strengthening efforts applied during the day to be more effective. Improvement in gait (enhanced tibialis anterior function, better balance, and improved gait pattern) has been demonstrated in a few studies (Hazlewood, Brown, Rowe, & Salter, 1994; Pape et al., 1993; Seifart, Unger, & Burger, 2009). However, the long-term effect of this treatment and any possible associated reduction in the subsequent need for surgical intervention have not yet been demonstrated.

Use of electronic stimulation incorporated as an assistance in daily ambulation has demonstrated improvement in ankle range, selective motor control and strength, and reduction in spasticity, toe drag, and falls (Pool, Blackmore, Bear, & Valentine, 2014), and increases cross-sectional areas of both agonist and antagonist muscles (Karabay et al., 2015). Lastly, the use of virtual reality–associated activities and robot-assisted devices, especially for a paretic upper extremity, show promise as therapeutic interventions (Fasoli, Ladenheim, Mast, & Krebs, 2012).

Given the multiple potential interventions and confounding clinical variables that exist, truly objective research design is extremely difficult. The use of standardized testing and functional scales may serve as an adjunct in such studies, permitting the patient to be compared to his or her own pretreatment performance. Such measurement tools include measurement of torque/resistance to passive stretch as an indicator of spasticity, the GMFM (Wei et al., 2006), the Wee-FIM (Functional Independence Measure for Children; Sanders et al., 2006), the PEDI (Hayley, Ludlow, & Coster, 1993), and the Ashworth scale for clinically reproducible measurement of spasticity (Clopton et al., 2005).

Surgical Options

Prevention of deformities resulting from inequalities in muscle tone and strength in association with fixed posturing due to the influence of retained positive primitive reflexes is the best treatment option; however, orthopedic surgery should not be perceived as a failure of previous treatment, but rather as an adjunct to achievement of therapeutic goals. The muscles of spastic patients with cerebral palsy are too short, with chronic increases in tone possibly resulting in reduced sarcomere length and abnormal connectin protein (Graham & Selber, 2003). With inability of the muscles to relax, imbalances occur between the growth of the long bones and the muscle tendons resulting in secondary structural deformities (Ziv, Blackborn, Rang, & Koresk, 1984). Subluxation and early-onset osteoarthritis with regression in function, not associated with an actual decline in neurological status, may occur. Hence, early and efficient surgical interventions are warranted (Frieden & Lieber, 2003) and may permit less invasive soft tissue rather than bony surgery (osteotomies) to be performed. Conversely, early tendon releases may initially interfere with acquisition of motor milestones and mobility, and may increase the need for repeat surgery as the child grows. Psychological support services to both parents and child to cope with fears and expectations are most important. At least 6 months of extensive postoperative physical rehabilitation may be required to see signs of functional improvement because of transient deconditioning (Reimers, 1990), with reduction of muscle strength and readjustment of the body to a new muscle length–tension ratio. The separation of the parent from the child and the financial burdens encountered are other factors to be considered.

A full discussion of the orthopedic deformities and their surgical treatment may be found in several excellent texts (Herring, 2013; Staheli, 2015). Common lower extremity deformities include hip flexion contractures, femoral anteversion with medial rotation of the legs, hip adduction with subluxation, pelvic asymmetry with secondary scoliosis, hamstring spasticity with kyphosis and knee flexion contractures, and equinovarus or equinvalgus deformities, with hemiplegia and diplegia, respectively. Typical upper extremity deformities include internal rotation contractures of the shoulders, flexion contractures at the elbows, wrist flexion contractures, ulnar deviation, finger flexion contractures, and thumb-in-palm deformities. For dependent patients, surgery may be performed to facilitate perineal care, reduce pain association with dislocation, and correct pelvic asymmetry that may exacerbate scoliosis and reduce supported sitting tolerance (Carr & Gage, 1987; Cooperman, Bartucci, Dietrick, & Miller, 1987). For children with better gross motor function, surgery is indicated to improve lower extremity alignment and correct a progressively crouched gait, scissoring, and other gait abnormalities that result in poor balance and easy fatigability due to excessive energy expenditure.

Procedures include adductor tenotomies and varus derotation osteotomies of the femurs. Previously, these patients were confined in extensive plaster casts postoperatively, but this is now less commonly used, resulting in fewer cases of secondary skin breakdown, and earlier mobilization, weight bearing, and rehabilitation without an increased rate of complication (Schaefer, McCarthy, & Josephic, 2007). Hamstring lengthenings are performed to correct knee flexion contractures, avoiding overlengthening, which could result in hyperextension at the knees (Gage, 1990) that would require another procedure (rectus femoris transfer) to be performed. Achilles tendon lengthenings are the most commonly performed procedure; with correction of the equinus deformity, toe walking is corrected, a stable base of support on a flat foot is established, and walking speed and stride length are increased (Shapiro & Susa, 1990). A posterior tibialis tendon transfer may be indicated to correct equinovarus and to elevate the foot when walking. For more resistant deformities at the foot, an extra-articular (Grice) procedure or other arthrodesis may be required (Fulford, 1990). Computerized gait analysis may be utilized to assess surgical indications and outcomes (Narayanan, 2007). The techniques of the lower extremity surgical procedures have not changed considerably in the recent past, but surgeries are more frequently performed at multiple levels at the same time to reduce both anesthetic exposures and rehabilitation admissions, while maximizing functional correction (Graham & Harvey, 2007). With growth, there may be a recurrence of deformities necessitating reoperation with an overall recurrence rate of about 10% to 15% per level.

Computerized gait analysis may facilitate this decision-making process (Thomason, Rodda, Sangvex, Seiber, & Kerr, 2012) and prevent the development of a progressive crouch gait (Vuillermin et al., 2011).

Bony procedures around the hips are associated with the development of heterotopic ossification (bone growth outside of skeletal tissue) in about 25% of cases, and the hardware usually needs to be removed after 1 year to prevent stress fractures and pain.

Surgery for the upper extremities is performed less frequently, as improved outcomes may be limited by cognitive and sensory impairments and may exceed the benfit of Botox and/or occupational therapy (VanHeest, Bagley, Molitard, & James, 2015). Procedures include release of the internal rotators of the shoulder, release of the biceps tendon and anterior capsulotomy to correct elbow flexion contractures, transfer of wrist flexors to function as wrist extensors, and release of the thumb-in-palm deformity (Mital & Sakellarides, 1981). Spinal fusion may be required to control scoliosis. Luque and other newer, segmental spinal instrumentations permit some patients to forego prolonged immobilization in a body jacket (Lonstein & Akbamia, 1983).

Neurosurgical procedures to restore function and to control associated intractable seizures by resection of localized focus of electrical abnormalities are newer adjuncts in the care of the patient with cerebral palsiy. Implantation of a cerebellar pacemaker had been utilized in the past for tone modulation, but is not currently used in any large numbers (Penn, Mykleburst, Gottlieb, Agarwal, & Etzel, 1980).

The selective dorsal rhizotomy procedure to decrease lower extremity tone and to secondarily permit for development of isolated lower extremity tone and improvement in gait has been utilized for almost 30 years. Spinal nerve rootlets that have been determined as being electrically abnormal are surgically lesioned in children who are purely spastic without clinical evidence of a progressive neurological disorder. With modulation of abnormal sensory input, there is a resetting of muscle spindle sensitivity with a reduction in tone. Electromyographic monitoring is used intraoperatively to assess which of the spastic rootlets should be lesioned, although responses may be less consistent than previously thought. In conjunction with a well-delineated postoperative program, improvements in tone, range, posture, sitting balance, and gait occurs in 85% to 90% of appropriately selected candidates (Abbott, Johann-Murphy, & Gold, 1991; Peacock & Staudt, 1991) to a greater extent than would be anticipated on the basis of physical therapy intervention alone (Steinbok, Reiner, Beauchamp, Armstrong, & Cochrane, 1997). Improvement in gait is characterized by increased dynamic range-of-motion at the hips, improved velocity of ambulation, and improved stride length (Thomas, Aiona, Pierce, & Piatt, 1996). Over time, this may result in a decreased need for Achilles tendon lengthenings, adductor releases, and hamstring releases, and may not affect the subsequent rates of ankle-foot operations, femoral osteotomies (Silva et al., 2012), and iliopsoas releases in these patients (Chicoine, Park, & Kaufman, 1997). An improvement of 12.1 versus 4.4 points in children treated with physical therapy alone has been documented on the GMFM at 6 to 12 months postoperatively. Although not a specific indication for performance of the procedure, secondary improvements in upper extremity function and reduction in bladder spasticity may also result (Sweetser, Badell, Schneider, & Badlin, 1995). Energy efficiency is improved in over one half of the patients. Recurrence of spasticity and deterioration of gait with adolescence is prevented in a majority of cases (Dudley et al., 2013; Nordmark et al., 2008). Complications may include dysesthesias, sensory deficits, and, on long-term follow-up, spinal stenosis (Gooch & Walker, 1996). Despite the documented improvements, 66% to 75% of patients undergoing rhizotomy will still require additional orthopedic surgery.

Rhizotomy, when compared to ITBP, provided a greater reduction in tone and improvement in gross motor function (Kan et al., 2008) although it is generally utilized for patietns with GMFCS scale of III or less.

The effect of anoxia on the spinal cord has been described (Clancy, Sladsky, & Rorke, 1989; Harrison, 1988), thus lending credence to the use of baclofen (Young & Delwaide, 1981). Baclofen is a derivative of the inhibitory neurotransmitter gamma-aminobutyric acid, which inhibits excitatory neurotransmission in the brain and spinal cord. This results in secondary inhibition of excitatory neurotransmitters and reduces muscle tone. This medication may also be administered intrathecally (Albright, Cervi, & Singletary, 1991), via a surgically implantable and programmable pump, allowing for titration and reversal of dosage with reduced risk of medication-induced side effects (Albright, 1996). The implementation of this treatment is more suitable in patients with less satisfactory underlying strength, which may require some spasticity for antigravity/ambulatory activities, and in older patients. Documented benefits in hamstring motion, upper extremity function, ambulation (Gertszten, 1997), and activities of daily living (ADL) have been associated with this treatment (Albright, Barron, Fasisck, Polinko, & Janosky, 1993), and possibly a reduction in the need for subsequent orthopedic surgical interventions from 58% to 21% in one population studied (Armstrong, Steinbok, & Cochrane, 1997). It may be implanted even when there is anticipated need for subsequent posterior spinal fusion for scoliosis treatment (Borowski, Shah, Littleton, Dabney, & Miller, 2008). Complications of this device include long-term reliance upon the device with need for approximately monthly refills of the reservoir in which the medication is housed, risk of catheter breakage and infection, risk of acute baclofen withdrawal if the pump is not refilled on a timely and regular basis or because of pump failure, risk of exacerbation of seizure disorders, loss of ability to assume and maintain antigravity positions, and possibly an increased risk of aspiration pneumonia when utilized in the most physically involved patients (Borowski et al., 2010; Sgoros & Seri, 2002). Selective dorsal rhizotomy, which reduces tone by surgical lesioning of sensory input at the spinal cord level (Fasano, Barolat-Romana, Zeme, & Squazzi, 1979), may also be utilized to this goal, as detailed earlier, and does not require ongoing services and pump replacement.

Psychological, Vocational, and Medical Problems of Adults

Therapeutic services may enhance acquisition of gross motor skills, but cognitive improvement and emotional maturity are more elusive to treat. The severity of the physical disability does not correlate with the physical or psychological health of the parents (Wallender, Babani, Varni, Banis, & Wilcox, 1989). Sibling and spousal support are pertinent predictors of achieving mental health and improvement in physical performance (Craft, Lakin, Oppliger, Clancy, & Vanderlinder, 1990). Despite similar interest and enjoyment in extracurricular activities as their typically developing peers, activities are significantly limited in children with cerebral palsy (Engel-Yeter, Jarus, Anaby, & Law, 2009). Lives of 50% to 90% of adolescents with cerebral palsy (and spina bifida) may be characterized by dependence on parents for personal care, lack of responsibility for home chores, lack of information about sexuality, and limited participation in social activities and sexual relationships (Blum, Resnick, Nelson, & St. Germaine, 1991; Hirtz, 1989; Murphy, Molnar, & Lankasky, 2000). This does not encourage independent living, marriage, or employment. In one optimistic study, up to 68% of adults with cerebral palsy were able to live independently (Michelsen, Uldall, Hansen, & Madsen, 2006). Only 30% to 50% of patients with cerebral palsy are employed full-time at maturity; patients with diplegia and hemiplegia are more successful (Bleck, 1987; Michelsen, Uldall, Mette, & Madsen, 2005). Other positive factors relating to employability include independence in ADL, ability to ambulate, being female, and enrollment in a nonrestrictive high school setting (Magill-Evans & Restall, 1991; Sillanpaa, Piekkala, & Pisira, 1982; Tobimatsu & Nakamura, 2000). Therefore, it is important to assess the ability of adult patients to perform instrumental ADL, which include money management, travel training, and meal planning (van der Dussen, Nieuwstraten, Roebroeck, & Stam, 2001).

Transition to adulthood for patients with cerebral palsy and those with other chronic diseases of childhood is extremely difficult as services are lacking and physicians treating adult patients may be unfamiliar with their disorders. This is a happy situation for which planning had not occurred, as 90% of patients with cerebral palsy will now live into adulthood. Education of both patients to familiarize themselves with the details of their history and to learn advocacy skills when parents are no longer able to provide these services may take years to learn (Donkervoort, Wiegerink, van Meeteren, Stam, & Roebroeck, 2009; Young, 2007).

It has not been established what therapeutic services are necessary for adult patients with cerebral palsy to maintain their function. It is sobering to acknowledge that deterioration in gait in the presence of a static encephalopathy may begin prior to 14 years of age, and is manifested by an increase in double-support time and a decrease in knee, ankle, and pelvic motion (Johnson, Damiano, & Abel, 1997). Because of this deterioration, only 20% of adult patients with cerebral palsy will be independent ambulators, 40% will ambulate with assistance, and 40% will be nonambulatory, although 75% of these patients will retain their independence in ADL (Andersson & Mattson, 2001; Brown, Bontempo, & Turk, 1992). Medical complications in an aging population (Bachrach & Greenspun, 1990) include cervical and lumbar radiculopathies (Ebara et al., 1990; Reese, Msall, & Owens, 1991), carpal tunnel syndrome (Alvarez, Larkin, & Roxborough, 1981), and arthritis at major joints, each of which may require surgical intervention for restoration of function. Specifically, cervical disc disease is eight times more frequent in the adult patient with athetoid cerebal palsy than in the general patient (Harade et al., 1996). There is an overall 63% incidence of degenerative arthritis, especially at the hips, in patients with cerebral palsy younger than 50 years (Bajelidze, Beithur, Littlerton, Dabney, & Miller, 2008). Chronic pain may occur in up to 84% of the adult population, which may require direct and indirect management, including treatment of increased spasticity (Engel, Kartin, & Jensen, 2002; Turk, Scandale, Rosenbaum, & Weber, 2001). Seizure disorders persist into adulthood. Neurogenic bladder and unrecognized problems with toileting accessibility may also be problematic. Referral sources for provision of gynecologic care, especially in provision of mammograms to nonambulatory patients, may be sorely lacking. Little in the way of organized and proactive treatment is available for this population (Murphy, Molnar, & Lankasky, 1995). As activity decreases, there may be a greater mortality in this population owing to ischemic heart disease, compounded by difficulty with communication and lack of family supervision once placement options have been sought (Strauss, Cable, & Shavelte, 1999), and an increased incidence of deep vein thromboses also related to inactivity (Rapp & Torres, 2000).

Despite potential complications, 90% survival into adulthood is seen with cerebral palsy (Day, Reynolds, & Kush, 2015; Evans, Evans, & Alberman, 1990). Earlier demise occurs in patients who have severe mental deficiency, are totally dependent, have poorly controlled seizures, require gastrostomy feeding, have no means of communication, and whose secondary illnesses are primarily respiratory in nature (Evans & Alberman, 1990; Maudsley, Hultor, & Pharoah, 1999). Recently, the poor prognostic implication of gastrostomy tube placement has come under review, and does not appear to auger quite the dire prognosis as when placed in the elderly. One study indicated that 83% of the pediatric population in whom gastrostomy placement occurs survive 2 years, 75% survive 7 years, and there is family satisfaction with quality of life in 90% (Smith, Camfield, & Camfield, 1999). There have been some studies to suggest that an increased susceptibility to infection exists not only on a neuromuscular basis, but on a biological basis as well. Some patients have been noted to have fewer soluble interleukin-2 receptors and lymphocyte proliferative and lytic responses, resulting in reduced resistance to an infectious agent. Demise is often coincident with the "aging-out" of parents and relocation from the home to an institutional facility (Eyman & Grossman, 1990). These findings should prompt the reexamination of public policies for provision of medical benefits to handicapped adults whose parents wish them to retain the family domicile and other financial assets that would permit home-based care.

SPINA BIFIDA

Spina bifida, or myelomeningocele, denotes a condition in which there are congenital abnormalities of the vertebral elements in association with extrusion of abnormally formed neural elements. Patients present with various degrees of lower-extremity motor and sensory deficits concomitant with variable bowel and bladder control, hydrocephalus, and other medical problems. The resultant condition impinges on normal motor development and may alter fine motor, perceptual, linguistic, and cognitive function. A discussion of treatment strategies reflects not only technical advancements but also the changes in the advocacy for the treatment of the physically challenged child. This is a congenital but not a static disorder, in which progressive neurological dysfunctions may occur over time in up to 40% of patients (Spindel, Bauer, & Dryon, 1987).

Anatomical Abnormalities

Failure of fusion of the posterior elements of the lumbosacral spine without associated neurological abnormalities is known as spina bifida occulta and occurs in 20% to 25% of the general population (without overt or open spina bifida). Should such findings be noted in a patient with incontinence, cavus (high-arched) feet, and/or hairy tuft or hemangioma over the lower spine, an associated malformation of the spinal cord may be present, which can readily be documented on an MRI study. A terminal myelocystocele is a closed defect that presents with a lumbosacral fat-containing mass comprised of cerebrospinal fluid and neural tissue, which will require surgical intervention. It may be associated with abnormal development of the lower spine, genitalia, bowel, bladder, kidneys, and opening of the abdominal wall, such as an omphalocele. It is not generally associated with hydrocephalus. Ambulatory compromise may require interventions similar to those in the more typical form of spinal dysraphism (Choi & McComb, 2000).

In the most severe of open spina bifida, there are abnormally formed neural elements with cystic structures within the spinal cord. Patients present with findings of both upper and lower motor neuron dysfunction, such as weakness, spasticity, and low tone. Defects at the lumbosacral level are the most common; thoracic and cervical lesions occur less frequently. Because of the resultant lack of normal innervation, varying degrees of paralysis of the lower extremities occur, and there are secondary and often severe orthopedic deformities that occur due to the imbalance of muscular forces. Such congenital problems include kyphosis, hemivertebrae, teratologic hip dislocation, clubfoot, and vertical talus (Chambers, 2014).

The Lorber Criteria and Their Abandonment

In the past, severely deformed infants with myelomeningocele died, without treatment, from meningitis, hydrocephalus, and/or renal failure because of the desire not to prolong the lives of children who were cognitively subnormal, nonambulatory, and chronically ill. The mortality rate within the first month of life was 63% and 89% by the sixth month. Lorber (1971) advised no treatment for those infants who would be totally plegic in the lower extremities, had severe hydrocephalus, had severe kyphoscoliosis that would not permit an erect posture, and/or had severe congenital malformations such as exstrophy of the bladder or congenital heart disease. He felt that only 18% of the population would be ambulatory, cognitively normal, and able to earn an income. The initial study did not recognize that the survivors would be more compromised than necessary (McLaughlin & Shurtleff, 1979), or that there was an inability to predict which of the cognitively normal patients would be sacrificed by the lack of treatment. Adoption of these criteria implied that a life in a wheelchair was one without quality. These and other assumptions have recently proved invalid with more advanced treatments, as noted subsequently (Khoury, Erickson, & James, 1982; McClone, Dias, Kaplan, & Sommers, 1985).

Neurosurgery in the neonate to drain the collection of excessive cerebrospinal fluid associated with hydrocephalus can result in restoration of a relatively normal head circumference and reexpansion of the cerebral mantle. With appropriate treatment, a 5-year survival rate of 86% has been reported; however, patients with brainstem dysfunction had a greater mortality (Worley, Schuster, & Oakes, 1996). The severe gibbus deformity (sharply angulated toward flexion of the spine) associated with kyphoscoliosis may be surgically corrected (Lintner & Lindseth, 1994), as may other congenital anomalies. Mental retardation is not intrinsic to spina bifida or to the Arnold–Chiari malformation, which results in hydrocephalus. Up to 75% of patients with spina bifida manifesta have normal intelligence (McClone, Czyzewski, Raimondi, & Somers, 1985), but the incidence of learning disabilities will be high, with arithmetic and design copying skills frequently being compromised (Wills, Holmbeck, Dillon, & McClone, 1990). Functional bowel and bladder continence may ideally be achieved in 80% of school-aged children. Eighty percent of school-aged children will be community ambulators. Only 10% to 15% of patients will require supportive care as adults. The emotional and psychological costs for delaying treatment are high. Hence, early and aggressive treatment of these infants is now the rule.

Incidence, Embryology, and Etiology

The incidence of spina bifida manifesta in the United States is approximately two cases per 10,000 births, which represents a decline of more than 27% to 50% over the past decades (Lary & Edmonds, 1996; Meyer & Siega-Riz, 2002; Timbolschi et al., 2015). This is largely attributable to the supplementation of grain products, such as cereal, with folic acid for women of child-bearing age. The decline has been greatest in mothers older than 30 years, those who have had a high school education, whose medical care was not Medicaid funded, and who were non-Hispanic Caucasians.

Although folic acid supplementation and possibly vitamin B_{12} plays a role in prevention, the etiology for neural tube defects is likely multifactorial, including a genetic basis. The undefined insult to the embryo occurs at 21 to 26 days of gestation, when the neural tube that will become the central nervous system is invaginating. Early theories suggested that there was a failure of fusion or disruption of the tissue columns caused by abnormalities in the cerebral spinal fluid pressure (Streeter, 1942). More recently, studies from animal models have revealed a group of developmental genes, termed homeobox genes, which direct the segmental development of the nervous system. In mammals, the Hox genes have been demonstrated to encode positions from the top of the brain to the lower spinal cord. Another similar group of genes has been described as assisting in differentiation of the ventral from the dorsal spinal cord. Mechanisms that damage gene function may affect the process of nervous system development, resulting in myelomeningocele and the related Chiari II malformation responsible for hydrocephalus; clinically, this may explain the mechanism in at least 15% of patients with spina bifida (McClone, 1998). Other genes that may be associated with myelomeningocele include the glucose transporter 3 (*GLUT 3*) gene (Connealy, Northrup, & Au, 2014), *PAX 5* and *T*, and *FZD3* genes (Shangguan et al., 2015).

The incidence of neural tube defects can be reduced by up to 86% by the intake of 0.4 mg/day folic acid in the periconceptual period. Decreased folate and increased total homocystiene levels have been documented in the mothers of such patients. This metabolically may result in a decrease in methionine formation, which results in abnormal gene transcription and impairment of neural tube differential and closure (Botto & Yang, 2000; Veland, Hosted, Schneede, Refsum, & Vollset, 2001).

Control of obesity (maternal weight less than 31 kg/m^2) prior to conception may play a role in this and other congenital anomalies, which does not appear to be directly related to dietary deficiencies (Stothard, Tennant, Bell, & Rankin, 2009). Other factors that have been implicated include maternal hyperthermia, other dietary deficiencies, use of valproate by epileptic women during pregnancy, and presence of certain chronic maternal diseases, such as diabetes (Khoury et al., 1982; Leck, 1974; Padmanabhan, 2006). There is a 5% risk of recurrence of another infant with spina bifida with subsequent pregnancies, and in all patients with spina bifida who produce offspring.

Prenatal diagnosis can be made by ultrasound (Robinson, Hood, Adam Gibson, & Ferguson-Smith, 1980). Prenatal anatomical levels as determined on high-resolution ultrasound can be reliably utilized to discuss functional motor outcome with the parents (Coniglio, Anderson, & Ferguson, 1996). Diagnosis can be further supported by documentation of posterior fossa changes in association with the Chiari malformation (Qin et al., 2014). Analysis of amniotic fluid and/or maternal serum for elevated alpha-fetoprotein, a substance that is liberated by fetal blood vessels of the uncovered neural elements, is also indicative of the disorder. Analyses are performed in the second trimester so that termination of pregnancy, if desired, is possible. False-positive results may occur in association with gastrointestinal malformations (Milunsky & Alpert, 1976a, 1976b). Anencephaly and skin-covered lesions cannot be identified by chemical analysis, so ultrasound is very important. These tests were not consistently performed in pregnancy so that in previous decades, the majority of cases were not diagnosed in utero. Of all neural tube defects so identified, 39.9% result in termination of pregnancy. For those pregnancies that go to completion, a cesarian section is indicated in fetuses with functional lower-extremity movements to lessen the risk of trauma to the exposed neural elements and hydrocephalus head.

Antenatal and Neonatal Treatment

In utero repair of myelomeningocele is a more contemporary option for attempting to reduce subsequent neurological dysfunction. Interposition of latissimus dorsi flaps over the neurological lesion or other techniques may prevent further in utero damage to the spinal cord and nerve roots, or damage that occurs at the time of delivery, hence improving lower extremity motor function (Meuli et al., 1997; Meuli-Simmen, Meuli, Adzick, & Harrison, 1997; Moldenhauer, 2014). Interventions have been attempted both laparoscopically and by robotic intervention (Bruner & Tulipan, 2005). The procedure may also lessen the risk for subsequent ventriculoperitoneal placement. Infusion of neural stem cells at the site of the open neural placode has been utilized in animal models (Fauza, Jennings, Teng, & Synder, 2008), and more recently human placenta–derived mesenchymal stromal cells have been used in utero surgical repair of ovine models, which supply neuroprotective and anti-inflammatory factors (Wang et al., 2015). In utero treatment of hydrocephalus has also been attempted. Both these treatment options may result in premature delivery, so there is a risk of trading one developmental disability for another given the current state of the art (Chervenak & McCullough, 2002; Committee opinion No. 550, 2013).

The deformities of spina bifida manifesta are obvious at birth. The spinal defect is generally closed at 24 to 48 hours, and a ventriculoperitoneal shunt is required in a total of 80% of patients at a variable time thereafter. In the period preceding surgical intervention, the infant should be transferred to a tertiary care facility where a multidisciplinary team is available, kept abdomen-down in a warmer, and placed on prophylactic intravenous antibiotics to prevent central nervous system infection. The patient should be assessed for other congenital abnormalities, and urologic and orthopedic assessments should also be performed (Alexander & Steig, 1989). The hiatus from birth to surgical treatment permits parents to be supplied with information about their child's condition, which will facilitate their ability to select suitable treatment options (Charney, 1990). Pediatricians who are unfamiliar with the diagnosis may offer an unnecessarily dire prognosis (Siperstein, Wolraich, Reed, & O'Keefe, 1988). Parents should handle the infant as soon as possible and be familiarized with range-of-motion techniques, learn how to deal with the infant's insensate skin, and be instructed in intermittent urinary catheterization if this is indicated (Boytim, Davidson, Charney, & Melchionne, 1991).

The Arnold–Chiari Malformation and Hydrocephalus

The Arnold–Chiari II malformation, seen in up to 90% of patients with spina bifida (Badell-Ribera, Swinyeard, Greenspan, & Deaver, 1964), is characterized by a downward displacement of a portion of the cerebellum through the foramen magnum into the spina canal, with secondary compression of the fourth ventricle and development of hydrocephalus. Untreated, this condition results in progressive expansion of the ventricles, with compression of cerebral tissue, spasticity, retardation, blindness, dysphagia, apnea, and death (Charney, Rorke, Sutton, & Schut, 1991). A shunt is placed from the ventricles into the peritoneal space to decompress the hydrocephalus. Patients with shunts, and those in whom shunting is not required, have normal IQs of 95 and 102, respectively. However, for each episode of bacterial ventriculitis, there is a 10 to 15 point decrement in the IQ, with an average score of 72 (Hunt & Holmes, 1976). Shunt surgery may also be complicated by breakage, distal blockage, nephritis, and hydrocele. Patients requiring shunt revision after the age of 2 years may have a poorer prognosis for overall cognitive function (Hunt, Oakeshold, & Kerry, 1999) and for memory skills that correlate with subsequent functional independence and quality of life.

New imaging studies of the brain, such as diffusion tensor tractography (DTT), may be of value in providing noninvasive estimation of potential intellectual involvement (Hasan, Sankar et al., 2008) and have demonstrated abnormalities of the association pathways needed for sustained concentration to task and higher intellectual function in some patients (Hasan, Eluvathingal et al., 2008). This is important information to derive and needs to be correlated with psychometric testing, given the risk for learning disabilities and modifications of therapeutic and school program, which may subsequently be indicated for these patients (Burmeister et al., 2005; Vinck, Maassen, Mullaart, & Rotteveel, 2006).

A newly developed alternative for the management of hydrocephalus is endoscopic third ventriculostomy. At present, its application may be best suited for patients older than 6 months up to 3.5 years. Long-term shunt dependence with later complications may thereby be avoided (Lam, Harris, Rocque, & Ham, 2014; Teo & Jones, 1996).

Seizures may occur in up to 21% of patients with spina bifida. Underlying additional structural anomalies of the brain such as encephalomalacia, agenesis of the corpus callosum, and/or calcifications predispose to this complication (Talwar, Baldwin, & Hornblatt, 1995; Yoshida et al., 2006).

Neurological Level: Functional Implications

The performance of a neurological examination in the neonate is challenging because of lack of cooperation and existence of spinal shock. Stimulation of the arms and the upper trunk rather than of the lower extremities may more reliably evoke volitional rather than reflexogenic movements. Somatosensory-evoked potentials may also be used to document the level of innervation. Determination of neuromuscular innervation can also be amplified by the use of muscle ultrasound (Verbeek et al., 2014). Discerning a sensory level of below L3 versus a T11 level may be a tool for determination of survival (71% vs. 61%, respectively), need for supportive daily care (22% vs. 71%), and ability to ambulate (61% vs. 0%; Oakeshott, Hunt, Poulton, & Reid, 2012). This determination is crucial, as it will indicate, with good reliability, ambulatory status and risk for the development of orthopedic deformities; those patients with the lowest sacral levels of spinal involvement having the best prognosis (De Souza & Carroll, 1976). Further delineation of prognosis involves the determination of strength of the musculature at a given level (McDonald, Jaffe, Mosca, Shurtleff, & Menalaus, 1991a, 1991b), especially the strength of the hip flexors and knee extensors and the presence of scoliosis, which may occur in up to 50% of this population (Drennan, 1976). Factors of lesser importance include age, sitting balance, height, sex, motivation, presence of spasticity, adequacy of bracing, appropriateness of orthopedic surgery, and motor planning abilities (Asher & Olsen, 1983). Infants with a thoracic level lesion will have no voluntary movements in their lower extremities. With training and correction of lower extremity contractures, 50% of this group become therapeutic or community ambulators in childhood, with extensive bracing (Charney, Melchionni, & Smith, 1991; Shafer & Dias, 1983). As the child matures, increasing weight, upward displacement of the center of gravity, and underlying trunk and respiratory muscle dysfunction cause increasing energy expenditure (Findley & Agre, 1988). By adulthood, this group is usually reliant on wheelchairs for mobility but is capable of independent transfers, dressing, bowel and bladder management, and being employed (Carroll, 1977). Despite the transient nature of their ambulation, walking should be attempted to provide patients with vertical orientation, permit performance of tabletop activities in standing, improve respiratory excursion and urinary drainage, and lessen the possibilities of skin breakdown, contractures, and osteoporosis-related fractures (Dosa et al., 2007).

Patients with innervation at the first three lumbar levels have motor power in hip flexors and adductors (which bring the legs to midline), and to a variable degree in the knee extensors. There is no ability to extend or abduct the hips or to move the feet. At this level, there is the highest risk of hip dislocation, given the imbalance of muscle pull. Hip dislocation may be an impediment to continued ambulation, especially if the hips are stiff or if the dislocation is unilateral resulting in leg-length discrepancy, pelvic obliquity, and progressive scoliosis (Crandall, Birkeback, & Wintor, 1989; Curtis, 1973). Iliopsoas transfers (Sharrard, 1964) were routinely performed in the past to prevent hip flexion contractures, but this limited patients' abilities to flex at hips and ascend stairs, and therefore it is currently rarely performed. Osteotomies of the femoral heads for treatment of subluxation are performed to restore symmetry around the hips, but are not obligatory for ambulation to be achieved (Sherk, Uppal, Lane, & Melchionni, 1991). Release of hip flexion contractures of greater than 30° can also be considered in this group (Frawley, Broughton, & Menalaus, 1996). Infants may be provided with foot drop splints to prevent progressive equinus deformities and may require hip abduction devices to maintain stability at those joints.

In nonambulatory children with high-level lesions, unilateral hip dislocations may cause little functional disability, and surgical intervention is less frequently indicated than in the years past. In ambulatory patients with lower-level lesions, leg-length discrepancy and its effect on functional problems mandate surgical correction (Fraser, Bourke, Broughton, & Menalaus, 1995). Patients with higher-level lesions are generally braced with full-control devices necessitated not only by their lower extremity weakness, but also by their hydrocephalus-related hypotonia. They can be supplied with a standing device known as a parapodium at about 18 months (Letts, Fulford, Eng, & Robinson, 1976). A spina bifida cart can also be provided for independent mobility (Charney, Rorke, et al., 1991). By 2 to 3 years of age, hip-knee-ankle-foot orthoses can be provided and gait training with a rollator commenced (Lough & Nielsen, 1986). Alternatively, an Orlau parawalker (a type of standing frame with a swivel base) can be considered (Major, Stollard, & Farmer, 1997). Depending on praxis and eye-hand coordination, crutches may be supplied at 4 to 5 years of age, with household and some community ambulation anticipated. Reciprocating gait orthosis (with cables) may help to facilitate ambulation and reduce energy consumption by up to 50% in this group when compared with the use of traditional knee-ankle-foot orthoses used with a four-point gait (Cuddeford et al., 1997).

With full innervation at the fourth lumbar level, knee extensors are stronger, and patients may be advanced to knee-ankle-foot orthoses. Some patients may have imbalance between knee flexors and extensors, requiring surgical release of the hamstrings to improve gait (Marshall, Broughton, Menelaus, & Graham, 1996). With innervation at the fifth lumbar level, muscle power around the hips is more balanced. The ankle dorsiflexors, but not the plantar flexors, are functioning, usually resulting in calcaneal deformities with ambulation occurring on insensate feet that increases the risk of skin breakdown at these sites. Thus, an indication arises for transfer of the tibialis anterior muscles, which normally dorsiflex the foot, to a more posterior location, so that weight bearing can be achieved in a plantargrade manner (Aydin, Topal, Tuncer, Canbek, & Kose, 2013). Foot deformities, such as clubfoot deformities and planovalgus, may occur at this and other levels. Although more commonly reserved for idiopathic clubfoot deformities, the Ponseti method of complete posteriormedial and lateral releases have met with success in the treatment of the stiff, teratologic deformities associated with this disorder (Funk, Lebek, Seidi, & Placzek, 2012).

Triple arthrodesis (subtalar fusion to stabilize inversion/eversion) may be performed at about 12 years of age, when the feet are relatively grown. Other surgical procedures considered for correction of valgus deformities provide correction with less rigidity (Abraham, Lubicky, Sanger, & Millar, 1996).

Patients with such lower-lumbar lesions can be anticipated to pull to standing by 1 year of age and ambulate in the community with or without orthoses despite gait deviations. For patients with sacral-level lesions, only minor foot deformities are anticipated. These patients may require shoe modifications or ankle-foot orthoses, but would be able to ambulate without them. They are, however, expected to have bowel and bladder incontinence because of involvement of nerves that normally regulate these functions. It is very important to follow up patients with such low lesions as almost one third may show a decline in ambulatory abilities over time, occurring because of skin breakdown, osteomyelitis, and the need for amputation in association with underrecognized tethering of the spinal cord and syringomyelia, as discussed subsequently (Brinker et al., 1994).

At all levels, especially higher ones, patients with myelomeningocele are at risk for fracures. Although there is not a strict correlation with ambulatory status, decreased serum 25-hydroxyl vitamin D are demonstrated in up to 97% of patients. Most patients also have elevated serum osteocalcin and phosphorus concentrations which correlate with the prescence of osteopenia. Monitoring of these laboratory parameters should be considered in patients who have pathologic fractures and may present with fever as a general systemic response, which warrants investigation.

Scoliosis and Tethering of the Spinal Cord

Management of a paralytic spinal curvature is difficult. As posterior vertebral elements are lacking, surgical fixation with traditional metal rods usually had to be performed both anteriorly and posteriorly (Banta & Park, 1983). Surgical procedures require a period of immobilization, but less so with the development of newer hardware systems which permit segmental fusion. Patients need to be observed postoperatively for further neurological compromise and the development of pseudoarthroses (movement in areas where bones should be solid). Unchecked, scoliosis causes restrictive pulmonary disease with decreased endurance. The uneven posture that results causes a disturbance in the sitting balance, necessitating the use of the upper extremities as tripods. The listing to one side, especially in tandem with hip dislocation, may result in formation of intractable skin breakdown due to asymmetries of pressure distribution.

As scoliosis often occurs before the achievement of skeletal maturity, there is a risk of compromise of total height in a population who is already short. Newer technical advancements to preserve growth potential such as the vertical expandable prosthetic titanium rib (VEPTR) permits correction without fusion so that growth can continue (Abol & Stuecker, 2014).

Scoliosis may occur in response to unequal innervation of the paraspinal muscles and may be compounded by vertebral abnormalities, but rapid progression may herald the development of neurological complications. Prior to the development of MRI, many of these conditions went undetected, and many childhood ambulators used wheelchairs by adolescence. Other factors that may negatively affect ambulatory performance include obesity, joint stiffness with arthritic changes, and lack of motivation.

The two primary conditions responsible for the deterioration in function and often seen with progression of scoliosis are tethering of the spinal cord and syringomyelia. Tethering is caused by scar tissue that holds the spinal cord firmly in place, placing it at risk for repeated microtrauma brought on by spinal flexion and extension (Yamada, Zinke, & Saunders, 1981). Patients exhibit decreased lower extremity strength, spasticity frequently associated with a crouched gait, dysesthesias or progressive sensory deficit, pain over the neural placode (site of the residual spinal deformity), and/or decompensation of a previously well-managed neurogenic bowel and bladder (Peacock, Arens, & Berman, 1987). MRI studies and somatosensory-evoked potentials may be helpful in providing objective evidence of the changes noted on physical examination (Li, Albright, Sclabassi, & Pang, 1996). Urodynamics and perineal-evoked potentials are also useful diagnostic tools in demonstrating change in neurological function (Torre et al., 2002). Surgical release of the tether can result in restoration of function or can stop further neurological progression in most cases (Clancy et al., 1989; Reigel, 1983). Surgical techniques should permit the neural elements to remain free in the cerebrospinal fluid, preventing the risk of retethering (Zide, Constantini, & Epstein, 1995). An expanding fluid-filled cyst may distend the cord at any level, and may be associated with increasing weakness and sensory deficits, frequently involving the upper extremities. This is known as syringomyelia; it can be treated by surgical drainage of the cyst and placement of a shunt at that level into the peritoneum.

Therapeutic Assessment and Intervention

Assessment should include evaluation and description of joint contractures and deformities; neurological level and muscle power; presence, location, and extent of pressure sores; and mobility and ability of patients to perform self-care skills. Treatment includes gentle, active-assistive range-of-motion exercises for the lower extremities, strengthening of innervated musculature, transfer training, gait training, and instruction in self-care skills. Physical activity programs aimed at improving cardiovascular fitness and strength may improve the self-image of the physically challenged child or adolescent (Andrade, Kramer, Garber, & Longmuir, 1991).

In general, infants with myelomeningocele are less active (Morrow, 1995). This coupled with low tone, weakness, and upper extremity dysfunction provides compelling reasons for referral to an early intervention program. Initial studies of patients so referred suggest subsequent enhancement of functional ambulatory and cognitive abilities so that educational mainstreaming is more likely to occur.

Hypotonia or hypertonia may exist in the trunk and upper extremities in association with hydrocephalus. Even children with sacral lesions may present in this manner and require early institution of therapeutic services. The infant should be encouraged to assume antigravity positions, such as quadruped with weight bearing on extended forearms. These attempts may have to be augmented by placing the child over a bolster in prone position and/or by provision of a scooter board. Care must be taken that devices are padded so that secondary skin irritation does not occur. As the child progresses, a bolster can be utilized to work on trunk and abdominal strengthening and sitting balance. Later, a standing table can be used. Depending on the neurological level, the child can then progress to rising from sitting to half-kneeling, and from half-kneeling to standing, utilizing adaptive equipment, as needed.

Newer interventions for physical therapy treatment in patients with myelomeningocele include the use of treadmill training to improve ambulatory skills and cardiovascular conditioning (Christensen & Lowes, 2014); potential use of serial casting in lieu of stretching to treat knee flexion contractures (Al-Oraibi & Tariah, 2013); and the use of the whole body vibration to improve ambulation (Stark et al., 2015).

Appropriate orthoses are either of metal and leather or of the newer custom-molded plastic variety (Krebs, Edelstein, & Fishman, 1988). Whereas the former devices permit accommodation for dependent edema if problematic, the latter are lighter and often considered more cosmetic. Ambulation, especially with hip-knee-ankle-foot orthoses, is energy inefficient, with caloric expenditures about six times greater than normal. The use of reciprocating gait orthoses should therefore be considered to reduce energy consumptions and improve endurance (McCall & Schmidt, 1986). More recently, it has been felt that use of such devices is a trade-off, and more conventional bracing might permit for rapid increases in speed required for activities such as crossing the street.

Upper extremity dysfunction and perceptual-motor problems correlate with both the severity of hydrocephalus and the level of the lesion. With the development of increased intracranial pressure, there is stretching of the motor and sensory fibers that surround the enlarged ventricles seen with the Arnold–Chiari malformation, and this may be compounded by abnormalities of the cervical nerve roots (Hwang, Kentish, & Burns, 2002). Hand function should be assessed in terms of preference, tactile discrimination, kinesthetic awareness, ability to conform to certain positions, and to perform activities including page turning, stacking of blocks and checkers, and the speed with which these activities are carried out, grasp, manipulation of small objects, handling of feeding utensils, graphesthesia, and two-point discrimination (Brunt, 1980; Grimm, 1976; Wallace, 1973). Older children must be assessed in terms of figure copying, graphomotor skills, and academic difficulties. Letter reversals and difficulty in sequencing of tasks are not uncommon. Visual problems of astigmatism, nystagmus, and hyperopia seen in association with hydrocephalus may be contributory factors (Mankinen-Heikkinen & Mustonene, 1987). Remediation of perceptual-motor difficulties may require use of occupational therapy and special education services (Gluckman & Barling, 1980). Upper extremity dysfunction may adversely affect the ability to use crutches (Radke & Gosky, 1981; Wallace, 1973), accounting for discrepancies in ambulation, which occur among patients of the same neurological level.

ADL skills in patients with spina bifida are likely to be below age-level norms (Sousa, Gordon, & Shurtleff, 1976). This may be related to dysfunction of praxis, motor planning, parental overprotection, and time constraints. Preparation for adulthood and independent living may be restricted by these factors rather than by lack of intelligence. The development of standardized assessments of self-care, such as the Functional Independence Measure for Children (Wee-FIM; Granger, Hamilton, & Kayton, 1987) and the PEDI (Feldman, Haley, & Coryell, 1990), help to pinpoint deficiencies that require remediation.

Up to 61% of patients with spina bifida may have strabismus. There is a high incidence of amblyopia as well, likely related to the presence of hydrocephalus. Such deficits require treatment, and their amelioration may permit better upper extremity and perceptual motor function (Bigan, 1995). Exacerbation of such findings may indicate need for reassessment of ventriculoperitoneal shunt malfunction.

Respiratory problems may occur as a result of brainstem dysfunction, either on the basis of a congenital malformation or as a result of repeated traction on that area. Loss of central ventilatory function may present with stridor, intermittent loss of consciousness, and apnea. Initially, stridor may be misinterpreted as a manifestation of reactive airway disease. Sleep studies with an analysis of respiratory gases document the lack of chemoregulatory ability, which can result in hypercarbia and anoxia (Swaminathan et al., 1989). In a recent study, up to 50% of patients with myelomeningocele exhibited mild sleep apnea. Most of these (57%) patients could be treated with oxygen supplementation (Patel, Rocque, & Hoson, 2015). Positive pressure or frank respiratory support may be required, in association with a tracheotomy necessitated by vocal cord paralysis, noting that some children gradually improve over time. Some centers advocate a posterior decompression of the cervical spine, although ultimate survival may not be improved with this intervention (Worley et al., 1996). Similarly, brainstem dysfunction may lead to oromotor incoordination, feeding difficulties, and aspiration.

Speech and language dysfunction arises from the various central structural abnormalities associated with spina bifida. Developmental as well as acquired lesions of the cerebellum result in a disruption of motor speech skills. There is resultant dysfluency, ataxia, dysarthria, and abnormality in the rate of speech or prosody, and alteration of intelligibility and vocal intensity. Abnormalities of the corpus callosum may result in difficulty in comprehension and in pragmatic speech, language skills, and use of idioms (Huber-Okrainec, Blaser, & Dennis, 2004) with relative preservation of grammar and lexicon (Fletcher, Barnes, & Dennis, 2002). More specifically, these deficits are characterized by echolalia/repetition, excessive use of social phrases in conversation, and overfamiliarity, in what has been termed the "cocktail party syndrome" (Tew, 1979). These patients may appear to function on a superficial basis better than they actually perform. Therapeutic efforts are indicated in these children to develop pragmatic, step-by-step verbal skills. These skills are prerequisites for instruction in dressing, learning the sequencing required to master self-catheterization, and other ADL tasks.

Bowel and bladder incontinence results from lack of innervation at the sacral levels, with paralysis and incoordination of the bladder and urinary sphincter on the basis of upper and lower motor neuron involvement (Verhoef, Lurvink, et al., 2005). Urinary incontinence, stasis, and reflux of urine back into the kidneys may result in chronic infections with a potential for urosepsis, chronic renal acidosis, hypertension, renal failure, and death (Mundy, Shah, Borzyskowski, & Saxton, 1985). Until about 30 years ago, upper urinary tract deterioration as characterized by hydronephrosis, hypertension, and decreased renal function was felt to be inevitable, resulting in surgical correction with an ileal conduit (an interposed loop of bowel to serve as a biological reservoir in which to contain urine). Currently, intermittent catheterization is the mainstay of treatment, decreasing the risk of infection and stasis, and permitting functional urinary continence (Petersen, 1987) and maintenance of good renal function (Pecker, Damber, Hjalman, Sjodin, & Von Zeigbergk, 1997). Catheterization may be required in infancy to prevent hydronephrosis, which can be present in up to 81% of patients by 5 years of age (Charney, Synder, & Melchionni, 1991; Kari, Safdar, Jamjoon, & Anshasi, 2009; Stein et al., 2015). Earlier initiation of catheterization may also prevent irreversible bladder dysfunction and reduce the number of children requiring bladder augmentation from 27% to 11% (Iwu, Baskin, & Kogan, 1997). Dependent upon sitting balance, hand function, and cognitive skills, self-catheterization can begin as early as 5 years of age (Smith, 1991). Perceptual problems may make the technique difficult to learn; anatomically correct dolls, coloring books, and other simple visual aids can facilitate training.

Continence can be further enhanced by use of uropharmacological agents. Drugs can be used that relax bladder tone to prevent uncontrolled and untimely voiding whereas other medications improve contraction of the urinary sphincter that prevents leakage. Low-dose oral antibiotic therapy may be clinically indicated to prevent recurrent infections, although research support of this recommendation is lacking. In males, external collecting devices can be used as a back-up measure, but females must rely upon diapers or pads. Attention should be paid to the development of latex allergies that may occur in up to 50% of patients with spina bifida, possibly related to prolonged and repeated exposures to the material from multiple surgeries and intermittent catheterizations (Buenodesa, Camiland, Cavalheiro, Cavalho-Mallozi, & Sole, 2013; Slater, 1989), as well as a disease-associated propensity for latex sensitization (Eiwegger et al., 2006). Allergic manifestations are not only those of reactive airway disease, but include urticaria and anaphylaxis. The average time from exposure to development of symptoms is from 1.5 to 9 years of age, with an average of 5.6 years of age, with the incidence being proportionate to the number of prior surgical procedures (Obojoski et al., 2002). Avoidance of latex-containing items in this population and the maintenance of a latex-free operating room in major medical centers are advised. Patients should be provided with emergency identification bracelets that denote their allergies and other relevant medical problems. When emergent procedures need to be performed under less than optimal circumstances, premedication with steroids and gastrointestinal prophylaxis should occur.

Yearly renal ultrasound studies and blood tests to monitor renal function are mandatory. Surgical techniques include bladder augmentation to increase bladder capacity between catheterizations and the placement of an artificial urinary sphincter (Kaplan, 1985). In patients with some residual sensation, biofeedback techniques may also be successful (Kaplan & Richard, 1988). Low-intensity transcutaneous therapeutic electrical stimulation may be a method for achieving urinary and fecal continence (Balcom, Wintrak, Blifield, Rauen, & Langenstroer, 1997; Kajbalzadeh, Sharifi-Rad, Ladi, & Masoumi, 2014). Most recently, injection of botulinum A toxin into the bladder may transiently modify bladder capacity and assist in achieving transient functional continence (Horts, Weber, Bodmer, & Gobet, 2011).

Patients with spina bifida have been reported to present with advanced bladder cancer. This is another reason for annual urological evaluations. Changes in status including leakage, pain, recurrent urinary tract infections and/or gross hematuria are indications for evaluation with visualization and biopsy, as needed (Mirkin, Casey, Mukhejee, & Kielle, 2013).

Bowel continence is generally managed by the use of stool softeners, diet, and suppositories or enemas given at a consistent time. The olfactory stigma of an incontinent child may result in ostracism and is a compelling reason for the early implementation of an effective bowel and bladder program. If the regimen is not successful, surgical interventions such as performance of a modified antegrade continence enema procedure utilizing the appendix for the stoma in a majority of cases is also a possibility (Sinha, Grewal, & Ward, 2008).

Endocrinological dysfunction has been overlooked in this population. Up to 15% of patients may have reduction in growth hormone levels as manifested by a decrease in longitudinal height and arm span. This is likely hydrocephalus-related, with secondary pressure effects being exerted on the hypothalamus, and/or pituitary gland (Hochhaus, Butenandl, Schwarz, & Ring-Mrozik, 1997). Higher-level spina bifida lesions may result in a greater degree of growth impairment (Rotenstein & Riegel, 1996). Not only are such reductions in height stigmatizing, but the associated changes in bony maturation may alter the standard surgical timetable. Supplementation of growth hormone is a treatment option, although its long-term effect in terms of accentuating linear growth, elevating the center of gravity, and increasing the incidence of symptomatic tethering of the spinal cord has not yet been determined (Gold, 1996).

General pediatric care may be compromised in this group given the 20-fold increase in frequency of hospitalizations for surgery, acute intercurrent infections, and other medical problems. Up to 25% of pediatric patients may be deficient in routine immunizations despite provision of multiple subspecialty medical services, augmented by parental concern with regard to pertussis vaccine administration due to coexistent neurological dysfunction. Accordingly, an immunization history is an important part of each clinic visit (Raddish, Goldman, Kaplan, & Perrin, 1998).

Given the increased longevity of the patient with spina bifida and the possibility of late complications, it is essential that team management is continued throughout the adult years (Lee & Mukherjee, 2015). Without such transdisciplinary services, well over one half of the patients might not receive any specialized services, and some patients might receive no medical care at all (Kaufman et al., 1994). With consistent, ongoing care, potentially preventable complications including pyelonephritis, sepsis, progressive paralysis due to cord-tethering, and osteomyelitis and amputation may be prevented (Calado & Loff, 2002; Rowe & Jadhav, 2008). With comprehensive care for adult patients that includes monitoring for these and other problems, such as cardiovascular diseases, upper extremity dysfunction due to prolonged wheelchair use–induced rotator cuff injuries, and possible increased risk of colorectal cancer (Tomlinson & Sugarman, 1995), specific interventions can be performed that decrease their impact on overall health and function. However, provision of care is not idealized, and transition issues that include instruction in medical conditions and self-advocacy skills are difficult to access and require preparation over many years (Greenley, Coakley, Holmbeck, Jandasek, & Wills, 2006). Parents should be proactive and develop a system of home-based medical records and treatment timelines that can be transferred to their teen or adult children when appropriate (Osterlund, Dosa, & Smith, 2005).

Considerations for Adults

In the setting of multiple physical and medical problems, it is admirable that patients with spina bifida can function as well as has been described. Acknowledgment of psychological differences in patients with myelomeningocele may be seen as early as in the preschool period. Figure drawings by such children reveal fewer portrayals of lower extremities than in the general population. Children tend to rate themselves as significantly different in terms of physical and cognitive competence, but not on maternal or peer acceptance (Mobley, Harless, & Miller, 1996). Most patients without hydrocephalus are independent in ADL skills except for bladder control regardless of their neurological level, as are patients with neurological levels at L2 or below, despite the presence of hydrocephalus (Verhoeft et al., 2006).

The secondary disability of social isolation results from the time allocated to medical care and hospitalizations, augmented by parental overprotectiveness, with mothers exhibiting this tendency to a greater extent than the fathers (Hombeck et al., 2002). Thus, by mid-childhood, children so afflicted have up to a fourfold risk of developing a psychiatric disorder, primarily neurotic in nature. Hence, early intervention, socialization, and family counseling are warranted (Connell & McConnel, 1981). Dorner (1976, 1977) detailed the social dysfunction of the group. Teenagers were found to be lonely and unhappy, and have limited exposure to the typically developing population, sexual experiences, and community resources. Despite attempts at comprehensive interventions and care, newer studies reflect similar findings (Buran, Mc Daniel, & Bree, 2002; Cate, Kennedy, & Stevenson, 2002), although some life satisfaction studies are more promising (Barf et al., 2007). Academic achievement may be somewhat improved on the basis of mainstreaming (Borjeson & Logergren, 1990; Lord, Varzis Behrman, Wicks, & Wicks, 1990). Participation in sport activities is also limited (Buffart et al., 2008).

Instruction in sexual and reproductive function by physicians is reported to occur in only 25% of male and 68% of female patients (Cardenas, Topolski, White, McLaughlin, & Walker, 2008). Adult males with spina bifida have decreased understanding of sexual function, decreased fertility, and difficulty in maintaining erections, with only 52% of such patients reporting sexual satisfaction (Verhoef et al., 2005). Attempts at direct treatment are being developed with two cases of penile reinnervation by the ilio-inguinal to dorsal penile nerve neurorrhaphy being performed to provide local restoration of sensation (Jacobs, Aveilino, Shurtleff, & Lendvay, 2013). Conversely, females often achieve fertility early because of their hydrocephalus. Pregnant females may be predisposed to premature labor owing to a contracted pelvis and urinary tract abnormalities. Ventriculoperitoneal shunts may have an increased incidence of dysfunction during this period. If a C-section is indicated for delivery, then prophylactic antibiotics should be given and peritoneal irrigation should be performed (Rietberg & Lindhout, 1993). Sexual education in either circumstance is exceedingly important.

Despite good cognitive skills and educational opportunities, it is not uncommon for more than 60% of patients to remain in the homes of their parents past maturity (Young et al., 2006). This may not only be a sign of prolonged emotional dependence, but may be an economic necessity as well, for less than 50% of adults are likely to be employed (Castree & Walker, 1981; Magill-Evans, Galambos, Darrah, & Nickerson, 2008), with about 20% being placed in a sheltered workshop environment (van Mechelen, Verheof, van Asbeck, & Post, 2008). Functional numeracy but not functional literacy skills appear to be correlated with a better chance for employment (Dennis & Barnes, 2002) and for quality of life, in general (Hetherington, Dennis, Barnes, Drake, & Gentili, 2006). The survival rate for the majority of patients with spina bifida now exceeds 90% of the total population. This provided the medical community with a mandate to expand the range of services available to such adults.

General Psychological and Neuropsychological Considerations

Although there are certainly psychological and neuropsychological issues that are unique to the individual diagnoses of cerebral palsy and spina bifida (as enumerated previously), there are also some general considerations that apply to both diagnoses.

As with all aspects of children's care, discussion of medical interventions must also address relevant psychological issues. Family expectations, relationships, and reactions clearly play a significant role in the trajectory of the child's development of sense of self, resilience, and adjustment to disability and medical interventions (Aran, Shalev, Biran, & Gross-Tsur, 2007). Family dynamics, support networks, coping resources, and adaptations to disability must be carefully assessed and addressed on an individualized basis as families react and respond to illness and disability in a myriad of ways (Greening & Stoppelbein, 2007).

With children who have congenital and/or developmental disabilities, families may need guidance regarding when they should realistically expect more from their child in terms of autonomy and resilience. This is especially difficult with children and adolescents who are actually dependent on their caregivers for so many basic ADL. Medical and therapeutic staff need to understand the familial perspective by including them as members of the team, by modifying their preconceived notions of absolute "right and wrong," and by avoiding the use of such judgmental labels as "enmeshed" and "infantilizing" (Zaccario, Salsberg et al., 2010). Connecting with parents and patients psychologically and emotionally and helping them move forward appropriately will ultimately culminate in a better treatment outcome for the child (Spates et al., 2007). It is not uncommon for parents to be reluctant to push their children toward independence as a mixed result of fear, protection, and doubt. An adolescent developmental level is especially challenging as separation and individuation issues become particularly salient during that time for even typically developing children. For example, adolescents with a developmental disability may no longer be comfortable with their parents assisting them with toileting and bathing skills, despite years of compliance and continued necessity (Zaccario, Salsberg, Gordon, & Bilginer, 2010). Although children and adolescents can be remarkably resilient and deficits in self-concept cannot be assumed just by the presence of a disability (Shields, Murdoch, Loy, Dodd, & Taylor, 2006), careful consideration does need to be given to their emotional functioning.

The medical and therapeutic staff must be attuned to the goals and expectations of a child with a disability, as well as those of their parents, even when these goals may not coincide with what seems medically or therapeutically important. For example, a teenager with spina bifida who is integrated into the community and quite functional with the motorized wheelchair, may not share the therapeutic goal of working on upright ambulation, partly because his awkward gait and slower speed could actually make him feel more disabled (Zaccario, Salsberg, Gordon, & Bilginer, 2010).

Given the unique stressors associated with pediatric illness and disability, it is not unusual for young patients and their parents to require repeated instructions and an integrated effort among treatment team members to appropriately and clearly understand disseminated information. Single meetings may not give families enough time to process information and to ask appropriate follow-up questions. Emotionally, they may be too angry, sad, stressed, depressed, and/or overwhelmed to properly understand information stated by a clinician on a single occasion (Brel, Woodrome, Fasterau, Buran, & Sawin, 2014). Consistent repetition of diagnostic, prognostic, and treatment information by multiple members of a treatment team can be an effective means of communicating information more thoroughly and respectfully to a family in crisis (Zaccario, Salsberg, Gordon, & Bilginer, 2010).

Commensurate with the rehabilitation model approach to treatment, it is also essential to consider cultural factors and multicultural perspectives when working with pediatric populations and their families (Hanson & Kerkhoff, 2007) as these perspectives can also affect how families deal with such issues as regarding authority, assertiveness, emotional expressiveness, and reactions to pain. Overall, understanding and appreciating the emotional and psychological issues of the individual child and family in the context of cultural background are critical for the delivery of optimal patient care and treatment outcome. Patient care also needs to be appropriately formulated based upon the individual child's developmental level and needs. Referrals to mental health professionals (depending on the medical setting, this could include the departments of child-life, psychology, psychiatry, and/or social work) should be made as appropriate to assist a family and the medical team; but these referrals also need to be made in a supportive, well-timed, and culturally sensitive manner. The therapeutic value of these referrals should be explained thoroughly to the family and framed not in the context of psychopathology, but rather as additional tools to promote optimal care of the affected child (Zaccario et al., 2010).

A neuropsychological consultation and evaluation should be considered for children diagnosed with spina bifida or cerebral palsy at various intervals throughout their childhood and adolescence (Gordon, Salsberg, & McCaul, 2001). Specifically, academic transitions, school-mandated triennial evaluations, postsurgical follow-ups, and reintegration of hospitalized patients into the community setting are examples of appropriate occasions for neuropsychological assessments. A properly trained psychologist (Warschausky, Kaufman, & Steirs, 2008) should be able to choose and adapt testing batteries to best serve these medically complex patients; to consider medical, neuropsychological, and psychiatric diagnoses when formulating cases and making recommendations; and to write reports that will be informative to referring physicians, treating therapists, patient families, and school personnel. When a full neuropsychological assessment is indicated for either pediatric inpatients or outpatients, the following neurocognitive domains are surveyed: intellectual abilities; verbal and language skills; visual–spatial, sensorimotor, and visuomotor skills; attention, memory, and learning; executive functioning; adaptive skills; and preacademic and/or academic abilities (Baron, 2000). In addition, but just as essential, an analysis of social–emotional functioning for the comprehensive assessment of medically fragile, neurologically impaired, and/or developmentally challenged patients is required. Specifically, an evaluator needs to consider the following domains: mood and affect; clarity of thinking and reality testing; self-perception and self-esteem;

interpersonal relatedness and perception of others; and coping resources and stress tolerance (Zaccario et al., 2010).

A crucial aspect of testing, with regard to this population, for an evaluating psychologist is the creation of appropriate and salient recommendations to parents, physicians, treating therapists, and school personnel in feedback sessions and in comprehensive neuropsychological reports. The neuropsychological report is often the primary tool utilized in aftercare programs and schools to reintegrate the recovering child or adolescent in the home and school environment. Therefore, recommendations need to be relevant, clearly written, and feasible for implementation (Maedgen & Semrud-Clikeman, 2007). They typically include educational placement suggestions; academic and classroom modifications; assistive technology; aftercare rehabilitative treatment (occupational, physical, and speech and language therapy); psychotherapy; counseling and group therapy; behavior modification plans; cognitive remediation; medical or professional follow-up; and suggestions for future assessments and reevaluations. It is crucial that the evaluating psychologist be not only well versed with the child's myriad of needs but also prepared to practically advise the family and the school system on implementation of recommendations (Zaccario et al., 2010). As such, a psychologist should understand the rights afforded to children by federal law governing special education, namely the Individuals with Disabilities Education Act (IDEA, 1990, 1997, 2004).

REFERENCES

Abbott, R., Johann-Murphy, M., & Gold, J. T. (1991). Selective functional rhizotomy for the treatment of spasticity in children. In M. Sindou (Ed.), *Neurosurgery for spasticity* (pp. 149–157). New York, NY: Springer-Verlag.

Abol, O. N., & Stuecker, R. (2014). Bilateral rib-to-pelvis Eiffel Tower VEPTR contruct for children with neuromuscular scoliosis. *A Preliminary Report Spine Journal, 14*, 1183–1191.

Abraham, E., Lubicky, J. P., Sanger, M. N., & Millar, E. A. (1996). Supramalleolar osteotomy for angle valgus in myelomeningocele. *Journal of Pediatric Orthopaedics, 16*, 774–781.

Albright, A. L. (1996). Baclofen in the treatment of cerebral palsy. *Journal of Child Neurology, 11*, 77–83.

Albright, A. L., Barron, W. B., Fascik, D., Polinko, P., & Janosky, J. (1993). Continuous intrathecal baclofen infusion for spasticity of cerebral origin. *Journal of the American Medical Association, 270*, 2475–2477.

Albright, A. L., Cervi, A., & Singletary, J. (1991). Intrathecal baclofen for spasticity in cerebral palsy. *Journal of the American Medical Association, 265*, 1418–1422.

Alexander, M. A., & Steig, N. L. (1989). Myelomeningocele: Comprehensive treatment. *Archives of Physical Medicine and Rehabilitation, 70*, 637–641.

Al-oraib, S., Tariah, H. A. (2013). Serial casting verus stretching techniques to treat knee flexion contracture in ch ildren with soina bifida: A comprehensive study. *Journal of Pediatric Rehabilitation Medicine, 6*, 147–153.

Alvarez, N., Larkin, C., & Roxbrough, J. (1981). Carpal-tunnel syndrome in athetoid-dystonic cerebral palsy. *Archives of Neurology, 39*, 311–326.

Andersson, C., Grooten, W., Hellsten, M., Kaping, K., & Mattson, E. (2003). Adults with cerebral palsy: Walking ability after progressive strength training. *Developmental Medicine and Child Neurology, 45*, 220–228.

Andersson, C., & Mattson, E. (2001). Adults with cerebral palsy: Survey describing problems, needs, and resources with special emphasis on locomotion. *Developmental Medicine and Child Neurology, 43*, 76–82.

Andrade, C. K., Kramer, J., Garber, M., & Longmuir, P. (1991). Changes in self-concept, cardiovascular endurance, and muscle strength of children with spina bifida aged 8 to 13 years in response to a 10-week physical activity program: A pilot study. *Child Care Health Development, 17*, 183–196.

Ansved, T., Odergren, T., & Borg, K. (1997). Muscle fiber atrophy in leg muscles after botulinum type A treatment of cervical dystonia. *Neurology, 48*, 1440–1442.

Aran, R., Shalev, S., Biran, G., & Gross-Tsur, V. (2007). Parenting style impacts on quality of life in children with cerebral palsy. *Journal of Pediatrics, 151*, 56–60.

Armstrong, R. W., Steinbok, P., & Cochrane, D. D. (1997). Intrathecally administered baclofen for the treatment of children with spasticity of cerebral origin. *Journal of Neurosurgery, 87*, 409–414.

Arpino, C., Vescio, M. F., DeLuca, A., Curatob, P. (2010). Efficiency of intensive versus non intensive physiotherapy in children with cerebral palsy: A meta-analysis. *International Journal of Rhebailitation Research, 33*, 165–171.

Asher, M., & Olsen, J. (1983). Factors affecting the ambulatory status of patients with spina bifida cystica. *Journal of Bone and Joint Surgery, 65-A*, 350–356.

Ashton, B., Piper, M. C., Warren, S., Stewin, L., & Byrne, P. (1991). Influence of medical history of assessment of at-risk infants. *Developmental Medicine and Child Neurology, 33*, 412–418.

Aydin, A., Topal, M., Tuncer, K., Canbek, U., & Kose, M. (2013). Extramembranous transfer of the tibialis posterior tendon for the treatment of drop foot deformity in children. *Archives of Iranian Medicine, 16*, 647–651.

Bachrach, S., & Greenspun, B. (1990). Care of the adult with myelomeningocele. *Delaware Medical Journal, 62*, 1287–1295.

Badell-Ribera, A., Swinyeard, C., Greenspan, L., & Deaver, G. (1964). Spina bifida with myelomeningocele: Evaluation of rehabilitation potential. *Archives of Physical Medicine and Rehabilitation, 45*, 443–453.

Bajelidze, G., Beithur, M., Littlerton, A. G., Dabney, K., & Miller, F. (2008). Diagnostic evaluation using whole-body technetium bone scan in children with cerebral palsy and pain. *Journal of Pediatric Orthopaedics, 28*, 112–117.

Bakheit, A. M. (2010). The use of botulinum toxin for the treatment of muscle spasticity in the first two years of life. *International Journal of Rehabilitation Research, 33*, 104–108.

Balaban, B., Tok, F., Tan, A., & Mathews, D. J. (2012). Botulinum toxin A treatment in children with Cerebral Palsy it's effects on walking and energy expenditure. *American Journal of Physical Medicine & Rehabilitation, 91*, 53–65.

Balcom, A. H., Wintrak, M., Blifeld, T., Rauen, K., & Langenstroer, P. (1997). Initial experience with home therapeutic electrical-stimulation for continence in the myelomeningocele population. *Journal of Urology, 158*, 1272–1276.

Banta, J. V., & Park, S. M. (1983). Improvement in pulmonary function in patients having combined anterior and posterior spine fusion for myelomeningocele scoliosis. *Spine, 8*, 765–770.

Barf, H. A., Post, M. W. M., Verhoef, M., Jennekens-Schickel, A., Gooskens, R., & Prevo, A. (2007). Life satisfaction of young adults with spina bifida. *Developmental Medicine and Child Neurology, 49*, 458–463.

Baron, I. S. (2000). Clinical implications and practical applications of child neuropsychological evaluations. In K. O. Yeates, M. D. Ris, & H. G. Taylor (Eds.), *Pediatric neuropsychology: Research, theory, and practice*. New York, NY: Guilford.

Bar-Haim, S., Harries, N., Belokopytov, M., Frank, A., Copeliovitch, L., Kaplanski, J., & Lahat, E. (2006). Comparison of efficacy of Adeli suit and neurodevelopmental treatment of children with cerebral palsy. *Developmental Medicine and Child Neurology, 48*, 325–330.

Bax, M., Tydeman, C., & Flodmark, O. (2006). Clinical and MRI correlates of cerebral palsy: The European cerebral palsy study. *Journal of the American Medical Association, 296*, 1602–1608.

Bell, M. J., & Hallenbeck, E. (2002). Effects of intrauterine inflammation on developing rat brain. *Journal of Neuroscience Research, 70*, 570–579.

Benedict, M. I., White, R. B., Wulff, L. M., & Hall, B. J. (1990). Reported maltreatment in children with multiple disabilities. *Child Abuse Neglect, 14*, 207–217.

Bergen, A. F., & Colangelo, C. (1982). *Positioning of the client with central nervous system deficits: The wheelchair and other adaptive equipment.* Valhalla, NY: Valhalla Rehabilitation.

Bigan, A. W. (1995). Strabismus associated with meningomyelocele. *Journal of Pediatric Ophthalmology Strabismus, 32*, 309–314.

Blair, E., & Stanley, F. (1990). Intrauterine growth retardation and spastic cerebral palsy: I. Association with birth weight for gestational age. *American Journal of Obstetrics and Gynecology, 162*, 229–237.

Bleck, E. E. (1987). Orthopedic management of cerebral palsy. In *Clinical developmental medicine* (Vol. 99/100). Oxford, England: MacKeith.

Blum, R. W., Resnick, M. D., Nelson, R., & St. Germaine, A. (1991). Familiar and peer issues among adolescents with spina bifida and cerebral palsy. *Pediatrics, 88*, 280–285.

Bobath, B., & Bobath, K. (1975). *Motor development in the different types of cerebral palsy*. London, England: Heineman.

Borjeson, M. C., & Logergren, J. (1990). Life conditions of adolescents with myelomeningocele. *Developmental Medicine and Child Neurology, 32*, 698–706.

Borowski, A., Littleton, A. G., Borkhuu, B., Presedo, A., Shah, S., Dabney, K., . . . Miller, F. (2010). Complications of intrathecal baclofen pump therapy in pediatric patients. *Journal Pediatric Orthopaedics, 30*, 76–81.

Borowski, A. E., Shah, S., Littleton, A., Dabney, K., & Miller, F. (2008). Baclofen pump implantation and spinal fusion in children: Techniques and complications. *Spine, 33*, 1995–2000.

Botto, L. D., & Yang, Q. (2000). Ethylene tetrahydrofolate reductase gene variants and congenital anomalies. A HuGE review. *American Journal of Epidemiology, 151*, 862–877.

Boyle, C. A., Boulet, S. L., Schieve, L. A., Cohen, R. A., Blumberg, S. J., Yeargin-Allsopp, M., . . . Kogan, M. D. (2011). Trends in the prevalence of developmental disabilities in U.S. children, 1997–2008. *Pediatrics, 127*(6), 1034–1042.

Boytim, M. J., Davidson, R. S., Charney, E., & Melchionne, J. B. (1991). Neonatal fractures in myelomeningocele patients. *Journal of Pediatric Orthopaedics, 11*, 28–30.

Brel, T. J., Woodrome, S. E., Fastenau, P. S., Buran, C. F., & Sawin, K. J. (2014). Depressive symtopms in parents of adolescents with myelomeningocele: The associated clinical adolescent neuropsychological functioning and family protective factors. *Journal of Pediatric Rehabilitation Mediicne, 7*, 341–352.

Brinker, M. R., Rosenfeld, S. R., Feiwell, R., Granger, S. P., Mitchell, D. C., & Rice, J. C. (1994). Myelomeningocele at the sacral level. *Journal of Bone and Joint Surgery, 76-A*, 1293–1300.

Bronkhorst, A. J., & Lamb, G. A. (1987). Orthosis to aid in the reduction of lower extremity spasticity. *Orthotics and Prosthetics, 41*, 23–28.

Brown, M. C., Bontempo, A., & Turk, M. A. (1992). *Secondary consequences of cerebral palsy: Adults with cerebral palsy in New York state.* Albany, NY: Developmental Disabilities Planning Council.

Bruggink, L. M., Einspieler, C., Butcher, P. R., Stremmelaar, E. F., Prechtl, H., & Bos, A. F. (2008). Quantitative aspects of the early motor repertoire in preterm infants: Do they predict minor neurological dysfunction at school age? *Early Human Development, 85*, 25–36.

Bruner, J. P., & Tulipan, N. (2005). Intrauterine repair of spina bifida. *Clinical Obstetrics and Gynecology, 48*, 942–955.

Brunt, A. (1980). Characteristics of upper limb movements in a sample of myelomeningocele children. *Perceptual Motor Skills, 51*, 431–437.

Buenodesa, A., Camiloaraujo, R. F., Cavalheiro, S., Cavalho-Mallozi, M., & Sole, D. (2013). Profile of Latex sensitization and allergies in children and adolescents with myelomenigocele in Sao Paulo, Brazil. *Journal of Investigational Allergology & Clinical Immunology,* 23, 43–49.

Buffart, L. M., van der Ploeg, H., Bauman, A. E., Van Asbeck, F. W., Stam, H. J., Roebroeck, M. E., & van den Berg-Emons R. J. (2008). Sports participation in adolescents and young adults with myelomeningocele and its role in total physical activity behaviour and fitness. *Journal of Rehabilitation Medicine, 40*, 702–708.

Buran, C. F., Mc Daniel, A., & Bree, T. J. (2002). Needs assessment in a spina bifida program: A comparison of the perceptions by adolescents with spina bifida and their parents. *Clinical Nurse Specialist, 16*, 256–262.

Burmeister, R., Hannay, H. J., Copeland, K., Fletcher, J. M., Boudousquale, A., & Dennis, M. (2005). Attention problems and executive functions in children with spina bifida and hydrocephalus. *Child Neuropsychology, 11*, 265–283.

Butler, J. M., Scianni, A., & Ado, L. (2010). Effect of cardiorespiratory training on aerobic fitness and carryover to activity in children with cerebral palsy: A systematic review. *Internationl Journal of Rehabilitation Research, 33*, 97–103.

Calado, E., & Loff, C. (2002). The "failures" of spina bifida transdisciplinary care. *European Journal of Pediatric Surgery, 12*, 525–526.

Capute, A. J. (1978). *Primitive reflex profile.* Baltimore, MD: University Park Press.

Capute, A. J., Shapiro, B. K., & Palmer, F. B. (1981). Spectrum of developmental disabilities. *Orthopedic Clinics of North America, 12*, 3–22.

Cardenas, D. D., Topolski, T. D., White, C. J., McLaughlin, J. F., & Walker, W. O. (2008). Sexual functioning in adolescents and young adults with spina bifida. *Archives of Physical Medicine and Rehabilitation, 89*, 31–35.

Carlson, W. E., Vaughn, C. L., Damiano, D. L., & Abel, M. F. (1997). Orthotic management of gait in spastic diplegia. *American Journal of Physical Medicine and Rehabilitation, 76*, 216–225.

Carlsson, M., Hagberg, G., & Olssom, I. (2003). Clinical and etiological aspects of epilepsy in children with cerebral palsy. *Developmental Medicine and Child Neurology, 45*, 371–376.

Carlsson, M., Olsson, I., Hagberg, G., & Beckung, E. (2008). Behavior in children with cerebral palsy with and without epilepsy. *Developmental Medicine and Child Neurology, 50*, 784–789.

Carr, C., & Gage, J. R. (1987). The fate of the non-operated hip in cerebral palsy. *Journal of Pediatric Orthopaedics, 7*, 262–267.

Carroll, N. C. (1977). The orthotic management of spina bifida children: Present status, future goals. *Prosthetics and Orthotics International, 1*(1), 39–42.

Castree, J., & Walker, J. H. (1981). The young adult with spina bifida. *British Medical Journal, 283*, 1040–1042.

Cate, I. M. P., Kennedy, C., & Stevenson, J. (2002). Disability and quality of life in spina bifida and hydrocephalus. *Developmental Medicine and Child Neurology, 44*, 317–322.

Chambers, H. (2014). Update on neuromuscular disorders in pediatric orthopaedics. *Journal of Pediatric Orthopaedics, 34*, S44–S48.

Charney, E. B. (1990). Parental attitudes toward management of newborns with myelomeningocele. *Developmental Medicine and Child Neurology, 32*, 14–19.

Charney, E. B., Melchionni, J. B., & Smith, D. R. (1991). Community ambulation by children with myelomeningocele and high-level paralysis. *Journal of Pediatric Orthopaedics, 11*, 579–582.

Charney, E. B., Rorke, L. B., Sutton, L. N., & Schut, L. (1991). Management of Chiari II complications in infants with myelomeningocele. *Journal of Pediatrics, 111*, 371–374.

Charney, E. B., Synder, H. M., & Melchionni, J. B. (1991). Upper urinary tract deterioration with myelomeningocele. *Developmental Medicine and Child Neurology, 33*(Suppl. 64), 18–37.

Chervenak, R. A., & McCullough, L. B. (2002). A comprehensive ethical framework for fetal research and its application to fetal surgery for spina bifida. *American Journal of Obstetrics and Gynecology, 187*, 10–14.

Chicoine, M. R., Park, T. S., & Kaufman, B. A. (1997). Selective dorsal rhizotomy and rates of orthopaedic surgery in children with spastic cerebral palsy. *Journal of Neurosurgery, 86*, 34–39.

Choi, S. H., & McComb, J. G. (2000). Long-term outcome of terminal myelocystocele patients. *Pediatric Neurosurgery, 32*, 86–91.

Christensen, C., & Lowes, L. P. (2014). Treadmill training for a child with Spina Bifida without functional ambulation. *Pediatric Physical Therapy, 26*, 265–272.

Chrysagis, N., Skordilis, E., Stavrov, N., Grammatopoulou, E., & Kootsouki, D. (2012). The effect of treadmill training on gross motor function and walking speed in ambulatory adolescents with cerebral palsy: A randomized controlled trial. *American Journal of Physical Medicine & Rehabilitation, 91*, 747–760.

Clancy, R. R., Sladsky, J. T., & Rorke, L. B. (1989). Hypoxic-ischemia spinal cord injury following perinatal asphyxia. *Annals of Neurology, 25*, 185–189.

Clopton, N., Dutton, J., Featherston, T., Grigsby, A., Mobley, J., & Melvin, J. (2005). Interrater and intrarater reliability of the Modified Ashworth Scale in children with hypertonia. *Pediatric Physical Therapy, 17*, 268–274.

Committee Opinion No. 500. (2013). Maternal fetal surgery for myelomeningocele. *Obstetrics & Gynecology, 121*, 218–219.

Coniglio, S. J., Anderson, S. M., & Ferguson, J. E. (1996). Functional motor outcome in children with myelomeningocele. Correlation with anatomic prenatal ultrasound. *Developmental Medicine and Child Neurology, 38*, 675–680.

Connell, H. M., & McConnel, T. S. (1981). Psychiatric sequelae in children treated operatively for hydrocephalus in infancy. *Developmental Medicine and Child Neurology, 23*, 505–517.

Connealy, B. D., Northrup, H., & Au, K. (2014). Genetic variations in the GLUT 3 gene associated with myelomeningocele. *American Journal of Obstetrics & Gynecology, 211*, e1–e8.

Cooperman, D. R., Bartucci, E., Dietrick, E., & Millar, E. A. (1987). Hip dislocation in spastic cerebral palsy: Long-term consequences. *Journal of Pediatric Orthopaedics, 7*, 268–276.

Coorsen, E. A., Msall, M. E., & Duffy, L. C. (1991). Multiple minor manifestations as a marker for prenatal etiology of cerebral palsy. *Developmental Medicine and Child Neurology, 33*, 730–736.

Cosgrove, A. P., & Graham, H. K. (1994). Botulinum toxin A prevents the development of contractures in the hereditary spastic mouse. *Developmental Medicine and Child Neurology, 36*, 379–385.

Craft, M. J., Lakin, J. A., Oppliger, R. A., Clancy, G. M., & Vander Linden, D. W. (1990). Siblings as change agents for promoting the functional status of children with cerebral palsy. *Developmental Medicine and Child Neurology, 32*, 1049–1057.

Crandall, R. C., Birkeback, C. R., & Wintor, B. R. (1989). The role of hip location and dislocation in the functional status of the myelodysplastic patient. *Orthopedics, 12*, 675–683.

Crenshaw, S., Herzog, R., Castagno, P., Richards, J., Miller, F., Michaloski, G., & Moran, E. (2000). The efficacy of tone-reducing splints in children with spastic diplegic cerebral palsy. *Journal of Pediatric Orthopaedics, 20*, 210–216.

Cuddeford, T. J., Freeling, R. P., Thomas, S. S., Aniona, M. D., Rex, D., Sirolli, H., . . . Magnusson, M. (1997). Energy consumption in children with myelomeningocele: A comparison between reciprocating gait orthosis and hip-knee-ankle-foot orthosis ambulators. *Developmental Medicine and Child Neurology, 39*, 239–242.

Curtis, B. H. (1973). The hip in the myelomeningocele child. *Clinical Orthopaedics and Related Research, 90*, 11–21.

Day, S. M., Reynolds, R. J., & Kush, S. J. (2015). Extrapolating published survivial curves to obtain evidence-based estimates of life expectancy in cerebral palsy. *Developmental Medicine and Chid Neurology, 57*, 1105–1118.

Damiano, D. L., Kelly, L. E., & Vaughn, C. L. (1995). Effects of quadriceps femoris muscle strengthening on crouch gait in children with spastic diplegia. *Physical Therapy, 75*, 658–667.

Damiano, D. L., Vaughn, C. L., & Abel, M. F. (1995). Muscle response to heavy resistance exercise in children with spastic cerebral palsy. *Developmental Medicine and Child Neurology, 37*, 731–739.

Deaver, G. (1956). Cerebral palsy: Methods of beating the neuromuscular disability. *Archives of Physical Medicine and Rehabilitation, 37*, 363–378.

Dennis, N., & Barnes, M. (2002). Math and numeracy in young adults with spina bifida and hydrocephalus. *Developmental Medicine and Child Neurology, 41*, 141–155.

De Souza, L. L., & Carroll, N. (1976). Ambulation of the braced myelomeningocele patient. *Journal of Bone and Joint Surgery, 58-A*, 1112–1118.

Diamond, N. (1986). Rehabilitation strategies for the child with cerebral palsy. *Pediatric Annals, 15*, 230–236.

Dieruf, K., Burtner, P., Provost, B., Phillips, J., Bernitsky-Beddingfield, A., & Sullivan, K. J. (2009). A pilot study of quality of life in children with cerebral palsy after intensive body weight-supported treadmill training. *Pediatric Physical Therapy, 21*, 45–52.

Donkervoort, M., Wiegerink, D., van Meeteren, J., Stam, H., & Roebroeck, M. (2009). Transition to adulthood: Validation of the rotterdam transition Profile for young adults with cerebral palsy and normal intelligence. *Developmental Medicine and Child Neurology, 51*, 53–62.

Dorner, S. (1976). Adolescents with spina bifida: How they view their situation. *Archives of Disease in Childhood, 51*, 439–444.

Dorner, S. (1977). Sexual interest and activity in adolescents with spina bifida. *Journal of Child Psychology, 18*, 220–237.

Dosa, N. P., Eckrich, M., Katz, D. A., Turk, M., & Liptak, G. S. (2007). Incidence, prevalence, and characteristic of fractures in children, adolescents, and adults with spina bifida. *Journal of Spinal Cord Medicine, 30*, S5–S9.

Drennan, J. C. (1976). Orthotic management of the myelomeningocele spine. *Developmental Medicine and Child Neurology, 18*, 97–103.

Druschel, C., Althuizes, H. C., Funk, J. M., Placzek, R. (2013). Off label use of botulinum toxin in children under two years of age. *A Systematic Review: Toxins, 5*, 60–72.

Dudley, R. W., Pardin, M., Gagnon, B., Saluja, R., Yap, R., Montpetit, K., . . . Farmer, J. P. (2013). Long-term functional benefits of selective dorsal rhizotomy for spastic cerebral palsy. *Journal of Neurosurgical Pediatrics, 12*, 142–150.

Duncan, R., Barton, I., Edmonds, E., & Blashill, B. M. (2004). Parental perceptions of the therapeutic efficacy of osteopathic manipulation or acupuncture in children with spastic cerebral palsy. *Clinical Pediatrics, 43*, 349–353.

Ebara, S., Yamazaki, Y., Harada, T., Hosono, N., Morimoto, Y., Tang, L., . . . Ono, K. (1990). Motion analysis of the cervical spine in athetoid cerebral palsy. *Spine, 15*, 1097–1103.

Eicher, D. J., Wagner, C. L., & Katikaneni, L. P. (2004). Moderate hypothermia in neonatal encephalopathy: Efficacy outcomes. *Journal of Pediatric Neurology, 32*, 11–17.

Eisenberg, S., Zuk, L., Carmeli, E., & Katz-Leuer, M. (2009). Contribution of stepping while standing to function and secondary conditions among children with cerebral palsy. *Pediatric Physical Therapy, 21*, 79–85.

Eiwegger, T., Dehlink, E., Schwindt, J., Popmberger, G., Reider, N., Frigo, E., . . . Szépfalusi, Z. (2006). Early exposure to latex products mediates latex sensitization in spina bifida but not in other diseases with comparable latex exposure rates. *Clinical and Experimental Allergy, 36*, 1242–1246.

Ellenberg, J. H., & Nelson, K. B. (1981). Early recognition of infants at risk for cerebral palsy. Examination at age 4 months. *Developmental Medicine and Child Neurology, 23*, 705–714.

Engel, J. M., Kartin, D., & Jensen, M. D. (2002). Pain treatment in persons with cerebral palsy. Frequency and helpfulness. *Journal of Physical Medicine and Rehabilitation, 81*, 291–296.

Engel-Yeger, B., Jarus, T., Anaby, D., & Law, M. (2009). Differences in patterns of participation between youth with cerebral palsy and typically developing peers. *American Journal of Occupational Therapy, 63*, 96–104.

Erkin, G., Cilha, C., Ozel, S., & Kirbiyik, E. G. (2010). Feeding and gastrointestinal problems in children with cerebral palsy. *Internationl Journal of Rehabilitation Research, 33*, 218–224.

Evans, D. M., & Alberman, E. (1990). Certified cause of death in children and young adults with cerebral palsy. *Archives of Disease in Childhood, 66*, 325–329.

Evans, D. M., Evans, J. W., & Alberman, E. (1990). Cerebral palsy: Why we must plan for survival. *Archives of Disease in Childhood, 65*, 1329–1333.

Eyman, R. K., & Grossman, H. J. (1990). The life expectancy of profoundly handicapped people with mental retardation. *New England Journal of Medicine, 323*, 584–589.

Facchin, P., Rosa-Rizzotlo, M., Visona Dlia Pozza L., Torconi, A. C., Pagliano, E., Sighorini, S., . . . Fedrizzi, E. (2011). Multisite trial comparing the efficiency of constraint induced movement therapy with that of bimanual intensive training in children with Hemiplegic cerbral palsy: Post intervention results. *American Journal of Physical Medicine & Rehabilitation, 90*, 539–553.

Farmer, S. F., Harrison, L. M., Ingram, D. A., & Stephens, J. A. (1991). Plasticity of central motor pathways in children with hemiplegic cerebral palsy. *Neurology, 41*, 1505–1510.

Fasano, V. A., Barolat-Romana, G., Zeme, S., & Suazzi, A. (1970). Electrophysiological assessment of spinal circuits in spasticity by direct dorsal root stimulation. *Neurosurgery, 4*, 146–151.

Fasoli, S., Ladenheim, B., Mast, J., & Krehs, I. T. (2012). New horizons for robot–assisted therapy in pediatrics. *American Journal of Physical Medicine, 11*, s280–s289.

Fauza, D. O., Jennings, R. W., Teng, Y. D., & Synder, E. Y. (2008). Neural stem cell delivery to the spinal cord in an ovine model of fetal surgery for spina bifida. *Surgery, 144*, 367–373.

Feldman, A. B., Haley, S. M., & Coryell, J. (1990). Concurrent and construct validity of the Pediatric evaluation of disability inventory. *Physical Therapy, 70*, 602–610.

Findley, T. W., & Agre, J. C. (1988). Ambulation of the adolescent with spina bifida: Oxygen costs of mobility. *Archives of Physical Medicine and Rehabilitation, 69*, 855–861.

Finnie, N. R. (1974). *Handling the young cerebral palsied child at home*. New York, NY: E.P. Dutton.

Fletcher, J. M., Barnes, M., & Dennis, M., (2002). Language development in children with spina bifida. *Seminars in Pediatric Neurology, 9*, 201–208.

Ford, G. W., Kitchen, W. H., Doyle, L. W., Richards, A. L., & Kelly, E. (1990). Changing diagnosis of cerebral palsy in very low birth weight children. *American Journal of Perinatology, 7*, 178–181.

Fragala-Pinkham, M., Dumas, H., Barlow, C., & Pasternak, A. (2009). An aquatic physical therapy program at a pediatric rehabilitation hospital: A case series. *Pediatric Physical Therapy, 21*, 68–78.

Fraser, R. K., Bourke, H. M., Broughton, N. S., & Menalaus, M. B. (1995). Unilateral dislocation of the hip in spina bifida: A long-term follow-up. *Journal of Bone and Joint Surgery, 77-B*, 299–302.

Frawley, P. A., Broughton, N. S., & Menalaus, M. B. (1996). Anterior release for fixed flextion deformity of the hip in spina bifida. *Journal of Bone and Joint Surgery, 78-B*, 299–302.

Frieden, J., & Lieber, R. (2003). Spastic muscle cells are shorter and stiffer than normal cells. *Muscle and Nerve, 26*, 157–164.

Fulford, G. E. (1990). Surgical management of ankle and foot deformities in cerebral palsy. *Clinical Orthopaedics and Related Research, 253*, 55–61.

Funk, J. F., Lebek, S., Seidi, T., & Plazczek, R. (2012). Comparison of treatment results of Idiopathic and Non-idiopathic congenital clubfoot. *Prospective Evaluation of the Ponseti Therapy Orthopade, 41*, 977–983.

Gage, J. R. (1990). Surgical treatment of knee dysfunction in cerebral palsy. *Clinical Orthopaedics and Related Research, 253*, 45–54.

Galvin, K. A. (1998). Postinjury magnesium sulfate treatment is not markedly neuroprotective for striatal medium spiny neurons after perinatal hypoxic/ischemia in the rat. *Pediatrics Research, 44*, 740–745.

Gerring, J. P., Brady, K. D., Chen, A., Vasa, R., Grados, M., Bandeen-Roche, K. J., . . . Denckla M. B. (1998). Premorbid prevalence of ADHD and development of secondary ADHD after closed head injury. *Journal of the American Academy of Child and Adolescent Psychiatry, 37*, 647–654.

Gertszten, P. C. (1997). Effect on ambulation of continuous intrathecal baclofen infusion. *Pediatric Neurosurgery, 27*, 40–44.

Gibson, C. S., Mac Lennan, A. H., Goldwater, P. N., & Dekker, G. A. (2003). Antenatal causes of cerebral palsy: Association between inherited thrombophilias, viral, and bacterial infections, and inherited susceptibilities to infection. *Obstetric and Gynecological Surgery, 58*, 209–220.

Glantzman, A. M., Kim, H., Swaminathan, K., & Beck, T. (2004). Efficacy of botulinum toxin A, serial casting, and combined treatment for spastic equinus: A retrospective analysis. *Developmental Medicine and Child Neurology, 46*, 807–811.

Gluckman, S., & Barling, J. (1980). Effect of remedial program on visual-motor perception in spina bifida children. *Journal of General Psychology, 136*, 195–200.

Gold, J. T. (1996). Growth hormone treatment of children with neural tube defects (Letter; comment). *Journal of Pediatrics, 129*, 177.

Gooch, J. L., & Walker, M. L. (1996). Spinal stenosis after total lumbar laminectomy for selective dorsal rhizotomy. *Pediatric Neurosurgery, 25*, 28–30.

Gordon, R., Salsberg, D., & McCaul, P. (2001). Neuropsychological assessment of childhood stroke. *Loss, Grief & Care, 9*, 61–82.

Gorter, H., Holty, L., Rameckers, E., Hans, J., & Rob, O. (2009). Changes in endurance and walking ability through functional physical therapy training in children with cerebral palsy. *Pediatric Physical Therapy, 21*, 31–37.

Gosechel, J., Wohlfarth, K., Frevert, J., Dengler, R., & Bilgalke, T. T. (1997). Botulinum A toxin therapy: Neutralizing and non-neutralizing antibodies—Therapeutic consequences. *Experimental Neurology, 147*, 96–102.

Graham, H. K., & Harvey, A. (2007). Assessment of mobility after multi-level surgery for cerebral palsy. *Journal of Bone and Joint Surgery, 89*, 993–994.

Graham, H. K., & Selber, P. (2003). Musculoskeletal aspects of cerebral palsy. *Journal of Bone and Joint Surgery, 85-B*, 157–166.

Graham, L., Levene, M. I., & Trounce, J. Q. (1987). Prediction of cerebral palsy in very low birth weight infants: Prospective ultrasound study. *The Lancet, 2*, 593–596.

Granger, C. V., Hamilton, B. B., & Kayton, R. (1987). *Guide to the use of the functional independence measure for children (WeeFIM) of the uniform data set for medical rehabilitation.* Buffalo, NY: Research Foundation, State University of New York.

Grant, A., O'Brien, N., Joy, M. T., Hennessy, E., & Mac Donald, D. (1989). Cerebral palsy among children born during the Dublin randomized trial of intrapartum monitoring. *The Lancet, 2*, 1233–1236.

Grecco, L. A., Mendonca, E., Duarte, N. A., Zsinon, N., & Olivelra, C. S. (2014). Transcranial direct current stimulation combined with treadmill gait training in delayed neuro- psychomotor development. *Journal of Physical Therapy Science, 26*, 945–950.

Greening, L., & Stoppelbein, L. (2007). Brief report: Pediatric cancer, parental coping style, and risk for depressive, posttraumatic stress and anxiety symptoms. *Journal of Pediatric Psychology, 32*, 1272–1277.

Greenley, R. N., Coakley, R. M., Holmbeck, G. N., Jandasek, B., & Wills, K. (2006). Condition-related knowledge among children with spina bifida: Longitudinal changes and predictors. *Journal of Pediatric Psychology, 31*, 828–839.

Grimm, R. A. (1976). Hand preference and tactile perception in a group of children with myelomeningocele. *American Journal of Occupational Therapy, 30*, 234–250.

Guyatt, G., Sackett, D., Taylor, D. W., Chong, J., Roberts, R., & Dugsley, S. (1986). Determining optimal therapy: Randomized trials in individual patients. *New England Journal of Medicine, 314*, 889–892.

Hack, M., & Costello, D. W. (2008). Trends in the rates of cerebral palsy associated with neonatal intensive care of preterm children. *Clinical Obstetrics and Gynecology, 51*, 763–774.

Hagberg, B., & Hagberg, G. (1989). The changing panorama of cerebral palsy in Sweden: 5 The birth year period 1979–1982. *Acta Paediatrica Scandinavica, 78*, 283–290.

Hagberg, B., & Hagberg, G. (1996). The changing panorama of cerebral palsy: Bilateral spastic forms in particular. *Acta Paediatrica Scandinavica, 415*, 48–52.

Halpern, D. (1982). Duration of relaxation after intramuscular neurolysis with phenol. *Journal of the American Medical Association, 247*, 1473–1476.

Halpern, D. (1984). Therapeutic exercises for cerebral palsy. In J. V. Basmajiani (Ed.), *Therapeutic exercises* (pp. 118–143). Baltimore, MD: Lippincott Williams & Wilkins.

Hanson, S. L., & Kerkhoff, T. R. (2007). Ethical decision making in rehabilitation: Consideration of Latino cultural factors. *Rehabilitation Psychology, 52*, 409–420.

Harade, T., Ebara, S., Anwar, M. M., Okawa, A., Kajiura, I., Kiroshima, K., & Ono, K. (1996). The cervical spine in athetoid cerebral palsy: A radiological study of 180 patients. *Journal of Bone and Joint Surgery, 78-B*, 613–619.

Harris, S. R. (1989). Early diagnosis of spastic diplegia, spastic hemiplegia, and quadriplegia. *American Journal of Disease in Childhood, 143*, 1356–1360.

Harrison, A. (1988). Spastic cerebral palsy: Possible interneuronal contributions. *Developmental Medicine and Child Neurology, 30*, 760–780.

Hasan, K. M., Eluvathingal, T. J., Kramer, L. A., Ewing-Cobbs, L., Dennis, M., & Fletcher, J. M. (2008). White matter microstructural abnormalities in children with spina bifida myelomeningocele and hydrocephalus: A diffusions tensor tractography study of the association pathways. *Journal of Magnetic Resonance Imaging, 27*, 700–709.

Hasan, K. M., Sankar, A., Halphen, C., Kramer, L. A., Ewing-Cobbs, L., Dennis, M., & Fletcher, J. M. (2008). Quantitative diffusion tensor imaging and intellectual outcomes in spina bifida. *Journal of Neurosurgery and Pediatrics, 2*, 75–82.

Hayek, S., Gershon, A., Weintrioub, S., & Yizhar, Z. (2010). The effect of injections of Botulinumtoxin A combines with casting on the equinus gait of children with cerebral palsy. *Journal of Bone and Joint Surgery, 92-B*, 1152–1159.

Hayley, S. M., Ludlow, L. H., & Coster, W. J. (1993). Pediatric evaluation of disability inventory. *Physical Medicine and Rehabilitation of North America, 4*, 529–540.

Haynes, R., Xu, G., Folkerth, R. D., Trachtenberg, F. L., Volpe, J. J., & Kinney, H. C. (2011). Potential neuronal repair in cerebral white matter injury in the human neonate. *Pediatric Research, 69*, 62–67.

Hazlewood, M. I., Brown, J. K., Rowe, P. J., & Salter, P. M. (1994). The use of therapeutic electrical stimulation in the treatment of hemiplegic cerebral palsy. *Developmental Medicine and Child Neurology, 36*, 661–673.

Henderson, R. C., Lark, R. K., & Kecskemethy, H. (2002). Bisphosphonates to treat osteopenia in children with quadriplegic cerebral palsy: A randomized clinical trial. *Journal of Pediatrics, 141*, 644–651.

Herring, J. (2013). *Tachdjian's pediatric orthopedics*. Philadephia, PA: Elsevier.

Hetherington, R., Dennis, M., Barnes, M., Drake, J., & Gentili, F. (2006). Functional outcome in young adults with spina bifida and hydrocephalus. *Child's Nervous System, 22*, 117–124.

Hill, A. E. (1990). Conductive education for physically handicapped children. *Ulster Medical Journal, 59*, 41–45.

Hinderer, K. A., & Harris, S. R. (1988). Effects of tone reducing versus standard plaster casts on gait improvement in children with cerebral palsy. *Developmental Medicine and Child Neurology, 30*, 370–377.

Hirtz, D. G., & Nelson, K. (1998). Magnesium sulfate and cerebral palsy in premature infants. *Current Opinion in Pediatrics, 10*, 131–137.

Hirtz, M. (1989). Patterns of impairment and disability related to social handicap in young people with cerebral palsy and spina bifida. *Journal of Biosocial Science, 21*, 1–12.

Hochhaus, R., Butenandl, O., Schwarz, H. P., & Ring-Mrozik, E. (1997). Auxological and endocrinological evaluation of children with hydrocephalus and/or meningomyelocele. *European Journal of Pediatrics, 156*, 597–601.

Holm, V. A. (1982). The causes of cerebral palsy. *Journal of the American Medical Association, 247*, 1473–1475.

Hombeck, G. N., Johnson, S. Z., Wills, K. E., McKernon, W., Rose, B., Erklin, S., & Kemper, T. (2002). Observed and perceived parental overprotection in relation to psychosocial adjustment in preadolescents with a physical disability: The mediation role of behavioral autonomy. *Journal of Consulting and Clinical Psychology, 70*, 96–110.

Horts, M., Weber, D. M., Bodmer, C., & Gobet, R. (2011). Repeated botulinum A toxin injection in the treatment of neuropathic bladder dysfunction and poor bladder compliance in children with myelomeningocele. *Neurology and Urodynamics, 30*, 1546–1549.

Huber-Okrainec, J., Blaser, S. E., & Dennis, M. (2004). Idiom comprehension deficits in relation to corpus callosum agenesis and hypoplasia in children with spina bifida meningomyelocele. *Brain Language, 93*, 349–368.

Hunt, G. M., & Holmes, A. E. (1976). Factors relating intelligence in treated cases of spina bifida cystica. *American Journal of Disease in Children, 130*, 823–827.

Hunt, G. M., Oakesholt, P., & Kerry, S. (1999). Link between the CSF shunt and achievement in adults with spina bifida. *Journal of Neurology, Neurosurgery, and Psychiatry, 67*, 591–595.

Hurvitz, E. A., Leonard, C., Ayyangar, R., & Nelson, V. S. (2003). Complementary and alternative medicine use in families of children with cerebral palsy. *Developmental Medicine and Child Neurology, 45*, 364–370.

Hwang, R., Kentish, M., & Burns, Y. (2002). Hand positioning in children with spina bifida myelomeningocele. *Australian Journal of Physiotherapy, 48*, 17–22.

Individuals with Disabilities Education Act of 1990, Public Law 101–476. U.S. Statutes at Large (1990).

Individuals with Disabilities Education Act of 1997, Public Law 105–17. (IDEA Reauthorized), U.S. Statutes at Large (1997).

Individuals with Disabilities Education Improvement Act of 2004, Public Law 108–446. (IDEA Reauthorized), U.S. Statutes at Large 118 (2004):2647.

Ingram, T. S. S. (1955). Early manifestations and course of diplegia in childhood. *Archives of Disease in Childhood, 30*, 244–250.

Iwu, H. Y., Baskin, L. S., & Kogan, B. A. (1997). Neurogenic bladder dysfunction due to myelomeningocele: Neonatal versus childhood treatment. *Journal of Urology, 157*, 2295–2297.

Jacobs, M. A., Avelino, A. M., Shurtleff, D., & Lendvay, T. S. (2013). Reinnervating the penis in spina bifida patients in the United States: Illioinguinal to dorsal-penile neurorrhaphy in two cases. *Journal of Sexual Medicine, 10*, 2593–2597.

Jones, M., McEvwan, I., & Neas, B. (2012). Effects of power wheelchairs on the development and function of young children with severe motor impairments. *Pediatric Physical Therapy*, *24*, 131–140.

Johnson, D. C., Damiano, D. L., & Abel, M. F. (1997). The evolution of gait in childhood and adolescent cerebral palsy. *Journal of Pediatric Orthopaedics, 17*, 392–396.

Kajbalzadeh, A. M., Sharifi-Rad, L., Ladi Seyedian, S. S., & Masoumi, A. (2014). Functional electrical stimulation for management of urinary incontinenece in children with myelomeningocele: *A Random Trial Pediatric Surgery International*, *30*(6), 663–668.

Kan, P., Cooch, J., Amini, A., Ploeger, D., Grmas, B., Oberg, W., . . . Keslte, J. (2008). Surgical treatment of spasticty in children. Comparison of selective dorsal rhizotomy and Intrathecal baclofen pumo implantation. *Childs Nervous System*, *24*, 239–243.

Kaplan, W. E. (1985). Management of myelomeningocele. *Urologic Clinics of North America, 12*, 930191.

Kaplan, W. E., & Richard, I. (1988). Intravesicle bladder stimulation in myelodysplasia. *Journal of Urology, 140*, 1282–1284.

Kari, J. A., Safdar, O., Jamjoon, R., & Anshasi, W. (2009). Renal involvement in children with spina bifida. *Saudi Journal of Kidney Disease Transplant, 20*, 102–105.

Karabay, I., Ozturk, G. T., Malas, F., Kara, M., Tiftik, T., Ersoz, M., & Ozcakar, L. (2015). Short term effect of neuromuscular electrical stimulation on muscle architecture of the tibialis anterior and gastrocnemius in children with cerebral palsy. *American Journal of Physical Medicine and Rhebailitation, 94*, 726–733.

Kassover, M., Tauber, C., Au, J., & Pugh, J. (1986). Auditory biofeedback in spastic diplegia. *Journal of Orthopedics Research, 4*, 246–249.

Kaufman, B. A., Terbrock, A., Winters, N., Ito, J., Klosterman, A., & Park, T. S. (1994). Disbanding a multidisciplinary clinic: Effects on health care of myelomeningocele patients. *Pediatric Neurology, 21*, 36–44.

Keating, J. C., McCarron, K., James, J., Gruenberg, J., & Lonczak, R. S. (1985). Urobehavioral intervention in the rehabilitation of lower urinary tract dysfunction: A case report. *Journal of Manipulative and Physiological Therapeutics, 8*, 185–189.

Kelly, B., MacKay-Lyons, M. J., Berryman, S., Hyndman, J., & Wood, E. (2008). Assessment protocol for serial casting after botulinum toxin A injections to treat equinus gait. *Pediatric Physical Therapy, 20*, 233–241.

Khoury, M. J., Erickson, J. D., & James, L. M. (1982). Etiologic heterogenicity of neural tube defects: Clues from epidemiology. *American Journal of Epidemiology, 115*, 538–548.

King, W., Levin, R., Schmidt, R., Oestreich, A., & Heubi, J. E. (2003). Prevalence of reduced bone mass in children and adults with spastic quadriplegia. *Developmental Medicine and Child Neurology, 45*, 12–16.

Korman, L. A., Mooney, J. F., Smith, B., Goodman, A., & Mulvaney, T. (1993). Management of cerebral palsy with botulinum-A toxin: Preliminary investigations. *Journal of Pediatric Orthopaedics, 13*, 489–495.

Kottke, F. J., Halpern, D., Easton, J. K. M., Ozel, A. T., & Burrill, C. A. (1978). The training of coordination. *Archives of Physical Medicine and Rehabilitation, 59*, 567–578.

Krageloh-Mann, I. (2015). Grey matter injury in cerebral palsy –pallidum for the role of the predicting severity. *Developmental Medicne & Child Neurology, 57*, 1089–1090.

Kraus, F. T. (1997). Cerebral palsy and thrombi in placental vessels of the fetus: Insights from litigation. *Human Pathology, 28*, 246–248.

Krebs, D. E., Edelstein, J. E., & Fishman, S. (1988). Comparison of plastic/metal and leather/metal knee-ankle-foot orthoses. *American Journal of Physical Medicine, 67*, 175–185.

Kurz, M., Wilson, T., Corr, B., Volkman, K. G. (2012). Neuromagnetic activity of the somatosensory cortices assoiciated with body weights supported & treadmill training in children with cerebral palsy. *Journal of Neurologic Physical Therapy*, *36*, 166–172.

Lam, S., Harris, D., Rocque, B. G., Ham, S. A. (2014). Pediatric endoscopic third ventriculostomy: A population based study. *Journal of Neurosurgery: Pediatrics*, *14*, 455–464.

Lary, J. M., & Edmonds, L. D. (1996). Prevalence of spina bifida at birth—United States 1983–1990: A comparison of two surveillance systems. *Morbidity Mortality Weekly Reports CDC Surveillance Summaries, 45*, 15–26.

Leck, I. (1974). Causation of neutral tube defects; Clues from epidemiology. *British Medical Bulletin, 30*, 158–163.

Lee, J. T., Mukherjee, S. (2015). Transition to adult care for patients with spina bifida. *Physical Medicine & Rehabilitaion Clinics of North America*, *26*, 29–38.

Letts, R. M., Fulford, D., Eng, B., & Robinson, D. A. (1976). Mobility aids for the paraplegic child. *Journal of Bone and Joint Surgery, 58-A*, 38–41.

Levine, M. S. (1980). Cerebral palsy diagnosis in children over 1 year of age: Standard criteria. *Archives of Physical Medicine and Rehabilitation, 61*, 385–392.

Li, V., Albright, A. L., Sclabassi, R., & Pang, D. (1996). The role of somatosensory evoked potentials in the evaluation of spinal cord retethering. *Pediatric Neurosurgery, 24*, 126–133.

Lin, S. C., Margolis, B., Yu, S. M., & Adirim, T. A. (2014). The role of medical home in emergency department use for children with developmental disabilities in the United States. *Pediatric Emergency Care*, *30*, 534–539.

Lintner, S. A., & Lindseth, R. E. (1994). Kyphotic deformity in patients—Who have myeloemingocele: Operative treatment and long-term follow-up. *Journal of Bone and Joint Surgery*, *76*(9), 1301–1307.

Lonstein, J. E., & Akbamia, B. (1983). Operative treatment of spinal deformities in patients with cerebral palsy or mental retardation. *Journal of Bone and Joint Surgery, 63-A*, 43–57.

Lorber, J. (1971). Results of treatment of myelomeningocele: An analysis of 524 selected cases with special reference to possible selection for treatment. *Developmental Medicine and Child Neurology, 13*, 279–303.

Lord, J. P. (1984). Cerebral palsy: A clinical approach. *Archives of Physical Medicine and Rehabilitation, 65*, 542–556.

Lord, J. P., Varzos, N., Behrman, B., Wicks, J. G., & Wicks, D. (1990). Implications of mainstream classrooms for adolescents with spina bifida. *Developmental Medicine and Child Neurology, 32*, 20–29.

Lough, L. K., & Nielsen, D. J. (1986). Ambulation of children with myelomeningocele: Parapodium versus parapodium with Orlau swivel modification. *Developmental Medicine and Child Neurology, 28*, 489–497.

Maedgen, J. W., & Semrud-Clikeman, M. (2007). Bridging neuropsychological practice with education. In S. J. Hunter & J. Donders (Eds.), *Pediatric neuropsychological intervention: A critical review of science and practice*. Cambridge: Cambridge University Press.

Magill-Evans, J., Galambos, N., Darrah, J., & Nickerson, C. (2008). Predictors of employment for young adults with developmental motor disabilities. *Work, 31*, 433–442.

Magill-Evans, J. E., & Restall, G. (1991). Self-esteem of persons with cerebral palsy: From adolescence to adulthood. *American Journal of Occupational Therapy, 45*, 819–825.

Major, R. E., Stollard, J., & Farmer, S. E. (1997). A review of 42 patients of 16 years and over using the orlau parawalker. *Prosthetics and Orthotics International, 21*, 147–152.

Maltais, D. B., Robitaille, N. M., Dumas, F., Boucher, N., & Richarsd, C. L. (2012). Measuring steady state oxygen uptake during the 6 min. walk test inadults with cerebral palsy feasibility and construct validity. *Internatinal Journal of Rehabilitation Research*, *35*, 181–183.

Mankinen-Heikkinen, A., & Mustonene, E. (1987). Ophthalmologic changes in hydrocephalus. *Acta Ophthalmologica, 65*, 81–86.

Mannino, F. L., & Traunor, D. (1983). Stroke in neonates. *Journal of Pediatrics, 102*, 605–609.

Marshall, P. D., Broughton, N. S., Menelaus, M. B., & Graham, H. K. (1996). Surgical release of knee flexion contractures in myelomeningocele. *Journal of Bone and Joint Surgery, 78-B*, 912–916.

Martin, J. E., & Epstein, L. H. (1976). Evaluating treatment effectiveness in cerebral palsy. *Physical Therapy, 56*, 285–293.

Martinez-Biarge, M., Diaz- Sebastian, J., Kapellou, O., Ginder, D., Allsop, J. M., Ruhterford, N. A., & Cowan, F. M. (2011). Predicting motor outcome and death in term hypoxic-ischemic encephalopathy. *Neurology*, *76*, 2055–2061.

Mathew, A., Mathew, C., Thomas, M., & Antonisamy, B. (2005). The efficacy of diazepam in enhancing motor function in children with spastic cerebral palsy. *Journal of Tropical Medicine and Hygiene, 51*, 109–113.

Matthews, D. (1988). Controversial therapies in the management of cerebral palsy. *Pediatric Annals, 17*, 762–765.

Maudsley, G., Hultor, J. L., & Pharoah, P. (1999). Cause of death in cerebral palsy: A descriptive study. *Archives of Disease in Childhood, 81*, 390–394.

Max, J. E., Mathews, K., Lansing, A. E., Robertson, B. A. M., Fox, P. T., Lancaster, J. L., . . . Smith, J. (2002). Psychiatric disorders after childhood stroke. *Journal of the American Academy of Child and Adolescent Psychiatry, 41*, 555–562.

McCall, R. E., & Schmidt, W. T. (1986). Clinical experiences with the reciprocating gait orthosis in myelodysplasia. *Journal of Pediatric Orthopaedics, 16*, 157–161.

McClone, D. G. (1998). The biological resolution of malformations of the central nervous system. *Neurosurgery, 43*, 1375–1380.

McClone, D. G., Cyzewski, D., Raimondi, A., & Sommers, M. (1985). Central nervous system infections as a limiting factor in the intelligence of children with myelodysplasia. *Pediatrics, 70*, 338–342.

McClone, D. G., Diaz, L., Kaplan, W., & Sommers, R. (1985). Concepts in the management of spina bifida. *Concepts in Pediatrics and Neurosurgery, 5*, 97–106.

McDonald, C. M., Jaffe, K. M., Mosca, V. S., Shurtleff, D. B., & Menalaus, M. B. (1991a). Ambulatory outcome of children with myelomeningocele: Effect of lower extremity strength. *Developmental Medicine and Child Neurology, 33*, 482–490.

McDonald, C. M., Jaffe, K. M., Mosca, V. S., Shurtleff, D. B., & Menalaus, M. B. (1991b). Modifications to the traditional description of neurosegmental innervation in myelomeningocele. *Developmental Medicine and Child Neurology, 33*, 473–481.

McLaughlin, J. F., & Shurtleff, D. B. (1979). Management of the newborn with myelodysplasia. *Clinical Pediatrics, 18*, 463–476.

McLellan, A., Cipparone, C., Giancola, D., Armstrong, D., & Bartlett, D. (2012). Medical and surgical procedures experienced by young children with cerebral palsy. *Pediatric Physical Therapy, 24*(3), 268–277.

McNeal, D., Hawtry, C. E., Wolraich, M. L., & Mapel, J. R. (1983). Symptomatic neurogenic bladder in a cerebral palsy population. *Developmental Medicine and Child Neurology, 25*, 612–621.

Mockford, M. M., & Caulton, J. M. (2010). The pathophysiological basis of weakness in children with cerebral palsy. *Pediatric Physcial Therapy*, 22, 222–233.

Mesples, B., Plaisant, F., & Gressens, P. (2003). Effects of interleukin-10 on neonatal excitotoxic brain lesions in mice. *Brain Research, 141*, 25–32.

Meuli, M., Meuli-Simmens, C., Hutchins, G. M., Seiler, M. J., Marrison, M. R., & Adzick, N. S. (1997). The spinal cord lesion in human fetuses with myelomeningocele. Implications for fetal surgery. *Journal of Pediatric Surgery, 32*, 448–452.

Meuli-Simmens, C., Meuli, M., Adzick, N. S., & Harrison, M. R. (1997). Latissimus dorsi flap procedures to cover myelomeningocele in utero: A feasibility study in human fetuses. *Journal of Pediatric Surgery, 32*, 1154–1156.

Meyer, R. E., & Siega-Riz, A. M. (2002). Sociodemographic patterns in spina bifida with prevalence trends—North Carolina, 1995–1999. *Morbidity Mortality Weekly Report, 51*, 12–15.

Michelsen, S. I., Uldall, P., Hansen, T., & Madsen, M. (2006). Social integration of adults with cerebral palsy. *Developmental Medicine and Child Neurology, 48*, 643–649.

Michelsen, S. I., Uldall, P., Mette, A., & Madsen, M. (2005). Education and employment prospects in cerebral palsy. *Developmental Medicine and Child Neurology, 47*, 511–517.

Milunsky, A., & Alpert, E. (1976a). Prenatal diagnosis of neural tube deficits: l. Problems and pitfalls: Analysis of 2495 cases using the alpha-fetoprotein assay. *Journal of Obstetrics and Gynecology, 48*, 1–5.

Milunsky, A., & Alpert, E. (1976b). Prenatal diagnosis of neural tube deficits: 2. Analysis of false positive and false negative alpha-fetoprotein results. *Journal of Obstetrics and Gynecology, 48*, 6–12.

Mirkin, C., Casey, J. T., Mukherjees, S., & Kielb, S. J. (2013). Risk of bladder cancer in patients with spina bifida: Case reports and review of the literature. *Journal of Pediatric Rehabiltation Medicine, 6*, 155–162.

Missuna, C., & Pollack, N. (1991). Play deprivation in children with physical disabilities: The role of the occupational therapist in preventing secondary disability. *American Journal of Occupational Therapy, 45*, 882–888.

Mital, M. A., & Sakellardies, H. (1981). Surgery of the upper extremity in the retarded individual with spastic cerebral palsy. *Orthopedic Clinics of North America, 12*, 127–136.

Mobley, C. E., Harless, L. S., & Miller, K. L. (1996). Self-perception of preschool children with spina bifida. *Journal of Pediatric Neurosurgery, 11*, 217–224.

Moldenhauer, J. S. (2014). In utero repair of Spina Bifida. *American Journal of Perinatology, 31*, 595–604.

Molenaers, G., Desloovere, K., & DeCat, J. (2001). Single event multi-level botulinum toxin type A treatment and surgery: Similarities and differences. *European Journal of Neurology, 8*, 88–97.

Molnar, G. E. (1979). Cerebral palsy prognosis and who to judge it. *Pediatric Annals, 8*, 10–24.

Molnar, G. E., & Taft, L. T. (1977). Pediatric rehabilitation: Part I. Cerebral palsy and spinal cord injuries. *Current Problems in Pediatrics, 7*, 6–11.

Morison, J. E., Bromfield, L. M., & Cameron, H. J. (2003). A therapeutic model for supporting families of children with a chronic illness or disability. *Child and Adolescent Mental Health, 8*, 125–130.

Morris, P. J. (2008). Physical activity recommendations for children and adolescents with chronic disease. *Current Sports Medicine Reports, 7*, 353–358.

Morrow, J. D. (1995). Temperament in the infant with myelomeningocele. *Journal of Pediatric Nursing, 10*, 99–104.

Mossberg, K. A., Linton, K. A., & Friske, K. (1990). Ankle-foot orthoses: Effect on energy expenditure of gait in spastic diplegic children. *Archives of Physical Medicine and Rehabilitation, 71*, 490–494.

Mundy, A. R., Shah, P. J. R., Borzyskowski, M., & Saxton, H. M. (1985). Sphincter behavior in myelomeningocele. *British Journal of Urology, 57*, 647–651.

Murphy, K. P., Molnar, G. E., & Lankasky, K. (1995). Medical and functional status of adults with cerebral palsy. *Developmental Medicine and Child Neurology, 37*, 1075–1084.

Murphy, K. P., Molnar, G. E., & Lankasky, K. (2000). Employment and social issues in adults with cerebral palsy. *Archives of Physical Medicine and Rehabilitation, 81*, 807–811.

Naeye, R. L., & Peter, E. C. (1989). Origins of cerebral palsy. *American Journal of Disease in Childhood, 143*, 1154–1160.

Narayanan, U. G. (2007). The role of gait analysis in the orthopaedic management of ambulatory cerebral palsy. *Current Opinion in Pediatrics, 19*, 38–43.

Nelson, K. B. (1989). Relationship of intrapartum and delivery events to long-term neurologic outcome. *Clinical Perinatology, 16*, 995–1007.

Nelson, K. B. (1998). Neonatal cytokines and coagulation factors in children with cerebral palsy. *Annals of Neurology, 44*, 665–675.

Nelson, K. B. (2008). Causative factors in cerebral palsy. *Clinical Obstetrics and Gynecology, 51*, 749–762.

Nelson, K. B., & Ellenberg, J. H. (1979). Neonatal signs as a predictor of cerebral palsy. *Pediatrics, 64*, 2–14.

Nelson, K. B., & Ellenberg, J. H. (1981). Apgar scores as predictors of cerebral palsy. *Pediatrics, 68*, 36–46.

Nelson, K. B., & Ellenberg, J. H. (1986). Antecedents of cerebral palsy. *New England Journal of Medicine, 315*, 81–86.

Nordmark, E., Josenby, A. L., Lagergren, J., Anderson, G., Stromblad, L. G., & Westbom, L. (2008). Long-term outcomes five years after selective dorsal rhizotomy. *BMC Pediatrics, 8*, 54–69.

Nwaobi, O. M., & Smith, P. D. (1986). Effects of adaptive seating on pulmonary function in children with cerebral palsy. *Developmental Medicine and Child Neurology, 28*, 351–354.

Oakeshott, P., Hunt, G. M., Poulton A., & Reid, I. (2012). Open Spina Bifida Birth Findings predict long term outcome. *Archives of Disease in childhood, 97*, 474–476.

Obojoski, A., Chodorski, J., Borg, W., Medal, W., Fal, A. M., & Malolepsz, Y. (2002). Latex allergy and sensitization in children with spina bifida. *Pediatrics Neurosurgery, 37*, 262–266.

O'Callaghan, M. E., MacLennan, A. H., Gibson, C. S., Haan, E., Broadbent, J. L., Goldwater, P. N., & Dekker, G. A. (2011). Epidemilogic assoications with cerebral palsy. *Obstetrics & Gynecology, 118*, 576–582.

Osterlund, C. S., Dosa, N. P., & Smith, C. A. (2005). Mother knows best: Medical record management for patients with spina bifida during the transition from pediatric to adult care. *AMIA Proceedings*, 580–584.

Padmanabhan, R. (2006). Etiology, pathogenesis, and prevention of neural tube defects. *Congenital Anomalies, 46*, 55–67.

Palisano, R., Rosenbaum, P., Walter, S., Russell, D., Wood, E., & Galuppi, B. (1997). Development and reliability of a system to classify gross motor function in children with cerbralpalsy. *Developmental Medicine and Child Neurology, 39*, 214–223.

Palisano, R. J., Rosenbaum, P., & Bartlett, P. (2008). Content validity of the expanded and revised gross motor function classfication system. *Developmental Medicine and Child Neurology, 50*, 744–750.

Palisano, R. J., Rosenbaum, P. L., Walter, S. D., & Hanna, S. (1997). Development and reliability of a system to classify gross motor function in children with cerebral palsy. *Developmental Medicine and Child Neurology, 39*, 214–223.

Palmer, F. B., Shapiro, B. K., Allen, M. C., Mosher, B. S., Bilker, S. A., Harryman, S. E., . . . Capute, A. J. (1990). Infant stimulation curriculum for infants with cerebral palsy: Effects on infant temperament, parent infant interaction and home environment. *Pediatrics, 85*, 411–415.

Palmer, F. B., Shapiro, B. K., & Wachtel, R. C. (1988). Effects of physical therapy on cerebral palsy. *New England Journal of Medicine, 318*, 803–808.

Pape, K. E., Kirsch, S. E., Galil, A., Boultron, J. E., White, M. A., & Chipman, M. (1993). Neuromuscular approach to the motor deficits of cerebral palsy: A pilot study. *Journal of Pediatric Orthopaedics, 13*, 628–633.

Patel, D. M., Rocque, B. G., Hopsom, B., Arynchyna, A., Bishop, E. R., Lozano, D., & Blount, J. P. (2015). Sleep-Disordered breathing in patients with myelomenigcele. *Journal of Neurosurgery Pediatrics, 16*, 30–35.

Peacock, W. J., Arens, L. J., & Berman, B. (1987). Cerebral palsy spasticity: Selective posterior rhizotomy. *Pediatric Neuroscience, 13*, 61–66.

Peacock, W. J., & Staudt, L. A. (1991). Functional outcomes following selective posterior rhizotomy for children with cerebral palsy. *Journal of Neurosurgery, 74*, 380–385.

Pecker, R., Danver, J. E., Hjalmas, K., Sjodin, J. G., & Von Zweibergk, M. (1997). The urological fate of young adults with myelomeningocele: A three decade follow-up study. *European Urology, 32*, 213–217.

Pellock, J. M. (2004). Defining the problem: Psychiatric and behavioral comorbidity in children and adolescents with epilepsy. *Epilepsy & Behavior, 5*(Suppl. 3), 3–9.

Penn, R. D., Mykleburst, B. M., Gottlieb, G. L., Agarwal, G. C., & Etzel, M. E. (1980). Chronic cerebellar stimulation for cerebral palsy. *Journal of Neurosurgery, 53*, 160–169.

Petersen, T. (1987). Management of urinary incontinence in children with myelomeningocele. *Acta Neurologica Scandinavica, 75*, 52–55.

Petrini, J., Dias, T., McCormick, M., Massolo, M., Green, N., & Escobar, G. (2009). Increased risk of adverse neurological development of later preterm infants. *Journal of Pediatrics, 154*, 169–176.

Pierce, S. R., Daly, K., Gallagher, K. G., Gershkoff, A. M., & Schaumburg, S. W. (2002). Constraint-induced therapy for a child with hemiplegic cerebral palsy: A case report. *Archives of Physical Medicine and Rehabilitation, 83*, 1462–1463.

Pool, D., Blackmore, A. M., Bear, N., & Valentine, J. (2014). Effects of short term daily community walk aide use on children with spastic cerebral palsy. *Pediatric Physical Therapy*, *26*, 308–317.

Preiss, R. A., Condie, D. N., Rowley, D. I., & Graham, H. K. (2003). The effects of botulinum toxin (BTX-A) on spasticity of the lower limb and gait in cerebral palsy. *Journal of Bone and Joint Surgery, 85-B*, 943–948.

Paleg, G. S., Smith, B. A., & Glickman, L. B. (2013). Systematic review and evidence-based cinical recommendations for closing of pediatric supported standing programs. *Pediatric Physical Therapy*, *25*, 232–247.

Qin, F. Z., Li, S. L., Wen, H. X., Ouyang, Y. R., Zheng, Q., & Bi, J. R. (2014). Ultrasound measurement of fetal posterior fossa at 11 to 13 gestational weeks for screening open spina bifida. *Journal of Southern Medical University*, *34*, 950–955.

Raddish, M., Goldman, D. A., Kaplan, D. C., & Perin, J. M. (1998). The immunization status of children with spina bifida. *American Journal of Diseases of Children, 147*, 849–853.

Radke, J., & Gosky, G. A. (1981). Hearing and speech screening in a hydrocephalus myelodysplasia population. *Spina Bifida Therapy*, *3*, 25–26.

Rapp, C. E., & Torres, M. M. (2000). The adult with cerebral palsy. *Archives of Family Medicine, 9*, 466–472.

Reese, M. E., Msall, M. E., & Owens, S. (1991). Acquired cervical spine impairment in young adults with cerebral palsy. *Developmental Medicine and Child Neurology, 33*, 153–156.

Reigel, D. H. (1983). Tethered spinal cord. *Concepts of Pediatric Neurosurgery*, *4*, 142–164.

Reimers, J. (1990). Functional changes in the antagonists after lengthening of the agonists in cerebral palsy. *Clinical Orthopaedics and Related Research, 253*, 3037.

Resnick, M. B., Eyler, F. D., Nelson, R. M., Eitman, D. V., & Bucciarelli, R. L. (1987). Developmental intervention for low birth weight infants: Improved early developmental outcome. *Pediatrics, 80*, 68–74.

Rezaie, P., & Dean, A. (2002). Periventricular leukomalacia, inflammation and white matter lesions within the developing nervous system. *Neuropathology, 22*, 106–132.

Rietberg, C. C., & Lindhout, D. (1993). Adult patients with spina bifida cystica. *European Journal of Obstetrics, Gynecological Reproductive Biology, 52*, 63–70.

Robinson, H. P., Hood, V. D., Adam, H. D., Gibson, A. A. M., & Ferguson-Smith, M. A. (1980). Diagnostic ultrasound: Early detection of fetal neural tube defects. *Obstetrics and Gynecology, 56*, 705–710.

Robinson, R. O. (1973). The frequency of other handicaps in children with cerebral palsy. *Developmental Medicine and Child Neurology, 15*, 305–316.

Ronan, S., & Gold, J. T. (2007). Nonoperative management of spasticity in children. *Children's Nervous System, 23*, 943–956.

Rosenbaum, P., Paneth, N., Leviton, A., Goldstein, M., Bax, M., Damiano, D., . . . Jacobsson, B. (2006). A report: The definition and classification of cerebral palsy. *Developmental Medicine & Child Neurology, 49*, 1098–1114.

Rosenstein, S. N. (1982). *Dentistry in cerebral palsy and related handicapping conditions*. Springfield, IL: Charles. C. Thomas.

Rotenstein, D., & Riegel, D. H. (1996). Growth hormone treatment of children with neural tube defects; Results from 6 months to 6 years. *Journal of Pediatrics, 128*, 184–189.

Rothman, J. G. (1978). Effects of respiratory exercise on the vital capacity and forced volume in children with cerebral palsy. *Physical Therapy, 58*, 421–425.

Rouse, D., Hirtz, D., Thom, E., Varner, M., Spong, C. Y., Mercer, B. M., . . . Eunice kennedy shriver NICHD maternal-fetal medicine units network. (2008). A randomized controlled trial of magnesium sulfate for the prevention of cerebral palsy. *New England Journal of Medicine, 359*, 895–905.

Rousset, C. I., Kassem, J., Olivier, P., Chalon, S., Gressens, P., & Saliba, E. (2008). Antenatal bacterial endotoxin sensitizes the immature rat brain to postnatal excitotoxic injury. *Journal of Neuropathology and Experimental Neurology, 67*, 994–1000.

Rowe, D. E., & Jadhav, A. L. (2008). Care of the adolescent with spina bifida. *Pediatric Clinics of North America, 55*, 1359–1374.

Rutz, E., Tirosh, O., Thomason, P., Barg, A., & Graham, H. K. (2012). Stability of the gross motor function classification system after single event multilevel surgery in cerrbral palsy. *Developmental Medicine and Child Neurology*, *54*, 1109–1113.

Sala, D. A., & Grant, A. D. (1995). Prognosis for ambulation in cerebral palsy. *Developmental Medicine and Child Neurology, 37*, 1020–1026.

Salakor, P. T., Sajaniemi, N., Hallvack, H., Kari, A., Rila, H., & von Wednt, L. (1997). Randomization study of the effects of antenatal dexamethasone on growth and development of premature children at the corrected age of two years. *Acta Paediatrica, 86*, 294–298.

Sanders, J. O., McConnell, S. L., King, R., Landford, A., Montpetit, K., Gates, P., . . . Curry, D. B. (2006). A prospective evaluation of the Wee FIM in patients with cerebral palsy undergoing orthopaedic surgery. *Journal of Pediatric Orthopaedics, 26*, 542–546.

Sankey, R. J., Anderson, D. M., & Young, J. A. (1989). Characteristics of ankle-foot orthoses for management of the spastic lower limb. *Developmental Medicine and Child Neurology, 31*, 466–471.

Satila, H., Pietkainen, T., Hsalo, T., Lehtonen-Katy, P., Salu, M., Haataja, R., . . . Autti-Rämö, I. (2008). Botulinum toxin type A injections into the calf muscles for treatment of spastic equinus in cerebral palsy: A randomized trial comparing single and multiple injection sites. *American Journal of Physical Medicine and Rehabilitation, 87*, 386–394.

Schaefer, M. K., McCarthy, J. J., & Josephic, K. (2007). Effects of early weight bearing on the functional recovery of ambulatory children with cerebral palsy after bilateral proximal femoral osteotomy. *Journal of Pediatric Orthopaedics, 27*, 668–670.

Seifart, A., Unger, M., & Burger, M. (2009). The effect of lower limb functional electrical stimulation on gait of children with cerebral palsy. *Pediatric Physical Therapy, 21*, 23–30.

Sgoros, S., & Seri, S. (2002). The effect of intrathecal baclofen on muscle co-contraction in children with spasticity of cerebral origin. *Pediatric Neurosurgery, 37*, 225–230.

Shafer, M. F., & Dias, L. S. (1983). *Myelomeningocele: Orthopaedic treatment*. Baltimore, MD: Lippincott Williams & Wilkins.

Shah, P. S., Ohlsson, A., & Perlman, A. (2007). Hypothermia to treat neonatal hypoxic ischemic encephalopathy. *Archives of Pediatrics and Adolescent Medicine, 161*, 951–958.

Shangguan, S., Wang, L., Chang, S., Lu, X., Wang, Z., Wu, L., . . . Zhang, T. (2015). DNA methylation aberrations rather than poly morphisms of FZD3 gene increase the risk of spina bifida in high risk region for neural tube defects. *Birth Defects Research, 103*, 37–44.

Shapiro, A., & Susa, K. Z. (1990). Pre-operative and post-operative gait evaluation in cerebral palsy. *Archives of Physical Medicine and Rehabilitation, 71*, 236–240.

Sharrard, W. J. W. (1964). Posterior iliopsoas transplantation in the treatment of paralytic dislocation of the hip. *Journal of Bone and Joint Surgery, 46-B*, 426–444.

Sherk, H. H., Uppal, G. S., Lane, G., & Melchionni, J. (1991). Treatment versus non-treatment of hip dislocations in ambulatory patients with myelomeningocele. *Developmental Medicine and Child Neurology, 33*, 491–494.

Shields, N., Murdoch, A., Loy, Y., Dodd, K. J., & Taylor, N. F. (2006). A systematic review of the self-concept of children with cerebral palsy compared with children without disability. *Developmental Medicine & Child Neurology, 48*, 151–157.

Sigurdardottir, S., Halldorsdottir, M., Thorkelsson, T., Thorarensen, O., & Vik, T. (2009). Trends in prevalence and characteristics of cerebral palsy among Icelandic children born 1990 to 2003. *Developmental Medicine and Child Neurology, 51*, 356–363.

Sillanpaa, M., Piekkala, P., & Pisira, H. (1982). The young adult with cerebral palsy and his chances of employment. *International Journal of Rehabilitation Research, 5*, 467–476.

Silva, S., Nowick, P., Caird, M. S., Hurvitz, E. A., Ayyangar, R. N., Farley, F. A., . . . Craig, C. L. (2012). A comparison of hip dislocation rates and hip containment procedures after selective dorsal ehizotomy versus Intrathecal Baclofen pump insertion in non ambulatory patients. *Journal of Pediatric Othropaedics, 32*, 853–856.

Sinha, C. K., Grewal, A., & Ward, H. C. (2008). Antegrade continence enema (ACE): Current practice. *Pediatric Surgery International, 24*, 685–688.

Siperstein, G. N., Wolraich, M. L., Reed, D., & O'Keefe, P. (1988). Medical decisions and prognostications of pediatricians for infants with myelomeningocele. *Journal of Pediatrics, 113*, 835–840.

Siracusa, C., Taylor, M., Geletka, B., & Overby, A. (2005). Effectiveness of biomechanical intervention in children with cerebral palsy. *Pediatric Physical Therapy, 17*, 83–84.

Slater, J. E. (1989). Rubber anaphylaxis. *New England Journal of Medicine, 320*, 1126–1129.

Smith, K. A. (1991). Bowel and bladder management of the child with myelomeningocele in the school setting. *Journal of Pediatric Health Care, 4*, 175–180.

Smith, S., Camfield, C., & Camfield, D. (1999). Living with cerebral palsy and tube feeding: A population-based follow-up study. *Journal of Pediatrics, 135*, 307–310.

Sotiriadis, A., Tsiami, A., Papatheodoroo, S., Bascaht, A., Sarafidis, K., & Makrydimas, G. (2015). Neurodevelopmental outcome after a singe course of antenatal steroids in children born preterm. A systematic review and meta-analysis. *Obstetrics & Gynecology, 125*, 1385–1396.

Sousa, J. C., Gordon, L. H., & Shurtleff, D. B. (1976). Assessing the development of daily living skills in patients with spina bifida. *Developmental Medicine and Child Neurology, 37*(Suppl. 18), 134–143.

Spates, C. R., Samaraweera, N., Plaiser, B., Souza, T., & Otsui, K. (2007). Psychological impact of trauma on developing children and youth. *Primary Care: Clinics in Office Practice, 34*, 387–405.

Spindel, M. R., Bauer, S. B., & Dyron, I. M. (1987). The changing lesion in myelodysplasia. *Journal of the American Medical Association, 258*, 1630–1633.

Spittle, A. M., Orton, J., Anderson, P. J., Boyd, R., & Doyle, L. W. (2015). Early developmental intervention programmes provided post hospital discharge to prevent motor and cognitive impairment in preterm infants. *Cochrane Database of Sytematic Reviews, 24*(11), CD005495.

Staheli, L. T. L. (2015). *Fundamentals of pediatric orthopedics* (5th ed.). New York, NY: Lippincott Williams & Wilkins.

Staheli, L. T. L., Duncan, W. R., & Schaefer, E. (1960). Growth alterations in the hemiplegic child. *Clinical Orthopaedics and Related Research, 60*, 205–212.

Stark, C., Heyer- Kuhn, H. -K., Semler, O., Hoebing, L., Dura, I., Cremer, R., & Schoenau, E. (2015). Neuromuscular training based on whole body vibration in children with spina bifida: A retrospective analysis of a new physiotherapy treatment program. *Child's Nervous System,* 31, 301–309.

Stallard, J., Major, R. E., & Farmer, S. E. (1996). The potential for ambulation by severely handicapped cerebral palsy patients. *Prosthetics and Orthototics International, 20*, 122–128.

Stanley, F., & Blair, E. (1991). Why we have failed to reduce the frequency of cerebral palsy? *Medical Journal of Australia, 154*, 623–626.

Stein, R., Assion, C., Beetz, R., Burst, M., Cremer, R., Ermert, A., . . . Wagner, W. (2015). Neurogenic bladder function disorders in patients with myelomemingocele S2k guidelines and therapy. *Urology,* 54, 239–253.

Steinbok, P., Reiner, A. M., Beauchamp, R., Armstrong, R. W., & Cochrane, D. D. (1997). A randomized clinical trial to compare selective posterior rhizotomy plus physiotherapy with physiotherapy alone in children with spastic diplegic cerebral palsy. *Developmental Medicine and Child Neurology, 39*, 178–184.

Stothard, K. J., Tennant, P., Bell, R., & Rankin, J. (2009). Maternal overweight and obesity and the risk of congenital anomalies. A systemic review and meta-analysis. *Journal of the American Medical Association, 301*, 636–650.

Strauss, D., Cable, W., & Shavelte, R. (1999). Causes of excess mortality in cerebral palsy. *Developmental Medicine and Child Neurology, 41*, 580–585.

Streeter, G. L. (1942). Developmental horizons in human embryos: Description of age group XI: 13 to 20 somites, and age group XII, 21–29 somites. *Contributions in Embryology, 30*, 211–245.

Strobi, W., Theologis, T., Bronner, R., Kocer, S., Viehwgwer, E., Pascual, I., & Placzek, R. (2015). Best clinical practice in botulinum toxin treatment for children with cerebral palsy. *Toxins*, 7, 1629–1648.

Sutherland, D. H. (1984). *Gait disorders of childhood and adolescence*. Baltimore, MD: Williams & Wilkins.

Swaminathan, S., Patton, J. Y., Ward, S. D. L., Jacobs, R. A., Sargent, C. W., & Keens, T. G. (1989). Abnormal control of ventilation in adolescents with myelodysplasia. *Journal of Pediatrics, 115*, 898–903.

Sweetser, P. M., Badell, A., Schneider, S., & Badlin, G. H. (1995). Effects of sacral dorsal rhizotomy on bladder function in patients with spastic cerebral palsy. *Neuroradiology and Urodyanamics, 14*, 57–64.

Szalay, E. A., Harriman, D., Eastlund, B., & Mercer, D. (2008). Quantifying postoperative bone loss in children. *Journal of Pediatric Orthopaedics, 28*, 320–323.

Talwar, D. D., Baldwin, N. A., & Hornblatt, C. (1995). Epilepsy in children with myelomeningocele. *Pediatric Neurology, 13*, 29–32.

Tanaka, H. M., Fukada, I., Miyamoto, A., Oka, R., Cho, K., & Fujieda, K. (2004). Effects of tizanidine for refractory sleep disturbance in disabled children with spastic quadriparesis. *No to Hattatsu, 36*, 455–460.

Tardieu, C., de la Tour, H., Bret, N. D., & Tardieu, G. (1982). Muscle hypoextensibility in children with cerebral palsy. *Archives of Physical Medicine and Rehabilitation, 63*, 97–110.

Tardieu, C., & Lespargot, A. (1988). For how long must the soleus muscle be stretched each day to prevent contracture? *Developmental Medicine and Child Neurology, 30*, 3019.

Tardorf, K. (1986). Spontaneous remission in cerebral palsy. *Neuropediatrics, 17*, 19–22.

Teo, C., & Jones, R. (1996). Management of hydrocephalus by endoscopic third ventriculostomy in patients with myelomeningocele. *Pediatric Neurosurgery, 25*, 57–63.

Tew, B. (1979). The "cocktail party syndrome" in children with hydrocephalus and spina bifida. *British Journal of Disorders of Communication, 14*, 89–101.

Thomas, S. S., Aiona, M. D., Pierce, R., & Piatt, J. H. (1996). Gait changes in children with spastic diplegia after selective dorsal rhizotomy. *Journal of Pediatric Orthopaedics, 16*, 474–452.

Thomason, P., Rodda, J., Sangeux, M., Seiber, P., & Kerr, G. (2012). Management of children with ambulatory cerebral palsy. *Journal of Pediatric Orthopaedics, 32*, s182–s186.

Timbolschi, D., Schafer, E., Monga, B., Fattori, D., Dott, B., Favre, R., Kohler, M., . . . Doray, B. (2015). Neural tube defects the experience of the registry of congenital malformation of fetal diagnosis and therapy. Alsace, France 1995-2009. *Fetal Diagnosis and Therapy*, 37, 6–17.

Tirosh, E., & Rabino, S. (1989). Physiotherapy for children with cerebral palsy. *American Journal of Diseases in Childhood, 143*, 551–553.

Tobimatsu, Y., & Nakamura, R. (2000). Retrospective study of factors affecting employability of individuals with cerebral palsy in Japan. *Tohoku Journal of Experimental Medicine, 192*, 291–299.

Tomlinson, P., & Sugarman, I. D. (1995). Complications in shunts in adults with spina bifida. *American Journal of Diseases in Childhood, 143*, 551–553.

Torre, M., Planche, D., Louis-Borrione, C., Sabiani, F., Lena, G., & Guys, J. M. (2002). Value of electrophysiological assessment after surgical treatment of spinal dysraphism. *Journal of Urology, 168*, 1759–1763.

Tscharnuter, I. (2002). Clinical application of dynamic theory concepts according to Tscharnuter Akademie for Movement Organizations (TAMO) therapy. *Pediatric Physical Therapy, 14*, 29–37.

Turk, M., Scandale, J., Rosenbaum, P. F., & Weber, R. J. (2001). The health of women with cerebral palsy. *Physical Medicine and Rehabilitation Clinics of North America, 12*, 153–166.

Unnithan, V., Katsmanis, G., Evangelinou, C., Kosmas, C., Kandrali, I., & Kellis, E. (2007). Effect of strength and aerobic training in children with cerebral palsy. *Medicine and Science in Sports and Exercise, 39*, 1902–1909.

Valvano, J. (2004). Activity-focused motor interventions for children with neurological conditions. *Physical and Occupational Therapy in Pediatrics, 24*, 79–107.

Van der Dussen, L., Nieustraten, W., Roebroeck, M., & Stam, H. J. (2001). Functional level of young adults with cerebral palsy. *Clinical Rehabilitation, 15*, 84–91.

VanHeest, A. E., Bagley, A., Molitar, F., & James, M. A. (2015). Tendon transfer surgery in upper extremity cerebral palsy is more effective than Botlinum injections or regular ongoing therapy. *Journal of Bone and Joint Surgery, 97-A*, 529–536.

Van Mechelen, M. C., Verheof, M., van Asbeck, F., & Post, M. W. M. (2008). Work participation among young adults with spina bifida in the Netherlands. *Developmental Medicine & Child Neurology, 50*, 772–777.

Vannucci, R. C. (1990). Experimental biology of cerebral hypoxic ischemia: Relationship of perinatal brain damage. *Pediatric Research, 27*, 317–326.

Veland, P. M., Hosted, S., Schneede, J., Refsum, H., & Vollset, S. (2001). Biological and clinical implications of MTHFR C677T polymorphism. *Trends in Pharmacological Science, 22*, 195–201.

Verbeek, R. I., Hoving, E. W., Mauritis, N. M., Brouwer, O. F., Vanderhoevern, J. H., & Sival, D. A. (2014). Muscle ultrasound quantifies segmental neuromuscular outcome in pediatric myelomeningocele. *Ultrasound in Medicine & Biology, 40*, 71–77.

Verhoef, M., Barf, H. A., Post, M. W. M., van Asbeck, F., Rob, H., & Arie, J. H. (2006). Functional independence among young adults with spina bifida, in relation to hydrocephalus and level of lesion. *Developmental Medicine and Child Neurology, 48*, 114–119.

Verhoef, M., Barf, H. A., Vroege, J. A., van Asbeck, F. W., Gooskens, R. H., & Prevo, A. J. (2005). Sex education, relationships, and sexuality in young adults with spina bifida. *Archives of Physical Medicine and Rehabilitation, 86*, 979–987.

Verhoef, M., Lurvink, M., Barf, H. A., Post, M. W. M., van Asbeck, F. W. A., Gooskens, R. H. J. M., & Prevo, A. J. (2005). High prevalence of incontinence among young adults with spina bifida: Description, prediction and problem perception. *Spinal Cord, 43*, 331–340.

Vinck, A., Maassen, B., Mullaart, R., & Rotteveel, J. (2006). Arnold-Chiari II malformation and cognitive functioning in spina bifida. *Journal of Neurology, Neurosurgery, and Psychiatry, 77*, 1083–1086.

Vohr, B. R., & Msall, M. E. (1997). Neuropsycholgical and functional outcomes of very low birth weight infants. *Seminars in Perinatology, 21*, 202–220.

Vuillermin, C., Rodda, J., Utz, E., Shore, B., Smith, K., & Graham, J. (2011). Severe crouch gait in spastic diplegia can be prevented. *Journal of Bone and Joint Surgery, 93-B*, 1670–1675.

Wagner, K., Risnes, I., Berntsen, T., Skaro, A., Ramberg, B., Vandvik, I. H., . . . Svennevig, J. L. (2007). Clinical and psychosocial follow-up of children treated with extracorporeal membrane oxygenation. *Annals of Thoracic Surgery, 84*, 1349–1355.

Wallace, S. J. (1973). The effect of upper-limb function on mobility of children with myelomeningocele. *Developmental Medicine and Child Neurology, 15*, 84–91.

Wallender, J. K., Babani, L., Varni, J. W., Banis, H. T., & Wilcox, K. T. (1989). Family resources as resistance factors for psychological maladjustment in chronically ill and handicapped children. *Journal of Pediatric Psychology, 14*, 157–173.

Wang, A., Brown, E. G., Lankford, K., Kellier, B. A., Pivetti, C. D., Sitkin, N. A., . . . Farmer, D. L. (2015). Placental mesenchymal stromal cells rescue ambulation in ovine myelomenigocele. *Stem Cells Translational Medicine, 4*, 659–669.

Warschausky, S., Kaufman, J. P., & Stiers, W. (2008). Training requirements and scope of practice in rehabilitation psychology and neuropsychology. *Journal of Pediatric Rehabilitation Medicine: An Interdisciplinary Approach, 1*, 61–65.

Wei, S., Su-juan, W., Yuan-Gui, L., Hong, Y., Xiu-Juan, X. U., & Xiao-Mei, S. (2006). Reliability and validity of the GMFM-66 in 0–3-year old children with cerebral palsy. *American Journal of Physical Medicine and Rehabilitation, 85*, 141–147.

Williams, M. D., Lewandowski, L. J., Coplan, J., & D'Eugenio, D. B. (1987). Neurodevelopmental outcome of preschool children born preterm with and without intracranial hemorrhage. *Developmental Medicine and Child Neurology, 29*, 243–249.

Wills, K. E., Holmbeck, G. N., Dillon, K., & McClone, D. G. (1990). Intelligence and achievement in children with myelomeningocele. *Journal of Pediatrics Psychology, 15*, 161–176.

Wilson, H., Haideri, M. E., Song, K., & Telford, D. (1997). Ankle foot orthosis for preambulatory children with spastic diplegia. *Journal of Pediatric Orthopaedics, 17*, 370–376.

Worley, G., Rosenfeld, L. R., & Lipscomb, J. (1991a). Financial counseling for families of children with chronic disabilities. *Developmental Medicine and Child Neurology*, 679–689.

Worley, G., Rosenfeld, L. R., & Lipscomb, J. (1991b). Influence on survival of cervical laminectomy for children with meningomyelocele who have potentially lethal brainstem dysfunction due to the Chiari II malformation. *Developmental Medicine and Child Neurology, 33*(Suppl. 64), 19–26.

Worley, G., Schuster, J. M., & Oakes, W. J. (1996). Survival at 5 years of a cohort of newborn infants with myelomeningocele. *Developmental Medicine and Child Neurology, 38*, 816–822.

Wu, Y. W., Croen, L. A., Vanderwerf, A., Geifand, A. A., & Torres, A. R. (2011). Candidate genes and risk for CP: A population-based study. *Pediatric Research, 70*, 642–646.

Yamada, S., Zinke, D. E., & Saunders, D. (1981). Pathophysiology of tethered cord syndrome. *Journal of Neurosurgery, 54*, 494–503.

Yokochi, K. (1997). Thalamic lesions revealed by MRI associated with periventricular leukomalacia and clinical profiles of suspect. *Acta Paediatrica Scandinavica, 86*, 493–496.

Yoshida, F., Morioka, T., Hashiguchi, K., Kawamura, T., Miyagi, Y., Nagata, S., . . . Sasaki, T. (2006). Epilepsy in patients with spina bifida in the lumbosacral region. *Neurosurgical Review, 29*, 327–332.

Young, N. L. (2007). The transition to adulthood for children with cerebral palsy: What do we know about their health care needs? *Journal of Pediatric Orthopaedics, 27*, 476–479.

Young, R. R., & Delwaide, P. J. (1981). Drug therapy: Spasticity. *New England Journal of Medicine, 304*, 28–43.

Young, N. L., Mc Cormick, A., Mills, W., Barden, W., Law, M., Wedge, J., . . . Williams, J. I. (2006). The transitions study: A look at youth and adults with cerebral palsy, spina bifida, and acquired brain injury. *Physical and Occupational Therapy in Pediatrics, 26*, 25–45.

Zaccario, M., Salsberg, D., Gordon, R., & Bilginer, L. (2010). Psychological and neuropsychological issues in the care of children with disabilities. *Journal of Pediatric Rehabilitation Medicine*, 2(2), 93–99.

Zarfonte, R., Lornard, L., & Elovic, E. (2004). Antispasticity medications: Uses and limitations of enteral therapy. *American Journal of Physical Medicine and Rehabilitation, 83*, s50–s66.

Zhao, X., Xiao, N., Li, H., & Du, S. (2013). Day vs. Day –Night use ankle foot orthosis in young children with spastic diplegia: A randomized controlled study. *American Journal of Physical Medicine Rehabilitation, 92*, 905–911.

Zide, B., Constantini, S., & Epstein, F. J. (1995). Prevention of recurrent tethered spinal cord. *Pediatric Neurosurgery, 22*, 111–1143.

Ziv, I., Blackborn, N., Rang, M., & Koresk, J. (1984). Muscle growth in normal and spastic mice. *Developmental Medicine and Child Neurology, 26*, 94–99.

CHAPTER

Geriatric Rehabilitation

Adrian Cristian, Armando Iannicello, Joan Y. Hou, Laurentiu I. Dinescu, Kirill Alekseyev, Nnabugo Ozurumba, and Andrew Brash

INTRODUCTION

The goals of geriatric rehabilitation are to maximize function and minimize activity limitations and restrictions on participation in daily life for older adults. This is accomplished in a variety of settings including acute inpatient rehabilitation facilities, skilled nursing facilities, outpatient rehabilitation clinics, and the home of the older adult. It is common for older adults to have multiple comorbid conditions such as diabetes mellitus, hypertension, coronary artery disease, congestive heart failure, and chronic obstructive pulmonary disease, pointing to the need for an individualized program with adequate precautions that minimizes the risk of injury to the person undergoing a rehabilitation program.

This chapter begins with a description of the demographic changes facing the U.S. population and the impact of these changes on the delivery of health care. It is then followed by a description of the physiological and anatomic changes associated with the aging process and key points to consider in the clinical assessment of the older adult. This is then followed by sections on exercise in the elderly, delirium and dementia, frailty, falls and fractures, traumatic brain injury, and pain management—all important topics for the practicing clinician providing care to the geriatric individual.

THE "GRAYING" OF THE UNITED STATES

Demographics

The United States is currently experiencing a twofold shift in demographics. The part of the population that "boomed" in the 1950s and 1960s are entering their senior years (Halaweish & Alam, 2015). As life expectancy increases, the number of persons aged 65 years and older will increase from 12.4% in 2000 to 20.2% in 2050 (Halaweish & Alam, 2015). Within the segment of the population aged 65 years and older, 50% of women and 60% of men are in the 65 to 74 age group, 33.3% of both men and women are aged 75 to 84 years, and 16.6% of women and 10% of men are aged 85 years and older.

Women constitute most of the older population. However, the gap between male and female life expectancies has been steadily narrowing. As of 2008, the difference in life expectancy was 5 years. The life expectancy of men and women aged 65 and older is reduced to less than 3 years, and only one-year difference by the age of 85. Changes in the demographics associated with aging will also be reflected along ethnic and racial lines (Halaweish & Alam, 2015).

Aging and Disease

While advances in modern medicine have helped enhance the quality of life and foster longevity, the risk of developing complex disease states still increases with age. The prevalence of comorbidities is significantly higher in the geriatric population, with each older person experiencing an average of two or three multiple chronic conditions (Halaweish & Alam, 2015). Almost half of Americans in the geriatric population report having hypertension and nearly 25% of both men and women report as afflicted with a coronary artery disease. Other common comorbidities of the elderly include obesity, arthritis, diabetes, stroke, cancer, and dementia. The prevalence of diabetes among geriatric Americans varies from 22% to 33%. This is associated with decreased functional status and is projected to have a 4.5-fold increase in adults older than 65 years (Halaweish & Alam, 2015).

Chronic conditions such as arthritis, injury related to falls, and coronary artery disease are common causes of disability. Survival with cardiovascular disease and cancers might have improved, but no evidence exists that their incidence is actually decreasing. Since the incidence of musculoskeletal disorders and arthritis is increasing, this expansion of life with disease is in concurrence with a steady rise of activities of daily living (ADLs) and instrumental activities of daily living (IADL) limitations in the older population (Chatterji et al., 2015).

Increased life expectancy also means an increase in the likelihood of developing cancer as a consequence of modern life. While the life expectancy in 1900 was only 48 years for men and 51 for women, the increase in longevity today provides for prolonged carcinogen exposure and thus increased cancer burden (Franceschi & La Vecchia, 2001). Similarly, earlier detection and lifestyle are related to increased cancer incidence in the elderly. More than 60% of new cancers occur in people over 65 years of age.

As of 2007, 60% of the 10 million cancer survivors were 65 years or older (Avis & Deimling, 2008). For newly diagnosed and long-term survivors, the presence of comorbidities at older ages can have a detrimental effect on physical and psychological quality of life with and after cancer. Reports of pain and weakness are common complaints with regard to function, while fears of new or recurring cancers can have a significant psychological effect (Avis & Deimling, 2008).

Aging and Disability

The cumulative impact of age-related comorbidities often results in disability and has a negative impact on the ability to perform essential activities of daily living (ADL; Rajan et al., 2012). Difficulty in performing ADLs such as dressing and bathing are very prevalent, with more than 50% of adults over the age of 65 reporting limitations. The number approaches 90% in those over the age of 85 (Halaweish & Alam, 2015).

According to a 2010 population report by the U.S. Census Bureau, National Health Interview Survey data found the prevalence of doctor-diagnosed arthritis to be 50% among the population aged 65 and older. For every 1,000 persons aged 65 to 74, 122 reported activity limitations caused by arthritis or other musculoskeletal disorders. The rate rose to 167 per 1,000 people for those aged 75 to 84 and to 281 per 1,000 people for those aged 85 and older. Researchers have found that women have a higher prevalence of arthritis than men (West, Cole, Goodkind, & He, 2010).

Another big contributor to disability is stroke. As of 2011, reports indicated that 75% to 89% of strokes occur in individuals over 65 years of age. Of these strokes, 50% occur in people who are age 70 years or older and nearly 25% in individuals who are aged over 85 years. Stroke is the largest cause of adult disability, with up to half of all patients who survive a stroke failing to regain independence and needing long-term health care (Chen et al., 2010).

The Health and Retirement Study (HRS), a longitudinal cohort study among the elderly in the United States, found a greater incidence of disabilities affecting physical function during retirement than in full-time work when aged 65 years or older. Work provides the structure, social relationships, and satisfaction of accomplishment vital to a full, active life. Previous studies have shown that social participation, social support, and social capital are associated with better physical functioning (Stenholm et al., 2014).

Aging and Mental Illness

Overall, 20% of people aged 55 years or older express symptoms of mental illness. Conditions such as cognitive impairment, mood disorders, and anxiety are most commonly reported (Centers for Disease Control and Prevention [CDC] and National Association of Chronic Disease Directors, 2008).

Older men have the highest rate of suicide among any group. Men aged 85 years or older have a suicide rate of 45.23 per 100,000 persons compared to an overall rate of 11.01 per 100,000. Adults aged 65 or older reported more frequently that they "rarely" or "never" received the social and emotional support they needed compared to younger adults (CDC and National Association of Chronic Disease Directors, 2008).

With a projected growth of the older population, an increasing prevalence of dementia will have a deep impact on the geriatric population and the health care system. As of 2014, 5.2 million Americans were diagnosed with Alzheimer's disease, the most common form of dementia. Five million of these persons are aged 65 years or older (Halaweish & Alam, 2015). Comorbidities result in more frequent hospitalizations and health care assistance, resulting in substantial costs to society (Halaweish & Alam, 2015).

Impact of Aging on Health Care Delivery

The most significant change in the future will be the substantial growth of the geriatric population, specifically those aged 85 years and older, the oldest-old. This population has high rates of disability and need for long-term care, hence the financial costs associated with the care of the oldest-old will be high (Halaweish & Alam, 2015). It has been reported that the cost of health care for persons older than 65 years is three to five times higher than the cost of providing care to a younger population. Costs associated with health care are expected to increase by 25% over the next 15 years due to medical needs of the aging U.S. population (Harris-Kojetin, Sengupta, Park-Lee, & Valverde, 2013).

The service side of health care is also witnessing an age-related impact on both its nature and its numbers. There is a direct relationship between increasing age and number of physician visits. On average, persons aged 75 years and older have more than 7 visits per person per year (Halaweish & Alam, 2015). Persons older than 65 years also account for a high percentage of hospitalizations, which result in longer lengths of stay and higher incurred costs compared to younger populations. The most common reasons for hospitalizations in the elderly are the treatment of heart disease, pneumonia, stroke, cancer, and fractures (Halaweish & Alam, 2015).

Medication is another sphere of health care affected by the trends seen in older adults. Americans aged 65 and older account for the purchase of 30% of all prescriptions and 40% of over-the-counter drugs. The average nursing home patient receives four to seven different medications daily. Thirty percent of elderly patients are taking eight or more prescription drugs daily, and the elderly population as a whole takes an average of 18 prescription drugs per year.

Here, too, we see pitfalls that highlight a need for reform. A large study of patients 65 and older found that 20% were provided at least one prescription for an inappropriate medicine. Over 175,000 people in the United States aged 65 or older will visit an emergency department due to an adverse reaction to commonly prescribed medications ("Statistics," 2012).

Among persons who need long-term care services, those aged 65 and older are more likely than younger adults to receive financial assistance (Harris-Kojetin et al., 2013). As of 2012, there were nearly 1.4 million people in nursing homes and about 4.7 million patients receiving services from home health agencies. California, New York, New Jersey, and Texas had the highest rates of enrollment for adult day-service centers. The recipient population of these long-term care services in the geriatric population were overwhelmingly female (Harris-Kojetin et al., 2013).

PHYSIOLOGICAL CHANGES ASSOCIATED WITH AGING

Aging precipitates numerous structural and mechanical changes that affect all organ systems. Although normal, these changes can predispose an individual to development of disease and disability. There are many theories about the mechanisms that drive the aging process. These include theories related to genetic programming, suggesting that our life span is predetermined, and theories related to the accumulation of physiologic wear-and-tear from harmful events. Aging is a process that begins from birth and involves several physiological phenomena such as a decrease in metabolic rate, paucity of tissue proteins, tissue atrophy, and decrease in cell counts. These lead to impaired functioning in immunity, the cardiopulmonary system, and the neurological and endocrine systems. Normal changes in the human body associated with aging are briefly discussed in the following sections.

Homeostenosis

Homeostenosis is a concept that refers to the inability of the body and its normal processes to maintain homeostasis when faced with stressors.

As the aging process continues, the physiologic reserves, which buffer the function of all organ systems, become depleted. Therefore, the elderly are prone to loss of homeostasis when faced with challenges demanding a greater physiologic reserve. This leads to increased vulnerability to disease and eventual frailty.

Cardiovascular System

A number of anatomical and physiological changes occur with aging. Anatomical changes occur to a greater degree in the left side of the heart than the right, with enlarging of the left atrium and stiffening of the left ventricle. Left ventricular wall thickness increases by an average of 10% (Gates, 2003). Thickening of the aortic valve and mitral annulus are seen, along with development of calcific deposits (Kitzman, 1988). There is a reduction in cardiac myocytes through apoptosis and necrosis. Cell loss also occurs at the sinoatrial and atrioventricular nodes. This may be related to the sensitivity to calcium channel blockers in the elderly.

There is a marked decrease in the maximum heart rate when undergoing exercise or facing other stressors. Intrinsic heart rate (without sympathetic/parasympathetic input) decreases by five or six beats per minute each decade after 25 years of age (Taffet, 2015). The adaptations to exercise such as increased stroke work, cardiac output, left ventricular function, and peripheral arterio-venous oxygen difference do not occur as efficiently in the elderly (Jaramillo, 2015).

With regard to hypertension, the elderly show a greater increase in systolic blood pressure than diastolic. There is decreased arterial compliance. Myocardial stiffness is seen due to increased interstitial fibrosis. Amyloid deposition in the myocardium occurs. Increased afterload due to thoracic aorta thickening causes outflow tract stiffness (Rughwani, 2011).

Also seen is the irregularity of endothelial cells, increased amount of connective tissue, and lipid deposits in the blood vessels contributing to atherosclerosis. These changes can lead to hypertension, cardiac arrhythmia, and increased susceptibility to myocardial infarction and stroke even though the cardiac output of the aging heart remains normal at rest. The elderly have a decreased inotropic (force of cardiac contraction) response to catecholamines and cardiac glycosides. There is an increased prevalence in atrial premature beats and ventricular ectopic beats.

Pulmonary System

There is a decrease in the number of alveoli and lung capillaries in the aging process. The alveoli enlarge because of loss of elastic fibers, resulting in less surface area for gas exchange. Approximately one third of the surface area per volume of lung tissue is lost as aging progresses (Janssens, 2005).

Age-related anatomic and functional changes of the respiratory system lead to increased likelihood of acquiring pneumonia and decreased oxygen uptake. Also of concern is an increase in chest wall stiffness, impaired intercostal muscle contraction, and less effective ventilation assistance from abdominal muscles, especially in the seated or supine positions. The diaphragm is less efficient due to flattening and decreased compliance of the muscle, thereby contributing to the increased work of breathing (Polkey, 1997).

Pulmonary function testing reveals additional changes associated with aging. There is an increase in the residual volume, decrease in vital capacity (40%–50%) by age 70, and a decrease in the forced expiratory volume in 1 second (particularly in the seventh and eighth decade; Kuster, 2008; Rughwani, 2011). The cough mechanism becomes weakened and is less effective at mucociliary clearance.

Digestive System

Aging-related changes in the digestive system include pharyngeal muscle weakness, reduction in stomach acid production, delay in emptying time, and reduction in the absorption of calcium, vitamin D, and iron. Constipation is common and diverticulosis can be seen in about one third of healthy adults older than 65 years and two thirds of adults over 80 years old. These changes can result in malabsorption and malnutrition.

Nutrition intake involves both peripheral and central mechanisms. There is a diminished central feeding drive, impaired thirst sensation, and, combined with changes in odor and taste, malnutrition becomes common among the elderly.

Decreased saliva production (decreased acinar cells), particularly involving saliva production from the parotid gland, is seen. There is thinning of the epithelium of the oral mucosa. Receding of the gum line leads to decay and dental caries (Taffet, 2015).

Increased resistance to flow across the upper esophageal sphincter leads to less effective food clearance in the pharynx. This elevates the risk for aspiration. With regard to motility, there is a decreased peristaltic response, increased esophageal transit time, and impaired relaxation of the lower esophageal sphincter.

Early satiety further impairs nutrition in the elderly. In the stomach, nitric oxide production decreases in the fundus, decreasing relaxation. This leads to a more rapid stretch and earlier satiety (Morley et al., 1996). Cholecystokinin release is greater in response to a fat load (McIntosh et al., 1999). Atrophic gastritis is common in the elderly. Acid production in the stomach decreases, leading to impaired absorption of vitamin B_{12}, calcium, zinc, and folic acid (Rosenberg, 1994). Women older than 75 years absorb 25% less calcium than younger women (Salles, 2007).

In the large intestine, a decrease in myenteric plexus neurons results in reduced motility. The elderly have an increased sensitivity to opioids, predisposing them to drug-induced constipation. Diverticuli are common, particularly in Western populations.

Liver mass decreases between 20% and 40% with age and hepatic blood flow is reduced by 50% (Mclean, 2004). Lipofuscin accumulates in hepatocytes. Although general liver function declines with age, liver function test values are minimally affected by aging. Low-density lipoprotein (LDL) cholesterol metabolism decreases, leading to increased serum levels of LDL. Cytochrome P450 activity decreases with age affecting drug clearance. There is decreased synthesis of vitamin K-dependent clotting factors. This contributes to a greater sensitivity when using vitamin K antagonists for anticoagulation (Taffet, 2015).

Genitourinary System

Aging has multiple effects on the renal system. These changes are important as they predispose the elderly to impaired clearance of toxins and drug metabolites. Kidney size decreases accompanied by a 25% to 30% reduction in weight. The majority of this decline is apparent after age 50 (Taffet, 2015). Cortical volume, as well as the number of glomeruli, decreases. Glomerular filtration rate (GFR) and renal tubule function are lowered. GFR is reduced by 50% by age 80. This is a consequence of a decrease in renal cells, hardening of the renal vessels, and diffuse sclerosis of the glomeruli with 30% destroyed by age 75 (Nyengaard, 1992). Renal blood flow decreases by 40% in healthy normotensive older men, further magnified by conditions that stimulate renal vasodilation (Fuiano, 2001).

Vasodilating prostaglandins are increased at baseline in older adults, contributing to risk of renal injury with nonsteroidal anti-inflammatory drug (NSAID) use (Whelton, 1999). There is decreased production of creatinine in aging (decreased muscle mass) associated with increased tubular secretion of creatinine.

The kidneys have decreased ability to eliminate toxins, medications, and drugs, with increased risk of perioperative ischemic damage, nephrotoxicity related to medications, and IV contrast-induced nephropathy. Other impairments involve the kidney's ability to retain water, solute, amino acids, and glucose. There is a reduction in the ability to acidify the urine, leading to inability to effectively excrete acid buildup in the body. There is decreased vitamin D activation, contributing to its deficiency.

Aging of the genitourinary system is often associated with urinary incontinence, urinary tract infections, erectile dysfunction, and dyspareunia (pain during sexual activity). Urinary incontinence is more common in women until age 80. Thereafter the prevalence is equalized between the genders. This process is related to weakening of the detrusor muscle, decreased bladder capacity (500–600 cc in younger populations compared to 250–600 cc in older populations), increased postvoid residual (volume of urine remaining in the bladder after voluntary voiding) and central changes (Tadic, 2012). The sensation of bladder fullness is diminished as is impaired control over voluntary voiding.

Sexual activity impairment is common in the elderly. There are multiple processes associated with the sexual act that are impaired, which result as a consequence of a number of vascular, neurological, and endocrine changes. Prostate gland enlargement due to hyperplasia is common in older men.

Integumentary System

Normal aging processes along with environmental factors such as "photo-aging" influence skin aging.

The moisture content of the skin, rate of epidermal renewal, elasticity, sebum secretion, vascular supply, hair and nail growth, sensitivity to touch, pain, and temperature all decrease, making the skin more vulnerable to damage and disease. Decreased subcutaneous fat and poor capillary function increase the risk of developing pressure ulcers. The skin also becomes more susceptible to shearing forces. This is related to epidermal thinning and decrease of the dermal layers. Decreased skin elasticity is also seen. The skin's ability to function as a protective barrier is impaired, leading to increased susceptibility to injury, infection, poor wound healing, and weak scar formation. Xerosis is also common among the elderly as is a decrease in Langerhans cells in the skin.

Furthermore, thermoregulation is affected by a decrease in sweat glands in the skin, decreased subdermal fat, and vasoconstrictive ability. Loss of Meissner's and Pacinian corpuscles leads to impaired touch and vibratory sensation. The skin's role in vitamin D synthesis is also impaired (Rughwani, 2011; Taffet, 2015).

Endocrine System

In general, as we age, hormone production is reduced and the response to hormones is also blunted. The function of the hypothalamus, pituitary gland, and end organs like the thyroid, parathyroid, adrenal glands, pancreas, and gonads change with age. Decreased feedback inhibition of the hypothalamic–pituitary–adrenal axis can result in imbalance of growth hormone, thyroid production, and a decrease in estrogen, progesterone, and testosterone production. Age-related endocrine dysfunctions put elderly people at risk for osteoporosis, osteoarthritis (OA), and diabetes. Other changes are seen in skin, hair, bone, and body fat composition. The anabolic response is impaired, with decreased production of growth hormone and insulin-like growth factor, leading to decreased protein synthesis. Insulin sensitivity and glucose tolerance are hindered.

Hematologic System

In the hematopoietic system, bone marrow mass decreases with increased fat deposition within the marrow. Total circulating white cell counts are stable in aging; however, these cells demonstrate increased clonal expansion, leading to greater chance for developing hematologic malignancies. Platelet count remains stable; however, there is an increase in responsiveness leading to decreased bleeding time. The levels of fibrinogen, Factor V, Factor VII, Factor IX, kininogen, prekallikrein, fibrin degradation fragments, D-dimer, and plasminogen activator inhibitor-1 are all increased with aging (Taffet, 2015). An increased risk for venous thromboembolism is also seen (Silverstein, 2007).

Immune System

The impact of aging on the immune system is known as immunosenescence. Impairments in the immune system associated with aging lead to increased rates of malignancies, infections, and autoimmune diseases. Some of the changes seen include a decreased T and B cell function, as well as a decreased response of naïve B cells to new antigens. Dysregulation of the inflammatory process leads to a different cytokine release profile seen in the elderly. This response has similarities to a low-grade, chronic type response. This phenomenon is also called "inflammaging" (Franceschi, 2014).

Neurological System

Aging-related changes involve both the central and peripheral nervous systems. Anatomic, physiologic, cognitive, and behavioral changes are associated with normal aging. Visual, auditory, motor, and sensory system changes are important as they cause changes in the quality of life and limitation of function. Of note, changes in cognitive function associated with aging include a decline in processing speed of cognitive activity, selective and divided attention, ability to encode new information into memory, and memory retrieval (Harada, Natelson Love, & Triebel, 2013).

The eyes may exhibit small irregular pupils with a diminished reaction to light and near reflexes, as well as reduced ocular range of motion on convergence and upward gaze. Motor changes include the presence of tremors, short-stepped and/or broad-based gait with diminished associated movement, dysmetria, dysdiadochokinesia (inability to perform rapid alternating movements), and prolonged reaction time. Sensory changes are manifested by diminished vibratory sense in the feet and hands in addition to reduced proprioception and increased threshold for light touch, pain, and temperature. Muscle stretch reflexes are often either reduced or absent with impaired righting reflexes.

Total brain volume decreases after age 65 with the loss being most prominent in the frontal and temporal lobes (Driscoll, 2009). Cerebral blood volume decreases by approximately 20% (Rughwani, 2011). Decreased number and impaired functioning of nerve cells is seen. The largest neuron loss is seen in the cerebral cortex and cerebellum. Neuronal axon and dendrite formation becomes impaired (Rughwani, 2011). Alteration in neurotransmitters occurs with age. Acetylcholine decreases due to impaired synthesis, reduced release, and decreased cholinergic and muscarinic neurons (Taffet, 2015). Dopamine and the respective receptors in the striatum and substantia nigra are also decreased.

Changes in the Senses

With regard to vision, loss of periorbital fat, laxity of the eyelids (leading to either ectropion or entropion), thickening and yellowing of the lens, lipid accumulations (arcus senilus), lacrimal gland impairment (decreased lacrimation), fibrosis of the iris, decreased pupil diameter, and thinning of the retina, are all common findings in the aging eye. These changes lead to presbyopia and macular degeneration. The ability of the eye to adapt to changes in lighting is also impaired. Color contrast sensitivity is also impaired (Rughwani, 2011).

Hearing is impaired in the elderly because of changes related to the accumulation and hardening of cerumen, thickening and loss of elasticity of the tympanic membrane, loss of articulation between the middle ear bones, and deterioration of central processing (Rughwani, 2011). Inner ear changes include loss of hair cells in the organ of corti, degeneration of neurons innervating the cochlea and auditory centers, impaired endolymph filtration, stiffening of the basilar membrane, and spiral ligament degeneration (Taffet, 2015). These changes result in presbycusis, sensorineural hearing loss at high frequencies, difficulty with source location of the sound, and impaired discrimination of the target sound from background noise.

The aging process impairs the senses of taste and smell. Smell detection is decreased by 50% by age 80 (Taffet, 2003). Loss of taste is strongly influenced by impaired olfaction. This results in decreased enjoyment during eating.

Muscular System

The cross-sectional area of muscles decreases with age (Kent-Braun, Ng, & Young, 2000). This is thought to be due to a reduction in fiber size, number, and morphological changes in the composition of the muscle itself. This is often investigated using microscopic imaging and muscle biopsies. Studies of the microscopic cross-sectional differences of vastus lateralis muscles between young and elderly subjects revealed that reduction in the total number of fibers within the muscle was more directly correlated with sarcopenia rather than reduction in fiber size (Lexell, 1988).

The morphological structure of muscles in the elderly has been shown to contain less contractile tissues and increased amounts of noncontractile tissue such as adipose, lipofuscin, and connective tissue (Kent-Braun et al., 2000). There is also evidence for selective atrophy of the fiber type. There is a greater proportion of type II (fast twitch) fiber degeneration than type I (slow twitch) fibers (Morley, 2001).

There is a decrease in the number of α-motor neurons associated with the aging process. This, in turn, leads to fewer motor units available. There is an increase in the size of the motor units due to collateral reinnervation to support an increased number of muscle fibers (Roos, Rice, & Vandervoort, 1997). These fibers are typically from denervated type II fibers being reinnervated by type I motor units. The result is a less distinct separation of fast- and slow-twitch fibers.

The decline in protein synthesis leads to a decrease in muscle mass with aging. This decline is more pronounced within the mitochondria, and thought to be due to the accumulation of genetic mutations associated with aging (Nair, 2000). There is also decreased synthesis of myosin heavy chains (MHC), which correlates with a decline in muscle strength. In addition, there is an increased expression of type I and II MHC isoforms. Since these structures are involved in cross-bridging with actin filaments, this ultimately affects the speed of muscle contractions.

Calcium homeostasis within the muscle is also affected in the aging process. Aged skeletal muscle shows reduced depolarization of the sarcoplasmic reticulum due to uncoupling between the SR excitation and calcium release. This results in diminished skeletal muscle force production (Delbono,

Renganathan, & Messi, 1997). The number of existing capillaries in the muscle is diminished in the elderly as compared to younger populations. This could be improved with endurance exercise programs, which can increase the number of new capillaries formed (Coggan et al., 1992).

Loss of muscle may also be caused by a shift in balance between anabolic and catabolic factors. An increase in catabolic factors such as inflammatory cytokines (i.e., IL-1β, TNF-α, & IL-6) may be responsible for some changes seen in sarcopenia. Anabolic factors such as neural growth factors, growth hormones, estrogens, and androgens decrease with aging and lead to muscle loss.

Skeletal System

The maintenance of bone mass is sustained through load-bearing by our body weight, and the forces generated by skeletal muscle on bone. With decreased activity, insufficient load-bearing leads to bone demineralization (Giangregorio, 2002). Bone density is seen to decrease in both cortical and trabecular bone. Decreased vitamin D absorption leads to decreased osteoblastic activity. In addition, there is an imbalance between osteoblastic and osteoclastic activity, leading to impaired bone remodeling and weakening of bone. Women also display further bone loss through changes in the endocrine system associated with menopause.

Physiologic Rhythms

Aging affects physiologic rhythms such as the circadian patterns of body temperature, plasma cortisol, and sleep. Pulsatile secretion of hormones (gonadotropins, growth hormone [GH], thyrotropin, melatonin, adrenocorticotropic hormone [ACTH]) is attenuated with age. This is related, in part, to the loss of neurons in the suprachiasmatic nucleus of the hypothalamus (Veldhuis, 1997).

CLINICAL ASSESSMENT OF THE OLDER ADULT

A comprehensive assessment consists of the chief complaint, history of present illness, medical history, and review of systems, allergies, a psychosocial assessment (including an evaluation for substance abuse), functional history, and comprehensive physical examination. History taking is a critical component of patient assessment. A careful and comprehensive evaluation of the older adult is imperative to both identifying the clinical problems and subsequently determining the appropriate rehabilitation plan. Various age-related sensory limitations (such as vision and hearing) can present a challenge in obtaining histories directly from older patients. Interview sessions should be individualized based on the patient's ability; however, information from other sources (physician, family members, or home aide) may be needed. It is equally important to include an evaluation for the presence of depression since the incidence of depression is 10% to 15% in community-dwelling elderly and even higher in the institutionalized segment of the population. The Geriatric Depression Screen is helpful in identifying underlying depression (Brink et al., 1982). Medications should be routinely reviewed on a routine basis since "polypharmacy" in the elderly can be associated with adverse side effects and drug–drug interactions.

Many older adults live with the consequences of various disabilities acquired over the span of a lifetime such as amputation of a lower extremity, stroke, brain injury, and multiple sclerosis. In assessing them, clinicians should also obtain a disability history with emphasis on the following elements: (a) disability-related symptoms such as impaired communication and swallowing, insomnia, pain, falls and near falls, bowel/bladder dysfunction, and spasticity; (b) disability-associated psychosocial issues such as anxiety, depression, aging caregivers, financial difficulties; (c) gaps in home health care and ability to manage their finances; (d) assessment of mobility aids such as prostheses, orthotics, and wheelchairs and the presence of adaptive equipment in the home such as grab bars, raised toilet seat, and tub bench (Cristian, 2006).

Physical Examination

A thorough physical examination should include the patient's vital signs, and an assessment of essentially all systems previously mentioned in the age-related changes section. Neurological evaluation should include examination of cognition, cranial nerves, sensation, proprioception, motor strength, reflexes, muscle tone, balance, and gait. The Mini-Mental Status Examination is useful and an easily administered screening tool at the bedside (Folstein, Folstein, & McHugh, 1975). A score of 24 or greater out of

30 is considered normal in the population aged 65 years and older. A score of less than 24 is associated with delirium, dementia, or severe depression.

Musculoskeletal examination should focus on presence of deformities, range of motion limitations, muscle strength, contractures, and tender areas in the spine and extremities.

Functional Assessment

As part of a comprehensive assessment, it is important for clinicians to evaluate and treat the older adult's ability to participate and maintain independence with regard to ADL, such as those involved in self-care, mobility, and community activities. Areas where it is feasible to address deficiency or inefficiency in function are identified and appropriate treatment goals and plans are made to improve the functional level of independence.

EXERCISE IN THE ELDERLY

Benefits of Exercise in the Elderly

An exercise program has been shown to improve daily function, reduce disability, reduce blood pressure, improve lipid profiles, lower cardiac mortality, reduce stroke-associated weakness, reduce pain and improve function in OA and rheumatoid arthritis, and reduce the risk of falling (Frankel, Bean, & Frontera, 2006).

Individuals who are physically active on a regular basis display better health, incur lower health care costs, and are less limited in mobility over time than sedentary individuals. The elderly possess an important residual, but latent, physical potential, which can be mobilized by physical training (Beyer et al., 2007). In the elderly, physical activity has been shown to reduce disease and disability while improving the quality of life. However, as of 2008, less than half (48%) of adults met the physical activity guidelines set forth by the U.S. Department of Health and Human Services, and 28% to 34% of adults aged 65 to 74 years of age are inactive (Elsawy & Higgins, 2010).

When prescribing an exercise program, the prescriber should focus on improvement of strength, flexibility, mobility, balance and aerobic capacity. Reasons for promoting exercise in the elderly include the reduced likelihood of falls and related injuries delaying onset of mobility impairments, reducing risk, and onset of chronic diseases such as cardiovascular disease, diabetes, hypertension, osteoporosis, stroke, and obesity. Other important benefits are improvements in mood, sleep quality, chronic pain, and constipation.

There are significant benefits of exercise in preventing illness and injury, and limiting functional loss and disability in older adults. Exercise in the elderly has been shown to lower mortality and increase independence in adults older than 85 (Frankel et al., 2006; Stressman, 2009). Whole body vibration has been linked with the greatest increase in muscle size and may be of use with individuals unable to participate in standard exercise programs (Stewart, Saunders, & Greig, 2014).

Two recent studies demonstrated that patients with knee osteoarthritis participating in resistance training displayed improvement in muscle strength/morphology, functional performance, pain, and balance (Ciolac, Silva, & Greve, 2015; Hernandez, 2015). Exercise programs should be individualized and take into consideration the patient's level of fitness and any comorbidities.

Precautions and Contraindications to Exercise in the Elderly

Whereas there are many benefits to exercise in the elderly, clinicians should be aware that exercise can pose dangers as well. Contraindications to exercise in the older adult include (a) acute medical illness; (b) unstable angina (a condition in which the heart does not get enough blood flow and oxygen, a prelude to a heart attack); (c) end-stage congestive heart failure; (d) severe cardiac valve disease; (e) unstable arrhythmia; (f) systolic blood pressure at baseline of 200 mmHg or greater and/or diastolic blood pressure of 110 mmHg or greater; (g) large or expanding abdominal aneurysm; (h) cerebral aneurysm; (i) acute retinal hemorrhage or recent eye surgery; (j) severe behavioral disturbance; or (k) severe dementia. It is prudent to obtain appropriate medical clearance for these conditions prior to the start of a exercise program.

Once an older patient has been medically cleared to participate in exercise, appropriate precautions in high-risk patients are recommended. Examples include the following: (a) monitoring vital signs (pulse, heart rate, and oxygen saturation) before, during, and immediately after exercise;

(b) maintaining heart rate at 60% to 70% of maximal heart rate (ideally determined via cardiac stress test); (c) maintaining a moderate level of intensity; (d) use of supplemental oxygen in patients that require it; (e) monitoring for fatigue and providing judicious rest periods; and (f) controlling pain prior to exercise. Treating therapists should also be made aware if a patient is at risk for fracture, falls, seizure, or hypoglycemia. They should also be informed of any weight-bearing precautions or restrictions to range of motion.

Progressive Resistance Strength Training

Progressive resistance strength training (PRST) consists of moving the major joints repeatedly through the full range of motion several times weekly, with or without some form of resistance. A typical program is performed two to three times per week and ranges from low intensity in deconditioned patients to moderately high intensity in more active older adults. Key muscle groups to focus on include those in the lower extremities such as the hip flexors, hip extensors, knee extensors, ankle dorsiflexors, ankle plantar flexors, and the triceps in the upper extremities. It is also important to add task-specific exercises that mimic real-life scenarios and improve functionality. Liu and Latham (2009) reviewed 121 trials with 6,700 participants to evaluate progressive resistance strength training for improving physical function in older adults. Overall, this review suggests that PRST has a small but significant effect on improving physical function, a small to moderate effect on decreasing some impairments and functional limitations, and a large effect on increasing strength. In addition, some preliminary evidence suggests that PRST might reduce pain in older people with OA (Liu and Latham, 2009).

PRST has been shown to increase muscle strength and muscle hypertrophy in individuals older than 75 years (Stewart et al., 2014). Short duration (12 weeks) high-intensity PRST programs (defined as 70% to 89% of one repetition maximum [RM]) have a greater benefit than lesser intense programs in improving the strength of muscles in the lower limbs and are relatively safe to perform with only minor musculoskeletal injuries reported. Additional benefits in flexibility and level of function have also been reported (Raymond, Bramley-Tzerefos, Jeffs, Winter, & Holland, 2013).

The benefits of PRST have also been associated with improved level of function in ADLs for older adults, including those residing in long-term care institutions (Valenzuela, 2012; Weening-Dijksterhuis, de Greef, Scherder, Slaets, & van der Schans, 2011). Recommendations for PRST for frail institutionalized older adults is to start with a weight that is 40% to 80% of the maximal weight that can be lifted once. The individual performs eight repetitions per set; one to three sets per session; three sessions per week for a duration of 10 weeks.

There is also accumulating evidence that PRST with amino acid/protein supplementation increases muscle hypertrophy and decreases the onset of sarcopenia in the elderly (Makanae, 2015). Impairment of balance is common among the elderly. Balance exercises help to protect against falling and fall-related injuries. Balance exercises should challenge gait patterns, improve awareness of one's center of gravity, and enhance sensory processing in balance. These should be performed thrice per week for 3 months (Weening-Dijksterhuis et al., 2011). Furthermore, several reviews have demonstrated that tai chi can be beneficial in improving balance in older adults and minimize the risk of falling (Schleicher, Wedam, & Wu, 2012; Song, Ahn, So, Lee, Chung, & Park, 2015).

SELECTED TOPICS

Delirium and Dementia

Delirium is a common and potentially serious acute neuropsychiatric syndrome with core features of inattention and global cognitive dysfunction. Clinical experience and recent research have shown that delirium can become chronic or result in permanent sequelae (Fong, Tulebaev, & Inouye, 2009). In elderly individuals, delirium can begin or be a key factor in a cascade of events that ultimately leads to a downward spiral of functional decline, loss of independence, institutionalization, and possibly death. It affects about 14% to 56% of all hospitalized elderly patients.

Delirium has important implications from both a functional and an economic standpoint. It is estimated to cost more than $143 billion annually, mostly due to longer hospitalizations. Older adults, when acutely ill, can present with symptoms atypical of a given illness, including delirium.

For instance, urinary tract infection, myocardial infarction, pneumonia, pain, and even constipation can lead to delirium or cognitive changes. When delirium is diagnosed or suspected, the clinician should seek an underlying cause. However, in a small percentage of older adults, no cause for delirium can be identified. Delirium is potentially preventable and treatable, but major barriers, including under-recognition of the syndrome and poor understanding of the underlying pathophysiology, have hampered the development of successful therapies. Rehabilitation team members must be able to recognize acute delirium in a timely manner and administer proper treatment to prevent further deterioration. Recognizing delirium can make the difference between successful rehabilitation and a poor outcome for older adults.

Dementia affects memory, executive function, and ADLs. Alzheimer's disease is the most common cause of a progressive dementia. Many types of dementia are irreversible but some causes may be reversible. The risk of dementia increases with age older than 60 years. It is imperative to evaluate for early signs of dementia in high-risk individuals. As function deteriorates, it is not uncommon for people with dementia to withdraw from more complex activity and social environments and for family and friends to want to step in to perform tasks for them. There is some evidence that adults with dementia can benefit from exercise programs to prevent falls in the community and improve cognitive function (Burton et al., 2015; Groot et al., 2015).

There are several differences between dementia and delirium as outlined in Table 16.1. Two tools that can be used to assist in differentiating between the two are the Confusion Assessment Method (CAM) and the Mini-Cog. The CAM can identify the presence or absence of delirium. It seeks to identify four key features that distinguish delirium from other types of cognitive impairment. These are: (a) acute onset and fluctuating course, (b) inattention, (c) disorganized thinking, and (d) altered level of consciousness. The diagnosis of delirium requires the presence of features a and b, and either c or d (Waszynski, 2004).

The Mini-Cog is a screening tool composed of a three-item recall and a clock drawing test. It is used to easily and quickly detect dementia. Unsuccessful recall of three items after the clock drawing distractor is classified as probable dementia. The Mini-Cog takes approximately 3 minutes to administer. It is not influenced by the patient's education, culture, or language. A positive Mini-Cog indicates the need for further assessment (Borson, Scanlan, Brush, Vitaliano, & Dokmak, 2000).

Although delirium and dementia have different characteristics, they both share the presence of cognitive impairment. Delirium can occur in patients with dementia, so it is vital to recognize the symptoms of delirium in these individuals. This is commonly known as delirium on superimposed dementia (DSD). The prevalence of DSD has been reported in acute hospitals, nursing homes, and community populations, but there are few studies in rehabilitation facilities. Both delirium and dementia affect functional recovery. The occurrence of delirium alone has been shown in rehabilitation hospitals to be linked to worse functional outcomes while the effect of dementia alone is still controversial. One study showed that individuals with DSD were significantly more functionally impaired in comparison to those with dementia

TABLE 16.1

CHARACTERISTICS OF DELIRIUM AND DEMENTIA

Delirium	Dementia
Acute onset	Slow, gradual onset
Identifiable time of onset	Time of onset not clear, typically note changes over months
Cause is usually treatable such as infection, medication, pain, constipation, and myocardial infarction	Due to chronic disorder such as Alzheimer's
Usually reversible	Progressive process
Attention impaired	Attention not impaired until late stages
Consciousness ranges from lethargic to hyper-alert	No effect on consciousness until late stages
Effect on memory varies	Loss of memory especially for recent events
Medical attention required immediately to prevent dire consequences	Medical attention required, less urgently

alone, delirium alone, or neither of these conditions. DSD was also a predictor of an increased risk of institutionalization (Elie, Cole, Primeau, & Bellavance, 1998). DSD in rehabilitation settings is an important predictor of 1-year mortality in older adults and of institutionalization upon discharge (Morandi et al., 2014).

Frailty and Sarcopenia

Frailty is a state of vulnerability to homeostasis after a stressor event and is a consequence of cumulative decline in many physiological systems over a course of a lifetime. This cumulative decline depletes homoeostatic reserves until such time that minor stressor events trigger disproportionate changes in health status. In landmark studies, the investigators have developed valid models of frailty and these models have allowed epidemiological investigations that show the association between frailty and adverse health outcomes (Clegg, Young, Iliffe, Rikkert, & Rockwood, 2013).

As the population ages, the prevalence of frailty increases. Statistics show that 25% of all adults older than 85 years old are frail. Frailty can occur in as much as 12% of all adults that are older than 65 years of age. Women have a higher percentage of frailty than men, with the African American population having a higher frailty percentage than the Caucasian population. As people are living longer, the number of frail individuals is also increasing.

Frailty is a disorder involving multiple inter-related physiological systems. There is a gradual decline in physiological reserve with aging but, in frailty, this decline is accelerated and homeostatic mechanisms start failing (Cruz-Jentoft et al., 2010; Ferrucci et al., 2002). It is therefore important to consider how the complex mechanisms of aging promote cumulative decline in multiple physiological systems, consequent erosion of homeostatic reserve, and vulnerability to disproportionate changes in health status following relatively minor stressor events. These complex aging mechanisms are influenced by underlying genetic and environmental factors (Taffett, 2003) in combination with epigenetic mechanisms, which regulate the differential expression of genes in cells and may be especially important in aging (Kirkwood, 2005; McGowan & Szyf, 2010).

Aging is considered to result from the lifelong accumulation of molecular and cellular damage caused by multiple mechanisms under the regulation of a complex maintenance and repair network (Taffett, 2003). There is uncertainty regarding the precise level of cellular damage required to cause impaired organ physiology but, importantly, many organ systems exhibit considerable redundancy, which provides the physiological reserve required to compensate for age and disease-related changes (Kahn & Fraga, 2009). For example, the brain contains more neurons and skeletal muscle more myocytes than are required for survival (Kahn & Fraga, 2009). Therefore, a key question is whether there is a critical threshold of age-related, cumulative decline in multiple physiological systems beyond which frailty becomes evident.

The brain, endocrine system, immune system, and skeletal muscle are intrinsically interrelated and are currently the organ systems best studied with regard to the development of frailty (Manini & Clark, 2012). It is important to recognize that frailty has been associated with the loss of physiological reserve in the respiratory (Gaczynska, Rock, Spies, & Goldberg, 1994), cardiovascular (Vaz Fragoso, Enright, McAvay, Van Ness, & Gill, 2012), renal (Afilalo et al., 2009), and hemopoietic and clotting systems (Abadir, 2011; Chaves et al., 2005), and that nutritional status can also be a mediating factor (Lang et al., 2010; Payette, Coulombe, Boutier, & Gray-Donald, 2000; Sullivan, Patch, Walls, & Lipschitz, 1990; Walston et al., 2006).

Sarcopenia has been defined as progressive loss of skeletal muscle mass, strength, and power and is considered a cornerstone characteristic of frailty (Howard et al., 2007; Walston et al., 2006). Loss of muscle strength and power may be more important than changes to muscle mass (Fried et al., 2001). Under normal circumstances, homeostasis in muscle is maintained in a delicate balance between new muscle cell formation, hypertrophy, and protein loss. This delicate balance is coordinated by the brain, endocrine system, and immune system and is influenced by nutritional factors and level of physical activity. The effects of frailty on the neurological, endocrine, and immune systems have the potential to upset this delicate homeostatic balance and accelerate the development of sarcopenia.

The mechanism of sarcopenia is quite complex. Several contributing causes include malnutrition, physical inactivity, muscle apoptosis, oxidative stress, and dysregulation of inflammatory cytokines and hormones. Inflammatory cytokines such as IL-6 and TNFα have also been reported to activate muscle breakdown (Lipsitz, 2002). Sarcopenia has been associated with decreased power and in elbow extension can be as high as 40%. Fast type 2 fibers seem to be more affected than type 1 fibers. Individuals with sarcopenia experience a delay in activating hip flexors and knee extensors during their swing phase of the gait cycle. A decreased thigh muscle cross-sectional area (CSA) and knee extension torque have been associated with an increased risk of hip fracture by 50% to 60% (Lang et al., 2010).

In order to assess an older adult for frailty, one must understand the frailty cycle, which proceeds as follows: (a) weakness (loss of muscle strength that starts in midlife), (b) slowness (low physical activity), (c) exhaustion, and (d) weight loss (Jones, Song, & Rockwood, 2004). There are several tools available to assist the clinician in diagnosing frailty: (a) the timed up and go test (TUGT) (Newman et al., 2001), (b) hand grip strength (Podsiadlo & Richardson, 1991), and (c) gait speed (Syddall, Cooper, Martin, Briggs, & Aihie Sayer, 2003). The Comprehensive Geriatric Assessment (CGA) can be used to detect frailty in older individuals. It is a multidisciplinary diagnostic process to determine an individual's medical, psychological, and functional status and used to develop a plan for treatment and follow-up (Studenski et al., 2011). The process, provided that it is closely linked to interventions, is associated with superior outcomes (Ellis, Whitehead, Robinson, O'Neill, & Langhorne, 2011; Extermann et al., 2005; Harari et al., 2007; Rockwood et al., 2005; Rubenstein, Stuck, Siu, & Wieland, 1991). The practical limitation of CGA is the time and expertise required for the process. Treatment options for frailty and sarcopenia include nutritional therapy, resistive exercise training, and hormone replacement with testosterone and estrogen. Nutritional therapy includes supplements, nutrients, vitamins, snacks, and drinks to offset frailty (Ho et al., 2011).

Falls and Fractures

According to the Centers for Disease Control and Prevention, one out every three adults older than 65 falls each year and one out of every five falls is associated with a significant injury such as a fracture or a head injury. Each year, 700,000 people are hospitalized for one of these injuries, and 250,000 for a hip fracture. Fall injuries are one of the 20 most expensive medical conditions to treat, with an average hospital cost of $35,000. The direct medical cost for fall injuries in the United States is $34 billion per year (Centers for Disease Control and Prevention, National Center for Injury Prevention and Control, Division of Unintentional Injury Prevention, n.d.).

A report by the World Health Organization (WHO) has found that: (a) in long-term institutions, 30% to 50% of residents fall each year and 40% of them experience multiple falls; (b) most falls occur during the day and outside the home; however, falls occur indoors more often for older, more frail adults; (c) falls that occur in the home typically occur in bedrooms, kitchens, and dining rooms; (d) men fall more often outdoors and women indoors; (e) approximately 10% to 20% of falls lead to fractures; (f) women are more likely to sustain nonfatal falls and men more likely to sustain fatal falls; (g) women are more likely to sustain fractures; and (h) adults with Parkinson's disease, depression, diabetes, incontinence, Alzheimer's disease, lower extremity weakness, cognitive impairment, and foot deformities have an increased risk of falling (WHO, n.d.).

Medication use by elderly individuals has also been linked with an increase in falls. According to the same WHO report, medications associated with an increased risk of falling include benzodiazepines, sedative-hypnotics, antipsychotics, antidepressants, diuretics, nitrates, NSAIDs, opioids, and antihistamines. Antihypertensives and cardiac medications have been linked with increased risk of postural hypotension, whereas commonly used analgesic medications have been linked with sedation and confusion.

Falls can lead to loss of independence and admission to a nursing home. Falls have also been linked with an increase in mortality. According to WHO, one out of every five hip fractures can lead to death within 6 months (WHO: "A global report"). Alcoholism in the elderly has been linked with both an increased risk of falls as well as increased risk of hip fracture (WHO: "A global report" . . .).

There is evidence that multifactorial interventions including home evaluations and modifications for environmental safety can reduce falls in both community dwelling of older adults and those in long-term care institutions (Cameron et al., 2012; Stubbs, Brefka, & Denkinger, 2015; Vlaeyen et al., 2015). Exercise that focuses on gait, balance, and functional activities has been shown to reduce the rate of falls, falls associated with injuries, and fear of falling. It has been recommended that a balanced program emphasizing endurance, balance, and strength is most effective (El-Khoury, Cassou, Charles, & Dargent-Molina, 2013; Gillespie et al., 2012; Kendrick et al., 2014; Stubbs et al., 2015). Other reported interventions that are beneficial in reducing falls include tai chi, first eye cataract surgery, pacemakers in people with carotid sinus hypersensitivity, withdrawal of psychotropic medications, and wearing an antislip shoe device in icy conditions (Gillespie et al., 2012).

Traumatic Brain Injury in the Elderly

Traumatic brain injury (TBI) is a significant problem in older adults. Presentation of TBI in the elderly differs from that of younger adults in many ways, including incidence, mechanism of injury, complications, comorbidities, length of hospitalization, functional outcomes, and mortality. It presents unique issues and challenges to the health care system as a result.

Epidemiology

Although the incidence of TBI is highest in the very young (age under 4 years old) and in adolescents and young adults (15–24 years old), a second peak incidence occurs in the elderly (Rutland-Brown, Langlois, Thomas, & Xi, 2006). There are 155,000 cases of TBI per year in persons aged 65 and older, leading to 12,000 deaths (Richmond et al., 2011). TBI in the elderly is responsible for more than 80,000 emergency department visits each year with 75%of these visits resulting in hospitalization as a result of the TBI (Thompson, McCormick, & Kagan, 2006). In 2003, the cost for treating a principal diagnosis of TBI in patients aged 65 and older exceeded $2.2 billion (H-CUPnet, 2006).

Etiology

Falls are the leading cause of TBI in the elderly. They account for more than half of TBIs (51%), followed by motor vehicle accidents (MVAs) (pedestrian or driver/passenger) (9%). Assaults account for 1% of TBIs in older adults, and all other known causes account for 17% (Langlois, Rutland-Brown, & Thomas, 2004).

Compared with adults aged 65 years or younger, the elderly are more likely to be hospitalized with a TBI-related fall. In 2002, the overall U.S. age-adjusted incidence rate of hospitalization from fall-related TBI was 29.6 per 100,000 population. For adults aged 65 to 74, this rate was almost double (58.6/100,000 population), and in adults aged 75 and older, the rate was more than six times higher (203.9/100,000). Older persons averaged a significantly longer rehabilitation length of stay, higher total rehabilitation charges, and a lower rate of change on functional measures (Cifu et al., 1996).

Pathophysiology of TBI in the Elderly

The pathophysiology of TBI is divided into two categories: primary brain injury and secondary brain injury; current approaches to the management of TBI focus on these two aspects of brain injury. Primary brain injury is the direct disruption of the brain parenchyma by the trauma and occurs at the time of trauma. Reversal of the primary damage is not possible, and therefore is not amenable to medical intervention; however, much of the brain injury in trauma patients is secondary to this primary brain injury, occurring as a cascade of biochemical, cellular, and molecular events that are initiated at the time of initial trauma and continue for hours or days, which will lead to neuronal cell death as well as secondary cerebral edema and increased intracranial pressure that can further exacerbate the brain injury. Secondary damage may be reduced with proper monitoring and treatment. The identification, prevention, and treatment of secondary brain injury are the principal foci of neurointensive care management for patients with severe TBI (Kass Cottrell, Abramowicz, Hou, & Lei, 2015).

Extra-axial hemorrhages are common after TBI and include epidural, subdural, and subarachnoid hemorrhages. Elderly individuals are particularly vulnerable to subdural hemorrhages (SDH) because bridging veins become more susceptible to shearing forces as the brain naturally atrophies with advancing age. A large acute SDH manifests as a rapid deterioration of arousal or development of focal neurologic impairments. However, a SDH may not be clinically evident during the acute stages in older adults, because of the enlargement of the subdural space that naturally occurs with aging. SDH frequently occurs in older adults after apparently trivial trauma and is often related to a fall in which there was no direct trauma to the head. An SDH may slowly expand in the elderly as a result of abnormalities of blood vessels, increased fibrinolysis, and abnormal coagulation, which partially account for the late deterioration of mental abilities often observed in elderly people who have SDH (Flanagan, Hibbard, Riordan, & Gordon, 2006).

Comorbidities and TBI in the Elderly

There is a significant increase in comorbidity in the elderly. One study found that 73% of elderly TBI patients had a medical condition before injury, compared with 28% of younger adults. In the United States, 48% of community-dwelling elderly have arthritis, 36% have hypertension, 27% have coronary disease, 10% have diabetes mellitus, and 6% have had a cerebrovascular accident. A higher number of medical comorbidities have been associated with longer rehabilitation stays in older adults. Some preexisting conditions place the elderly trauma patient at greater risk for secondary complications. These complications increase the hospital length of stay and are associated with an increased mortality. It has been also reported that 9% to 20% of older adult patients with TBI had been taking warfarin preinjury. This has been associated with a more severe TBI and a higher rate of mortality as is the case with antiplatelet agents (Mak et al., 2012; Thompson et al., 2006).

Comorbid dementia or mild cognitive impairment, whether from Alzheimer's disease or a consequence of other etiologies, is a risk factor for TBI and for slower recovery following TBI. However, it is often difficult to separate what part of cognitive impairment is due to preexisting dementia and what is due to TBI. Preexisting cognitive impairment confounds the diagnosis of TBI in such patients following trauma (Thompson et al., 2006).

Outcomes Following a TBI in the Elderly

Older age has long been recognized as an independent predictor of worse outcome from TBI (Coronado et al., 2011). Elderly individuals suffering a TBI have been shown to have poorer outcomes than younger persons across all severity levels. Rosenthal et al. reported both increased mortality and decreased functional status for patients 65 years and older with severe TBI. Mortality as a consequence of TBI has been shown to be two to three times higher in the elderly than in their younger counterparts (Susman et al., 2002). Elderly individuals with TBI tend to have poorer functional outcomes and longer length of hospital stay than younger patients (Mosenthal et al., 2002).

Management of TBI in the Elderly

Acute care management of TBI involves (a) lowering intracranial pressure (ICP) (ICP; a reasonable target is below 20), (b) maintaining adequate cerebral perfusion pressure (CPP) (the difference between mean arterial pressure and ICP), (c) reducing vasospasm, and (d) removing blood from the extradural space. Cerebral ischemia was a common finding in histologic studies of terminal trauma cases. It is of great importance to prevent the secondary ischemia that frequently follows brain trauma (Kass et al., 2015). In elderly individuals who experience a severe TBI, the primary focus of acute care management is on preventing secondary brain injury that may arise as a result of diffuse cerebral ischemia. Increased intracerebral pressure resulting from intracranial hemorrhages or brain swelling often impedes cerebral blood flow, particularly in instances of systemic hypotension (Flanagan et al., 2006).

Rehabilitation following TBI is ideally initiated shortly after hospitalization, often while the patient resides in an intensive care setting. The immediate goal of rehabilitation is to prevent the complications associated with a prolonged period of immobilization, such as joint contractures, skin breakdown, venous stasis, and pulmonary compromise, and to preserve joint mobility of paralyzed limbs; this is achieved by ranging all limbs through a full range of motion several times daily. Rehabilitative intervention plans include initiation of neuropsychological, physical, occupational, and speech therapies.

Prevention of TBI in the Elderly

Any effective strategy for reducing the burden of TBI among elderly populations must begin with prevention. As falls are overwhelmingly the leading cause of injury leading to TBI, interventions aimed specifically at fall reduction would have the greatest effect on TBI incidence and related mortality among the elderly. There are numerous extrinsic and intrinsic risk factors for falls and many interventions can be instituted to prevent a fall. Periodic assessment of vision, medication use, and the evaluation of gait and balance and of the home environment can have a significant impact on the prevention of falls among the elderly (Michael et al., 2010).

Suicidal Ideation and TBI in the Elderly

Adults aged 65 and older show the highest incidence of either suicidal ideation or behavior across all age groups. Suicide attempts in this age group commonly involve the use of a firearm and jumping from a height. In older adults, White males are at highest risk; other risk factors include a history of depression, chronic pain, or illness; and social isolation. About 70% of older adults who completed suicide had seen their primary care provider within the previous month, denoting a crucial opportunity for intervention by the provider (Thompson et al., 2006).

Pain in Older Adults

The prevalence of persistent pain increases with age with a majority of older adults reporting that their pain is undertreated. Twenty-five to 40% of older cancer patients report daily pain. Low back pain is among the most common complaints along with headache and joint pain. Almost three fifths of adults aged 65 and older reported that their pain had lasted for 1 or more years. Women report severely painful joints more often than men (10% versus 7%). Nearly one in two people may develop symptomatic knee OA by age 85 years; one in four people may develop painful hip arthritis by age 85 years ([CDC]/National Center for Health Statistics, 2006a, 2006b).

Assessment of Pain in the Elderly

The history should focus on the pain characteristics surrounding the chief complaint (location, radiation, onset, duration, intensity, character, aggravating/alleviating factors, associated symptoms), previous workup completed, previous treatments, and their success in relieving the pain. The practitioner should not overlook "red flags," which can be misinterpreted as being of musculoskeletal origin. Examples include (a) neck and left shoulder pain may stem from an acute myocardial infarction, pericarditis, aortic dissection, and tumors; (b) right shoulder pain may be caused by gallstones, cholecystitis, Pancoast tumors, or even pancreatitis; (c) back pain may be caused by aortic dissection, pancreatitis, pyelonephritis, kidney/ureteral stones; (d) chest and back pain may be caused by pneumonia, pleuritis, esophageal, or cardiovascular problems; and (e) abdominal pain may be of gastrointestinal, genitourinary, or gynecological etiology.

The physical examination should document appearance, gait, pain behaviors, posture, and anatomic abnormalities (e.g., amputations, asymmetries, contractures). A focused neurological exam should include mental status, affect, cranial nerve evaluation, motor strength, sensation, muscle stretch reflexes, and coordination testing. This focused exam can help differentiate between central pain conditions and peripheral sources of pain. Musculoskeletal examination can help identify and localize pain generators in various structures including skin, subcutaneous tissue, tendons, joints, ligaments, muscle, or the periosteum.

Lab and imaging testing should be done in a stepwise approach taking the cost of tests into consideration and their importance in guidance of treatment plan.

Treatment Options

Older adults with pain require comprehensive individualized approach that takes into account personal and caregiver goals, as well as functional, physiologic, and neuropsychologic considerations (sleep, mood, behavior).

Pain prevention can begin with helping the patient set realistic pain treatment goals and then developing a written pain management plan. The plan should include regular and frequent pain assessments and should anticipate and aggressively treat for pain before, during, and after painful diagnostic/therapeutic interventions or any activities known to elicit pain. The patient and caregiver should be educated about the pain medication use, side effects, and issues of addiction, dependence and tolerance, as well as other nonpharmacological strategies such as physical and occupational therapy, relaxation, massage, acupuncture, yoga, or other modalities (Alan, Kaye, Baluch, Jared, & Scott, 2010).

Pharmacological approach in older patients should be well documented and consistent among health care providers in order to avoid the risk of "polypharmacy" or drug interactions. Pain drugs should be administered on a regular basis to maintain therapeutic levels and on an as needed (PRN) basis for breakthrough pain. Oral administration is preferable over parenteral and intravenous over intramuscular. Opioid medications can be used for moderate-to-severe pain and nonopioids for mild-to-moderate pain (Alan et al., 2010).

According to the American Geriatric Society and WHO, the following are recommended with respect to medications for the treatment of pain conditions (Agency for Healthcare Research and Quality, 2012).

1. Acetaminophen should be considered as initial and ongoing treatment of persistent pain, particularly musculoskeletal pain. Guidelines recommend not exceeding 4 g/day (max 3 g/day in frail older adults) and a 50% to 75% dose reduction in adults with reduced hepatic function or history of alcohol abuse.
2. NSAIDs and cyclooxygenase 2 selective inhibitors (COX-2i) should be used with caution in the elderly, and monitored frequently due to the risk of bleeding, nephrotoxicity, delirium, and cardiovascular adverse events. Proton pump inhibitors should be considered to reduce gastrointestinal irritation, especially when the patient is taking COX-2i with aspirin. Patients should not take more than one nonselective NSAID or COX-2i for pain control. Ibuprofen should not be used if patient is taking aspirin for cardioprophylaxis.
3. Opioids should be considered for patients with moderate to severe pain, pain-related functional impairment, or diminished quality of life secondary to pain. Around-the-clock opioid treatment may be used for complaints of daily frequent or continuous pain. Long-acting opioid preparations should be used together with short-acting immediate release opioids for breakthrough pain. All patients on opioid medications should be reassessed for adverse effects, safe and responsible use of medications, and attainment of therapeutic goals.
4. Adjuvant analgesics are indicated for all patients with refractory pain or with neuropathic pain. The analgesic effects are enhanced when adjuvants are combined with other analgesics. "Start low and go slow" is a recommended approach in the elderly, wherein therapy is begun with the lowest possible dose and increased slowly based on response and side effects. Examples of adjuvant medications are antidepressants, anticonvulsants, alpha-2 adrenergic agonists, local anesthetics, corticosteroids, muscle relaxants, calcitonin, antihistamines, and N-methyl-d-aspartate (NMDA) receptor agonists.

Systemic corticosteroids are reserved for patients with pain associated with inflammatory disorders or metastatic bone pain. Topical lidocaine can be used for patients with localized neuropathic and non-neuropathic pain. Topical NSAIDs can be used for other localized non-neuropathic persistent pain. Alternative topical agents (capsaicin, menthol) have been used for regional pain syndromes.

Tertiary tricyclic antidepressants should be avoided in the elderly due to higher risk of adverse effects (anticholinergic effect, cognitive impairment). Other agents (e.g., glucosamine, chondroitin, botulinum-toxin, cannabinoids, alpha-2 adrenergic agonists, calcitonin, vitamin D, ketamine, bisphosphonates) should be used with caution in older adults and merit further research.

Although increasingly accepted and incorporated by Western medicine, the complementary and alternative medicine approach is generally still lacking extensive and rigorous evidence-based support. This type of treatment should be recommended in accordance with the physician's knowledge of and level of comfort with these interventions. See Chapter 27 on Integrative Medicine for more information.

Interventional procedures may help determine the underlying pain originator. Nerve blocks, chemical neurolysis, radiofrequency lesioning, cryoneurolysis, neuraxial drug delivery, and the implantation of spinal cord stimulators are some interventions that can improve pain and often reduce the need for heavy medication use, thereby decreasing undesirable side effects.

FUNCTIONAL OUTCOMES AND SITE OF POSTACUTE REHABILITATION

There is evidence that the site of postacute care can make a difference in recovery following a stroke.

Better functional outcomes have been reported 6 months post-stroke for persons who received acute inpatient rehabilitation compared to those in skilled nursing facilities and those receiving home health/outpatient care (Chan, Sandel, Jette, & Appelman, 2013).

One study following patients after repair of a hip fracture did not find such site-specific advantages to be significant immediately post- discharge (Mallinson, Deutsch, Bateman, Tseng, & Manheim, 2014). Another study, however, showed persons rehabilitated in an inpatient rehabilitation facility following a hip fracture were more likely to attain most of their prefracture functional status by 6 months postdischarge than those receiving care in a skilled nursing facility (Munin, Begley, Skidmore, & Lenze, 2006).

A review of 13 trials involving 2,498 older adults with hip fracture examined the effects of multidisciplinary rehabilitation, in either inpatient or ambulatory care settings, for older patients and found a nonstatistically significant tendency toward a better overall result in patients receiving multidisciplinary inpatient rehabilitation, which was also not harmful to those participating (Handoll, Cameron, Mak, & Finnegan, 2009). Functional outcomes at discharge for joint replacements between skilled nursing facilities and inpatient rehabilitation facilities have been compared, with the latter reporting better motor functional outcomes, though not by a large margin. Earlier and more intensive rehabilitation was associated with better outcomes (Dejong, 2009).

Older persons receiving postacute rehabilitation for medical and surgical conditions have greater premorbid disability, but are more likely to recover their premorbid functional level when compared to those who sustained a hip fracture or stroke. However, their 1-year mortality is significantly greater. Cognitive impairment and the presence of a pressure ulcer at rehabilitation admission are associated with a poorer functional recovery (Johnson, Kramer, Lin, Kowalsky, & Steiner, 2000).

CONCLUSION

As the number of older adults continues to increase, rehabilitation will continue to play a significant role in their overall health and improvement of the quality of their lives. The goals of geriatric rehabilitation are to maximize function and minimize disability in a population with multiple comorbidities. An interdisciplinary team approach that uses the principles described in this chapter provides an important cornerstone of a geriatric rehabilitation program.

ACKNOWLEDGMENT

The editorial contribution of Thomas Pascal, BS, to this chapter is very much appreciated.

REFERENCES

Abadir, P. M. (2011). The frail renin-angiotensin system. *Clinics in Geriatric Medicine*, *27*(1), 53–65.

Afilalo, J., Karunananthan, S., Eisenberg, M. J., Alexander, K. P., & Bergman, H. (2009). Role of frailty in patients with cardiovascular disease. *The American Journal of Cardiology*, *103*(11), 1616–1621.

Agency for Healthcare Research and Quality. (2012). Pain management in older adults (Guideline summary NGC-9720). In *Evidence-based geriatric nursing protocols for best practice*. Rockville, MD: Author. Retrieved from https://www.guideline.gov/summaries/summary/43932/pain-management-in-older-adults-in-evidencebased-geriatric-nursing-protocols-for-best-practice

Alan, D., Kaye, M. D., Baluch, A., Jared, T., & Scott, M. D. (2010). Pain management in the elderly population: A review. *The Ochsner Journal, 10*(3), 179–187.

Avis, N. E., & Deimling, G. T. (2008). Cancer survivorship and aging. *Cancer, 113*(Suppl. 12), 3519–3529.

Beyer, N., Simonsen, L., Bülow, J., Lorenzen, T., Jensen, D. V., Larsen, L., . . . Kjaer, M. (2007). Old women with a recent fall history show improved muscle strength and function sustained for six months after finishing training. *Aging Clinical and Experimental Research, 19*(4), 300–309.

Borson, S., Scanlan, J., Brush, M., Vitaliano, P., & Dokmak, A. (2000). The mini-cog: A cognitive 'vital signs' measure for dementia screening in multi-lingual elderly. *International Journal of Geriatric Psychiatry, 15*(11), 1021–1027.

Brink, T. L., Yesavage, J. A., Lum, O., Heersema, P., Adey, M. B., & Rose, T. L. (1982). Screening tests for geriatric depression. *Clinical Gerontologist, 1*, 37–44.

Burton, E., Cavalheri, V., Adams, R., Browne, C. O., Bovery-Spencer, P., Fenton, A. M., . . . Hill, K. D. (2015). Effectiveness of exercise programs to reduce falls in older people with dementia living in the community: A systematic review and meta-analysis. *Clinical Interventions in Aging, 10*, 421–434. doi:10.2147/CIA.S71691

Cameron, I. D., Gillespie, L. D., Robertson, M. C., Murray, G. R., Hill, K. D., Cumming, R. G., & Kerse, N. (2012). Interventions for preventing falls in older people in care facilities and hospitals. *Cochrane Database of Systematic Reviews, 12*, CD005465. doi:10.1002/14651858.CD005465.pub3

Centers for Disease Control and Prevention/National Center for Health Statistics. (2006a, November). New report finds pain affects millions of Americans. Retrieved from http://www.cdc.gov/nchs/pressroom/06facts/hus06.htm

Centers for Disease Control and Prevention/National Center for Health Statistics. (2006b, November). Health, United States, 2006: With chartbook on trends in the health of Americans (DHHS Pub No. 2006-1232). Retrieved from http://www.cdc.gov/nchs/data/hus/hus06.pdf

Centers for Disease Control and Prevention, National Center for Injury Prevention and Control, Division of Unintentional Injury Prevention. (n.d.). Retrieved from https://www.cdc.gov/injury

Centers for Disease Control and Prevention/National Association of Chronic Disease Directors. (2008). *The state of mental health and aging in America issue brief 1: What do the data tell us?* Atlanta, GA: National Association of Chronic Disease Directors.

Chan, L., Sandel, M. E., Jette, A. M., & Appelman, J. (2013). Does postacute care site matter? A longitudinal study assessing functional recovery after a stroke. *Archives of Physical Medicine and Rehabilitation, 94*(4), 622–629.

Chatterji, S., Byles, J., Cutler, D., Seeman, T., & Verdes, E. (2015). Health, functioning, and disability in older adults: Present status and future implications. *The Lancet, 385*(9967), 563–575.

Chaves, P. H., Semba, R. D., Leng, S. X., Woodman, R. C., Ferrucci, L., Guralnik, J. M., & Fried, L. P. (2005). Impact of anemia and cardiovascular disease on frailty status of community-dwelling older women: The women's health and aging studies I and II. *The Journals of Gerontology. Series A, Biological Sciences and Medical Sciences, 60*(6), 729–735.

Chen, R., Balami, J. S., Esiri, M. M., Chen, L., & Buchan, A. M. (2010). Ischemic stroke in the elderly: An overview of evidence. *Nature Reviews Neurology, 6*(5), 256–265.

Cifu, D. X., Kreutzer, J. S., Marwitz, J. H., Rosenthal, M., Englander, J., & High, W. (1996). Functional outcomes of older adults with traumatic brain injury: A prospective, multicenter analysis. *Archives of Physical Medicine and Rehabilitation, 77*(9), 883–888.

Ciolac, E. G., Silva, J. M., & Greve, J. M. (2015). Effects of resistance training in older women with knee osteoarthritis and total knee arthroplasty. *Clinics, 70*(1), 7–13.

Clegg, A., Young, J., Iliffe, S., Rikkert, M. O., & Rockwood, K. (2013). Frailty in elderly people. *The Lancet, 381*(9868), 752–762. doi:10.1016/s0140-6736(12)62167-9

Coggan, A. R. Spina, R. J., King, D. S., Rogers, M. A., Brown, M., Nemeth, P. M., & Holloszy, J. O. (1992). Skeletal muscle adaptations to endurance training in 60- to 70-yr-old men and women. *Journal of Applied Physiology, 72*, 1780–1786.

Coronado, V. G., Xu, L., Basavaraju, S. V., McGuire, L. C., Wald, M. M., Faul, M. D., . . . Centers for Disease Control and Prevention. (2011). Surveillance for traumatic brain injury related deaths-United States 1997–2007. *Surveillance Summaries: Morbidity and Mortality Weekly Report, 60*, 1–32.

Cristian, A. (2006). The Assessment of the older adult with a physical disability: A guide for clinicians. *Clinics in Geriatric Medicine, 22*, 221–238.

Cruz-Jentoft, A. J., Baeyens, J. P., Bauer, J. M., Boirie, Y., Cederholm, T., Landi, F., . . . Zamboni, M. (2010). Sarcopenia: European consensus on definition and diagnosis: Report of the European working group on sarcopenia in older people. *Age & Ageing, 39*(4), 412–423.

Dejong, G., Horn, S. D., Smout, R. J., Tian, W., Putman, K., & Gassaway, J. (2009). Joint replacement rehabilitation outcomes on discharge from skilled nursing facilities and inpatient rehabilitation facilities. *Archives of Physical Medicine and Rehabilitation, 90*(8), 1284–1296. doi:10.1016/j.apmr.2009.02.009

Delbono, O., Renganathan, M., & Messi, M. L. (1997). Excitation-Calcium release contraction coupling in single aged human skeletal muscle fiber. *Muscle & Nerve, 20*(Suppl. 5), 88–92.

Driscoll, I. (2009). Longitudinal pattern of regional brain volume change differentiates normal aging from MCI. *Neurology, 72*, 1906.

Elie, M., Cole, M. G., Primeau, F. J., & Bellavance, F. (1998). Delirium risk factors in elderly hospitalized patients. *Journal of General Internal Medicine, 13*(3), 204–212. doi:10.1046/j.1525-1497.1998.00047.x

El-Khoury, F., Cassou, B., Charles, M. A., & Dargent-Molina, P. (2013, October 29). The effect of fall prevention exercise programmes on fall induced injuries in community dwelling older adults: Systematic review and meta-analysis of randomised controlled trials. *British Journal of Sports Medicine, 347*, f6234. doi:10.1136/bmj.f6234

Ellis, G., Whitehead, M. A., Robinson, D., O'Neill, D., & Langhorne, P. (2011). Comprehensive geriatric assessment for older adults admitted to hospital: Meta-analysis of randomised controlled trials. *British Journal of Sports Medicine, 343*, d6553.

Elsawy, B., & Higgins, K. E. (2010). Physical activity guidelines for older adults. *American Family Physician, 81*(1), 55–59.

Extermann, M., Aapro, M., Bernabei, R., Cohen, H. J., Droz, J. P., Lichtman, S., . . . Topinkova, E. (2005). Use of comprehensive geriatric assessment in older cancer patients: Recommendations from the task force on CGA of the International society of geriatric oncology (SIOG). *Critical Reviews in Oncology/Hematology, 55*(3), 241–252.

Ferrucci, L., Cavazzini, C., Corsi, A., Bartali, B., Russo, C. R., Lauretani, F., . . . Guralnik, J. M. (2002). Biomarkers of frailty in older persons. *Journal of Endocrinological Investigation, 25*(Suppl. 10), 10–15.

Flanagan, S. R., Hibbard, M. R., Riordan, B., & Gordon, W. A. (2006). Traumatic brain injury in the elderly: Diagnostic and treatment challenges. *Clinics in Geriatric Medicine, 22*(2), 449–468.

Folstein, M. F., Folstein, S. E., & McHugh, P. R. (1975). Mini-mental state. A practical method for grading the cognitive state of patients for the clinician. *Journal of Psychiatric Research, 12*, 189–198.

Fong, T. G., Tulebaev, S. R., & Inouye, S. K. (2009). Delirium in elderly adults: Diagnosis, prevention and treatment. *Nature Reviews. Neurology, 5*(4), 210–220. doi:10.1038/nrneurol.2009.24

Franceschi, C. (2014). Chronic inflammation (inflammaging) and its potential contribution to age-associated diseases. *The Journals of Gerontology. Series A, Biological Sciences and Medical Sciences, 69*, 4–9.

Franceschi, S., & La Vecchia, C. (2001). Cancer epidemiology in the elderly. *Critical Reviews in Oncology/Hematology, 39*(3), 219–226.

Frankel, J. E., Bean, J. F., & Frontera, W. R. (2006). Exercise in the elderly: Research and clinical practice. *Clinics in Geriatric Medicine, 22*, 239–256.

Fried, L. P., Tangen, C. M., Walston, J., Newman, A. B., Hirsch, C., Gottdiener, J., . . . McBurnie, M. A. (2001). Frailty in older adults: Evidence for a phenotype. *The Journals of Gerontology. Series A, Biological Sciences and Medical Sciences, 56*(3), M146–M156.

Fuiano, G. (2001). Renal hemodynamic response tp maximal vasodilating stimulus in healthy older subjects. *Kidney International, 59*, 1052–1058.

Gaczynska, M., Rock, K. L., Spies, T., & Goldberg, A. L. (1994). Peptidase activities of proteasomes are differentially regulated by the major histocompatibility complex-encoded genes for LMP2 and LMP7. *Proceedings of the National Academy of Sciences of the United States of America, 91*(20), 9213–9217.

Gates, P. (2003). Left ventricular structure and diastolic function with human aging. Relation to habitual exercise and arterial stiffness. *European Heart Journal, 24*, 2213–2220.

Giangregorio, L. (2002). Skeletal adaptations to alterations in weight-bearing activity: A comparison of models of disuse osteoporosis. *Sports Medicine, 32*, 459.

Gillespie, L. D., Robertson, M. C., Gillespie, W. J., Sherrington, C., Gates, S., Clemson, L. M., & Lamb, S. E. (2012). Interventions for preventing falls in older people living in the community. *Cochrane Database of Systematic Reviews*, (9), CD007146. doi:10.1002/14651858.CD007146.pub3

Groot, C., Hooghiemstra, A. M., Raijmakers, P. G., van Berckel, B. N., Scheltens, P., Scherder, E. J., . . . Ossenkoppele, R. (2015). The effect of physical activity on cognitive function in patients with dementia: A meta-analysis of randomized control trials. *Ageing Research Reviews, 25*, 13–23. doi:10.1016/j.arr.2015.11.005

Halaweish, I., & Alam, H. B. (2015). Changing demographics of the American population. *Surgical Clinics of North America, 95*(1), 1–10. doi:10.1016/j.suc.2014.09.002

Handoll, H. H., Cameron, I. D., Mak, J. C., & Finnegan, T. P. (2009, October 7). Multidisciplinary rehabilitation for older people with hip fractures. *Cochrane Database of Systematic Reviews*, (4), CD007125. doi:10.1002/14651858.CD007125.pub2

Harada, C. N., Natelson Love, M. C., & Triebel, K. L. (2013). Normal cognitive aging. *Clinics in Geriatric Medicine, 29*(4), 737–752. doi:10.1016/j.cger.2013.07.002

Harari, D., Hopper, A., Dhesi, J., Babic-Illman, G., Lockwood, L., & Martin, F. (2007). Proactive care of older people undergoing surgery ('POPS'): Designing, embedding, evaluating and funding a comprehensive geriatric assessment service for older elective surgical patients. *Age & Ageing, 36*(2), 190–196.

Harris-Kojetin, L., Sengupta, M., Park-Lee, E., & Valverde, R. (2013). Long-term care services in the United States: 2013 overview. National Center for Health Statistics. *Vital and Health Statistics, Series, 3*(37), 1–107.

H-CUPnet. (2006). Healthcare cost and utilization project. *Agency for healthcare quality and research* [Online]. Retrieved from http://hcupnet.ahrq.gov

Hernandez, H. J. (2015). Progressive resistance exercise with eccentric loading for the management of knee osteoarthritis. *Frontiers in Medicine, 2*, 45.

Ho, Y.-Y., Matteini, A. M., Beamer, B., Fried, L., Xue, Q.-l., Arking, D. E., . . . Walston, J. (2011). Exploring biologically relevant pathways in frailty. *The Journals of Gerontology Series A: Biological Sciences and Medical Sciences, 66A*(9), 975–979. doi:10.1093/gerona/glr061

Howard, C., Ferrucci, L., Sun, K., Fried, L. P., Walston, J., Varadhan, R., . . . Semba, R. D. (2007). Oxidative protein damage is associated with poor grip strength among older women living in the community. *Journal of Applied Physiology, 103*(1), 17–20.

Janssens, J. (2005). Aging of the respiratory system: Impact on pulmonary function tests and adaptation to exertion. *Clinics in Chest Medicine, 26*, 469.

Jaramillo, C. (2015). The geriatric patient. In D. X. Cifu (Ed.), *Braddom's physical medicine and rehabilitation* (p. 653). Richmond, VA: Elsevier.

Johnson, M. F., Kramer, A. M., Lin, M. K., Kowalsky, J. C., & Steiner, J. F. (2000). Outcomes of older persons receiving rehabilitation for medical and surgical conditions compared with hip fracture and stroke. *Journal of the American Geriatrics Society, 48*(11), 1389–1397.

Jones, D. M., Song, X., & Rockwood, K. (2004). Operationalizing a frailty index from a standardized comprehensive geriatric assessment. *Journal of the American Geriatrics Society, 52*(11), 1929–1933.

Kahn, A., & Fraga, M. F. (2009). Epigenetics and aging: Status, challenges, and needs for the future. *The Journals of Gerontology. Series A, Biological Sciences and Medical Sciences, 64*(2), 195–198.

Kass, I. S., Cottrell, J. E., Abramowicz, A. E., Hou, J. Y., & Lei, B. (2015). Brain metabolism, the pathophysiology of brain injury, and potential beneficial agents and techniques. In *Cottrell and Patel's neuroanesthesia* (6th ed., p. 1). Philadelphia, PA: Mosby Elsevier.

Kendrick, D, Kumar, A., Carpenter, H., Zijlstra, G. A., Skelton, D. A., Cook, J. R., . . . Delbaere, K. (2014). Exercise for reducing fear of falling in older people living in the community. *Cochrane Database of Systematic Reviews*, (11), CD009848. doi:10.1002/14651858.CD009848.pub2

Kent-Braun, J. A., Ng, A. V., & Young, K. (2000). Skeletal muscle contractile and noncontractile components in young and older women and men. *Journal of Applied Physiology, 88*, 662–668.

Kirkwood, T. B. (2005). Understanding the odd science of aging. *Cell, 120*(4), 437–447.

Kitzman, D. (1988). Age-related changes in normal human hearts during the first ten decades of life. *Mayo Clinic Proceedings, 63*, 137–146.

Kuster, S. (2008). Reference equations for lung equations for lung function screening of healthy never-smoking adults aged 18–80 years. *European Respiratory Journal, 31*, 860.

Lang, T., Streeper, T., Cawthon, P., Baldwin, K., Taaffe, D. R., & Harris, T. B. (2010). Sarcopenia: Etiology, clinical consequences, intervention, and assessment. *Osteoporosis International, 21*(4), 543–559. doi:10.1007/s00198-009-1059-y

Langlois, J. A., Rutland-Brown, W., & Thomas, K. E. (2004). *Traumatic brain injury in the United States: Emergency department visits, hospitalizations, and deaths*. Atlanta, GA: National Center for Injury Prevention and Control.

Lexell, J. T. C. (1988). What is the cause of the ageing atrophy? Total number, size, and proportion of different fiber types studied in whole vastus lateralis muscle from 15 to 83 yr old men. *Journal of the Neurological Sciences, 84*, 275–294.

Lipsitz, L. A. (2002). Dynamics of stability: The physiologic basis of functional health and frailty. *The Journals of Gerontology. Series A, Biological Sciences and Medical Sciences, 57*(3), B115–B125.

Liu, C. J., & Latham, N. K. (2009). Progressive resistance strength training for improving physical function in older adults. *Cochrane Database of Systematic Reviews*, (3), CD002759.

Mak, C. H. K., Wong, S. K. H., Wong, G. K., Ng, S., Wang, K. K. W., Lam, P. K., & Poon, W. S. (2012). Traumatic brain Injury in the elderly: Is it as bad as we think? *Current Translational Geriatrics and Experimental Gerontology Reports, 1*(3), 171–178. doi:10.1007/s13670-012-0017-2

Makanae, Y. (2015). Role of exercise and nutrition in preventing sarcopenia. *Journal of Nutritional Science and Vitaminology, 61*, s125–s127.

Mallinson, T., Deutsch, A., Bateman, J., Tseng, H. Y., & Manheim, L. (2014). Comparison of discharge functional status after rehabilitation in skilled nursing, home health, and medical rehabilitation settings for patients after hip fracture repair. *Archives of Physical Medicine and Rehabilitation, 95*(2), 209–217. doi:10.1016/j.apmr.2013.05.031

Manini, T., & Clark, B. (2012). Dynapenia and aging: An update. *The Journals of Gerontology. Series A, Biological Sciences and Medical Sciences, 67A*(1), 28–40.

McGowan, P. O., & Szyf, M. (2010). Environmental epigenomics: Understanding the effects of parental care on the epigenome. *Essays Biochem, 48*(1), 275–287.

McIntosh, C. G., Andrews, J. M., Jones, K. L., Wishart, J. M., Morris, H. A., Jansen, J. B., . . . Chapman, I. M. (1999). Effects of age on concentrations of plasma cholecystokinin, glucagon-like peptide 1, and peptide YY and their relation to appetite and pyloric motility. *American Journal of Clinical Nutrition, 69*, 999–1006.

Mclean, A. (2004). Aging biology and geriatric clinical pharmacology. *Pharmacological Reviews, 56*, 163–184.

Michael, Y., Whitlock, E., Lin, J., Fu, R., O'Connor, E., & Gold, R. (2010). Primary care-relevant interventions to prevent falling in older adults: A systematic evidence review for the U.S. Preventative Services Task Force. *Annals of Internal Medicine, 153*, 815.

Morandi, A., Davis, D., Fick, D. M., Turco, R., Boustani, M., Lucchi, E., . . . Bellelli, G. (2014). Delirium superimposed on dementia strongly predicts worse outcomes in older rehabilitation inpatients. *Journal of the American Medical Directors Association, 15*(5), 349–354. doi:10.1016/j.jamda.2013.12.084

Morley, J. B. R. (2001). Sarcopenia. *The Journal of Laboratory and Clinical Medicine, 137*, 231–243.

Morley, J. E., Kumar, V. B., Mattammal, M. B., Farr, S., Morely, P. M. K., & Flood, J. F. (1996). Inhibition of feeding by a nitric oxide synthase inhibitor: Effects of aging. *European Journal of Pharmacology, 311*, 15–19.

Mosenthal, A. C., Lavery, R. F., Addis, M., Kauls, S., Ross, S., Marburger, R., . . . Livingston, D. H. (2002). Isolated traumatic brain injury: Age is an independent predictor of mortality and early outcome. *Journal of Trauma, 52,* 907–911.

Munin, M. C., Begley, A., Skidmore, E. R., & Lenze, E. J. (2006). Influence of rehabilitation site on hip fracture recovery in community-dwelling subjects at 6-month follow-up. *Archives of Physical Medicine and Rehabilitation, 87*(7), 1004–1006.

Nair, K. (2000). Age related changes in muscle. *Mayo Clinic Proceedings, 75,* 8–14.

Newman, A. B., Yanez, D., Harris, T., Duxbury, A., Enright, P. L., & Fried, L. P. (2001). Weight change in old age and its association with mortality. *Journal of the American Geriatrics Society, 49*(10), 1309–1318.

Nyengaard, J. (1992). Glomerular number and size in relation to age, kidney weight, and body surface in normal man. *The Anatomical Record, 232,* 194–201.

Payette, H., Coulombe, C., Boutier, V., & Gray-Donald, K. (2000). Nutrition risk factors for institutionalization in a free-living functionally dependent elderly population. *Journal of Clinical Epidemiology, 53*(6), 579–587.

Podsiadlo, D., & Richardson, S. (1991). The timed "Up & Go": A test of basic functional mobility for frail elderly persons. *Journal of the American Geriatrics Society, 39*(2), 142–148.

Polkey, M. (1997). The contractile properties of the elderly human diaphragm. *American Journal of Respiratory and Critical Care Medicine, 155,* 1560.

Rajan, K. B., Hebert, L. E., Scherr, P., Dong, X., Wilson, R. S., Evans, D. A., & Mendes de Leon, C. F. (2012). Cognitive and physical functions as determinants of delayed age at onset and progression of disability. *The Journals of Gerontology. Series A: Biological Sciences and Medical Sciences, 67*(2), 1419–1426.

Raymond, M. J., Bramley-Tzerefos, R. E., Jeffs, K. J., Winter, A., & Holland, A. E. (2013). Systematic review of high-intensity progressive resistance strength training of the lower limb compared with other intensities of strength training in older adults. *Archives of Physical Medicine and Rehabilitation, 94*(8), 1458–1472. doi:10.1016/j.apmr.2013.02.022

Richmond, R., Aldaghlas, T. A., Burke, C., Rizzo, A. G., Griffen, M., & Pullarkat, R. (2011). Age: Is it all in the head? Factors influencing mortality in elderly patients with head injuries. *The Journal of Trauma: Injury, Infection, and Critical Care, 71*(1), E8–E11.

Rockwood, K., Song, X., MacKnight, C., Bergman, H., Hogan, D. B., McDowell, I., & Mitnitski, A. (2005). A global clinical measure of fitness and frailty in elderly people. *Canadian Medical Association Journal, 173*(5), 489–495.

Roos, M. R., Rice, C. L., & Vandervoort, A. A. (1997). Age-related changes in motor unit function. *Muscle & Nerve, 20,* 679–690.

Rosenberg, I. (1994). Nutrition and Aging. In W. R. Hazzard (Ed.), *Principle of geriatric medicine and gerontology* (3rd ed.). New York, NY: McGraw-Hill.

Rubenstein, L. Z., Stuck, A. E., Siu, A. L., & Wieland, D. (1991). Impacts of geriatric evaluation and management programs on defined outcomes: Overview of the evidence. *Journal of the American Geriatrics Society, 39*(9, Pt. 2), 8S–16S; discussion, 7S–8S.

Rughwani, N. (2011). Normal anatomic and physiologic changes with aging and related disease outcomes: A refresher. *Mount Sinai Journal of Medicine, 78,* 509–514.

Rutland-Brown, W., Langlois, J. A., Thomas, K. E., & Xi, Y. L. (2006). Incidence of traumatic brain injury in the United States, 2003. *The Journal of Head Trauma Rehabilitation, 21,* 544.

Salles, N. (2007). Basic mechanisms of the aging gastrointestinal tract. *Digestive Diseases, 25,* 112–117.

Schleicher, M. M., Wedam, L., & Wu, G. (2012). Review of Tai Chi as an effective exercise on falls prevention in elderly. *Research in Sports Medicine, 20*(1), 37–58. doi:10.1080/15438627.2012.634697

Silverstein, R. (2007). Venous thromboembolism in the elderly: More questions than answers. *Blood: American Society of Hematology, 110*(9), 3097.

Song, R., Ahn, S., So, H., Lee, E. H., Chung, Y., & Park, M. (2015). Effects of T'ai Chi on balance: A population-based meta-analysis. *The Journal of Alternative and Complementary Medicine, 21*(3), 141–151. doi:10.1089/acm.2014.0056

"Statistics." (2012). *Polypharmacy initiative.* Louisville, Kentucky: University of Louisville. Retrieved from http://www.polypharmacyinitiative.com

Stenholm, S., Westerlund, H., Salo, P., Hyde, M., Pentti, J., Head, J., . . . Vahtera, J. (2014). Age-related trajectories of physical functioning in work and retirement: The role of sociodemographic factors, lifestyle and disease. *Journal of Epidemiology and Community Health, 68*(6), 503–509.

Stewart, V. H., Saunders, D. H., & Greig, C. A. (2014). Responsiveness of muscle size and strength to physical training in very elderly people: A systematic review. *Scandinavian Journal of Medicine & Science in Sports, 24*(1), e1–e10. doi:10.1111/sms.12123

Stressman, J. (2009). Physical activity, function, and longevity among the very old. *Archive of Internal Medicine, 169,* 1476.

Stubbs, B., Brefka, S., & Denkinger, M. D. (2015). What works to prevent falls in community-dwelling older adults? Umbrella review of meta-analyses of randomized controlled trials. *Physical Therapy, 95*(8), 1095–1110. doi:10.2522/ptj.20140461

Studenski, S., Perera, S., Patel, K., Rosano, C., Faulkner, K., Inzitari, M., . . . Guralnik, J. (2011). Gait speed and survival in older adults. *Journal of the American Medical Association, 305*(1), 50–58.

Sullivan, D. H., Patch, G. A., Walls, R. C., & Lipschitz, D. A. (1990). Impact of nutrition status on morbidity and mortality in a select population of geriatric rehabilitation patients. *The American Journal of Clinical Nutrition, 51*(5), 749–758.

Susman, M., DiRusso, S. M., Sullivan, T., Risucci, D., Nealon, P., Cuff, S., . . . Benzil, D. (2002). Traumatic brain injury in the elderly: Increased mortality and worse functional outcome at discharge despite lower injury severity. *Journal of Trauma, 53*, 219–223; discussion, 223–224.

Syddall, H., Cooper, C., Martin, F., Briggs, R., & Aihie Sayer, A. (2003). Is grip strength a useful single marker of frailty? *Age & Ageing, 32*(6), 650–656.

Tadic, S. (2012). Brain activity underlying impaired continence control in older women with overactive bladder. *Neurourology and Urodynamics, 31*, 652–658.

Taffett, G. (2003). Physiology of aging. In C. Cassell (Ed.), *Geriatric medicine: An evidence based approach*. New York, NY: Springer-Verlag.

Taffet, G. (2015). Normal aging. Retrieved from http://www.uptodate.com/contents/normal-aging

Thompson, H., McCormick, W., & Kagan, S. (2006). Traumatic brain injury in older adults: Epidemiology, outcomes, and future implications. *Journal of the American Geriatrics Society, 54*, 1590–1595. doi:10.1111/j.1532-5415.2006.00894.x

Valenzuela, T. (2012). Efficacy of progressive resistance training interventions in older adults in nursing homes: A systematic review. 1. *Journal of the American Medical Directors Association, 13*(5), 418–428. doi:10.1016/j.jamda.2011.11.001

Vaz Fragoso, C. A., Enright, P. L., McAvay, G., Van Ness, P. H., & Gill, T. M. (2012). Frailty and respiratory impairment in older persons. *The American Journal of Medicine, 125*(1), 79–86.

Veldhuis, J. (1997). Altered pulsatile and coordinate secretion of pituitary hormones in aging: Evidence of feedback disruption. *Aging, 9*, 19–20.

Vlaeyen, E., Coussement, J., Leysens, G., Van der Elst, E., Delbaere, K., Cambier, D., . . . Milisen, K. (2015). Center of expertise for fall and fracture prevention flanders. characteristics and effectiveness of fall prevention programs in nursing homes: A systematic review and meta-analysis of randomized controlled trials. *Journal of the American Geriatrics Society, 63*(2), 211–221. doi:10.1111/jgs.13254

Walston, J., Hadley, E. C., Ferrucci, L., Guralnik, J. M., Newman, A. B., Studenski, S. A., . . . Fried, L. P. (2006). Research agenda for frailty in older adults: Toward a better understanding of physiology and etiology: Summary from the American geriatrics society/National institute on aging research conference on frailty in older adults. *Journal of the American Geriatrics Society, 54*(6), 991–1001.

Waszynski, C. M. (2004). Confusion assessment method. *Medsurg Nursing, 13*(4), 269–270.

Weening-Dijksterhuis, E., de Greef, M. H., Scherder, E. J., Slaets, J. P., & van der Schans, C. P. (2011). Frail institutionalized older persons: A comprehensive review on physical exercise, physical fitness, activities of daily living, and quality-of-life. *American Journal of Physical Medicine & Rehabilitation, 90*(2), 156–168. doi:10.1097/PHM.0b013e3181f703ef

West, L. A., Cole, S., Goodkind, D., & He, W. (2010). *65+ in the United States*. United States Census Bureau. U.S. Department of Commerce, June 2014. Retrieved from https://www.census.gov/content/dam/Census/library/publications/2014/demo/p23-212.pdf

Whelton, A. (1999). Nephrotoxicity of NSAID drugs: Physiologic foundations and clinical implications. *The American Journal of Medicine, 106*, 13s–24s.

World Health Organization. (n.d.). *A global report on falls prevention-epidemiology of falls*. Retrieved from http://www.who.int/ageing/projects/1.Epidemiology%20of%20falls%20in%20older%20age.pdf

Vascular Disorders

17

CHAPTER

Aleksandra Policha and Glenn R. Jacobowitz

Peripheral vascular disease (PVD) encompasses not only diseases of arteries and veins but also multiple underlying medical conditions such as coronary artery disease, diabetes, and renal insufficiency that are associated with, and are often the cause of, the vascular pathology. Such a broad range of diseases involves the entire body, literally from the head to toe. The brain, abdominal viscera, lungs, and upper and lower extremities are all end organs affected by vascular disease. It is not uncommon for one patient to manifest different aspects of the vascular disease. There are various functional presentations that must be recognized. After treatment of PVD, patients are often left with disabilities that require extensive rehabilitation, both physical and psychological. Ambulation and activities of daily living must often be relearned after either revascularization or amputation of an extremity. Cerebrovascular disease may lead to central cognitive and/or motor deficits. A wide range of services may be required for these patients, including physical therapy, occupational therapy, and psychosocial support. In addition, rehabilitation physicians and staff must be aware of the chronic nature of PVD. In the rehabilitation phase of recovery, these patients may have recurrence of their disease (e.g., leg ischemia and transient ischemic attack), which must be recognized and expeditiously treated. Therefore, it is critical for the rehabilitation physician and other rehabilitation providers to have an understanding of the functional presentation and treatment of PVD.

The broad scope of PVD may be separated into several areas. A practical organization may include (a) lower extremity peripheral arterial occlusive disease, (b) cerebrovascular disease, (c) venous disease, and (d) peripheral and abdominal arterial aneurysmal disease. All these entities are associated with specific medical presentations, indications for operation, treatment modalities, recovery regimens, and disabilities that warrant separate attention and will therefore be reviewed individually, noting that cerebrovascular diseases is also reviewed in the stroke chapter (Chapter 25) of this textbook.

FUNCTIONAL PRESENTATION

Lower Extremity Peripheral Arterial Occlusive Disease

There are several disease processes, associated disorders, and degrees of disability related to lower extremity PVD. The most common is atherosclerotic occlusive disease. Patients with chronic lower extremity ischemia can be divided into two groups. The first group includes patients with intermittent claudication (pain in the muscles of the lower extremity with ambulation), who are considered to have a good prognosis and low rate of amputation or need for surgical intervention. In contrast, the second group includes patients with limb-threatening ischemia. Limb-threatening ischemia is manifested by limb pain while at physical rest or the presence of ulceration or gangrene in the extremity. If left untreated, these patients have a poor prognosis with a very high likelihood of requiring an amputation.

In the past, the presence of limb-threatening ischemia was the primary indication for surgical intervention and appropriate angiographic studies. However, because the diagnostic and interventional armamentarium has expanded in recent years, previous indications for intervention and imaging have been reevaluated. The advent of balloon angioplasty, intra-arterial stenting, thrombolytic agents, and endovascular prostheses has revolutionized the treatment of PVD. Imaging techniques, including both conventional angiography and magnetic resonance angiography (MRA), have significantly improved. Now, there are many treatment options for vascular disease, including noninvasive modalities that carry less risk for the debilitated patient. Physicians caring for patients with vascular disease should be aware of these options and the indications for their use.

The term "claudication" is derived from the Latin verb "to limp" or "to be lame." Claudication occurs when there is inability to mount an appropriate augmentation of blood supply in response to exercise. Claudicaton symptoms classically occur in muscle groups distal to the affected arterial segment. Claudication consists of three essential features: The pain is in a functional muscle unit; it is reproducibly precipitated by a consistent amount of exercise; and it is promptly relieved by cessation of exercise. At least 10% of the population above the age of 70 and 1% to 2% of younger patients have intermittent claudication (Society for Vascular Surgery Lower Extremity Guidelines Writing Group et al., 2015). However, the majority of these patients can be treated nonoperatively. A thorough understanding of the natural history of lower extremity ischemia and the available treatment options form the basis of sound clinical decision making.

The most important studies on the natural history of intermittent claudication have focused not only on patient history but also on objective evidence of arterial obstruction by arteriography or noninvasive means such as ankle-brachial blood pressure indices (ABIs). Some of these studies document that up to 80% of such patients remain stable or improve over time (Cronenwett et al., 1984; Imparato, Kim, Davidson, & Crowley, 1975; Jonason & Ringquiest, 1985; Rosenbloom et al., 1988). One study showed that for claudicants, the cumulative 10-year risk of development of ischemic ulceration and ischemic rest pain was 23% and 30%, respectively (Aquino et al., 2001).

Risk factors for worsening ischemia include cigarette smoking and diabetes. The single worst prognostic factor is the severity of arterial occlusive disease at the time of initial presentation (Cronenwett et al., 1984; Imparato et al., 1975; Jonason & Ringquiest, 1985; Rosenbloom et al., 1988). Limb-threatening ischemia occurs when arterial occlusion is severe enough to restrict blood flow to a level that is insufficient to meet baseline metabolic demands during the periods of inactivity. Clinically, this presents as rest pain (typically in the most distal portion of the extremity such as the forefoot or toes), ulceration, or gangrene. The degree of pain is typically dependent on how the limb is oriented in relation to the body. It is worse when the limb is relatively elevated, exacerbating the low arterial blood flow that has to fight the effects of gravity. Pain is usually alleviated by placing the leg in a dependent or lower position, thus using gravity to increase blood supply to the ischemic limb. Ischemic ulceration may occur when minor traumatic lesions fail to heal because of inadequate blood flow. Gangrene occurs when arterial blood flow is so poor that areas with the least perfusion undergo spontaneous necrosis (Figure 17.1).

The assumption that rest pain or tissue loss results in uniform limb loss is not entirely valid, as shown by several studies using nonoperative therapy (Rivers, Veith, Ascer, & Gupta, 1986; Schuler et al., 1984). Chronic ischemia represents a spectrum of levels of disease from fairly benign, mild intermittent claudication to the gangrenous extremity. The likelihood of limb loss remains related to

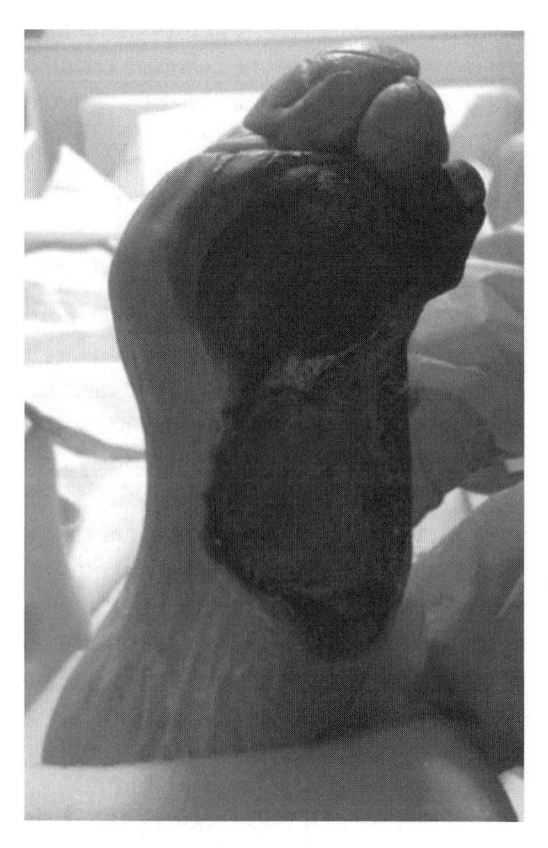

FIGURE 17.1 Left foot dry gangrene in a patient with peripheral arterial disease who previously underwent amputation of the fourth and fifth toes.

the severity of ischemia at initial presentation, as measured both angiographically (injecting contrast dye into the artery and visualizing the areas of blockage) and through arterial Doppler signals (noninvasive measurements of blood pressure at the ankle). Absent Doppler signals carry a poor prognosis for the limb in question if no intervention is performed (Felix, Siegel, & Gunther, 1987).

The success of exercise and cessation of smoking make this nonoperative therapy the first treatment option in patients with intermittent claudication. Most exercise programs involve supervised activity such as treadmill or track walking, which is of sufficient intensity to bring on claudication pain (Lauret et al., 2014). Exercise is alternated with rest over the course of a 30- to 60-minute session. Such sessions should be performed at least three times per week. For patients not capable of completing the exercise protocol because of concomitant comorbidities, an adjusted protocol or alternative exercise regime, such as cycling, strength training, and upper extremity ergometry is recommended. An additional reason is the observation (although controversial) that a failed bypass graft may acutely induce limb-threatening ischemia or ultimately obligate a higher level of amputation than a nonoperated limb (Dardik, Kahn, Dardik, Sussman, & Ibrahim, 1982; Schlenker & Wolkoff, 1975). Antiplatelet agents, such as aspirin and clopidogrel, and cholesterol-lowering statins are an important pharmacological adjuct to lifestyle modification in the treatment of claudication. Additionally, the phosphodiesterase inhibitor, cilostazol, has been shown to be of significant benefit in improving walking distance in individuals with intermittent claudication secondary to PVD (Bedenis et al., 2014; Society for Vascular Surgery Lower Extremity Guidelines Writing Group et al., 2015). Operative management is thus reserved for threatened limb loss as determined by clinical and angiographic parameters.

The less invasive modalities of percutaneous angioplasty and stent placement have significantly broadened the scope of treatable conditions, particularly for debilitated patients. Limb-threatening ischemia can often be treated with these measures, frequently with the patient under local anesthesia, which minimizes risk. Advancements in catheter and stent technology have allowed vascular specialists to treat lesions in the popliteal and tibial arteries, as well as more proximal lesions in the iliac and femoral vessels. These included smaller-diameter balloons and stents as well as wires and devices that can effectively cross long areas of chronic occlusion in vessels. Several studies have shown that amputation-free survival in patients with critical limb ischemia is similar in patients treated with balloon angioplasty compared with those treated with open bypass (Adam et al., 2005; Romiti et al., 2008). Furthermore, a recent study demonstrated that, among patients with femoropopliteal disease, angioplasty with a paclitaxel-coated balloon may result in improved vessel patency in comparison to angioplasty with a standard balloon (Rosenfield et al., 2015). Such novel drug-eluting balloons, as well as drug-coated stents, will serve to further improve the outcomes for patients treated with endovascular therapy for PVD. Finally, advancements in closure devices now allow for most endovascular procedures to be performed percutaneously (through only a needle puncture in the skin). Using a percutaneous closure device, sutures are delivered to the access artery before the start of the procedure. At the completion of the operation, the sutures are used to close the artery puncture site, thus entirely eliminating the need for incisions. This technology allows many peripheral endovascular interventions to be performed in an outpatient setting.

Extracranial Cerebrovascular Disease

Cerebrovascular disease may include disease of the aortic arch, carotid arteries, or the vertebrobasilar system. Although individuals with cerebrovascular disease may be asymptomatic, functional presentations may include a transient ischemic attack (e.g., amaurosis fugax—a temporary blindness in one eye resulting from plaque embolization from the carotid artery to the ophthalmic artery supplying the eye—or other neurological deficit resolving within 24 hours) or a completed stroke. Depending on the degree of disability, patients may require varying degrees of rehabilitation and support services. It is extremely important to evaluate the extracranial circulation in patients presenting for rehabilitation after strokes so that further strokes may be prevented, when possible, by surgical or medical intervention.

The diagnosis and treatment of extracranial cerebrovascular disease begins at the aortic valve. Historically, the decrease in annual stroke rate in the United States paralleled the increase in the frequency of carotid endarterectomy (Lamparello & Riles, 1975). Currently, approximately 135,000 carotid endarterectomies are performed annually in this country (Ricotta et al., 2011). During the past 40 years, the safety of carotid surgery has improved, with most large centers reporting perioperative morbidity and mortality rates of less than 2%. Indications for extracranial cerebral revascularization have been well defined for both symptomatic and asymptomatic patients in large prospective, randomized trials. The North American Symptomatic Carotid Endarterectomy Trial established that symptomatic patients with more than 70% diameter reduction of the internal carotid artery have a significant reduction in the incidence of stroke with surgery when compared with medical management alone (North American Symptomatic Carotid Endarterectomy Trial Collaborators, 1991). Similarly, the Asymptomatic Carotid Atherosclerosis Study demonstrated better stroke prevention in patients with more than 60% stenosis treated with endarterectomy versus those treated medically (The Executive Committee for the Asymptomatic Carotid Atherosclerosis Study, 1995). As noted above, these patients may present after completed strokes, with a history of a transient ischemic attack, or they may be asymptomatic, with carotid stenoses detected on duplex examinations performed as part of a workup for a bruit heard on physical examination or for nonspecific neurological symptoms.

Upper extremity ischemia is also often related to aortic arch disease. Emboli (blood clots that travel from one part of the body to another) to the hands or fingers may originate in the chambers of the heart, aortic arch, or axillary and subclavian arteries. Transesophageal echocardiography and aortic arch and upper extremity angiography are the tests of choice for identifying a potential source of emboli. MRA may also be useful. Functional presentation is similar to that in the lower extremity with sudden onset of pain and cyanosis of the distal hand or fingers. Pulses may be absent. Collateral circulation of the upper extremity is usually excellent, often allowing the hand to remain viable during workup. In the last decade, significant advancements have been made in the technology and efficacy of carotid artery stenting. This is a less invasive procedure that can be performed under local anesthesia by means of a femoral arterial puncture. The development of balloon- and umbrella-type cerebral protection devices, which are temporarily deployed during the procedure to prevent distal embolization of plaque material, has significantly reduced the periprocedural stroke rate observed with carotid stenting. Although carotid endarterectomy remains the gold standard treatment for carotid artery disease, carotid stenting may be favored in certain patient populations. This includes patients with significant medical comorbidities, prior cervical operations, anatomically inaccessible lesions, and radiation-induced carotid stenosis (Veith et al., 2001).

It is not uncommon for patients undergoing rehabilitation to have significant medical comorbidities, and the risks and benefits of carotid stenting versus carotid endarterectomy should be considered. The Carotid Revascularization Endarterectomy vs. Stenting Trial (CREST) demonstrated that among patients with symptomatic or asymptomatic carotid stenosis, the risk of the composite primary outcome of any stroke, myocardial infarction, or death during the periprocedural period or ipsilateral stroke within 4 years after randomization did not differ significantly in the group undergoing carotid-artery stenting (CAS) and the group undergoing carotid endarterectomy (CEA) (7.2% and 6.8%, p = .51, respectively). During the periprocedural period, the rates of the individual endpoints did, however, differ between the CAS and CEA groups. There was a higher risk of stroke in the CAS group compared to the CEA group (4.1% vs. 2.3%, respectively; p = .01). Conversely, there was a higher rate of myocardial infarction (MI) in the CEA group than in the CAS group (2.3% vs. 1.1%, respectively; p = .03). Additionally, the 4-year rate of stroke or death was 6.4% in the CAS group as compared with 4.7% in the CEA group p = .03). Finally, the effect of stroke on the patients' overall physical and mental health was more debilitating than was the effect of MI (Brott et al., 2010). Because the original carotid intervention studies, including North American Symptomatic Carotid Endarterectomy Trial (NASCET) and Asymptomatic Carotid Atherosclerosis Study (ACAS), were conducted before the advent of statins and potent antiplatelet agents including clopidogrel, the CREST-2 study is currently being conducted to compare 21st century best medical management alone with best medical management and either CEA or CAS.

Venous Disease

Patients with venous disorders frequently exhibit a chronic course and are not often markedly improved by surgical procedures. Chronic venous insufficiency (CVI) is the most common form of venous disease, and nonoperative therapy remains the mainstay of treatment. The other form of venous disease seen commonly, especially in the nonambulatory patient, is acute deep venous thrombosis. This is more sudden in onset and requires systemic anticoagulation or, occasionally, placement of a vena-caval filter, and more rarely, mechanical or pharmacological thrombolysis with catheter-directed therapy. These two forms of venous disease will be discussed separately.

CVI: Anatomy, Etiology, Function, and Treatments

The venous anatomy consists of a superficial and a deep system. In the lower extremity, the longest superficial vein, the great saphenous vein, is located anterior to the medial malleolus and courses along the medial aspect of the leg until it reaches the saphenofemoral junction in the medial aspect of the proximal thigh. The short saphenous vein is located in the posterior calf and most commonly drains into the popliteal vein. Connecting the superficial system to the deep system are the perforating veins. The functional presentation of CVI includes swelling, pain, and ulceration of the lower extremity. This is due to valvular incompetence of the venous system, resulting in increased hydrostatic pressure. Typically, CVI presents as swelling of the distal lower extremity with thickening of the subcutaneous tissue in the perimalleolar "gaiter" distribution. Mild CVI is associated with mild-to-moderate ankle edema. Often, the patients complain of a feeling of heaviness or pain in the legs. This mild form of insufficiency is usually limited to the superficial veins. Moderate CVI has hyperpigmentation of the skin caused by hemosiderin deposition in the subcutaneous tissue, moderate nonpitting edema, and subcutaneous fibrosis without ulceration. Severe CVI is associated with ulceration, eczematoid skin changes (stasis dermatitis), and severe edema. Extensive involvement of the deep venous system and diffuse loss of valvular function are present. These different stages of venous disease are now well described in a uniform classification system called the CEAP classifications, which includes Clinical, Etiology, Anatomical, and Pathophysiologic descriptions (Eklof et al., 2004). The clinical classifications are listed in Table 17.1, and examples are shown in Figures 17.2A and 17.2B.

TABLE 17.1

CEAP CLINICAL CLASSIFICATION	
Class 0	No venous disease
Class 1	Telangiectasias of reticular veins
Class 2	Varicose veins
Class 3	Edema
Class 4	Skin changes
Class 5	Healed ulcer
Class 6	Open ulcer

Bed rest and limb elevation have universally been accepted as effective therapy for CVI. However, they are impractical for most patients, particularly those in a rehabilitation program promoting ambulation. Effective therapy must control the symptoms of CVI, promote healing, and prevent recurrence of venous stasis ulcers while allowing for normal ambulation.

Several studies have shown the benefits of compression stockings in the treatment of CVI and venous ulceration (Dinn & Henry, 1992; Mayberry, Moneta, & Taylor, 1991). Cellulitis may be associated with CVI and often requires oral or intravenous antibiotic therapy. Hydrocortisone cream may help surround stasis dermatitis. Typical compression stockings have 30–40 Torr of elastic compression at the level of the ankle, which gradually decreases more proximally. This type of stocking may be used with normal arterial circulation. If arterial circulation is compromised, a stocking with less compression must be used to permit adequate circulation. In addition, elastic bandages may be used. There are multiple brands of compression stockings in the market, with different designs to make application possible for the patient with disability. Additionally, new graduated pneumatic compression devices are available for patients who do not tolerate wearing compression stockings (Betz, 2009; Harding, Vanscheidt, Partsch, Caprini, & Comerota, 2014; Vanscheidt, Ukat, & Partsch, 2009).

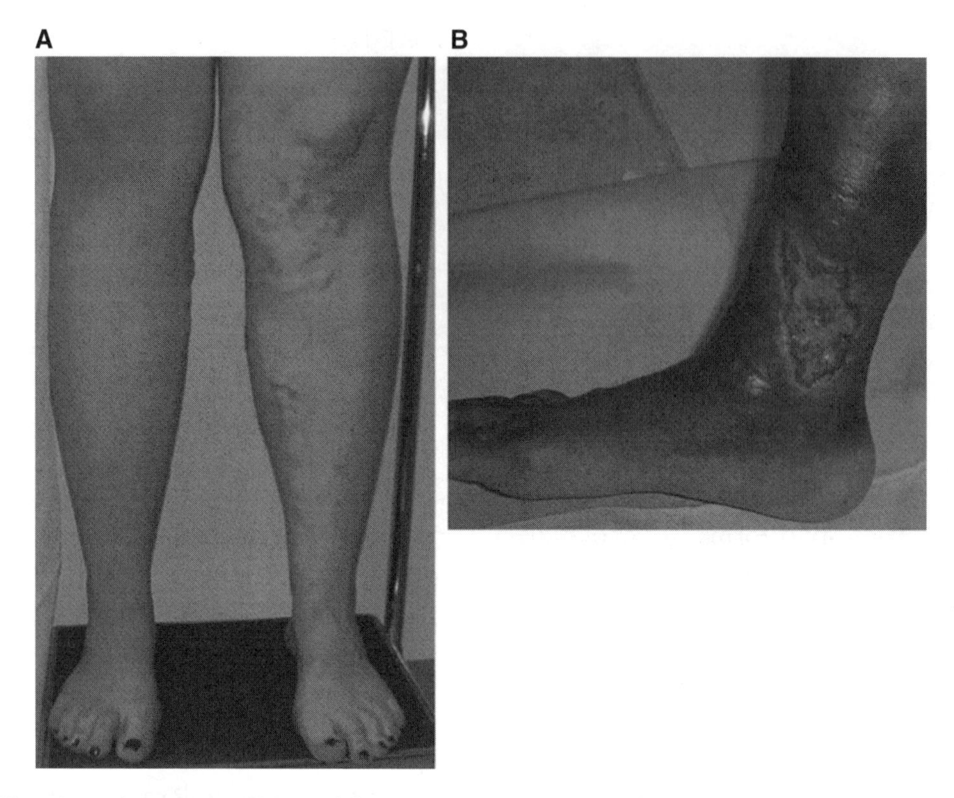

FIGURE 17.2 Manifestations of venous insufficiency. (A) Varicose veins and edema of the left lower extremity (CEAP classification C3); (B) Active ulceration (CEAP classification C6).

Acute Deep Venous Thrombosis

Acute deep venous thrombosis may occur in the upper or, more commonly, the lower extremity. In the upper extremity, thrombus may occur in the axillosubclavian vein, and the most common causes are thoracic outlet syndrome and catheter-related thrombosis. Under most circumstances, one or more of the features of Virchow's triad for venous thrombosis is present. The triad includes endothelial injury (as by a catheter), stasis (as by thoracic outlet obstruction), or a hypercoagulable state (as with some malignancies).

Functional presentation of upper extremity deep venous thrombosis includes swelling of the extremity, usually to the level of the axilla, and prominence of the subcutaneous veins over the shoulder girdle and the anterior chest wall, which become engorged with collateral venous flow due to obstruction of the deep vein (Figure 17.3). Pain of an aching or stabbing type may include the shoulder and axilla but can also be felt in the arm. These classic symptoms are particularly common in patients who thrombose acutely because of thoracic outlet compression. This can occur after weightlifting or similar exertional activity with the upper extremity. Axillosubclavian vein thrombosis may also present after sleeping, probably because of sleeping with the arm overhead (with the thoracic outlet partially obstructed).

Initial diagnosis of axillosubclavian vein thrombosis is by venous duplex examination. If this is

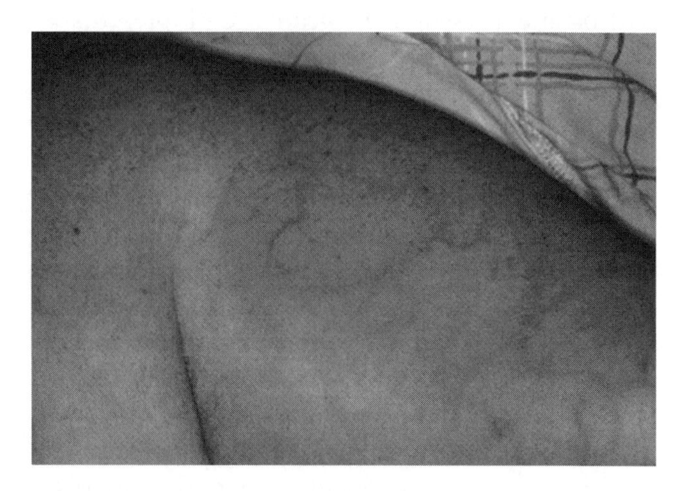

FIGURE 17.3 Left upper extremity edema and prominent collateral veins in a patient with subclavian vein deep venous thrombosis.

negative and there is a high clinical index of suspicion, then a venogram should be performed. Similarly, if the duplex is positive and thrombolytic therapy is being considered, venography is indicated. The reported incidence of pulmonary embolism with untreated upper extremity deep venous thrombosis is about 9% to 12% (Becker, Philbrick, & Walker, 1991). Patients should be treated with heparin anticoagulation followed by a 3- to 6-month course of warfarin or other oral anticoagulants. Persistent symptoms are least likely to develop in patients with catheter-related thrombosis. Chronic symptoms (arm swelling with exercise) occur in about 38% of the patients treated with anticoagulation and 15% receiving thrombolytic therapy (intra-arterial urokinase infusion) compared with 64% receiving no therapy (Becker et al., 1991). When axillosubclavian vein thrombosis is recognized, a vascular surgeon should be consulted to further direct therapy. Unless contraindicated, anticoagulation should be started promptly to prevent further propagation of thrombus. If thrombolysis is performed, currently available techniques include mechanical thrombectomy catheters and tissue plasminogen activator infusion.

The signs and symptoms of lower extremity deep venous thrombosis are similar to those of upper extremity deep venous thrombosis. They include swelling of the limb, prominence of superficial veins, and pain that is usually dull in character. Unfortunately, physical examination is often false-negative in patients with acute deep venous thrombosis and false-positive in patients with symptoms related to conditions other than deep venous thrombosis (Goodacre, Sutton, & Sampson, 2005).

The acute complication of deep venous thrombosis is pulmonary embolism, and the late complication is the post-thrombotic syndrome. This syndrome is that of chronic swelling and venous insufficiency due to valvular damage, which occurs from the thrombus. Anticoagulation will reduce the risk for pulmonary embolus from approximately 25%, if left untreated, to less than 5% (Hyers, Hull, & Weg, 1992). In patients with a contraindication to anticoagulation, a vena-caval filter may be placed (usually percutaneously), which prevents the embolus from reaching the pulmonary vessels. These devices will lower the incidence of pulmonary embolus to 2% to 4%.

Abdominal Aortic and Peripheral Arterial Aneurysmal Disease

Abdominal aortic aneurysm (AAA) is defined as a focal dilation of the aorta of at least 50% greater than the expected normal diameter (Johnston, Rutherford, & Tilson, 1991; Figure 17.4). The main complication of AAA is rupture, for which the mortality may exceed 90%. The 5-year risk of rupture for AAA 5 cm or greater in diameter ranges from 25% to 40%. This may be as high as 20% per year for aneurysms more than 7 cm in diameter. Aneurysms measuring between 4 and 5 cm in diameter have lower 5-year rupture rates of about 3% to 12% (Brown, Pattenden, & Gutelius, 1992). Aneurysms less than 4 cm in diameter have a rupture rate of about 2%. Overall elective surgical mortality is about 2% to 4% (Ernst, 1993).

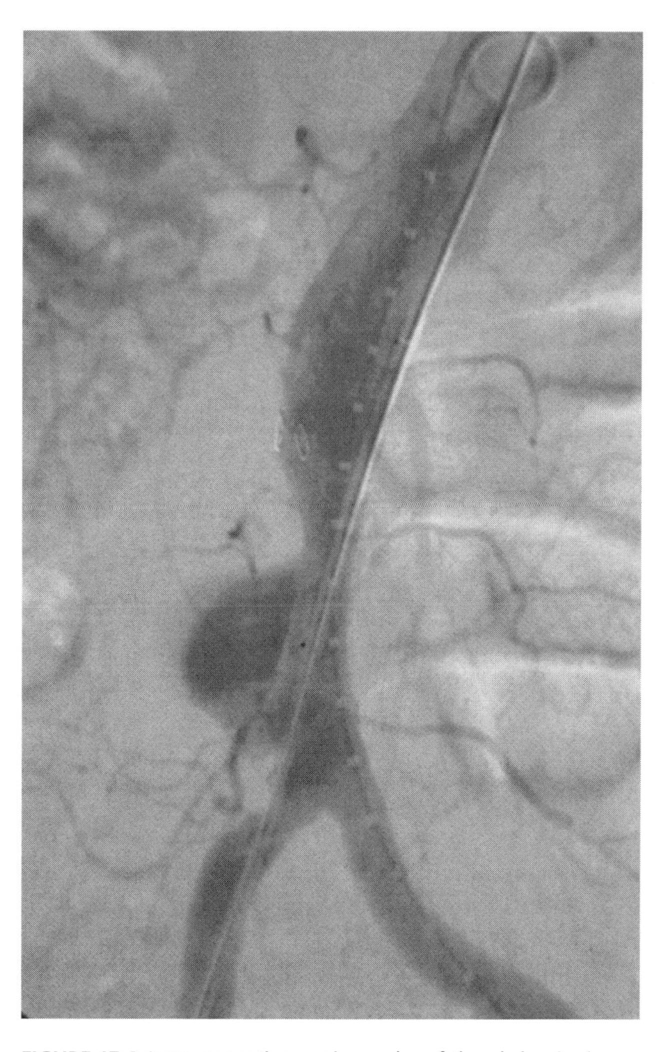

FIGURE 17.4 Intra-operative angiography of the abdominal aorta demonstrating infra-renal abdominal aortic aneurysm.

Therefore, repair of AAA is reserved for asymptomatic aneurysms more than 5 cm in diameter, symptomatic aneurysms (abdominal or back pain), or a ruptured AAA. Rarely, laminated thrombus from the inner lining of an aneurysm sac may embolize to the lower extremities. This is also an indication for repair regardless of aneurysm diameter. Open surgical repair involves replacement of the aneurysmal segment with a synthetic graft, usually Dacron. Today, however, most aortic aneurysms are repaired via an endovascular approach. An endograft is delivered transfemorally under fluoroscopic guidance to exclude the aneurysmal segment from arterial pressure. This method of endovascular aortic repair (EVAR) has been shown to be effective in preventing AAA rupture with reduced patient morbidity and mortality (Arko et al., 2002; Zarins et al., 1999). Debilitated patients who were at prohibitive risk for standard surgical repair are now often considered for the less invasive endovascular repair. Hospital stay is often as short as one day. Long-term complications include endoleaks that occur when the endovascular graft does not completely seal off the aneurysm sac. These endoleaks can often be treated with additional endovascular maneuvers. The number of patients treated with EVAR has risen exponentially since the late 1990s and early 2000s. Conversely, the number of patients treated with open aortic surgery has decreased dramatically. For instance, one study reported that in 2000, 2,358 cases of AAA were treated with EVAR, while in 2011, this number rose to 35,028. During this interval, the number of open aortic surgeries decreased from 42,872 to 10,039 (Dua, Upchurch, Lee, Eidt, & Desai, 2014).

Several large, randomized clinical trials have demonstrated that although EVAR may offer a short-term survival benefit (up to 2–3 years) over open AAA repair, the long-term survival appears similar between patients treated with open and endovascular aortic repair. Furthermore, EVAR is associated with a increased number of reinterventions following repair, mandating a need for continued surveillance with imaging studies such as computed tomography (CT) or ultrasound (De Bruin et al., 2010; Lederle et al., 2012; United Kingdom EVAR Trial Investigators, 2010).

Traditionally, EVAR was reserved for patients with infrarenal aortic aneurysms. When an aneurysm occurs in a segment of aorta close to the renal arteries, standard EVAR is contraindicated, since there will be an inadequate length of suitable aorta for endograft attachment. The development of new endografts, which contain fenestrations (windows) and scallops in the proximal portion of the grafts, has expanded the applicability of EVAR to a larger patient population. These fenestrations and scallops, which are customized to fit each patient's unique anatomy, allow for continued perfusion of the renal arteries and superior mesenteric artery while excluding flow in the aneurysm and allowing for an appropriate seal to be formed at the proximal portion of the graft, above the renal arteries. Patients who would have previously been treated with open surgery can now undergo endovascular treatment with fenestrated endovascular aortic repair (FEVAR). Early data on outcomes for patients undergoing FEVAR appears favorable. For instance, Oderich and colleagues evaluated 67 patients with juxtarenal AAAs who were prospectively enrolled in 14 centers in the United States from 2005 to 2012. A total of 178 visceral arteries required incorporation with small fenestrations in 118, scallops in 51, and large fenestrations in nine. Technical success was 100%. There was one postoperative death within 30 days (1.5%). Mean length of hospital stay was 3.3 ± 2.1 days. No aneurysm ruptures or conversions were noted during a mean follow-up of 37 ± 17 months. Fifteen patients (22%) required secondary interventions for renal artery stenosis/occlusion or endoleak treatment. At 5 years, patient survival was 91% ± 4%, and freedom from major adverse events was 79% ± 6% (Oderich et al., 2014).

AAA usually presents as a finding on routine physical examination (pulsatile abdominal mass) or as an incidental finding on a radiological study (abdominal ultrasound, CT scan, or magnetic resonance imaging scan) obtained for other reasons. Any aneurysm more than 3 cm in diameter should be brought to the attention of an internist or vascular surgeon who can follow-up the patient with yearly ultrasound examination to monitor the aneurysm size. The average annual growth of AAA is about 0.4 cm in diameter per year.

Popliteal artery aneurysms (PAA) are the most common peripheral artery aneurysm. There is a strong association of PAA with AAA. A patient with a unilateral PAA has a 50% chance of having a contralateral PAA and a 30% chance of having an AAA. More than 90% of PAAs occur in men (Szilagyi, Schwartz, & Reddy, 1981). A popliteal artery is considered aneurysmal if its diameter exceeds 2 cm or 1.5 times the diameter of the proximal, nonaneurysmal segment. The clinical presentation is variable. Almost 30% of PAAs are symptomatic. They are usually found on physical examination (pulsatile mass or wide pulse at the popliteal fossa) or incidentally on ultrasound, CT scan, or magnetic resonance imaging of the popliteal fossa. The results of surgical management in this group of patients are excellent. Although ruptures are rare, symptomatic PAAs usually present with distal embolization to the tibial arteries. This embolization is often severe, with lower-limb ischemia occurring in up to 70% of patients and amputation rates as high as 30% (Mousa et al., 2006). Elective repair of all PAAs is recommended because of the high rate of limb loss once these aneurysms become symptomatic. Advances in available devices and techniques have also made endovascular repair of PAAs possible with short- and mid-term results comparable to those for open repair, albeit with higher rates of reintervention in order to maintain patency (von Stumm, Teufelsbauer, Reichenspurner, & Debus, 2015).

PSYCHOLOGICAL AND VOCATIONAL IMPLICATIONS

PVD can leave patients with severe vocational impairment and psychological stress. Partial or complete amputation of a limb, and the ramifications of strokes, can be tremendously disabling, both physically and psychologically.

Two-thirds of all lower extremity amputations are currently performed as a result of complications of PVD or diabetes. As a result, a majority of lower extremity amputations are performed by vascular surgeons. The purpose of amputation is to remove gangrenous tissue, relieve pain, obtain primary healing of the most distal amputation possible, and obtain maximum rehabilitation after amputation.

It has been shown that the greatest chance of successful ambulation is with expeditious rehabilitation, either by immediate postoperative prosthesis or by accelerated conventional programs using temporary prosthesis until a permanent prosthesis can be made (Folsum, King, & Rubin, 1992). Advantages of early ambulation include decreased hospital time, increased rates of rehabilitation, a reduction in the complications of amputation, and an improvement in the psychological outcome of the patient after amputation (Bradway, Racy, & Malone, 1984). Early ambulation alleviates a sense of loss and inadequacy experienced by many amputees.

It is clear that a full rehabilitation team provides the best outcome. This should include the rehabilitation physician, prosthetist, patient's family, physical and occupational therapists, social services, and community services.

PVD is present in many patients who have had strokes, and it is the common underlying cause of those strokes. Fortunately, the perioperative stroke rate for carotid endarterectomy in most major centers is less than 3%. However, many patients present with a completed stroke before carotid endarterectomy, and the operation serves only to prevent further infarction. As a result, many patients with PVD, and in particular those with extracranial cerebrovascular disease, may require rehabilitation for stroke.

The major factors affecting rehabilitation of stroke victims include motivation and family support (Evans & Northwood, 1983). In addition, depression may be a significant complication of stroke that can inhibit patient motivation (Parikh, Lipsey, & Robinson, 1987). Anxiety and fear are also common among stroke victims, which can be eased by an empathetic rehabilitation team. The recovery of physical function and motor skills is often enhanced by emotional stability of the patient. In turn, the return of function enhances psychosocial functioning. Thus, psychosocial, recreational, and vocational interventions must all be provided. Peer support may also be extremely helpful. All of these services should be provided in the setting of a directed stroke rehabilitation program, which has been shown to enhance functional ability beyond that of natural recovery (Kalra, 1994).

Age alone probably does not play a major role in determining the recovery of a patient with stroke. However, it may be associated with significant medical comorbidities (such as PVD), which may make recovery more difficult. Consequently, older patients may have longer recovery times and require increased psychosocial support.

CONCLUSION

Patients with PVD usually have multiple medical problems, and the nature of their disease may be chronic and involve multiple organ systems. The high incidence of limb surgery, limb loss, and stroke makes patients with PVD in particular need of rehabilitation medicine and services. The chronic nature of PVD requires the rehabilitation team to be keenly aware of its functional presentation because recurrences or progression of disease are not uncommon. In addition, advances in minimally invasive endovascular techniques have increased treatment options for debilitated patients who are not candidates for conventional open surgical interventions. These advances have continued to expand treatment options in recent years. It is only with a full range of physical and psychological rehabilitation services that patients with PVD may be completely treated.

REFERENCES

Adam, D. J., Beard, J. D., Cleveland, T., Bell, J., Bradbury, A. W., Forbes, J. F., . . . BASIL trial participants. (2005). Bypass versus angioplasty in severe ischemia of the leg (BASIL): Multicentre, randomized controlled trial. *The Lancet, 366*, 1925–1934.

Aquino, R., Johnnides, C., Makaroun, M., Whittle, J. C., Muluk, V. S., Kelley, M. E., & Muluk, S. C. (2001). Natural history of claudication: Long-term serial follow-up study of 1244 claudicants. *Journal of Vascular Surgery, 34*, 962–770.

Arko, F. W., Lee, W. A., Hil, B. B., Olcott, C., Dalman, D. L., Harris, E. J., . . . Zarins, C. K. (2002). Aneurysm-related death: Endpoint analysis for comparison of open and endovascular repairs. *Journal of Vascular Surgery, 36*, 297–304.

Becker, D. M., Philbrick, J. T., & Walker, F. B. (1991). Axillary and subclavian venous thrombosis: Prognosis and treatment. *Archives of Internal Medicine, 151*, 1934–1943.

Bedenis, R., Stewart, M., Cleanthis, M., Robless, P., Mikhailidis, D. P., & Stansby, G. (2014). Cilostazol for intermittent claudication. *Cochrane Database of Systematic Reviews, 10*, CD003748.

Betz, C. (2009). Flexitouch- using a programmable pneumatic device with truncal therapy to facilitate wound healing: A case series. *Ostomy Wound Management, 55*, 34–40.

Bradway, J. P., Racy, J., & Malone, J. M. (1984). Psychological adaptation to amputation. *Orthotics and Prosthetics, 38*, 46–50.

Brott, T. G., Hobson, R. W., Howard, G., Roubin, G. S., Clark, W. M., Brooks, W., . . . CREST Investigators. (2010). Stenting versus endarterectomy for treatment of carotid-artery stenosis. *New England Journal of Medicine, 363*, 11–23.

Brown, P. M., Pattenden, R., & Gutelius, J. R. (1992). The selective management of small abdominal aortic aneurysms: The Kingston study. *Journal of Vascular Surgery, 15*, 21–27.

Cronenwett, J. L., Warner, K. G., Zelenock, G. B., Whitehouse, W. M., Graham, L. M., Lindenhauser, S. M., & Stanley, J. C. (1984). Intermittent claudication: Current results of non-operative management. *Archives of Surgery, 119*, 430–436.

Dardik, H., Kahn, M., Dardik, I., Sussman, B., & Ibrahim, I. (1982). Influence of failed bypass procedures on conversion of below-knee to above-knee amputation levels. *Surgery, 91*, 64–69.

De Bruin, J. L., Baas, A. F., Buth, J., Prinssen, M., Verhoeven, E. L., Cuypers, P. W., . . . DREAM Study Group. (2010). Long-term outcome of open or endovascular repair of abdominal aortic aneurysm. *New England Journal of Medicine, 362,* 1881–1889.

Dinn, E., & Henry, M. (1992). Treatment of venous ulceration by injection sclerotherapy and compression hosiery. *Phlebology, 7*, 23–26.

Dua, A., Upchurch, G. R., Lee, J. T., Eidt, J., & Desai, S. S. (2014). Predicted shortfall in open aneurysm experience for vascular surgery trainees. *Journal of Vascular Surgery, 60*, 945–949.

Eklof, B., Rutherford, R. B., Bergan, J. J., Carpentier, P. H., Gloviczki, P., Kistner, R. L., . . . American Venous Forum International ad hoc committee for revision of the CEAP classification. (2004). Revision of the CEAP classification for chronic venous disorders: Consensus statement. *Journal of Vascular Surgery, 40*, 1248–1252.

Ernst, C. B. (1993). Abdominal aortic aneurysm. *New England Journal of Medicine, 328*, 1167–1173.

Evans, R. L., & Northwood, L. (1983). Social support needs in adjustment to stroke. *Archives of Physical Medicine and Rehabilitation, 64*, 61–64.

The Executive Committee for the Asymptomatic Carotid Atherosclerosis Study. (1995). Endarterectomy for asymptomatic carotid artery stenosis. *Journal of the American Medical Association, 273*, 1421–1428.

Felix, W. R. Jr., Siegel, B., & Gunther, N. L. (1987). The significance for morbidity and mortality of Doppler absent pedal pulses. *Journal of Vascular Surgery, 5*, 849–855.

Folsum, D., King, T., & Rubin, J. (1992). Lower extremity amputation with immediate postoperative prosthetic placement. *American Journal of Surgery, 164*, 320–323.

Goodacre, S., Sutton, A. J., & Sampson, F. C. (2005). Meta-analysis: The value of clinical assessment in the diagnosis of deep venous thrombosis. *Annals of Internal Medicine, 143*, 129–139.

Harding, G. K., Vanscheidt, W., Partsch, H., Caprini, J. A., & Comerota, A. J. (2014). Adaptive compression therapy for venous leg ulcers: A clinically effective, patient-centered approach. *International Wound Journal, 11*, 1–9.

Hyers, T. M., Hull, R. D., & Weg, J. G. (1992). Antithrombotic therapy for venous thromboembolic disease. *Chest, 102*(Suppl.), 408–425.

Imparato, A. M., Kim, G. E., Davidson, T., & Crowley, J. G. (1975). Intermittent claudication: Its natural course. *Surgery, 78*, 795–799.

Johnston, K. W., Rutherford, R. B., & Tilson, M. D. (1991). Suggested standards for reporting on arterial aneurysms. *Journal of Vascular Surgery, 13*, 452–458.

Jonason, T., & Ringquiest, I. (1985). Factors of prognostic importance for subsequent rest pain in patients with intermittent claudication. *Acta Medica Scandinavica, 218*, 27–33.

Kalra, L. (1994). The influence of stroke unit rehabilitation on functional recovery from stroke. *Stroke, 25*, 821–825.

Lamparello, P. J., & Riles, T. S. (1975). MR angiography in carotid stenosis: A clinical perspective. *MRI Clinics of North America, 3*, 455–465.

Lauret, G. J., Fakhry, F., Fokkenrood, H. J., Hunink, M. G., Teijink, J. A., & Spronk, S. (2014). Modes of exercise training for intermittent claudication. *Cochrane Database of Systematic Reviews,* (7).

Lederle, F. A., Freischlag, J. A., Kyriakides, T. C., Matsumara, J. S., Padberg, F. T., Kohler, T. R., . . . OVER Veterans Affairs Cooperative Study Group. (2012). Long-term comparison of endovascular and open repair of abdominal aortic aneurysm. *New England Journal of Medicine, 367*, 1988–1997.

Mayberry, J. C., Moneta, G. L., & Taylor, L. M. (1991). Fifteen-year results of ambulation compression therapy for chronic venous ulcers. *Surgery, 109*, 573–581.

Mousa, A. Y., Beauford, R. B., Henderson, P., Patel, P., Faries, P. L., Flores, L., & Fogler, R. (2006). Update on the diagnosis and management of popliteal aneurysm and literature review. *Vascular, 14*, 103–108.

North American Symptomatic Carotid Endarterectomy Trial Collaborators. (1991). Beneficial effect of carotid endarterectomy in symptomatic patients with high-grade stenosis. *New England Journal of Medicine, 325*, 445–453.

Oderich, G. S., Greenberg, R. K., Farber, M., Lyden, S., Sanchez, L., Fairman, R., . . . Bharadwaj, P. (2014). Results of the United States multicenter prospective study evaluating the Zenith fenestrated endovascular graft for treatment of juxtarenal abdominal aortic aneurysms. *Journal of Vascular Surgery, 60*, 1420–1428.

Parikh, R. M., Lipsey, J. R., & Robinson, R. G. (1987). Two-year longitudinal study of post-stroke mood disorders: Dynamic changes in correlates of depression at one and two years. *Stroke, 18*, 579–584.

Ricotta, J. J., AbuRahma, A., Ascher, E., Eskandari, M., Faries, P., & Lal, B. K. (2011). Updated Society for Vascular Surgery guidelines for management of extracranial carotid disease. *Journal of Vascular Surgery, 54*, e1–e31.

Rivers, S. P., Veith, F. J., Ascer, E., & Gupta, S. K. (1986). Successful conservative therapy of severe limb threatening ischemia: The value of nonsympathectomy. *Surgery, 99*, 759–762.

Romiti, M., Albers, M., Brochado-Neto, F. C., Durazzo, A. E., Pereira, C. A., & De Luccia, N. (2008). Meta-analysis of infrapopliteal angioplasty for chronic critical limb ischemia. *Journal of Vascular Surgery, 47*, 975–981.

Rosenbloom, M. S., Flanigan, D. P., Schuler, J. J., Meyer, J. P., Durham, J. P., Edrup-Jorgensen, J., & Schwarcz, T. H. (1988). Risk factors affecting the natural history of claudication. *Archives of Surgery, 123*, 867–870.

Rosenfield, K., Jaff, M. R., White, C. J., Rocha-Singh, K., Mena-Hurtado, C., Metzger, D. C., . . . LEVANT 2 Investigators. (2015). Trial of a paclitaxel-coated balloon for femoropopliteal artery disease. *New England Journal of Medicine, 373*, 145–153.

Schlenker, J. D., & Wolkoff, J. S. (1975). Major amputation after femoropopliteal bypass procedures. *American Journal of Surgery, 129*, 495–499.

Schuler, J. J., Flanigan, D. P., Holcroft, J. W., Ursprung, J. J., Mohrland, J. S. A., & Pyke, J. (1984). Efficacy of prostaglandin E1 in the treatment of lower extremity ischemic ulcers secondary to peripheral vascular occlusive disease: Results of a prospective randomized double-blind multicenter clinical trial. *Journal of Vascular Surgery, 1*, 160–170.

Society for Vascular Surgery Lower Extremity Guidelines Writing Group, Conte, M. S., Pomposelli, F. B., Clair, D. G., Geraghty, P. J., McKinsey, J. F., . . . Sidawy, A. N. (2015). Society for Vascular Surgery practice guidelines for atherosclerotic occlusive disease of the lower extremities: management of asymptomatic disease and claudication. *Journal of Vascular Surgery, 61*, 2S–41S.

Szilagyi, D. E., Schwartz, R. I., & Reddy, D. L. (1981). Popliteal arterial aneurysms. *Archives of Surgery, 116*, 724–728.

United Kingdom EVAR Trial Investigators. (2010). Endovascular versus open repair of abdominal aortic aneurysm. *New England Journal of Medicine, 326*, 1862–1871.

Vanscheidt, W., Ukat, A., & Partsch, H. (2009). Dose-response of compression therapy for chronic venous edema-higher pressures are associated with greater volume reduction: Two randomized clinical studies. *Journal of Vascular Surgery, 49*, 395–402.

Veith, F. J., Amor, M., Ohki, T., Beebe, H. G., Bell, P. R., Bolia, A., . . . Yadav, S. S. (2001). Current status of carotid bifurcation angioplasty and stenting based on a consensus of opinion leaders. *Journal of Vascular Surgery*, *33*(Suppl. 2), S111–S116.

von Stumm, M., Teufelsbauer, H., Reichenspurner, H., & Debus, E. S. (2015). Two decades of endovascular repair of popliteal artery aneurysm: A meta-analysis. *European Journal of Vascular and Endovascular Surgery, 50*, 351–359.

Zarins, C. K., White, R. A., Schwarten, D., Kinney, K., Dietrich, E. B., Hodgson, K. J., . . . Investigators of the Medtronic AneuRx Multicenter Clinical Trial. (1999). AneuRx stent graft vs. open surgical repair of abdominal aneurysm: Multicenter prospective clinical trial. *Journal of Vascular Surgery, 29*, 292–308.

18

CHAPTER

Limb Deficiency

Jeffrey M. Cohen, Joan E. Edelstein, Claribell Bayona, and Christopher J. Kort

INTRODUCTION

Limb deficiency is a complete or partial loss of an upper or lower limb. It can be congenital (present at birth) or acquired. In the first section of the chapter, we focus on lower-limb deficiency. Specifically, we discuss etiology, levels of amputation, pre- and postoperative management, lower-limb prostheses, prosthetic rehabilitation, and outcome studies. The second portion of the chapter concerns individuals with an upper-limb deficiency, focusing on etiology, amputation levels, pre- and postoperative management, prostheses, and prosthetic training.

Amputation surgery dates to prehistoric times (Murdoch & Wilson, 1996). In 1754 BCE, the Babylonian code of Hammurabi discusses punitive amputation. Plato's *Symposium* (385 BCE) mentions therapeutic amputation of the hand and foot (Plato, 2016). Hippocrates's 4th century BCE *De Articulis* provides the earliest description of amputation for dysvascular gangrene, cautioning that amputation should be at the edge of the ischemic tissue, with the wound left open to allow healing by secondary intent. The ensuing centuries have led to refinements in surgery technique, hemostasis (control of bleeding), perioperative management, and anesthesia. Today, approximately 140,000 new amputations are performed annually in the United States. The number of persons estimated to be living with limb loss in this country is 1.7 million (Morris, Potter, Athanasian, & Lewis, 2015). This number is projected to be 3.6 million by the year 2050 (Ziegler, MacKenzie, Ephraim, Travison, & Brookmeyer, 2008).

LOWER-LIMB DEFICIENCY

Etiology

In the United States, major etiologies of lower-limb deficiency are vascular disease (pertaining to the blood vessels), trauma, malignancy, and congenital absence (Dillingham, Pezzin, & MacKenzie, 2002). Most new amputations result from complications of the vascular system. Over the past 30 years, the proportion of dysvascular amputations has increased by 27%. In contrast, amputations secondary to trauma and cancer have decreased by 50% as a result of advanced surgical and oncologial technologies and treatments. The incidence of congenital limb deficiency has remained stable.

Dysvascular Disease

Lower-limb deficiency is most commonly due to vascular disease (82%; Dillingham et al., 2002). An episode of acute arterial insufficiency can lead to gangrene. Small-vessel occlusion may also progress to ulcers over pressure points, infection of the skin (cellulitis) and bone (osteomyelitis), as well as gangrenous changes in the distal lower limbs. Individuals with vascular disease often undergo several procedures in an attempt to salvage the involved limb (e.g., attempts at revascularization, multiple debridements, toe and foot amputations). Ultimately, limb removal may be required for uncontrollable soft tissue or bone infection, nonreconstructable disease with persistent tissue loss, or unrelenting rest pain due to muscle ischemia.

An estimated 65,000 lower-limb amputations are performed each year in the United States for adults with vascular disease. Most are due to complications from diabetes mellitus (Boulton, Kirsner, & Vileikyte, 2004). Diabetes mellitus has a prevalence of 14% in the general population and the prevalence increases in those older than age 60 (Menke, Casagrande, Geiss, & Cowie, 2015). A twofold increased risk for leg lesions, including gangrene, exists among persons with diabetes. About 85% of all lower-limb amputations in diabetics are preceded by a foot ulcer. Pickwell et al. (2015) prospectively studied 575 patients with an infected diabetic foot ulcer, of whom 159 (28%) underwent an amputation. Independent risk factors for amputation were: periwound edema, foul smell, nonpurulent exudate, deep ulcer, positive probe-to-bone test, pretibial edema, fever, and elevated C-reactive protein. The more proximal the amputation, the higher the mortality. In 1965, the ratio of transfemoral to transtibial amputations was 70:30. By 1990, the ratio had become 30:70, as better diagnostic and surgical procedures increased the probability of retaining the knee joint. Of those with a dysvascular amputation, 15% to 28% undergo a contralateral limb amputation within 3 years. In recent years, the proportion of diabetic patients undergoing amputation has declined markedly (Alvarsson, Sandgren, Wendel, Alvarsson, & Brismar, 2012; Duhon, Hand, Howell, & Reveles, 2015).

Trauma

Trauma is the primary etiology in 18% of cases of lower-limb deficiency (Dillingham et al., 2002). Traumatic limb loss is most often secondary to motor vehicle or industrial accidents. It usually occurs among young men. Such accidents can result in a direct limb transsection or an open fracture with associated nerve injury, soft tissue loss, and ischemia. Limb-salvage techniques, if feasible, are attempted; however, salvage may require multiple surgical procedures at very high cost in time and money. Despite such attempts, the individual may be left with a painful, nonfunctional limb that ultimately will require amputation surgery.

Malignancy

In 0.9% of persons with lower-limb deficiency, malignancy is the primary etiological factor (Dillingham et al., 2002). For persons with malignant bone tumors, advanced limb-salvage surgery has replaced amputation as the initial treatment. The patient is referred for amputation only if limb salvage has been excluded as an option.

Congenital Absence

In children, congenital limb deficiencies outnumber acquired deficiencies. Congenital limb deficiencies comprise 0.8% of cases of lower-limb deficiency. They usually result from failure of the formation of part or all of a limb bud. The first trimester is the critical time for limb formation with the bud occurring at 26 days and differentiation through the 8th week of gestation (Rossi, Alexander, & Cuccurullo, 2004). Precise etiology is often unclear, but teratogenic agents, for example, thalidomide and radiation exposure, and maternal diabetes are risk factors.

Levels of Amputation

The International Standards Organization (ISO, 1989) adopted a series of standards for terminology intended for descriptive use in prosthetics and orthotics (Schuch & Pritham, 1994). This standard applies to acquired amputation levels. It consists of terms relating to external limb prostheses and wearers of these prostheses. The standards replace terms "above," "below," or "through" the involved joint, for example, above knee and below knee. The current terminology uses "trans," "disarticulation," and "partial" to describe amputation levels. The prefix "trans" is used when the amputation is across the axis of a long bone, for example, transfemoral/transhumeral. Where the amputation is through two contiguous bones, for example, tibia and fibula, only the larger bone is identified, for example, transtibial. When the amputation is through the center of a joint (between long bones), the descriptor is disarticulation, for example, knee disarticulation. The term "partial" describes amputations of the foot distal to the ankle joint and amputations of the hand distal to the wrist. In current terminology, any amputation distal to the ankle level is referred

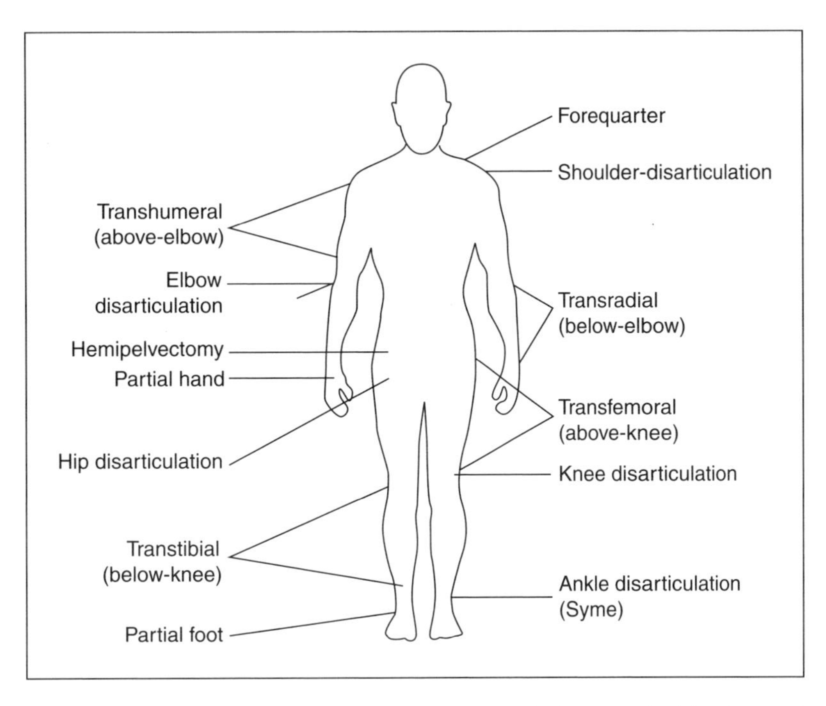

FIGURE 18.1 A depiction of acquired amputation levels, the new ISO terms, and where applicable, the previously accepted standards. *Source:* Schuch and Pritham (1994). Reprinted by permission of the publisher.

to as a partial foot amputation. The single exception is the use of the term "forequarter amputation" for amputations of the upper limb at the scapulothoracic and the sternoclavicular joints. Figure 18.1 (Schuch & Pritham, 1994) depicts acquired amputation levels, the ISO terms, and, where applicable, the previous terms. Table 18.1 (Uustal & Baerga, 2004) provides a detailed description of levels of amputation.

Management of Lower Limb Deficiency

Management of a person undergoing lower-limb amputation surgery can be divided into pre- and postoperative phases. The preoperative phase helps to prepare the patient both physically and psychologically for the upcoming surgery. The postoperative phase focuses on wound healing, edema control, contracture prevention, pain management, and postoperative rehabilitation. This is the time to prepare the patient and the residual limb for prosthetic fitting.

Preoperative Management

The time to start thinking about rehabilitation is the day that amputation is considered. When an amputation is anticipated, rehabilitation clinicians have an opportunity to help prepare the patient physically and psychologically. Ideally, discussions should involve the surgeon, physiatrist, physical therapist, occupational therapist, prosthetist, psychologist, and social worker. If possible, a visit by a rehabilitated person with a similar level of amputation can be of tremendous benefit, reducing anxiety and fear for the patient and family (Marzen-Groller & Bartman, 2005).

Due to the increased comorbidities in patients with dysvascular disease, preoperative rehabilitation evaluation by a multidisciplinary team is crucial to ensure optimal patient outcomes (Hakimi, Eftekhari, & Czerniecki, 2008).

Preoperative assessment of the patient includes an evaluation of the individual's strength, endurance, range of motion, and ambulatory status. The presence of any joint contracture (shortening of a muscle or tendon making passive stretching difficult) should be noted. A major component of the preoperative management is patient education. The likely exercise program is reviewed and a series of range of motion and strengthening exercises is initiated. Training in ambulation with crutches or a walker on level surfaces and stairs is also begun if the patient is medically stable. In addition, education about prostheses is helpful. Early involvement of a psychologist is critical. New amputees' feelings

TABLE 18.1

LEVELS OF AMPUTATION: LOWER LIMB

Level	Anatomical Description	Details
Partial foot	Amputation distal to the ankle level	• Preserves the ankle dorsiflexors and plantarflexors allowing for a functional weightbearing foot.
Ankle disarticulation	Amputation through the ankle joint	• Maintains nearly all limb length and preserves the heel pad, providing an excellent weightbearing limb. • Bulbous residual limb. • May not be appropriate for dysvascular patients as requires healthy plantar heel skin.
Transtibial	Amputation through the tibia and fibula	• Lower mortalities and higher healing rate (80%–90%) compared with the transfemoral level.
Knee disarticulation	Amputation through the knee joint	• Patient supports weight through the end of the amputation limb. • Slight difference in thigh lengths when the patient sits.
Transfemoral	Amputation through the femur	• Higher mortality rates and lower healing rate compared with the transtibial level.
Hip disarticulation	Amputation through the hip joint	• Most patients are adolescents or young adults with bone tumors.
Transpelvic	Amputation through any portion of the pelvis	• Most patients are adolescents or young adults with bone tumors.

Source: Adapted from Cuccurullo (2004). Copyright 2004 by Demos Medical Publishing. By permission of the publisher.

run the gamut of apprehension, depression, and anger, with adjustment and grief reactions common. Stages of survival, recovery, and reintegration are common (Van Dorsten, 2004).

Many amputees report that the preoperative meeting with the rehabilitation team was critical to their making informed decisions and adjusting to life postoperatively. Patient education with exposure to prostheses and amputee peers reduces fear, shortens recovery time, and maximizes the rehabilitation effort (Hakimi et al., 2008).

Postoperative Medical Management

The postoperative medical management of persons undergoing lower-limb amputation surgery focuses on promoting wound healing, controlling edema, and managing pain.

Wound Healing

Wound healing requires scrupulous attention to wound cleanliness and optimal nutrition. Well-nourished patients have an 86% success rate for wound healing after amputation, while malnourished individuals have an 85% failure rate (Dickhaut, DeLee, & Page, 1984). In addition, anemia should be corrected, along with optimizing glycemic control in diabetic patients.

Edema Control

Controlling limb edema (swelling due to excessive accumulation of fluid in body tissues) is necessary to facilitate wound healing, reduce pain, and prepare the limb for prosthetic fitting. The ideal shape for a transtibial residual limb is cylindrical, whereas the ideal shape for a transfemoral residual limb is somewhat conical. To control edema and promote limb shaping, various dressings (i.e., rigid, semirigid, and soft) are used.

Rigid Dressing

A rigid dressing is a cast made of plaster or fiberglass that is suspended by a waist belt or shoulder harness. A removable rigid dressing (RRD) is made in two pieces so it can be removed easily to allow for wound inspection. If removed, however, the dressing must be replaced within minutes to prevent edema reaccumulation. The rigid dressing promotes healing by protecting the residual limb from trauma and helps to desensitize the limb. In the case of transtibial amputations, the dressing also prevents knee flexion contractures. Rigid dressings help control edema, leading to rapid residual limb volume stabilization and a reduction in postoperative pain (Hakimi et al., 2008). They have been shown to lead to a significantly quicker healing time, as measured by the time to be cast for a prosthesis, when compared with a soft dressing (Churilov, Churilov, & Murphy, 2014; Sumpio, Shine, Mahler, & Sumpio, 2013).

Rigid dressings may remain on the patient's amputation limb until healing is presumed to have occurred. Alternatively, the dressing may have provision for brief periods of wound inspection (Taylor, Cavenett, Stepien, & Crotty, 2008).

Semirigid Dressing

Several types of semirigid postoperative dressings are available to control edema and facilitate healing. The Unna paste dressing uses a bandage permeated with zinc oxide, gelatin, glycerin, and calamine lotion. It is generally applied directly on the skin, although it may be wrapped over a soft elastic dressing (Hakimi et al., 2008). Unna semirigid dressings are more effective than elastic dressings in facilitating healing and preparing the limb for prosthetic fitting. Transfemoral amputees treated with an Unna dressing are more likely to ambulate with a prosthesis upon discharge from a rehabilitation facility than those treated with soft dressings (Wong & Edelstein, 2000). Air splints are an easily applied alternative semirigid dressing; however, they are bulky, vulnerable to puncture, and promote perspiration at the amputation limb.

Soft Dressing

Soft dressings are of two forms: elastic bandages and elastic shrinker socks. Elastic bandages are inexpensive and lightweight, but must be reapplied multiple times daily because the bandage loosens as the patient moves about. Bandages are ineffective if patients fail to master the proper wrapping technique. The preferred technique is a figure-of-eight method, which uses diagonal turns. If poorly applied, elastic bandages can cause circumferential constriction with distal edema. Elastic shrinker socks are easier to apply and provide uniform compression. If not adequately suspended by a waist belt, however, they too can lead to skin damage and limb constriction.

Pain Management

Amputation is followed by both painful and nonpainful phantom phenomena in many amputees. Nonpainful phantom sensations rarely pose any clinical problem, but 60% to 80% of all amputees also experience painful sensations (i.e., phantom pain referable to the missing limb). The severity of phantom pain usually decreases with time, but severe pain persists in 5% to 10% of patients (Nikolajsen, 2012).

Pain can lead to significant disability, difficulty performing daily living skills, and a diminished ability to tolerate a prosthesis. A careful evaluation to determine the source of pain is necessary as it may originate from bone, muscle, nerve, or skin. Pain can be categorized as residual limb pain or phantom limb pain (PLP).

Residual Limb Pain

Residual limb pain is a local pain that originates from the residual limb. It may be due to pressure on adherent scars or a neuroma (nerve ending left exposed during surgery). It may also originate from bone spurs or from a poorly fitting prosthesis. In addition, it may represent intermittent claudication (pain that is caused by inadequate blood flow to the leg muscles). Residual limb pain may also be an indication of a local tumor recurrence in patients who had undergone an amputation for tumor removal. Incisional pain tends to resolve as the wound heals.

Phantom Sensation and Phantom Limb Pain

In addition to postoperative pain, most patients experience phantom sensations, the feeling that all or parts of the amputated limb are still present. These sensations are produced by brain networks that are normally triggered by continuous input from the extremity prior to its amputation. Once the limb is removed, this input is replaced by phantom sensations. These sensations manifest as painless tingling. They are common, with an incidence of 80% to 100% in amputees immediately postoperatively. Only 10% of patients develop it after 1 month (Hakimi et al., 2008). The phenomenon of "telescoping," the sensation that the phantom limb has shrunk, e.g., the toes are at the ankle or the foot is at the knee, often accompanies phantom sensations. The intensity of phantom sensation typically diminishes over time, but some awareness can persist throughout the patient's lifetime.

PLP is the sensation of pain originating from the amputated portion of the extremity. It may be related to neuronal deafferentiative hyperexcitability. Deafferentiation is a loss of sensory input from a portion of the body due to the elimination or interruption of sensory-nerve fibers. After deafferentiation, alterations in the functional properties of the dorsal horn of the spinal cord occur, and may underlie the occurrence of abnormal sensations referred to the denervated body part (Ovelmen-Levitt, 1988). PLP is most often characterized as a cramping, squeezing, burning, or a sharp, shooting pain (Flor, 2002). It may accompany phantom sensation. PLP usually develops within the first postoperative month, and it is most intense immediately after the amputation. It may be diffuse, through the phantom limb, or localized to a single-nerve distribution. It is usually worse at night or after the limb has been in a dependent position and can be exacerbated by anxiety and stress. PLP tends to diminish over time, and chronic PLP is rare, reported by less than 5% of the amputee population. Of those complaining, only 14% report it is severely limiting (Ehde et al., 2000).

Many treatments for PLP have varying levels of success. Overall, therapeutic regimens have less than a 30% long-term efficacy (Czerniecki & Ehde, 2003). The mainstay of treatment for PLP is pharmacological. McCormick, Chang-Chien, Marshall, Huang, and Harden (2014) reviewed current evidence-based pharmacotherapy for PLP. They found that the best evidence exists for the use of IV ketamine and IV morphine for the short-term perioperative treatment of PLP and oral morphine for an intermediate to long-term treatment effect (8 weeks to 1 year). The evidence was mixed for the efficacy of perioperative epidural anesthesia with morphine and bupivacaine for short- to long-term pain relief (perioperatively up to 1 year) as well as for the use of gabapentin for pain relief of intermediate duration (6 weeks). Other authors have found that morphine, gabapentin, and ketamine demonstrate trends toward short-term analgesic efficacy (Alviar, Hale, & Dungca, 2011).

Oral gabapentin in patients aged 18 years or older may decrease phantom limb pain. Nevertheless, a strong recommendation for the effectiveness of gabapentin in PLP cannot be made until more methodologically sound studies are executed in this population (Abbass, 2012).

Antidepressants (duloxetine, nortriptyline, amitryptyline) can be effective and also improve sleep. Interventional treatments such as nerve blocks, epidural blocks, chemical sympathectomy, or other neurosurgical procedures are reserved for refractory cases. They have poor long-term success.

Although the mainstay treatments for PLP are pharmacological, there is increasing acknowledgment of the need for nondrug interventions. In light of this, an interdisciplinary approach to the treatment of PLP encompassing physical, pharmacological, and psychological means is often utilized. Treatment measures that create increased peripheral input can provide at least temporary relief. Such measures include desensitization techniques (massaging or gently tapping the residual limb), consistent wearing of a prosthesis as well as the use of transcutaneous electrical nerve stimulation (TENS), the application of electrical current through the skin for pain control. A Cochrane database systematic review to assess the analgesic effectiveness of TENS for the treatment of PLP and stump pain following amputation in adults was conducted by Mulvey, Bagnall, Johnson, and Marchant (2010). They concluded that there were no randomized controlled trials (RCTs) on which to judge the effectiveness of TENS for the management of PLP and stump pain and that further RCT evidence was required before such a judgment can be made. Anecdotal reports, however, suggest that treatment aimed at reducing neuromas and infections diminishes PLP.

A literature search by Hu et al. (2014) revealed some evidence for the use of acupuncture and TENS for the treatment of PLP. In two controlled studies, acupuncture significantly improved pain compared with usual care. Two studies using TENS showed significant improvement in pain compared with sham TENS. However, the authors concluded that insufficient high-quality evidence was available. They also noted that no studies evaluated the cost-effectiveness or adverse effects of these treatments.

Mirror therapy (MT) can reduce PLP experienced by unilateral limb amputees. The visual feedback of observing a limb moving in the mirror is critical for its therapeutic efficacy. Brenda et al. (2007) conducted a randomized, sham-controlled trial of MT versus imagery therapy involving patients with PLP. MT reduced PLP, but such pain was not reduced by either a covered-mirror or mental-visualization treatment. Pain relief associated with MT may be due to the activation of mirror neurons in the hemisphere of the brain that is contralateral to the amputated limb. Alternatively, visual input of what appears to be movement of the amputated limb might reduce the activity of systems that perceive protopathic pain. Nevertheless, compelling evidence supporting MT for PLP is lacking (Rothgangel, Braun, Beurskens, Seitz, & Wade, 2011).

Psychological interventions such as watching an experimenter move his or her own limbs to mimic the patient's phantom limb (Tung et al., 2014), hypnosis, biofeedback, behavioral therapy, relaxation therapy, and voluntary control of the phantom limb (mental imaging) have also met with varying levels of success.

Postoperative Rehabilitation Management

Early aggressive, comprehensive rehabilitation after amputation is necessary for an optimal functional and psychological outcome. Rehabilitation that begins soon after surgery has many advantages, including minimizing residual and PLP and improving prosthetic ambulation and overall function.

■ Physical Therapy

Contractures compromise prosthetic fitting and patient mobility. Maintaining range of motion, especially in the proximal joints of the affected limb, is critical to a successful, functional outcome. Full joint excursion in the residual limb correlates with successful prosthetic ambulation (Munin et al., 2001). For the transtibial amputee, the focus is on preventing a knee-flexion contracture. To accomplish this, strategies include avoiding placing a pillow under the knee, limiting sitting for prolonged periods, and maintaining aggressive pain control. Patients benefit from wearing a soft- or rigid-knee splint when sitting. They should keep the knee extended on a board placed under the wheelchair cushion; the board extends to the distal end of the amputation limb. The transfemoral amputee is prone to the development of hip flexion, abduction, and external rotation contractures. Transfemoral amputation results in the unopposed pull of the iliopsoas, gluteus medius/minimus, and deep external rotator muscles, pulling the hip into a position of flexion, abduction, and external rotation. The patient should avoid placing a pillow under the thigh or between the thighs or standing with the residual limb resting on a crutch handle. Other preventive strategies include lying in a prone or side-lying position on a firm mattress, three times daily for 15 minutes each, if clinically feasible. The patient should be encouraged to extend the hip on the amputated side actively while flexing the contralateral limb.

Physical conditioning is essential, especially for those with cardiovascular or peripheral vascular compromise. Improving aerobic capacity has a positive impact on the potential for functional ambulation, even for the frailest patients. Endurance activities such as wheelchair propulsion, single-limb ambulation with an appropriate assistive device and upper-limb ergometry improve the patient's cardiovascular status in preparation for prosthetic training.

To function successfully with a prosthesis requires good upper-body strength, adequate hip and knee stability, as well as good posture and balance. Strengthening programs for the upper body focus on the biceps, triceps, and latissimus dorsi. A lower-limb strengthening regimen for the transfemoral amputee emphasizes the gluteal muscles on both the intact and amputated sides. Transtibial amputees should focus on strengthening the gluteal muscles, hamstrings, and quadriceps. Strengthening exercises help facilitate transfers from the sitting to standing position and ambulation with assistive devices prior to fitting with a prosthesis (Rheinstein, Wong, & Edelstein, 2006).

■ Occupational Therapy

Occupational therapy helps the patient achieve functional independence in activities of daily living. Occupational therapists evaluate patients for appropriate assistive and adaptive equipment. They assess the patient's home environment to maximize independence and safety. Wheelchair prescription emphasizes the importance of ordering a chair with a posteriorly placed rear axle to prevent rearward tipping and swing-out leg rests to facilitate transferring in and out of the wheelchair.

Psychological Therapy

Continued involvement of a psychologist is necessary throughout the postoperative period. The psychologist should follow the patient through the immediate postamputation period, through the prosthetic training period, and as the patient attempts to reintegrate into society. New amputees have to deal with the physical ordeal of the amputation and its impact on interpersonal relationships, careers, and the stresses of daily living. The patient must learn to accept a permanently altered self-image. The psychologist helps the new amputee cope with these realities and recognize that he or she is still basically the same person as prior to the surgery.

Vocational Rehabilitation

Not only is training for physical mobility and independence in activities of daily living necessary post amputation, but return to school or work, especially in the younger population, is also important. Employment is central to well-being, as it enlarges one's social environment and can provide a stable income. The aims of vocational rehabilitation should be to shorten the time between the amputation and the return to work and to adapt the workplace to any limitations imposed by the amputation.

Success in job reintegration is associated with younger age, higher educational level, and wearing a more comfortable prosthesis (Schoppen et al., 2001). Amputees who changed to a physically less-demanding type of work following surgery have a greater success rate in returning to work. In addition, those who have returned to work have been noted to experience greater job satisfaction than their able-bodied peers (Schoppen et al., 2002). Job satisfaction among unilateral lower-limb amputees could be improved by workplace modifications, depending on the functional capabilities of the person and the functional demands of the job. Vocational satisfaction can also be improved by engaging the patient in vocational rehabilitation programs, especially for those people with additional medical problems.

Prosthetics

Candidacy

When evaluating a patient as a potential prosthetic candidate, multiple factors must be considered. This is especially true in the elderly dysvascular patient who may have such comorbidities as diabetes mellitus, kidney disease, cardiovascular disorder, respiratory disease, arthritis, neuropathy, and impaired vision. Each patient should undergo a thorough musculoskeletal and functional evaluation to assess the person's suitability for prosthetic wear and use. Amputation level, cardiovascular status, cognition, as well as the person's mobility goals, are considered in determining whether the patient will benefit from prosthetic rehabilitation.

Energy Requirements

In assessing a lower-limb amputee's potential for prosthetic ambulation, one must be aware of the energy requirements involved. As the level of amputation proceeds from distal (e.g., transtibial) to more proximal, (e.g., transfemoral), the energy required to walk increases while walking speed decreases. Table 18.2 (Uustal & Baerga, 2004) depicts the increased energy requirements above normal required for traumatic amputees of different amputation levels to ambulate a fixed distance. Of note, traumatic bilateral transtibial amputees actually exert less extra effort to ambulate than do unilateral transfemoral amputees. This finding

TABLE 18.2

ENERGY EXPENDITURE OF TRAUMATIC AMPUTEES BY LEVEL OF AMPUTATION

Level of Amputation	Increased Energy Expenditure Above Normal (%)
Transtibial	20–25
Bilateral transtibial	41
Transfemoral	60–70
Transtibial/transfemoral	118
Bilateral transfemoral	>200

Source: Adapted from Cuccurullo (2004). Copyright 2004 by Demos Medical Publishing. By permission of the publisher.

emphasizes the importance of retaining the anatomical knee whenever possible.

Vllasolli et al. (2014) evaluated the physiological cost index and comfortable walking speed at transfemoral, transtibial, and Syme levels in nonvascular patients and the relationship of these physiological variables to prosthetic ambulation. Higher levels of amputation were associated with less energy-efficient walking and slower walking speed.

The etiology of the amputation also influences energy cost (Table 18.3; Uustal & Baerga, 2004). Individuals whose amputations are due to trauma walk faster and use less energy than dysvascular amputees (Dougherty, McFarland, Smith, & Reiber, 2014; Su, Gard, Lipschutz, & Kuiken, 2010). Persons with a vascular amputation walk at a substantially higher (45.2%) relative aerobic load than those with an amputation due to trauma. However, the preferred walking speed in both groups of amputees is slower than that of able-bodied controls and below their most economical walking speed (Wezenberg, van der Woude, Faber, de Haan, & Houdijk, 2013).

Difference in performance may result partly from age-related changes and partly from concurrent cardiovascular disease. Dysvascular amputees tend to be older and have lower energy reserves (Mac Neill, Devlin, Pauley, & Yudin, 2008). In the dysvascular amputee, the energy source for walking may be anaerobic rather than the more efficient aerobic metabolic pathways. Due to the increased energy demands, long-term use of bilateral transfemoral prostheses in the dysvascular population is rare. In contrast, the typically younger traumatic amputee has a larger cardiac and respiratory functional reserve. A significant number of traumatic bilateral transtibial amputees are successful prosthetic users.

A well-fitting prosthesis that results in a satisfactory gait, not requiring crutches or a walker, significantly decreases physiological energy demands. For individuals with unilateral transtibial or transfemoral amputations, regardless of their age or etiology of amputation, the energy cost of walking with a well-fitted prosthesis is less than that expended when walking without a prosthesis using crutches or a walker (Waters & Mulroy, 1999). Adults with a transtibial amputation using a prosthesis (and no assistive device) walked with 21% more efficiency in terms of VO_2 uptake rate and 92% more efficiency in terms of EE/min as compared to walking with crutches without a prosthesis (Mohanty, Lenka, Equebal, & Kumar, 2012).

TABLE 18.3

ENERGY EXPENDITURE—TRAUMATIC VS. VASCULAR AMPUTATIONS

Level of Amputation	Increased Energy Expenditure Above Normal (%)
Transtibial	
Traumatic	25
Vascular	40
Transfemoral	
Traumatic	68
Vascular	100

Source: Adapted from Cuccurullo (2004). Copyright © 2004 by Demos Medical Publishing.

Terminology

A prosthesis is a replacement for a body part, including false teeth, heart valves, hip replacements, and artificial limbs. Limb prostheses are made by prosthetists who are skilled in prosthetic design, materials, and methods of fitting so that patients are comfortable and obtain the maximum function from their prostheses. The prosthetist works closely with the physician and physical therapist.

The major purpose of a limb prosthesis is to restore the appearance and function of the missing limb. Because no prosthesis fulfills these goals completely, the patient and the rehabilitation team must determine which compromises are most acceptable. Nevertheless, Medicare regulations (HCFA, 2001), which are not limited to the elderly, specify which components will be reimbursed, depending on the physician's assessment of the patient's current or anticipated level of function. Medicare requires the physician to categorize the amputee's potential by designating a K level. The K level will limit the amputee to certain prosthetic components, depending on their potential activity level. The following K levels apply to persons with unilateral transtibial and transfemoral amputations.

- **Level 0:** The amputee does not have the ability or potential to ambulate or transfer safely. Prosthesis is not appropriate, usually because of dementia or very poor cardiopulmonary function.
- **Level 1:** Household ambulator. Ability or potential to use a prosthesis for transfers or ambulation on level surfaces at a fixed speed. SACH (solid ankle, cushion heel) or single-axis foot for transtibial and transfemoral prostheses and knee units, excluding fluid-controlled ones, are covered.
- **Level 2:** Limited community ambulator. Ability or potential for traversing low environmental barriers, such as curbs, stairs, and uneven surfaces. Flexible keel or a multiaxial foot, as well as an axial rotation unit, are covered for transtibial and transfemoral prostheses. Knee units excluding fluid-controlled units are covered.
- **Level 3:** Community ambulator. Ability or potential for ambulation with various speeds; ability to traverse most environmental barriers, involves vocational, therapeutic, or exercise activity beyond simple walking. Energy storing feet, including Flex-Foot, and a rotation unit are permitted. Pneumatic and hydraulic knee units, with or without electronic control, are covered.
- **Level 4:** Child, active adult, or athlete. Ability or potential to exceed basic ambulation skills, and participate in activities of high impact, stress, or energy levels. Any of the feet, rotators, and knee units are covered.

Transtibial Prostheses

The transtibial prosthesis (Figure 18.2) consists of four parts, namely, a prosthetic foot, shank, socket, and suspension. Many options are available for each of these parts. The unique combination for each patient should enable the individual to stand and walk with reasonable comfort, appearance, and efficiency. Walking involves supporting weight on the prosthesis during stance phase when all or a part of the foot contacts the floor, as well as clearing the floor during the swing phase.

All prosthetic feet share several characteristics. They resemble the size and general shape of the human foot, in sizes suitable for young children to large adults. They enable the wearer to stand. Feet enable stance phase, providing a slight amount of plantar flexion when the wearer first contacts the floor; this motion contributes to stability when balancing over the prosthesis. Later in the stance phase, feet simulate dorsiflexion, which normally occurs at the metatarsophalangeal joints. In the swing phase, feet remain in neutral position, allowing the wearer to clear the floor without dragging the prosthetic forefoot. No prosthetic feet permit tip toeing, nor do they provide sensory feedback.

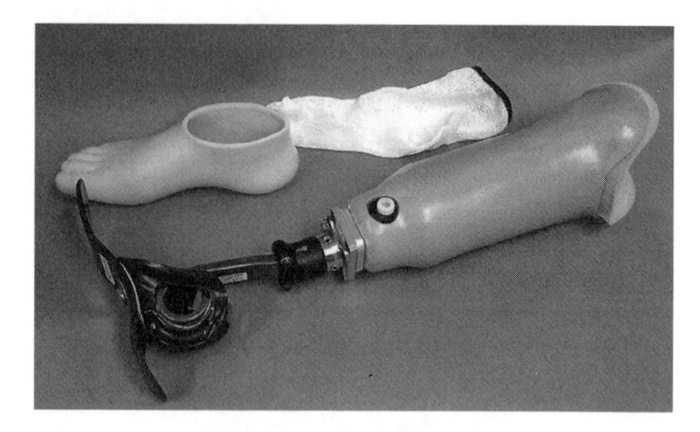

FIGURE 18.2 Transtibial prosthesis.

The most frequently used foot is the SACH (solid ankle, cushion heel) foot (Figure 18.3) developed in 1957. The solid portion, known as the keel, is usually wooden; it extends from the top of the foot to a point corresponding to the base of the toes. This basic foot suits people who limit their walking to moving about the home. Other feet substitute flexible material for the keel; such feet adapt more readily to irregular terrain. The single-axis foot has a transverse axle that enables slight plantar flexion and dorsiflexion during the stance phase; the ease of motion is influenced by rubber bumpers in front and in back of the axle (Figure 18.4).

Some prosthetic feet store energy in early- and mid-stance and return the stored energy to the wearer in late stance. These dynamic,

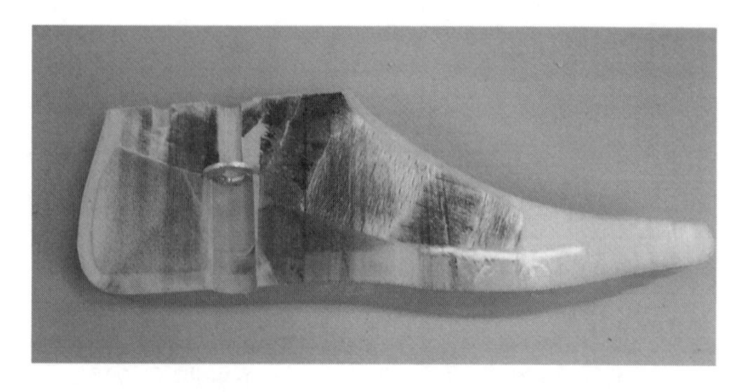

FIGURE 18.3 SACH (solid ankle, cushion heel) foot.

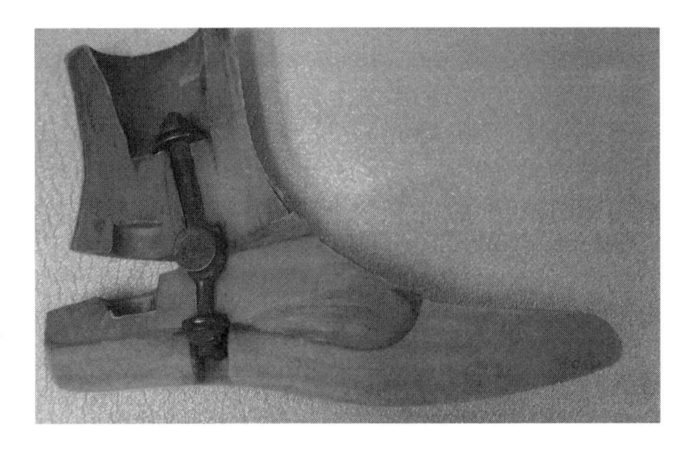

FIGURE 18.4 Single-axis foot. Posterior bumper removed.

energy-responsive feet, such as the Seattle foot, which has a synthetic keel, and the Flex-Foot with a carbon graphite keel extending proximally, contribute to a springy, lively walking pattern appropriate for people who walk vigorously indoors and outdoors (Hsu, Nielsen, Lin-Chan, & Shurr, 2006; Zmitrewicz, Neptune, Walden, Rogers, & Bosker, 2006). Newer feet include those made of fiberglass and those with hydraulic ankles that have microprocessor control. The development of the bionic foot has led to further reductions in energy expenditure during ambulation for the transtibial amputee. Powered feet facilitate walking on level surfaces, stair ascent, and ramp descent (Agrawal, Gailey, Gaunaurd, O'Toole, & Finnieston, 2013; D'Andrea, Wilhelm, Silverman, & Grabowski, 2014; Delussu et al., 2013).

A few prosthetic feet are multiaxial, providing mediolateral and transverse plane motion, in addition to limited plantar and dorsiflexion; they adapt well to cobblestones and similar surfaces (Marinakis, 2004). Some feet permit adjustments to accommodate shoes having various heel heights.

The portion of the prosthesis located immediately above the foot is the *shank* (shin). An exoskeletal shank is a hard shell shaped and colored to resemble the intact leg. An endoskeletal shank is a central pylon covered with foam material carved to duplicate the contours of the opposite leg; it is covered with hosiery that matches the patient's skin color. The endoskeletal shank permits minor adjustments after the prosthesis is fabricated and is somewhat lighter in weight as compared with the exoskeletal version. The foam cover, however, is not as durable as the hard shell. Recently, 3-D printed shank covers have become available; they can duplicate the appearance of the sound lower limb (Gretsch et al., 2015). Whether exo- or endoskeletal, the shank may include an axial rotation unit which absorbs shock in the transverse plane. A vertical shock absorber may also be included in an endoskeletal shank. Shock absorbers shield the skin and anatomic joints on the amputated side from impact (Berge, Czerniecki, & Klute, 2005; Segal, Kracht, & Klute, 2014).

The most important part of any prosthesis is the socket, which encases the amputation limb. The upper part of an exoskeletal shank terminates in the socket. If the prosthesis has an endoskeletal shank, the socket is placed above the pylon. Sockets are custom made of plastic, either a combination of flexible thermoplastic and rigid plastic, or entirely rigid. The traditional design is the patellar tendon bearing (PTB) socket that features a marked indentation in the upper part of the anterior surface intended to support a fair amount of load on the patellar tendon (ligament). Other areas that tolerate pressure are the interosseous region, the proximal portion of the tibia (pes anserinus, also known as medial tibial flare), and the gastrocnemius-soleus belly. Socket reliefs (concavities) are located over the fibular head, femoral condyles, tibial crest, and distal tibia. Total surface weight-bearing (TSWB) sockets are gaining popularity. The TSWB socket has slightly smoother contours (Selles, Janssens, Jongenengel, & Bussmann, 2005). Both socket types contact all portions of the amputation limb to maximize the contact area, thus minimizing unit pressure. Sockets are frequently equipped with a resilient liner to cushion the amputation limb. Patients often wear cotton or wool socks inside the socket. Alternatively, vigorous walkers may prefer a silicone or urethane liner, which reduces friction that occurs as the amputation limb moves slightly within the socket during walking (Baars & Geertzen, 2005).

In order that the prosthesis may stay securely on the patient's limb during the swing phase of walking and when the wearer is climbing stairs, some form of suspension is required. A leather or fabric cuff may be attached to the socket; the cuff wraps around the lower portion of the thigh. A popular option is a silicone sheath, which the wearer rolls onto the amputation limb, and then dons the socket. The sheath has external ridges which cling to the socket interior. This suspension mode minimizes pistoning of the amputation limb in the socket (Baars & Geertzen, 2005; Gholizadeh, Abu Osman, Eshraghi, Ali, & Razak, 2014). Pin suspension requires wearing a silicone liner that has a metal pin at the lower end. The pin locks into a receptacle at the bottom of the socket. Some individuals utilize an elevated vacuum suspension. Vacuum suspension includes a resilient polyurethane or silicone socket liner, an air-expulsion mechanism in the distal end of the socket, and a knee sealing sleeve. This type of suspension reduces vertical motion of the amputation limb in the socket and enhances circulation within the amputation limb. Vacuum suspension enables lower peak positive pressures in stance phase and higher peak negative pressures in swing phase. This is because with vacuum suspension, fluid is pushed out of the limb in stance phase and drawn back into the limb in swing phase, thereby maintaining volume fluctuation within the residual limb more appropriately (Beil, Street, & Covey, 2002; Gerschutz, Hayne, Colvin, & Denune, 2015; Klute et al., 2009). Some people augment suspension with an elastic sleeve that extends from the lower thigh to the upper part of the socket. Others attach a forked strap to the socket; the upper part of the strap has elastic webbing that attaches to a waist belt. Two other modes of suspension are extensions of the socket, namely, supracondylar and supracondylar/suprapatellar, both of which cover more of the upper part of the amputation limb. A few patients require a thigh corset that is attached to the socket by a pair of metal side bars.

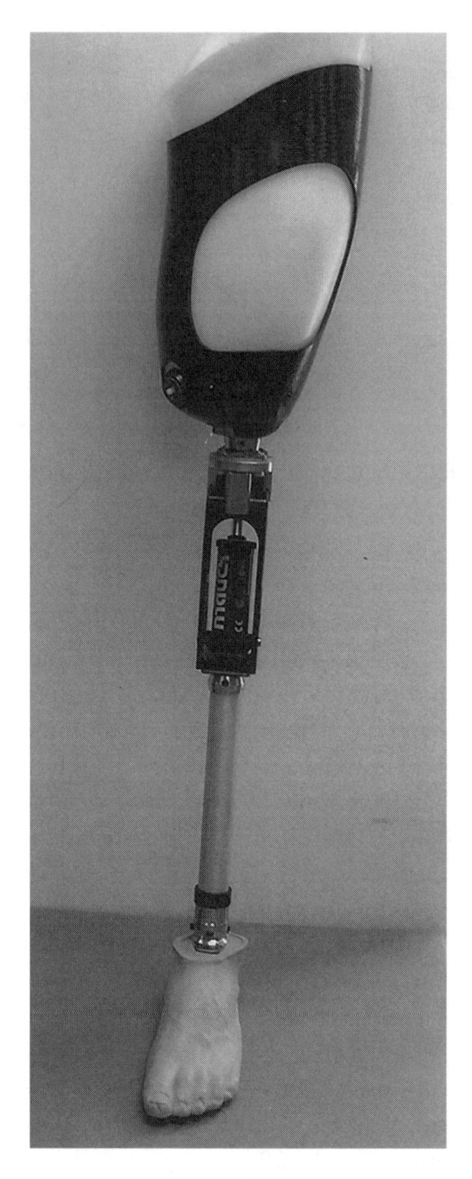

FIGURE 18.5 Transfemoral prosthesis.

Transfemoral Prostheses

The transfemoral prosthesis consists of five parts: a prosthetic foot, shank, knee unit, socket, and suspension (Figure 18.5). As with the transtibial prosthesis, many options are available for each of these parts.

Most choices of prosthetic foot and shank as previously described are available for the transfemoral prosthesis. Athletically inclined patients walk more efficiently with energy-storing feet (Graham, Datta, Heller, Howitt, & Pros, 2007). Newer components are microprocessor-controlled hydraulic foot-knee units.

All knee units bend to permit patients to sit comfortably. Most units also allow the shank to oscillate during the swing phase of walking. The critical parts of knee units relate to the wearer's stability when standing and during stance phase, and the individual's ease of progressing through swing phase. Stance-phase stability is influenced by the alignment of the prosthesis. A patient who is very unsteady may require a manually locked knee unit (Devlin et al., 2002). The prosthesis will be stiff-kneed during the stance phase, maximizing stability. A locked knee presents an unnatural appearance during the swing phase. The wearer unlocks the knee when sitting. The alternative means of providing stance stability include various braking mechanisms. These resist knee flexion during early stance, but permit knee flexion during late stance and swing phase.

During the swing phase, most knee units (except manually locked units) contain a friction mechanism to resist extreme knee flexion during early swing and abrupt knee extension at late swing. The individual who is expected to walk on a limited basis, primarily at home, will be well served by a friction mechanism consisting of a pair of clamps around the axle (knee bolt) that can be tightened or loosened according to the patient's walking style. The clamps affect the ease with which the shank swings. People who are more active benefit from the relatively expensive pneumatic (air) and hydraulic (oil) units. Because air and oil are fluids, the units adjust automatically when the patient walks slowly or rapidly. Some hydraulic units incorporate stance control, providing very high resistance when the patient first strikes the floor with the prosthetic heel (Sapin, Goujon, de Almeida, Fode, & Lavaste, 2008). The most sophisticated hydraulic units, such as the C-Leg and the newer Genium unit, have electronic sensors that detect the wearer's walking speed, shank position, and the contour and texture of the walking surface. Wearers of microprocessor units exhibit smoother, more efficient gait, and report greater activity (Eberly et al., 2014; Kahle, Highsmith, & Hubbard, 2008; Kannenberg, Zacharias, & Probsting, 2014; Kaufman et al., 2008; Sawers & Hafner, 2013; Segal et al., 2006; Uchytil, Jandacka, Zahradnik, Farana, & Janura, 2014). Microprocessor knee units enable the wearer to recover from a potential stumble, and facilitate step-over-step stair descent. The newest microprocessor units incorporate magnetized fluid rather than oil, with good clinical results (Johansson, Sherrill, Riley, Bonato, & Herr, 2005). Several electronic knee units enable the patient to ascend stairs step-over-step (Aldridge Whitehead, Wolf, Scoville, & Wilken, 2014).

Sockets, as always, are the most crucial part of the prosthesis. Custom made to fit the individual patient, sockets are generally made of flexible thermoplastic in a rigid plastic frame. A popular design is the ischial containment socket that covers the ischial tuberosity; this socket features a narrow mediolateral width. The older design is quadrilateral, named for its four-sided contour. In this design, the anteroposterior width is relatively narrow, while the mediolateral dimension is wide. The patient supports a fair amount of weight on the posterior brim of the socket, via the ischial tuberosity. Both socket types contact the entire amputation limb.

Most transfemoral sockets are suspended with suction. Pressure within the socket is lower than atmospheric pressure. Suction sockets have a one-way air expulsion valve to maintain the pressure difference. Full-suction suspension does not require any straps or other attachments and thus permits the freest hip motion. In order to obtain good suspension with suction, the patient must have an amputation limb that does not fluctuate in volume. A newer alternative is some form of a silicone socket liner; various liner designs include a single large seal, multiple smaller seals, and adjustable seals. As noted earlier, the liner has external ridges, which cling to the socket interior. As a group, silicone socket liners are easier to don than sockets with suction suspension. Another mode of suspension, which is relatively easy to don, has a lanyard strap at the end of the silicone socket liner. The patient dons the silicone liner, places the strap through a slit in the outer socket, and fastens the strap to a fixture on the exterior of the outer socket. Some people wear an elastic belt over the top of the prosthesis for extra suspension. Those who have varying amounts of edema require additional suspension devices such as a Silesian webbing belt attached to the socket and surrounding the lower torso. The most rigid suspension is provided by a pelvic band, generally used with a more loosely fitting socket. The pelvic band is a belt with a rigid portion to which is attached a hinged metal or plastic upright joining the belt to the socket. The pelvic band limits mediolateral and rotational hip motions and is the heaviest suspension option. Rather than a socket with suction or other suspension mode, the prosthesis may be attached to the distal femur via a surgical procedure known as percutaneous osseous integration. In this procedure, a direct attachment is created between the amputee's residual femur and the surface of the implanted prosthesis. Patients demonstrate improved function (Hagberg, Hansson, & Branemark, 2014). The drawbacks of osseous integration include extended rehabilitation duration, and risk of infection and fracture (Gholizadeh et al., 2014).

Other Prostheses

Prostheses for people with hip disarticulation or transpelvic amputation (formerly known as hemipelvectomy) consist of a socket, hip unit, thigh section, knee unit, shank, and foot. The socket encases the lower torso and, depending on the extent of loss, may encroach on the lower ribs. The hip unit permits sufficient hip flexion so the individual can sit, as well as slight hip extension, important when the wearer is walking. Although most hip units do not allow other motions, recently developed units permit motion in all planes for a more natural appearing gait. The thigh section is a foam-covered endoskeletal connection between the hip unit and the knee unit. Knee units, shanks, and feet are the same as used in transtibial and transfemoral prostheses.

The knee disarticulation prosthesis has a socket that may have an opening in the front, a knee unit similar to that used for transfemoral prostheses, and a shank and a foot that resemble those used for transfemoral prostheses.

Partial foot prostheses range from a toe filler in the shoe of the person who is missing one or more toes, to a full socket for those who have more extensive amputation. The ideal transmetatarsal prosthesis consists of a socket fitted to a modified prosthetic foot. A similar approach is used for individuals whose foot has been severed in the intertarsal region, such as Lisfranc (disarticulation between the metatarsals and the tarsals) and Chopart (disarticulation through the midtarsal joints). The Syme's prosthesis, for an amputation through the distal tibia and fibula with preservation of the calcaneal fat pad, consists of a socket covering most of the leg and a specially designed prosthetic foot.

Bilateral prostheses resemble those for single amputations, except for foot size and leg length. The patient will achieve greater stability by wearing a pair of prosthetic feet that are shorter and wider than the preamputation shoe size. Shorter prosthetic feet facilitate transferring weight forward during the stance phase of walking; wider feet aid mediolateral stability. Reducing the height of the shanks also contributes to stability, placing the individual's center of gravity closer to the floor; this advantage, however, must be balanced against the cosmetic implications of reducing the wearer's height (Mac Neill et al., 2008).

Once the components of the prosthesis are selected, the prosthetist measures the patient's limb in order to construct the socket. The limb may be wrapped in plaster of Paris to form a cast that the prosthetist will use to create a model of the limb as the basis of the socket. Alternatively, the prosthetist may take electronic measurements to enable computer-aided design and computer-aided manufacture of the socket. In either case, the resulting socket should fit comfortably, protecting sensitive areas from excessive loading. The prosthetic foot is then fitted to a temporary shank, and the socket is attached to the shank. The temporary shank enables the prosthetist to align the prosthesis, that is, altering the relation of the parts of the prosthesis. Alignment contributes to the comfort and stability that the patient will achieve with the prosthesis. The alignment is then transferred to the permanent shank. Finally, the suspension is attached, unless it is part of the upper contour of the socket.

Prosthetic Training

The basic elements of training are donning and doffing the prosthesis, standing and sitting in various chairs, and walking on a level surface, as well as caring for the amputation limb and the prosthesis. The patient can sit while donning the transtibial prosthesis, first applying a sock, then the socket liner, if present, and then placing the residual limb in the socket and securing the suspension. Pin suspension requires that the individual apply a silicone liner that has a distal pin onto the residual limb and then add socks as needed for a snug socket fit. The patient then pushes the residual limb into the socket so that the pin engages the locking mechanism. Donning the transfemoral socket is easiest if the patient wears a silicone liner, and then lodges the thigh in the socket. Alternatively, the individual may remove the suction valve, lubricate the thigh with lotion, push the amputation limb into the socket, and install the valve. Another method has the patient apply tubular stockinet onto the thigh, then draw the end of the stockinet through the valve hole, and pull on the fabric while flexing and extending the contralateral hip and knee. After the stockinet has been pulled from the limb, the patient installs the valve and fastens any additional suspension, such as a Silesian belt or pelvic band.

To rise from a chair, the patient should place the sound (or stronger) leg closer to the chair, regardless of level of amputation. By extending both hips and knees, the individual comes to the standing position. Sitting also is easiest with the sound leg closer to the chair, so that the individual can feel the chair with the intact leg and can maneuver the center of gravity most easily.

Walking requires the ability to shift weight to the prosthesis in order to control the prosthetic foot. The transfemoral amputee learns to flex the prosthetic knee by flexing the hip and to extend the knee unit by hip extension (Nolan & Lees, 2000; Rau, Bonvin, & de Bie, 2007; Vrieling et al., 2008a, 2008b). Beyond rudimentary activities, more agile patients learn to climb stairs and ramps and maneuver over irregular terrain (Paysant, Beyaert, Datie, Martinet, & Andre, 2006; Vickers, Palk, McIntosh, & Beatty, 2008), step over obstacles (Vrieling et al., 2007), drive a car (Boulias, Meikle, Pauley, & Devlin, 2006), and engage in a wide range of sports (Nolan, Patritti, & Simpson, 2012; Nolan, Patritti, Stana, & Tweedy, 2011; Yazicioglu, Taskaynatan, Guzelkucuk, & Tugcu, 2007).

■ Special Considerations for Children

Congenital limb deficiencies are classified as transverse, similar in appearance to acquired amputation, and longitudinal, with both proximal absence and distal presence of portions of the limb (Fisk & Smith, 2004; ISO, 1989). Prenatal vascular disruption may be a significant causative factor (Boonstra, Rijnders, Groothoff, & Eisma, 2000).

Children's prostheses are simplified versions of adult ones, with a more limited selection of components. The choice of components is governed by the developmental level of the child as well as the need to accommodate growth. Very young children begin walking by striking the ground with the entire sole, unlike the mature pattern of making initial contact with the heel, and then transferring weight over the rest of the foot. Consequently, the first foot is likely to be the SACH foot, fitted to infants as early as 6 months. The first transtibial prosthesis will also have an exoskeletal shank, custom-made socket, and cuff suspension. Typically, the first transfemoral prosthesis does not have a knee unit and is usually suspended with a harness. Toddlers have a wider choice of feet. The smallest, more sophisticated foot and knee unit designs suit 10- to 12-year-olds. Electronic knee units are appropriate for older adolescents.

Increase in height can be accommodated with an endoskeletal shank and, for transfemoral prostheses, the shank and thigh sections. The outgrown pylon can be exchanged for a longer unit. Planning for the increasing girth and length of the amputation limb often includes initially fitting the child with one or two concentric sockets. When the innermost socket becomes tight, it can be discarded, extending the duration of use of the prosthesis. An alternative approach involves fitting the child with a thermoplastic socket in an extra thick frame. Thermoplastic can be remolded by heating it and the thick walls of the frame ground slightly to accommodate the larger socket. Growth also requires periodically exchanging the prosthetic foot for one that matches the sound foot size. Functional outcome is excellent, with most children wearing their prostheses full time and engaging in age-appropriate activities (Nagarajan et al., 2003).

Functional Outcomes

Multiple studies demonstrate an improved functional outcome among those with more distal amputations and those with a traumatic, rather than dysvascular, etiology (Asano, Rushton, Miller, & Deathe, 2008; Bilodeau, Hebert, & Destrosiers, 2000; Bussmann, Schrauwen, & Stam, 2008; Christiansen, Fields, Lev, Stephenson, & Stevens-Lapsley, 2015; Davies & Datta, 2003; Deans, McFadyen, & Rose, 2008; Dillingham, Pezzin, MacKenzie, & Burgess, 2001; Dougherty, 2003; Gailey, Allen, Castles, Kucharik, & Roeder, 2008; Gauthier-Gagnon, Grise, & Potvin, 1999; Karmarkar, et al., 2014; MacKenzie et al., 2004; Nehler et al., 2003; Pezzin, Dillingham, & MacKenzie, 2000; Pezzin, Dillingham, MacKenzie, Ephraim, & Rossbach, 2004; Schoppen et al., 2001, 2002, 2003; Wright, Marks, & Payne, 2008).

The functional outcome of patients who sustained tumor-related amputations is very positive (Kauzlarić, Kauzlarić, & Kolundzić, 2007). Most were independent ambulators, with employment, income, marital status, and health comparable to the general nondisabled population.

Functional, social, and emotional outcomes for persons with vascular-related amputations who receive care at an inpatient rehabilitation facility (IRF) are better than for those treated at other postacute care settings, such as at a skilled nursing facility (SNF). An inpatient rehabilitation facility is an inpatient rehabilitation hospital that provides an intensive rehabilitation program (minimum of 3 hours of rehabilitation therapy daily) to inpatients. In contrast, a skilled nursing facility is an inpatient health care facility that provides rehabilitation services to patients at a lesser intensity of service than an IRF. Patients at a SNF need nursing care, but do not require hospitalization. Sauter, Pezzin, and Dillingham (2013) examined the effect of the postacute rehabilitation setting on functional outcomes among patients who underwent major dysvascular lower extremity amputations. Two hundred ninety-seven patients were analyzed on the basis of postacute care rehabilitation setting: IRF, SNF, or home. On the Short Form-36 subscales, significantly improved outcomes were observed for the patients receiving postacute care at an IRF relative to those cared for at a SNF. Patients receiving postacute care in IRFs also experienced better outcomes compared with those discharged directly home. Lower activity of daily living impairment was observed in IRF patients compared with SNF.

Patients receiving postacute care at an IRF were significantly less likely to experience depressive symptoms or to report low emotional functioning as compared with those receiving postacute care at a SNF or home. They also reported better social functioning than did those who received postacute care in SNFs (Pezzin, Padalik, & Dillingham, 2013).

UPPER-LIMB DEFICIENCY

Etiology

In the United States, only 10% of all amputations involve the upper limb, most frequently below the elbow (Hakimi et al., 2008). Trauma is the leading cause of upper limb amputations. Accidents involving machinery include power tools, firearms, and motor vehicle accidents. The second most common etiology for upper-limb deficiency is congenital absence. Among children, however, this is the most common cause of upper-limb deficiency. The third most common etiology is oncological, particularly osseous tumors at the distal end of the humerus followed by vascular disorders (Meier & Atkins, 2004).

Levels of Amputation

The level of amputation may be determined by the type of traumatic injury or by the nature of the disease process such as a tumor or infection.

Consistent with lower-limb amputation terminology, terms adopted by the International Standards Organization in 1989 apply to the upper extremity (Schuch & Pritham, 1994). Table 18.4 describes the levels of upper limb amputation (Uustal & Baerga, 2004).

Management of Upper-Limb Deficiency

Upper-limb amputees experience a loss of function in prehensile activities, the ability to use sensation, and a means of communication. Care of the patient with an upper-limb amputation is similar to that described for the lower limb. The major distinctions relate to the different functions performed by the arms and legs. The upper-limb amputation wound is generally smaller and thus faster to heal than a wound through the thigh or lower leg. Arms are rarely used to support weight, unlike standing on the legs. Most functional activities can be performed with one hand.

■ Preoperative Management

Most upper-limb amputations occur suddenly, without an extended preoperative period. The rehabilitation team should meet with the patient and family as early as possible to discuss the likely course of rehabilitation. In a few instances, reimplantation of the hand may be attempted (Alolabi, Chuback, Grad, & Thoma, 2015; Elliott, Tintle, & Levin, 2014). If the decision to amputate is made after attempts to salvage the limb, the amount of residual neurovascular damage should be determined. Discussion with the patient and family regarding surgical level and plans for postoperative prosthetic fitting should be conducted during this period. Peer support is especially valuable to enable the patient to realize the functional implications of upper-limb loss. After amputation, the range of motion and strength of both arms and the trunk should be assessed (Meier & Atkins, 2004).

■ Postoperative Medical Management

Postoperative management focuses on promoting wound healing, edema minimization, and pain control. It also focuses on increasing strength of both arms and the trunk. Although edema is much less a problem with the smaller body part and the generally younger age of the patient, some form of limb

TABLE 18.4

LEVELS OF AMPUTATION—UPPER LIMB

Level	Anatomical Description	Details
Partial hand	Amputation distal to wrist level	• Rarely fitted with a prosthesis. • Surgical reconstruction may be a more appropriate choice to preserve or enhance function, while maintaining sensation in the residual partial hand.
Wrist disarticulation	Amputation through the wrist joint, preserving the distal radius-ulnar articulation	• Preserves full forearm supination and pronation. • Long bony leverage for lifting. • Poor cosmesis due to a bulbous residual limb.
Transradial	Amputation through the forearm: 1. Very short-residual limb length (<35%) 2. Short-residual limb length (35%–55%) 3. Long-residual limb length (55%–90%)	• Allows a high level of functional recovery in the majority of cases. • Suitable for body-powered or externally powered prosthesis. • Suitable for physically demanding work. • Residual limb length of 60%–70% is preferred for using an externally powered prosthesis.
Elbow disarticulation	Amputation through the elbow joint	• Rapid surgery with decreased blood loss. • Improved prosthetic self suspension. • Good control of socket rotation on residual limb. • Poor cosmesis as needs external elbow mechanism.
Transhumeral	Amputation through the humerus: 1. Humeral neck-residual limb length (<30%) 2. Short-residual limb length (30%–50%) 3. Standard-residual limb length (50%–90%)	• Longer residual length associated with better prosthetic function.
Shoulder disarticulation	Amputation through the shoulder joint	• Difficult to fit with a functional prosthesis.
Forequarter	Amputation of the entire arm and a portion of the shoulder girdle, thorax, or both	• Difficult to fit with a functional prosthesis.

Source: Adapted from Cuccurullo (2004). Copyright 2004 by Demos Medical Publishing. By permission of the publisher.

dressing is required. Rigid and semirigid dressings are effective in controlling edema, thereby accelerating healing and reducing pain. Some patients have a soft elastic bandage or shrinker dressing. Pain is likely to be a greater issue with loss of any portion of the upper limb. In addition to residual limb pain, the patient is likely to complain about phantom pain and sensation. The hand is much more emotionally significant than the foot and the brain has a larger cortical representation for the hand. The same treatments to control pain, as described for the lower limb, are used.

Postoperative Rehabilitation Management

The team approach is crucial in order to achieve the best outcomes for the upper-limb amputee. Members of the team include, but are not limited to, physiatrist, occupational therapist, physical therapist, prosthetist, social worker, and psychologist.

Ideally, the patient should be treated in a rehabilitation facility that specializes in the care of persons with upper-limb deficiency (Gajewski & Granville, 2006). Most clinicians see many fewer such patients; thus, it is difficult to acquire substantial experience. The psychologist and social worker play a major role in rehabilitating children born with limb loss and the adults who acquire an upper-limb amputation. Establishing emotional support during this time is important for successful rehabilitation. Team members should provide education to the patient and family regarding the rehabilitation process, and show empathy and support for the patient's and family's feelings. Contact with an amputee peer visitor or support group is very helpful in addressing the patient's concerns and questions about returning to previous roles and activities.

Preprosthetic Training Phase

During the preprosthetic training phase, goals of treatment include managing pain and edema, improving range of motion of the residual limb, and promoting independence in activities of daily living (ADL) skills training (without and later with a prosthesis). Treatment aims to enable the patient to regain maximum self-sufficiency. Education during this phase focuses on skin hygiene to promote wound healing and to maintain skin integrity. If the amputation limb does not have a rigid or semirigid dressing, the patient will be instructed in applying an elastic bandage to control edema and reduce postoperative pain. Desensitization techniques reduce the sensitivity of the amputation limb. During this phase, the patient should be taught exercises to strengthen all joints of the upper limbs and trunk, as well as procedures to maintain range of motion in the amputation limb.

The transradial amputee is vulnerable to elbow flexion contractures. Focus in therapy must be on maintaining elbow range of motion. With transhumeral amputations, preprosthetic management focuses on maintaining maximum shoulder and shoulder girdle range of motion and strength. High-level amputations alter posture, compromising appearance and respiration (Meier & Atkins, 2004).

If the patient has lost the dominant hand, change of hand dominance should be initiated during this phase. Regardless of prosthesis, the anatomic hand retains greater dexterity and sensation. One-handed techniques and maintaining proper body mechanics are taught during this period. Adaptive/assistive equipment can facilitate independent performance of self-care tasks. A simple temporary prosthesis can maximize activity in the early stage of rehabilitation.

Upper-Limb Prosthetics

Types of Prostheses

Passive Prostheses

A passive prosthesis has no parts that the patient can control with a harness or electrodes. It resembles the appearance of the hand and enables the patient to hold bulky objects bimanually. For amputations below the elbow, the prosthesis has a socket, which fits over the forearm. Transhumeral passive prostheses may have a socket for the amputation limb or may be suspended with a harness; such prostheses have a hinge at the elbow so that the wearer can place the prosthesis in the desired angle. Passive prostheses are lighter in weight and less expensive than other prostheses (Ritchie, Wiggins, & Sanford, 2011). Inasmuch as most daily activities can be performed with one hand, the person who wears a passive hand can present a convincing appearance. Occasionally, the prosthesis is suspended by osseointegration (Jonsson, Caine-Winterberger, & Branemark, 2011).

Body-Powered Prostheses

These prostheses have a harness and cable mechanism enabling the patient to transmit shoulder motion to control the replacement of the anatomic hand (terminal device [TD]) and elbow unit.

Myoelectric Prostheses

Myoelectric prostheses are externally powered by a battery. Electromyographic (EMG) surface electrodes are imbedded in the prosthetic socket. The patient wears the socket over the bare skin. The electrodes detect muscular contractions and transmit the signal to a processor, which amplifies and rectifies the signal. The processed signal causes a motor to respond, whether to open or close the TD or operate the wrist unit or elbow unit (Biddiss & Chau, 2007; Otr, Reinders-Messelink, Bongers, Bouwsema, & Van Der Sluis, 2010; van der Niet, Bongers, & van der Sluis, 2013; Williams, 2004). The socket may be fabricated in a manner similar to that used for lower-limb prostheses, or made with a 3-D printer (Gretsch et al., 2015).

Electric TDs are activated by a battery-powered motor. Electric hands and hooks give most wearers the versatility of directly controlling both the opening and closing of the TD. The motor is usually activated with a switch placed in the harness that suspends the prosthesis. As compared with cable-operated TDs, electric ones are considerably heavier, more expensive, more fragile, and require periodic battery recharging (Edelstein & Berger, 1993; Pylatiuk, Schulz, & Doderline, 2007). Nevertheless, children and adults fitted with myoelectric prostheses tend to wear them for most of the day and prefer them to cable-operated ones.

Body-powered prostheses are more durable, less expensive, lighter in weight, easier to learn, require less maintenance, while externally powered prostheses offer more motion options in the TD (van der Niet, Bongers, & van der Sluis, 2013) and, for the transradial prosthesis, may eliminate the harness (Carey, Lura, & Highsmith, 2015; Williams, 2011).

Emerging technology in upper-limb prosthetics is focusing on sensory feedback so the wearer can discern the texture and weight of the held object (Antfolk, et al., 2012, 2013; Schofield, Evans, Carey, & Hebert, 2014; Nghiem et al., 2015). Implanted electrodes, especially for prostheses for individuals with shoulder amputation, also show promise (Cheesborough, Smith, Kuiken, & Dumanian, 2015; Cipriani, Segil, Birdwell, & Weir, 2014; Hebert et al., 2014; Kung et al., 2013; Pasquina et al., 2015; Resnik et al., 2012; Resnik, Klinger, & Etter, 2014).

Hybrid Prostheses

Typically used for transhumeral amputees, the hybrid prosthesis has both body-powered and externally powered components. It allows for increased grip force via a myoelectrically controlled TD, yet is lighter than a fully electric prosthesis. With a hybrid prosthesis, the patient can control the elbow, wrist, and TD at the same time (Biddiss & Chau, 2007).

Activity-Specific Prostheses

Some individuals prefer a prosthesis fitted with a TD designed for a particular vocational or recreational activity, such as carpentry, biking, kayaking, lifting weights, and golfing (Radocy & Furlong, 2004; Walker, Coburn, Cottle, Burke, & Talwalkar, 2008; Webster, Levy, Bryant, & Prusakowski, 2001). Work-related TDs, which function as tools, include hammers, wrenches, screw drivers, and gardening tools. Alternative prostheses can make a strong positive impact on the amputee's psychosocial well-being (Biddiss & Chau, 2007).

Transradial Prostheses

The transradial prosthesis includes a TD, wrist unit, socket, suspension, and control system (Figure 18.6). These prostheses are suitable for people with wrist disarticulations as well as forearm absence to a point just below the anatomic elbow. The TD may be a prosthetic hand, which is passive or active with three or more moving fingers. Usually, the hand is covered with a silicone glove in a color matching the wearer's skin tone. Active hands have a mechanism that allows the wearer to open and close three or more fingers. In most models, the thumb, index, and middle finger move at the base of the finger; the ring and little fingers are passive. Interphalangeal joints usually do not move. An active hand may be operated by a cable, a switch-controlled electric motor, or electrodes.

Alternatively, the TD may be a hook that the patient can open and close by applying tension to the harness. Hook TDs have two fingers, one or both of which can move. Hook fingers are

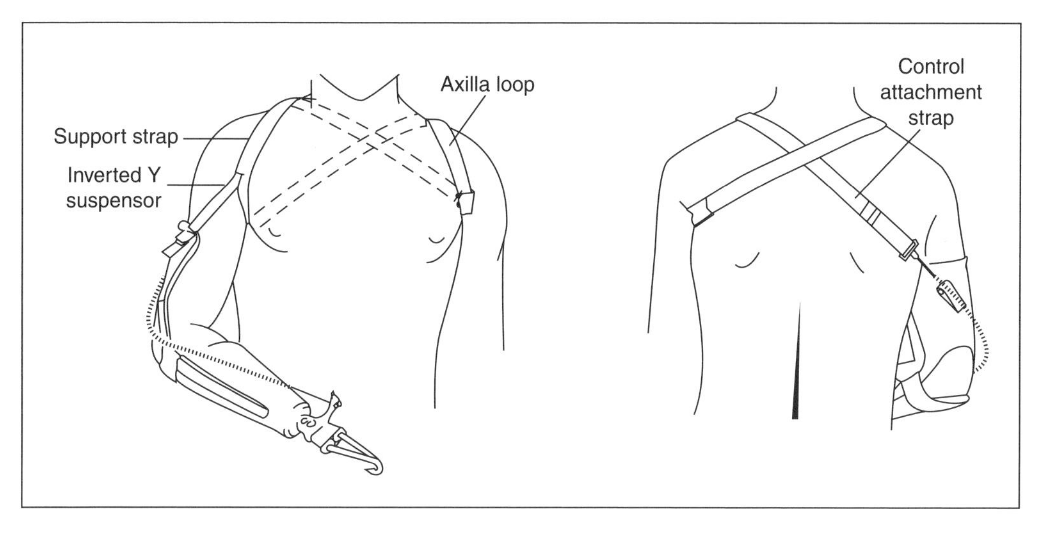

FIGURE 18.6 Transradial prosthesis.

more slender than prosthetic hand fingers, thus making it easier for the wearer to see the object being handled. Hooks are usually made of aluminum or steel, with several shape options. Some hooks come with a vulcanized rubber material to increase friction and give the user increased control. The two most common shapes for hooks are canted and lyre. The canted shape hook provides a finer precision grip and allows the user to have greater visual feedback. The lyre-shaped hook is more beneficial for gripping larger cylindrical objects such as cans. In addition to these standard shapes, there are specialized work hooks that are optimal for stabilizing work tools. These hooks are less expensive than hands, more durable, and lighter in weight. Grasping small objects is less difficult with a hook, while larger items are easier to manage with the larger surface area of the hand. In daily use, most people learn to function with either type of TD.

Body-powered TDs are either voluntary opening (VO) or a voluntary closing (VC). Ipsilateral shoulder flexion or scapular protraction applies tension to the cable, which connects the harness to the TD. The patient voluntarily opens the VO version; rubber bands or springs close it when the wearer releases tension on the harness. Grasp force is determined by the TD mechanism. When using a VC TD, the patient uses tension to close the TD and maintain it closed. Harness tension determines the grasp force. Both hands and hooks may be either VO or VC (Berning, Cohick, Johnson, Miller, & Sensinger 2014; Sensinger, Lipsey, Thomas, & Turner, 2015; Smit, Bongers, Van der Sluis, & Plettenburg, 2012). Neither hand nor hook provides tactile feedback, nor the near infinite variety of anatomic finger motions.

A wrist unit is the receptacle for the TD. A quick disconnect wrist unit permits interchanging TDs if the wearer has several of them. Wrist units enable the wearer to rotate the TD to place it in any angle of pronation, midposition, and supination. Some patients require a wrist flexion unit, in addition to the basic wrist unit. The flexion unit offers several positions of palmar flexion, facilitating placing the TD at the midline of the body. Patients who can abduct and rotate the shoulder can position the TD at the head and torso and thus generally do not need a flexion unit. Most wrist units and flexion units are passive, without cable or electrode control. The wearer uses the opposite hand or leans against a rigid surface to nudge the unit into the desired position. A wrist flexion unit on one prosthesis is especially useful for those with bilateral amputations.

The transradial socket encases the amputation limb. If the limb is relatively long, the upper margin of the socket lies below the elbow. A shorter limb requires a supracondylar socket that covers the lower part of the arm. A socket utilizing the supracondylar design provides suspension by obtaining a bony lock above the humeral epicondyles. People who wear myoelectric TDs may also be fitted with a supracondylar socket, which eliminates the need for a harness to suspend the prosthesis. A new development is 3-D printing of a socket (Gretsch et al., 2015).

A provision for suspension is essential. Either the patient will have a supracondylar socket or a Dacron webbing harness to resist the weight of the prosthesis. The most common harness is called figure-of-eight because it resembles the numeral. In addition to suspending the prosthesis, the harness provides an attachment for a cable leading to the TD, if the prosthesis is body-powered. Because a myoelectric TD incorporates electrodes rather than a cable, there is no need for a cable attachment to a harness. Other methods for transradial suspension include roll-on silicone liners, similar to that used with a transtibial prosthesis. This method utilizes a locking pin at the end of the liner and a locking receptacle mechanism inside the distal end of the prosthetic socket.

The transradial control system enables the wearer to operate the TD. Cable control is achieved when the wearer puts tension on the cable connecting the TD to the harness. In addition to the figure-of-eight harness, a figure-of-nine harness can be utilized solely for connection to the cable control for TD actuation. A figure-of-nine harness does not provide any suspension, thus it lacks an anterior support strap and inverted Y suspensor strap. Its main components are the axilla loop and control attachment strap. With either harness, flexing the shoulder on the amputation side causes the TD to move, whether VO or VC. Relaxing the shoulder muscles produces the opposite action. When buttoning a shirt or performing other activities close to the body, the patient will abduct the scapula on the amputation side to tense the cable. Electric switch control is similar, because the switch is usually located in the harness. Myoelectric control involves contracting the appropriate muscle, usually the forearm extensor muscles to open the TD and the forearm flexor muscles to close the TD.

Transhumeral Prostheses

Prostheses for the arm (above-elbow, transhumeral) amputations include a TD, wrist unit, forearm section, elbow unit, socket, suspension, and control system.

TD and wrist unit options are identical to those for transradial prostheses. The forearm section is a rigid shell that replaces the length of the missing forearm. Its lower end is attached to the wrist unit and the upper end joins the elbow unit.

With transhumeral prostheses, component weight becomes more important because the patient has to lift the forearm section, the TD, plus the weight of the object being held.

The elbow unit is a hinge that permits the patient to place the TD as needed for a particular activity. Most elbow units have a cable-controlled locking mechanism. The mechanism alternates locking and unlocking in the same manner that a light switch alternates lighting and darkening a lamp. The transhumeral prosthesis also has a passive turntable with which the wearer can rotate the forearm to the desired position.

As with all sockets, the transhumeral socket is plastic, or carbon composite, custom made, and makes contact with all portions of the amputation limb. For those with a relatively long amputation limb, the upper margin of the socket lies near the shoulder. Shorter amputation limbs need a socket that covers part of the chest.

Transhumeral prostheses are ordinarily suspended with a harness, usually a figure-of-eight harness similar to that used on transradial prostheses. The transhumeral harness has additional straps to aid suspension and to enable controlling more components. An alternate suspension is osseous integration (Jonsson et al., 2011).

Control of the transhumeral prosthesis is usually dual control, with two cables attached to the harness. The longer cable extends from the back of the harness, past the elbow, to the TD. When the elbow unit is unlocked, tension on this cable causes the elbow hinge to flex. Ballistic motion can also be used to achieve elbow flexion while the unit is unlocked. When the elbow unit is locked, the same cable operates the TD, whether VO or VC. A shorter cable runs from the front of the harness to the elbow lock cable. Most patients exert tension on this cable by depressing and simultaneously extending the ipsilateral shoulder in order to lock the elbow. The first motion locks the elbow; the second motion in the same direction unlocks the elbow, in an alternating manner. When the patient wishes to move an object from the table to a shelf, the first step is to flex the elbow with the long cable, angling the prosthesis so the TD reaches the shelf. The next step is to lock the elbow with the short cable. The final step is to lean over the table, grasp the object with the long cable, stand upright, and release the object on the shelf. Fortunately, most practical activities do not require elbow motion. The patient flexes and locks the elbow unit and then can perform many TD maneuvers in the same way as someone wearing a transradial prosthesis.

A recent development is targeted muscle reinnervation involving the surgical implantation of electrodes to control a transhumeral or higher prosthesis (Cheesborough et al., 2015; Cipriani et al., 2014; Hebert et al., 2014; Kuiken et al., 2009; Kung et al., 2013; Pasquina et al., 2015; Resnik et al., 2012; Resnik, Klinger, & Etter, 2014). The technology is still experimental; components are not yet available commercially.

Other Prostheses

Partial Hand Prostheses

Most people who have finger loss do not wear a prosthesis because the prosthesis covers sensate areas. Surgical reconstruction may be preferred. For example, if the thumb is missing, the second digit may be rotated and stabilized to oppose the other fingers. Technological developments, however, in the prosthetics and engineering fields have made it possible for the partial hand amputee to have options for using a prosthesis to perform functional activities. Depending on the level of injury, the patient now has options ranging from static silicone restoration fingers to myoelectric powered digits. These choices give the partial hand amputee the ability to add length to a digit(s) and increase surface area of the hand without compromising proximal joints during task performance.

Elbow Disarticulation Prostheses

Elbow disarticulation prostheses are similar to transhumeral ones, except that the elbow unit is simpler. The patient has the full length of the upper arm and thus can transmit shoulder rotation to the rest of the prosthesis, eliminating the need for a turntable. The prosthesis still requires dual control to operate the elbow hinge, elbow lock, and TD.

Humeral Neck, Shoulder Disarticulation, Forequarter and Bilateral Prostheses

Humeral neck (a very small portion of the upper arm remains), shoulder disarticulation, and forequarter (absence of the entire arm and some portion of the shoulder girdle and rib) prostheses are cumbersome because they must cover part of the chest. Except for humeral neck amputations, the prostheses also include a passive shoulder joint. Other components and control systems are similar to those for the transhumeral prosthesis. Those with unilateral amputations have a very high rejection rate for these prostheses.

The principal difference between unilateral and bilateral prostheses is, in addition to two prostheses, the design of the harness. The unilateral figure-of-eight harness is modified so that the cables from both prostheses can be attached to the harness, thereby enabling the wearer to control both prostheses. Some people prefer to wear matching TDs, while others trade the functional versatility of having two different TD designs for the abnormal appearance. The only contraindicated fitting is a pair of passive hands. People have been successfully fitted with one or both active hands, whether controlled via cable or myoelectrically, as well as various pairs of hooks or hook–hand combinations. The remainder of each prosthesis, including the control system, is the same as for unilateral fitting. Individuals who have a very high amputation may prefer to wear only a prosthesis on the longer amputation limb (Uellendahl, 2004).

Physically, most people with well-healed upper-limb amputations are candidates for a prosthesis. Nevertheless, the individual's emotional status must be considered, as well as available funding, particularly if an electric or myoelectric prosthesis is sought.

Prosthetic Training Phase

The goal of prosthetic training is to teach the patient how to care for and use the prosthesis and ultimately to incorporate it in every aspect of the person's life. Education on donning/doffing, skin care, cleaning the prosthesis, and controlling it increase the patient's compliance with using the prosthesis to perform desired tasks (Johnson & Mansfield, 2014).

Training may begin with a temporary prosthesis, which restores some bimanual function and helps the patient to adjust to his or her new reality. If the dominant hand has been amputated, then efforts to change dominance should begin as early as possible. Although some people choose to write with the prosthesis, other tasks involving fine manipulation, such as buttoning, are easier to accomplish with the remaining hand. If both hands are amputated, then early restoration of independent function with or without temporary prostheses is imperative for the patient's emotional health and self-care. The patient learns to depend on visual cues rather than the tactile and proprioceptive feedback that prostheses lack.

Two principal stages of training are controls training and use training:

1. Controls Training:
The goal of controls training is to educate the upper limb amputee to effectively operate the prosthesis (Veterans Administration, 2014). Education includes training on proper prepositioning of the prosthesis as well as on training on how to grasp and release objects. The consistent incorporation of proper body mechanics during this time to minimize compensatory movements is stressed.

a. Body Powered Control Training
Transradial level: The body controls necessary to operate a body powered prosthesis for the transradial amputee are scapular abduction, chest expansion, shoulder depression, extension, abduction, and flexion (Meier & Atkins, 2004). It is also important for the transradial amputee to maintain full range of motion in elbow flexion/extension in order to facilitate reaching in different planes without using poor body mechanics

The transradial prosthesis has two mechanisms that the patient must control, namely, the TD and the wrist unit. If the TD is cable operated, the patient should flex the shoulder on the amputation side to apply tensile stress to the cable that, in turn, transmits the stress to the TD, whether voluntary opening or voluntary closing (Atkins, 2004). After this skill is well established, the patient learns to operate the TD by scapular abduction; this motion is essential for using the TD close to the body.

Most wrist units are passively operated. The patient learns to turn the unit to position the TD in the desired position, whether pronation, mid-position, or supination. If the unit has a locking mechanism, the wearer is taught how to unlock it, turn the unit, then lock it. Wrist flexion units are also generally passive, requiring the patient to nudge its control lever to position the terminal device in the appropriate degree of palmar flexion. Patients are trained on prepositioning of the TD and opening/closing of the TD to grasp and release objects from different height levels In addition, they are trained on how to don/doff the harness.

Transhumeral Level: A transhumeral amputee with a body-powered prosthesis learns to use shoulder movements to lock and unlock the elbow and then close and open the TD to grasp or release an object. The patient should first learn how to operate the TD with the elbow unit locked by the therapist. Wrist unit instruction then follows. The third step is learning to flex and extend the elbow with the same body movements as used to control the TD. The fourth step is operating the elbow lock with scapular depression augmented by slight abduction. Controls training culminates with flexing the elbow, then locking it, and finally positioning the TD and operating it.

b. Myoelectric Control Training

In preparation for training the upper-limb amputee in the use of a myoelectric prosthesis, it will be important to identify which muscle signals the patient will be using to control the prosthesis. The patient, prosthetist, and therapist will work together to identify which muscles will send signals to operate the motions at the elbow, wrist, and hand of a myoelectric prosthesis. Once the muscles have been identified, training in isolating those muscles to provide signals for each control mode (elbow, wrist, or hand) will begin (Powell, Kaliki, & Thakor, 2014). The transradial amputee ordinarily uses the bellies of wrist and finger extensors to open the TD and the wrist and finger flexors to close the TD. The myoelectric user will be educated on how to charge the battery, turn the prosthesis on and off, and how to perform basic controls of opening and closing of the TD.

For the transhumeral amputee, the most commonly used muscle sites are the biceps and the triceps muscles. These will be used to control the externally powered elbow, wrist and hand. The patient will use repetitive drills, including picking up objects of different sizes and weights from varying height surfaces to work on improving control of the prosthesis. Subsequent to this, proportional control training will begin.

c. Proportional Control Training

Achieving proportional control of the body-powered system or the externally powered system will be crucial in order for the patient to use the prosthesis successfully during ADL. During proportional control training, the upper limb amputee learns how to control the speed and force necessary to operate the TD to grasp and release objects of different sizes and and weights during a given amount of time. An example of good proportional control is demonstrating the ability to apply enough pressure to pick up a plastic cup with either the body powered or externally powered TD and not crush it. Mastering proportional control leads to increasing efficiency in using the upper limb prosthesis and reduces the possibility of damaging or causing injury during grasping of items with the TD. The patient will benefit from a hierarchical progression when training to control the prosthesis to achieve the best outcomes.

2. Use Training

When training upper limb amputees in using a prosthesis, it is important to have them perform bimanual ADL and instrumental activities of daily living (IADL) tasks. This will increase their ability to incorporate the prosthesis during functional tasks and optimize the features of the prosthesis. The unilateral upper-limb amputee will need to be able to use the prosthesis as a gross assist and stabilizer of objects while the sound hand interacts with the object. The intact upper limb will always be the dominant extremity for all bimanual activities (Meier & Atkins, 2004). For the bilateral upper-limb amputee, the training will take more time and the patient will rely on the use of a prosthesis for all ADL and IADL tasks. Generally, the longer, stronger amputation limb will be dominant. ADL tasks to include when training the patient are dressing, feeding, opening containers, cutting foods, meal preparation, and folding clothing. IADL tasks to include during training with a prosthesis are grocery shopping (placing items in a bag and carrying bag), performing laundry (placing and removing clothing from washer/dryer and then folding clothing), home management (cleaning of countertops, doing dishes, vacuuming), and tool management (using tools for home repairs and leisure tasks). Focus on energy conservation and the proper body mechanics will minimize excess stress (Carey, Jason-Highsmith Maitland, & Duey, 2008).

Vocational and Avocational Activities

Young adults who sustain an upper-limb amputation should be directed to specialized vocational training. This enables the individual either to return to his or her original job or be trained for a new occupation with minimal dependence on adaptive equipment (Fernández, Isusi, & Gómez, 2000). Amputation is not a deterrent to driving an automobile (Boulias et al., 2006). Simple adaptations in technique or equipment enable many people to engage in a wide range of sports, from archery to windsurfing (Radocy & Furlong, 2004; Vasluian, van Wijk, Dijkstra, Reinders-Messelink, & Van Der Sluis, 2015).

Special Considerations for Children

As compared with adults, children grow in size and maturity (Le & Scott-Wyard, 2015). Infants are likely to be fitted with a passive hand or a plastic-coated hook at approximately 6 months of age. The first transradial prosthesis will lack a wrist unit, while the initial transhumeral prosthesis will have a passive elbow unit. Both will be suspended with a harness designed to prevent the youngster from removing the prosthesis. Early fitting accustoms the child to bimanual function, such as holding a large stuffed toy or ball. The prosthesis also prevents the infant from relying on the tactile sensation of the anatomic limb. Passive hands with flexed fingers are manufactured to facilitate crawling. At about 12 months of age, most children can learn to operate TD cable control. Those as young as 18 months old can control a myoelectric TD. The delicate mechanism needs to be shielded from such hazardous environments as water, sand, and high-impact play. Most 3-year-olds can use a cable-controlled elbow unit (Shaperman, Landsberger, & Setoguchi, 2003).

Provision for enlarging the socket is important for children's prostheses. As with the lower-limb counterpart, the socket may be either several concentric encasements or a thermoplastic socket in a thick frame. Socket fit is particularly important for those fitted with myoelectric control. The thermoplastic socket is heated to enlarge it and the frame thickness is reduced to receive the larger socket. Maintaining length symmetry is not as critical for upper-limb prostheses as compared with lower-limb devices. Nevertheless, for aesthetic reasons, the prosthesis should approximate the length of the sound arm. A forearm section resembling an endoskeletal shank facilitates lengthening.

Training the infant involves establishing a consistent wearing schedule, providing opportunities for bimanual usage, and recognizing when prosthetic adjustments are needed (Patton, 2004). Older children engage in a wide range of sports, sometimes utilizing specialized terminal devices (Walker et al., 2008; Webster et al., 2001).

One outcome study suggests that children are likely to wear multiple prostheses to perform specific activities and may prefer simpler prostheses to myoelectric ones (Crandall & Tomhave, 2002). Another report indicates greater preference for the transradial prosthesis with a myoelectric hand as compared with a body-powered VO hand (Edelstein & Berger, 1993).

Functional Outcome

Upper-limb prostheses are much more likely to be rejected, as compared with lower-limb prostheses (Raichle et al., 2008). Prosthetic restoration of the appearance and function of the hand is much less successful than that of the leg and foot. With usual clothing, the hand is more visible than the leg. Individuals with bilateral amputations or unilateral transradial amputation are more likely to wear prostheses than those with unilateral transhumeral or higher amputations (Dabaghi-Richerand, Haces-Garcia, & Capdevila-Leonori, 2015; McFarland et al., 2010; Wright, Hagen, &

Wood, 1995). Those with a congenital limb deficiency are more likely to wear a prosthesis than those with an acquired amputation (Gaine, Smart, & Bransby-Zachary, 1997). One investigator noted that fewer than half of patients wore their prostheses (Davidson, 2002), while others report higher utilization (Biddiss & Chau, 2007). Greater acceptability of transradial and wrist disarticulation prostheses (Ostlie et al., 2012) suggests that patients derive sufficient function from them, while those with higher amputations dislike the weight of the prosthesis, the relative complexity of operating the elbow unit, and may prefer to function unimanually.

SUMMARY

Loss of a limb produces a permanent disability that can have a devastating effect on a persons's self-image, self-care, and mobility. New amputees have to deal not only with the physical ordeal of the amputation but also its impact on interpersonal relationships, careers, and the stresses of daily living. To handle these challenges, the amputee requires a devoted interdisciplinary team of experts, with each member playing a vital role in the amputee's recovery. This team of physicians, nurses, physical and occupational therapists, psychologists, recreational therapists, vocational counselors, social workers, and prosthetists helps the amputee overcome the many physical and emotional barriers he or she faces. Rehabilitation following an amputation helps the amputee come to terms with an altered self-image, live with the new realities, and return to the highest level of function and independence possible.

REFERENCES

Abbass, K. (2012). Efficacy of gabapentin for treatment of adults with phantom limb pain. *Annals of Pharmacotherapy, 46*, 1707–1711.

Agrawal, V., Gailey, R. S., Gaunaurd, I. A., O'Toole, C., & Finnieston, A. A. (2013). Comparison between microprocessor–controlled ankle/foot and conventional prosthetic feet during stair negotiation in people with unilateral transtibial amputation. *Journal of Rehabilitation Research & Development, 50*, 941–950.

Aldridge Whitehead, J. M., Wolf, E. J., Scoville, C. R., & Wilken, J. M. (2014). Does a microprocessor–controlled prosthetic knee affect stair ascent strategies in persons with transfemoral amputation? *Clinical Orthopaedics & Related Research, 472*, 3093–3101.

Alolabi, N., Chuback, J., Grad, S., & Thoma, A. (2015). The utility of hand transplantation in hand amputee patients. *Journal of Hand Surgery (American), 40*, 8–14.

Alvarsson, A., Sandgren, B., Wendel, C., Alvarsson, M., & Brismar, K. (2012). A retrospective analysis of amputation rates in diabetic patients: Can lower extremity amputations be further prevented? *Cardiovascular Diabetology, 11*, 18.

Alviar, J. J., Hale, T., & Dungca, M. (2011). Pharmacologic intervention for treating phantom limb pain. *The Cochrane Database of Systemic Reviews, 7*(12), CD006380.

Antfolk, C., Bjorkman, A., Frank, S. O., Sebelius, F., Lundborg, G., & Rosen, B. (2012). Sensory feedback from a prosthetic hand based on air–mediated pressure from the hand to the forearm skin. *Journal of Rehabilitation Medicine, 44*, 702–707.

Antfolk, C., D'Alonzo, M., Rosen, B., Lundborg, G., Sebelius, F., & Cipriani, C. (2013). Sensory feedback in upper limb prosthetics. *Expert Review of Medical Devices, 10*, 45–54.

Asano, M., Rushton, P., Miller, W. C., & Deathe, B. A. (2008). Predictors of quality of life among individuals who have a lower limb amputation. *Prosthetics and Orthotics International, 32*, 231–243.

Atkins, D. (2004). Functional skills training with body–powered and externally powered prostheses. In R. H. Meier & D. J. Atkins (Eds.), *Functional restoration of adults and children with upper extremity amputation* (pp. 139–158). New York, NY: Demos Medical Publishing.

Baars, E. C., & Geertzen, J. H. (2005). Literature review of the possible advantages of silicon liner socket use in trans–tibial prostheses. *Prosthetic and Orthotics International, 29*, 27–37.

Beil, T. L., Street, G. M., & Covey, S. J. (2002). Interface pressures during ambulation using suction and vacuum–assisted prosthetic sockets. *Journal of Rehabilitation Research and Development, 39*, 693–700.

Berge, J. S., Czerniecki, J. M., & Klute, G. K. (2005). Efficacy of shock–absorbing versus rigid pylons for impact reduction in transtibial amputees based on laboratory, field, and outcome metrics. *Journal of Rehabilitation Research and Development, 42*, 795–808.

Berning, K., Cohick, S., Johnson, R., Miller, L. A., & Sensinger, J. W. (2014). Comparison of body–powered voluntary opening and voluntary closing prehensor for activities of daily life. *Journal of Rehabilitation Research and Development, 51*, 253–261.

Biddiss, E. A., & Chau, T. T. (2007). Upper limb prosthesis use and abandonment: A survey of the last 25 years. *Prosthetics and Orthotics International, 31*, 236–257.

Bilodeau, S., Hébert, R., & Desrosiers, J. (2000). Lower limb prosthesis utilisation by elderly amputees. *Prosthetics and Orthotics International, 24*, 126–132.

Boonstra, A. M., Rijnders, L. J., Groothoff, J. W., & Eisma, W. H. (2000). Children with congenital deficiencies or acquired amputations of the lower limbs: Functional aspects. *Prosthetics and Orthotics International, 24*, 19–27.

Boulias, C., Meikle, B., Pauley, T., & Devlin, M. (2006). Return to driving after lower-extremity amputation. *Archives of Physical Medicine and Rehabilation, 87*, 1183–1188.

Boulton, A. J., Kirsner, R. S., & Vileikyte, L. (2004). Clinical practice: Neuropathic diabetic foot ulcers. *New England Journal of Medicine, 351*, 48–55.

Brenda, L., Chan, B. A., Witt, R., Charrow, A. P., Magee, A., Howard, R., & Pasquina, P. F. (2007). Mirror therapy for phantom limb pain. *New England Journal of Medicine, 357*, 2206–2207.

Bussmann, J. B., Schrauwen, H. J., & Stam, H. J. (2008). Daily physical activity and heart rate response in people with a unilateral traumatic transtibial amputation. *Archives of Physical Medicine and Rehabilitation, 89*, 430–434.

Carey, S. L., Jason-Highsmith, M., Maitland, M. E., & Duey, R. V. (2008). Compensatory movements of transradial prosthesis users during common tasks. *Clinical Biomechanics, 23*, 1128–1135.

Carey, S. L., Lura, D. J., & Highsmith, M. J. (2015). Differences in myoelectric and body-powered upper-limb prostheses: Systematic literature review. *Journal of Rehabilitation Research and Development, 52*, 247–262.

Cheesborough, J. E., Smith, L. H, Kuiken, T. A., & Dumanian, G. A. (2015). Targeted muscle reinnervation and advanced prosthetic arms. *Seminars in Plastic Surgery, 29*, 62–72.

Christiansen, C. L., Fields, T., Lev, G., Stephenson, R. O., & Stevens-Lapsley, J. E. (2015). Functional outcomes after the prosthetic training phase of rehabilitation after dysvascular lower extremity amputation. *PM& R: The Journal of Injury, Function, and Rehabilitation, 11*, 1118–1126.

Churilov, I., Churilov, L., & Murphy, D. (2014). Do rigid dressings reduce the time from amputation to prosthetic fitting? A systematic review and meta-analysis. *Annals of Vascular Surgery, 28*, 1801–1808.

Cipriani, C., Segil, J. L., Birdwell, J. A., & Weir, R. F. (2014). Dexterous control of a prosthetic hand using fine-wire intramuscular electrodes in targeted extrinsic muscles. *IEEEE Transactions on Neural Systems and Rehabilitation Engineering, 22*, 828–836.

Crandall, R. C., & Tomhave, W. (2002). Pediatric unilateral below-elbow amputees: Retrospective analysis of 34 patients given multiple prosthetic options. *Journal of Pediatric Orthopedics, 22*, 380–383.

Cuccurullo, S. J. (2004). *Physical medicine and rehabilitation board review*. New York, NY: Demos Medical Publishing.

Czerniecki, J. M., & Ehde, D. M. (2003). Chronic pain after lower extremity amputation. *Critical Reviews in Physical and Rehabilitation Medicine, 15*, 3–4.

Dabaghi-Richerand, A., Haces-Garcia, F., & Capdevila-Leonori, R. (2015). Prognostic factors of a satisfactory functional result in patients with unilateral amputations of the upper limb above the wrist that use an upper limb prosthesis. *Revista Espanola de Cirugia Ortopedica y Traumatologia, 59*, 343–347.

D'Andrea, S., Wilhelm, N., Silverman, A. K., & Grabowski, A. M. (2014). Does use of a powered ankle–foot prosthesis restore whole-body angular momentum during walking at different speeds? *Clinical Orthopaedics and Related Research, 472*, 3044–3054.

Davidson, J. (2002). A survey of the satisfaction of upper limb amputees with their prostheses, their lifestyles, and their abilities. *Journal of Hand Therapy, 15*, 62–70.

Davies, B., & Datta, D. (2003). Mobility outcome following unilateral lower limb amputation. *Prosthetics and Orthotics International, 27*, 186–190.

Deans, S. A., McFadyen, A. K., & Rowe, P. J. (2008). Physical activity and quality of life: A study of a lower-limb amputee population. *Prosthetics and Orthotics International, 32*, 186–200.

Delussu, A. S., Brunelli, S., Paradisi, F., Iosa, M., Pellegrini, R., Zenardi, D., & Traballesi, M. (2013). Assessment of the effects of carbon fiber and bionic foot during overground and treadmill walking in transtibial amputees. *Gait & Posture, 38*, 876–882.

Devlin, M., Sinclair, L. B., Colman, D., Parsons, J., Nizio, H., & Campbell, J. E. (2002). Patient preference and gait efficiency in a geriatric population with transfemoral amputation using a free-swinging versus a locked prosthetic knee joint. *Archives of Physical Medicine and Rehabilitation, 83*, 246–249.

Dickhaut, S. C., DeLee, J. C., & Page, C. P. (1984). Nutritional status: Importance in predicting wound-healing after amputation. *Journal of Bone and Joint Surgery American, 66*, 71–75.

Dillingham, T. R., Pezzin, L. E., & MacKenzie, E. J. (2002). Limb amputation and limb deficiency: Epidemiology and recent trends in the United States. *Southern Medical Journal, 95*, 875–883.

Dillingham, T. R., Pezzin, L. E., MacKenzie, E. J., & Burgess, A. R. (2001). Use and satisfaction with prosthetic devices among persons with trauma-related amputations: A long-term outcome study. *American Journal of Physical Medicine and Rehabilitation, 80*, 563–571.

Dougherty, P. J. (2003). Long-term follow–up of unilateral transfemoral amputees from the Vietnam war. *Journal of Trauma, 54*, 718–723.

Dougherty, P. J., McFarland, L. V., Smith, D. G., & Reiber, G. E. (2014). Bilateral transfemoral/transtibial amputations due to battle injuries: A comparison of Vietnam veterans with Iraq and Afghanistan servicemembers. *Clinical Orthopaedics and Related Research, 472*, 3010–3016.

Duhon, B., Hand, E., Howell, C., & Reveles, K. (2015). Retrospective cohort study evaluating the incidence of diabetic foot infections among hospitalized adults with diabetes in the United States from 1996–2010. *American Journal of Infection Control, 44*, 199–202.

Eberly, V. J., Mulroy, S. J., Gronley, J. K., Perry, J., Yule, W. J., & Burnfield, J. M. (2014). Impact of a stance phase microprocessor–controlled knee prosthesis on level walking in lower functioning individuals with a transfemoral amputation. *Prosthetics and Orthotics International, 38*, 447–455.

Edelstein, J. E., & Berger, N. (1993). Performance comparison among children fitted with myoelectric and body-powered hands. *Archives of Physical Medicine and Rehabilitation, 74*, 376–380.

Ehde, D. M., Czerniecki, J. M., Smith, D. G., Campbell, K. M., Edwards, W. T., Jensen, M. P., & Robinson, L. R. (2000). Chronic phantom sensations, phantom pain, residual limb pain, and other regional pain after lower limb amputation. *Archives of Physical Medicine and Rehabilitation, 81*, 1039–1044.

Elliott, R. M., Tintle, S. M., & Levin, L. S. (2014). Upper extremity transplantation: Current concepts and challenges in an emerging field. *Current Review of Musculoskeletal Medicine, 71*, 83–86.

Fernández, A., Isusi, I., & Gómez, M. (2000). Factors conditioning the return to work of upper limb amputees in Asturias, Spain. *Prosthetics and Orthotics International, 24*, 143–147.

Fisk, J. R., & Smith, D. G. (2004). The limb-deficient child. In D. G. Smith, J. W. Michaels, & J. H. Bowker (Eds.), *Atlas of amputations and limb deficiencies* (3rd ed., pp. 773–777). Rosemont, IL: American Academy of Orthopaedic Surgeons.

Flor, H. (2002). Phantom–limb pain: Characteristics, causes and treatment. *Lancet Neurology, 1*, 182–189.

Gailey, R., Allen, K., Castles, J., Kucharik, J., & Roeder, M. (2008). Review of secondary physical conditions associated with lower-limb amputation and long-term prosthetic use. *Journal of Rehabilitation Research and Development, 45*, 15–30.

Gaine, W. J., Smart, C., & Bransby-Zachary, M. (1997). Upper limb traumatic amputees: Review of prosthetic use. *Journal of Hand Surgery British, 22*, 73–76.

Gajewski, D., & Granville, R. (2006). The United States Armed Forces amputee patient care program. *Journal of the American Academic of Orthopaedic Surgeons, 14*, S183–S187.

Gauthier-Gagnon, C., Grisé, M. C., & Potvin, D. (1999). Enabling factors related to prosthetic use by people with transtibial and transfemoral amputation. *Archives of Physical Medicine and Rehabilitation, 80*, 706–713.

Gerschutz, M. J., Hayne, M. L., Colvin, J. M., & Denune, J. A. (2015). Dynamic effectiveness evaluation of elevated vacuum suspension. *Journal of Prosthetics & Orthotics, 27*, 161–165.

Gholizadeh, H., Abu Osman, N. A., Eshraghi, A., & Ali, S. (2014). Transfemoral prosthesis suspension systems: A systematic review of the literature. *American Journal of Physical Medicine and Rehabilitation, 93*, 809–823.

Graham, L. E., Datta, D., Heller, B., Howitt, J., & Pros, D. (2007). A comparative study of conventional and energy-storing prosthetic feet in high-functioning transfemoral amputees. *Archives of Physical Medicine and Rehabilitation, 88*, 801–806.

Gretsch, K. F., Lather, H. D., Peddada, K. V., Deeken, C. R., Wall, L. B., & Goldfarb, C. A. (2015). Development of novel 3D-printed robotic prosthetic for transradial amputees. *Prosthetics and Orthotics International, 40*, 400–403.

Hagberg, K., Hansson, E., & Brånemark, R. (2014). Outcome of percutaneous osseointegrated prostheses for patients with unilateral transfemoral amputation at two-year follow-up. *Archives of Physical Medicine and Rehabilitation, 95*, 2120–2127.

Hakimi, K., Eftekhari, N., & Czerniecki, J. (2008). Amputation rehabilitation: Epidemiology, preprosthetic management and complications. In B. J. O'Young, M. A. Young, & S. A. Stiens (Eds.), *Physical medicine and rehabilitation secrets* (3rd ed., pp. 267–276). Philadelphia, PA: Mosby Elsevier.

Health Care Financing Administration, Department of Health and Human Services, 2001.

Hebert, J. S., Olson, J. L., Morhart, M. J., Dawson, M. R., Marasco, P. D., Kuiken, T. A., & Chan, K. M. (2014). Novel targeted sensory reinnervation technique to restore functional hand sensation after transhumeral amputation. *IEEE Transactions on Neural Systems and Rehabilitation Engineering, 22*, 765–773.

Hsu, M. J., Nielsen, D. H., Lin–Chan, S. J., & Shurr, D. (2006). The effects of prosthetic foot design on physiologic measurements, self–selected walking velocity, and physical activity in people with transtibial amputation. *Archives of Physical Medicine and Rehabilitation, 87*, 123–129.

Hu, X., Trevelyan, E., Yang, G., Lee, M. S., Lorenc, A., Liu, J., & Robinson, N. (2014). The effectiveness of acupuncture/TENS for phantom limb syndrome. I: A systematic review of controlled clinical trials. *European Journal of Integrative Medicine, 6*, 355–364.

International Organization for Standardization, Geneva, Switzerland (1989).

Johansson, J. L., Sherrill, D. M., Riley, P. O., Bonato, P., & Herr, H. (2005). A clinical comparison of variable-damping and mechanically passive prosthetic knee devices. *American Journal of Physical Medicine and Rehabiilitation, 84*, 563–575.

Johnson, S. S., & Mansfield, E. (2014). Prosthetic training: Upper limb. *Physical Medicine and Rehabilitation Clinics of North America, 25*, 133–151.

Jonsson, S., Caine-Winterberger, K., & Branemark, R. (2011). Osseointegration amputation prostheses on the upper limbs: Methods prosthetics and rehabilitation. *Prosthetics and Orthotics International, 35*, 190–200.

Kahle, J. T., Highsmith, M. J., & Hubbard, S. L. (2008). Comparison of nonmicroprocessor knee mechanism versus C-Leg on prosthesis evaluation questionnaire, stumbles, falls, walking tests, stair descent, and knee preference. *Journal of Rehabilitation Research and Development, 45*, 1–14.

Kannenberg, A., Zacharias, B., & Probsting, E. (2014). Benefits of microprocessor–controlled prosthetic knees to limited community ambulators: Systematic review. *Journal of Rehabilitation Research and Development, 51*, 1469–1496.

Karmarkar, A. M., Graham, J. E., Reistetter, T. A., Kumar, A., Mix, J. M., Niewczyk, P., & Ottenbacher K. J. (2014). Association between functional severity and amputation type with rehabilitation outcomes in patients with lower limb amputation. *Rehabilitation Research and Practice, 2014*, 1–7.

Kaufman, K. R., Levine, J. A., Brey, R. H., McCrady, S. K., Padgett, D. J., & Joyner, M. J. (2008). Energy expenditure and activity of transfemoral amputees using mechanical and microprocessor–controlled prosthetic knees. *Archives of Physical Medicine and Rehabilitation, 89*, 1380–1385.

Kauzlarić, N., Kauzlarić, K. S., & Kolundzić, R. (2007). Prosthetic rehabilitation of persons with lower limb amputations due to tumour. *European Journal of Cancer Care (England), 16*, 238–243.

Klute, G. K., Kantor, C., Darrouzet, C., Wild, H., Wilkinson, S., Iveljic, S., & Creasey, G. (2009). Lower-limb amputee needs assessment using multistakeholder focus-group approach. *Journal of Rehabilitation Research and Development, 46*, 293–304.

Kuiken, T. A., Li, G., Lock, B. A., Lipschultz, R. D., Miller, L. A., Stubblefield, K. A., & Englehart, K. B. (2009). Targeted muscle reinnervation for real-time myoelectric control of multifunction artificial arms. *Journal of the American Medical Association, 301*, 619–628.

Kung, T. A., Bueno, R. A., Alkhalefah, G. K., Langhals, N. B., Urbanchek. M. G., & Cederna, P. S. (2013). Innovations in prosthetic interfaces for the upper extremity. *Plastic and Reconstructive Surgery, 132*, 1515–1523.

Le, J. T., & Scott-Wyard, P. R. (2015). Pediatric limb differences and amputations. *Physical Medicine and Rehabilitation Clinics of North America, 26*, 95–108.

Mac Neill, H. L., Devlin, M., Pauley, T., & Yudin, A. (2008). Long-term outcomes and survival of patients with bilateral transtibial amputations after rehabilitation. *American Journal of Physical Medicine and Rehabilitation, 87*, 189–196.

MacKenzie, E. J., Bosse, M. J., Castillo, R. C., Smith, D. G., Webb, L. X., Kellam, J. F., . . . McCarthy, M. L. (2004). Functional outcomes following trauma-related lower-extremity amputation. *Journal of Bone and Joint Surgery American, 86*, 1636–1645.

Marinakis, G. N. (2004). Interlimb symmetry of traumatic unilateral transtibial amputees wearing two different prosthetic feet in the early rehabilitation stage. *Journal of Rehabilitation Research and Development, 41*, 581–590.

Marzen-Groller, K., & Bartman, K. (2005). Building a successful support group for post-amputation patients. *Journal of Vascular Nursing, 23*, 42–45.

McCormick, Z., Chang-Chien, G., Marshall, B., Huang, M., & Harden, R. N. (2014). Phantom limb pain: A systematic neuroanatomical-based review of pharmacologic treatment. *Pain Medicine, 15*, 292–305.

McFarland, L. V., Hubard Winkler, S. L., Heinemann, A. W., Jones, M., & Esquenazi, A. (2010). Unilateral upper–limb loss: Satisfaction and prosthetic-device use in veterans and service members from vietnam and OIF/OEF conflicts. *Journal of Rehabilitation Research and Development, 47*, 299–316.

Meier, R. H., & Atkins, D. J. (Eds.). (2004). *Functional restoration of adults and children with upper extremity amputation*. New York, NY: Demos Medical Publishing.

Menke, A., Casagrande, S. l., Geiss, L., & Cowie, C. C. (2015). Prevalence of and trends in diabetes among adults in the United States, 1988–2012. *Journal of the American Medical Association, 314*, 1021–1029.

Mohanty, R. K., Lenka, P., Equebal, A., & Kumar, R. (2012). Comparison of energy cost in transtibial amputees using prosthesis and crutches without prosthesis for walking activities. *Annals of Physical and Rehabilitation Medicine, 55*, 252–262.

Morris, C. D., Potter B. K., Athanasian, E. A., & Lewis, V. O. (2015). Extremity amputations: Principles, techniques, and recent advances. *Instructional Course Lecture, 64*, 105–117.

Mulvey, M. R., Bagnall, A. M., Johnson, M. I., & Marchant, P. R. (2010). Transcutaneous electrical nerve stimulation (TENS) for phantom pain and stump pain following amputation in adults. *The Cochrane Database of Systemic Reviews, 12*(5), CD007264.

Munin, M. C., Espejo-De Guzman, M. C., Boninger, M. L., Fitzgerald, S. G., Penrod, L. E., & Singh, J. (2001). Predictive factors for successful early prosthetic ambulation among lower-limb amputees. *Journal of Rehabilitation Research and Development, 38*, 379–384.

Murdoch, G., & Wilson, A. B. (Eds.). (1996). *Amputation: Surgical practice and patient management*. St. Louis, MO: Butterworth-Heinemann Medical.

Nagarajan, R., Neglia, J. P., Clohisy, D. R., Yasui, Y., Greenberg, M., Hudson, M., & Robison, L. L. (2003). Education, employment, insurance, and marital status among 694 survivors of pediatric lower extremity bone tumors: A report from the childhood cancer survivor study. *Cancer, 97*, 2554–2564.

Nehler, M. R., Coll, J. R., Hiatt, W. R., Regensteiner J. G., Schnickel, G. T., Klenke, W. A., . . . Krupski, W. C. (2003). Functional outcome in a contemporary series of major lower extremity amputations. *Journal of Vascular Surgery, 38*, 7–14.

Nghiem, B. T., Sando, I. C., Gillespie, R. B., McLaughlin, B. L., Gerling, G. J., Langhals, N. B., . . . Cederna, P. S. (2015). Providing a sense of touch to prosthetic hands. *Plastic and Reconstructive Surgery, 135*, 1652–1663.

Nikolajsen, L. (2012). Postamputation pain: Studies on mechanisms. *Danish Medical Journal, 59*, B4527.

Nolan, L., & Lees, A. (2000). The functional demands on the intact limb during walking for active trans-femoral and trans-tibial amputees. *Prosthetics and Orthotics International, 24*, 117–125.

Nolan, L., Patritti, B. L., & Simpson, K. J. (2012). Effect of take-off from prosthetic versus intact limb on transtibial amputee long jump technique. *Prosthetics and Orthotics International, 36*, 297–305.

Nolan, L., Patritti, B. L., Stana, L., & Tweedy, S. M. (2011). Is increased residual shank length a competitive advantage for elite transtibial amputee long jumpers? *Adaptive Physical Activity Quarterly, 28*, 267–276.

Ostlie, K., Lesio I. M., Franklin, R. J., Garfelt, B., Skjeldal, O. H., & Magnus, P. (2012). Prosthesis rejection in acquired major upper-limb amputees: A population-based survey. *Disability and Rehabilitation: Assistive Technology, 7*, 294–303.

Otr, O. V., Reinders-Messelink, H. A., Bongers, R. M., Bouwsema, H., & Van Der Sluis, C. K. (2010). The i-LIMB hand and the DMC plus hand compared: A case report. *Prosthetics and Orthotics International, 34*, 216–220.

Ovelmen-Levitt, J. (1988). Abnormal physiology of the dorsal horn as related to the deafferentation syndrome. *Applied Neurophysiology, 51*, 104–116.

Pasquina, P. F., Evangelista, M., Carvalho, A. J., Lockhart, J., Griffin, S., Nanos, G., . . . Hankin, D. (2015). First-in-man demonstration of a fully implanted myoelectric sensors system to control an advanced electromechanical prosthetic hand. *Journal of Neuroscience Methods, 244*, 85–93.

Patton, J. G. (2004). Training the child with a unilateral upper-extremity prosthesis. In R. H. Meier & D. G. Atkins (Eds.), *Functional restoration of adults and children with upper extremity amputation* (pp. 297–316). New York, NY: Demos Medical Publishing.

Paysant, J., Beyaert, C., Datié, A. M., Martinet, N., & André, J. M. (2006). Influence of terrain on metabolic and temporal gait characteristics of unilateral transtibial amputees. *Journal of Rehabilitation Research and Development, 43*, 153–160.

Pezzin, L. E., Dillingham, T. R., Mackenzie, E. J., Ephraim, P., & Rossbach, P. (2004). Use and satisfaction with prosthetic limb devices and related services. *Archives of Physical Medicine and Rehabilitation, 85*, 723–729.

Pezzin, L. E., Dillingham, T. R., & MacKenzie, E. J. (2000). Rehabilitation and the long-term outcomes of persons with trauma-related amputations. *Archives of Physical Medicine and Rehabilitation, 81*, 292–300.

Pezzin, L. E., Padalik, S. E., & Dillingham, T. R. (2013). Effect of postacute rehabilitation setting on mental and emotional health among persons with dysvascular amputations. *Physical Medicine and Rehabilitation, 5*, 583–590.

Pickwell, K., Siersma, V., Kars, M., Apelqvist, J., Bakker, K., Edmonds, M., & Schaper, N. (2015). Predictors of lower-extremity amputation in patients with an infected diabetic foot ulcer. *Diabetes Care, 38*, 852–857.

Plato. (2016). *Plato: The Complete Works*. e-artnow. Amazon Digital Services.

Powell, M. A., Kaliki, R. R., & Thakor, N. V. (2014). User training for pattern recognition-based myoelectric prostheses: Improving phantom limb movement consistency and distinguishability. *IEEE Transactions on Neural Systems and Rehabilitation Engineering, 22*, 522–532.

Pylatiuk, C., Schulz, S., & Döderlein, L. (2007). Results of an Internet survey of myoelectric prosthetic hand users. *Prosthetics and Orthotics International, 31*, 362–370.

Radocy, R., & Furlong, A. (2004). Recreation and sports adaptations. In R. H. Meier & D. J. Atkins (Eds.), *Functional Restoration of adults and children with upper extremity amputation* (pp. 251–274). New York, NY: Demos Medical Publishing.

Raichle, K. A., Hanley, M. A., Molton, I., Kadel, N. J., Campbell, K., Phelps, E., & Smith, M. D. (2008). Prosthesis use in persons with lower-and upper-limb amputation. *Journal of Rehabilitation Research and Development, 45*, 961–972.

Rau, B., Bonvin, F., & de Bie, R. (2007). Short-term effect of physiotherapy rehabilitation on functional performance of lower limb amputees. *Prosthetics and Orthotics International, 31*, 258–270.

Resnik, L., Klinger, S. L., & Etter, K. (2014). The DEKA arm: Its features, functionality, and evolution during the veterans affairs study to optimize the DEKA arm. *Prosthetics and Orthotics International*, *38*, 492–504.

Resnik, L., Meucci, M. R., Lieberman-Klinger, S., Fantini, C., Kelty, D. L., Disla, R., & Sasson, N. (2012). Advanced upper limb prosthetic devices: Implications for upper limb prosthetic rehabilitation. *Archives of Physical Medicine and Rehabilitation*, *93*, 710–717.

Rheinstein, J., Wong, C. K., & Edelstein, J. E. (2006). Post-operative management. In K. Carroll & J. E. Edelstein (Eds.), *Prosthetics and patient management: A comprehensive clinical approach* (pp. 15–31). Thorofare, NJ: Slack.

Ritchie, S., Wiggins, S., & Sanford, A. (2011). Perceptions of cosmesis and function in adults with prostheses: A systematic literature review. *Prosthetics and Orthotics International*, *35*, 332–341.

Rossi, R., Alexander, M., & Cuccurullo, S. (2004). Pediatric rehabilitation. In S. J. Cuccurullo (Ed.), *Physical medicine and rehabilitation board review* (pp. 645–741). New York, NY: Demos Medical Publishing.

Rothgangel, A. S., Braun, S. M., Beurskens, A. J., Seitz, R. J., & Wade, D. T. (2011). The clinical aspects of mirror therapy in rehabilitation: A systematic review of the literature. *International Journal of Rehabilitation Research*, *34*, 1–13.

Sapin, E., Goujon, H., de Almeida, F., Fode, P., & Lavaste, F. (2008). Functional gait analysis of transfemoral amputees using two different single-axis prosthetic knees with hydraulic swing-phase control: Kinematic and kinetic comparison of two prosthetic knees. *Prosthetics and Orthotics International*, *32*, 201–218.

Sauter, C. N., Pezzin, L. E., & Dillingham, T. R. (2013). Functional outcomes of persons who underwent dysvascular lower extremity amputations: Effect of postacute rehabilitation setting. *American Journal of Physical Medicine and Rehabilitation*, *92*, 287–296.

Sawers, A. B., & Hafner, B. J. (2013). Outcomes associated with the use of microprocessor-controlled prosthetic knees among individuals with unilateral transfemoral limb loss: A systematic review. *Journal of Rehabilitation Research and Development*, *50*, 273–314.

Schofield, J. S., Evans, K. R., Carey, J. P., & Hebert, J. S. (2014). Application of sensory feedback in motorized upper extremity prosthesis: A review. *Expert Review of Medical Devices*, *11*, 499–511.

Schoppen, T., Boonstra, A., Groothoff, J. W., deVries, J., Goeken, L. N., & Eisma, W. H. (2001). Factors related to successful job reintegration of people with a lower limb amputation. *Archives of Physical Medicine and Rehabilitation, 82*, 1425–1431.

Schoppen, T., Boonstra, A., Groothoff, J. W., deVries, J., Goeken, L. N., & Eisma, W. H. (2002). Job satisfaction and health experience of people with a lower-limb amputation in comparison with healthy colleagues. *Archives of Physical Medicine and Rehabilitation*, *83*, 628–634.

Schoppen, T., Boonstra, A., Groothoff, J. W., deVries, J., Goeken, L. N., & Eisma, W. H. (2003). Physical, mental, and social predictors of functional outcome in unilateral lower-limb amputees. *Archives of Physical Medicine and Rehabilitation, 84*, 803–811.

Schuch, C. M., & Pritham, C. H. (1994). International forum—International Standards Organization terminology: Application to prosthetics and orthotics. *Journal of Prosthetics and Orthotics, 6*, 29–33.

Segal, A. D., Kracht, R., & Klute, G. K. (2014). Does a torsion adapter improve functional mobility pain, and fatigue in patients with transtibial amputation? *Clinical Orthopaedics and Related Research, 472*, 3085–3092.

Segal, A. D., Orendurff, M. S., Klute, G. K., MacDowell, M. L., Pecoraro, J. A., & Shofer, J. (2006). Kinematic and kinetic comparisons of transfemoral amputee gait using C-Leg and Mauch SNS prosthetic knees. *Journal of Rehabilitation Research and Development, 43*, 857–870.

Selles, R. W., Janssens, P. J., Jongenengel, C. D., & Bussmann, J. A. (2005). A randomized controlled trial comparing functional outcome and cost efficiency of a total surface-bearing socket versus a conventional patellar tendon-bearing socket in transtibial amputees. *Archies of Physical Medicine and Rehabilitation, 86*, 154–161.

Sensinger, J. W., Lipsey, J., Thomas, A., & Turner, K. (2015). Design and evaluation of voluntary opening and voluntary closing prosthetic terminal device. *Journal of Rehabilitation Research and Development, 52*, 63–76.

Shaperman, J., Landsberger, S., & Setoguchi, Y. (2003). Early upper limb prosthetic fitting: When and what do we fit? *Journal of Prosthetics and Orthotics, 15*, 11–19.

Smit, G., Bongers, R. M., van der Sluis, C. K., & Plettenburg D. H. (2012). Efficiency of voluntary opening hand and hook prosthetic devices: 24 years of development? *Journal of Rehabilitation Research and Development*, *49*, 523–534.

Su, P. F., Gard, S. A., Lipschutz, R. D., & Kuiken, T. A. (2010). The effects of increased prosthetic ankle motions on the gait of persons with bilateral transtibial amputations. *American Journal of Physical Medicine and Rehabilitation, 89*, 34–47.

Sumpio, B., Shine, S. R., Mahler, D., & Sumpio, B. E. (2013). A comparison of immediate postoperative rigid and soft dressings for below-knee amputations. *Annals of Vascular Surgery*, *27*, 774–780.

Taylor, L., Cavenett, S., Stepien, J. M., & Crotty, M. (2008). Removable rigid dressings: A retrospective case-note audit to determine the validity of post-amputation application. *Prosthetics and Orthotics International*, *32*, 223–230.

Tung, M. L., Murphy, I. C., Griffin, S. C., Alphonso, A. L., Hussey-Anderson, L., Hughes, K. E., . . . Tsao, J. W. (2014). Observation of limb movements reduces phantom limb pain in bilateral amputees. *Annals of Clinical and Translational Neurology, 1*, 633–638.

Uchytil, J., Jandacka, D., Zahradnik, D., Farana, R., & Janura, M. (2014). Temporal-spatial parameters of gait in transfemoral amputees: Comparison of bionic and mechanically passive knee joints. *Prosthetics and Orthotics International, 38*, 199–203.

Uellendahl, J. E. (2004). Bilateral upper limb prostheses. In D. G. Smith, J. W. Michael, & J. H. Bowker (Eds.), *Atlas of amputations and limb deficiencies* (3rd ed., pp. 311–326). Rosemont, IL: American Academy of Orthopedic Surgeons.

Uustal, H., & Baerga, E. (2004). Prosthetics and orthotics. In S. J. Cuccurullo (Ed.), *Physical medicine and rehabilitation board review* (pp. 409–487). New York, NY: Demos Medical Publishing.

van der Niet, O., Bongers, R. M., & van der Sluis, C. K. (2013). Functionality of i-LIMB and i-LIMB pulse hands: Case report. *Journal of Rehabilitation Research and Development, 50*, 1123–1128.

Van Dorsten, B. (2004). Integrating psychological and medical care: Practice recommendations for amputation. In R. H. Meier & D. J. Atkins (Eds.), *Functional restoration of adults and children with upper extremity amputation* (pp. 73–88). New York, NY: Demos Medical Publishing.

Vasluian, E., van Wijk, I., Dijkstra, P. U., Reinders-Messelink, H. A., & Van Der Sluis, C. K. (2015). Adaptive devices in young people with upper limb reduction deficiencies: Use and satisfaction. *Journal of Rehabilitation Medicine, 47*, 346–355.

Veterans Affairs, Department of Defense. (2014). *Evidence based practice guideline for the management of upper extremity amputation rehabilitation.* Washington, DC: Department of Veterans Affairs, Department of Defense

Vickers, D. R., Palk, C., McIntosh, A. S., & Beatty, K. T. (2008). Elderly unilateral transtibial amputee gait on an inclined walkway: A biomechanical analysis. *Gait and Posture, 27*, 518–529.

Vllasolli, T. O., Zafirova, B., Orovcanec, N., Poposka, A., Murtezani, A., & Krasniqi, B. (2014). Energy expenditure and walking speed in lower limb amputees: A cross sectional study. *Ortopedia, Traumatologia Rehabilitacja, 16*, 419–426.

Vrieling, A. H., van Keeken, H. G., Schoppen, T., Otten, E., Halbertsma, J. P., Hof, A. L., & Postema, K. (2007). Obstacle crossing in lower limb amputees. *Gait & Posture*, 26, 587–594.

Vrieling, A. H., van Keeken, H. G., Schoppen, T., Otten, E., Halbertsma, J. P., Hof, A. L., & Postema, K. (2008a). Gait initiation in lower limb amputees. *Gait & Posture, 27*, 423–430.

Vrieling, A. H., van Keeken, H. G., Schoppen, T., Otten, E., Halbertsma, J. P., Hof, A. L., & Postema, K. (2008b). Uphill and downhill walking in unilateral lower limb amputees. *Gait & Posture, 28*, 235–242.

Walker, J. L., Coburn, T. R., Cottle, W., Burke, C., & Talwalkar, V. R. (2008). Recreational terminal devices for children with upper extremity amputations. *Journal of Pediatric Orthopedics, 28*, 271–273.

Waters, R. L., & Mulroy, S. (1999). The energy expenditure of normal and pathological gait. *Gait & Posture, 9*, 207–231.

Webster, J. B., Levy, C. E., Bryant, P. R., & Prusakowski, P. E. (2001). Sports and recreation for persons with limb deficiency. *Archives of Physical Medicine and Rehabilitation, 82*, S38–S44.

Wezenberg, D., van der Woude, L. H., Faber, W. X., de Haan, A., & Housijk, H. (2013). Relation between aerobic capacity and walking ability in older adults with a lower-limb amputation. *Archives of Physical Medicine and Rehabilitation, 94*, 1714–1720.

Williams, T. W. (2004). Control of powered upper extremity prostheses. In R. H. Meier & D. J. Atkins (Eds.), *Functional restoration of adults and children with upper extremity amputation* (pp. 207–224). New York, NY: Demos Medical Publishing.

Williams, T. W. (2011). Progress on stabilizing and controlling powered upper-limb prostheses. *Journal of Rehabilitation Research and Development, 48*, ix–xix.

Wong, C. K., & Edelstein, J. E. (2000). Unna and elastic postoperative dressings: Comparison of their effect on function of adults with amputation and vascular disease. *Archives of Physical Medicine and Rehabilitation, 81*, 191–198.

Wright, D. A., Marks, L., & Payne, R. C. (2008). A comparative study of the physiological costs of walking in ten bilateral amputees. *Prosthetics and Orthotics International, 32*, 57–67.

Wright, T. W., Hagen, A. D., & Wood, M. B. (1995). Prosthetic usage in major upper extremity amputations. *Journal of Hand Surgery, 20*, 619–622.

Yazicioglu, K., Taskaynatan, M. A., Guzelkucuk, U., & Tugcu, I. (2007). Effect of playing football (soccer) on balance, strength, and quality of life in unilateral below-knee amputees. *American Journal of Physical Medicine and Rehabilitation, 86*, 800–805.

Ziegler, G. K., MacKenzie, E. J., Ephraim, P. L., Travison, T. G., & Brookmeyer, R. (2008). Estimating the prevalence of limb loss in the United States: 2005–2050. *Archives of Physical Medicine and Rehabilitation, 89*, 422–429.

Zmitrewicz, R. J., Neptune, R., Walden, J. G., Rogers, W. E., & Bosker, G. W. (2006). The effect of foot and ankle prosthetic components on braking and propulsive impulses during transtibial amputee gait. *Archives of Physical Medicine and Rehabilitation, 87*, 1334–1339.

19

CHAPTER

Organ Transplantation and Rehabilitation: Process and Interdisciplinary Interventions

Jeffrey M. Cohen, Mark Young, Bryan O'Young, and Steven A. Stiens

INTRODUCTION

Life-saving treatment of disease by organ transplantation has become a standard part of medical practice. The past 30 years have seen considerable advances in the field of organ transplantation. This has been the result of advances in surgical techniques, technological improvements, and the discovery of potent immunosuppressive drugs that reduced rejection of the grafted organ (Young, Stiens, O'Young, & Mayer, 2011). Today, there are more than 19 transplantable organ systems. The focus of this chapter is on the four most common solid organ transplants seen in rehabilitation medicine: liver, renal, cardiac, and pulmonary.

The challenge of rehabilitation after organ transplantation is that the rehabilitation professional (Stiens, O'Young, & Young, 2008) joins the care team in consultation and must help the team overcome the myth that replacement of the organ cures the impairment and makes everything well again (Stiens, Reyes, & Svircev, 2008). The most successful intervention comes from the rediscovery of the person that makes up the patient, focusing on immediate and long-term patient and family-centered goals (Young, Stiens, O'Young, & Mayer, 2011). The treatment plan is then designed using a biopsychosocial model, with a problem-based assessment that starts with the multiple effects of the organ failure on associated body systems. The rehabilitation team's job is to dissect out the secondary effects (weakness, malnutrition, decreased endurance, depression) and sort them into goals. Focusing interventions on each goal produces the most synergistic effect.

What is most intriguing about transplantation rehabilitation is that in contrast to all other rehabilitation cases, the impairment is in fact remediated if all goes well. Many associated systems rejuvenate themselves after the organ is replaced and the patient is reanimated. With proper design and modulation of rehabilitation interventions, the interaction between these body systems can be maximized and the process can be most efficient. The design of the interventions can start with the conceptual environmental model (Figure 19.1). During the pretransplant period, low-level conditioning of the patient and maximization of function of the diseased organs are emphasized. These interventions occur in the internal environment (within the person). Adaptations to the patient's immediate and intermediate environment maximize function in spite of the patients' low exercise tolerance and strength. After transplantation, immunomodulators and their side effects are active in the internal environment while the replacement organ and rehabilitation interventions improve the function of secondary systems compromised by organ failure before transplantation. Emphasis is then on normalizing the interactions between the patient and the intermediate, community, and natural environments through vocational and recreational therapy.

LIVER TRANSPLANTATION

Liver transplantation is considered a life-saving procedure. Over the past 50 years, the world has witnessed evolving strategies in surgical techniques,

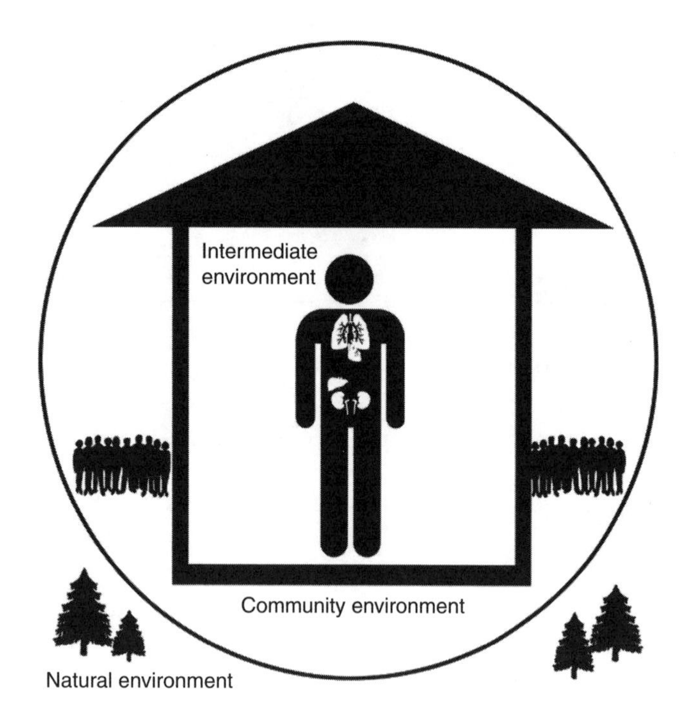

FIGURE 19.1 Conceptual environmental model.
The physical environment can be divided into concentric sectors for the analysis of rehabilitation interventions. The internal environment (inside the person) includes all organ systems and their interactions. Solid organs with pathology (pretransplant) or fully functioning (posttransplant) are depicted with icons. The immediate environment is from the patient's surface out and may be adapted with mechanical heart support devices, dialysis machines, braces, crutches, or wheelchairs needed to support patient function. The intermediate environment is adapted specifically for the inhabitant and may include environmental controls in the home. The community environment includes not only the physical structures, but also includes people and the institutions governed by a common culture or laws. The natural environment is not modified and may require adaptations for access as required by the activity limitations of the patient.
Source: Stiens, Shamberg, and Shamberg (2008).

immunosuppressive drugs, intensive pre- and postoperative care, and, the prevention of disease recurrence. This has led to the present state of liver transplantation, a well-established procedure that has saved innumerable lives worldwide. Today, there are hundreds of liver transplant centers in over 80 countries (Song, Avelino-Silva, Pecora, D'Albuquerque, & Abdala, 2014).

Liver transplantation is the therapeutic option of choice for patients with acute and chronic end-stage liver disease. Liver disease can be either acute (fulminant or subfulminant failure) or chronic (decompensated cirrhosis). In the pretransplantation era, liver failure was nearly universally fatal, with mortalities from fulminant hepatic failure of 80% to 90% and 1-year mortality in decompensated cirrhosis of more than 50%. The first attempts at human liver transplantation were made in 1963 by Starzl and colleagues (see also Keeffe, 2001; Starzl, Klintmalm, Porter, Iwatsuki, & Schroter, 1981). However, the first successful liver transplantation was not achieved until 1967 (Keeffe, 2001). In the 1970s, the overall 1-year survival was approximately 30%, and the majority of patients died from rejection and/or infection. Over the past several decades, liver transplantation has evolved from being primarily an experimental procedure with limited success, to a routine operation that provides excellent survival rates for patients with irreversible acute or chronic end-stage liver disease. Presently, 1-year patient survival rates exceed 80% and outcomes continue to improve (Zarrinpar & Busuttil, 2013). Ten-year survival rates may exceed 70% for many indications (Song et al., 2014).

The development of immunosuppressive agents was a critically important step in the growth of solid organ transplantation. The early 1980s witnessed the discovery of cyclosporine, which led to an increased survival rate after liver transplantation, from 30% to more than 70% (Starzl et al., 1981). The development of newer immunosuppressive agents such as tacrolimus was associated with further improvements in 1-year graft and patient survival rates. Its use was associated with fewer episodes of acute cellular and steroid-resistant rejection (The U.S. Multicenter FK 506 Liver Study Group, 1994). From 1988 to 2009, liver transplantation in the United States grew 3.7-fold, from 1,713 to 6,320 transplants annually. The expansion of liver transplantation has been driven chiefly by scientific breakthroughs that have extended patient and graft survival well beyond those expected 50 years ago. The success of liver transplantation is now its primary obstacle, as the pool of donor livers fails to keep pace with the growing number of patients added to the national liver transplant waiting list (Wertheim, Petrowsky, Saab, Kupiec-Weglinski, & Busuttil, 2011).

Indications

Patients with liver failure who undergo liver transplantation fall into two major categories: acute fulminant hepatic failure and chronic liver failure

(Table 19.1; Rudow & Goldstein, 2008). This population varies greatly in terms of the extent of their debility. Acute fulminant hepatic failure may be the result of a toxic ingestion (e.g., acetaminophen overdose) or secondary to viral hepatitis. As the liver failure occurs suddenly, in otherwise healthy patients, these patients often present with limited functional deficits. In contrast, patients experiencing chronic liver failure have usually lived with their disease for a number of years. They have experienced a generalized decline in their functional abilities, resulting in a state of severe deconditioning and fatigue. Cirrhosis and chronic liver failure are leading causes of morbidity and mortality in the United States. The majority of preventable cases are attributed to excessive alcohol consumption, viral hepatitis, or nonalcoholic fatty liver disease (Heidelbaugh & Bruderly, 2006). Other etiologies of chronic liver failure include primary biliary cirrhosis, primary sclerosing cholangitis, autoimmune hepatitis, cholestatic disorders (disorders in which the excretory function of the liver is compromised), metabolic diseases such as hemochromatosis and Wilson's disease, and hepatocellular carcinoma. In the pediatric population, the most common indications for liver transplantation are biliary atresia and alpha 1-antitrypsin deficiency.

Liver transplantation is indicated for acute liver failure, chronic liver failure leading to cirrhosis, inherited metabolic liver diseases, hepatocellular carcinoma (HCC), and other hepatic cancers. The indications for liver transplantation have changed over the years. In the past, patients with unresectable, large, or multinodular tumors were selected for liver transplantation. This resulted in low survival rates and high rates of recurrence. Presently, it is felt that the best candidates are patients with small and uninodular or binodular tumors. In addition, transplantation for primary biliary cirrhosis has decreased over time, whereas transplantation for alcoholic and hepatitis C cirrhosis has increased, both in the United States and Europe. The survival rate for patients undergoing liver transplantation is better for those with primary biliary cirrhosis and autoimmune cirrhosis, whereas those with malignant liver tumors and hepatitis C have worse outcomes, due to high rates of recurrence. Despite improved survival rates, liver transplantation recipients have an estimated loss of 7 years compared with an age- and sex-matched general population, with increasing differences for recipients at younger age (Song et al., 2014).

As alcoholic cirrhosis remains the second most common indication for liver transplantation, most transplant centers worldwide need a minimum of 6 months of alcohol abstinence for listing these patients. Patients with alcohol dependence are at high risk for relapse to alcohol use after transplantation (recidivism). These patients need to be identified and require alcohol rehabilitation treatment before transplantation. Recidivism to the level of harmful drinking is reported in about 15% to 20% cases (Singal, Chaha, Rasheed, & Anand, 2013).

TABLE 19.1

INDICATIONS FOR LIVER TRANSPLANT
1. Acute liver failure
Drug induced
Toxin hypersensitivity
Fulminant hepatitis/necrosis
2. Chronic liver failure
Cholestatic disorders
Primary biliary cirrhosis
Biliary atresia
Alagille syndrome
Familial cholestasis
Secondary biliary cirrhosis
Primary sclerosing cholangitis
Parenchymal cirrhosis
Cryptogenic cirrhosis
Chronic hepatitis B and C
Alcoholic cirrhosis
Congenital hepatic fibrosis
Autoimmune hepatitis
Metabolic liver disease
Metabolic defect in the liver resulting in end-stage liver disease:
Alpha-1 antitrypsin deficiency
Wilson's disease
Tyrosinemia
Cystic fibrosis
Familial amyloidosis
Malignancies
Hepatocellular carcinoma
Hepatoblastoma
Hemangioendothelioma (confined to the liver)
Cholangiocarcinoma (new research protocols)
Vascular disease
Budd–Chiari syndrome
Portal vein thrombosis
Giant hepatic hemangioma

Source: Rudow and Goldstein (2008).

Types of Liver Transplantation

Liver transplantation involves the replacement of a diseased or injured liver with a new organ (allograft). The allograft can involve taking a whole organ from a deceased donor, a split liver graft from a deceased donor, or a partial graft from a live donor. As organ shortage is a major problem worldwide, split liver transplantation and living donor liver transplantation (LDLT) have been developed to expand sources of grafts. A split liver transplantation involves obtaining two grafts from a unique single deceased donor. Traditionally, the liver is split for an adult and a child. Survival for split liver transplantation has been found to be similar to that of whole organ recipients (Doyle et al., 2013). LDLT is a planned surgical procedure in which a healthy donor donates part of his or her liver. Beyond its technical complexity, a major concern about LDLT is the morbidity and risk of death for the donors (Song et al., 2014).

Selection for Liver Transplantation

The following factors are assessed in order to determine whether a patient is suitable for liver transplantation: etiology and stage of the liver disease, patient's psychosocial status, and potential contraindications to surgery. Clinically, the following conditions warrant consideration for liver transplantation (Lopez & Martin, 2006):

1. Fulminant hepatic failure (severe impairment of liver function in the absence of preexisting liver disease)
2. Intractable ascites (an abnormal accumulation of fluid in the abdomen)
3. Refractory encephalopathy (changes in consciousness, mentation, and behavior seen in patients with advanced liver disease due to the accumulation of wastes from protein breakdown)
4. Recurrent variceal bleeding (bleeding from dilated or variceal veins, usually esophageal varices, due to end-stage liver failure)
5. Severe deficits in the ability of the liver to perform its synthetic functions (production of the protein albumin and clotting factors). This leads to severe malnutrition and defects in the ability of the blood to clot in the usual time period.

Since 2002, the Model of End Stage Liver Disease (MELD) score has been the basis for the liver transplant allocation system. It has resulted in lower waiting list death rates among recipients in comparison to the pre-MELD era (Malines, Chen, Allore, & Quagliarello, 2014). The MELD score is calculated from three objective variables: the international normalized ratio (INR) of the prothrombin time, the serum bilirubin, and creatinine. It is used worldwide for listing and transplanting patients with end-stage liver disease, allowing for transplanting sicker patients first, irrespective of the wait time on the list (Singal & Kamath, 2013).

Contraindications to liver transplantation include uncontrolled infection, metastatic hepatobiliary or extrahepatic cancers, multiorgan failure, and irreversible brain damage (Koffron & Stein, 2008; Table 19.2). Over time, the contraindications for liver transplantation have also evolved. In the past, it was believed that HIV infection constituted an absolute contraindication; however, with the advent

TABLE 19.2

CURRENT ABSOLUTE AND RELATIVE CONTRAINDICATIONS IN LIVER TRANSPLANTATION
Absolute contraindications
Active extrahepatic malignancy
Hepatic malignancy with macrovascular or diffuse tumor invasion
Uncontrolled infection, except infection of the hepatobiliary system
Active substance or alcohol abuse
Severe comorbid conditions
Noncompliance or insufficient motivation
Technical impediment
Brain death
Relative contraindications
Advanced age
Human immunodeficiency virus (HIV) infection
Cholangiocarcinoma
Portal vein thrombosis
Psychosocial problems

Source: Koffron and Stein (2008).

of highly active antiviral therapy and the evolving knowledge of drug interactions, these patients are regarded as potential candidates (Samuel, Duclos Vallee, Teicher, & Vittecoq, 2003). Portal vein thrombosis had previously been an absolute contraindication to liver transplantation. However, with the use of operative strategies such as simple thrombectomy, extra-anatomic venous graft, arterialization of the portal vein, and cavoportal hemitransposition, this is no longer the case. Advanced age is another relative contraindication in which there has been a change over the years. In the 1990s, the population of patients over 60 years old accounted for approximately 10% of all transplanted patients, whereas more recently, they constitute almost 20% of the procedures (Adam & Hoti, 2009). Presently, there is no universally accepted age limit for considering transplantation, and centers deal with this issue on a case-by-case basis.

Medical Issues Pre–Liver Transplantation

Laboratory abnormalities commonly associated with hepatocellular dysfunction include anemia and leukopenia (a lower-than-normal amount of white blood cells, also known as leukocytes, in the blood), which places an individual at an increased risk of infection. Other laboratory abnormalities include thrombocytopenia (abnormally low number of platelets in the bloodstream) and an increased prothrombin time—a measure of the amount of time it takes for the liquid portion of one's blood (plasma) to clot.

Whereas a minority of patients (e.g., those with acute fulminant liver failure) will have only a few days of physical inactivity prior to transplantation, the majority live with their diseased liver for a prolonged period of time before transplantation occurs. They present as severely malnourished and deconditioned. The following are some of the salient features to watch out for when working with chronically debilitated liver-failure patients prior to transplantation.

■ Cachexia

The etiology of cachexia (severe muscle wasting) in liver disease is multifactorial. Cirrhosis of the liver is considered a catabolic disease and can lead to profound loss of muscle mass. The prevalence of cachexia has been found to be as high as 80% in patients with cirrhosis (Harrison, McKiernan, & Neuberger, 1997). Because of the dysfunction of the diseased liver in glycogen storage and gluconeogenesis (the formation of glucose from noncarbohydrate sources, such as protein and fat), muscle protein and fat are broken down for energy use. These result in weakness and weight loss because the need to use protein and fat for energy further decreases protein's availability for muscle maintenance. Other contributing factors to cachexia and protein-energy malnutrition are anorexia (decreased dietary intake) and malabsorption (steatorrhea). Diseased bile ducts results in reduced synthesis and secretion of bile salts into the intestines, making fat and fat-soluble vitamin absorption difficult. Fat malabsorption, or steatorrhea, occurs and is prevalent in 40% to 50% of cirrhotic patients (Munoz, 1991). Cachexia has been found to be predictive of poor outcomes after liver transplantation (Vintro, Krasnoff, & Painter, 2002).

■ Osteoporosis

Osteoporosis is a disease characterized by a decrease in bone mass and density. It is the most common bone disorder in persons with chronic liver disease, with a prevalence documented as 15% to 40% (Crosbie, Freaney, McKenna, & Hegarty, 1999). Ingestion of alcohol can directly and indirectly promote bone loss. In addition, poor diet and physical inactivity contribute further to the deterioration of bone. Absorption of vitamin D and calcium may be reduced in liver disease (Li et al., 2000). The incidence of fractures has been reported to be as high as 30% in persons awaiting liver transplantation (Diamond, Stiel, Wilkinson, & Posen, 1990). Persons who have a low bone mineral density (BMD) prior to liver transplantation are at an even greater risk of fracture after transplantation, which results in significantly increased morbidity and mortality (Keogh et al., 1999).

■ Exercise Limitations

Patients with chronic liver disease experience a prolonged period of weakness and fatigue resulting in deconditioning. This is expressed as decreased oxygen uptake, decreased muscle strength, and poor endurance. These patients have been found to have a reduced VO_2 max (the maximal volume of oxygen that can be utilized in 1 minute during maximal exercise). Patients with chronic liver disease have been found to have a VO_2 max that is 40% less than predicted for sedentary healthy individuals of the same age and sex (Beyer et al., 1999). In addition, muscle strength in these patients has been found to be 30% of age-predicted levels (Beyer, Aadahl, Strange, Mohr, & Kjaer, 1995). Inactivity and bed rest results in the disuse of muscles (primarily postural and weight-bearing muscles), which leads to a deterioration of muscle structure and function (Saltin et al., 1968). In addition, patients with cirrhosis often have severe edema (swelling of soft tissues as a result of excess water accumulation) and ascites that negatively affect their ability to move in bed, to transfer, and to ambulate. The adverse effects of physical inactivity and bed rest not only exacerbate the complications of cachexia/muscle wasting and bone loss but also have been correlated with posttransplant success (Carithers, 2000).

Pre–Liver Transplantation—Rehabilitation Program

■ Goals of Therapy

Rehabilitation therapy in patients with end-stage liver disease is directed at improving a patient's physical functioning and quality of life (QOL). This must be supplemented by appropriate nutritional care. It is critical to institute rehabilitation therapy as soon as possible to maintain relatively healthy levels of physical functioning and to improve survival before and after transplantation. Patients who have been wasting muscle at a higher rate have a poorer prognosis after transplantation (Selberg et al., 1997).

■ Physical Activity

To prevent the significant physical deconditioning associated with reduced physical activity while waiting for a transplant, a pretransplantation rehabilitation program is instituted. Disuse weakness and atrophy are most effectively treated by prevention. Therefore, a program of graded isometric exercises aimed at restoring muscle mass and strength is employed. Contraction of a muscle at 20% to 30% of maximal strength for a few seconds daily will maintain its strength (Kohzuki et al., 2000). Contractures of joints are best prevented by the institution of an exercise program that involves range of motion and gentle stretching exercises. Exercise programs instituted in the preoperative period can reduce the cardiovascular risk and the extent of osteoporosis and muscle wasting after liver transplantation (Vintro et al., 2002). The introduction of a respiratory physiotherapeutic program for liver transplantation candidates has been found to significantly improve respiratory parameters preoperatively (Limongi et al., 2014). The program consists of diaphragmatic breathing exercises, diaphragmatic isometric exercises, as well as upper limb and abdominal strengthening exercises.

■ Nutrition

Careful nutritional monitoring, frequent nutritional reassessment, and provision of adequate calories are essential in the preliver transplantation patient. Individualized dietary counseling should be offered to all patients. Nutrient-dense foods, nutritional supplements, and smaller, more frequent meals during the day are recommended. Megestrol acetate has been used successfully in patients with end-stage liver disease for appetite stimulation (Gurk-Turner, 1997). Parenteral nutrition may be indicated in some cases. Liver-transplant candidates should be encouraged to consume foods high in calcium and vitamin D, and if consumption is low, supplementation is recommended.

■ Psychological Issues

Psychological and social work support services play an important role in the pretransplantation assessment. Assessment of the patient's lifestyle, psychological stability, and family support are key factors that can help predict a patient's ability to function following liver transplantation. This is particularly true in patients with a history of drug and alcohol abuse. As noted previously, recidivism to the level of harmful drinking is reported in about 15% to 20% cases (Singal et al., 2013). The ability of a patient to abstain from alcohol posttransplantation is predicted by an ability to abstain from alcohol for at least 6 months before transplantation, a stable employment history, and a strong family/friend support structure (Koffron & Stein, 2008). In light of the high relapse rate, the need for continued psychological support posttransplant is essential.

Medical Issues Post–Liver Transplantation

Complications of Liver Transplantation

Most life-threatening complications associated with liver transplantation occur within the perioperative period and include primary graft malfunction (graft failure in the immediate postoperative period with no obvious cause), acute rejection episodes (process in which a transplant recipient's immune system attacks the transplanted organ or tissue), severe infections, and technical complications such as hepatic artery thrombosis (formation of a blood clot within a blood vessel causing a partial or total obstruction) and biliary leaks (Table 19.3). Long-term morbidity and mortality after liver transplantation, in contrast, are mainly the result of the adverse effects of the immunosuppressive medications prescribed to prevent rejection (Benten, Staufer, & Sterneck, 2009).

Rejection

The risk of liver rejection is highest (40%) during the first 3 to 6 months after transplantation and decreases significantly afterward (Lopez & Martin, 2006). Acute (cellular) hepatic allograft rejection typically occurs 7 to 14 days posttransplantation but can also occur earlier or later. Rejection is most commonly manifested by fever, malaise, right upper-quadrant pain or tenderness, graft enlargement, and diminished graft function. A rise in bilirubin and transaminase levels is observed. With early detection, most acute rejection episodes can be treated successfully by augmentation of existing immunosuppressive medications or high doses

TABLE 19.3

COMPLICATIONS OF LIVER TRANSPLANT	
Graft dysfunction Primary nonfunction Preservation injury Small for size Syndrome Rejection Vascular thrombosis Hepatic artery thrombosis Portal vein thrombosis Biliary complications Stricture Leaks Infection Bacterial Viral Fungal Opportunistic Nosocomial Latent Recurrent Gastrointestinal Ileus Ulcer Gastrointestinal bleeding Diarrhea Drug interactions Interference with cytochrome P 3A4	Neurologic complications Neuropathy Seizure Coma Encephalopathy Aphasia Tremors Central Pontine Myelinolysis Electrolyte imbalance Hyponatremia Hypokalemia Hyperkalemia Hypocalcemia Hypophosphoremia Hypoglycemia Hyperglycemia Hypomagnesium Pulmonary Mechanical ventilation Pneumonia Pleural Effusion Pneumothorax Pulmonary Hypertension Hypoxia

Source: Rudow and Goldstein (2008).

of steroids. Chronic rejection that occurs months to years posttransplantation results in progressive jaundice and graft dysfunction and may require retransplantation.

Electrolyte Imbalances

Electrolyte imbalances are a very common metabolic problem after liver transplantation. These include abnormally low concentrations of sodium, potassium, calcium, phosphorus, and magnesium in the blood. They can also manifest as abnormally high concentrations of potassium and glucose in the blood (Rudow & Goldstein, 2008). A low serum magnesium level potentiates cyclosporine and tacrolimus (immunosuppressive drugs) neurotoxicity and may result in seizures. As a result, efforts are made to keep the magnesium level high enough to prevent this complication. Careful laboratory monitoring of electrolytes is necessary.

Musculoskeletal Complications

Post liver transplantation, issues of continued muscle loss, osteoporosis, and fatigue continue. The most common posttransplantation complaints by patients include the following: muscle weakness, fatigue, and bone/joint discomfort (Beyer et al., 1995). A study by van Ginneken et al. (2007) found that of 96 liver-transplant patients, 66% were fatigued and 44% were severely fatigued during the posttransplantation phase. They noted that the patients experienced physical fatigue and reduced activity levels rather than mental fatigue and reduced motivation. They reasoned that fatigue after liver transplantation might be reduced by rehabilitation programs focusing on improving activity patterns and physical fitness.

Neurological Complications

Neurological complications are a relatively common effect of posttransplantation (Rudow & Goldstein, 2008). Pretransplant encephalopathy can manifest postoperatively as disorientation and somnolence. This condition typically resolves as liver function returns to normal. Additional neurological manifestations include headaches, seizures, delirium, coma, and stroke. In addition, patients who have undergone liver transplantation are prone to developing neuropathies. The frequency and causes of generalized neuromuscular weakness after liver transplantation has been studied (Campellone, Lacomis, Giuliani, & Kramer, 1998). The authors prospectively performed detailed neurological examinations on 100 liver-transplant recipients and found that 10% of these individuals had developed focal peripheral nerve lesions during the postoperative period. Ulnar neuropathy was the most common mononeuropathy and was felt to result from intraoperative compression or postoperative trauma in the region of the elbow. It was felt that this finding warranted the use of empiric elbow padding intraoperatively. Of note, no incidences of brachial plexopathy were found in their patient population. Brachial plexopathy, which is the most common neurological complication in surgical patients, is felt to be due to excessive traction on the brachial plexus from hyperabduction of the arm during surgery. The authors felt that the absence of this complication in their series was due to the strict adherence to maintaining the patient's arms at less than 90° abduction during surgery.

■ Maintenance Immunosuppression and Complications

Maintenance immunosuppression is usually achieved by using the calcineuron inhibitors (cyclosporine A or tacrolimus) and corticosteroids. These may be combined with newer antimetabolite compounds (e.g., mycophenolate-cellcept) with the goal of decreasing steroid and/or calcineurin inhibitor use (Koffron & Stein, 2008). Side effects of some of the most frequently used antirejection agents are listed in Table 19.4. Monitoring parameters for immunosuppressive medications are listed in Table 19.5.

Cyclosporine toxicity is manifested by tremulousness, hypertension, hyperkalemia, and nephrotoxicity. The most common cause of a rise in blood urea nitrogen (BUN) and creatinine levels after transplantation is cyclosporine toxicity. This improves with a reduction in its dosage. Cyclosporine also has neurotoxic effects, including seizures, paranoid delusions, and hallucinations. As noted previously, a low serum magnesium level potentiates cyclosporine neurotoxicity and may result in seizures.

Tacrolimus is a macrolide antibiotic that shares many characteristics with cyclosporine. Like cyclosporine, tacrolimus toxicity is manifested by

TABLE 19.4

SYSTEMIC AND METABOLIC EFFECTS OF TRANSPLANT ANTI-REJECTION DRUGS		
Drug	**Adverse Effect**	**Clinical Manifestation**
Antithymocyte globulin (ATG)	Anaphylactic reactions	Hypotension, dyspnea, wheezing, fever, chills
	Serum sickness associated with antibody formation to foreign protein	Pain, redness, extreme muscle soreness, swelling
	Bone marrow suppression associated with prolonged use in conjunction with azathioprine	Anemia, leukopenia, thrombocytopenia, pancytopenia
	Local inflammatory reactions associated with IM administration	Inflammation
	Increased risk of malignancy when associated with high doses of multiple agents	Dependent on type and location of malignancy
Azathioprine (AZA)	Bone marrow suppression	Anemia, leukopenia, thrombocytopenia, pancytopenia
	Hepatotoxicity	Elevated bilirubin, alkaline phosphatase, AST, ALT levels; jaundice
	Increased risk of malignancy when associated with high doses of multiple agents	Dependent on type and location of malignancy
Corticosteroids	Aseptic necrosis of bone, osteoporosis	Pain in weight-bearing joints; pathologic fractures
	Hyperglycemia, steroid-induced diabetes mellitus	Elevated serum glucose; polydipsia, polyuria
	Salt and water retention	Weight gain/fluctuations
	Hypertension	Elevated blood pressure
	Skin alterations: acne, sun sensitivity, hirsutism	Rash or pimples on face and/or trunk; susceptibility to sunburn; excessive hair growth on face, trunk, extremities
	Growth retardation in children	Failure to reach normal height for age
	Gastritis/gastrointestinal ulcerations	Abdominal pain, dysphagia, hematemesis, guaiac-positive stools
	Cataracts	Visual acuity problems
Cyclosporine	Nephrotoxicity	Elevated BUN and serum creatinine levels; oliguria or anuria; weight gain, edema
	Hypertension	Elevated blood pressure
	Hepatotoxicity	Elevated bilirubin, alkaline phosphatase, AST, ALT levels; jaundice
	Hypertrichosis	Hirsutism
	Myopathy	Weakness, especially when given in combination with statins
	Tremors, seizures	Fine motor tremors, especially hands; associated paresthesias; seizure activity
	Gingival hyperplasia	Growth of gums over teeth, bleeding gums
	Increased risk of malignancy when associated with high doses of multiple agents	Dependent on type and location of malignancy
Muromonab-CD3	Pyrexia, malaise	Fever, chills, flu-like symptoms, headache, diarrhea
	Respiratory distress associated with initial doses and fluid overload	Chest tightness, dyspnea, wheezing
	Increased risk of malignancy when associated with high doses of multiple agents	Dependent on type and location of malignancy

(continued)

TABLE 19.4 (*continued*)

SYSTEMIC AND METABOLIC EFFECTS OF TRANSPLANT ANTI-REJECTION DRUGS		
Drug	**Adverse Effect**	**Clinical Manifestation**
Mycophenolate	Pancytopenia	Thrombocytopenia, leukopenia, anemia
	GI complaints	Diarrhea, nausea, abdominal pain
	Nephrotoxicity	Elevated BUN and creatinine; oliguria or anuria; weight gain, edema
Sirolimus	Vasculitis	Stroke
	Wound dehiscence	Rupture at incision
	Malignancy	Especially lymphoma
	Pancytopenia	Thrombocytopenia, leukopenia, anemia
	Tremor	Tremor
	Neuropathy	Pain, numbness, weakness
Tacrolimus (FK506)	Nephrotoxicity associated with high doses	Elevated BUN and creatinine levels; oliguria or anuria; weight gain, edema
	Hyperkalemia	Elevated potassium levels
	Insomnia	Sleep disturbances
	Malaise associated with IV administration	Headache, nausea and vomiting
	Neuropathy	Pain, numbness, weakness

ALT, alanine aminotransferase; AST, aspartate aminotransferase; BUN, blood urea nitrogen.

nephrotoxicity and neurotoxicity. Nephrotoxicity is related to high levels of the drug and improves with dosage reduction. Manifestations of neurotoxicity may range from mild symptoms (tremors, insomnia, somnolence, headaches) to severe complications (seizures, obtundation, coma). These symptoms are related to high doses of the drug and improve with dosage reduction. Tacrolimus levels are monitored daily by obtaining trough levels.

TABLE 19.5

IMMUNOSUPPRESSIVE MEDICATION MONITORING QUICK GUIDE		
Drug	**Side Effect**	**Monitoring**
Prednisone	GI irritability	Stool occult blood; hematocrit
	Fluid retention	Daily weight
	Diabetes mellitus	Fasting urine glucose
Cyclosporine	Nephrotoxicity	BUN; creatinine
	Hepatotoxicity	Bilirubin, alkaline phosphatase, AST, ALT levels
Azathioprine	Pancytopenia	CBC
	Hepatotoxicity	Bilirubin, alkaline phosphatase, AST, ALT levels

ALT, alanine aminotransferase; AST, aspartate aminotransferase; BUN, blood urea nitrogen; CBC, complete blood count.

Corticosteroids are routinely used following solid organ transplantation to prevent rejection. Long-term steroid use is associated with complications such as refractory hypertension, diabetes, osteoporosis, fractures, hip necrosis, cataracts, and obesity. The introduction of tacrolimus has enabled maintaining patients on lower doses of prednisone.

As noted, immunosuppressive agents have significant toxicities, and thus antiproliferative drugs such as azathioprine, mycophenolate mofetil, and sirolimus are added to decrease steroid and/or calcineurin inhibitor use. They work by inhibiting mitosis, and hence, proliferation of lymphocytes.

Maintenance Infection Prophylaxis

Maintenance prophylaxis for infections is instituted for 3 to 12 months posttransplantation. These medications include trimethoprim-sulfamethoxazole and dapsone (prophylactic antibiotics to prevent *Pneumocystis carinii* pneumonia), acyclovir (to inhibit herpes viruses), ganciclovir (to inhibit cytomegalovirus), and clotrimazole and/or nystatin (to control fungal infections such as *candida*).

Post–Liver Transplantation—Rehabilitation Program

Physical Rehabilitation

The goal of physical activity after liver transplantation is to reverse the musculoskeletal changes resulting from inactivity and bed rest. Physical therapy should be instituted immediately after the transplant recipient has been surgically stabilized. Restoration of muscle mass and strength begins with graded isometric exercises. In addition, aerobic conditioning exercises must be included in the rehabilitation program. The association between a patient's functional capacity and short-term survival (90-day mortality without transplantation) was measured by Ow et al. (2014). They found that a lower mean VO_2 max was a significant predictor of poorer short-term survival. Beyer et al. (1999) evaluated the effects of a fitness program on 23 men and 15 women before and at 6 months posttransplantation. Posttransplantation patients participated in a supervised exercise program that consisted of aerobic and muscle-strengthening exercises for 1 hour twice a week over 8 to 24 weeks. Exercise capacity increased 43% and knee extensor/flexor strength increased 60% to 100% by 6 months after transplantation. However, these patients still remained 10% to 20% below age-matched controls, an indication of how deconditioned they were pretransplantation. All patients were independent in functional activity of daily living skills at 6 months posttransplantation. The authors concluded that a supervised post-liver transplant exercise program improves physical fitness, muscle strength, and functional performance in persons with chronic liver disease. Garcia, Veneroso, Soares, Lima, and Correia (2014) investigated the effect of a physical exercise program on the functional capacity of liver transplantation patients. Patients were divided into two groups, the exercise group and a control group. After undergoing exercise training, patients in the exercise group showed a 19.4% increase in the distance walked as well as an increase in their resting energy expenditure, indicating an increase in their exercise capacity and metabolic improvements. The authors concluded that the exercise program promoted significant improvements in functional capacity and felt these findings have positive implications for the control of metabolic diseases, which are common in patients after liver transplantation.

An outpatient rehabilitation program consisting of exercise training and physical activity counseling has also been shown to be well tolerated and can reduce fatigue and improve fitness among recipients of liver transplants. Van den Berg-Emons et al. (2014) evaluated the role of a 12-week outpatient exercise program on 18 liver transplant recipients. The primary outcome measure was fatigue. After the program, participants were significantly less fatigued, and the percentage of individuals with severe fatigue was significantly lower than before the program. In addition, aerobic capacity and knee flexion strength were significantly higher, and body fat was significantly lower after the program. Participants were able to perform physical exercise at the target training intensity, no adverse events were registered, and attendance (93%) and mean patient satisfaction (8.5 out of 10, range = 7–10) were high. Studies have also shown that highly trained liver-transplant recipients are capable of achieving high levels of physical functioning. Sixteen liver-transplant recipients tested at the 1996 U.S. Transplant Games were found to achieve exercise capacities that were 101% of age-predicted normal levels (Painter et al., 1997). In addition, long-term liver-transplant recipients who reported participation in regular physical activity had higher scores on health-related QOL scales than those who were inactive. Also, physically active patients had less hypertension and fewer orthopedic complaints (Painter, Krasnoff, Paul, & Ascher, 2001).

Psychological Issues

As noted earlier, due to the high relapse rate in patients with a history of drug and alcohol abuse posttransplantation, close, continued psychological support is essential.

Nutrition

Following successful liver transplantation, the albumin level slowly rises to normal levels. As it normalizes, the generalized edema that patients experience posttransplantation begins to disappear. Posttransplantation nutritional therapy should include a diet that is moderate in protein intake. Nutritional recommendations should also include a diet that reduces the risk of osteoporosis and promotes bone synthesis. Osteoporosis is common after transplantation with the greatest amount of bone loss occurring between 3 and 12 months posttransplantation (McCaughan & Feller, 1994). Dietary calcium and vitamin D intakes should reach 1.0 to 1.5 g and 400 to 800 units/daily, respectively. In addition, diets should be low in fat, low in sodium, and high in vegetables and fruits (Weseman & McCashland, 1998).

Post–Liver Transplantation—Outcomes

As patient survival rates after liver transplantation continue to rise, there has been an increased emphasis on measuring successful outcomes by improvements in patient functional status and QOL. A retrospective study on 55 liver transplantation patients found that significant functional gains as measured by the Functional Independence Measure (FIM) instrument could be achieved in an acute inpatient rehabilitation program (Cortazzo, Helkowski, Pippin, Boninger, & Zafonte, 2005). All patients had improvements in their FIM scores with an average gain of 26 points. In addition, the majority of patients were discharged home after acute rehabilitation. The authors also found that patients admitted to the rehabilitation unit with lower albumin levels remained in rehabilitation longer and made less significant gains in therapy based on FIM efficiency (the amount of FIM gained per day in rehabilitation). They felt that this finding reinforces the need to emphasize good nutrition both before and after liver transplantation to potentially improve functional gains. In addition, the authors noted several comorbidities in their patient population that had rehabilitation implications. They found that 12 patients (22%) developed neuropathies with five requiring bracing (four ankle-foot orthoses and one volar wrist-extension splint). They also found that four patients (7%) had symptomatic osteoporotic spine compression fractures, with three of them requiring spinal bracing. The authors recommended weight-bearing exercises to help maintain/increase bone mass in this population.

A survey to determine the functional outcomes of patients 3 years post–liver transplantation at the University of Pittsburgh Medical Center found that 61% of patients reported severe impairments in endurance prior to transplantation (Robinson, Switala, Tarter, & Nicholas, 1990). However, only 6% reported endurance impairments after transplantation. Overall, the patients were largely independent in activities of daily living (ADL) skills and mobility. Another survey of 166 patients who underwent liver transplantation at Rush-Presbyterian-St. Lukes Medical Center in Chicago found that at 1 year posttransplantation, nearly all patients were able to perform basic ADL skills (Nicholas, Oleske, Robinson, Switala, & Tarter, 1994). In addition, the percentage of patients with severely impaired endurance had decreased from 43.9% pretransplantation to 8.0% following the transplant.

Despite these improved functional outcomes, there remains a high rate of unemployment among recipients of liver transplantation. Huda, Newcomer, Harrington, Blegen, and Keeffe (2012) performed an analysis of the employment status of 21,942 transplant recipients and found that only approximately one fourth of the recipients were employed within 24 months after transplantation. The demographic variables that were independently associated with post-transplant employment were an age of 18 to 40 years, male sex, a college degree, Caucasian race, and pretransplant employment. Patients with alcoholic liver disease had a significantly lower rate of employment than patients with other etiologies of liver disease. The recipients who were employed after transplantation had a significantly better functional status than those who were not employed. The authors concluded that in light of the low employment rate after LT, new national and individual transplant program policies are needed to assess the root causes of unemployment in recipients who wish to work following liver tansplantation.

Summary

Liver transplantation is the only definitive treatment modality for end-stage liver disease. There has been enormous progress over the past 50 years with advances in technical skills, improvements in immunosuppressive drugs, and the management of postoperative complications. Liver transplantation has become the standard treatment for many patients with acute fulminant liver failure and chronic liver disease. However, there is a continued need for improvement, especially in the prevention of complications that are associated with long-term immunosuppression use. Today, the major constraint to meeting the demand for liver transplants is the availability of donated (cadaver) organs. Continued efforts to raise public awareness to the worldwide problem of organ shortage are critical.

RENAL TRANSPLANTATION

Renal transplantation is the treatment of choice for patients with end-stage renal disease (ESRD). Renal or kidney transplantation is a surgical procedure during which a diseased kidney is replaced by a healthy kidney from another person. It is classified as deceased-donor (formerly cadaveric) or living-donor transplantation, depending on the source of the recipient organ. Living-donor transplantations are further classified as living related (if a biological relationship exists between the donor and recipient) or living unrelated. Since the first transplantation of a kidney from one human to another in 1954, renal transplantation has evolved from essentially an experimental procedure to one which is now commonplace and has excellent survival rates. In the United States, in 2011, first-time recipients of a living-donor transplant had 1-year patient- and graft-survival rates of 99% and 97%, respectively. The first-time recipients of a deceased-donor renal transplant had 1-year patient and graft survival rates of 96% and 92%, respectively (U.S. Renal Data System, 2014, p. 86).

Improvements in the success rate of renal transplantation reflect improvements in immunosuppressive regimens, antimicrobial prophylaxis, surgical and medical care, as well as improvements in cross-matching tests (pretransplantation in-vitro assays to detect donor antibodies to recipient human leukocyte antigens). Long-term graft survival (beyond the first year) has not improved to the same extent as early survival. The principal causes of renal allograft loss beyond the first transplantation year are cardiovascular disease, infection, and malignancy. As such, one primary area of research interest is on renal transplantation strategies that aim to improve long-term outcomes by preventing and treating cardiovascular disease, infection, bone disease, and neoplasia.

Indications

The indication for kidney transplantation is ESRD, regardless of the primary cause. This is defined as creatinine clearance of less than 15. Diabetes and hypertension are the two leading causes of ESRD in the United States and worldwide (U.S. Renal Data System, 2014, p. 82). Other diseases leading to serious kidney dysfunction and for which renal transplants may be required include glomerulonephritis, polycystic kidney disease, congenital renal obstructive disorders leading to hydronephrosis, congenital nephrotic syndrome, Alport syndrome, as well as autoimmune conditions such as systemic lupus erythematosus and Goodpasture's syndrome.

Prerenal Transplantation Rehabilitation Issues

■ Diminished Exercise Tolerance

Patients with compromised renal function have a markedly impaired exercise tolerance. This impaired physical performance not only interferes with their ability to perform physical tasks such as climbing stairs but also interferes with their ability to perform leisure-time exercise. A majority of patients with impaired renal function are unable to work due to their impaired energy status. Their reduced physical fitness is characterized by reduced flexibility, coordination disturbances, as well as decreased muscular strength and endurance (Fuhrmann & Krause, 2004). The mechanisms behind this reduced work capacity are not fully known, but are felt, in part, to be due to years of reduced activity level prior to transplantation. The decline in physical fitness parallels the progression of the renal disease. Patients with renal disease awaiting transplantation have been found to have a decreased maximal oxygen uptake (VO_2 max; Robertson et al., 1990). Oxidative metabolism is impaired in their skeletal muscles, which is most likely caused by impaired exchange of oxygen between muscle and blood (Young & Stiens, 2006). Erythropoetin treatment has been found to increase the VO_2 max by 20% to 30%. However, despite treatment with erythropoietin and a restoration of a normal hemoglobin concentration, the VO_2 max remained lower than normal (Kjaer et al., 1996).

■ Muscle Weakness and Atrophy

Patients with ESRD exhibit weakness in both their proximal and distal musculature. The cause of this weakness is felt to be a combination of muscle atrophy, a decreased ability of the muscle to generate strength, and a reduced capacity of the nervous system to activate motor units (Juskowa et al., 2006). These patients have been found to have a reduced muscle strength in their legs, which contributes to a reduced physical performance (Bohannon, Smith, Hull, Palmeri, & Barnhard, 1995). In addition, deficiencies of vitamin D and parathyroid hormone contribute to stiffening of periarticular soft tissue that additionally limits the motor capacity of these patients.

Prerenal Transplantation Rehabilitation Program

Studies of hemodialysis patients engaged in an exercise program have shown that training has multiple beneficial effects. Training has been shown to result in an increase in physical work capacity (VO_2 max) and muscle strength (Painter et al., 1986). The Borg Rating of Perceived Exertion (RPE) scale is a simple method of rating perceived exertion. The scale ranges from 6 to 20 (6 = no exertion at all to 20 = maximal exertion; Borg, 1982). The Borg RPE scale is recommended for monitoring the training of patients with ESRD (Fuhrmann & Krause, 2004). Physical exercise has also been shown to increase the hematocrit level, improve the lipid profile, lower the requirement for antihypertensive medications, and normalize insulin sensitivity (Goldberg et al., 1986). It essentially modifies factors known to be associated with atherogenesis and cardiovascular disease in hemodialysis patients. In addition to its physiological benefits, exercise has been found to improve depressed mood in hemodialysis patients (Carney et al., 1987).

Postrenal Transplantation Medical Issues

When working with the patient following renal transplantation, the rehabilitation team must be aware of the most common complications that occur during the postoperative period. These include the following.

■ Transplant Rejection

As discussed earlier in this chapter, rejection is the normal reaction of the body to a foreign object. When a new kidney is placed in the body, the body sees the kidney as a threat and the host immune system produces antibodies to reject the new organ. Kidney rejection is often preceded by symptoms of malaise and anorexia. Clinical signs of kidney transplant rejection that arise in the postoperative period include elevated temperature, decreased urine output, edema (usually beginning in the hands or feet), a sudden increase in weight (3–5 pounds in a 24-hour period) as well as tenderness at the graft site. Laboratory findings include a leukocytosis (elevation in the white blood cell count) as well as elevated BUN and creatinine levels (Young & Stiens, 2006).

To prevent rejection, immunosuppressants are used to suppress the immune system from rejecting the donor kidney. The most commonly used antirejection medications following renal transplantation are cyclosporine and tacrolimus. A combination of agents is often utilized to achieve adequate immunosuppression, without the need for toxic doses of any one agent (Colm & Pascual, 2004). As the risk of acute rejection is greatest in the early posttransplantation period, more intensive immunosuppression is given early and is progressively lowered in the following weeks and months. Immunosupressant medications must be taken for the rest of a patient's life.

Infections

The transplantation procedure and subsequent immunosuppression increase the risk of serious infections. In the first month after transplantation, infections of the surgical wound, lungs, urinary tract, and those involving vascular catheters are most common. Between 1 and 6 months posttransplantation, however, weeks of intense immunosuppresion increase the risk of opportunistic infections from microorganisms such as cytomegalovirus, Epstein–Barr virus, and *P. carinii.* Prophylactic measures for infections posttransplantation include antiviral prophylaxis (for 1–3 months) and prophylaxis against *P. carinii* (trimethoprim-sulfamethoxazole, for 6–12 months), similar to those with liver transplantation.

Bleeding

Bleeding is uncommon postrenal transplantation (Humar, Denny, Matas, & Najarian, 2003). When it occurs, it is usually due to small blood vessels in the renal hilum that had not been ligated during surgery. Meticulous hemostasis during the operation can help to prevent this complication. Close observation of a patient's vital signs and hematocrit is necessary in the early postoperative period to detect bleeding. A falling hematocrit, hypotension, or tachycardia can alert the clinician to the possibility of bleeding. Most small perirenal hematomas are asymptomatic. However, large hematomas can produce significant flank pain and lower-extremity swelling due to venous or ureteral obstruction and may require surgical exploration.

Postrenal Transplantation Rehabilitation Issues

When prescribing a rehabilitation program for a patient following a renal transplant, one must be aware of several important physiological factors in this patient population. The renal transplant recipient's capacity for exercise remains quite limited. This is due to the presence of anemia as well as increased stresses on the cardiovascular system. The presence of anemia results in a reduction in the patient's blood oxygen-carrying capacity. In addition, the sodium and water retention that accompanies renal failure results in an increase in circulatory volume. As this volume increases, it places greater stresses on the cardiovascular system (Young & Stiens, 2006). This leads to a worsening of hypertension and hypertrophy of the cardiac muscle, which in turn lead to a decrease in compliance and stiff ventricles. The VO_2 max decreases and is found to be in the range of only 75% to 80% of that observed healthy control-group subjects (Krull, Schulze-Neick, Hatopp, Offner, & Brodehl, 1994).

In addition, the patient's reduced BMD continues to be a major problem after transplantation. This is a result of suboptimal kidney function and the superimposed effects of steroids on bone. A reduction in BMD has been found in 60% of patients in the first 18 months after renal transplantation (Colm & Pascual, 2004), with pathological fractures commonly occurring postrenal transplantation. The estimated fracture rate after transplantation is 2% per year in nondiabetic patients, 5% per year in diabetic patients, and 12% per year in pancreas–kidney recipients. It is also important to note that there is a high incidence of muscle/tendon injuries in the posttransplant population (Agarwal & Owen, 1990), which is felt to be due to a combination of metabolic and immunological factors, as well as the administration of corticosteroids. Together, these factors impair the mechanical properties of connective tissue, placing patients at a higher risk for overuse injuries.

Postrenal Transplantation Rehabilitation Program

Rehabilitation after renal transplantation seeks to improve the patient's physical and psychological fitness. The goal is to achieve a level of activity that permits maintenance of an active lifestyle. The rehabilitation program focuses on stretching exercises, repetitive low-level resistance exercises, and aerobic exercises. The initiation of an exercise program posttransplantation can result in an improvement in an individual's exercise capacity and cardiac function (Kempeneers et al., 1988). It can also improve insulin resistance (Christiansen et al., 1996) and improve the quality and quantity of sleep and lipid profile in these patients (Pooranfar et al., 2014).

When prescribing a rehabilitation program for postrenal transplantation patients, care should be given to close monitoring of blood pressure. Although patients may be normotensive at rest, they respond to exercise with a higher-than-normal blood pressure, which indicates an inappropriately high systemic vascular resistance (Scott, Hay, Higenbuttam, Evans, & Calne, 1990). In addition, care should be taken during exercise training to not overload tendons in order to prevent tendon rupture (Agarwal & Owen, 1990).

Renal transplant patients who engaged in a structured rehabilitation program showed significant improvements in respiratory function (peak expiratory flow) as well as range of motion in the radiocarpal joint when compared with postrenal transplant controls (Korbiewska, Lewandowska, Juskowa, & Bialoszewski, 2007). The rehabilitation program focused on strengthening exercises for the abdominal muscles and upper and lower extremities, breathing exercises, coordination and relaxation exercises. The authors concluded that there is a need to establish rehabilitation programs for patients who have undergone successful renal transplantation.

Juskowa et al. (2006), in a randomized controlled clinical trial of exercise training after renal transplantation, found a positive correlation between muscle strength and improved graft function in the group receiving rehabilitation compared with the control group. A prospective, randomized controlled study by Painter et al. (2002b) examined the effects of exercise intervention on health-related fitness (exercise capacity, muscle strength, body composition) and QOL in patients following renal transplantation. Their data showed that the group undergoing an exercise training program exhibited improved cardiopulmonary fitness, increased muscle strength, and less limitations in physical functioning compared with the control group that persisted for at least 12 months posttransplantation. The authors felt that exercise recommendations should be part of the routine medical treatment of patients during the posttransplantation phase, in order to optimize overall health and achieve the best-possible outcomes.

Postrenal Transplantation Outcomes

Posttransplant, patients work hard to reestablish normality, albeit in a "reset" form (Boaz & Morgan, 2014). This normality is a very personal construct, shaped by a wide range of factors including age, gender, and personal circumstances. Some patients encounter significant challenges in regaining normality, both at 3 months for those experiencing acute and distressing side effects, and later relating to the long-term side effects of transplant medication and comorbidities. However, the most dramatic threat to normality (disrupted normality) has been found to be due to episodes of rejection leading to transplant failure.

Better adherence to immunosuppressives in the first year postransplantation produces better outcomes. Factors associated with full adherence to immunosuppressives in the first year posttransplantation include female sex, higher education, higher perceived side effects of corticosteroids, better perceived cardiac and renal function, and higher perceived family social support. Alternatively, poor adherence to immunosuppressive therapy led to a higher likelihood of death (Prihodova et al., 2014).

As the survival rate following renal transplantation continues to improve, there has been an increased focus on health-related quality of life (HRQL). It has been shown that patients following successful transplantation exhibit a significantly higher HRQL compared to patients on dialysis (Fujisawa et al., 2000). Overbeck et al. (2005) evaluated QOL in 76 transplant patients compared with 65 patients with ESRD and awaiting transplantation. Their data demonstrated a considerable improvement in the QOL in the transplant patients. However, despite the improved QOL, levels of unemployment remained high, emphasizing the need for vocational rehabilitation in this patient population. Neipp et al. (2006), in a retrospective study, found that 15 years posttransplantation, patients continued to exhibit a satisfactory HRQL. Renal transplant patients who were employed reported a significantly improved HRQL in areas such as physical functioning, physical pain, vitality, social functioning, and mental health. The authors stress that vocational rehabilitation following transplantation is of utmost importance among long-term survivors and is associated with improved HRQL.

QOL is improved greatly by kidney transplantation, immunosuppresives, and exercise. However, it is apparent that not everyone has a positive experience and there is a need to identify individual factors that make certain individuals have a more positive experience. A correlational study from

Ireland (White & Gallagher, 2010) found that participants who perceived that they had a good QOL used more problem solving than avoidance-coping strategies. Avoidance-coping strategies were associated with statistically significantly lower QOL following transplantation. Being younger, attaining a higher education level, being employed, and being married were associated with a higher quality of life following transplantation (White & Gallagher, 2010). Assessment of coping strategies among the transplant population in clinical practice should be further explored to promote adaptive coping strategies to maximize QOL after transplantation.

Summary

Renal transplantation extends a typical patient's life by 10 to 15 years longer than one maintained on dialysis (Wolfe et al., 1999). This gain in years of life has been found to be even greater for younger patients. However, even 75-year-old recipients gain an average 4 more years of life. Patients who have undergone a kidney transplant have been found to have more energy, a less restricted diet, and fewer complications compared with those who stay on conventional dialysis. Studies have also shown that the longer a patient is on dialysis prior to transplantation, the less time the kidney transplant will survive. Thus, there is a need for the rapid referral to a transplant program for the population of patients with ESRD.

CARDIAC TRANSPLANTATION

Cardiac transplantation is a major surgical procedure utilized for persons with cardiomyopathy, coronary artery disease, congenital heart disease, retrotransplant/graft failure, valvular heart disease, and other serious cardiac conditions unresponsive to other forms of medical management. Scientific and procedural innovations in the fields of immunology, surgery, care plans, and cardiac rehabilitation have extended life considerably for heart transplant survivors, therefore creating an ever-growing role for physical medicine and rehabilitation specialists (Cohen, Young, & Stiens, 2012). Rehabilitation through all phases of the cardiac transplant process prevents complications, enhances performance, and enriches QOL (Young & Stiens, 2002). The person-centered rehabilitation of persons who have undergone cardiac transplantation is guided by an evidence-based approach designed with research conducted internationally (Young & O'Young, 2012).

Since the first cardiac transplant procedure performed in 1967, the 90-day survival rate has increased dramatically (Solomon et al., 2004). Overall 1-year survival rate for North American transplant recipients reported between April 1, 2010 and March 31, 2014 was approaching 91%, and 3-year survival rate in that same time period was around 84% (International Society for Heart & Lung Transplantation, 2014). Reports of 20-year survivors indicate a need for ongoing treatment of comorbid medical conditions, such as hypertension (87%), allograft vasculopathy (43%), diabetes (14%), and malignancy (44%) (Deuse et al., 2008; Kittleson & Kobashigawa, 2014).

Several factors have played a role in the growing success of cardiac transplantation. Improvements in organ availability and surgical capacity in the United States have contributed to a 45% decline in the cardiac transplant waiting list (from 2,414 in 1997 to 1,327 in 2006), and the downward trend is continuing (Mulligan et al., 2008). Technological advancements have provided inventive methods of "buying time." Continued innovation in augmentation of cardiac output with medication regimens and mechanical pumps has increased survivorship. For example, left ventricular assist devices (LVAD) and the temporary artificial heart (TAH), have led to decreases in morbidity and mortality (Copeland et al., 2004; Lahpor, 2009). Another advancement, the introduction of a "wearable" pneumatic driver technology that powers an artificial heart outside of the hospital setting, has improved outcomes and creates a "bridge to life" (International Society for Heart & Lung Transplantation, 2009). A total of 1,091 Jarvik-7 type TAHs have been placed between 1985 and 2012 and devices such as the Syncardia 50/50 are smaller and can be used in small children (Ryan, Jefferies, Zafar, & Morales, 2015). Newer models, such as the Freedom Driver, and the totally implantable AbioCor, allow patients to leave the hospital (Ryan, Jefferies, Zafar, & Morales, 2015). Judicious patient selection, continued improvements in surgical techniques and technology, reduced rejection rates, and ongoing and innovative rehabilitation efforts create a positive forecast for continued improvement of post-cardiac transplant survival rates.

According to International Society for Heart and Lung Transplantation (ISHLT) statistics, a total of 2,614 heart transplants were performed throughout North America in 2013. Demographically, 69.7% of cardiac transplant recipients were male and 30.3% female; the largest number of recipients were in the 50 to 64 age range (1,043), while 455 recipients were in both the 35 to 49 and 65+ age ranges (International Society for Heart & Lung Transplantation, 2014).

Indications

End-stage congestive heart failure (CHF), which has proven refractory to traditional medical therapy, is a major indication for heart transplantation. Often end-stage CHF necessitating transplant is preceded by a history of idiopathic cardiomyopathy, viral myocarditis, ischemic heart disease, or valve dysfunction (Joshi & Kevorkian, 1997; Latlief & Young, 1994). Absolute indications for transplant set forth by the 2009 American College of Cardiology/American Heart Association (ACC/AHA) heart failure guidelines include hemodynamic compromise due to heart failure, refractory cardiogenic shock, documented dependence on IV inotropic support to maintain adequate organ perfusion, peak VO_2 less than 10 mL/kg per minute with achievement of anaerobic metabolism, severe symptoms of ischemia that consistently limit routine activity, and are not amenable to coronary artery bypass surgery or percutaneous coronary intervention and recurrent symptomatic ventricular arrhythmias refractory to all therapeutic modalities. Relative indications from ACC/AHA (2009) include peak VO_2 11 to 14 mL/kg per minute (or 55% predicted) and major limitation of the patient's daily activities; recurrent unstable ischemia not amenable to other intervention; or recurrent instability of fluid balance/renal function not due to patient noncompliance with the medical regimen.

Selection

Cardiac transplantation remains the best treatment option for patients with end-stage New York Heart Association (NYHA) class IV heart failure that have failed conventional therapy (Heroux & Pamboukian, 2014). Multiple criteria are thoroughly evaluated when selecting a transplantation candidate, including assessment of circulatory impairments and exercise intensity endurance, as well as an evaluation of conditions that affect heart function and physical functionality (D'Amico, 2005; Tayler & Bergin, 1995). A comprehensive interdisciplinary team approach is vital for improvement in functional performance and QOL in this population. Cardiologists, transplant surgeons, physiatrists, nurses, nutritionists, physical therapists, occupational therapists, psychologists, and social workers all synergistically enhance outcomes with varied and distinct interventions. This assessment also necessitates patient-centered and family perspectives of expectations so that the rehabilitation program can be custom designed to maximize the patient's potential. Successful cardiac transplant outcomes are often dependent on identifying candidates who demonstrate sufficient physical capacity and endurance reserves. Patients with achievable surgical, medical, and rehabilitation goals attain maximal physical performance, QOL, and productivity (Solomon et al., 2004). During the period of heart procurement, implantation of LVAD and other "bridge-to-transplant" devices such as the TAH can improve tolerance for activity and allow preliminary rehabilitation (Gammie, Edwards, Griffith, Pierson, & Tsao, 2004; Rao et al., 2003; Ryan et al., 2015). Risk factors for coronary artery disease need to be minimized.

Postcardiac Transplantation Complications

The major causes of mortality associated with cardiac transplantation include rejection, infection, malignancy, and transplant coronary artery disease; associated morbidity includes renal dysfunction, hypertension, diabetes, dyslipidemia, gout, and osteoporosis. Advances in noninvasive monitoring of immune status, including AlloMap gene expression profile for monitoring of rejection and Cylex immune monitoring of immunosuppression, aid in minimizing toxicity (Kittleson & Kobashigawa, 2014). Complications associated with cardiac transplantation surgery must be intimately known and understood by the entire rehabilitation team, enabling safe and timely recognition and treatment of any complications that arise. Comprehensive and longitudinal coordination of care, as well as effective communication between rehabilitation team members, including the cardiac surgeon, cardiologist, and physiatrist, is essential for successful rehabilitation outcomes.

Rejection

One major posttransplant complication is allograft failure due to organ rejection. Acute rejection in heart transplantation may be predicted by fulminant exacerbation of CHF, increased peripheral edema, premature atrial contractions, a diastolic gallop, and a sudden, marked reduction in exercise capacity. After the posttransplant patient has achieved circulatory and vascular stability, prevention of rejection becomes a continued goal. It is important to remember that the cardiac-transplant recipient is less immunologically depressed than the kidney transplant patient. Prolonged uremia associated with renal failure accounts for this difference.

Chronic rejection can also progress with accelerated allograft vasculopathy, a process similar to atherosclerosis, but different due to lack of intimal lining damage but accumulation of subintimal matrix and inflammatory cell infiltrate, which narrows blood vessels (Dandel et al., 2003; Von Scheidt, Kembes, Reichart, & Erdmann, 1993). At 1-year posttransplantation, 10% to 15% of patients have developed accelerated graft atherosclerosis, which increases to 35% to 50% by the fifth postoperative year (Drexler & Schroeder, 1994; Shiba et al., 2004). After heart transplantation, the heart is no longer innervated by the autonomic nervous system, causing a cardiac muscle process called denervation. Denervation produces an upregulation of muscarinic receptors, which facilitates increased calcium influx in the coronary arteries of the transplanted heart. This causes diffuse, circumferential narrowing of the arterial luminal diameters. Vasculopathy progresses due to conventional coronary artery disease risk factors as well as alloimmunity with production of donor-specific antibodies (Pober, Jane-wit, Qin, & Tellides, 2014). Pathology shows concentric intimal expansion with extracellular matrix and mononuclear cell infiltrates, but luminal endothelial cell lining remains intact (Seki & Fishbein, 2014). This type of coronary artery disease has a major negative effect on the long-term survival of cardiac transplant patients. In order to reduce the instance and/or prevent the complication of graft atherosclerosis, the treatment plan should include educating the patient about the complication, regular arterial monitoring, and proper use of immunosuppressive medication. Scientific investigations have suggested this condition can be prevented and improved with calcium channel blockers (Shiba et al., 2004; Schroeder et al., 1993).

Pulmonary Hypertension

A frequently encountered complication during the early postoperative phase is the inability of the transplanted right ventricle to cope with preexisting pulmonary hypertension. Pulmonary hypertension can be due to chronic right-sided heart failure or to cyclosporine-induced renal vasoconstriction (Greenberg et al., 1987; McGiffin, Kirklin, & Nafiel, 1985; O'Connell et al., 1992). Medical management of pulmonary hypertension includes using alternative cyclosporine dosing regimens, as well as the use of calcium-channel antagonists and angiotensin-converting enzyme inhibitors to promote arteriolar dilation (Bunke & Ganzel, 1992; Legault, Olgilvie, Cardella, & Leenen, 1993; Valentine et al., 1992). Throughout the physical restoration process, blood pressures should be closely monitored and used as a guide for antihypertensive therapy (Painter et al., 2002a). In most cases, this is achievable without interrupting the exercise therapy regimen. Timely and appropriate medical management of the hypertensive state encourages full participation in the rehabilitative process to achieve functional improvements in patients.

Infection

Infection is the leading cause of death in post-cardiac transplant patients (Miller et al., 1994; Vaska, 1993). Common types include mediastinitis, pneumonia, cytomegalovirus, urinary tract infections, and intravenous catheter-induced sepsis (Hosenpud, Novick, Breen, & Daily, 1994; Miller et al., 1994; Vaska, 1993). Most infections develop during the first 2 years following cardiac transplant (Braith et al., 2000; Mills, 1994). Bacterial and viral infections account for 47% and 41% of the infections, respectively, while infections caused by fungus and protozoa comprise 12% of posttransplant morbidity (Espinoza & Bertolet, 1997).

Neurological Complications

Neurological complications following cardiac transplantation often are divided into central versus peripheral and early versus late (Heroux & Pamboukian, 2014). Central sequelae present during the acute posttransplant period, though they can also occur during the rehabilitative/restorative phase, long after the original transplant surgery (Sliwa & Blendonohy, 1988). These complications include metabolic encephalopathy, posterior reversible encephalopathy syndrome, stroke, central nervous system infection, seizures, and psychosis. Drug toxicities lower the seizure threshold. Common etiologies for stroke soon after transplantation include particulate embolism, air embolism, or inadequacy of perfusion arising from the transplantation procedure. Infections and malignancies such as posttransplant lymphoproliferative disorder (PTLD) may have neurological sequelae. Neurological sequelae also may include side effects caused by immunosuppressive agents (Heroux & Pamboukian, 2014). The physiatrist and rehabilitation team should evaluate neurological integrity during the postoperative phase through careful review of the patient's mental status, sensory perception, and motor functions. Table 19.6 lists posttransplant neuromusculoskeletal complications and possible etiologies.

In a study of cardiac transplant recipients on an inpatient rehabilitation unit, several treatable secondary complications were identified, including hypertension, nutritional limitations, neuromuscular deficits, and compression fractures (Joshi & Kevorkian, 1997). Stress fractures of the weight-bearing extremities have also been observed, which, in most cases, are attributable to steroid-induced osteoporosis (Lucas & Einhorn, 1993). The likelihood of this complication can be reduced through monitoring vitamin D levels and preventive supplementation of vitamin D (1,000–5,000 units/daily).

Postcardiac Transplantation: Rehabilitation Factors

■ Physiology and Function of a Transplanted Heart

Developing a rehabilitation program for a transplant patient requires a thorough understanding of the physiology of the transplanted heart and the impact of exercise on cardiac dynamics. The normal heart is innervated and strongly influenced by both the autonomic nervous system, which exerts chronotropic (affecting the heart rate) and inotropic (affecting the force of muscular contractions) effects, and the sympathetic nervous system, which serves to enhance venous return, stroke volume, and cardiac output (Auerbach et al., 1999; Beck, Barnard, & Schrire, 1969). Stroke volume is the amount of blood pushed out of the left ventricle with one beat of the heart and can be affected by preload (the volume of blood pushed into the

TABLE 19.6

POST HEART TRANSPLANT NEUROMUSCULOSKELETAL COMPLICATIONS

Complication	Possible Etiologies
Delirium	ICU psychosis, transplant medications, hyponatremia, hypernatremia, hypoglycemia, sepsis, hypotension, hypoxia, encephalitis (bacterial, fungal, or viral)
Stroke	Embolism, watershed infarct from hypotension, mycotic aneurysm, vasculitis (medication-induced)
Paraparesis	Spinal cord infarction, myelopathy
Peripheral neuropathy	Critical illness, transplant medications, metabolic or endocrine disorders, nerve impingements (brachial plexus, accessory, axillary, median, ulnar, femoral, sciatic, peroneal)
Tremor	Transplant medications
Myopathy	Critical illness, transplant medications
Contracture	Positioning/immobility, graft vs. host disease, nephrogenic diabetes insipidus
Osteoporotic fracture	Immobility, transplant medications

ventricle befor systole), ventricular wall contractility, and valve function. With orthotropic heart transplantation, there is complete denervation of the heart, which leads to a loss of the autonomic nervous system control mechanism. Since the transplanted heart is denervated, it consequently achieves a maximal heart rate more slowly in response to circulating epinephrine. The transplanted heart modulates its heart rate primarily through a response to circulating catecholamines and to a limited extent via partial and inconsistent, gradual, sympathetic reinnervation (Bernardi et al., 2007; Wenting et al., 1987). The denervated heart has a higher than normal resting heart rate, which can be lowered with carotid massage, the Valsalva maneuver, and body inclination (Leenen, Davies, & Fourney, 1995; Wechsler, Giardina, Sciacca, Rose, & Barr, 1995). The physiological explanation for the higher-than-normal heart rate is the loss of vagal tone associated with denervation (Savin, Haskell, Schroeder, & Stinson, 1980). Following an exercise session or mobility activity, the heart-transplant patient experiences a more gradual return to baseline. Despite the denervated status of the transplanted heart, cardiac output will typically increase in response to dynamic total body activity, promoting venous return, and increasing stroke volume through increased preload volume of blood filling the left ventricle (Bernardi et al., 2007). Refer to Box 19.1 for a summary of cardiac output following orthotopic heart transplant.

BOX 19.1 ORTHOTOPIC HEART TRANSPLANT AND CARDIAC OUTPUT

- Resting heart rate (HR) higher due to autonomic denervation
- HR increases with circulating catecholamines from adrenal glands
- HR and stroke volume increase with a greater preload (Frank Sterling effect)
- HR increases with Valsalva maneuver due to increased venous return
- HR increases with lower extremity venous distention (Bainbridge reflex)
- HR increases with recumbent leg raise, returning increased preload
- HR decreases with carotid massage (vagal effect) postreinnervation
- Cardiac output primarily increased due to larger stroke volumes

For the cardiac transplant patient participating in rehabilitation, there are a host of physiological adaptations that take place. As the patient gradually begins exercise, a slight increase in heart rate (HR) is immediately observable and can be attributed to the Bainbridge reflex triggered by right atrial distention (Shaver, Leon, Gray, Leonard, & Bahnson, 1969). This is an increase in heart rate in response to increased pressure in the veins entering the right heart or the increased rate of ventricular work, which continues for 3 to 5 minutes. This gradual, ongoing increase in heart rate continues into the recovery period and may contribute to a slower-than-normal return to preexercise heart rate (Martin, Gaucher, Pupa, & Seaworth, 1994). Advising the patient that he or she should first warm up and then gradually increase the intensity of activities is thus essential. It is generally recognized that the peak HR achieved during maximal exercise is significantly lower in cardiac transplant recipients than in age-matched control participants (Leenen et al., 1995; Martin et al., 1994). The transplanted heart compensates for output demand primarily by increasing stroke volume. The resting stroke volume of patients with transplanted hearts is less than that of individuals without transplantation (Kavanagh et al., 1988). Despite this, cardiac output is virtually normal (Kavanagh et al., 1988; Kavanagh & Yacoub, 1992; Meyer et al., 1994). Most heart recipients experience a rapid increase in stroke volume of about 20% when they begin their exercise regimen (Leenen et al., 1995; Meyer et al., 1994). Subsequent increases in stroke volume or cardiac output during prolonged submaximal exercise are mediated by inotropic responses to circulating catecholamines (Kao et al., 1995; Kavanagh & Yacoub, 1992; Keteyian et al., 1994; Leenen Davies, & Fourney, 1995). Following gradual conditioning, higher-intensity training can be completed over 15 months to achieve athletic capabilities in some younger transplant recipients (Rajendran, Pandurangi, Mullasari, Gomathy, & Rao, 2006).

Since heart-transplant patients display an unusual catecholamine-driven cardioacceleratory response to exercise, empiric exercise prescriptions based on target heart rates have limited utility and are not recommended (Borg, 1982; Greenberg et al., 1987; Kavanagh & Yacoub, 1992). The effect of transplantation on blood pressure is that both systolic and diastolic blood pressures are higher than expected, but pulse pressure (the difference between the maximum systolic blood pressure and the minimum diastolic blood pressure in one heart beat) is essentially normal at rest (Greenberg et al., 1985). Diastolic blood pressure may decline early in submaximal exercise because of reduced peripheral resistance (Greenberg et al., 1985; Griepp, Stinson, Dong, Clark, & Shumway, 1971; Joshi & Kevorkian, 1997; Kao et al., 1995). The peak systolic blood pressure is less than that of individuals without cardiac transplants, but diastolic blood pressure is not significantly different.

Following heart transplantation, patients consume less oxygen during submaximal exercise than do normal controls (Kavanagh & Yacoub, 1992; Keteyian et al., 1994; Paterson, Cunningham, Pickering, Babcock, & Boughner, 1994; Squires, 1991). Oxygen consumption at the anaerobic threshold is also considerably lower than that of age-matched normal individuals (Kavanagh & Yacoub, 1992; Paterson et al., 1994; Squires, 1991). According to Braith and Edwards (2000), the decrease in peak oxygen consumption seen in transplant recipients is due, in part, to architectural alterations in the skeletal muscle. Skeletal-muscle myopathy associated with the heart failure syndrome produces atrophy, decreased mitochondrial counts, and decreased oxidative enzymes. Post transplant, corticosteroids and cyclosporine cause thinning of the primarily Type II fibers and decrease oxidative enzymes (Braith & Edwards, 2000). See Table 19.7 for transplantation effects on selected cardiovascular variables at rest and during exercise that serve as guides for rehabilitation planning.

Postcardiac Transplantation Rehabilitation Outcomes

When cardiac transplantation was first emerging, it was considered inadvisable to start a patient on an exercise protocol immediately following surgery. New research, however, suggests exercise therapy, beginning within a month after transplant surgery, is vitally important in the rehabilitative process (Braith & Edwards, 2000; Valentine et al., 1992). Benefits from early exercise therapy include improved strength, enhancement of aerobic capacity, and extended endurance in physical work capability (Lampert, Mettauer, Hoppeler, Charloux, & Charpentier, 1998; Ville et al., 2002).

TABLE 19.7

EFFECT OF CARDIAC TRANSPLANTATION ON CARDIOVASCULAR VARIABLES

Condition	Heart Rate	Stroke Volume	Systolic BP	Diastolic BP	Pulmonary Arterial Pressure	VO_2 Max	Serum Lactate
Rest	> normal	< normal (Bainbridge reflex)	> normal	> normal	Slightly > normal (but typically lower than pre-transplant)	–	> normal
Submaximal exercise	Little or no immediate increase; delayed, slow rise	Initial increase (Frank-Starling mechanism); late increase (circulating catecholamines)	> normal	Initial decrease (reduced peripheral resistance)	> normal (rate of change)	< normal (absolute value)	> normal
Maximal exercise	Blunted peak (25% < normal)	Peak 40%–50% > than most	Peak < normal	About the same	–	< normal (absolute value); relative anaerobic threshold slightly > normal	No marked difference

Increasing evidence suggests supervised exercise programs should be a standard of care for heart transplant patients (Stewart, Badenhop, Brubaker, Keteyian, & King, 2003; Kobashigawa et al., 1999; Le Jemtel, 2003). Studies in the rehabilitation literature have focused on the hemodynamic responses to upright exercise after cardiac transplantation, as well as the cardiovascular response to gait training and ambulation in hemiparetic heart recipients (Sliwa, Andersen, & Griffin, 1990; Sliwa & Blendonohy, 1988). Kobashigawa et al. (1999) evaluated 27 cardiac-transplant patients, randomly divided into structured exercise and nonstructured exercise groups. The 14 patients in the exercise group worked with a physical therapist and had a customized program of muscular strength and aerobics training. They participated in a 6-month aerobics exercise program involving sitting-to-standing exercises. The 13 patients in the nonstructured exercise group received only written instructions about exercises to do at home, with no supervised sessions. All 27 patients were tested for muscle strength, aerobic capacity, and flexibility within 1 month of receiving a heart transplant, and again 6 months later. Although all patients showed improvement in all areas, those in the structured-exercise group showed significantly better results. Muscle strength, measured by the number of times a patient could stand from a sitting position repetitively for 1 minute, improved 125% for the structured-exercise group (from a mean of 10.6 times per minute to a mean of 23.9 times per minute). The nonstructured exercise group showed only an 18% gain, increasing from 10.4 times per minute to 12.3 times per minute. Aerobic capacity, tested by peak oxygen consumption, increased 49% in the group receiving formal exercise training, compared to just 18% in the nonstructured exercise group.

Aerobic capabilities, as measured by VO_2 max, have been shown to increase from 12% to 49%, with cardiovascular exercises done three times per week over 7 to 11 months (Braith et al., 2000). Training with a cycle ergometer and limiting intensity to 15 on the Borg scale prevents excessive exertion. As an alternative, exercise can be dosed by time and rate on the cycle ergometer (Shephard, Kavanagh, Mertens, & Yacoub, 1996). It is generally held that cardiac transplant survivors can perform exercise and physical training routines, achieving improvements comparable to those by normal individuals of similar age (Kjaer, Beyer, & Secher, 1999). Aerobic cardiovascular conditioning programs and exercise regimens emphasizing endurance tasks have also been shown to improve the ability of heart transplant patients to achieve higher levels of participation in AOL skills (Mettauer et al., 2005). Supervised high-intensity (80%–90% maximal heart rate) treadmill training in four intervals of 4 minutes, three times per week, over a 1-year period has also been found to be well tolerated. Reduced heart rates and average increases of 89% of VO_2 max have been observed with high-intensity exercise (Nytrøen & Gullestad, 2013). A regularly scheduled practical exercise regimen that can be carried out in a group setting is generally suggested for heart transplant recipients. With ongoing sympathetic reinnervation continuing beyond 1 year, return to athletic activity is possible for some. Fellowship and support occurring within group exercise is valuable in the rehabilitation process.

Progressive resistance training also proves to be beneficial following cardiac transplantation (Kobashigawa et al., 1998; Oliver et al., 2001; Quittan et al., 2001; Shephard et al., 1996; Tegtbur, Pethig, Machold, Haverich, & Busse, 2003; Wiesinger et al., 2001). Resistance training should not begin until 6 to 8 weeks after transplantation, permitting time for sternum healing and corticosteroid tapering (Tegtbur, Busse, Jung, Pethig, & Haverich, 2005). A controlled study designed to determine the effect of resistance exercise training on bone metabolism in heart transplant recipients revealed that as soon as two months after heart transplantation, about 3% of whole-body BMD has been lost, due to decreases in trabecular bone (Streiff et al., 2001). Six months of resistance exercise, consisting of low-back exercises that isolate the lumbar spine, and a regimen of variable resistance exercises, restored BMD toward pretransplantation levels. Further research concurs, suggesting resistance exercise is osteogenic and should be incorporated into the rehabilitation program after heart transplantation (Braith & Edwards, 2000). Progressive resistance exercise with lumbar extension and upper- and lower-limb resistance machines has been demonstrated to limit muscle mass loss, with initial training resistance set at 50% of the one repetition maximum, and repetitions being limited to 15 per session (Braith, Welsch, Mills, Keller, & Pollock, 1998). Tomczak,

Tymchak, and Haykowski (2013) have shown programs of alternating daily aerobic (60%–80% peak heart rate) and resistance (50% one repetition maximal) exercise for the upper and lower extremities completed over 12 weeks lead to improvement in lean muscle mass and further increased VO_2 maximum (more than expected with aerobic exercise alone).

Although almost every cardiac transplant patient faces the specter of graft rejection, it is rarely necessary to curtail the patient's exercise regimen during episodes of moderate rejection. However, if the patient shows signs of new arrhythmias, hypotension, or fever, the physiatrist may need to abruptly adjust the exercise regimen in order to balance medical management with restorative rehabilitative services (Braith et al., 2000; Kevorkian, 1999). The patient's long-term prognosis generally becomes worse as rejection episodes increase in frequency and severity. Clinical and physiological monitoring of the patient, and regular review of personal life and family goals is essential to maximizing the patient's prognosis, life plans, and family function (Moro et al., 2008). Patient and family education play a critical role in transplantation rehabilitation and should be considered a mainstay of medical management (Hummel, Michauk, Hetzer, & Fuhrmann, 2001). Pertinent patient/family transplant education topics are included in Box 19.2.

BOX 19.2 PATIENT/FAMILY TRANSPLANT EDUCATION TOPICS

- Basic immune system function
- Purpose of immunosuppression
- Activities related to immunosuppression
- Avoiding crowds
- Wearing a mask in hospital and clinic
- Caring for cuts and wounds
- Oral care/dental visits
- Notifying transplant team of any disease exposure
- Other activities
- Exercise
- Sternal precautions (6 weeks postoperative)
- Sexual activity/birth control
- Medications (proper administration, side effects, purpose)
- Immunosuppressants
- Prophylactics (antivirals, antibiotics, antifungals, antacids)
- Others (antihypertensives, vitamins, etc.)
- Home monitoring
- Blood pressure readings
- Temperature
- Stool (occult blood; quality—tan/clay colored, black, maroon, normal)
- Urine (glucose or blood; quality—cloudy, dark, normal)
- Weight (daily)
- Diet
- Restrictions (fat, sugar, salt)
- Balanced/low-calorie snacks
- Expected increase in appetite and fat deposition (due to steroids)
- Signs and symptoms of complications
- Infection/rejection
- What to do and whom to notify
- Medical follow-up
- Biopsies (typically 3 and 6 months, then yearly; with dysfunction)
- Transplant clinic visits (blood work, radiographic testing)
- Routine checkups with referring and transplant physicians
- Cancer monitoring (annual PAP smear, self-breast exam, testicular exam, mammogram; stool monitoring for occult blood)
- Routine dental visits (prophylactic antibiotics)

Summary

Cardiac transplantation is an essential and lifesaving surgical intervention used for persons with severe heart muscle disease, end-stage heart failure, and irreversible coronary artery disease associated with multiple myocardial infarctions, which have proven unresponsive to maximal medical and surgical management. Equally as important is the comprehensive and systematic rehabilitation aftercare of this population (Young & O'Young, 2012). Recent research has demonstrated the critical importance of the application of early exercise initiation following heart transplantation. As outlined in this section, a variety of important benefits result from cardiac rehabilitation transplant programs, which include optimization of aerobic capacity, enhanced physical endurance and vocational capability, as well as improved psychosocial outlook. Rehabilitation team professionals play an important role in this life-extending activity.

LUNG TRANSPLANTATION

Application of a structured pulmonary rehabilitation (PR) program following lung transplantation is regarded to be an essential component of "best practice management" (Munro, Holland, Bailey, Button, & Snell, 2009). Physical restoration of persons who have undergone complex transplant procedures is an important priority of the rehabilitation team and has emerged as a global rehabilitation priority (Cohen et al., 2012).

Role of Pretransplant Rehabilitation: Anticipatory Therapy

Recent clinical investigations have demonstrated the utility of structured pulmonary rehabilitation programs during the pretransplant phase as well. Studies have shown exercise capacity and training volumes to be well preserved among lung transplant candidates participating in pulmonary rehabilitation, even in the circumstance of severe, progressive lung disease. Pulmonary rehabilitation participants with greater exercise capacity prior to transplantation demonstrate more favorable outcomes after transplantation (Li, Mathur, Chowdhury, Helm, & Singer, 2013).

Brief Overview of Pulmonary Physiology

Lungs serve a "bellows-like" function with a bronchial tree for ventilation, capillaries for circulation, and alveoli for gas exchange. Lungs acquire oxygen from the atmosphere and eliminate carbon dioxide (CO_2) from the blood. In respiratory failure, the level of oxygen in the blood becomes dangerously low and/or the level of CO_2 becomes dangerously high. This can happen in two ways: the process by which oxygen and CO_2 are exchanged between blood and the alveoli can be compromised; or the movement of air into and out of the lungs can become dysfunctional. Either process, resulting in chronic respiratory failure, can lead to multiple impairments, including severe dyspnea and fatigue that can interfere with the person's ability to participate in ADLs. In cases of progressive end-stage lung disease refractory to medical and rehabilitation management, lung transplantation becomes an essential and viable option not only to prolong life, but also to improve patients' ability to live meaningfully.

Historical Perspective: Lung Transplant

In 1963, James Hardy performed the first single-lung transplant at the University of Mississippi (Hardy, Webb, Dalton, & Walker, 1963). Although the patient died in 18 days, the transplant was considered a tremendous success after several decades of animal studies promising the feasibility of human lung transplants. Since then, innovations in surgical techniques and transplant technology have led to an increase in the number of lung transplant surgeries conducted each year. Bilateral lung transplants have more than doubled in the past decade to represent 64% of the lung transplants performed in 2008 (887 total) (Mulligan et al., 2008). The International Society for Heart and Lung Transplantation reports 1-year survival rates of 87.5 % for double lung recipients and 83% to 84% for single lung recipients; 3-year survival rates were 68.4% for double lung recipients and 59 to 60% for single lung recipients between April 1, 2010 and March 31, 2014. The median wait list time has dropped by 87% over the last decade to 132 days in 2006 (Mulligan et al., 2008). Improved screening methods for infection and tissue-matching techniques for tissue compatibility in organ donors have been developed to prevent or minimize transplant-related infection and organ rejection. This has resulted in marked improvements in the survival rate of organ recipients (American Transplant Congress, 2003). In addition, state-of-the-art developments in pharmacotherapy, including novel solutions for achieving immunosuppression by employing drugs with greater potency and diminished side effects, have notably improved patient outcomes. Within many medical centers, overall improvement in postsurgical transplantation care, and antirejection and anti-infection treatment modes, has allowed earlier transfer to acute rehabilitation venues.

Indications

Lung transplants are reserved for qualified candidates with Stage IV lung disease based on the Global Initiative for Chronic Obstructive Lung disease (GOLD) Severity Scale. Table 19.8

TABLE 19.8

INDICATIONS FOR LUNG TRANSPLANTATION	
Single Lung Transplant	Chronic obstructive pulmonary artery disease (COPD) Idiopathic pulmonary fibrosis (IPF)
Bilateral Lung Transplant	Cystic fibrosis (CF) Pulmonary hypertension (PHTN)

BOX 19.3 COMMON DIAGNOSES OF PULMONARY TRANSPLANT PATIENTS

Pulmonary Vascular Disease
Primary pulmonary hypertension (PPH)
Eisenmenger syndrome
Cardiomyopathy with congestive heart failure

Obstructive Lung Disease
Idiopathic giant bullous emphysema (vanishing lung syndrome)
Alpha-1 antitrypsin deficiency induced emphysema
Cystic fibrosis (CF)
Bronchiectasis
Posttransplant obliterative bronchiolitis
Rejection (acute and chronic)
Side effects of immunosuppressive therapy

summarizes the common indications for single and bilateral lung transplantation. Chronic obstructive pulmonary disease and idiopathic pulmonary fibrosis are the most common indications for single-lung transplants. Cystic fibrosis and pulmonary hypertension can necessitate bilateral lung transplants. Common diagnoses for patients undergoing lung transplantation are shown in Box 19.3. Criteria for lung transplantation include shortness of breath on mild exertion, right heart failure, cyanosis, and a forced expiratory volume at 1 second (FEV_1) (the volume of air that can forcibly be blown out in 1 second, after full inspiration), which is less than 30% of predicted (Rabe et al., 2007). Pulmonary function testing (PFT) criteria for lung transplantation are shown in Box 19.4. Workup for lung transplant candidacy includes chest x-rays, CT scans, and ventilation–perfusion scans. To assess for ischemia, cardiac assessment with catheterization or a chemical stress test (persantine thallium) is used.

BOX 19.4 PULMONARY FUNCTION TESTING CRITERIA FOR LUNG TRANSPLANTATION

Lung transplantation referrals are generally considered for patients with one of the following criteria:

- FEV_1 values of less then 30% of predicted
- Hypoxia manifested by $PO_2 < 60$ mmHg
- Hypercarbia marked by $PCO_2 > 50$ mmHg

Pre–Lung Transplantation Rehabilitation Program

A pulmonary rehabilitation program is established to document baseline functions and maximize performance prior to surgery. Using variable flow tanks and ambulatory oxygen saturation meters, oxygen saturations and optimized flow rates at rest and with exercise are determined. Manual muscle testing is used to localize weak areas and guide a program of resistance exercises. Careful review of patient body mass index (BMI), diet, prealbumin and albumin levels are also essential, as maximal protein and vitamin nutritional intake in these patients helps to improve postoperative outcomes (Hasse, 1997).

In order to assess pulmonary functional capacity, the rehabilitation team should quantify ventilatory effort, vital capacity, FEV_1, and performance with the incentive spirometer. Effectiveness of bronchodilators, mucociliary clearance, and expectoration efficiency can be assessed by auscultation of the chest for wheezing and bronchial breath sounds (Downs, 1996). The six-minute walk test (6MWT) is a standard assessment tool used to measure exercise tolerance in patients with various pulmonary diseases, in which the patient is instructed to ambulate as fast as possible over a flat measured course for 6 minutes (American Thoracic Society, 2002). Adjusting oxygen saturations to stay above 90% and utilization of the most efficient ambulation are used to maximize performance. The cycle ergometer or treadmill provide a larger workload for patients that have improved strength and endurance.

After an individualized plan is designed, patients are initially encouraged to exercise repeatedly for short intervals to avoid prolonged breathlessness. Incentive spirometry strengthens the diaphragm, prevents atelectasis, promotes cough and estimates forced vital capacity (FVC). Interval exercise training, rather than continuous training, is often more successful for lung transplant candidates with end-stage pulmonary disease because it requires less ventilatory demand. The goal of therapy is to gradually and incrementally decrease the number of required rest periods, and thus enable the patient to achieve longer exercise durations and to reduce the amount of exercise-limiting symptoms. In general, each program should include instructions on efficient ventilation, expectoration, stretching, strengthening, and low-level aerobic endurance. Target heart rates can also be applied to patients with lung disease, much like the procedure followed for patients with cardiac disease, however, the high resting-heart rates for this population must be taken into account. According to Downs (1996), an exercise program that gradually approaches and maintains 60% of peak heart rate can very effectively condition patients. Exercise regimens using 60% of peak heart rate as a target, as determined by an exercise test, have been demonstrated to increase exercise tolerance (Biggar, Malen, Trulock, & Cooper, 1993; Bunzel & Laederach-Hofmann, 1999). Patients with severe lung disease, however, typically do not attain predicted maximal heart rates, as exercise is limited by pulmonary rather than cardiac function. Traditional cardiac rehabilitation target exercise formulas do not universally apply to the pulmonary rehabilitation patient (Butler, 1995). Identifying the optimal level of exercise intensity suitable for each patient is an important goal of the rehabilitation team.

Upper-limb exercise has been safely and effectively utilized in pulmonary rehabilitation programs as well, although it can sometimes contribute to dyspnea. In patients with severe pulmonary disease, upper-limb exercise can result in decreased exercise duration and dyssynchronous thoracoabdominal breathing, and hence should be prescribed cautiously.

Inspiratory muscle exercise training can also help to optimize function (Reid & Dechman, 1995). Energy conservation techniques and equipment may help the patient adjust to the low functional capacity caused by advanced pulmonary disease. An occupational therapist can help formulate work-simplification strategies and energy-conservation measures. The "dyspnea index" is a helpful and simple clinical tool for monitoring and prescribing exercise intensity in patients with dyspnea (Karam et al., 2003). This five-level index, based on the number of breaths the patient must take to count to 15, runs from Level 0 (patient can count to 15 in one breath), to Level 4 (patient is too short of breath to count). An alternative measure is the "dyspnea scale" in which the patient rates the degree of dyspnea during exercise (Biggar et al., 1993). A third alternative is the Borg RPE scale, which requires the patient to evaluate self-perceived effort during exercise (Borg, 1982).

Deteriorating disease can cause alterations in the patient's health status during the acute pretransplant period. As pulmonary reserves worsen, the pre–lung transplant patient might require abrupt cessation of exercise until he or she is deemed clinically stable enough to resume (Biggar et al., 1993). Hospitalization might be required if the patient's lung function continues to decline. Clinical deterioration can move the patient's name closer to the top of the transplant waiting list. Some lung transplant programs even require the patient to move closer to the operating center in order to be more closely monitored (Egan, Kaiser, & Cooper, 1989; Egan et al., 1992).

Post–Lung Transplantation Complications

Infection

Infection is the most common complication post–lung transplantation and can lead to premature death if not properly recognized and treated (Yun & Mason, 2009). As such, it is extremely important for clinicians to be aware of common pathogens associated with infection. Cytomegalovirus is a common viral pathogen that generally appears 14 to 100 days postoperatively. Its diagnosis can be made with bronchoscopic lavage and biopsy. Typical fungal pathogens include *Candida, Aspergillus*, and *Pneumocystis* (Arthurs et al., 2009).

Rejection

A majority of acute rejection episodes occur during the initial three months following transplantation. Lower acute rejection rates were reported with tacrolimus-based regimens compared with cyclosporine regimens (George & Guttendorf, 2011). Chronic rejection can also occur and manifest as a sudden decrease in FEV_1 (De Vito Dabbs et al., 2004). Histologically, this is known as bronchiolitis obliterans, which may be exacerbated by gastroesophageal reflux (Corris & Christie, 2008). In order to prevent acute and chronic rejection, patients are commonly placed on triple drug immunosuppressant induction regimens, such as basiliximab, daclizumab, and antithymocyte globulin. Discharge baseline therapy typically includes corticosteroids, tacrolimus, and an antimetabolite, such as azathioprine. The newer generation of immunosuppressant medications—tacrolimus, rapamycin, and leflunomide—are very helpful in averting acute and/or chronic rejection, but often have significant side effects (McShane & Garrity, 2009; Ng, Madsen, Rosengard, & Allan, 2009).

Nerve Injury

Diaphragmatic paralysis from phrenic nerve damage has been reported with an incidence ranging from 3% to 30%. Injury to the vagus or recurrent laryngeal nerves can cause swallowing dysfunction. Raising the head of the bed reduces refluxing (George & Guttendorf, 2011).

The Transplanted Lung—Physiology and Function

On implantation of the allograft, a bronchial anastomosis is made but autonomic nerves, blood supply, and lymphatic drainage are interrupted. The transplanted lung is denervated, which leads to impairments of the cough reflex, gas exchange, circulatory autoregulation, mucociliary clearance, and fluid balance. This can result in ineffective clearance of airway secretions, necessitating chest physical therapy. Lymphatic disruption contributes to fluid retention and congestion that hinders gas exchange and reduces lung compliance. Electrodiagnostic studies can be used to evaluate diaphragmatic dysfunction, which can also be present in lung transplant recipients (Biggar et al., 1993; Bunzel & Laederach-Hofmann, 1999; Chlan et al., 1998). Bed rest in these patients can cause orthostatic intolerance, reduced ventilation, increased resting heart rate, and decreased oxygen uptake (Saltin et al., 1968).

Post–Lung Transplantation Rehabilitation Program

Immediate goals of postoperative rehabilitation are to minimize atelectasis, clear airway secretions, and normalize gas exchange. Decreased mucociliary clearance associated with denervated lungs, can contribute to increased susceptibility to infection in the early postoperative period (Dolovich et al., 1987). If a patient's position can be altered from supine to side-lying or upright, it can increase drainage from chest tubes and promote drainage of pulmonary secretions. Therefore, the patient should be assisted with airway clearance, beginning on the first postoperative day, if the patient is stable. Patients who are mechanically ventilated can benefit from a combination of shaking (Pneumovest), hyperinflation with a manual ventilation bag, and assisted cough with the mechanical insufflator-exsufflator (Webber & Pryor, 1993).

Following extubation, the patient can use the active-cycle-of-breathing technique or a flutter-valve device. The active-cycle-of-breathing technique utilizes alternate periods of breathing control, thoracic expansion exercises, and huffing with an open glottis (in place of coughing) to mobilize secretions. A flutter valve is a pipe-like device used to interrupt expiratory airflow and promote secretion mobilization with a combination of positive expiratory pressure and airway oscillation.

Secretion expectoration requires an effective cough, but such efforts are often hampered by incisional pain and bronchial sensory defects from denervation (Egan et al., 1989; Richard et al., 1955). Pain at the incision can also interfere with activity progression and deep-breathing exercises (Webber & Pryor, 1993). By using adequate pain control measures and optimal positioning, coughing technique can be improved (Lannefors & Wollmer, 1992). The patient should be encouraged to sit upright during coughing to achieve the greatest expiratory flow rates (Lannefors & Wollmer, 1992; Webber & Pryor, 1993). Huffing produces a lower sound, vibrates the pharynx less, and patients may find it more comfortable than normal coughing after surgery. Huff coughing is performed without closing the glottis and has been shown to produce a larger volume of expired air at a higher flow rate of secretions than conventional coughing (Hietpas, Roth, & Jensen, 1979). For patients unable to generate substantial airflow, the techniques of stacking breaths or positive pressure breathing (before the expulsion phase) can increase the effectiveness of a cough. Splinted coughing, with a pillow against the incision, may also help reduce incisional pain. Patients complaining of pain originating from chest tube sites may benefit from epidural analgesia, which can help with pain management and allow the patient to participate more enthusiastically in rehabilitation.

Progressive activity should be initiated on the first postoperative day, beginning with range of motion exercises (Palmer & Tapson, 1998). These can be advanced to transfers out of bed to a chair, and then to ambulation. After the patient leaves the intensive care unit, rehabilitation should continue to focus on lung ventilation, mobilizing pulmonary secretions, and ventilation–perfusion matching to optimize the concentration of oxygen in the blood. Thoracic mobility can be improved by instructing the patient in chest and upper-extremity mobilization exercises (Butler, 1995; Downs, 1996). Breathing exercises should be incorporated into thoracic mobility, cardiovascular exercise programs, coughing, airway clearance techniques, and general activities.

As a patient progresses, treadmill and cycle ergometer exercises can be introduced, aiding the patient with cardiovascular endurance and strength, and reducing infection risk. Pulmonary transplant recipients can often reach exercise intensities comparable to fully able-bodied patients of similar ages (Palmer & Tapson, 1998). Denervation of the lungs does not impair the ability to increase ventilation during physical exertion, and most studies show that physical training results in improved endurance and strength (Kjaer et al., 1999). In fact, systematic exercise training in lung transplant rehabilitation has been demonstrated to improve participation in ADL's in a randomized trial (Langer, 2015). Before discharge from the hospital, the patient should progress to stair climbing. This is the hallmark of recovery, as advanced pulmonary disease typically makes it impossible for most patients to do this for a period of weeks to years pretransplant.

Cardiopulmonary exercise testing has demonstrated areas of limitation in assessing exercise capacity after lung transplantation. Aerobic capacity, judged by maximal oxygen uptake, typically remains reduced by 32 to 60% of the predicted value in this patient population (Williams, Grossman, & Maurer, 1990). This reduction in aerobic capacity is thought to underlie the exercise limitations in lung transplant patients. Abnormalities of gas exchange and ventilation perfusion are not thought to play a major role in the reduced exercise capacity of single-lung-transplant patients. Many other factors can contribute to reduced exercise reserve, including chronic deconditioning, muscle atrophy with decreased mitochondrial density, and reduced oxidative enzyme capacity. Peripheral muscle strength and endurance is reduced following lung transplantation and is the primary component limiting performance of patients while exercising (Walsh et al., 2013).

Post–Lung Transplantation Outcomes

Scientific studies have definitively shown that durations of structured exercise training can improve maximal and functional exercise capacity, skeletal muscle strength, and lumbar bone mineral density in lung transplant recipients. Additional investigations are required to determine the potential for exercise training to optimize functional outcomes, and to formulate guidelines for exercise prescription among lung transplant patients (Wickerson, Mathur, & Brooks, 2010). A considerable restoration of functional ability is usually achieved after lung transplantation (Duarte et al., 2008). Compared to education alone, pulmonary rehabilitation has been shown to further increase exercise performance, decrease muscle fatigue and reduce shortness of breath (Ries, Kaplan, Limberg, & Prewitt, 1995). Improvement in exercise tolerance through pulmonary rehabilitation has been demonstrated by an increase in six-minute walk distances after transplantation (Biggar et al., 1993; Egan et al., 1992; Mal et al., 1994; Williams et al., 1990). One center reported that none of their lung transplant recipients had to terminate a maximal symptom-limited exercise test because of dyspnea, as the main complaint was lower-limb discomfort or pain (Howard, Iademarco, & Trulock, 1994).

Return to work is the logical next step for a lung transplant patient after surgery and the successful recuperative process to that point. Quite often, returning to work or homemaking duties aids in restoring a critical sense of normalcy, and helps to significantly bolster self-esteem and wellness (Petrucci et al., 2007). More than 90% of lung transplantation patients report satisfaction with their health while performing these tasks (Craven, Bright, & Dear, 1990). One leading study revealed a 37% employment rate among lung transplant survivors (Paris et al., 1998). Type of lung transplantation (single or bilateral) has not been shown to be correlated with employment status (Huddleston et al., 2002).

QOL after lung transplantation has been recently reviewed (Singer & Singer, 2013). The most commonly used generic measure was the SF-36. Longitudinal studies with this 100-point scale show subjects with improvements of 3 to 20 points primarily in the physical functioning, physical role, and general health domains in the first six months. From six to twelve months, little additional improvement was observed (Kugler et al., 2010). Various authors have determined that bronchiolitis obliterans syndrome, lack of family support, failure to return to work, anxiety, and depression are associated with low quality of life scores (Singer & Singer, 2013).

Summary

Rehabilitation following lung transplant is an essential component of restorative aftercare that can facilitate marked improvements in ADLs and functional independence. The early goals of post–lung transplant rehabilitation are largely physiological, that is, promotion of normalized gas exchange, clearing of airway secretions, and minimization of atelectasis. During the more advanced phase of pulmonary rehabilitation, patients are remobilized, and encouraged to regain proficiency in ADLs, build endurance, achieve functional self-sufficiency, and demonstrate consistent community reintegration. Ultimately, the lung transplant patient is provided with opportunities for vocational development adaptations and employment as a component of advanced rehabilitation. Essentially, the goal of lung transplant is to lengthen life, improve function and increase QOL.

CONCLUSION

Within the past 25 years, advances in medical care, surgical techniques, and technology have significantly reduced morbidity and mortality in post-transplantation patients. Success can no longer be measured by the number of years after transplantation, but must instead be measured by the quality of life in those years. Rehabilitation plays a pivotal role in maximizing the potential of these patients, now more than ever (Ataneloy, Stiens, & Young, 2015). Transplant rehabilitation can add "life to years," serving as a vital complement to transplant surgery that adds "years to life."

ACKNOWLEDGEMENTS

The authors would like to thank Bryn Thatcher for creation of the tables, updating citations and statistics, and general editing of this chapter.

REFERENCES

Adam, R., & Hoti, E. (2009). Liver transplantation: The current situation. *Seminars in Liver Disease, 29*(1), 3–18.

Agarwal, S., & Owen, R. (1990). Tendinitis and tendon rupture in successful renal transplant recipients. *Clinical Orthopaedics and Related Research, 252* 270–275.

American Heart Association. (2009). ACCF/AHA practice guideline: Full text. Retrieved from http://circ.ahajournals.org/content/119/14/e391.full.pdf+html

American Thoracic Society. (2002). ATS statement: Guidelines for the six-minute walk test. *American Journal of Respiratory and Critical Care Medicine, 166*, 111–117.

American Transplant Congress. (2003, May 30–June 4). *The fourth joint American transplant meeting.* Washington, DC.

Arthurs, S. K., Eid, A. J., Deziel, P. J., Marshall, W. F., Cassivi, S. D., Walker, R. C., & Razonable, R. R. (2009). The impact of invasive fungal diseases on survival after lung transplantation. *Clinical Transplantation, 24*, 341–348.

Ataneloy, L., Stiens, S. A., & Young, M. A. (2015). History of physical medicine and rehabilitation and its ethical dimensions. *American Medical Association Journal of Ethics, 17*(6), 568–574.

Auerbach, I., Tenenbaum, A., Motro, M., Stroh, C. I., Har-Zahav, Y., & Fisman, E. Z. (1999). Attenuated responses of doppler-derived hemodynamic parameters during supine bicycle exercise in heart transplant recipients. *Cardiology, 92*, 204–209.

Beck, W., Barnard, C. N., & Schrire, V. (1969). Heart rate after cardiac transplantation. *Circulation, 40*, 437–445.

Benten, D., Staufer, K., & Sterneck, M. (2009). Orthotopic liver transplantation and what to do during follow-up: Recommendations for the practitioner. *Gastroenterology and Hepatology, 6*, 23–36.

Bernardi, L., Radaelli, A., Passino, C., Falcone, C., Auguadro, C., Martinelli, L., . . . Finardi, G. (2007). Effects of physical training on cardiovascular control after heart transplantation. *International Journal of Cardiology, 118*, 356–362.

Beyer, N., Aadahl, M., Strange, B., Kirkegaard, P., Hansen, B. A., Mohr, T., & Kjaer, M. (1999). Improved physical performance after orthotopic liver transplantation. *Liver Transplant Surgery, 5*, 301–309.

Beyer, N., Aadahl, M., Strange, B., Mohr, T., & Kjaer, M. (1995). Exercise capacity of patients after liver transplantation. *Medicine & Science in Sports & Exercise, 6*, S84.

Biggar, D. G., Malen, J. F., Trulock, E. P., & Cooper, J. D. (1993). Pulmonary rehabilitation before and after lung transplantation. In R. Kasaburi & T. L. Petty (Eds.), *Principles and practice of pulmonary rehabilitation* (pp. 459–467). Philadelphia, PA: W. B. Saunders.

Boaz, A., & Morgan, M. (2014). Working to establish 'normality' post-transplant: A qualitative study of kidney transplant patients. *Chronic Illness, 10*(4), 247–258.

Bohannon, R. W., Smith, J., Hull, D., Palmeri, D., & Barnhard, R. (1995). Deficits in lower extremity muscle and gait performance among renal transplant candidates. *Archives of Physical Medicine and Rehabilitation, 76*, 547–551.

Borg, G. (1982). Psychophysical basis of perceived exertion. *Medicine & Science in Sports & Exercise, 14*, 377–381.

Braith, R. W., Clapp, L., Brown, T., Brown, C., Schofield, R., Mills, R. M., & Hill, J. A. (2000). Rate-responsive pacing improves exercise tolerance in heart transplant recipients: A pilot study. *Journal of Cardiopulmonary Rehabilitation, 20*, 377–382.

Braith, R. W., & Edwards, D. G. (2000). Exercise following heart transplantation. *Sports Medicine, 30*, 171–192.

Braith, R. W., Welsch, M. A., Mills, R. M. Jr., Keller, J. W., & Pollock, M. L. (1998). Resistance exercise prevents glucocorticoid-induced myopathy in heart transplant recipients. *Medicine & Science in Sports & Exercise, 30*, 483–489.

Bunke, M., & Ganzel, B. (1992). Effects of calcium antagonists on renal function in hypertensive heart transplant recipients. *Journal of Heart and Lung Transplantation, 2*, 1194–1199.

Bunzel, B., & Laederach-Hofmann, K. (1999). Long-term effects of heart transplantation: The gap between physical performance and emotional well-being. *Scandinavian Journal of Rehabilitation Medicine, 31*, 214–222.

Butler, B. B. (1995). Physical therapy in heart and lung transplantation. In E. Hillegas & S. Sadowski (Eds.), *Cardiopulmonary physical therapy* (3rd ed., pp. 404–422). St. Louis, MO: Mosby.

Campellone, J. V., Lacomis, D., Giuliani, M. J., & Kramer, D. J. (1998). Mononeuropathies associated with liver transplantation. *Muscle and Nerve, 21*, 896–901.

Carithers, R. L. Jr. (2000). Liver transplantation: American association for the study of liver diseases. *Liver Transplantation, 6*, 122–135.

Carney, R. M., Templeton, B., Hong, B. A., Harter, H. R., Hagberg, J. M., Schechtman, K. B., & Goldberg, A. P. (1987). Exercise training reduces depression and increases the performance of pleasant activities in hemodialysis patients. *Nephron, 47*, 194–198.

Chlan, L., Snyder, M., Finkelstein, S., Hertz, M., Edin, C., Wielinski, C., & Dutta, A. (1998). Promoting adherence to an electronic home spirometry research program after lung transplantation. *Applied Nursing Research, 11*, 36–40.

Christiansen, E., Vestergaard, H., Tibell, A., Hother-Nielsen, O., Holst, J. J., Pedersen, O., & Madsbad, S. (1996). Impaired insulin-stimulated non-oxidative glucose metabolism in pancreas-kidney transplant recipients. Dose-response characteristics of insulin on glucose turnover. *Diabetes, 45*, 1267–1275.

Cohen, J., Young, M. A., & Stiens, S. A. (2012, November). *Pulmonary transplantation rehabilitation.* Poster session presented at the AAPM&R annual meeting, Atlanta, GA.

Colm, C. M., & Pascual, M. (2004). Update in renal transplantation. *Archives of Internal Medicine, 164*, 1373–1388.

Copeland, J. G., Smith, R. G., Arabia, F. A., Nolan, P., Sethi, G. K., Tsau, P. H., & CardioWest Total Artificial Heart Investigators. (2004). CardioWest total artificial heart investigators: Bridge to transplantation. *New England Journal of Medicine, 351*, 859–867.

Corris, P. A., & Christie, J. D. (2008). Update in transplantation 2007. *American Journal of Respiratory and Critical Care Medicine, 177*, 1062–1067.

Cortazzo, M. H., Helkowski, W., Pippin, B., Boninger, M. L., & Zafonte, R. (2005). Acute inpatient rehabilitation of 55 patients after liver transplantation. *American Journal of Physical Medicine & Rehabilitation, 84*, 880–884.

Craven, J. L., Bright, J., & Dear, C. L. (1990). Psychiatric, psychosocial and rehabilitative aspects of lung transplantation. *Clinics in Chest Medicine, 11*, 247–257.

Crosbie, O., Freaney, R., McKenna, M., & Hegarty, J. (1999). Bone density, vitamin D status and disordered bone remodeling in end-stage chronic liver disease. *Calcified Tissue International, 64*, 295–300.

D'Amico, C. L. (2005). Cardiac transplantation: Patient selection in the current era. *Journal of Cardiovascular Nursing, 20*(Suppl. 5), S4–S13.

Dandel, M., Wellnhofer, E., Hummel, M., Meyer, R., Lehmkuhl, H., & Hetzer, R. (2003). Early detection of left ventricular dysfunction related to transplant coronary artery disease. *Journal of Heart and Lung Transplantation, 22*, 1353–1364.

De Vito Dabbs, A., Hoffman, L. A., Swigart, V., Happ, M. B., Iacono, A. T., & Dauber, J. H. (2004). Using conceptual triangulation to develop an integrated model of the symptom experience of acute rejection after lung transplantation. *Advances in Nursing Science, 27*, 138–149.

Deuse, T., Haddad, F., Pham, M., Hunt, S., Valantine, H., Bates, M. J., . . . Reitz, B. A. (2008). Twenty-year survivors of heart transplantation at stanford university. *American Journal of Transplantation, 8*, 1769–1774.

Diamond, T., Stiel, D., Wilkinson, M., & Posen, J. R. (1990). Osteoporosis and skeletal fractures in chronic liver disease. *Gut, 31*, 82–87.

Dolovich, M., Rossman, C., Chambers, C., Grossman, R. F., Newhouse, M., & Maurer, J. (1987). Mucociliary function in patients following single lung or lung/heart transplantation. *American Review of Respiratory Disease, 135*, A363.

Downs, A. M. (1996). Physical therapy in lung transplantation. *Physical Therapy, 76*, 626–642.

Doyle, M. B., Maynard, E., Lin, Y., Vachharajani, N., Shenoy, S., Anderson, C., . . . Chapman, W. C. (2013). Outcomes with split liver transplantation are equivalent to those with whole organ transplantation. *Journal of the American College of Surgeons, 217*(1), 102–112; discussion 113–114.

Drexler, H., & Schroeder, J. S. (1994). Unusual forms of ischemic heart disease. *Current Opinion in Cardiology, 9*, 457–464.

Duarte, A. G., Terminella, L., Smith, J. T., Myers, A. C., Campbell, G., & Lick, S. (2008). Restoration of cough reflex in lung transplant recipients. *Chest, 134*, 310–316.

Egan, T. M., Kaiser, L. R., & Cooper, J. D. (1989). Lung transplantation. *Current Problems in Surgery, 26*, 673–752.

Egan, T. M., Westerman, J. H., Lambert, C. J. Jr., Detterbeck, F. C., Thompson, J. T., Mill, M. R., . . . Wilcox, B. R. (1992). Isolated lung transplantation for end-stage lung disease: A viable therapy. *Annals of Thoracic Surgery, 53*, 590–596.

Espinoza, J. V., & Bertolet, B. D. (1997). Cardiac transplantation for the practicing clinical cardiologist. *ACC Current Journal Review*, 6(2), 65–69.

Fuhrmann, I., & Krause, R. (2004). Principles of exercising in patients with chronic kidney disease, on dialysis and for kidney transplant recipients. *Clinical Nephrology, 61*, S14–S25.

Fujisawa, M., Ichikawa, Y., Yoshiya, K., Isotani, S., Higuchi, A., Nagano, S., . . . Kamidono, S. (2000). Assessment of health-related quality of life in renal transplant and hemodialysis patients using the SF-36 health survey. *Urology, 56*, 201–206.

Gammie, J. S., Edwards, L. B., Griffith, B. P., Pierson, R. N, 3rd, & Tsao, L. (2004). Optimal timing of cardiac transplantation after ventricular assist device implantation. *Journal of Thoracic and Cardiovascular Surgery, 127*, 1789–1799.

Garcia, A. M., Veneroso, C. E., Soares, D. D., Lima, A. S., & Correia, M. I. (2014). Effect of a physical exercise program on the functional capacity of liver transplant patients. *Transplantation Proceedings*, *46*(6), 1807–1808.

George, E. L., & Guttendorf, J. (2011). Lung transplant. *Critical Care Nursing Clinics of North America, 23*(3), 481–503.

Goldberg, A. P., Geltman, E. M., Gavin, J. R. 3rd, Carney, R. M., Hagberg, J. M., Delmez, J. A., . . . Harter, H. R. (1986). Exercise training reduces coronary risk and effectively rehabilitates hemodialysis patients. *Nephron, 42*, 311–316.

Greenberg, A., Egel, J. W., Thompson, M. E., Hardesty, R. L., Griffith, B. P., Bahnson, H. T., . . . Puschett, J. B. (1987). Early and late forms of cyclosporine nephrotoxicity: Studies in cardiac transplant recipients. *American Journal of Kidney Diseases, 9*, 12–22.

Greenberg, M. L., Uretsky, B. F., Reddy, P. S., Bernstein, R. L., Griffith, B. P., Hardesty, R. L., . . . Bahnson, H. T. (1985). Long-term hemodynamic follow-up of cardiac transplant patients treated with cyclosporine and prednisone. *Circulation, 71*, 487–494.

Griepp, R. B., Stinson, E. D., Dong, E. Jr., Clark, D. A., & Shumway, N. E. (1971). Hemodynamic performance of the transplanted human heart. *Surgery, 70*, 88–96.

Gurk-Turner, C. (1997). Management of the metabolic complications of liver disease: An overview of commonly used pharmacological agents. *Support Line, 19*, 17–19.

Hardy, J. D., Webb, W. R., Dalton, M. L., & Walker, G. R., Jr. (1963). Lung homotransplantation in man. *Journal of the American Medical Association, 186*, 1065–1074.

Harrison, J., McKiernan, J., & Neuberger, J. M. (1997). A prospective study on the effect of recipient nutritional status on outcome in liver transplantation. *Transplant International, 10*, 360–374.

Hasse, J. M. (1997). Diet therapy for organ transplantation. A problem-based approach. *Nursing Clinics of North America, 32*, 863–880.

Heidelbaugh, J. J., & Bruderly, N. (2006). Cirrhosis and chronic liver failure: Part I. diagnosis and evaluation. *American Family Physician, 74*, 756–762.

Heroux, A., & Pamboukian, S. V. (2014). Neurological aspects of heart transplantation. *Handbook of Clinical Neurology, 121*, 1229–1236.

Hietpas, B., Roth, R., & Jensen, W. (1979). Huff coughing and airway patency. *Respiratory Care, 24*, 710–714.

Hosenpud, J. D., Novick, R. J., Breen, T. J., & Daily, O. P. (1994). Registry of the international society for heart and lung transplantation: Eleventh official report—1994. *Journal of Heart and Lung Transplantation, 13*, 561–570.

Howard, D. K., Iademarco, E. J., & Trulock, E. P. (1994). The role of cardiopulmonary exercise testing in lung and heart-lung transplantation. *Clinics in Chest Medicine, 15*, 405–420.

Huda, A., Newcomer, R., Harrington, C., Blegen, M. G., & Keeffe, E. B. (2012). High rate of unemployment after liver transplantation: Analysis of the united network for organ sharing database. *Liver Transplantation, 18*(1), 89–99.

Huddleston, C. B., Bloch, J. B., Sweet, S. C., de la Morena, M., Patterson, G. A., & Mendeloff, E. N. (2002). Lung transplant in children. *Annals of Surgery, 236*, 270–276.

Humar, A., Denny, R., Matas, A. J., & Najarian, J. S. (2003). Great and quality of life outcomes in older recipients of a kidney transplant. *Experimental and Clinical Transplantation, 1*, 69–72.

Hummel, M., Michauk, I., Hetzer, R., & Fuhrmann, B. (2001). Quality of life after heart and heart-lung transplantation. *Transplantation Proceedings, 33*, 3546–3548.

International Society for Heart & Lung Transplantation. (2009). *International society for heart and lung transplant ishlt- 29th annual meeting and scientific sessions*. Paris, France.

International Society for Heart & Lung Transplantation. (2014). *ISHLT Transplant registry quarterly reports for heart in North America*. Retrieved from http://www.ishlt.org/registries/quarterlyDataReportResults.asp?organ=LU&rptType=tx_char&continent=4

Joshi, A., & Kevorkian, C. G. (1997). Rehabilitation after cardiac transplantation. Case series and literature review. *American Journal of Physical Medicine & Rehabilitation, 76*, 249–254.

Juskowa, J., Lewandowska, M., Bartłomiejczyk, I., Foroncewicz, B., Korabiewska, I., Niewczas, M., & Sierdziński, J. (2006). Physical rehabilitation and risk of atherosclerosis after successful kidney transplantation. *Transplantation Proceedings, 38*, 157–160.

Kao, A. C., Van Trigt, P. R., Shaeffer-McCall, G. S., Shaw, J. P., Kuzil, B. B., Page, R. D., & Higginbotham, M. B. (1995). Allograft diastolic dysfunction and chronotropic incompetence limit cardiac output response to exercise two to six years after heart transplantation. *Journal of Heart and Lung Transplantation, 14*, 11–22.

Karam, V., Castaing, D., Danet, C., Delvart, V., Gasquet, I., Adam, R., . . . Bismuth, H. (2003). Longitudinal prospective evaluation of quality of life in adult patients before and one year after liver transplantation. *Liver Transplantation, 9*, 703–711.

Kavanagh, T., & Yacoub, M. H. (1992). Exercise training in patients after heart transplantation. *Annals Academy of Medicine Singapore, 21*, 372–378.

Kavanagh, T., Yacoub, M. H., Mertens, D. J., Kennedy, J., Campbell, R. B., & Sawyer, P. (1988). Cardiorespiratory responses to exercise training after orthotopic cardiac transplantation. *Circulation, 77*, 162–171.

Keeffe, E. B. (2001). Liver Transplantation: Current status and novel approaches to liver replacement. *Gastroenterology, 120*, 749–762.

Kempeneers, G. L. G., Myburgh, K. H., Wiggins, T., Adams, B., van Zyl-Smit, R., & Noakes, T. D. (1988). The effect of an exercise training program on renal transplant recipients. *Transplantation Proceedings, 20*(Suppl. 1), 381–386.

Keogh, J. B., Tsalamandris, C., Sewell, R. B., Jones, R. M., Angus, P. W., Nyulasi, I. B., & Seeman, E. (1999). Bone loss at the proximal femur and reduced lean mass following liver transplantation: A longitudinal study. *Nutrition, 15*, 661–664.

Keteyian, S., Marks, C. R., Levine, A. B., Fedel, F., Ehrman, J., Kataoka, T., & Levine, T. B. (1994). Cardiovascular responses of cardiac transplant patients to arm and leg exercise. *European Journal of Applied Physiology, 68*, 441–444.

Kevorkian, C. G. (1999). Stroke rehabilitation and the cardiac transplantation patient. *New England Journal of Medicine, 340*, 976.

Kittleson, M. M., & Kobashigawa, J. A. (2014). Long-term care of the heart transplant recipient. *Current Opinion in Organ Transplantation, 19*(5), 515–524.

Kjaer, M., Beyer, N., & Secher, N. H. (1999). Exercise and organ transplantation. *Scandinavian Journal of Medicine & Science in Sports, 9*, 1–14.

Kjaer, M., Kelding, S., Engfred, K., Rasmussen, K., Sonne, B., Kirkegård, P., & Galbo, H. (1996). Glucose homeostasis during exercise in humans with a liver or kidney transplant. *American Journal of Physiology, 268*, E636–E644.

Kobashigawa, J. A., Laks, H., Marelli, D., Moriguchi, J. D., Hamilton, M. A., Fonarow, G., . . . Kawata, N. (1998). The university of california at los angeles experience in heart transplantation. *Clinical Transplantation*, 303–310.

Kobashigawa, J. A., Leaf, D. A., Lee, N., Gleeson, M. P., Liu, H., Hamilton, M. A., . . . Laks, H. (1999). A controlled trial of exercise rehabilitation after heart transplantation. *New England Journal of Medicine, 340*(12), 976.

Koffron, A., & Stein, J. A. (2008). Liver transplantation: Indications, pre-transplant evaluation, surgery, and post-transplant complications. *Medical Clinics of North America, 92*, 861–888.

Kohzuki, M., Abo, T., Watanabe, M., Goto, Y., Ohkohchi, N., Satomi, S., & Sato, T. (2000). Rehabilitating patients with hepatopulmonary syndrome using living-related orthotopic liver transplant: A case report. *Archives of Physical Medicine and Rehabilitation, 81*, 1527–1530.

Korbiewska, L., Lewandowska, M., Juskowa, J., & Bialoszewski, D. (2007). Need for rehabilitation in renal replacement therapy involving allogeneic kidney transplantation. *Transplantation Proceedings, 39*, 2776–2777.

Krull, F., Schulze-Neick, I., Hatopp, A., Offner, G., & Brodehl, J. (1994). Exercise capacity and blood pressure response in children and adolescents after renal transplantation. *Acta Paediatrica, 83*, 1296–1302.

Kugler, C., Tegtbur, U., Gottlieb, J., Bara, C., Malehsa, D., Dierich, M., . . . Haverich, A. (2010). Heath-related quality of life in long term survivors after heart and lung transplantation: A prospective cohort study. *Transplantation, 90*, 451–457.

Lahpor, J. R. (2009). State of the art: Implantable ventricular assist devices. *Current Opinion in Organ Transplantation, 14*, 554–559.

Lampert, E., Mettauer, B., Hoppeler, H., Charloux, A., & Charpentier, A. (1998). Skeletal muscle response to short endurance training in heart transplant recipients. *Journal of the American College of Cardiology, 32*, 420–426.

Langer, D. (2015). Rehabilitation in patients before and after lung transplantation. *Respiration, 89*(5), 353–362.

Lannefors, L., & Wollmer, P. (1992). Mucus clearance with three chest physiotherapy regimens in cystic fibrosis: A comparison between postural drainage, PEP, and physical exercise. *European Respiratory Journal, 5*, 748–753.

Latlief, G. A., & Young, M. A. (1994). Cardiac transplant rehabilitation in a post-partum woman. *Archives of Physical Medicine and Rehabilitation, 75*, 1040.

Le Jemtel, T. H. (2003). Review of a controlled trial of exercise rehabilitation after heart transplantation. *Transplantation Proceedings, 35*, 1513–1515.

Leenen, F. H., Davies, R. A., & Fourney, A. (1995). Role of cardiac beta 2- receptors in cardiac responses to exercise in cardiac transplant patients. *Circulation, 91*, 685–690.

Legault, L., Olgilvie, R. I., Cardella, C. J., & Leenen, P. H. (1993). Calcium antagonists in heart transplant recipients: Effects on cardiac and renal function and cyclosporine pharmacokinetics. *Canadian Journal of Cardiology, 9*, 398–404.

Li, M., Mathur, S., Chowdhury, N. A., Helm, D., & Singer, L. G. (2013). Pulmonary rehabilitation in lung transplant candidates. *Journal of Heart and Lung Transplantation, 32*, 626–632.

Li, S., Lue, W., Mobarhan, S., Nadir, A., Van Thiel, D., & Hagety, A. (2000). Nutrition support for individuals with liver failure. *Nutrition Reviews, 58*, 242–247.

Limongi, V., dos Santos, D. C., da Silva, A. M., Ataide, E. C., Mei, M. F., Udo, E. Y., & Stucchi, R. S. (2014). Effects of a respiratory physiotherapeutic program in liver transplantation candidates. *Transplant Proceedings, 46*(6), 1775–1777.

Lopez, P. M., & Martin, P. (2006). Update on liver transplantation: Indications, organ allocation and long-term care. *Mount Sinai Journal of Medicine, 73*, 1056–1066.

Lucas, T. S., & Einhorn, T. A. (1993). Stress fracture of the femoral neck during rehabilitation after heart transplantation. *Archives of Physical Medicine and Rehabilitation, 74*, 1004–1006.

Mal, H., Sleiman, C., Jebrak, G., Messian, O., Dubois, F., Darne, C., & Kitzis, M. (1994). Functional results of single-lung transplantation for chronic obstructive lung disease. *American Journal of Respiratory and Critical Care Medicine, 149*, 1476–1481.

Malinis, M. F., Chen, S., Allore, H. G. & Quagliarello, V. J. (2014). Outcomes among older adult liver transplantation recipients in the model of end stage liver disease (MELD) era. *Annals of Transplantation, 19*, 478–487.

Martin, T. W., Gaucher, J., Pupa, L. E., & Seaworth, J. F. (1994). Response to upright exercise after cardiac transplantation. *Clinical Cardiology, 17*, 292–300.

McCaughan, G. W., & Feller, R. B. (1994). Osteoporosis in chronic liver disease: Pathogenesis, risk factors and management. *Digestive Diseases of Sciences, 12*, 223–231.

McGiffin, D., Kirklin, J. K., & Nafiel, D. C. (1985). Acute renal failure after heart transplantation and cyclosporine therapy. *Journal of Heart and Lung Transplantation, 4*, 396–399.

McShane, P. J., & Garrity, E. R. Jr. (2009). Minimization of immunosuppression after lung transplantation: Current trends. *Transplant International, 22*, 90–95.

Mettauer, B., Levy, F., Richard, R., Roth, O., Zoll, J., Lampert, E., . . . Geny, B. (2005). Exercising with a denervated heart after cardiac transplantation. *Annals of Transplantation, 10*, 35–42.

Meyer, M., Rahmel, A., Marconi, C., Grassi, B., Cerretelli, P., & Cabrol, C. (1994). Adjustment of cardiac output to step exercise in heart transplant recipients. *Zeitschrift für Kardiologie, 83*(Suppl. 3), 103–109.

Miller, L. W., Naftel, D. C., Bourge, R. C., Kirklin, J. K., Brozena, S. C., Jarcho, J., . . . Mills, R. M. (1994). Infection after heart transplantation: A multiinstitutional study. Cardiac Transplant Research Database Group. *Journal of Heart and Lung Transplantation, 13*(3), 381–393.

Mills, R. M. Jr. (1994). Transplantation and the problems afterward including coronary vasculopathy. *Clinical Cardiology, 17*, 287–290.

Moro, J. A., Almenar, L., Martńez-Dolz, L., Agüero, J., Sánchez-Lázaro, I., Iglesias, P., . . . Salvador, A (2008). Support program for heart transplant patients: Initial experience. *Transplantation Proceedings, 40*, 3039–3040.

Mulligan, M. S., Shearon, T. H., Weill, D., Pagani, F. D., Moore, J., & Murray, S. (2008). Heart and lung transplantation in the united states 1997–2006. *American Journal of Transplantation, 8*(Pt. 2), 977–987.

Munoz, S. (1991). Nutritional therapies in liver disease. *Seminars in Liver Disease, 11*, 278–289.

Munro, P. E., Holland, A. E., Bailey, M., Button, B. M., & Snell, G. I. (2009). Pulmonary rehabilitation following lung transplantation. *Transplantation Proceedings, 41*, 292–295.

Neipp, M., Karavul, B., Jackobs, S., Meyer zu Vilsendorf, A., Richter, N., Becker, T., . . . Klempnauer, J. (2006). Quality of life in adult transplant recipients more than 15 years after kidney transplantation. *Transplantation, 81*, 1640–1644.

Ng, C. Y., Madsen, J. C., Rosengard, B. R., & Allan, J. S. (2009). Immunosuppression for lung transplantation. *Frontiers in Bioscience, 1*, 1627–1641.

Nicholas, J. J., Oleske, D., Robinson, L. R., Switala, J. A., & Tarter, R. (1994). The quality of life after orthotopic liver transplantation: An analysis of 166 cases. *Archives of Physical Medicine and Rehabilitation, 75*, 431–435.

Nytrøen, K., & Gullestad, L. (2013). Exercise after heart transplantation: An overview. *World Journal of Transplantation, 3*(4), 78–90.

O'Connell, J. B., Bourge, R. C., Costanzo-Nordin, M. R., Driscoll, D. J., Morgan, J. P., Rose, E. A., & Uretsky B. F. (1992). Cardiac transplantation: Recipient selection, donor procurement, and medical follow-up—A statement for health professionals from the committee on cardiac transplantation of the council on clinical cardiology, american heart association. *Circulation, 86*, 1061–1079.

Oliver, D., Pflugfelder, P. W., McCartney, N., McKelvie, R. S., Suskin, N., & Kostuk, W. J. (2001). Acute cardiovascular responses to leg-press resistance exercise in heart transplant recipients. *International Journal of Cardiology, 81*, 61–74.

Overbeck, I., Bartels, M., Decker, O., Harms, J., Hauss, J., & Fangmann, J. (2005). Changes in quality of life after renal transplantation. *Transplantation Proceedings, 37*, 1618–1621.

Ow, M. M., Erasmus, P., Minto, G., Struthers, R., Joseph, M., Smith, A., . . . Cross, T. J. (2014). Impaired functional capacity in potential liver transplant candidates predicts short-term mortality before transplantation. *Liver Transplantation, 20*(9), 1081–1088.

Painter, P. L., Hector, L., Ray, K., Lynes, L., Dibble, S., Paul, S. M., . . . Ascher, N. L. (2002b). A randomized trial of exercise training after renal transplantation. *Transplantation, 74*, 42–48.

Painter, P. L., Luetkemeier, M. J., Moore, G. E., Dibble, S. L., Green, G. A., Myll, J. O., & Carlson, L. L. (1997). Health-related fitness and quality of life in organ transplant recipients. *Transplantation, 64*, 1795–1800.

Painter, P., Krasnoff, J., Paul, S., & Ascher, N. (2001). Physical activity and quality of life in long-term liver transplant recipients. *Liver Transplantation, 7*, 213–219.

Painter, P., Moore, G., Carlson, L., Paul, S., Myll, J., Phillips, W., & Haskell, W. (2002a). Effects of exercise training plus normalization of hematocrit on exercise capacity and health-related quality of life. *American Journal of Kidney Diseases, 39*, 257–265.

Painter, P. L., Nelson-Worel, J. N., Hill, M. M., Thornbery, D. R., Shelp, W. R., Harrington, A. R., . . . Weinstein A. B. (1986). Effects of exercise training during hemodialysis. *Nephron, 43*, 87–92.

Palmer, S. M., & Tapson, V. F. (1998). Pulmonary rehabilitation in the surgical patient. Lung transplantation and lung volume reduction surgery. *Respiratory Care Clinics of North America, 4*, 71–83.

Paris, W., Diercks, M., Bright, J., Zamora, M., Kesten, S., Scavuzzo, M., & Paradis, I. (1998). Return to work after lung transplantation. *Journal of Heart and Lung Transplantation, 17*, 430–436.

Paterson, D. H., Cunningham, D. A., Pickering, J. G., Babcock, M. A., & Boughner, D. R. (1994). Oxygen uptake kinetics in cardiac transplant recipients. *Journal of Applied Physiology, 77*, 1935–1940.

Petrucci, L., Ricotti, S., Michelini, I., Vitulo, P., Oggionni, T., Cascina, A., . . . Klersy, C. (2007). Return to work after thoracic organ transplantation in a clinically-stable population. *European Journal of Heart Failure, 9*, 1112–1119.

Pober, J. S., Jane-wit, D., Qin, L., & Tellides, G. (2014). Interacting mechanisms in the pathogenesis of cardiac allograft vasculopathy. *Arteriosclerosis, Thrombosis & Vascular Biology, 34*(8), 1609–1614.

Pooranfar, S., Shakoor, E., Shafahi, M., Salesi, M., Karimi, M., Roozbeh, J., & Hasheminasab, M. (2014). The effect of exercisetraining on quality and quantity of sleep and lipid profile inrenal transplant patients: A randomized clinical trial. *International Journal of Organ Transplantation Medicine, 5*(4), 157–165.

Prihodova, L., Nagyova, I., Rosenberger, J., Majernikova, M., Roland, R., Groothoff, J. W., & van Dijk, J. P. (2014). Adherence in patients in the first year after kidney transplantation and its impact on graft loss and mortality: A cross-sectional and prospective study. *Journal of Advanced Nursing, 70*(12), 2871–2883.

Quittan, M., Wiesinger, G. F., Sturm, B., Puig, S., Mayr, W., Sochor, A., . . . Global Initiative for Chronic Obstructive Lung Disease. (2001). Improvement of thigh muscles by neuromuscular electrical stimulation in patients with refractory heart failure: A single-blind, randomized, controlled trial. *American Journal of Physical Medicine & Rehabilitation, 80*, 206–214, 215–216, 224.

Rabe, K. F., Hurd, S., Anzueto, A., Barnes, P. J., Buist, S. A., Calverly, P., & Zielinski, J. (2007). Global strategy for the diagnosis, management, and prevention of chronic obstructive pulmonary disease: GOLD executive summary. *American Journal of Respiratory and Critical Care Medicine, 176*(6), 532–555.

Rajendran, A. J., Pandurangi, U. M., Mullasari, A. S., Gomathy, S., & Rao, K. V. (2006). High intensity exercise training programme following cardiac transplant. *Indian Journal of Chest Diseases & Allied Sciences, 48*, 271–273.

Rao, V., Oz, M. C., Flannery, M. A., Catanese, K. A., Argenziano, M., & Naka, Y. (2003). Revised screening scale to predict survival after insertion of a left ventricular assist device. *Journal of Thoracic & Cardiovascular Surgery, 125*, 855–862.

Reid, W. D., & Dechman, G. (1995). Considerations when testing and training the respiratory muscles. *Physical Therapy, 75*, 971–982.

Richard, C., Girard, F., Ferraro, P., Chouinard, P., Boudreault, D., Ruel, M., & Girard, D. C. (1955). Acute postoperative pain in lung transplant recipients. *Annals of Thoracic Surgery, 77*, 1951–1955.

Ries, A. L., Kaplan, R. M., Limberg, T. M., & Prewitt, L. M. (1995). Effects of pulmonary rehabilitation on physiologic and psychosocial outcomes in patients with chronic obstructive pulmonary disease. *Annals of Internal Medicine, 122*, 823–832.

Robertson, H. T., Haley, N. R., Guthrie, M., Cardenas, D., Eschbach, J. W., & Adamson, J. W. (1990). Recombinant erythropoietin improves exercise capacity in anemic hemodialysis patients. American Journal of Kidney Diseases. *American Journal of Physical Medicine & Rehabilitation, 15*, 325–332.

Robinson, L. R., Switala, J., Tarter, R. E., & Nicholas, J. J. (1990). Functional outcome after liver transplantation: A preliminary report. *Archives of Physical Medicine and Rehabilitation, 71*, 426–427.

Rudow, D. L., & Goldstein, M. J. (2008). Critical care management of the liver transplant recipient. *Critical Care Nursing Quarterly, 31*, 232–243.

Ryan, T. D., Jefferies, J. L., Zafar, F., & Morales, D. L. (2015). The evolving role of the total artificial heart in the management of end-stage congenital heart disease and adolescents. *American Society for Artificial Internal Organs Journal, 61*(1), 8–14.

Saltin, B., Blomqvist, G., Mitchell, J., Johnson, R. J., Wildenthal, K., & Chapman, C. (1968). Response to exercise after bed rest and after training. *Circulation, 38*(Suppl. 5), 1–80.

Samuel, D., Duclos Vallee, J. C., Teicher, E., & Vittecoq, D. (2003). Liver transplantation in patients with HIV infection. *Journal of Hepatology, 39*(1), 3–6.

Savin, W. M., Haskell, W. L., Schroeder, J. S., & Stinson, E. B. (1980). Cardiorespiratory responses of cardiac transplant patients to graded symptom limited exercise. *Circulation, 62*, 55–60.

Schroeder, J. S., Gao, S. Z., Alderman, E. L., Hunt, S. A., Johnstone, I., Boothroyd, D. B., . . . Stinson, E. B. (1993). A preliminary study of diltiazem in the prevention of coronary artery disease in heart transplant recipients. *New England Journal of Medicine, 328*, 164–170.

Scott, J. P., Hay, I. F., Higenbuttam, C., Evans, D., & Calne, R. Y. (1990). Hypertensive exercise responses in cyclosporine treated normotensive renal transplant recipients. *Nephron, 56*, 143–147.

Seki, A., & Fishbein, M. C. (2014). Predicting the development of cardiac allograft vasculopathy. *Cardiovascular Pathology, 23*(5), 253–260.

Selberg, O., Bottcher, J., Tusch, G., Pichlmayr, R., Henkel, E., & Muller, M. (1997). Identification of high and low-risk patients before liver transplantation: A prospective cohort study of nutritional and metabolic parameters in 150 patients. *Hepatology, 25*, 652–657.

Shaver, J. A., Leon, D. F., Gray, S. D., Leonard, J. J., & Bahnson, H. T. (1969). Hemodynamic observations after cardiac transplantation. *New England Journal of Medicine, 281*, 822–827.

Shephard, R. J., Kavanagh, T., Mertens, D. J., & Yacoub, M. (1996). The place of perceived exertion ratings in exercise prescription for cardiac transplant patients before and after training. *British Journal of Sports Medicine, 30*, 116–121.

Shiba, N., Chan, M. C., Kwok, B. W., Valantine, H. A., Robbins, R. C., & Hunt, S. A. (2004). Analysis of survivors more than 10 years after heart transplantation in the cyclosporine era: Stanford experience. *Journal of Heart and Lung Transplantation, 23*(2), 155–164.

Singal, A. K., Chaha, K. S., Rasheed, K., & Anand, B. S. (2013). Liver transplantation in alcoholic liver disease current status and controversies. *World Journal of Gastroenterology, 19*(36), 5953–5963.

Singal, A. K., & Kamath, P. S. (2013). Model for end-stage liver disease. *Journal of Clinical and Experimental Hepatology, 3*(1), 50–60.

Singer, J. P., & Singer, L. G. (2013). Quality of life in lung transplantation. *Seminars in Respiratory and Critical Care Medicine, 34*(3), 421–430.

Sliwa, J. A., & Blendonohy, P. M. (1988). Stroke rehabilitation in a patient with a history of heart transplantation. *Archives of Physical Medicine and Rehabilitation, 69*, 973–975.

Sliwa, J. A., Andersen, S., & Griffin, J. (1990). Cardiovascular responses to gait training and ambulation in a hemiparetic heart recipient. *Archives of Physical Medicine and Rehabilitation, 71*, 424–425.

Solomon, N. A., McGiven, J. R., Alison, P. M., Ruygrok, P. N., Haydock, D. A., Coverdale, H. A., & West, T. M. (2004). Changing donor and recipient demographics in a heart transplantation program: Influence on early outcome. *Annals of Thoracic Surgery, 77*, 2096–2102.

Song, A. T., Avelino-Silva, V. I., Pecora, R. A., D'Albuquerque, L. A., & Abdala, E. (2014). Liver transplantation: Fifty years of experience. *World Journal of Gastroenterology, 20*(18), 5363–5374.

Squires, R. W. (1991). Exercise training after cardiac transplantation. *Medicine & Science in Sports & Exercise, 23*, 686–694.

Starzl, T. E., Klintmalm, G. B., Porter, K. A., Iwatsuki, S., & Schroter, G. P. (1981). Liver transplantation with use of cyclosporin A and prednisone. *New England Journal of Medicine, 305*, 266–269.

Stewart, K. J., Badenhop, D., Brubaker, P. H., Keteyian, S. J., & King, M. (2003). Cardiac rehabilitation following percutaneous revascularization, heart transplant, heart valve surgery, and for chronic heart failure. *Chest, 123*, 2104–2111.

Stiens, S. A., Reyes, M. R., & Svircev, J. (2008). The Physiatric consultation: Acute treatment, immediate rehabilitation in future enablement. In B. J. O'Young, M. A. Young, & S. A. Stiens (Eds.), *Physical medicine and rehabilitation secrets* (3rd ed., pp. 93–100). St. Louis, MO: Mosby.

Stiens, S. A., Shamberg, S., & Shamberg, A. (2008). Environmental barriers: Solutions for participation, collaboration, and togetherness. In B. J. O'Young, M. A. Young, & S. A. Stiens (Eds.), *Physical medicine and rehabilitation secrets* (3rd ed., pp. 76–86). St. Louis, MO: Mosby.

Stiens, S. A., O'Young, B. J., & Young, M. A. (2008). Person-centered rehabilitation: Interdisciplinary intervention to enhance patient enablement. In B. J. O'Young, M. A. Young, & S. A. Stiens (Eds.), *Physical medicine and rehabilitation secrets* (3rd ed., pp. 118–125). St. Louis, MO: Mosby.

Streiff, N., Feurer, I., Speroff, T., Davis, S. F., Butler, J., Chomsky, D., . . . Wright Pinson, C. (2001). The effects of rejection episodes, obesity, and osteopenia on functional performance and health-related quality of life after heart transplantation. *Transplantation Proceedings, 33*, 3533–3535.

Tayler, A., & Bergin, J. (1995). Cardiac transplantation for the cardiologist not trained in transplantation. *Annals of Thoracic Surgery, 129*, 578–592.

Tegtbur, U., Busse, M. W., Jung, K., Pethig, K., & Haverich, A. (2005). Time course of physical reconditioning during exercise rehabilitation late after heart transplantation. *Journal of Heart & Lung Transplantation, 24*, 270–274.

Tegtbur, U., Pethig, K., Machold, H., Haverich, A., & Busse, M. (2003). Functional endurance capacity and exercise training in long-term treatment after heart transplantation. *Cardiology, 99*, 171–176.

Tomczak, C. R., Tymchak, W. J., & Haykowski, M. J. (2013). Effect of exercise training on pulmonary oxygen uptake kinetics in heart transplant recipients. *The American Journal of Cardiology, 112*(9), 1489–1492.

The U.S. Multicenter FK 506 Liver Study Group. (1994). A comparison of tacrolimus (FK 506) and cyclosporine for immunosuppression in liver transplantation. *New England Journal of Medicine, 331*, 1110–1115.

United States Renal Data System. (2014). *USRDS annual data report: Epidemiology of kidney disease in the United States* (Vol. 2). Bethesda, MD: National Institutes of Health, National Institute of Diabetes and Digestive and Kidney Diseases. Retrieved from https://www.usrds.org/2014/view

Valentine, H., Keogh, A., McIntosh, N., Hunt, S., Oyer, P., & Schroeder, J. (1992). Cost containment: Co-administration of diltiazem with cyclosporine, after heart transplantation. *Journal of Heart & Lung Transplantation, 2*, 1–7.

van den Berg-Emons, R. J., van Ginneken, B. T., Nooijen, C. F., Metselaar, H. J., Tilanus, H. W., Kazemier, G., & Stam, H. J. (2014). Fatigue after liver transplantation: Effects of a rehabilitation program including exercise training and physical activity counseling. *Physical Therapy, 94*(6), 857–865.

van Ginneken, B. T., van den Berg-Emons, R. J., Kazemier, G., Metselaar, H. J., Tilanus, H. W., & Stam, H. J. (2007). Physical fitness, fatigue and quality of life after liver transplantation. *European Journal of Applied Physiology, 100*, 345–353.

Vaska, P. L. (1993). Common infections in heart transplant patients. *American Journal of Critical Care, 2*, 145–156.

Ville, N. S., Varray, A., Mercier, B., Hayot, M., Albat, B., Chamari, K., . . . Mercier, J. (2002). Effects of an enhanced heart rate reserve on aerobic performance in patients with a heart transplant. *American Journal of Physical Medicine & Rehabilitation, 81*, 584–589.

Vintro, A. Q., Krasnoff, J. B., & Painter, P. (2002). Roles of nutrition and physical activity in musculoskeletal complications before and after liver transplantation. *AACN Clinical Issues, 13*, 333–347.

Von Scheidt, W., Kembes, B. M., Reichart, B., & Erdmann, E. (1993). Percutaneous transluminal coronary angioplasty of focal coronary lesions after cardiac transplantation. *Journal of Clinical Investigation, 71*, 524–530.

Walsh, J. R., Chambers, D. C., Davis, R. J., Morris, N. R., Seale, H. E., Yerkovich, S. T., & Hopkins, P. M. (2013). Impaired exercise capacity after lung transplantation is related to delayed recovery of muscle strength. *Clinical Transplant, 27*(4), E504–E511.

Webber, B. A., & Pryor, J. A. (1993). Physiotherapy skills: Techniques and adjuncts. In B. A. Webber & J. A. Pryor (Eds.), *Physiotherapy for respiratory and cardiac problems* (pp. 116–127). Edinburgh, Scotland: Churchill Livingstone.

Wechsler, M. E., Giardina, E. G., Sciacca, R. R., Rose, E. A., & Barr, M. L. (1995). Increased early mortality in women undergoing cardiac transplantation. *Circulation, 91*, 1029–1035.

Wenting, G. J., vd Meiracker, A. H., Simoons, M. I., Stroh, C. I., Har-Zahav, Y., & Fisman, E. Z. (1987). Circadian variation of heart rate but not of blood pressure after heart transplantation. *Transplantation Proceedings, 19*, 2554–2555.

Wertheim, J. A., Petrowsky, H., Saab, S., Kupiec-Weglinski, J. W., & Busuttil, R. W. (2011). Major challenges limiting liver transplantation in the United States. *American Journal of Transplantation, 11*(9), 1773–1784.

Weseman, R. A., & McCashland, T. M. (1998). Nutritional care of the chronic post-transplant patient. *Topics in Clinical Nutrition, 13*, 27–34.

White, C., & Gallagher, P. J. (2010). Effect of patient coping preferences on quality of life following renal transplantation. *Journal of Advanced Nursing, 66*(11), 2550–2559.

Wickerson, L., Mathur, S., & Brooks, D. (2010). Exercise training after lung transplantation: A systemic review. *Journal of Heart and Lung Transplantation, 29*, 497–503.

Wiesinger, G. F., Crevenna, R., Nuhr, M. J., Huelsmann, M., Fialka-Moser, V., & Quittan, M. (2001). Neuromuscular electric stimulation in heart transplantation candidates with cardiac pacemakers. *Archives of Physical Medicine and Rehabilitation, 82*, 1476–1477.

Williams, T. J., Grossman, R. F., & Maurer, J. R. (1990). Long-term functional follow-up of lung transplant recipients. *Clinics in Chest Medicine, 11*, 347–358.

Wolfe, R. A., Ashby, V. B., Milford, E. L., Ojo, A. O., Ettenger, R. E., Agodoa, L. Y., . . . Port, F. K. (1999). Comparison of mortality in all patients on dialysis, patients on dialysis awaiting transplantation and recipients of a first cadaveric transplant. *New England Journal of Medicine, 341*, 1725–1730.

Young, M. A., & O'Young B. J. (2012). Cardiac transplantation. In H. J. Stam, H. M. Buyruk, J. L. Melvin, & G. Stucki (Ed.), *Acute medical rehabilitation* (pp. 251–268). Muğla, Turkey: VitalMed.

Young, M. A., & Stiens, S. A. (2002). Rehabilitation of the transplant patient. In B. J. O'Young, M. A. Young, & S. A. Stiens (Eds.), *Physical medicine and rehabilitation secrets* (2nd ed., pp. 317–320). Philadelphia, PA: Hanley Belfus.

Young, M. A., & Stiens, S. A. (2006). Transplant rehabilitation. In R. H Braddom (Ed.), *Physical medicine and rehabilitation* (3rd ed., pp. 1443–1453). Philadelphia, PA: W. B. Saunders.

Young, M. A., Stiens, S. A., O'Young, B. J., Mayer, R. S. (2011). Transplantation of organs: Rehabilitation to maximize outcomes. In R. L. Braddom & L. Chan (Eds.), *Physical medicine and rehabilitation* (4th ed., pp. 1439–1457). Philadelphia, PA: Elsevier/Saunders.

Yun, J. J., & Mason, D. P. (2009). Lung transplantation: Past, present, and future. *Minerva Chirurgica, 64*, 37–44.

Zarrinpar, A., & Busuttil, R. W. (2013). Liver transplantation: Past, present and future. *Nature Reviews. Gastroenterology and Hepatology, 10*(7), 434–440.

CHAPTER

Psychiatric Disorders

Annalee V. Johnson-Kwochka and Gary R. Bond

Psychiatric disability refers to a psychiatric disorder associated with functional limitations that prevent achievement of age-appropriate goals. The nomenclature and diagnostic criteria for psychiatric disabilities vary widely, however, across the mental health, rehabilitation, and Social Security disability systems. Within the mental health field, serious mental illness is the most common term referring to the population of adults (18 years and older) with serious psychiatric disabilities. Serious mental illness is defined as a diagnosable mental, behavioral, or emotional disorder that causes serious functional impairment and substantially interferes with or limits one or more major life activities (e.g., those relating to employment, self-care, self-direction, interpersonal relationships, learning and recreation, independent living, and economic self-sufficiency; Kessler et al., 2003). According to this definition, approximately 5.5% of American adults have a serious mental illness (Hudson, 2009).

Currently, the diagnostic standards in the mental health field are codified in the International Classification of Diseases and Related Health Problems (ICD, 10th revision; World Health Organization [WHO], 2004), which is in wide use internationally, and the *Diagnostic and Statistical Manual of Mental Disorders, Fifth Edition (DSM-5)*, which is used in the United States (American Psychiatric Association [APA], 2013). Both diagnostic systems are critical sources of mental health and diagnostic information and they correspond closely in content. Both undergo periodic update and revision; ICD-11 is scheduled for release in 2018. Because the *DSM-5* is used in the United States, we will refer to it in this chapter.

The *DSM-5* uses a descriptive, atheoretical stance toward classifying disorders. It attempts to define symptoms of psychiatric disorders based on observable criteria. To increase specificity, the *DSM-5* uses a multiaxial system of diagnosis, with assessment on five distinct dimensions: clinical syndromes (Axis I), personality disorders and mental retardation (Axis II), general medical conditions (Axis III), psychosocial stressors (Axis IV), and current level of functioning (Axis V). Psychiatric disabilities include Axis I (excluding substance use disorders) and personality disorders, although individuals with psychiatric disorders often have co-occurring disorders, such as substance use disorders.

Psychiatric disorders are a leading contributor to the global burden of disease in both developed and developing countries (Whiteford et al., 2013). Common mental disorders refer to psychiatric disorders that are less disabling than serious mental illness but still impact role functioning. In some countries, increased rates of people with common mental disorders on disability rolls have raised concerns (Butterworth, Leach, McManus, & Stansfeld, 2013). This chapter describes both serious mental illness and common mental disorders.

People with psychiatric disabilities constitute one of the largest disability groups served by the state–federal vocational rehabilitation system in the United States, with nearly one fourth of clients receiving vocational rehabilitation services diagnosed with either a psychotic or affective disorder (Salzer, Baron, Brusilovskiy, Lawer, & Mandell, 2011). Similarly, people with psychiatric disabilities constitute approximately one third of all beneficiaries receiving income support from the two disability programs administered by the U.S. Social Security Administration, Social Security Disability Insurance (SSDI), and Supplemental Security Income (SSI; Danziger, Frank, & Meara, 2009).

KEY PSYCHIATRIC DIAGNOSES

The most reliable method for assessing psychiatric disorders is for a trained diagnostician with access to records of the patient's psychiatric history to administer a structured interview (APA, 2013). In practice, however, diagnoses are often given based on far less rigorous assessment procedures. Although important for treatment planning, particularly medication decisions, diagnosis is less relevant to rehabilitation planning than is a functional assessment of the individual's strengths and deficits in specific environments (Corrigan, Mueser, Bond, Drake, & Solomon, 2008).

Information on psychiatric diagnosis is widely available in many sources, ranging from technical manuals (APA, 2013) to less technical but detailed guides for the general public (Mueser & Gingerich, 2006; Solomon, 2000), and personal accounts from those with a psychiatric illness (Jamison, 1997; Styron, 1992).

Schizophrenia and Related Disorders

Schizophrenia is a diagnosis given to a heterogeneous group of disorders affecting every sphere of life, including cognition, emotion, and decision making. Difficulties in social functioning and deficits in social skills are also common features of the disorder (Green, Horan, & Lee, 2015). Schizophrenia is a psychotic disorder that typically includes episodes of impaired reality, as indicated by disorientation and confusion, odd sensory experiences (e.g., hallucinations), false beliefs (e.g., delusions), and/or impairments in the emotional domain (e.g., affect flattening or depression). Schizophrenia is also a thought disorder, as individuals often display distortions in thought content (e.g., delusions) and language and thought processes (e.g., disorganized speech). The course of the illness is highly individualized. For some, there are acute episodes interspersed with normal or near-normal adjustment. In still other instances, the disturbance is relatively continuous, punctuated by periods of temporary improvement and deterioration. Related diagnoses in the *DSM-5* include schizophreniform disorder, which applies when all the symptoms of schizophrenia are present, but the duration of the disorder is less than 6 months, and schizoaffective disorder, where symptoms of schizophrenia are accompanied by prominent affective symptoms (depression and/or mania).

■ Positive Symptoms

Delusions are sometimes bizarre beliefs that do not change in spite of conflicting evidence. Delusions range from innocuous confusions to extensive paranoid delusions involving perceived threats from conspiracies of seemingly unrelated people and events. Delusions often involve ideas of reference, where one attaches personal significance to unrelated activities of others (e.g., concluding that an overheard conversation between strangers refers to oneself). Paranoid delusions may be combined with delusions of grandeur, an exaggerated belief in one's own powers and sometimes the assumption of the identity of a famous person. Some people with schizophrenia believe that they are experiencing thought insertion (alien thoughts inserted into one's mind) or thought broadcasting (that anyone around them may be able to read their thoughts).

Hallucinations are involuntary, perception-like experiences that occur without an external stimulus. Hallucinations may occur in any sensory modality, but auditory hallucinations are the most common (Bauer et al., 2011); these are usually experienced as voices that are perceived as different from an individual's own thoughts. In an international study of schizophrenia, 75% of respondents reported auditory hallucinations, with 39% reporting visual hallucinations (Bauer et al., 2011).

■ Negative Symptoms

Negative symptoms of schizophrenia make up a pattern of nonresponse in people with the illness; passivity, a lack of spontaneity, flat affect (a lack of emotional expression), social withdrawal, a lack of motivation, and anhedonia (an inability to experience pleasure) are common symptoms (APA, 2013). Flat affect is especially common, present in about two thirds of individuals with schizophrenia (Sartorius, Shapiro, & Jablonsky, 1974). Ambivalence (difficulty making decisions) may perpetuate a pattern of inaction. Dysfunctional attitudes and low self-efficacy appear to contribute to negative symptoms in schizophrenia, and are particularly common in early-course patients (Ventura et al., 2014). Overall, negative symptoms are associated with poorer functional outcomes in schizophrenia (Fervaha, Foussias, Agid, & Remington, 2014).

■ Disorganized Symptoms

Disorganized behavior may include childlike silliness and/or unpredictable agitation, difficulty performing the activities of daily living (e.g., difficulties dressing appropriately leading to a disheveled appearance, deficits in personal hygiene) and impairments in goal-directed behavior. Disorganized speech includes loose associations (odd juxtaposition of topics and ideas), neologisms (invented words with private meanings), and poverty of speech (conversation conveying little information; APA, 2013). People with schizophrenia have difficulty with words that have more than one meaning; a word that they interpret with the wrong meaning may lead them off on a tangent. They are also often baffled by simple analogies, as suggested by their poor performance in diagnostic tests requiring that they interpret common proverbs. Transfer of training from one context to another (e.g., applying skills learned in a hospital setting to a community setting) is often poor (Stein & Test, 1980).

Cognitive Deficits

Schizophrenia is associated with notable impairments in the areas of verbal and nonverbal memory, working memory, attention, executive function, and processing speed. A review of empirical studies (including studies that utilized both performance-based measures and neuroimaging) found that people with schizophrenia display deficits in all of these areas as compared with healthy control participants, with the largest deficits found in episodic memory and executive functioning (Reichenberg & Harvey, 2007).

People with schizophrenia range widely in their capacity to apply their intellectual abilities. After the onset of schizophrenia, they often do not attain or regain the level of accomplishment expected by their premorbid educational achievement. When onset of symptoms occurs in adolescence, the educational process and peer-group affiliation are both significantly disrupted. Cognitive functioning in people with schizophrenia may also be a significant predictor of functioning in important areas of life, for example, gaining and keeping a job (McGurk & Mueser, 2004).

Prevalence

Although a commonly cited prevalence rate for schizophrenia has been 0.8% to 1.0% of the population at any given year (Torrey, 2006), more recent reviews suggest that the prevalence rate may be lower than previously thought (Eaton, 1985; Eaton, 1991; Goldner, Hsu, Waraich, & Somers, 2002). A recent systematic review of major epidemiological studies conducted between 1990 and 2013 found a median lifetime prevalence for schizophrenia of 0.48% in general populations, with a 12-month prevalence of 0.33% (Simeone, Ward, Rotella, Collins, & Windisch, 2015). The incidence rate has been estimated at a median value of 15.2 per 100,000 people (Saha et al., 2005).

Important differences in the incidence and prevalence of schizophrenia are found across cultures. In the United States, African Americans are significantly more likely to be diagnosed with schizophrenia, as compared with other ethnoracial groups (Schwartz & Blankenship, 2014). Cultural bias may influence the diagnosis of schizophrenia in African Americans (Schwartz & Blankenship, 2014). People who reside in an urban area or migrate from a rural area to an urban area are also more likely to be diagnosed with the disorder (Cantor-Graae & Selten, 2005; Pedersen & Mortensen, 2001).

Schizophrenia and related disorders rarely develop before adolescence, but show a marked increase in prevalence between ages 15 and 17 (Jacobi et al., 2004). It is most common for people to develop schizophrenia between the ages of 19 and 25; however, as many as 25% of people who develop schizophrenia do so after the age of 25 (Kessler et al., 2007). Women generally have a later age-at-onset than men (Eranti, MacCabe, Bundy, & Murray, 2013). The overall rate of schizophrenia is higher in males (McGrath et al., 2004).

Prognosis

The prognosis for schizophrenia is generally worse than for most other major psychiatric disorders. For many, it is a lifelong, disabling condition. However, contrary to an early misconception promulgated by Emil Kraepelin, the German psychiatrist who first identified a set of syndromes that served as a framework for the diagnosis, schizophrenia does not follow a relentlessly downward course (Harrow, Grossman, Jobe, & Herbener, 2005); rather, it is quite heterogeneous in course and outcome based upon patient-related factors (e.g., age of onset, type of symptoms, acuteness at onset) and other prognostic factors (Jobe & Harrow, 2005). Decline in psychosocial functioning typically plateaus approximately 5 to 10 years after onset of the disorder (McGlashan, 1988). Traditionally, the prognostic rule of thumb for schizophrenia has been that one third are expected to show a sharp decline in functioning, one third to achieve a marginal adjustment, and one third to recover to essentially former levels of functioning (Jobe & Harrow, 2005). With appropriate community support and rehabilitation, a substantially larger percentage may approach former levels of functioning (Harding, Strauss, Hafez, & Liberman, 1987). In addition, the introduction and widespread use of antipsychotic drugs helped to reduce relapse rates and decrease the severity of florid psychotic symptoms (Jobe & Harrow, 2005).

Swift intervention early in the course of psychosis is important for recovery. A longer duration of untreated first episode psychosis is associated with a poorer response to antipsychotic medications and a lower likelihood of functional and symptomatic recovery (Perkins, Gu, Boteva, & Lieberman, 2005; Marshall et al., 2005). Long-term use of antipsychotics, however, may not be the optimal treatment. Recent research found better long-term symptomatic and functional recovery when patients either reduced the dose of antipsychotics or discontinued entirely during the early stages after remission from a first episode of psychosis (Wunderink, Nieboer, Wiersma, Sytema, & Nienhuis, 2013).

Several factors predict the course of schizophrenia, including demographic variables, socioeconomic factors, family history, stress, and drug use (Liberman, Kopelowicz, Ventura, & Gutkind, 2002). For instance, people with schizophrenia who abuse illegal drugs and alcohol after their first psychotic episode are more likely to have future psychiatric hospitalizations and have more psychotic symptoms as compared with those who do not (Sobara, Liraud, Assens, Abalan, & Verdoux, 2003).

Mood Disorders

The two major types of mood disorders (also known as "affective disorders") are unipolar depressive disorders, and bipolar disorders, which also include episodes of mania.

Unipolar Disorders

Whereas disordered thought in schizophrenia is often bizarre and puzzling, the distortions accompanying major depression are usually coherent, albeit often magnifying difficulties and jumping to distorted conclusions from incomplete information or selective attention to details. The cognitive symptoms of depression include pessimistic beliefs, negative self-image (including feelings of guilt and worthlessness), suicidal thoughts, and trouble concentrating (APA, 2013).

Depression also includes physical symptoms such as lethargy, insomnia or hypersomnia, loss of appetite or overeating, and lack of sexual interest (APA, 2013). Severe depression can be termed psychotic when it includes hallucinations or delusions (e.g., "I am dead"). Depression is probably the widest-ranging psychiatric disorder in terms of severity and duration. There are vexing diagnostic problems, for example, in deciding if depressed feelings accompanying a difficult situation, such as physical disability or recent bereavement, qualify as a separate psychiatric diagnosis.

Bipolar Disorders

Bipolar disorder (previously known as "manic depression") differs from major depression primarily in the presence of mania, an episode of elevated or irritable mood. Manic episodes last from several days to several months. In its most severe form, bipolar disorder involves frequent alternation between manic and depressive episodes (rapid cycling), but there are many different patterns including those in which either mania or depression rarely occurs. People experiencing a manic episode are expansive, unrealistically happy (although they can also be irritable when thwarted), impulsive, and easily distracted. They often have an exaggerated belief in their own abilities and make reckless decisions (e.g., extravagant purchases). Another common symptom is nonstop talking (pressured speech), even when others try to break in, or when no one is listening. Their conversation may show flight of ideas in which they quickly shift from one unfinished topic to another.

Bipolar disorder is classified into two primary types: bipolar I disorder and bipolar II disorder. Bipolar I disorder is the more severe form, in which an individual experiences phases of depression and periods of severe, full-blown mania, which may include psychosis. Bipolar II disorder is marked by periods of depression and periods of hypomania, which is a less severe form of the mania characterized by extremely high-energy and mild euphoria, generally without the psychotic symptoms and grandiosity seen in full-blown mania (APA, 2013).

Prevalence

The 12-month prevalence rates of mood disorders are 7% for major depressive disorder, 2% for persistent depressive disorder (a chronically depressed mood for at least 2 years, sometimes also meeting the criteria for major depressive disorder), 0.6% for bipolar I disorder, and 0.8% for bipolar II disorder (APA, 2013). During a lifetime, 16.6% of people will be diagnosed with major depressive disorder; women are significantly more likely to be diagnosed with depression (Kessler et al., 2005). Bipolar disorders have a lifetime prevalence of 1.0% to 1.1% and affect men and women equally (Merikangas et al., 2007). The age of onset for depression is highly variable, while the onset of bipolar disorder is around 20 years of age for both men and women (Merikangas et al., 2007).

Prognosis

Most people with major depression recover, with or without treatment. One longitudinal study found that 60% and 80% of both clinical and nonclinical populations who developed a major depressive episode recovered by 6 months and 1 year, respectively (Coryell et al., 1994). Another study found that approximately half of participants with a depressive mood disorder (i.e., major depressive episode, dysthymic disorder) no longer reported symptoms that met the criteria for the diagnosis at the 3-year follow-up (Forsell, 2007). However, a substantial minority experience recurrent and chronic depression: the 2- and 6-month relapse rates are 20% and 30%, respectively (Belsher & Costello, 1988), and 22% of patients experience an episode persisting more than 1 year (Thornicroft & Sartorius, 1993). Another study found that between 42% (primary care patients) to 61% (psychiatric care patients) of participants with major depression reported experiencing at least one relapse across the 7-year follow-up period; 21% to 26%, respectively, of the two patient groups still met the criteria for major depressive disorder after 7 years (Poutanen et al., 2007).

Between depressive episodes, people with major depression may be highly functional and productive (e.g., as illustrated by the historical examples of Winston Churchill and Abraham Lincoln). With proper treatment, most people with major depression have a good prognosis. Among older adults, however, the prognosis is poorer, complicated by increasing medical conditions that come with aging, and by poorer response to antidepressant medications (Mitchell & Subramaniam, 2005).

Anxiety Disorders

In contrast to psychotic disorders, people with anxiety disorders usually recognize their symptoms, are not out of touch with reality, and are more likely to seek treatment. Hence, these disorders tend to be less severe (Kessler, Dupont, Berglund, & Wittchen, 1999). Anxiety disorders can often be distinguished from nonclinical anxiety through the presence of somatic symptoms (i.e., muscle tension, fatigue, nausea, accelerated heart rate) and the disruption of daily life. High levels of stress or anxiety arousal (muscle tension, rapid heartbeat, etc.) can impair the body's immune system, leading to an increased vulnerability to physical illness. Chronic anxiety also impacts sleep patterns, dietary practices, and exercise.

Prevalence

Affecting approximately 22.2% of the adult population in any given 12-month period and 33.7% over their lifetime (Kessler, Petukhova, Sampson, Zaslavsky, & Wittchen, 2012), anxiety disorders are the most prevalent of all psychiatric diagnoses. Several common anxiety disorders and their individual prevalence rates are listed in Table 20.1.

Prognosis

Long-term prognosis for anxiety disorders varies widely. Many people do achieve full recovery from symptoms. However, anxiety disorders—particularly social anxiety disorder and generalized anxiety disorder—can also take a chronic course, and long-term, moderate levels of impairment

TABLE 20.1

COMMON ANXIETY DISORDERS AND PREVALENCE ESTIMATES			
Diagnosis	**Characteristic Symptoms**	**12-Month Prevalence**	**Lifetime Prevalence**
Panic disorder	Sudden unanticipated attacks of an imminent sense of doom, accompanied by physical symptoms such as increased heart rate, dizziness, or difficulty breathing; in the *DSM-5*, diagnosed with or without agoraphobia.	2%–3%	5.2%
Generalized anxiety disorder	Excessive anxiety and worry across situations, often leading to fatigue, difficulty concentrating, muscle tension, and sleep disturbance.	2.9%	6.2%
Obsessive-compulsive disorder	Intrusive and recurring thoughts and impulses, called *obsessions*, and (in response to the obsession) ritualistic repetitions of illogical behaviors, called *compulsions*.	1.2%	2.7%
Posttraumatic stress disorder	Extreme emotional reaction to a life trauma (i.e., combat, rape, or an accident); the individual reexperiences the feared event in nightmares and flashbacks. Can include estrangement from others, poor concentration, and an inability to recall aspects of the trauma	3.5%	8.0%

Lifetime prevalence rates are from Kessler et al. (2012) and 12-month prevalence rates are from the *DSM-5* (APA, 2013).

associated with anxiety are not uncommon (Rhebergen et al., 2011). In a 7-year, community-based study of anxiety and depressive disorders, 10.9% of the participants experienced a chronic course of illness, while 37.3% were free of symptoms during the entire 7-year follow-up (Rhebergen et al., 2011). Other longitudinal studies have found higher percentages of chronic illness (Bruce et al., 2005; Fichter, Quadflieg, Fischer, & Kohlboeck, 2010). The presence of multiple, co-occurring disorders (i.e., social anxiety disorder and major depressive disorder) is associated with a poorer prognosis (Keller, Krystal, Hen, Neumeister, & Simon, 2005).

Eating Disorders

Eating disorders are characterized by serious and persistent disturbances in eating behavior that can significantly impair physical and psychosocial functioning. They frequently involve unhealthy systems of beliefs and fears about food and body image. Eating disorders are most often diagnosed during adolescence, and (with the exception of binge eating disorder) appear to be more common among women than men. The *DSM-5* includes diagnostic criteria for three main types of eating disorders: anorexia nervosa, bulimia nervosa, and binge eating disorder. Prevalence rates are shown in Table 20.2.

Prognosis

Many people with eating disorders recover over time, but it is also common for these illnesses to take a chronic course. In a 21-year outcome study of patients with anorexia nervosa, 51% of patients were fully recovered at the 21-year follow-up, 21% were partially recovered, 10% still met full diagnostic criteria for the illness, and 16% were deceased due to complications related to anorexia nervosa (Lowe et al., 2001). Meta-analyses have found mortality rates for anorexia and bulimia nervosa to be significantly higher than the general population, while bulimia nervosa generally has a lower mortality rate than anorexia nervosa (Arcelus, Mitchell, Wales, & Nielson, 2011; Birmingham, Su, Hlynsky, Goldmer, & Gao, 2005). There are limited data on the long-term outcome of binge eating disorder; remission rates in randomized controlled trials range from 19% to 65% across studies (Smink, van Hoeken, & Hoek, 2013). Little is known about the course and outcome of binge eating disorder.

Chronic eating disorders can result in long-term physical complications. Anorexia nervosa can result in severe fatigue, menstrual irregularity or permanent loss of menses, and heart complications (Mitchell & Crow, 2006). Bulimia nervosa can be associated with gastrointestinal and dental complications related to frequent vomiting. Individuals

TABLE 20.2

COMMON EATING DISORDERS AND PREVALENCE ESTIMATES

Disorder	Characteristic Symptoms	12-Month Prevalence	Lifetime Prevalence
Anorexia nervosa	• Intense fear of gaining weight • Restriction of food intake, sometimes leading to significantly low body weight	0.4%	4%
Bulimia nervosa	• Recurrent episodes of binge eating, often triggered by negative affect • "Purging" behaviors, i.e., vomiting or misuse of laxatives • Self-evaluation overly influenced by body shape and weight	1% to 1.5%	2%
Binge eating disorder	• Recurrent episodes of binge eating, accompanied by a sense of a lack of control over the behavior • Greater functional impairment and psychiatric comorbidity than weight-matched obese individuals without binge eating disorder	Females = 1.6% Males = 0.8%	2%

Prevalence rates for bulimia nervosa and anorexia nervosa are for women only from Keski-Rahkonen et al. (2007) and prevalence rates for binge eating disorder are from Kessler et al. (2013).

with bulimia nervosa are also at an elevated risk for suicide, substance abuse, major depressive disorder, and borderline personality disorder (Mehler, 2011; Mitchell & Crow, 2006). People with binge eating disorder have medical complications related to obesity and increased health care utilization even when compared with body mass index (BMI)-matched control subjects (Bulik, Sullivan, & Kendler, 2002).

Personality Disorders

Personality disorders are defined by the presence of inflexible and maladaptive personality traits that cause significant functional impairment or subjective distress. They are highly comorbid with other mental illnesses. Severe cases of personality disorders may be accompanied by brief psychotic symptoms. Personality disorders are grouped into three clusters in the *DSM-5* (see Table 20.3).

Diagnosis of most personality disorder subtypes is unreliable. Two of the better-researched personality disorders are borderline personality disorder (BPD) and antisocial personality disorder (ASPD).

■ Borderline Personality Disorder

BPD is associated with extreme difficulty in regulating emotions and thoughts, leading to impulsive, reckless behavior and difficulty in maintaining stable relationships (APA, 2013). Self-harm and suicidal behaviors are also common among people with BPD.

■ Antisocial Personality Disorder

ASPD is defined by a pattern of socially irresponsible, exploitative, and guiltless behavior. People with this disorder—which is more common among men—often fail to conform to the law, maintain employment, or develop stable relationships. ASPD is highly associated with co-occurring mental health, addictive, and medical disorders, and people with ASPD also tend to have high mortality rates due to accidents, suicides, and homicides (Black, 2015). Most people diagnosed with ASPD develop symptoms during childhood, and are diagnosed with conduct disorder prior to age 18 (Black, 2015). Symptoms usually continue through adulthood, although there is evidence that some people may improve with age; conflicts with law enforcement tend to cease around middle age, but trouble with relationships and employment continue (Black, 2015).

■ Prognosis

There is limited research literature on the prognosis of people living with personality disorders. We do not yet have many effective treatment strategies to

TABLE 20.3

PERSONALITY DISORDERS		
Cluster	**Diagnosis**	**Symptoms**
Odd/Eccentric Cluster	*Paranoid personality disorder*	Pervasive and unwarranted suspiciousness and mistrust of others
	Schizoid personality disorder	Detachment from social relationships and a restricted range of expression of emotions
	Schizotypal personality disorder	Eccentric behavior
Dramatic/Emotional/Erratic Cluster	*Antisocial personality disorder*	Violation of the rights of others without remorse
	Borderline personality disorder	Impulsivity and a pervasive pattern of instability of interpersonal relationships, self-image, and affects
	Narcissistic personality disorder	An exaggerated sense of self-importance and need for admiration
	Histrionic personality disorder	Excessive emotionality and attention seeking
Anxious/Fearful Cluster	*Avoidant personality disorder*	Extreme social discomfort
	Dependent personality disorder	Submissive behavior
	Obsessive-compulsive personality disorder	Pervasive orderliness and perfectionism

help such individuals "recover" from a personality disorder, although with targeted interventions, promising functional improvements have been shown for some diagnoses (Linehan & Armstrong, 1991). Specifically, in recent years, dialectical behavior therapy has been shown to be an effective treatment for BPD, particularly in regard to a reduction in suicide attempts (Linehan et al., 2006)

CO-OCCURRING CONDITIONS

Substance Abuse

Substance abuse disorder is among the most common co-occurring disorders in all psychiatric disabilities, affecting 50% of people with psychiatric disabilities at some point in their lifetime (Regier et al., 1990). Substance abuse is a complicating factor in psychiatric disability because of its interaction with the mental illness and with psychotropic medications. Presence of a dual diagnosis of substance abuse with psychiatric disabilities has consistently been associated with negative outcomes including increased relapses and hospitalizations, housing instability and homelessness, violence, economic burden on the family, serious infections such as HIV and hepatitis, treatment nonadherence (Drake, Mercer-McFadden, Mueser, McHugo, & Bond, 1998), as well as problems with the legal system, occupational dysfunction, and reduced access to health care (Compton, Weiss, West, & Kaslow, 2005).

Anxiety Disorders

Anxiety disorders are highly comorbid with other psychiatric diagnoses, including other anxiety disorders, mood and eating disorders, and schizophrenia spectrum disorders (Kaye, Bulik, Thornton, Barbarich, & Masters, 2004; Kroenke, Spitzer,

Williams, Monahan, & Lowe, 2007; Young et al., 2013). Research suggests that anxiety disorders may represent additional vulnerability to other psychiatric illnesses, since anxiety disorders often develop prior to other psychopathology, that is depression or anorexia nervosa (Kaye et al., 2004).

In particular, posttraumatic stress disorder (PTSD) is a common comorbid diagnosis in people with psychiatric disabilities, with prevalence rates for current PTSD diagnosis ranging between 29% and 43% in some studies (Mueser et al., 1998; Rosenberg et al., 2001). Exposure to trauma and the presence of PTSD are associated with poorer functioning in people with psychiatric disabilities, including more severe symptoms, poorer health, and higher rates of psychiatric and medical hospitalization (Switzer et al., 1999).

Medical Conditions and Early Mortality

Up to 75% of people with schizophrenia have at least one co-occurring medical condition. Compared to the general population, people with schizophrenia are at much higher risk for cardiometabolic conditions such as abdominal obesity, hypertension, low high-density lipoprotein cholesterol, hypertriglyceridemia, metabolic syndrome, and diabetes, compared to controls (Vancampfort et al., 2013). Substantially higher rates of tobacco use and addiction contribute to higher rates of medical morbidity and mortality in people with schizophrenia and other psychiatric disorders (Ziedonis et al., 2008). Epidemiological studies have increasingly documented higher mortality rates at younger ages for people with serious mental illness, with one meta-analysis estimating an average of 10 years lost for people with serious mental illness compared to the general population (Walker, McGee, & Druss, 2015).

FUNCTIONAL PRESENTATION OF PSYCHIATRIC DISABILITY

Interpersonal Issues

People with psychiatric disabilities generally have much smaller social networks than those with less serious or without mental health conditions. In one study of people with serious mental illness, participants identified an average of only four critical members of their social network who provided support in some capacity (Goldberg, Rollins, & Lehman, 2003). Often, an immediate family member or mental health professional provides the only continuous social contact (Pescosolido, Wright, & Lutfey, 1999). The prevalence of negative or depressive symptoms is associated with a smaller social network (Meeks & Hammond, 2001). People with psychiatric disabilities may avoid seeking contact with others, and their symptoms may strain existing family and caregiver relationships. In most studies of people with severe psychiatric disabilities, the rate of those currently married is 20% or less, with particularly low rates reported for men with schizophrenia (Rogers, Anthony, & Jansen, 1988).

In schizophrenia, the development of the illness has a complex relationship with the person's social network. It is common for people to become socially isolated during the prodromal phase of schizophrenia (before the initial onset of psychotic symptoms), which may in turn exacerbate the development of delusions (Mueser & Jeste, 2008). During the course of illness, negative symptoms appear to interfere most with the formation and maintenance of intimate relationships; in particular, avolition—a decrease in goal-directed behaviors—correlates with lower quality of life and a smaller social network (Rocca et al., 2014).

Disability in anxiety disorders may be partially explained by avoidance behavior (Hendriks et al., 2014). For example, among people with social anxiety disorder, many social or "performance" situations (i.e., participating in a group discussion at work) provoke an immediate anxiety response, and are later avoided. Avoidance behavior may significantly decrease a person's social engagement.

Vulnerability to Stress

Stress is an important mechanism in the underlying pathophysiology that influences the development of depression and anxiety disorders (Mineka & Zinbarg, 2006). Childhood experiences of diminished control in important situations may lead to the development of cognitive biases that cause people to respond maladaptively to common life stressors (i.e., perceiving things as out of one's control) and lead to the development of anxiety and depression (Chorpita & Barlow, 1998).

People with schizophrenia are much more likely to relapse into psychotic symptoms when living in families with high expressed emotion, that is, families who are hostile and critical (Butzlaff & Hooley, 1998). Similar findings have been reported for major depression and bipolar disorder (Mueser & Glynn, 1995).

Unemployment and Poverty

While the majority of adults with psychiatric disabilities want to work and feel that work is an important goal in their recovery, only 15% of clients with psychiatric disabilities enrolled in community mental health programs are competitively employed at any time (Bond & Drake, 2014). The most common reason given for not seeking work is the fear of losing the Social Security benefits and other entitlements (MacDonald-Wilson, Rogers, Ellison, & Lyass, 2003).

Poverty is another common consequence of psychiatric disability (Draine, Salzer, Culhane, & Hadley, 2002). Many people with psychiatric disabilities are unable to meet basic needs, such as those relating to housing, mental health care, transportation, and personal safety (Perese, 2007). Among people with severe psychiatric disabilities attending mental health programs, 80% or more typically have government entitlements as their main source of support (Rogers et al., 1988).

Living Situation

Many people with psychiatric disabilities are not well integrated in community life, and the majority of individuals are unsatisfied with their current living situation (Perese, 2007). Fortunately, relatively few spend years in psychiatric hospitals, as was the case a half-century ago. In the United States, at any given time only a minority of people with schizophrenia are living independently; perhaps a quarter or more (especially young adults) are living with their families; and the remainder live in supervised housing, hospitals, nursing homes, jails/prisons, shelters, or are experiencing homelessness (Torrey, 2006). In one large-scale study of mental health service users in San Diego County, about 20% of people with schizophrenia had experienced homelessness (Folsom et al., 2005). Men, African Americans, and people with comorbid substance abuse disorder were more likely to have been homeless. Among those counted as "living in the community" are many who lead isolated, barren lives without social or recreational outlets (Segal & Aviram, 1978). Unfortunately, "successful discharges" from psychiatric hospitals often include individuals transferred to nursing homes (Grabowski, Aschbrenner, Feng, & Mor, 2009) and supervised group home settings. Some observers have suggested that in this process, many patients have not been deinstitutionalized but are transinstitutionalized. Studies of homelessness further document the grim realities of psychiatric disabilities, as research has shown that homeless individuals with psychiatric disabilities are more likely to utilize inpatient and emergency services than outpatient services (Folsom et al., 2005).

Criminal Justice Involvement

In the United States, criminal justice involvement among people with serious mental illness now exceeds half those in the public mental health system (Frounfelker, Glover, Teachout, Wilkniss, & Whitley, 2010; Robertson, Swanson, Frisman, Lin, & Swartz, 2014). Arrests, court hearings, and other law enforcement actions undermine positive self-identity and decrease access to jobs, housing, and other community resources that promote recovery (Baron, Draine, & Salzer, 2013; Tschopp, Perkins, Hart-Katuin, Born, & Holt, 2007). Criminal justice involvement increases the likelihood of rearrest, stigma, reluctance of professionals to provide assistance, and difficulty accessing mental health and rehabilitation services (McGuire & Rosenheck, 2004; Osher, Steadman, & Barr, 2003). Incarceration further exacerbates the negative impact of criminal justice involvement.

The widely held belief that mental illness leads to increased risk of violent behavior is a damaging stereotype, reinforced by dramatic examples (e.g., the assassination attempt on President Reagan by John Hinkley, who has a diagnosis of schizophrenia). Although rates of violent behaviors in adults with psychiatric disabilities are slightly higher than those with no psychiatric diagnosis (Arseneault, Moffitt, Caspi, Taylor, & Silva, 2000; Swanson, Holzer, Ganju, & Jono, 1990), the vast majority of individuals with psychiatric disabilities do not commit violent acts. When violence does occur, it is often associated with substance abuse, medication nonadherence, past violent victimization, and violence in the surrounding environment (Steadman et al., 1998; Swanson et al., 2002; Swartz et al., 1998).

In schizophrenia, involvement with the criminal justice system is associated with the prevalence of disorganized symptoms (Fukunaga & Lysaker, 2013). Among people with schizophrenia, those with comorbid substance abuse have much higher rates of violence. Higher rates of violence have also been associated with the presence of particular delusional symptoms, including feeling threatened or controlled by external forces or people (Mueser & Jeste, 2008).

Victimization and Trauma

Victimization of people with psychiatric disabilities is a serious public health problem, as they are 11 times more likely to be victimized by violence and crime than the general population (Teplin, McClelland, Abram, & Weiner, 2005). Between 43% and 81% of people with psychiatric disabilities report some type of victimization over their lifetime (Rosenberg et al., 2001). Victimization of this group occurs in many forms, such as physical and sexual assaults, verbal abuse, exploitation, bullying, threats, and theft, often at the hands of others in the community, caregivers, and even family members (Perese, 2007). In a large-scale survey, one third of men and women with schizophrenia reported severe physical or sexual assault in the past year (Goodman et al., 2001). In addition, up to 53% of people with psychiatric disabilities report childhood sexual or physical abuse (Rosenberg et al., 2001). One study of people with schizophrenia living in the community found that participants were at least 14 times more likely to be victims of a violent crime than to be arrested for one (Brekke, Prindle, Woo Bae, & Long, 2001). Given the high prevalence, especially among homeless women, interpersonal violence can be considered a normative experience for people with psychiatric disabilities (Goodman, Dutton, & Harris, 1997).

Increased Risk for Suicide

People who die by suicide have very high rates of psychiatric disability (Cavanagh, Carson, Sharpe, & Lawrie, 2003). The yearly suicide prevalence rate for major depression is approximately 0.29%, with similar rates for bipolar disorder. Overall, the risk for suicide regarding mood disorders is 20 to 30 times that of the general population (Tondo, Isacsson, & Baldessarini, 2003). The lifetime suicide rate for people with schizophrenia has been estimated to be between 1.8% and 5.6% (Palmer, Pankratz, & Bostwick, 2005). The risk for suicide is especially great for those who are younger and newly diagnosed with the disorder, and is most often precipitated by a stressful life event like the death of a family member (Palmer et al., 2005).

A recent meta-analysis concluded that the onset of major depression is predictive of suicidal thoughts and urges, but not actual suicide attempts. Instead, commonly comorbid disorders characterized by anxiety, agitation, and poor impulse control (i.e., bipolar disorder, PTSD) are associated with carrying out a suicide attempt (Nock, Hwang, Sampson, & Kessler, 2003).

Environmental Influences

Although many of the characteristics already described are directly related to psychiatric symptoms, they are also influenced by external factors (e.g., institutionalization and societal attitudes). For example, the inhibiting effects of hospital and nursing homes undoubtedly reinforce the passivity and withdrawal so prominent in psychiatric disabilities (Goffman, 1961). At the societal level, the labeling process in mental illness is demoralizing and discriminatory (Estroff, 1989). Sometimes, individuals with psychiatric disabilities internalize social stigma, creating feeling of demoralization, reduced self-esteem, and barriers to self-empowerment and the attainment of important life goals (Corrigan et al., 2008). Moreover, employers attach more stigma to psychiatric disabilities than to physical disabilities (Thornicroft, 2006). In the housing domain, the NIMBY (Not In My Back Yard) prejudice against people with psychiatric disabilities is intense; group homes are especially likely to meet with community resistance if located in conservative, middle-class neighborhoods (Segal & Aviram, 1978). Stigma and discrimination continue to be significant barriers to community integration (Hall, Graf, Fitzpatrick, Lane, & Birkel, 2003; Wahl, 1997).

TREATMENT AND REHABILITATION

History of Treatment Approaches

Prior to the 1950s, numerous somatic treatments were used for schizophrenia and other serious mental illnesses (Isaac & Armat, 1990). With the exception of electroconvulsive therapy, none of these proved to be effective and many were harmful. Psychiatric hospitalization in large state-run facilities providing little more than custodial care (and often neglect) was standard practice. Beginning in the 1950s, a combination of economic, legal, and humanitarian factors in addition to the widespread use of antipsychotic medications led to deinstitutionalization, the process of releasing patients from state hospitals (Talbott, 1978). The resident population of state and county mental hospitals, which peaked at 558,922 in 1955, declined to 52,000 by 2005 (Manderscheid, Atay, & Crider, 2009). In 1963, the Community Mental Health Centers Act authorized the creation of a network of community mental health centers (CMHCs) with a broad mission to address the mental health needs of the nation including the care and treatment of discharged patients with mental disorders (U.S. Congress, 1963). Altogether, 789 CMHCs were eventually funded, providing public mental health services for people with psychiatric disabilities (Torrey, 2006).

Initially, most CMHCs were unprepared to serve the intended population, for reasons including unrealistic expectations about the efficacy of medications (i.e., the assumption that medications alone would allow individuals to function in the community), poor planning (e.g., too few CMHCs to serve the large numbers of patients being released from hospitals), poor coordination and execution of services (e.g., lack of communication between hospitals and CMHCs; CMHCs were not taking responsibility for patients upon hospital discharge), and funding irregularities (Torrey, 2006). Finally, CMHCs failed to address a wide range of needs relating to housing, employment, socialization, and other areas of functioning discussed previously. The phenomenon of revolving-door clients—clients repeatedly readmitted to psychiatric hospitals—was one consequence of this limited treatment focus. Periodically, state and local governments have cut mental health budgets, eliminating funding for psychiatric beds, which has in turn typically led to increased emergency department use (Nesper, Morris, Scher, & Holmes, 2015).

Pharmacological Treatments

■ Medications for Schizophrenia

About two thirds of people with schizophrenia benefit from antipsychotic medications, which include chlorpromazine (Thorazine), thioridazine (Mellaril), and haloperidol (Haldol). The efficacy of antipsychotic medications in reducing the relapse rate and the positive symptoms of schizophrenia is well established (Dixon, Lehman, & Levine, 1995). Unfortunately, antipsychotics have troubling side effects that usually increase with long-term use. One of the most serious side effects, tardive dyskinesia, involves stereotyped, involuntary movements of the mouth and face and is usually irreversible. Other common, difficult side effects include significant weight gain, drowsiness, sexual dysfunction, and low blood pressure. Another limitation of antipsychotics is their lack of impact on negative symptoms.

Beginning in 1990, several atypical antipsychotic drugs were developed and approved for use in the United States by the Food and Drug Administration (FDA), including clozapine (Clozaril), risperidone (Risperdal), and aripiprazole (Abilify). Atypicals were heavily marketed (with great success) by pharmaceutical companies (Wang, West, Tanielian, & Pincus, 2000). Early optimistic reports of significantly greater effectiveness with fewer side effects for atypical antipsychotics as compared to the traditional drugs generally have not been borne out (Lieberman et al., 2005). The one exception has been clozapine, which is the most effective of the newer antipsychotics. Clozapine has shown benefits for patients who do not respond to other antipsychotic medications (McEvoy et al., 2006). One major drawback of atypicals is that they are priced many times higher than traditional antipsychotics. Some atypical antipsychotics (especially clozapine and olanzapine) have also been associated with clinically significant bodyweight gain (Allison et al., 1999), increasing the risk of medical comorbidity including diabetes, hypertension, cardiovascular disease, and high cholesterol (Geddes, Freemantle, Harrison, & Bebbington, 2000).

Medications for Mood Disorders

A range of drugs have been used in the treatment of mood disorders. Lithium is used to treat bipolar disorder, particularly during the manic phases, although it is also used by patients who have never had manic episodes. It is highly effective in preventing manic episodes (Prien, Klett, & Caffey, 1973). Lithium is lethal in high doses, so patients require careful blood monitoring. More recently, anticonvulsant medications (e.g., Depakote and Lamictal), and atypical antipsychotic medications have been prescribed as treatments for acute and mixed phases in bipolar disorders, particularly for those patients who do not respond to or cannot tolerate lithium.

Various antidepressant drugs have been used for major depression. Before the 1990s, the most common were the tricyclics, including amitriptyline (Elavil) and monoamine oxidase inhibitors (MAOIs), such as tranylcypromine (Parnate). These drugs are rarely prescribed today because they have serious side effects, including irregularities in the cardiovascular system (for tricyclics) and life-threatening hypertension facilitated by the interaction between MAOIs and certain foods.

A group of antidepressants known as selective serotonin reuptake inhibitors (SSRIs) including fluoxetine (Prozac), and sertraline (Zoloft) have favorable side effect profiles (Glod, 1996; Möller & Volz, 1996) and are prescribed for major depression and a wide array of other psychiatric disorders. Evidence of publication bias in clinical trials of SSRIs cast doubt on the strength of the findings for these medications (Turner, Matthews, Linardatos, Tell, & Rosenthal, 2008).

Recently, mixed reuptake inhibitors that block the reuptake of serotonin and norepinephrine in the brain (e.g., venlafaxine [Effexor] and duloxetine [Cymbalta]) and drugs that inhibit dopamine and norepinephrine uptake (e.g., bupropion [Wellbutrin]) have been developed.

Medications for Anxiety Disorders

People with anxiety disorders are often prescribed benzodiazepines, including diazepam (Valium) and alprazolam (Xanax). These drugs have major drawbacks in that they may lead to physical and psychological dependence and are dangerous if taken in combination with alcohol (Brunette, Noordsy, Xie, & Drake, 2003). Because of this, SSRIs are also commonly prescribed to treat anxiety disorders.

Medication Nonadherence

Medication nonadherence is a major barrier to effective treatment of psychotic disorders, with at least half of patients not taking drugs as prescribed (Lacro, Dunn, Dolder, Leckband, & Jeste, 2002). One review concluded that patients on antipsychotics took an average of 58% of the recommended amount, with higher adherence rates for patients on antidepressants (Cramer & Rosenheck, 1998). In mood disorders, a review of empirical studies found that the median prevalence rate for medication nonadherence ranges from 41% to 53%. Risk factors for nonadherence in affective disorders include self-stigma or negative attitudes about their illness, the degree of "choice" in treatment options, the quality of the doctor–patient relationship, and comorbid drug and alcohol use (Lingam & Scott, 2002).

Nonadherence to treatment regimens in psychiatric disabilities has serious consequences, often resulting in higher rates of relapse and rehospitalization and poorer community adjustment. Fundamental to any medication treatment is the identification of the optimal dosage level. With careful monitoring, the use of much lower dosage levels than usually prescribed can reduce side effects while retaining the positive effects of antipsychotics (Hogarty et al., 1988). Medication education (Wallace, Liberman, MacKain, Blackwell, & Eckman, 1992) and behavioral tailoring (i.e., fitting medication-taking into daily routines; Mueser et al., 2002) are strategies used to increase adherence. Another strategy to ensure adherence to antipsychotic medication is to substitute long-acting injectable forms of medications such as fluphenazine decanoate (Prolixin) for the usual oral administration (Kane, Woerner, & Sarantakos, 1986).

Trends in Psychopharmacology

A variety of psychotropic medications, especially antidepressants and antipsychotics, have been prescribed off-label for psychiatric illnesses (i.e., prescribed for conditions, or for patient subgroups, such as children, for which they have not been approved) (Alexander, Gallagher, Mascola,

Moloney, & Stafford, 2011; Thomas, Conrad, Casler, & Goodman, 2006). While off-label prescriptions can be clinically useful, in practice their usage often has no scientific support (Stafford, 2008) and is associated with adverse outcomes (Maher et al., 2011). In addition, many doctors prescribe multiple psychotropic medications in the same class (e.g., two antipsychotics) to one patient—a phenomenon called polypharmacy; 60% of patients in outpatient psychiatry settings are prescribed two or more medications (Mojtabai & Olfson, 2010). Polypharmacy increases the potential for adverse drug–drug interactions (Mojtabai & Olfson, 2010). These trends suggest an over-reliance on medication for the treatment of mental illness.

Psychotherapy

Psychotherapy is another method of treating people with serious mental illness; medications and "talk" therapies are often used in concert. Like medication, there are many different psychotherapeutic approaches, and there is no single "best" approach. Research has consistently found that the quality of the therapeutic alliance between therapist and patient has a significant impact on treatment outcome and may be more critical than the specific psychotherapy model (Krupnick et al., 1996). The therapeutic alliance is characterized by mutual respect, empathy, honesty, and unconditional positive regard (Turkington, Kingdon, & Weiden, 2006). Furthermore, effective psychotherapies have been found to share several common factors (Wampold, 2015). Effective interventions for people with psychiatric disabilities entail direct, unambiguous communication, supportive, noncritical attitudes, and a focus on problem-solving and skills training (Mueser & Gingerich, 2006). In the following we briefly outline two broad orientations to psychotherapy, as well evidence for and against their efficacy.

■ Cognitive-Behavioral Therapies

The central tenet of cognitive-behavioral therapy (CBT) contends that it is possible to ameliorate emotional distress by correcting maladaptive patterns of cognition and behavior. For example, CBT for depression might involve making "thought records" designed to test the validity of a client's negative beliefs such as, "I made a mistake, and now my supervisor thinks I'm useless." The therapist might ask the client to make a list of evidence for and against this belief; evidence against the belief might include "my supervisor asks me for feedback." Making "thought records" can help clients develop more balanced beliefs, such as, "Making mistakes is normal. I can learn from this. My supervisor will be impressed to see me learning from my mistakes and incorporating her feedback." CBT leads to symptom reduction in adult and childhood depression, generalized anxiety disorder, panic disorder, social phobia, and PTSD, and is hallmarked by large effects (Butler, Chapman, Forman, & Beck, 2006). CBT is also an effective adjunct to pharmacological treatment in schizophrenia. Empirical reviews have found that CBT results in decreases in positive symptoms and fewer psychotic relapses (Turkington, Kingdon, & Weiden, 2006), as well as a reduction in negative symptoms that may persist across time. There are many different varieties and adaptations of CBT tailored to particular theoretical orientations or specific diagnoses. Mindfulness and awareness training has been added to some forms of CBT (Segal, Williams, & Teasdale, 2002). Dialectical behavior therapy (DBT) was developed specifically for the treatment of borderline personality disorder (Linehan et al., 2006).

■ Client-Centered and Psychodynamic Therapies

In contrast to cognitive and behaviorally based therapies, client-centered and psychodynamic therapies attempt to resolve emotional distress by uncovering the patient's underlying emotions and internal conflicts. Psychodynamic therapies, in particular, are controversial because of their historical association with hierarchical, paternalistic, and sometimes damaging techniques. Client-centered therapy (also known as person-centered therapy) focuses on enabling the client to actualize their full human potential through nondirective responses from the therapist (Rogers, 1951). Today, a reasonable body of evidence suggests that revised forms of short-term psychodynamic and client-centered therapies are effective for a wide variety of disorders, including personality, anxiety, mood, and eating disorders (Bogels, Wijts, Oort, & Sallaerts, 2014; Driessen et al., 2015; Leichsenring, Rabung, & Leibing, 2004).

Intensive psychotherapeutic approaches emphasizing insight and exploration of childhood experiences, however, are not helpful and are sometimes harmful for individuals with schizophrenia (Drake & Sederer, 1986). The Schizophrenia Patient Outcomes Research Team (PORT) specifically recommended that psychodynamic therapies emphasizing transference and regression not be used for people with schizophrenia (Lehman, Steinwachs, & PORT Co-Investigators, 1998).

Group Therapy

Community mental health centers often provide psychotherapy, counseling, and skills training in a group format. Group approaches differ fundamentally from individual (dyadic) psychotherapy by virtue of "therapeutic factors," such as cohesiveness, universality, acceptance by the group, and vicarious learning (Yalom & Leszcz, 2005). Many of these therapeutic mechanisms can only be experienced within a group format. Group approaches are also more cost-effective than individual approaches, and on balance, the evidence suggests that group approaches are as effective as individual approaches with a wide range of psychiatric disorders, including serious mental illness (McRoberts, Burlingame, & Hoag, 1998). Group approaches are not suited to all clients, however. Some clients have strong preferences regarding group versus individual formats, and these preferences are crucial considerations for determining which format would be a better option.

Telemedicine

The ever-increasing prevalence of technology in daily life represents an opportunity to expand mental health services to areas and populations that have been historically underserved. Recent research suggests that using videoconferencing, mobile technology, and other technology-based tools may expand access to diagnostic and therapeutic care of comparable quality to in-person services (Hilty et al., 2013). A trial of a technology-based collaborative care model in rural mental health clinics (without access to onsite psychiatrists) has suggested that telemedicine may be an effective model of care for depression (Fortney et al., 2007). This is a new field, and additional research is necessary to establish the efficacy of and best-practices for treatment via these new technologies.

Other Psychotherapeutic Approaches

Effective treatments for mood disorders include mindfulness-based therapies (Kuyken et al., 2008), interpersonal therapy (de Mello, de Jesus Mari, Bacaltchuk, Verdeli, & Neugebauer, 2005), and behavioral activation techniques (Cuijpers, Van Straten, & Warmerdam, 2007). Other evidence-based therapeutic interventions for anxiety disorders include behavioral techniques, such as exposure-based therapies (i.e., for the treatment of PTSD; Foa et al., 1999) and systematic desensitization (i.e., for the treatment of specific phobias; Choy, Fyer, & Lipsitz, 2007).

Psychiatric Rehabilitation

Psychiatric rehabilitation refers to interventions to help people with psychiatric disabilities achieve optimal functioning and full integration into society ". . . so that they are successful and satisfied in their environments of choice with the least amount of ongoing professional intervention" (Anthony, Cohen, Farkas, & Gagne, 2002, p. 2.) Psychiatric rehabilitation addresses the many psychosocial challenges associated with psychiatric disabilities, such as unemployment, cognitive impairment, deficits in interpersonal functioning, isolation, difficulties managing personal affairs, vulnerability to stress, independent living, and housing instability. Psychiatric rehabilitation services focus on both enhancing client skills and providing supports to help clients overcome barriers to community integration.

Psychiatric rehabilitation services are most effective when closely integrated with mental health treatments (Corrigan et al., 2008). Unfortunately, in many countries, including the United States, mental health and rehabilitation services are funded by separate agencies, leading to segregation of services in different service systems. Starting in the 1970s, community mental health centers began expanding their role in providing employment, residential, and case management services (Turner & TenHoor, 1978), while stand-alone psychiatric rehabilitation centers, common in an earlier era (Dincin, 1995), have had a diminishing role in the

United States. Integrating rehabilitation services with mental health treatment has been challenging.

Most psychiatric rehabilitation approaches embrace a common set of evidence-based principles including individualized and comprehensive assessment, planning, and intervention; community integration (helping clients exit patient roles, treatment centers, segregated housing arrangements, and/or sheltered work); pragmatism (helping clients with the practical problems in everyday life, with services organized around specific, tangible goals); client choice (empowering clients to set personally meaningful goals and make informed decisions in their treatment and rehabilitation, and basing services on shared decision making); building on client strengths; promoting hope (building self-confidence and optimism); and integration of treatment and rehabilitation (Corrigan et al., 2008). These principles mirror the guiding principles for the field of rehabilitation in general.

Numerous psychiatric rehabilitation approaches have been developed over the last half-century (Corrigan et al., 2008). In an effort to identify best practices, a variety of research groups have issued guidelines based on expert recommendations, consisting mostly of practices that have been systematically evaluated in randomized controlled trials and consequently been designated as evidence-based (Drake, Goldman, et al., 2001). One such guideline development is the Schizophrenia PORT psychosocial treatment recommendations (Dixon et al., 2010). In this section, we describe several widely disseminated evidence-based psychiatric rehabilitation practices.

Assertive Community Treatment

In the 1970s Stein and Test (1980) developed and evaluated a service model for serious mental illness known as assertive community treatment (ACT) that deeply influenced psychiatric rehabilitation practice. Test and Stein (1976) had concluded that hospital training programs to prepare psychiatric patients for community living after discharge were ineffective, and that providing training and support within community settings after discharge was superior. The principle of in vivo assessment, training, and support is a cornerstone of the model. Most ACT team contacts occur in clients' homes and neighborhoods, rather than in agency offices. ACT emphasizes a holistic approach to services, helping with illness management, medication management, housing, finances, and anything else critical to an individual's community adjustment. With the locus of contact in the community, ACT uses assertive outreach to engage clients who do not keep clinic appointments. Low client–staff ratios permit multiple contacts each week with clients needing intensive support. ACT employs a multidisciplinary team of mental health professionals representing various disciplines (e.g., psychiatry, nursing, case management, vocational, and substance abuse specialists), providing intensive, timely, and personalized services, facilitated through frequent team meetings to review treatment plans and services. ACT is a direct service model, with practitioners providing most needed services themselves rather than referring to other providers. Another ACT innovation was integration of services, which has demonstrated advantages over brokered approaches (i.e., referring clients to other programs for many services). ACT teams integrate mental health treatment, housing, rehabilitation, and many other services, and tailor them to the needs and goals of each client.

ACT was originally developed for patients being discharged from psychiatric hospitals but quickly evolved into a service model for people with frequent psychiatric hospitalizations. As an intensive and therefore expensive service model, ACT is most appropriate for clients who do not benefit from office-based services. ACT teams also serve clients with mental illness who are homeless, have co-occurring substance use disorders, and/or have criminal justice involvement (Bond & Drake, 2015). In 1999, the Supreme Court, citing the Americans with Disabilities Act, handed down the Olmstead decision. This decision stipulated that states must provide community services to enable people with disabilities to live in their own homes rather than in institutions or in congregate facilities. Subsequently, the U.S. Department of Justice has led successful class action suits against numerous states to conform to this decision (Burnim, 2015). In many cases, these suits have led to settlements committing state departments of mental health to implement large-scale dissemination of ACT teams to assist patients exiting hospital and nursing homes.

Dozens of randomized controlled trials of ACT have shown that ACT is more effective than standard services in reducing hospital use and increasing community tenure. These studies have demonstrated improved outcomes for ACT clients in residential stability, symptom management, and quality of life. ACT is strongly effective and cost-effective for clients who return repeatedly to psychiatric hospitals, but not so for infrequently hospitalized clients (Bond, Drake, Mueser, & Latimer, 2001). Several large-scale evaluations in the United Kingdom failed to show any advantage for ACT over standard services, suggesting that ACT is effective only in communities with inadequate community mental health systems and an overutilization of psychiatric hospitals (Burns, 2010).

Housing First

Psychiatric rehabilitation programs often focus on housing issues and on independent living. The general approach most congruent with psychiatric rehabilitation principles is called supported housing, which aims at helping clients find regular community housing (not group homes) that is safe, affordable, and meets their preferences; supported housing also provides ongoing support to empower clients to live independently (e.g., managing finances, cooking, housekeeping, and relationships with landlords; Rog et al., 2014). The supported housing model with the strongest evidence is called Housing First. It is an approach that was originally developed for homeless people with mental illness and substance use disorders (Tsemberis & Eisenberg, 2000). Defying conventional wisdom, Housing First programs do not require clients to prove they are clean and sober before they are eligible for independent housing; instead, Housing First programs offer supported housing without preconditions. Client preferences and shared decision making guide the process of selecting a place to live. Several research studies, including a multisite-controlled trial in Canada, have found that clients enrolled in Housing First attain greater improvements in housing stability, quality of life, and community functioning than clients receiving usual services, which typically offer homeless shelters as a first step in the rehabilitation process (Aubry et al., 2015).

Supported Employment

Defined as paid employment in normal work settings with ongoing job coaching, supported employment was developed originally for people with intellectual disabilities as a more effective, humane, and cost-effective alternative to sheltered workshops (Wehman & Moon, 1988). Individual Placement and Support (IPS) is an evidence-based model of supported employment developed for people with serious mental illness (Becker & Drake, 2003). IPS is based on eight principles: eligibility based solely on client choice (no screening for "readiness"); integration of employment services with mental health treatment; exclusive focus on competitive employment as the goal; attention to client preferences; rapid job search (i.e., no requirements for completing extensive preemployment assessment and training); systematic job development; personalized benefits planning; and ongoing follow-along support (Drake, Bond, & Becker, 2012). Over 20 controlled studies comparing IPS to traditional vocational approaches (e.g., skills training preparation, sheltered workshops, transitional employment, and day treatment) have found overwhelming support favoring IPS. About two thirds of IPS participants succeed in competitive employment, more than twice the rate as for clients not receiving IPS. IPS participants start working sooner, earn more from employment, have longer job tenure, and report greater job satisfaction than control participants (Bond, Drake, & Becker, 2012; Marshall et al., 2014). Long-term studies show that about half of IPS participants maintain steady employment for up to 10 years after enrolling (Hoffmann, Jäckel, Glauser, Mueser, & Kupper, 2014). IPS helps people with different diagnoses, age groups, educational levels, ethno-racial backgrounds, and prior work histories (Drake et al., 2012). It is also effective for people with co-occurring mental illness and substance use disorders (Mueser, Campbell, & Drake, 2011). A large multisite controlled trial of IPS for Social Security disability beneficiaries with schizophrenia or affective disorders found better competitive employment outcomes for IPS participants compared to controls, but participants did not exit the disability rolls (Drake et al., 2013). Because IPS is effective for young adults experiencing early psychosis (Bond, Drake, & Luciano, 2015), some have hypothesized that providing IPS to this group might help forestall entry into the Social Security disability system. IPS programs targeted to young adults typically include supported education, which aims at helping clients obtain education and training in order to have the skills and credentials necessary for obtaining jobs with career potential (Manthey, Holter, Rapp, Davis, & Carlson, 2012).

Other Psychiatric Rehabilitation Practices

The Schizophrenia PORT (Dixon et al., 2010) recommended family-based services to educate family members, reduce stress in the family, teach coping skills, and promote client outcomes (Dixon et al., 2001). Family psychoeducation approaches include both those focusing exclusively on psychoeducation (Lyman et al., 2014) as well as those that also include behavioral management techniques teaching communication skills (Dixon et al., 2001). Nonprofessionals often facilitate family psychoeducation classes; an example is the Family-to-Family program sponsored by the National Alliance on Mental Illness. Several family behavior management models have been developed and these approaches are typically professionally led. Family-based services reduce relapse rates and psychiatric hospitalization rates, and may also decrease expressed emotion in families and increase treatment adherence (Pfammatter, Junghan, & Brenner, 2006).

Many guidelines recommend integrating treatment for mental health issues with co-occurring conditions, such as substance use (Drake, Goldman, et al., 2001) and co-occurring general medical conditions, including obesity, cardiovascular disorders, and other common medical conditions (Shiers, Rafi, Cooper, & Holt, 2014). The critical ingredients of integrated dual disorders treatment approaches include assertive outreach, motivational interventions, and a comprehensive, long-term, individualized approach providing interventions specific to each patient's stage of change (Drake, Goldman, et al., 2001). It is too early to tell whether the Affordable Care Act will successfully promote integration between primary care and mental health treatment, as its provisions intend (Olfson, Pincus, & Pardes, 2013).

Because of cognitive deficits common in people with psychiatric disabilities, especially in schizophrenia, many research groups have developed cognitive remediation interventions. These skills training approaches often use computer exercises and both individualized and structured teaching strategies aimed at improving cognitive functioning. A meta-analysis found modest impacts for cognitive remediation on reducing symptoms and improving general functioning; cognitive remediation appears to be more effective when used as an adjunct to other rehabilitation interventions, such as supported employment (Wykes, Huddy, Cellard, McGurk, & Czobor, 2011).

Self-Management and Consumer-Led Approaches

Self-help groups and advocacy groups led by people with psychiatric disabilities (often referred to as "consumers") have a long history. Since the 1980s, the consumer movement has prompted major changes in psychiatric rehabilitation services. Advocates insisted that people with mental illness should have equal access to societal and environmental resources in places where people live, work, play, and pray (New Freedom Commission on Mental Health, 2003; Ralph & Corrigan, 2005).

Self-management of one's disability is an important theme within the consumer movement. Mental health consumers have advocated for the illness self-management approach in order to gain control over their lives and reduce dependence on professional services. The Wellness Action Recovery Plan is a consumer-developed manual that provides systematic tools for coping with symptoms and developing relapse prevention plans (Copeland, 1997). A randomized controlled trial of this program found it reduced symptoms of anxiety and depression and increased self-reported recovery (Cook et al., 2012).

Recent advocacy work by organizations such as the National Alliance on Mental Illness (NAMI) has focused on educating the public about the biological nature of mental illness—essentially, equating mental illness with physical illness in order to reduce the blame and guilt associated with mental health conditions. However, research now suggests that focusing on biological origins may backfire, because (while reducing blame) the public may come to believe that mental health conditions are innate and therefore untreatable (Read, Haslam, Sayce, & Davies, 2006; Rusch, Todd, Bodenhausen, & Corrigan, 2010).

Combining treatment information with biological explanations may be a more effective form of mental health education (Lebowitz & Ahn, 2012).

Access to Treatment and Rehabilitation

Unfortunately, while research has established the effectiveness of a variety psychiatric rehabilitation practices, many people needing these services do not receive them (Mojtabai et al., 2009). There are several reasons for the gap. First, mental health and vocational rehabilitation services are seriously underfunded in the United States and elsewhere. Second, many people who have needs have concluded that the treatments that the mental health centers offer are not acceptable or not useful. Third, implementation of evidence-based practices is often inadequate; despite wide consensus on effective practices, most mental health centers do not provide them (Lehman et al., 1998; West et al., 2005). In an effort to disseminate the best practices of psychiatric rehabilitation, the National Implementing Evidence-Based Practices Project developed standardized guidelines and training materials, and demonstrated that the toolkits in conjunction with systematic training and consultation can facilitate faithfully implementing evidence-based practices in routine mental health service settings (McHugo et al., 2007).

CONCLUSION

Psychiatric disorders can look very different from one another in terms of symptom presentation, course, and treatment. An encouraging shift in the collective mindset regarding the treatment of psychiatric disabilities has occurred, with an emphasis on the right and ability of individuals to pursue meaningful goals comparable to nondisabled people.

Like individuals with other types of long-term illnesses, people with psychiatric disabilities want to manage their own illnesses, form and maintain meaningful social relationships, work in the community, and live in normal housing situations. With the help of pharmacological treatments, psychotherapy, and psychosocial rehabilitation services, clients can attain these goals. Hence, the focus of psychiatric rehabilitation is not only to keep clients stable and out of the hospital, but also to assist and empower them in pursuing their personal aspirations, management of their illnesses, independence, and self-fulfillment. Progress has been made toward realizing these objectives, although many changes are needed in the mental health system before exemplary services are available to everyone who could benefit from them.

REFERENCES

Alexander, G. C., Gallagher, S. A., Mascola, A., Moloney, R. M., & Stafford, R. S. (2011). Increasing off-label use of antipsychotic medications in the United States, 1995-2008. *Pharmacoepidemiology & Drug Safety, 20*, 177–184. doi:10.1002/pds.2028

Allison, D. B., Mentore, J. L., Heo, M., Chandler, L. P., Cappelleri, J. C., Infante, M. C., & Weiden, P. J. (1999). Antipsychotic-induced weight gain: A comprehensive research synthesis. *American Journal of Psychiatry, 156*, 1686–1696.

Anthony, W. A., Cohen, M., Farkas, M. D., & Gagne, C. (2002). *Psychiatric rehabilitation* (2nd ed.). Boston, MA: Center for Psychiatric Rehabilitation.

Arcelus, J., Mitchell, A. J., Wales, J., & Nielsen, S. (2011). Mortality rates in patients with anorexia nervosa and other eating disorders: A meta-analysis of 36 studies. *Archives of General Psychiatry, 68*, 724–731. doi:10.1001/archgenpsychiatry.2011.74

Arseneault, L., Moffitt, T. E., Caspi, A., Taylor, P. J., & Silva, P. (2000). Mental disorders and violence in a total birth cohort: Results from the Dunedin study. *JAMA Psychiatry, 57*, 979–986. doi:10.1001/archpsych.57.10.979

American Psychiatric Association. (2013). *Diagnostic and statistical manual of mental disorders* (5th ed.). Arlington, VA: American Psychiatric Publishing.

Aubry, T., Tsemberis, S., Adair, C. E., Veldhuizen, S., Streiner, D., Latimer, E., . . . Goering, P. (2015). One-year outcomes of a randomized controlled trial of housing first with ACT in five Canadian cities. *Psychiatric Services, 66*, 463–469. doi:10.1176/appi.ps.201400167

Baron, R. C., Draine, J., & Salzer, M. S. (2013). "I'm not sure that I can figure out how to do that": Pursuit of work among people with mental illnesses leaving jail. *American Journal of Psychiatric Rehabilitation, 16*, 115–135.

Bauer, S. M., Schanda, H., Karakula, H., Olajozzy-Hilkesberger, L., Rudaleviciene, P., Okribelashvili, N., . . . Stompe, T. (2011). Culture and the prevalence of hallucinations in schizophrenia. *Comprehensive Psychiatry, 52*, 319–325. doi:10.1016/j.comppsych.2010.06.008

Becker, D. R., & Drake, R. E. (2003). *A working life for people with severe mental illness*. New York, NY: Oxford University Press.

Belsher, G., & Costello, C. G. (1988). Relapse after recovery from unipolar depression: A critical review. *Psychological Bulletin, 104*, 84–96.

Birmingham, C. L., Su, J., Hlynsky, J. A., Goldmer, E. M., & Gao, M. (2005). The mortality rate from anorexia nervosa. *International Journal of Eating Disorders, 38*, 143–146.

Black, D. M. (2015). The natural history of antisocial personality disorder. *Canadian Journal of Psychiatry, 60*, 309–314.

Bogels, S. M., Wijts, P., Oort, F. J., & Sallaerts, S. J. (2014). Psychodynamic psychotherapy versus cognitive behavior therapy for social anxiety disorder: An efficacy and partial effectiveness trial. *Depression and Anxiety, 31*, 363–373. doi:10.1002/da.22246

Bond, G. R., & Drake, R. E. (2014). Making the case for IPS supported employment. *Administration and Policy in Mental Health and Mental Health Services Research, 41*, 69–73.

Bond, G. R., & Drake, R. E. (2015). The critical ingredients of assertive community treatment: An update. *World Psychiatry, 14*, 240–242.

Bond, G. R., Drake, R. E., & Becker, D. R. (2012). Generalizability of the individual placement and support (IPS) model of supported employment outside the U.S. *World Psychiatry, 11*, 32–39.

Bond, G. R., Drake, R. E., & Luciano, A. (2015). Employment and educational outcomes in early intervention programs for early psychosis: A systematic review. *Epidemiology and Psychiatric Sciences, 24*, 446–457.

Bond, G. R., Drake, R. E., Mueser, K. T., & Latimer, E. (2001). Assertive community treatment for people with severe mental illness: Critical ingredients and impact on patients. *Disease Management & Health Outcomes, 9*, 141–159.

Brekke, J., Prindle, C., Woo Bae, S., & Long, J. (2001). Risks for individuals with schizophrenia who are living in the community. *Psychiatric Services, 52*, 1358–1366. doi:10.1176/appi.52.10.1358

Bruce, S. E., Yonkers, K. A., Otto, M. W., Eisen, J. L., Weisberg, R. B., Pagano, M., . . . Keller, M. B. (2005). Influence of psychiatric comorbidity on recovery and recurrence in generalized anxiety disorder, social phobia, and panic disorder: A 12-year prospective study. *American Journal of Psychiatry, 162*, 1179–1187.

Brunette, M. F., Noordsy, D. L., Xie, H., & Drake, R. E. (2003). Benzodiazepine use and abuse among patients with severe mental illness and co-occurring substance use disorders. *Psychiatric Services, 54*, 1395–1401.

Bulik, C. M., Sullivan, P. F., & Kendler, K. S. (2002). Medical and psychiatric morbidity in obese women with and without binge eating. *International Journal of Eating Disorders, 32*, 72–78. doi:10.1002/eat.10072

Burnim, I. (2015). The promise of the Americans with Disabilities Act for people with mental illness. *Journal of the American Medical Association, 313*, 2223–2224.

Burns, T. (2010). The rise and fall of assertive community treatment? *International Review of Psychiatry, 22*, 130–137.

Butler, A. C., Chapman, J. E., Forman, E. M., & Beck, A. T. (2006). The empirical status of cognitive-behavioral therapy: A review of meta-analyses. *Clinical Psychology Review*, *26*, 17–31.

Butterworth, P., Leach, L. S., McManus, S., & Stansfeld, S. A. (2013). Common mental disorders, unemployment and psychosocial job quality: Is a poor job better than no job at all? *Psychological Medicine, 43*, 1763–1772.

Butzlaff, R. L., & Hooley, J. M. (1998). Expressed emotion and psychiatric relapse: A meta-analysis. *Archives of General Psychiatry*, *55*, 547–552.

Cantor-Graae, E., & Selten, J. P. (2005). Schizophrenia and migration: A meta-analysis and review. *American Journal of Psychiatry, 162*, 12–24. doi:10.1176/appi.ajp.162.1.12

Cavanagh, J. T., Carson, A. J., Sharpe, M., & Lawrie, S. M. (2003). Psychological autopsy studies of suicide: A systematic review. *Psychological Medicine, 33*, 395–405.

Chorpita, B. F., & Barlow, D. H. (1998). The development of anxiety: The role of control in the early environment. *Psychological Bulletin, 124*, 3–21. doi:10.1037/0033-2909.124.1.3

Choy, Y., Fyer, A. J., & Lipsitz, J. D. (2007). Treatment of specific phobia in adults. *Clinical Psychology Review*, *27*, 266–286.

Compton, M. T., Weiss, P. S., West, J. C., & Kaslow, N. J. (2005). The associations between substance use disorders, schizophrenia-spectrum disorders, and axis IV psychosocial problems. *Social Psychiatry & Psychiatric Epidemiology, 40*, 939–946. doi:10.1007/s00127-005-0964-4

Cook, J. A., Copeland, M. E., Floyd, C. B., Jonikas, J. A., Hamilton, M. M., Razzano, L., . . . Boyd, S. (2012). A randomized controlled trial of effects of wellness recovery action planning on depression, anxiety, and recovery. *Psychiatric Services, 63*, 541–547.

Copeland, M. E. (1997). *Wellness recovery action plan*. Brattleboro, VT: Peach Press.

Corrigan, P. W., Mueser, K. T., Bond, G. R., Drake, R. E., & Solomon, P. (2008). *Principles and practice of psychiatric rehabilitation: An empirical approach*. New York, NY: Guilford Press.

Coryell, W., Akiskal, H. S., Leon, A. C., Winokur, G., Maser, J. D., Mueller, T. I., & Keller, M. B. (1994). The time course of nonchronic major depressive disorder. Uniformity across episodes and samples. National institute of mental health collaborative program on the psychobiology of depression—clinical studies. *Archives of General Psychiatry, 51*, 405–410.

Cramer, J. A., & Rosenheck, R. (1999). Enhancing medication compliance for people with serious mental illness. *Journal of Nervous and Mental Disease, 187*, 53–55.

Cuijpers, P., Van Straten, A., & Warmerdam, L. (2007). Behavioral activation treatments of depression: A meta-analysis. *Clinical Psychology Review, 27*, 318–326.

Danziger, S., Frank, R. G., & Meara, E. (2009). Mental illness, work, and income support programs. *American Journal of Psychiatry, 166*, 398–404.

de Mello, M. F., de Jesus Mari, J., Bacaltchuk, J., Verdeli, H., & Neugebauer, R. (2005). A systematic review of research findings on the efficacy of interpersonal therapy for depressive disorders. *European Archives of Psychiatry and Clinical Neuroscience, 255*, 75–82.

Dincin, J. (1995). A pragmatic approach to psychiatric rehabilitation: Lessons from Chicago's thresholds program. *New Directions for Mental Health Services, 68*(Whole Issue).

Dixon, L. B., Dickerson, F., Bellack, A. S., Bennett, M., Dickinson, D., Goldberg, R. W., . . . Kreyenbuhl, J. (2010). The 2009 schizophrenia PORT psychosocial treatment recommendations and summary statements. *Schizophrenia Bulletin, 36*, 48–70.

Dixon, L. B., Lehman, A. F., & Levine, J. (1995). Conventional antipsychotic medications for schizophrenia. *Schizophrenia Bulletin, 21*, 567–577.

Dixon, L. B., McFarlane, W. R., Lefley, H., Lucksted, A., Cohen, M., Falloon, I., . . . Sondheimer, D. (2001). Evidence-based practices for services to families of people with psychiatric disabilities. *Psychiatric Services, 52*, 903–910.

Draine, J., Salzer, M. S., Culhane, D. P., & Hadley, T. R. (2002). Role of social disadvantage in crime, joblessness, and homelessness among persons with serious mental illness. *Psychiatric Services, 53*, 565–573. doi:10.1176/appi.ps.53.5.565

Drake, R. E., Bond, G. R., & Becker, D. R. (2012). *Individual placement and support: An evidence-based approach to supported employment*. New York, NY: Oxford University Press.

Drake, R. E., Essock, S. M., Shaner, A., Carey, K. B., Minkoff, K., Kola, L., . . . Rickards, L. (2001). Implementing dual diagnosis services for clients with severe mental illness. *Psychiatric Services, 52*, 469–476.

Drake, R. E., Frey, W. D., Bond, G. R., Goldman, H. H., Salkever, D. S., Miller, A. L., . . . Milford, R. (2013). Assisting social security disability insurance beneficiaries with schizophrenia, bipolar disorder, or major depression in returning to work. *American Journal of Psychiatry, 170*, 1433–1441.

Drake, R. E., Goldman, H. H., Leff, H. S., Lehman, A. F., Dixon, L. B., Mueser, K. T., & Torrey, W. C. (2001). Implementing evidence-based practices in routine mental health service settings. *Psychiatric Services, 52*, 179–182.

Drake, R. E., Mercer-McFadden, C., Mueser, K. T., McHugo, G. J., & Bond, G. R. (1998). Review of integrated mental health and substance abuse treatment for patients with dual disorders. *Schizophrenia Bulletin, 24*, 589–608.

Drake, R. E., & Sederer, L. I. (1986). Inpatient psychosocial treatment of chronic schizophrenia: Negative effects and current guidelines. *Psychiatric Services, 37*, 897–901.

Driessen, E., Hegelmaier, L. M., Abbass, A. A., Barber, J. P., Dekker, J. J., Van. H. L., . . . Cuijpers, P. (2015). The efficacy of short-term psychodynamic psychotherapy for depression: A meta-analysis update. *Clinical Psychology Review, 42*, 1–15. doi:10.1016/j.cpr.2015.07.004

Eaton, W. W. (1985). Epidemiology of schizophrenia. *Epidemiological Review, 7*, 105–126.

Eaton, W. W. (1991). Update on the epidemiology of schizophrenia. *Epidemiological Review, 13*, 370–378.

Eranti, S. V., MacCabe, J. H., Bundy, H., & Murray, R. M. (2013). Gender difference in age at onset of schizophrenia: A meta-analysis. *Psychological Medicine, 43*, 155–167. doi:10.1017/S003329171200089X

Estroff, S. E. (1989). Self, identity, and subjective experiences: In search of the subject. *Schizophrenia Bulletin, 15*, 189–196.

Fervaha, G., Foussias, G., Agid, O., & Remington, G. (2014). Impact of primary negative symptoms on functional outcomes in schizophrenia. *European Psychiatry, 29*, 449–455.

Fichter, M. M., Quadflieg, N., Fischer, U. C., & Kohlboeck, G. (2010). Twenty-five-year course and outcome in anxiety and depression in the upper bavarian longitudinal community study. *Acta Psychiatrica Scandinavica, 122*, 75–85.

Foa, E. B., Dancu, C. V., Hembree, E. A., Jaycox, L. H., Meadows, E. A., & Street, G. P. (1999). A comparison of exposure therapy, stress inoculation training, and their combination for reducing posttraumatic stress disorder in female assault victims. *Journal of Consulting and Clinical Psychology, 67*, 194–200.

Folsom, D. P., Hawthorne, W., Lindamer, L., Gilmer, T., Bailey, A., Golshan, S., . . . Jeste, D. V. (2005). Prevalence and risk factors for homelessness and utilization of mental health services among 10,340 patients with serious mental illness in a large public mental health system. *American Journal of Psychiatry, 162*, 370–376.

Forsell, Y. (2007). A three-year follow-up of major depression, dysthymia, minor depression and subsyndromal depression: results from a population-based study. *Depression and Anxiety, 24*, 62–65. doi:10.1002/da.20231

Fortney, J. C., Pyne, J. M., Edlund, M. J., Williams, D. K., Robinson. D. E., Mittal, D., & Henderson, K. L. (2007). A randomized trial of telemedicine-based collaborative care for depression. *Journal of General Internal Medicine, 22*, 1086–1093.

Frounfelker, R. L., Glover, C., Teachout, A., Wilkniss, S., & Whitley, R. (2010). Access to supported employment for consumers with criminal justice involvement. *Psychiatric Rehabilitation Journal, 34*, 49–56.

Fukunaga, R., & Lysaker, P. H. (2013). Criminal history in schizophrenia: associations with substance use and disorganized symptoms. *Journal of Forensic Psychiatry and Psychology, 24*, 293–308. doi:10.1080/14789949.2013.776617

Geddes, J., Freemantle, N., Harrison, P., & Bebbington, P. (2000). Atypical antipsychotics in the treatment of schizophrenia: Systematic overview and meta-regression analysis. *British Medical Journal, 321*, 1371–1376.

Glod, C. A. (1996). Recent advances in the pharmacotherapy of major depression. *Archives of Psychiatric Nursing, 10*, 355–364.

Goffman, E. (1961). *Asylums: Essays on the social situation of mental patients and other inmates.* Chicago, IL: Aldine.

Goldberg, R. W., Rollins, A. L., & Lehman, A. F. (2003). Social network correlates among people with psychiatric disabilities. *Psychiatric Rehabilitation Journal, 26*, 393–402.

Goldner, E. M., Hsu, L., Waraich, P., & Somers, J. M. (2002). Prevalence and incidence of schizophrenic disorders: A systematic review of the literature. *Canadian Journal of Psychiatry, 47*, 833–843.

Goodman, L. A., Dutton, M. A., & Harris, M. (1997). The relationship between violence dimensions and symptom severity among homeless, mentally ill women. *Journal of Traumatic Stress, 10*, 51–70.

Goodman, L. A., Salyers, M. P., Mueser, K. T., Rosenberg, S. D., Swartz, M., Essock, S. M., . . . Swanson, J. (2001). Recent victimization in women and men with severe mental illness: Prevalence and correlates. *Journal of Traumatic Stress, 14*, 615–632.

Grabowski, D. C., Aschbrenner, K. A., Feng, Z., & Mor, V. (2009). Mental illness in nursing homes: Variations across states. *Health Affairs, 28*, 689–700.

Green, M. F., Horan, W. P., & Lee, J. (2015). Social cognition in schizophrenia. *Nature Reviews: Neuroscience, 16*, 620–631.

Hall, L. L., Graf, A. C., Fitzpatrick, M. J., Lane, T., & Birkel, R. C. (2003). *Shattered lives: Results of a national survey of NAMI members living with mental illnesses and their family members TRIAD report.* Bethesda, MD: Stanley Medical Group.

Harding, C. M., Strauss, J. S., Hafez, H., & Liberman, P. B. (1987). Work and mental illness. I. Toward an integration of the rehabilitation process. *Journal of Nervous and Mental Disease, 175*, 317–326.

Harrow, M., Grossman, L. S., Jobe, T. H., & Herbener, E. S. (2005). Do patients with schizophrenia ever show periods of recovery? A 15-year multi-follow-up study. *Schizophrenia Bulletin, 31*, 723–734. doi:10.1093/schbil/sbi026

Hendriks, S. M., Spijker, J., Licht, C. M., Beekman, A. T., Hardeveld, F., de Graaf, R., . . . Penninx, B. W. (2014). Disability in anxiety disorder. *Journal of Affective Disorders, 166*, 227–233. doi:10.1016/j.jad.2014.05.006

Hilty, D. M., Ferrer, D. C., Parish, M. B., Johnston, B., Callahan, E. J., & Yellowlees, P. M. (2013). The effectiveness of telemental health: A 2013 review. *Telemedicine and e-Health, 19*, 444–454. doi:10.1089/tmj.2013.0075

Hoffmann, H., Jäckel, D., Glauser, S., Mueser, K. T., & Kupper, Z. (2014). Long-term effectiveness of supported employment: Five-year follow-up of a randomized controlled trial. *American Journal of Psychiatry, 171*, 1183–1190.

Hogarty, G. E., McEvoy, J. P., Munetz, M., DiBarry, A. L., Bartone, P., Cather, R., . . . Madonia, M. J. (1988). Dose of fluphenazine, familial expressed emotion, and outcome in schizophrenia: Results of a two-year controlled study. *Archives of General Psychiatry, 45*, 797–805.

Hudson, C. G. (2009). Validation of a model for estimating state and local prevalence of serious mental illness. *International Journal of Methods in Psychiatric Research, 18*, 251–264. doi:10.1002/mpr.294

Isaac, R. J., & Armat, V. C. (1990). *Madness in the streets: How psychiatry and the law abandoned the mentally ill.* New York, NY: Free Press.

Jacobi, F., Wittchen H., Hoting, C., Hofler, M., Pfister, H., Muller, N., & Lieb, R. (2004). Prevalence, co-morbidity and correlates of mental disorders in the general population: Results from the German health interview and examination survey (GHS). *Psychological Medicine, 34*, 597–611.

Jamison, K. R. (1997). *An unquiet mind: A memoir of moods and madness.* New York, NY: Knopf.

Jobe, T. H., & Harrow, M. (2005). Long-term outcome of patients with schizophrenia: A review. *Canadian Journal of Psychiatry, 50*, 892–900.

Kane, J. M., Woerner, M., & Sarantakos, S. (1986). Depot neuroleptics: A comparative review of standard, intermediate, and low-dose regimens. *Journal of Clinical Psychiatry, 47*, 30–33.

Kaye, W. H., Bulik, C. M., Thornton, L., Barbarich, N., & Masters, K. (2004). Comorbidity of anxiety disorders with anorexia and bulimia nervosa. *American Journal of Psychiatry, 161*, 2215–2221. doi:10.1176/appi.ajp.161.12.2215

Keller, M. B., Krystal, J. H., Hen, R., Neumeister, A., & Simon, N. (2005). Untangling depression and anxiety: Clinical challenges. *Journal of Clinical Psychiatry, 66*, 1447–1487.

Keski-Rahkonen, A., Hoek, H. W., Susser, E. S., Linna, M. S., Sihvola, E., Raevuori, A., . . . Rissanen, A. (2007). Epidemiology and course of anorexia nervosa in the community. *American Journal of Psychiatry, 164*, 1259–1265.

Kessler, R. C., Amminger, P. G., Aguilar-Gaxiola, S., Alonso, J., Lee, S., & Ustun, T. B. (2007). Age of onset of mental disorders: A review of recent literature. *Current Opinion Psychiatry, 20*, 359–364. doi:10.1097/YCO.0b013e32816ebc8c

Kessler, R. C., Barker, P. R., Colpe, L. J., Epstein, J. F., Gfroerer, J. C., Howes, M. J., . . . Zaslavsky, A. M. (2003). Screening for serious mental illness in the general population. *Archives of General Psychiatry, 60*, 184–189.

Kessler, R. C., Berglund, P. A., Chiu, W. T., Deitz, A. C., Hudson, J., Shahly, V., . . . Xavier, M. (2013). The prevalence and correlate of binge eating disorder in the World Health Organization World Mental Health Surveys. *Biological Psychiatry, 73*, 904–914. doi:10.1016/j.biopsych.2012.11.020

Kessler, R. C., Berglund, P., Demler, O., Jin, R., Merikangas, K. R., & Walters, E. E. (2005). Lifetime prevalence and age-of-onset distributions of DSM-IV disorders in the National Comorbidity Survey replication. *Archives of General Psychiatry, 62*, 593–602. doi:10.1001/archpsyc.62.6.593

Kessler, R. C., DuPont, R. L., Berglund, P., & Wittchen, H. U. (1999). Impairment in pure and comorbid generalized anxiety disorder and major depression at 12 months in two national surveys. *American Journal of Psychiatry, 156*, 1915–1923.

Kessler, R. C., Petukhova, M., Sampson, N. A., Zaslavsky, A. M., & Wittchen, H. (2012). Twelve-month and lifetime prevalence and lifetime morbid risk of anxiety and mood disorders in the United States. *International Journal of Methods in Psychiatric Research, 21*, 169–184. doi:10.1002/mpr.1359

Kroenke, K., Spitzer, R. L., Williams, J., Monahan, P. O., & Lowe, B. (2007). Anxiety disorders in primary care: Prevalence, impairment, comorbidity, and detection. *Annals of Internal Medicine, 146*, 317–325.

Krupnick, J. L., Sotsky, S. M., Simmens, S., Moyer, J., Elkin, I., Watkins, J., & Pilkonis, P. A. (1996). The role of the therapeutic alliance in psychotherapy and pharmacotherapy outcome: Findings of the National Institute of Mental Health Treatment of depression collaborative research program. *Journal of Consulting and Clinical Psychology, 64*, 532–539. doi:10.1037/0022-006X.64.3.532

Kuyken, W., Byford, S., Taylor, R. S., Watkins, E., Holden, E., White, K., . . . Teasdale, J. D. (2008). Mindfulness-based cognitive therapy to prevent relapse in recurrent depression. *Journal of Consulting and Clinical Psychology, 76*, 966.

Lacro, J. P., Dunn, L. B., Dolder, C. R., Leckband, S. G., & Jeste, D. V. (2002). Prevalence of and risk factors for medication nonadherence in patients with schizophrenia: A comprehensive review of recent literature. *Journal of Clinical Psychiatry, 63*, 892–909.

Lebowitz, M. S., & Ahn, W. (2012). Combining biomedical accounts of mental disorders with treatability information to reduce mental illness stigma. *Psychiatric Services, 63*, 496–499.

Lehman, A. F., Steinwachs, D. M., Dixon, L. B., Postrado, L., Scott, J. E., Fahey, M., . . . Skinner, E. A. (1998). Patterns of usual care for schizophrenia: Initial results from the schizophrenia patient outcomes research team (PORT) client survey. *Schizophrenia Bulletin, 24*, 11–20.

Lehman, A. F., Steinwachs, D. M., & PORT Co-Investigators. (1998). Translating research into practice: The Schizophrenia patient outcomes research team (PORT) treatment recommendations. *Schizophrenia Bulletin, 24*, 1–10.

Leichsenring, F., Rabung, S., & Leibing, E. (2004). The efficacy of short-term psychodynamic psychotherapy in specific psychiatric disorders. *Archives of General Psychiatry, 61*, 1208–1216.

Liberman, R. P., Kopelowicz, A., Ventura, J., & Gutkind, D. (2002). Operational criteria and factors related to recovery from schizophrenia. *International Review of Psychiatry, 14*, 256–272. doi:10.1080/09540260210000016905

Lieberman, J. A., Stroup, T. S., McEvoy, J. P., Swartz, M. S., Rosenheck, R. A., Perkins, D. O., . . . Hsiao, J. K. (2005). Effectiveness of antipsychotic drugs in patients with chronic schizophrenia. *New England Journal of Medicine, 353*, 1209–1223. doi:10.1056/NEJMoa051688

Linehan, M., & Armstrong, H. (1991). Cognitive-behavioral treatment of chronically parasuicidal borderline patients. *Archives of General Psychiatry, 48*, 1060–1064.

Linehan, M., Comtois, K. A., Murray, A. M., Brown, M. Z., Gallop, R. J., Heard, H. L., . . . Lindenboim, N. (2006). Two-year randomized controlled trial and follow-up of dialectical behavior therapy vs. therapy by experts for suicidal behaviors and borderline personality disorder. *Archives of General Psychiatry, 63*, 757–766. doi:10.1001/archpsyc.63.7.757

Lingam, R., & Scott, J. (2002). Treatment non-adherence in affective disorders. *Acta Psychiatrica Scandinavica, 105*, 164–172.

Lowe, B., Zipfel, S., Buchholz, C., Dupont, Y., Reas, D. L., & Herzog, W. (2001). Long-term outcome of anorexia nervosa in a prospective 21-year follow-up study. *Psychological Medicine, 31*, 881–890.

Lyman, D. R., Braude, L., George, P., Dougherty, R. H., Daniels, A. S., Ghose, S. S., & Delphin-Rittmon, M. E. (2014). Consumer and family psychoeducation: Assessing the evidence. *Psychiatric Services, 65*, 416–428.

MacDonald-Wilson, K. L., Rogers, E. S., Ellison, M. L., & Lyass, A. (2003). A study of the Social Security Work Incentives and their relation to perceived barriers to work among persons with psychiatric disability. *Rehabilitation Psychology, 48*, 301–309.

Maher, A. R., Maglione, M., Bagley, S., Suttorp, M., Hu, J., Ewing, B., . . . Shekelle, P. G. (2011). Efficacy and comparative effectiveness of atypical antipsychotic medications for off-label uses in adults. *Journal of the American Medical Association, 306*, 1359–1369. doi:10.1001/jama.2011.1360

Manderscheid, R. W., Atay, J. E., & Crider, R. A. (2009). Changing trends in state psychiatric hospital use from 2002 to 2005. *Psychiatric Services, 60*, 29–34.

Manthey, T. J., Holter, M., Rapp, C. A., Davis, J. K., & Carlson, L. (2012). The perceived importance of integrated supported education and employment services. *Journal of Rehabilitation, 78*, 16–24.

Marshall, M., Lewis, S., Lockwood, A., Drake, R., Jones, P., & Croudace, T. (2005). Association between duration of untreated psychosis and outcome in cohorts of first-episode patients. *Archives of General Psychiatry, 62*, 975–983.

Marshall, T., Goldberg, R. W., Braude, L., Dougherty, R. H., Daniels, A. S., Ghose, S. S., . . . Delphin-Rittmon, M. E. (2014). Supported employment: Assessing the evidence. *Psychiatric Services, 65*, 16–23.

McEvoy, J. P., Lieberman, J. A., Stroup, T. S., Davis, S. M., Meltzer, H. Y., Rosenheck, R. A., . . . Severe, J. (2006). Effectiveness of clozapine versus olanzapine, quetiapine, and risperidone in patients with chronic schizophrenia who did not respond to prior atypical antipsychotic treatment. *American Journal of Psychiatry, 163*, 600–610.

McGlashan, T. H. (1988). A selective review of recent North American long-term followup studies of schizophrenia. *Schizophrenia Bulletin, 14*, 515–542.

McGrath, J., Saha, S., Welham, J., Saadi, O. E., MacCauley, C., Chant, D. (2004). A systematic review of the incidence of schizophrenia: the distribution of rates and the influence of sex, urbanicity, migrant status and methodology. *BMC Medicine, 2*, 13. doi:10.1186/1741-7015-2-13

McGuire, J. F., & Rosenheck, R. A. (2004). Criminal history as a prognosis indicator in the treatment of homeless people with severe mental illness. *Psychiatric Services, 55*, 42–48.

McGurk, S. R., & Mueser, K. T. (2004). Cognitive functioning, symptoms, and work in supported employment: A review and heuristic model. *Schizophrenia Research, 70*, 147–173. doi:10.1016/j.schres.2004.01.009

McHugo, G. J., Drake, R. E., Whitley, R., Bond, G. R., Campbell, K., Rapp, C. A., . . . Finnerty, M. T. (2007). Fidelity outcomes in the National implementing evidence-based practices project. *Psychiatric Services, 58*, 1279–1284.

McRoberts, C., Burlingame, G. M., & Hoag, M. J. (1998). Comparative efficacy of individual and group psychotherapy: A meta-analytic perspective. *Group Dynamics: Theory, Research, and Practice, 2*, 101–117. doi:10.1037/1089-2699.2.2.101

Meeks, S., & Hammond, C. T. (2001). Social network characteristics among older outpatients with long-term mental illness. *Journal of Mental Health and Aging, 7*, 445–464.

Mehler, P. S. (2011). Medical complications of bulimia nervosa and their treatments. *International Journal of Eating Disorders, 44*, 95–104. doi:10.1002/eat.20285

Merikangas, K. R., Akiskal, H. S., Angst, J., Greenberg, P. E., Hirschfeld, R., Petukhova, M., & Kessler, R. C. (2007). Lifetime and 12-month prevalence of bipolar spectrum disorder in the national comorbidity survey replication. *Archives of General Psychiatry, 64*, 543–552. doi:10.1001/archpsyc.64.5.543

Mineka, S., & Zinbarg, R. (2006). A contemporary learning theory perspective on the etiology of anxiety disorders: It's not what you thought it was. *American Psychologist, 61*, 10–26. doi:10.1037/0003-066X.61.1.10

Mitchell, A. J., & Subramaniam, H. (2005). Prognosis of depression in old age compared to middle age: A systematic review of comparative studies. *American Journal of Psychiatry, 162*, 1588–1601. doi:10.1176/appi.ajp.162.9.1588

Mitchell, J. E., & Crow, S. (2006). Medical complications of anorexia nervosa and bulimia nervosa. *Current Opinion Psychiatry, 19*, 438–443. doi:10.1097/01.yco.0000228768.79097.3e

Mojtabai, R., Fochtman, L., Chang, S., Kotov, K., Craig, T. J., & Bromet, E. (2009). Unmet need for care in schizophrenia. *Schizophrenia Bulletin, 35*, 679–695.

Mojtabai, R., & Olfson, M. (2010). National trends in psychotropic medication polypharmacy in office-based psychiatry. *Archives of General Psychiatry, 67*, 26–36. doi:10.1001/archdenpsychiatry.2009.175

Möller, H., & Volz, H. (1996). Drug treatment of depression in the 1990s: An overview of achievements and future possibilities. *Drugs, 52*, 625–638.

Mueser, K. T., Campbell, K., & Drake, R. E. (2011). The effectiveness of supported employment in people with dual disorders. *Journal of Dual Disorders, 7*, 90–102.

Mueser, K. T., Corrigan, P. W., Hilton, D. W., Tanzman, B., Schaub, A., Gingerich, S., . . . Herz, M. I. (2002). Illness management and recovery: A review of the research. *Psychiatric Services, 53*, 1272–1284.

Mueser, K. T., & Gingerich, S. (2006). *The complete family guide to schizophrenia: Helping your loved one get the most out of life.* New York, NY: Guilford Press.

Mueser, K. T., & Glynn, S. M. (1995). *Behavioral family therapy for psychiatric disorder.* Needham Heights, MA: Allyn & Bacon.

Mueser, K. T., Goodman, L. B., Trumbetta, S. L., Rosenberg, S. D., Osher, F. C., Vidaver, R., . . . Foy, D. W. (1998). Trauma and posttraumatic stress disorder in severe mental illness. *Journal of Consulting and Clinical Psychology, 66*, 493–499.

Mueser, K. T., & Jeste, D. V (Eds.). (2008). *Clinical handbook of schizophrenia.* New York, NY: Guilford Press.

Nesper, A. C., Morris, B. A., Scher, L. M., & Holmes, J. F. (2015). Effect of decreasing county mental health services on the emergency department. *Annals of Emergency Medicine*, *67*(4), 525–530. doi:10.1016/j.annemergmed.2015.09.007

New Freedom Commission on Mental Health. (2003). *Achieving the promise: Transforming mental health care in America*. Final Report. DHHS Pub. No. SMA-03-3832. Rockville, MD: Substance Abuse and Mental Health Services Administration.

Nock, M. K., Hwang, I., Sampson, N. A., & Kessler, R. C. (2010). Mental disorders, comorbidity and suicidal behavior: Results from the National comorbidity survey replication. *Molecular Psychiatry, 15*, 868–876.

Olfson, M., Pincus, H. A., & Pardes, H. (2013). Investing in evidence-based care for the severely mentally ill. *Journal of the American Medical Association, 310*, 1345–1346.

Osher, F., Steadman, H. J., & Barr, H. (2003). A best practice approach to community reentry from jails for inmates with co-occurring disorders: The APIC model. *Crime and Delinquency, 49*, 79–96.

Palmer, B. A., Pankratz, V. S., & Bostwick, J. M. (2005). The lifetime risk of suicide in schizophrenia: A reexamination. *JAMA Psychiatry, 62*, 247–253. doi:10.1001/archpsyc.62.3.247

Pedersen, C. B., & Mortensen, P. B. (2001). Evidence of a dose-response relationship between urbanicity during upbringing and schizophrenia risk. *Archives of General Psychiatry, 58*, 1039–1046. doi:10.1001/archpsych.58.11.1039

Perese, E. F. (2007). Stigma, poverty, and victimization: Roadblocks to recovery for individuals with severe mental illness. *Journal of the American Psychiatric Nurses Association, 13*, 285–295. doi:10.1177.1078390307307830

Perkins, D. O., Gu, H., Boteva, K., & Lieberman, J. A. (2005). Relationship between duration of untreated psychosis and outcome in first-episode schizophrenia: A critical review and meta-analysis. *American Journal of Psychiatry, 162*, 1785–1804.

Pescosolido, B. A., Wright, E. R., & Luftey, K. (1999). The changing hopes, worries, and community supports of individuals moving from a closing long-term care facility. *Journal of Behavioral Health Services and Research, 26*, 276–288.

Pfammatter, M., Junghan, U. M., & Brenner, H. D. (2006). Efficacy of psychological therapy in schizophrenia: Conclusions from meta-analyses. *Schizophrenia Bulletin*, *32*(Suppl. 1), S64–S80.

Poutanen, O., Mattila, A., Seppala, N. H., Groth, L., Koivisto, A. M., & Salokangas, R. K. (2007). Seven-year outcome of depression in primary and psychiatric outpatient care: Results of the TADEP (tampere depression) II study. *Nordic Journal of Psychiatry, 61*, 62–70. doi:10.1080/08039480601135140

Prien, R. F., Klett, C. J., & Caffey, E. M. (1973). Lithium carbonate and imipramine in prevention of affective episodes: A comparison in recurrent affective illness. *Archives of General Psychiatry, 29*, 420–425.

Ralph, R. O., & Corrigan, P. W (Eds.). (2005). *Recovery in mental illness: Broadening our understanding of wellness*. Washington, DC: American Psychological Association.

Read, J., Haslam, N., Sayce, L., & Davies, E. (2006). Prejudice and schizophrenia: A review of the 'mental illness is an illness like any other' approach. *Acta Psychiatrica Scandinavica, 114*, 303–318. doi:10.1111/j.1600-0447.2006.00824.x

Regier, D. A., Farmer, M. E., Rae, D. S., Locke, B. Z., Keith, S. J., Judd, L. L., & Goodwin, F. K. (1990). Comorbidity of mental disorders with alcohol and other drug abuse. Results from the epidemiologic catchment area (ECA) study. *Journal of the American Medical Association, 264*, 2511–2518.

Reichenberg, A., & Harvey, P. D. (2007). Neuropsychological impairments in schizophrenia: Integration of performance-based and brain imaging findings. *Psychological Bulletin, 133*, 833–858. doi:10.1037/0033-2909.133.5.833

Rhebergen, D., Batelaan, N. M., de Graaf, R., Nolen, W. A., Spijker, J., Beekman, A. T., & Penninx, B. W. (2011). The 7-year course of depression and anxiety in the general population. *Acta Psychiatrica Scandinavica, 123*, 297–306.

Robertson, A. G., Swanson, J. W., Frisman, L. K., Lin, H., & Swartz, M. S. (2014). Patterns of justice involvement among adults with schizophrenia and bipolar disorder: Key risk factors. *Psychiatric Services, 65*, 931–938.

Rocca, P., Montemagni, C., Zappia, S., Pitera, R., Sigaudo, M., & Bogetto, F. (2014). Negative symptoms and everyday functioning in schizophrenia: A cross-sectional study in a real world-setting. *Psychiatry Research, 218*, 284–289. doi:10.1016/j.psychres.2014.04.018

Rog, D. J., Marshall, T., Dougherty, R. H., George, P., Daniels, A. S., Ghose, S. S., & Delphin-Rittmon, M. E. (2014). Permanent supportive housing: Assessing the Evidence. *Psychiatric Services, 65*, 287–294.

Rogers, C. R. (1951). *Client-centered therapy: Its current practice, implications, and theory*. Boston, MA: Houghton Mifflin.

Rogers, E. S., Anthony, W. A., & Jansen, M. A. (1988). Psychiatric rehabilitation as the preferred response to the needs of individuals with severe psychiatric disability. *Rehabilitation Psychology, 33*, 5–14. doi:10.1037/h0091689

Rosenberg, S. D., Mueser, K. T., Friedman, M. J., Gorman, P. G., Drake, R. E., Vidaver, R. M., . . . Jankowski, M. K. (2001). Developing effective treatments for posttraumatic disorders among people with severe mental illness. *Psychiatric Services, 52*, 1453–1461.

Rusch, N., Todd, A. R., Bodenhausen, G. V., & Corrigan, P. W. (2010). Biogenetic models of psychopathology, implicit guilt, and mental illness stigma. *Psychiatry Research, 179*, 328–332. doi:10.1016/j.psychres.2009.09.010

Saha, S., Chant, D., Welham, J., & McGrath, J. (2005). A systematic review of the prevalence of schizophrenia. *PLoS Medicine, 2*, 413–433. doi:10.1371/journal.pmed.0020141

Salzer, M. S., Baron, R. C., Brusilovskiy, E., Lawer, L. J., & Mandell, D. S. (2011). Access and outcomes for persons with psychotic and affective disorders receiving vocational rehabilitation services. *Psychiatric Services, 62*, 796–799.

Sartorius, N., Shapiro, R., & Jablonsky, A. (1974). The international pilot study of schizophrenia. *Schizophrenia Bulletin, 2*, 21–35.

Schwartz, R. C., & Blankenship, D. M. (2014). Racial disparities in psychotic disorder diagnosis: A review of empirical literature. *World Journal of Psychiatry, 4*, 133–140. doi:10.5498/wip.v4.i4.133

Segal, S. P., & Aviram, U. (1978). *The mentally ill in community-based sheltered care: A study of community care and social integration*. New York, NY: John Wiley & Sons.

Segal, Z. V., Williams, J. M., & Teasdale, J. D. (2002). *Mindfulness-based cognitive therapy for depression: A new approach to preventing relapse*. New York, NY: Guilford Press.

Shiers, D. E., Rafi, I., Cooper, S. J., & Holt, R. I. (2014). *Positive cardiometabolic health resource: An intervention framework for patients with psychosis and schizophrenia. 2014 update*. London, England: Royal College of Psychiatrists.

Simeone, J. C., Ward, A. J., Rotella, P., Collins, J., & Windisch, R. (2015). An evaluation of variation in published estimates of schizophrenia prevalence from 1990-2013: A systematic literature review. *BMC Psychiatry, 15*, 193–207. doi:10.1186/s12888-015-0578-7

Smink, F., van Hoeken, D., & Hoek, H. W. (2013). Epidemiology, course, and outcome of eating disorders. *Current Opinion in Psychiatry, 26*, 543–548.

Sobara, F., Liraud, F., Assens, F., Abalan, F., & Verdoux, H. (2003). Substance use and the course of early psychosis: A 2-year follow-up of first-admitted subjects. *European Psychiatry, 18*, 133–136. doi:10.1016/S0924-9338(03)00027-0

Solomon, A. (2000). *The noonday demon: An atlas of depression*. New York, NY: Scribner.

Stafford, R. S. (2008). Regulating off-label drug use: Rethinking the role of the FDA. *New England Journal of Medicine, 358*, 1427–1429. doi:10.1056/NEJMp0802107

Steadman, H. J., Mulvey, E. P., Monahan, J., Robbins, P. C., Appelbaum, P. S., Grisso, T., . . . Silver, E. (1998). Violence by people discharged from acute psychiatric inpatient facilities and by others in the same neighborhoods. *Archives of General Psychiatry, 55*, 393–404.

Stein, L. I., & Test, M. A. (1980). An alternative to mental health treatment. I: Conceptual model, treatment program, and clinical evaluation. *Archives of General Psychiatry, 37*, 392–397.

Styron, W. (1992). *Darkness visible*. New York, NY: Vintage.

Swanson, J. W., Holzer, C. E., Ganju, V. K., & Jono, R. T. (1990). Violence and psychiatric disorder in the community: Evidence from the epidemiologic catchment area surveys. *Psychiatric Services, 41*, 761–770. doi:10.1176/ps.41.7.761

Swanson, J. W., Swartz, M. S., Essock, S. M., Osher, F. C., Wagner, H. R., Goodman, L. A., . . . Meador, K. G. (2002). The social-environmental context of violent behavior in persons treated for severe mental illness. *American Journal of Public Health, 92*, 1523–1531.

Swartz, M. S., Swanson, J. W., Hiday, V. A., Borum, R., Wagner, H. R., & Burns, B. J. (1998). Violence and severe mental illness: The effects of substance abuse and nonadherence to medication. *American Journal of Psychiatry, 155*, 226–231.

Switzer, G. E., Dew, M. A., Thompson, K., Goycoolea, J. M., Derricott, T., & Mullins, S. D. (1999). Posttraumatic stress disorder and service utilization among urban mental health center clients. *Journal of Traumatic Stress, 12*, 25–39.

Talbott, J. A. (Ed.). (1978). *The chronic mental patient*. Washington, DC: American Psychiatric Association.

Teplin, L. A., McClelland, G. M., Abram, K. M., & Weiner, D. A. (2005). Crime victimization in adults with severe mental illness: Comparison with the national crime victimization survey. *JAMA Psychiatry, 62*, 911–921. doi:10.1001/archpsyc.62.8.911

Test, M. A., & Stein, L. I. (1976). Practice guidelines for the community treatment of markedly impaired patients. *Community Mental Health Journal, 12*, 72–82.

Thomas, C. P., Conrad. P., Casler, R., & Goodman, E. (2006). Trends in the use of psychotropic medications among adolescents, 1994 to 2001. *Psychiatric Services, 57*, 63–69. doi:10.1176/appi.ps.57.1.63

Thornicroft, G. (2006). *Shunned: Discrimination against people with mental illness*. Oxford, England: Oxford University Press.

Thornicroft, G., & Sartorius, N. (1993). The course and outcome of depression in different cultures: 10-year follow-up of the WHO collaborative study on the assessment of depressive disorders. *Psychological Medicine, 23*, 1023–1032.

Tondo, L., Isacsson, G., & Baldessarini, R. J. (2003). Suicidal behavior in bipolar disorder. *CNS Drugs*, 17, 491–511.

Torrey, E. F. (2006). *Surviving schizophrenia: A manual for families, consumers, and providers* (5th ed.). New York, NY: Harper-Collins.
Tschopp, M. K., Perkins, D. V., Hart-Katuin, C., Born, D. L., & Holt, S. L. (2007). Employment barriers and strategies for individuals with psychiatric disabilities and criminal histories. *Journal of Vocational Rehabilitation, 26*, 175–187.
Tsemberis, S., & Eisenberg, R. F. (2000). Pathways to housing: Supported housing for street-dwelling homeless individuals with psychiatric disabilities. *Psychiatric Services, 51*, 487–493.
Turkington, D., Kingdon, D., & Weiden, P. J. (2006). Cognitive behavior therapy for schizophrenia. *American Journal of Psychiatry, 163*, 365–373.
Turner, E. H., Matthews, A. M., Linardatos, E., Tell, R. A., & Rosenthal, R. (2008). Selective publication of antidepressant trials and its Influence on apparent efficacy. *New England Journal of Medicine, 358*, 252–260.
Turner, J. C., & TenHoor, W. J. (1978). The NIMH community support program: Pilot approach to a needed social reform. *Schizophrenia Bulletin, 4*, 319–348.
U.S. Congress. (1963). *P. L. 88-164 -- Mental Retardation Facilities and Community Mental Health Centers Construction Act of 1963*, Washington, DC.
Vancampfort, D., Wampers, M., Mitchell, A., Correll, C. U., De Herdt, A., Probst, M., & De Hert, M. (2013). A meta-analysis of cardio-metabolic abnormalities in drug naıve, first-episode and multi-episode patients with schizophrenia versus general population controls. *World Psychiatry, 12*, 240–250.
Ventura, J., Subotnik, K. L., Ered, A., Gretchen-Doorly, D., Hellemann, G. S., Vaskinn, A., & Nuechterlein, K. H. (2014). The relationship of attitudinal beliefs to negative symptoms, neurocognition, and daily functioning in recent-onset schizophrenia. *Schizophrenia Bulletin, 40*, 1308–1318.
Wahl, O. F. (1997). *Media madness: Public images of mental illness*. New Brunswick, NJ: Rutgers University Press.
Walker, E. R., McGee, R. E., & Druss, B. G. (2015). Mortality in mental disorders and global disease burden implications: A systematic review and meta-analysis. *JAMA Psychiatry, 72*, 334–341.
Wallace, C. J., Liberman, R. P., MacKain, S. J., Blackwell, G., & Eckman, T. A. (1992). Modules for training social and independent living skills: Application and impact in chronic schizophrenia. *American Journal of Psychiatry, 49*, 654–658.
Wampold, B. E. (2015). How important are the common factors in psychotherapy? An update. *World Psychiatry, 14*, 270–277.
Wang, P. S., West, J. C., Tanielian, T., & Pincus, H. A. (2000). Recent patterns and predictors of antipsychotic medication regimens used to treat schizophrenia and other psychotic disorders. *Schizophrenia Bulletin, 26*, 451–457.
Wehman, P., & Moon, M. S. (Eds.). (1988). *Vocational rehabilitation and supported employment.* Baltimore, MD: Paul Brookes.
West, J. C., Wilk, J. E., Olfson, M., Rae, D. S., Marcus, S., Narrow, W. E., . . . Regier, D. A. (2005). Patterns and quality of treatment for patients with schizophrenia in routine psychiatric practice. *Psychiatric Services, 56*, 283–291.
Whiteford, H. A., Degenhardt, L., Rehm, J., Baxter, A. J., Ferrari, A. J., Erskine, H. E., . . . Vos, T. (2013). Global burden of disease attributable to mental and substance use disorders: Findings from the global burden of disease study 2010. *The Lancet, 382*, 1575–1586.
World Health Organization. (2004). *ICD 10 International statistical classification of diseases and related health problems: Tenth revision* (10th ed.). Geneva, Switzerland: Author.
Wunderink, L., Nieboer, R. M., Wiersma, D., Sytema, S., & Nienhuis, F. J. (2013). Recovery in remitted first-episode psychosis at 7 years of follow-up of an early dose reduction/discontinuation or maintenance treatment strategy: Long-term follow-up of a 2-year randomized clinical trial. *JAMA Psychiatry, 70*, 913–920.
Wykes, T., Huddy, V., Cellard, C., McGurk, S. R., & Czobor, P. (2011). A meta-analysis of cognitive remediation for schizophrenia: Methodology and effect sizes. *American Journal of Psychiatry, 168*, 472–485.
Yalom, I. D., & Leszcz, M. (2005). *Theory and practice of group psychotherapy* (5th ed.). New York, NY: Basic Books.
Young, S., Pfaff, D., Lewandowski, K. E., Ravichandran, C., Cohen, B. M., & Ongur, D. (2013). Anxiety disorder comorbidity in bipolar disorder, schizophrenia, and schizoaffective disorder. *Psychopathology, 46*, 176–185.
Ziedonis, D., Hitsman, B., Beckham, J. C., Zvolensky, M., Adler, L. E., Audrain-McGovern, J., . . . Riley, W. T. (2008). Tobacco use and cessation in psychiatric disorders: National institute of mental health report. *Nicotine and Tobacco Research, 10*, 1691–1715.

CHAPTER

Pulmonary Disorders

Frederick A. Bevelaqua and Anthony Steven Lubinsky

INTRODUCTION

Respiratory disease is one of the leading causes of death worldwide (World Health Organization [WHO], 2014). Lung infections, lung cancer, and chronic obstructive pulmonary disease (COPD) currently account for about one sixth of all deaths across the globe due to disease (WHO, 2014). WHO in 2008 estimated that pulmonary disease accounted for about 10% of the disability-adjusted life years (DALYs) lost worldwide in 2008 (WHO, 2008). This is a measure of the overall burden of disease expressed as the number of years lost due to illness, disability, or early death. According to a WHO fact sheet ischemic heart disease, stroke, lower respiratory tract infection, and COPD have been the major causes of death over the past decade (WHO, 2014). The Global Burden of Disease (GBD) Study (WHO, 2012) compared the contribution of major diseases to deaths and disability worldwide. COPD was ranked third in 2010, lower respiratory infections fourth, and lung cancer fifth. In terms of years lived with disability, COPD was ranked fifth in 2010 and asthma 14th. The GBD Study also presented rankings for years lived with disability. When premature deaths and disabilities were combined as DALYs lost, COPD was ranked ninth in 2010. In 2011, a Centers for Disease Control and Prevention (CDC) survey found that approximately 20.5 million (8.8%) of adults residing in the United States reported currently having asthma (CDC, 2013a). Another survey from the CDC in 2010 showed that asthma was linked to 3,404 deaths in 2010 (CDC, 2013b). Furthermore, nearly three out of every five asthmatics limited his or her usual activity because of asthma. These statistics serve to emphasize the fact that pulmonary disease is a major cause of death and disability throughout the world.

In this chapter, we review some of the basics of pulmonary anatomy, physiology, and pathophysiology as they relate to some of the more common chronic pulmonary disorders that cause long-term disability. We also review some the epidemiologic aspects associated with these disorders, morbidity and mortality issues, etiologies, clinical characteristics, functional limitations, medical evaluation, and methods to assess disability. Much of this material is beyond the scope of a single chapter in this text, but hopefully the material presented here provides significant insight into the issues concerning the medical aspects of pulmonary disability.

BASIC PULMONARY ANATOMY, PHYSIOLOGY, AND PATHOPHYSIOLOGY

In order to understand pulmonary disease it is necessary to understand the basic anatomy and physiology of the lungs. When you inhale, air travels through the nose and mouth down the trachea and into the bronchi. These bronchial passageways branch into a myriad of smaller bronchial tubes called *bronchioles*. These bronchioles end in clusters of tiny air sacs known as *alveoli*. The *alveoli* have very thin walls being only one cell thick and are surrounded by tiny blood vessels known as *capillaries*. It is through the alveoli and the capillaries that surround them that absorption of oxygen from the atmosphere and excretion of carbon dioxide produced by metabolism occur. When someone inhales, the muscles of the diaphragm, chest wall, and rib cage contract, thereby expanding the chest cavity, which draws air into the lungs. During normal unforced exhalation, the natural elasticity of the lungs, known as elastic recoil pressure, causes the lungs to deflate or contract, thereby expelling the air. However, in many pulmonary disorders such as COPD and asthma there is obstruction to airflow. There are many factors that combine to create this obstruction to airflow. Spasm of the smooth muscle lining the respiratory tract, edema or swelling of the airways, excessive mucus production, and compression or collapse of the bronchi and bronchioles all contribute to airflow obstruction particularly during expiration. Normally, the network of connective tissue and alveoli in the lungs provides a supporting framework or architecture that helps to maintain the patency of the bronchioles during respiration. Particularly during expiration this supporting framework helps to prevent premature closure or collapse of the smaller airways, the bronchioles. With the loss of alveoli that occurs in pathologic disorders such as emphysema there is a diminishment of this supporting framework, which prevents the bronchioles from resisting the compressive forces of exhalation. This causes premature collapse of the bronchioles during expiration, which results in obstruction to airflow. Therefore the reduction in airflow in obstructive lung diseases can be due to several factors depending on the underlying pathophysiology. For example, in patients whose predominant pathophysiology involves the loss of alveoli as occurs in emphysema, the primary causes for decreased airflow are the decrease in the elastic recoil pressure in the lung and the obstruction to airflow due to the premature closure of the distal airways on exhalation. In patients in whom the primary pathophysiology is that of hypertrophy of the smooth muscle lining the airways, edema of the airways due to inflammation, and mucus plugging due to excess mucus production as is seen in chronic bronchitis and asthma, the obstruction to airflow is primarily due to the narrowing and blockage of the bronchi and bronchioles.

Clinically and for the sake of simplicity COPD is often broken down into two major subtypes or categories: chronic bronchitis and emphysema depending on which type of airflow obstruction predominates; that is, airflow obstruction due primarily to airway disease (*chronic bronchitis*) or airflow obstruction due to alveolar disease (*emphysema*). Chronic bronchitis is sometimes called *Type B* chronic obstructive lung disease and emphysema *Type A* chronic obstructive lung disease. The key to both of these subcategories of COPD is the understanding that airflow is *chronic*. Although the severity of the airflow obstruction may vary from day to day in COPD based on a number of factors such as the degree of inflammation present in the airway at any given time, there is always a fixed obstructive component in COPD. On the other hand, in other types of obstructive lung disease, such as asthma, the degree of airflow obstruction may be very variable, so much so that in very well-controlled asthma there may be very little, if any, evidence of a fixed obstructive component. Airway inflammation in chronic bronchitis can be caused by a variety of infections and airway irritants, the most common of which is cigarette smoke. This airway inflammation results in damage to the lining of the respiratory tract. One result of this inflammation is mucus gland hypertrophy and the production of excess amounts of mucus that tend to clog the airways in chronic bronchitis. The mucociliary clearance mechanism of the tracheobronchial tree, which normally moves mucus up and out of the respiratory tract, is also impaired (Isawa, Techima, Hirano, Ebina, & Kono, 1984). Therefore, the normal protective function of mucus, which is to trap bacteria, viruses, and irritants, is compromised because of too much mucus buildup, which inhibits normal clearance mechanisms. Hypertrophy of the smooth muscle lining the respiratory tract also plays an important role in causing airflow obstruction in many types of lung disease. Excess mucus production and impaired clearance mechanisms contribute to airflow obstruction in COPD. Inflammation of the airways also stimulates the parasympathetic nervous system of the lungs causing spasm of the hypertrophic smooth muscle lining the airways. Therefore in *bronchitis*, which by definition is inflammation of the bronchial passages, there are two pathways to obstruction of airflow. One pathway involves direct mechanical obstruction to airflow due to inflammation and swelling of the respiratory mucosa with excess mucus accumulation in the airway. The other pathway of obstruction in *bronchitis* involves hypertrophy of the smooth muscle lining the airway and spasm of that smooth muscle triggered by inflammation and irritation.

Both types of bronchial obstruction occur in asthma, another type of obstructive lung disease, but in asthma there tends to be a much greater potential for reversibility of airflow obstruction such that between attacks of asthma airflow may be normal or very close to normal. In emphysema, yet another type of obstructive lung disease sometimes referred to as *Type A* chronic obstructive lung disease, the decrease in expiratory airflow results primarily from the loss of alveoli. This decrease in alveoli causes a loss of the supporting framework in the interstitial tissue of the lung, which in turn causes the bronchioles to collapse earlier in expiration resulting in premature closure of the distal airways, obstruction to airflow, and trapping of air in the lungs. The loss of alveoli in emphysema also results in decreased surface area for the exchange of carbon dioxide and oxygen with the atmosphere. Furthermore, the loss of alveoli contributes to the loss of elasticity of the lung tissue. Elasticity of the lung causes the lung to contract during normal exhalation much like an elastic rubber band contracts to its resting position after it is stretched and released. With loss of elasticity the lung tends to remain hyperinflated. So this loss of elasticity along with the premature closure of the airways during exhalation in patients with emphysematous lungs is what leads to hyperinflation. The bronchial obstruction that occurs in chronic bronchitis leads to a drop in arterial blood oxygen level (hypoxemia) and an increase in carbon dioxide retention (hypercapnia) because of a mismatch of ventilation of the lungs to blood perfusion of the lungs. Bronchial obstruction prevents inhaled air from effectively reaching alveoli, where the exchange of carbon dioxide for oxygen normally occurs. As a consequence, carbon dioxide builds up in the blood and oxygen levels fall. If the hypoxemia is chronic and severe enough, it may lead to pulmonary hypertension because hypoxemia causes constriction of blood vessels in the lung, resulting in increased pulmonary arterial pressure. This in turn increases the strain on the right ventricle of the heart, causing right ventricular hypertrophy or enlargement (cor pulmonale), and ultimately right ventricular failure. Low blood oxygen may also induce a syndrome referred to as *secondary polycythemia*, in which low blood oxygen levels stimulate the bone marrow to produce more red blood cells to carry oxygen to the tissues. This increase in red blood cell mass, if severe enough, can lead to increased risk of thrombosis and worsening pulmonary hypertension. Furthermore, the increased carbon dioxide retention (hypercapnia) seen in patients with severe COPD causes respiratory acidosis (a decrease in blood pH), which leads to a cycle of worsening pulmonary vasoconstriction, pulmonary hypertension, and bronchoconstriction. As the disease progresses, respiratory failure eventually ensues.

Patients with predominant emphysema tend to have less carbon dioxide retention earlier on than patients with predominant chronic bronchitis. This seems to occur for a variety of reasons, but one of these reasons may have to do with better preservation of the matchup between ventilation and perfusion in emphysema compared to chronic bronchitis. In emphysema there is a closer correlation between the loss of alveoli and the loss of capillary perfusion, whereas in patients with more predominant chronic bronchitis there tends to be a greater mismatch between ventilation and perfusion, which results in more carbon dioxide retention. However, as emphysema progresses so does the decrease in oxygenation and the increase in carbon dioxide retention.

Although it has been convenient and somewhat helpful in the past to characterize patients with *chronic* obstructive lung disease as emphysema (*Type A)* or chronic bronchitis (*Type B*), it should be emphasized that most patients with COPD have elements of both chronic bronchitis and emphysema although in any given patient one form or the other may predominate. Even some patients with severe, chronic asthma may develop pathologic lung changes that look like chronic bronchitis and emphysema so that the distinctions often tend to blur. The one unifying physiologic characteristic of all obstructive lung disease is obstruction to airflow although the predominating mechanism of obstruction may vary from type to type as might the degree of reversibility of obstruction. It is also important to remember that the old, classic *clinical* definition of chronic bronchitis—a chronic cough or mucus production for at least 3 months of the year for 2 consecutive years—is not really adequate to identify all patients with chronic bronchitis though it may be useful in helping to identify most patients with this disorder.

The term *asthmatic bronchitis* is sometimes seen in the medical literature and can be somewhat confusing because it is used to describe two different clinical situations. It is sometimes used to describe a variation of chronic bronchitis in which there is a more variable degree of airflow obstruction much like that seen in asthma, but unlike most cases of asthma this variability in airflow obstruction is superimposed on a more chronic, fixed degree of obstruction. Therefore, the airflow obstruction in this situation is somewhat similar to asthma in that there is potential for the reversal of the airflow obstruction that is due to acute inflammation of the respiratory tract. This acute inflammation causes spasm of the smooth muscle lining the respiratory tract, excess mucus production, and edema of the bronchial mucosa much like what happens in asthma. However, unlike most cases of asthma there is only limited reversibility of airflow obstruction because of the fixed obstruction to airflow that is due to the chronic inflammation and scarring characteristic of *chronic bronchitis*. Another way in which the term *asthmatic bronchitis* is sometimes used is in the clinical situation in which an episode of *acute bronchitis,* usually following a respiratory tract infection, is associated with a prolonged period of coughing, wheezing, and sputum production.

An understanding of the pathophysiology of obstructive lung diseases is critical to an understanding of what can be done to ameliorate symptoms, improve functional capacity, and prevent progression. It is important to identify patients early in the course of their disease in order to maximize the potential for improvement with pharmacologic therapy, physical therapy, exercise reconditioning, and the elimination of provocative factors such as cigarette smoking. It is also important to realize that COPD is associated with numerous extrapulmonary disorders. These so-called systemic comorbidities include cardiovascular disease, congestive heart failure, diabetes, lung cancer, osteoporosis, skeletal muscle weakness, and depression. Although tobacco smoke itself is a risk factor for many of these conditions, it is suspected that a "spillover" of lung derived inflammation in COPD may make an additional contribution to the development or severity of these conditions in COPD patients. Comorbid disease makes a significant contribution to morbidity and mortality in patients with COPD (Barnes & Celli, 2009).

EPIDEMIOLOGY OF COPD

Prevalence

Estimates regarding the prevalence of COPD and other obstructive lung diseases in the United States and around the world are likely to be imprecise because of a number of factors. Varying definitions of disease, underdiagnosis, underreporting, differences in survey techniques, and different criteria used to identify various obstructive lung diseases make it very difficult to get an accurate assessment of the prevalence, severity, and morbidity of various obstructive lung diseases (Halbert, Isonaka, George, & Iqbal, 2003). For example, lack of appropriate testing with pulmonary function studies is an important factor that underestimates the true prevalence of COPD. Nonetheless, COPD is generally recognized as being the most common of obstructive lung diseases and a leading cause of morbidity and mortality throughout the world. The economic and social implications of this worldwide disorder are staggering and likely to worsen in the future because of air pollution, tobacco smoking, and the aging of the world's population. As individuals live longer with continued exposure to risk factors, the likelihood of developing COPD will increase.

Although the estimates of the prevalence of COPD may vary, certain conclusions can be made based on the available data (Halbert et al., 2006). First, the prevalence of COPD is higher in smokers and ex-smokers than in those who have never smoked. Second, the prevalence is greater in individuals older than 40 years compared to those younger than 40. Third, although men previously were more likely to be diagnosed with the disease than women, the incidence in women appears to be increasing. In the past, most studies showed that COPD prevalence and mortality were greater among men than women, but more recent data from developed countries show that the prevalence of the disease is now almost equal in men and women, which may reflect the changing patterns of tobacco smoking.

Some studies have even suggested that women are more susceptible to the effects of tobacco smoke than men (GOLD Report, Global Initiative for Chronic Obstructive Lung Disease, 2016). Women are now about twice as likely to be diagnosed with chronic bronchitis as men. In a 2011 study, 3.3 million men (29.6 per 1,000 population) had a diagnosis of chronic bronchitis compared to 6.8 million women (56.7 per 1,000 population; CDC, 2011). Also, more women are now being diagnosed with emphysema than men. In another 2011 study, 2.6 million women (21.4 per 1,000 population) compared to 2.1 million men (19.0 per 1,000 population) were diagnosed with emphysema (CDC, 2011). In addition, more women appear to be dying from COPD than men. Over the past decade, women have exceeded men in the number of deaths attributable to COPD (American Lung Association COPD Fact Sheet, May 2014). When reviewing these statistics, the likelihood that COPD is really underdiagnosed should be kept in mind. According to another study done in 2011, 12.7 million U.S. adults (aged 18 and over) were estimated to have COPD (CDC, 2012). However, close to 24 million U.S. adults had evidence of impaired lung function on pulmonary function testing strongly suggesting that COPD is very underdiagnosed (Mannino et al., 2002).

Morbidity and Mortality

The term *pulmonary disorders* encompasses a wide variety of diseases and as such it is beyond the scope of this chapter to cover all the issues regarding morbidity and mortality for all pulmonary diseases. Therefore, we concentrate on the issues of morbidity and mortality insofar as they pertain to COPD, the most common of pulmonary diseases. In doing so, many of the issues concerning the morbidity and mortality of pulmonary disease in general can, by extension, be applied in varying degrees to other less common pulmonary disorders.

Parameters used to measure morbidity usually include factors such as the number of doctor visits, emergency department visits, and hospitalizations over a period of time. The data that are available from the National Heart, Lung, and Blood Institute based on these parameters indicate that the morbidity due to COPD increases with age and that it is greater in men than in women (National Heart, Lung, and Blood Institute, 1998). COPD is generally regarded as being one of the leading causes of hospitalization of adults in the United States, particularly among older adults (Sullivan, Strassels, & Smith, 1996). Moreover, deaths either directly related to or associated with COPD have been increasing steadily in the United States (Jemal, Ward, Hao, & Thun, 2005). Another indication of the importance of COPD as a disease entity is the years of life lost resulting from premature death as a consequence of this illness and the loss of functionality due to the disability it causes.

COPD is the third leading cause of death in the United States just behind cancer and heart disease (Minino, Xu, & Kochanek, 2010). While there is a considerable body of data concerning the number of deaths attributed each year to COPD throughout the developed world, particularly for the United States, there is a paucity of data for developing world regions. However, COPD is probably underdiagnosed, even in developed countries (Mannino, Xu, & Kochanek, 2002). The availability of accurate epidemiological data for COPD mortality is hampered by the expense involved in collecting and collating the information, misclassification of cause of death by attributing COPD-related deaths to other causes, or simply the underdiagnosis of COPD. All of these factors underestimate the true burden of COPD mortality. Also, misclassification potentially omits large categories of patients with other obstructive lung diseases by focusing only on chronic bronchitis and emphysema (Mannino & Kiri, 2006).

Etiologies and Pathogenesis of Obstructive Lung Diseases

A unifying factor in the development of all obstructive lung diseases is the occurrence of inflammation in the respiratory tract and the response of the lung to this inflammation in terms of bronchoconstriction (spasm of the smooth muscle lining the airway), excess mucus production, edema of the airways, destruction of alveoli, and bronchial smooth muscle hypertrophy. COPD (chronic bronchitis and emphysema) is by far the most common of the obstructive lung diseases, but other types of obstructive lung disease include bronchiectasis, bronchiolitis, asthma and reactive airways dysfunction syndrome (RADS), cystic fibrosis (CF), and more.

Cigarette smoking is by far the most important etiological factor in the development of COPD (chronic bronchitis and emphysema). However, exposure to various dusts, vapors, and other airborne irritants, often on an occupational basis, can also lead to the development of various obstructive airway diseases such as RADS and occupational asthma. Cigarette smoke and other inhalational toxins induce inflammation in the lungs as evidenced by increased numbers of white blood cells (neutrophils, lymphocytes, and macrophages) in the lumen of the airways (Barnes, 2004; Stockley, 2002).

This inflammatory response causes edema of the airway, constriction of the smooth muscles lining the airway, excess mucus production, scarring, loss of alveoli, and a host of other pathologic responses in the lung. Both viral and bacterial infections can contribute to the pathogenesis and progression of COPD and other obstructive lung diseases (Sethi, Maloney, Grove, Wrona, & Berenson, 2001). The normal clearance mechanisms of the tracheobronchial tree are also impaired in obstructive lung diseases leading to mucus plugging of the airways, which further facilitates the development of infection leading to a cycle of continuing inflammation (Burgel & Nadel, 2004).

Epidemiological data suggest a close correlation between the severity of air pollution and the development of obstructive lung disease (Abbey et al., 1998). However, genetic factors play an important role in any given individual's susceptibility to the development of obstructive lung disease. One of the best known and well documented of these predisposing genetic factors is that of α1-antitrypsin deficiency. Although this disorder occurs in only a very small percentage of cases of obstructive lung disease (Stoller & Aboussouan, 2005), its effects can be devastating. In this relatively rare genetic disorder, there is a deficiency of a proteolytic enzyme inhibitor in the blood known as α1-antitrypsin. In the presence of normal levels of this inhibitor, the enzymes that are normally released from blood leukocytes, alveolar macrophages, and bacteria during inflammation are prevented from causing excessive lung damage. However, when the levels of this proteolytic inhibitor are deficient, there is more extensive breakdown of lung tissue, with subsequent loss of alveoli and decreased elasticity of the lung. Without adequate levels of this proteolytic enzyme inhibitor, inflammation goes on unchecked for prolonged periods, leading to progressive alveolar destruction and loss of elastic lung tissue. Another genetic disorder associated with the development of obstructive lung disease is CF, which is discussed later in this chapter. This is a complicated genetic disorder that affects a variety of organs in addition to the lung including the pancreas, liver, kidneys, and intestines.

Clinical Characteristics of Chronic Bronchitis and Emphysema

Since we cannot cover the clinical characteristics of all the obstructive lung diseases in this brief review, we concentrate on the more common ones. As we discussed previously, chronic bronchitis and emphysema are the most common of the chronic obstructive lung diseases and in many ways the clinical characteristics of these disorders are similar to the other chronic obstructive lung diseases.

Although the clinical and pathophysiological features of chronic bronchitis and emphysema frequently overlap, some patients with COPD have characteristics that more clearly place them in one category or the other. The reason why some patients develop a predominantly chronic bronchitis pattern and others a predominantly emphysematous pattern is unclear, but it may have to do with genetic factors that influence the response of the lung to inflammation and the types of agents that induce the inflammation. For the sake of simplicity, patients are often labeled as having one form of COPD or the other. The patients who have predominantly chronic bronchitis are characterized by a more chronic cough and sputum production and are more likely to be hypoxic and hypercapnic. Low blood oxygen levels will cause these patients to look cyanotic, that is, to have a blue discoloration of the skin particularly in the nail beds and the lips. They are also more likely to develop cor pulmonale (enlargement of the right ventricle of the heart) secondary to the development of pulmonary hypertension. Furthermore, mucus gland hyperplasia, smooth muscle hypertrophy, and increased mucus production are likely to be more extensive in chronic bronchitis compared with emphysema leading to more pronounced cough and sputum production typically seen in chronic bronchitis.

Patients who more predominantly have the emphysematous form of COPD tend to have less cough and sputum production. They also tend to be less hypoxic and hypercapnic until the disease is very advanced. In emphysema, the loss of alveoli is more pronounced than in chronic bronchitis. This results in a decrease in elastic recoil of the lung that in turn results in greater hyperinflation. As a consequence, patients with emphysematous lungs tend to have a more flattened diaphragm that can be apparent on physical examination and x-ray. Flattening of the diaphragm also tends to impair the normal respiratory mechanics of breathing because the flattened diaphragm functions at a mechanical disadvantage. As discussed earlier, loss of lung elastic recoil also results in restricted airflow because it facilitates compression of the airways during expiration. In severe cases, airflow may be limited even when the individual is breathing at rest, causing an individual to appear to be short of breath (dyspneic) even when not engaged in any physical activity. The loss of alveoli in emphysematous lungs is also associated with the loss of alveolar capillaries. Therefore, emphysematous lungs contain many areas with a higher than normal ratio of ventilation to blood perfusion. This results in an increase of the so-called physiological dead spaces, which are areas of the lung that are ventilated with air but not well perfused by the blood so that gas exchange with the atmosphere is impaired. When this happens, the minute ventilation (liters per minute of air moved in and out of the lung) required to produce adequate levels of alveolar ventilation (liters of air actually involved with gas exchange in functioning alveoli) increases, thereby increasing the total work of breathing. As the disease progresses, the patient is less able to compensate even with the increased work required to breathe. A more severe impairment of gas exchange may occur in areas of the lung where there is underventilation in relation to perfusion. This results in so-called physiological shunting where blood passing through the lungs is exposed to poorly ventilated alveoli causing inadequate amounts of oxygen absorption, leading to hypoxemia and the clinical manifestation of cyanosis. This is a major cause of hypoxemia seen in COPD. Patients with emphysema may also have areas of low ventilation to perfusion similar to those with chronic bronchitis because inflammatory changes in the airways of emphysema patients may also contribute to airflow obstruction, resulting in decreased ventilation to perfusion. This is usually more striking in patients who present with acute bronchitis superimposed on preexisting emphysema. Interestingly, patients who predominantly have emphysema usually maintain an arterial oxygen level remarkably close to normal despite a marked degree of airflow limitation until their disease is far advanced. Such preservation of arterial oxygen level is unusual in patients who predominantly have severe chronic bronchitis. For an equivalent degree of airflow limitation, the patient with predominant emphysema is less likely to develop low blood oxygen and high carbon dioxide compared with the patient with predominant chronic bronchitis. This clinical characteristic also reflects the relatively well-preserved ventilatory response to carbon dioxide noted in the emphysema patient. In other words, the emphysema patient tends to maintain a greater degree of sensitivity to rising carbon dioxide levels as a stimulus to respiration compared with the patient with chronic bronchitis (Lane & Howell, 1970). The reason for this preservation of carbon dioxide responsiveness as a stimulus to respiration in emphysema patients and the apparently impaired responsiveness to increasing carbon dioxide levels in chronic bronchitis patients is not well understood. Although patients with emphysema tend to have less severe hypoxemia and hypercapnia than patients with chronic bronchitis, as emphysema progresses, both hypoxemia and hypercapnia are likely to develop, once again blurring the clinical distinctions between chronic bronchitis and emphysema.

When emphysema exists in relatively pure form there is dyspnea on exertion, but the patient is relatively free from the productive cough or bronchospasm associated with chronic bronchitis. Cyanosis and clubbing (bulbous enlargement of the fingertips and toes) are usually absent, but use of accessory muscles of respiration and pursed-lip breathing occur. In so-called pursed-lip breathing, the patient tends to breathe out against partially closed lips, similar to whistling. This maneuver tends to maintain pressure within the smaller airways during expiration helping to prevent the premature closure of these airways that is characteristic of emphysema. In the classic chronic bronchitis patient there is also dyspnea (shortness of breath) with minimal exertion, but the patient usually has a more productive cough frequently associated with bronchospasm. In such patients, cyanosis is also more common. Use of accessory muscles of respiration and pursed-lip breathing may also occur, but this is usually less pronounced than in the more emphysematous type patient.

On physical examination, the emphysematous patient tends to be more barrel-chested than the patient with predominantly chronic bronchitis because of the hyperinflation of the lung. Hyperinflation of the lung in emphysema also makes the lung of the emphysema patient more hyperresonant or drum-like when the chest wall is percussed or tapped during the physical examination. Diaphragmatic excursion in the emphysema patient is also diminished because the hyperinflation of the lung impairs movement of the diaphragm. On auscultation wheezes and rhonchi are less pronounced in patients with emphysema because these abnormal breath sounds are due to the type of airflow turbulence more likely caused by the pathophysiological changes in the airways associated with chronic bronchitis. Chest x-rays of a patient with emphysema usually demonstrate an increased front-to-back diameter of the chest, low lying or flat diaphragms, increased air space behind the sternum, prominent or enlarged pulmonary arteries, and an elongated mediastinum (central compartment of the chest in which the heart, blood vessels, and other structures lie). So-called bullae may also be noted, which are areas of the lung that have undergone degenerative change because of loss of alveoli resulting in thin-walled cystic areas filled with air. CT scanning gives an even more precise picture of the anatomical changes in the lung associated with both chronic bronchitis and emphysema. However, it must be remembered that the diagnostic evaluation of the patient with COPD, be it primarily emphysema or chronic bronchitis, relies on a combination of factors including patient history, physical examination, pulmonary function studies, and radiological findings.

Other Types of Chronic Obstructive Lung Disease

Asthma, CF, and bronchiectasis are examples of other lung diseases in which the major pathophysiological processes involve the airways. Asthma and CF are discussed in more detail later in this chapter. Bronchiectasis is characterized pathologically by chronic, irreversible dilatation and distortion of the bronchi. These abnormalities often develop following some sort of inflammatory or infectious injury to the respiratory tract (e.g., tuberculosis, severe pneumonia, or other respiratory tract infections). Anatomical bronchial abnormalities that are congenital in nature may also lead to the development of bronchiectasis. The clinical manifestations of bronchiectasis depend on the severity of the pathology and the degree of vascularity associated with the anatomical distortion of the bronchi. Patients with bronchiectasis usually have a chronic cough that is productive of excessive amounts of mucus that is often infected, although some patients may have minimal cough and sputum production. Hemoptysis (expectoration of blood) that at times may be severe and life-threatening can also occur. Chronic sinusitis and clubbing of the fingers are common clinical characteristics often associated with bronchiectasis.

Functional Disabilities

In regard to the chronic obstructive lung diseases in general the earliest clinical manifestations may be relatively mild. However, as time goes on, dyspnea usually becomes the predominant limiting factor. Other factors such as cough and sputum production may also become major limiting factors. Cough and sputum production are particularly troublesome when dealing with entities such as severe chronic bronchitis, bronchiectasis, and CF. However, years may pass before the dyspnea, cough, or sputum production is severe enough to limit routine daily activities such as stair climbing or walking. Until the underlying disease is very far advanced, relatively sedentary activities may be accomplished without too much difficulty. Even with fairly advanced disease driving may be possible, but walking short distances may not be possible if an incline or stairs are involved.

Nonetheless, there are some patients with severe obstructive lung disease who maintain a better than expected level of physical activity despite reduced oxygen saturation of the blood and elevated carbon dioxide levels. Such individuals may be able to remain at work if the work is sedentary in nature and transportation is not a problem. Therefore, assessment of a given patient's functional capability as it relates to occupational activities may be difficult to determine based on pulmonary function studies and blood gases alone. Much depends on the physical requirements of the job and transportation issues to and from work. In addition, depression, fear, and anxiety are potent ancillary factors that may further exacerbate the patient's physical limitations from a psychological standpoint. Recurrent respiratory tract infections and continued smoking greatly enhance the progression of the underlying disease process. Immobility in patients with COPD is associated with increased rates of hospitalization and decreased survival (Garcia-Rio et al., 2012). Once a diagnosis of obstructive lung disease is made, preparation for a more sedentary occupation would be wise even at the onset of relatively mild disease since the rate of progression can be variable.

Medical Evaluation and Disability Assessment

In general, patients with symptomatic respiratory disease should be examined and evaluated by a specialist in internal medicine or pulmonary disease. A complete medical history should be taken including information regarding symptom severity and duration. Factors that precipitate the onset of symptoms need to be identified as well as the occupational and environmental factors that might be involved in the pathogenesis of the patient's illness. A history of smoking should be noted as well as any family history of pulmonary disease, followed by a detailed physical examination. A chest x-ray should be obtained to rule out other associated medical problems such as cancer and infection. However, while a chest x-ray often shows changes characteristic of emphysema and chronic bronchitis, there is frequently a poor correlation between x-ray findings, a patient's functional capacity, and rehabilitation potential. Although dyspnea is often the most prominent symptom in a patient with pulmonary disease, it is not useful in determining the level of impairment. Dyspnea can be attributed to both pulmonary and nonpulmonary causes such as cardiac disease or anxiety. Additionally, there are limitations in both the specificity and sensitivity of scales used to rate levels of self-reported dyspnea (Balmes & Barnhart, 2005). The impact of pulmonary impairment on functional abilities and the ability to perform activities of daily living or maintain employment determines the degree of disability. Activity limitation and participation restriction are not as easy to quantify as impairment since they are affected by factors unique to each individual. These factors include age, gender, body mass index, educational level, economic status, social environment, and the physical or energy requirements of one's occupation (American Thoracic Society [ATS], 1986). The determination of activity limitation and participation restriction requires consideration of medical and nonmedical variables; therefore, individuals with similar levels of impairment may experience different levels of disability (ATS, 1993). Other tests such as blood studies and electrocardiogram may help identify nonpulmonary disorders that may be contributory to the patient's pulmonary symptoms. Pulmonary function tests (PFTs) are particularly important in evaluating a patient's functional capacity. Two important parameters that are followed in patients with obstructive lung disease are the forced vital capacity (FVC) and the forced expiratory volume in 1 second (FEV_1). The FVC is the maximum amount of air that can be exhaled after a full inspiration. The FEV_1 is the volume of air expired during the first second of the forced expiratory maneuver after a full inhalation. Table 21.1, taken from the Global Initiative for Chronic Obstructive Lung Disease (GOLD Report, Global Initiative for Chronic Obstructive Lung Disease, 2008), lists commonly used criteria for determining level of severity of COPD based on the FVC and FEV_1.

Global Initiative for Chronic Obstructive Lung Disease (GOLD)

Classification of COPD Severity

The volume exhaled with a forced expiratory maneuver during the second (FEV_2) and third

TABLE 21.1

GLOBAL INITIATIVE FOR CHRONIC OBSTRUCTIVE LUNG DISEASE (GOLD) CLASSIFICATION OF COPD SEVERITY

Stage	Lung Function[a]		Symptoms
	FEV_1 (%)	FEV_1/FVC	
I (Mild)	>80	<0.7	With or without cough, sputum
II (Moderate)	50–80	<0.7	With or without cough, sputum, dyspnea
III (Severe)	30–50	<0.7	With or without cough, sputum, dyspnea
IV (Very severe)	<30[b]	<0.7	Respiratory or right heart failure

[a]Based on postbronchodilator function.

[b]A postbronchodilator FEV_1 <30% predicted or FEV_1 <50% with respiratory failure.

Source: From GOLD Report, Global Initiative for Chronic Obstructive Lung Disease. Global strategy for the diagnosis, management, and prevention of chronic obstructive pulmonary disease (update 2015).

(FEV_3) seconds is also often measured during simple spirometry testing. The FVC, FEV_1, FEV_2, and FEV_3 are all reduced in obstructive lung diseases, but restrictive lung diseases (see the section "Interstitial Lung Diseases") can also reduce these parameters. However, in obstructive lung disease, the ratios of FEV_1, FEV_2, and FEV_3 to FVC are reduced, whereas in restrictive lung diseases, these ratios tend to be normal or at times above normal. Each agency that provides disability compensation will utilize its own specific rating scales for determining disability. Other scales that are often utilized include: the American Medical Association (AMA) *Guides to the Evaluation of Permanent Impairment*; Social Security (Disability Programs, Medical/Professional Relations, Disability Evaluation under Social Security, U.S. Department of Health and Human Resources); Workers' Compensation Insurance; and the Department of Veterans Affairs (Balmes & Barnhart, 2005).

It should be noted that PFTs are useful in evaluating a patient's performance only when patient cooperation is complete and a competent technician is performing the study. Arterial blood gas determinations, lung volume measurements using various methodologies, cardiopulmonary stress testing, and determination of airflow resistance are other types of PFTs that can be helpful in evaluating a patient's pulmonary limitations.

In the updated GOLD guidelines (GOLD Report, Global Initiative for Chronic Obstructive Lung Disease, 2016) the evaluation of severity of COPD has become more multifactorial based not only on spirometry but also symptoms, exacerbation risk, and the presence of comorbidities.

Cardiopulmonary stress testing is a further extension of pulmonary function testing during which the patient is actively exercised while ventilatory and cardiac monitoring is done to see if certain levels of exercise uncover pulmonary and/or cardiac limitations. Although exercise testing is not always necessary in the investigation of pulmonary impairment, it may be useful when the cause of shortness of breath cannot be determined by conventional PFTs done at rest or when the patient's complaints are out of proportion to lung function abnormalities found on conventional PFTs (AMA, 2008). Exercise testing provides more information about an individual's physiological responses to exercise and the maximal oxygen consumption (VO_2 max) attained during performance of a graded exercised protocol. Determining a person's VO_2 max can be helpful in estimating both exercise intensity and the general level of physical activity that can be safely performed. Such testing also provides a clearer picture of the patient's physical work capabilities.

Although PFTs and cardiopulmonary stress testing are helpful in assessing physical capabilities, it should be remembered that highly motivated, well-trained, and well-conditioned patients are likely to be more capable of performing physical activity compared with poorly motivated and deconditioned patients even though their pulmonary function studies may be comparable. After reviewing the medical history, physical examination, laboratory studies, radiological findings, PFTs, and, as needed, cardiopulmonary exercise testing, the physician is better able to categorize the level of impairment regarding an individual's pulmonary disorder.

Treatment

Many patients with chronic pulmonary disease have potential for some reversibility or improvement that can be achieved with proper medical management. Tobacco smoking cessation is a disease modifying intervention that improves lung function, slows the rate of disease progression, and improves survival in smokers and patients with COPD (Anthonisen et al., 1994).

Periodical acute exacerbations caused by a variety of factors including infection may also occur. Such exacerbations may cause an acute deterioration in function that will improve as the acute process is treated. A wide variety of antibiotics are available to treat respiratory infections. There are also a number of medications that can help alleviate the bronchospasm found in many patients with COPD. Theophylline-type drugs were commonly used in the past to alleviate bronchospasm, but they have been largely replaced by other more effective medications. Inhaled long-acting antimuscarinic agents (LAMAs) including tiotropium, aclidinium, and umeclidinium improve lung function and limit the rate of acute exacerbations (Tashkin et al., 2008). Inhaled corticosteroids (ICSs), often in combination with inhaled long-acting beta agonists (LABAs), are commonly used and have bronchodilating and anti-inflammatory properties that improve lung function and decrease rates of acute exacerbation of COPD (AECOPD; Claverly et al.,

2007). However, inhaled steroids may statistically increase the risk of pneumonia in this population. The oral phosphodiesterase-4 inhibitor roflumilast has been shown to improve lung function and decrease the rate of AECOPD, but its use is limited by gastrointestinal and psychiatric side effects (Fabbri et al., 2009). Prolonged use of the antibiotic azithromycin can decrease the risk of acute exacerbation in those prone to exacerbations, although there is some concern for hearing loss and antibiotic resistance with this treatment (Albert et al., 2011). Oral, intravenous, and intramuscular corticosteroid drugs have marked anti-inflammatory properties that can be extremely helpful in managing acute, severe bronchospasm. However, use of these drugs on a long-term basis can be associated with severe side effects such as osteoporosis, weight gain, muscle weakness, elevated blood sugar, cataract formation, and peptic ulcer disease. ICS-type drugs such as beclomethasone, budesonide, fluticasone, mometasone, ciclesonide, and others may be particularly helpful for long-term management of steroid responsive bronchospasm because of their minimal systemic side effects. However, inhaled steroids are usually not very useful for acute, severe bronchospasm. Antileukotriene-type drugs, which were primarily developed to reduce airway inflammation in asthma patients, may also be useful in reducing the inflammatory response in patients who have COPD with a bronchospastic component (Riccioni, DiIlio, Theoharides, & D'Orazio, 2004). Preventing dehydration in patients with COPD is also an important factor in treatment since it tends to thicken respiratory tract secretions, making it much more difficult for patients to clear their airways.

Hypoxemic patients with COPD benefit from supplemental oxygen. Continuous oxygen therapy to provide a blood oxygen saturation greater than 88% improves dyspnea and prolongs survival in these patients. The benefit of oxygen for patients with exercise hypoxemia is not as well defined, but is commonly provided and may improve symptoms (Stoller, Panos, Krachman, Doherty, & Make, 2010). The careful use of oxygen therapy may be very useful in helping the patient with chronic pulmonary disease and hypoxemia maintain a more active lifestyle. However, oxygen supplementation requires careful monitoring and supervision. Transcutaneous oxygen saturation should be monitored periodically to ensure that the desired level of oxygen saturation is being achieved. Also, arterial blood gas determinations may periodically be needed to make sure that the patient's carbon dioxide level is not too high and that the acid–base balance in the blood remains satisfactory. Monitoring nocturnal blood oxygen saturation is also helpful in patients who have underlying chronic pulmonary disease because they are at risk for developing hypoxemia as they sleep, which predisposes them to other complications including pulmonary hypertension and cardiac arrhythmias. Improvement in oxygen saturation may have beneficial effects on a patient's pulmonary circulation, cardiac function, and sense of general well-being.

Chest physical therapy and pulmonary rehabilitation (PR) programs can be very useful to patients with chronic pulmonary disease. Postural drainage (use of gravity assisted positioning) and percussion techniques (manual tapping on the thorax over different lung segments) can assist the patient with clearance of respiratory tract secretions. Breathing exercises, relaxation techniques, and occupational therapy may help the patient more efficiently perform activities of daily living. Exercise reconditioning programs can help increase a patient's physical endurance and work capacity. The benefits of exercise reconditioning include increased muscle strength and exercise tolerance, as well as decreased exertional dyspnea and fatigue (Nici et al., 2006; Troosters, Gosselink, Burtin, & DeCramer, 2008). PR following an episode of AECOPD is associated with a decreased rate of hospital readmission (Spruit et al., 2013). In graded exercise programs, patients should be monitored closely for cardiac arrhythmias, myocardial ischemia, and oxygen desaturation that may occur during exercise. Supplemental oxygen may be useful and necessary during such programs.

Vocational Implications

Although COPD is often considered a disease afflicting older adults, it also affects the working-age population (Sin, Stafinsk, Ng, Bell, & Jacobs, 2002). In a 2002 epidemiological survey (Eisner, Yelin, Trupin, & Blanc, 2002) individuals with COPD were both more likely to report a perceived inability to work and less likely to be currently employed compared with individuals with nonrespiratory chronic health conditions. Most studies indicate that individuals with COPD who stop working have greater airflow limitation, as demonstrated by a lower FEV_1, than those who continue to work (Kremer, Pal, & van Keimpema, 2006; Sin et al., 2002). Sin and colleagues also found that COPD was associated with decreased participation in the workforce: 3.4% for those with mild COPD, 3.9% for those with moderate COPD, and 14.4% for those with severe COPD. One study found that even though airflow limitation of equal severity was present in working and nonworking individuals with COPD, the quality of life was reported to be less satisfactory in those unable to work (Orbon et al., 2005).

To increase the likelihood of remaining in the workforce, it is imperative that individuals with COPD stop smoking and obtain optimal medical treatment for their lung disease including appropriate medications, exercise reconditioning, and secretion clearance techniques when needed. Once lung function is optimized, it is important to consider the energy requirements of different types of work. Individuals with COPD must be able to meet the energy demands of a job and work in an environment free of substances that pose a further risk of respiratory injury (ATS, 1986).

To estimate whether the energy demands of a particular job can be met, it is helpful to know the worker's VO_2 max. Oxygen consumption in the resting state is 3.5 mL/kg/minute (McArdle, Katch, & Katch, 1994). To sustain activity at increasing levels of intensity, more oxygen would be required. Generally, an individual can sustain a work level that is equal to 40% of his or her VO_2 max for an 8-hour time period (ATS, 1986; Gallagher, 1994), and for shorter periods of time, an individual can sustain a work level that is equal to 50% of his or her maximal oxygen consumption (ATS, 1986). Table 21.2 includes estimates of the energy requirements needed for the performance of different intensities of work.

TABLE 21.2

ESTIMATES OF ENERGY REQUIREMENTS FOR WORK

Type of Work	Required Oxygen Consumption
Office work	5–7 mL/kg/min
Moderate labor	15 mL/kg/min
Strenuous heavy labor	20–30 mL/kg/min

Source: From GOLD Report, Global Initiative for Chronic Obstructive Lung Disease. Global strategy for the diagnosis, management, and prevention of chronic obstructive pulmonary disease (update 2015).

If energy requirements of a particular job are unable to be met, individuals with COPD may need workplace accommodations, a change in employment setting, or possibly retirement. Workplace accommodations may be as simple as having access to supplemental oxygen to allow chronically hypoxic individuals or those who desaturate with exertion to remain employed in a sedentary occupation.

Other features of COPD may preclude working in certain occupations. If frequent coughing and expectoration are present, an individual may be unable to work in occupations that involve close personal interaction. If a protective mask is required in certain work environments, an individual with chronic bronchitis may be unable to wear it continuously because of the need to expectorate (Balmes & Barnhart, 2005). Finally, for individuals with COPD, the mode of travel to and from work must be considered, as this may pose a level of exertion that is beyond the individual's capacity. It is also extremely important that patients and their families develop a good understanding of the illness so that they can deal with it effectively. Frequently, proper use of medications results in significant symptom relief permitting resumption of some, if not all, routine activities. Smoking cessation is crucial in helping to delay disease progression. Proper nutrition, exercise reconditioning as part of a PR program, and chest physical therapy can sometimes provide great help to the patient trying to resume a more normal, active life. Psychological counseling can also help the patient deal with the anxiety and stress associated with chronic pulmonary disease. Anxiety and stress can symptomatically worsen the sense of shortness of breath associated with chronic pulmonary disease, thereby further compromising the patient's level of activity. However, learning to deal effectively with these symptoms and make satisfactory adaptations in lifestyle may make the difference between a productive life and a desperate one. In some cases, patients may have to change their employment goals. For patients who are severely compromised (e.g., FEV_1 of 1 or less), slow walking on a level surface may be possible, but stair climbing is likely to be very difficult. Likewise, resting hypoxemia (arterial oxygen level of 60 mmHg or lower) may be adequate for sedentary jobs, but even minimally strenuous activity may cause a significant drop in the oxygen level, which might preclude continued employment. Access to supplemental oxygen can often allow the chronically hypoxemia patient, or the patient who becomes hypoxemic with minimal exertion, to remain employed at a sedentary occupation. However, even sedentary activities may periodically require greater levels of activity that are not feasible. For example, traveling to and from work sometimes poses a level of exertion beyond the patient's capability.

PFTs are particularly important in evaluating pulmonary impairment, and criteria for impairment based on PFTs have been established by the Social Security Administration, other government agencies, and medical societies. Usually the degree of impairment based on PFTs is divided into mild, moderate, and severe, although the criteria for establishing these categories vary somewhat depending on which guidelines are selected. Mild impairment is usually not correlated with diminished ability to perform most jobs. Moderate impairment is correlated with a decreased ability to meet the demand of many jobs, particularly those that involve strenuous activity. Severe impairment prevents the patient from fulfilling the demands of most jobs. Formal exercise testing may be very helpful in more accurately estimating a patient's physical capacity to do work and as such may be very important in the evaluation of the patient's degree of disability.

ASTHMA

Etiology, Pathogenesis, and Clinical Characteristics

Asthma is an inflammatory airway disease that is characterized by a marked reversibility of airflow obstruction and bronchial hyperreactivity. It is often divided into allergic (extrinsic asthma) and nonallergic (intrinsic) asthma. The allergic or "extrinsic" type of asthma commonly has its onset in childhood, whereas intrinsic or nonallergic asthma usually has its onset in adulthood. In extrinsic asthma, exposure to an allergen such as pollen, dust, animal dander, mold, and certain foods may precipitate an attack. On the other hand, intrinsic asthma is more often precipitated by respiratory tract infection or by nonspecific airway irritation such as exposure to cold air. However, there is considerable overlap between the two groups, with many patients demonstrating clinical features of both. Because bronchial hyperreactivity or hyperresponsiveness is present in all asthmatics, attacks may be precipitated by many types of stimuli including extremes of temperature and humidity, inhaled chemicals, airborne particulate material, cigarette smoke, ozone, certain odors, aspirin, certain food additives (e.g., sulfites), and even exercise in many susceptible patients. When an asthma attack occurs, there is constriction of the bronchial smooth muscle lining the respiratory tract, which in conjunction with excessive mucus production leads to plugging of small airways. The end result of these processes is obstruction to airflow. The frequency, duration, and severity of asthmatic attacks vary markedly from patient to patient. An attack is typically characterized by shortness of breath and wheezing, which is often accompanied by cough and mucus production. In some individuals, cough may be the only symptom of asthma. During an acute attack, the patient breathes abnormally fast, often using accessory muscles of respiration in the neck and chest areas. Severe attacks may lead to exhaustion, with slowing of the respiratory rate causing hypoxemia, hypercapnia, and respiratory acidosis leading to respiratory arrest.

Reactive airways dysfunction syndrome (RADS; Brooks, Weiss, & Bernstein, 1985) and irritant-induced asthma (IIA) (Brooks, Hammad, Richards, Giovinco-Barbas, & Jenkins, 1998) are similar clinical entities caused by exposure to toxic irritants and characterized by the absence of asthma symptoms for at least 2 years prior to exposure, persistence of asthma symptoms for at least 3 months after exposure, and objective evidence of nonspecific bronchial hyperresponsiveness on PFTs. Perhaps the most noteworthy outbreak of RADS/IIA yet described is that reported in individuals exposed to the irritants associated with the World Trade Center disaster of 9/11. Although these disorders are in many ways similar to asthma, current scientific evidence appears to support the conclusion that RADS and IIA are distinct clinical entities whose pathogenesis of which different than that of asthma.

Functional Disability

During a severe asthmatic attack, the patient may be totally disabled. Even talking may be compromised because of severe breathlessness. The patient may be very restless and unable to lie flat. Eating and drinking may be difficult. Severe cough may ensue resulting in musculoskeletal pain of the chest wall. Depending on the severity of the patient's underlying asthma, the attack may be totally or partially reversible. Between acute attacks, the patient is typically able to resume normal activity. However, patients with severe, unremitting asthma may remain chronically symptomatic, resembling people with chronic bronchitis and emphysema in terms of disability.

Medical Evaluation

The standard evaluation of the asthmatic patient is similar to that of those with COPD. Essential components to the evaluation include obtaining a history of occupational and environmental exposure to irritants and toxins in addition to a thorough allergy assessment. Laboratory evaluation should assess for the presence of CF especially in children and young adults since the diagnosis of CF is associated with prognostic and management issues that are different from those of COPD and asthma. Psychological evaluation may be very important because emotional factors can precipitate asthmatic attacks. In children and young adults, a social service evaluation may be helpful in identifying developmental and environmental factors that contribute to asthma, such as the presence of dust mites, cats, dogs, or mold in the home.

As with COPD, PFTs are used in the diagnosis and management of asthma patients. An improvement of greater than 12% or 200 mL in FEV_1 and FVC following inhalation of a bronchodilator medication is indicative of reversible or partially reversible airflow obstruction (AMA, 2008). When reversibility of airway obstruction is present, asthma or an asthmatic component exists in the pulmonary impairment. In some cases, when an asthmatic component is suspected but reversible airflow limitation has not been demonstrated, a methacholine or histamine challenge may be administered to document airway hyperresponsiveness. Cardiopulmonary stress tests are not routinely performed in the investigation of asthma but may be useful in investigating complaints of dyspnea by comparing spirometry measures before and after exercise (ATS, 1993. In most individuals, exercise-induced bronchospasm can be controlled with appropriate medications.

Impairment or disability related to asthma may be temporary or permanent. Temporary impairment is used to describe an individual's status when improvement is expected in the future through avoidance of trigger factors, use of optimal therapy, or both. Permanent impairment describes an individual's status when optimal medical management has maximized improvement, but airflow limitations persist (Balmes & Barnhart, 2005). Therefore, an individual with asthma must be clinically stable with maximal and optimal medical therapy in place prior to performing spirometry testing for the purpose of impairment evaluation.

The AMA *Guides to the Evaluation of Permanent Impairment* 2008 uses three separate criteria reflecting airway function to determine impairment classification in asthma. The criteria for impairment take into consideration the type and amount of medication required to control asthmatic symptoms; spirometric evidence of airway obstruction following administration of a bronchodilator; and the degree of airway hyperresponsiveness present. Each of the three criteria is divided into five classes, with class 0 representing no disease and class 4 representing severe disease.

For disability compensation related to asthma, many agencies have established their own criteria for determining the presence of disability in asthmatic individuals. They include the following: Social Security (Disability Programs, Medical/Professional Relations, Disability Evaluation Under Social Security, U.S. Department of Health and Human Resources); Workers' Compensation Insurance; and the Department of Veterans Affairs, for military personnel with illnesses attributed to military service (Balmes & Bernhardt, 2005). Further information regarding the disability criteria of specific agencies can be obtained from their websites.

Treatment

Therapy is focused on the treatment and prevention of an asthmatic attack. The emphasis on prevention stems from the view that asthma is an inflammatory disease and that by controlling inflammation in the lung asthma can be controlled. Medical management of asthma has been greatly aided by the development of anti-inflammatory agents. Asthma medications are typically divided into "controller medications" and "reliever medications." The controller medications are primarily anti-inflammatory agents or long-acting bronchodilators that are taken on a regular basis. The reliever medications are used as needed to alleviate acute bronchospasm. Patients with very mild, intermittent asthma may be treated with rapid acting bronchodilators taken infrequently. However, patients with more frequent or chronic symptoms are usually treated with anti-inflammatory agents such as ICS sprays, antileukotriene drugs, and long-acting beta-agonist-type drug (so-called LABA drugs). Patients with severe asthma may require oral or parenteral corticosteroid type drugs given either intermittently or in the most severe cases on a more chronic basis. Self-monitoring with a home peak flow meter (a device that can measure airflow rates) can be helpful in determining the degree of airflow obstruction. Doing so can be useful to the patient and physician in recognizing the severity of an attack, adjusting treatment plans, and determining permitted levels of activity.

Careful monitoring of the asthmatic patient's status and making appropriate adjustments in outpatient management may help avoid emergency-room treatment and/or hospitalization. However, severe asthmatic attacks often require hospitalization despite appropriate outpatient treatment. Some patients with allergic (extrinsic) asthma may be helped by desensitization treatments in which the patient is exposed to very small amounts of the specific allergens to which he or she is sensitive, usually accomplished by subcutaneous injection. This treatment is designed to build up so-called blocking antibodies in the patient's body that attach themselves to the specific inhaled allergens to which the patient is sensitive. This inactivates the allergens before they can attach themselves to the antibodies that would otherwise trigger an allergic response. Careful avoidance of environmental allergens to which a patient is sensitive should be practiced at home and at work, thereby limiting the occurrences of asthmatic attacks. More recently, treatment for allergic asthma has centered on the use of omalizumab, a synthesized monoclonal antibody (IgG) that selectively binds to human immunoglobulin E antibody (IgE), thereby inactivating it and preventing it from attaching to an allergen that would trigger an allergic response.

Vocational Implications

The degree of disability in individuals with asthma can vary depending on the severity of the disease and on the effectiveness of prescribed treatment regimens in controlling attacks. Since asthma is characterized by variable airflow obstruction, a given individual's clinical status may change over time (Balmes & Barnhart, 2005). Individuals with asthma should avoid work situations where potential environmental irritants exist, including outdoor work and exposure to extremes of temperature, humidity, fumes, or cigarette smoke. Clinicians need to counsel individuals with asthma regarding the selection of appropriate work settings, which should include discussions pertaining to preventive, environmental, and behavioral factors that minimize risk and maximize function (ATS, 2004). In some instances, a worker with asthma may be able to continue employment with accommodations such as modification of the work required or changes in the work site (ATS, 2004).

Occupational asthma results from sensitization to agents found only in the workplace. Once diagnosed, occupational asthma is managed by removing the worker from further exposure and considering him or her unable to return to that job or any other job where exposure to the same causative agent could occur (ATS, 1993). Early diagnosis and immediate removal from exposure are the most important factors in improving long-term outcomes in individuals with occupational asthma (Venables & Chan-Yeung, 1997).

In general, the asthmatic patient is younger than the patient with COPD and therefore has more potential for pursuing career changes through job retraining or additional education. Vocational rehabilitation interventions that train workers with chronic diseases, including COPD and asthma, help develop feelings of self-confidence in dealing with work-related problems and are effective in maintaining employment (Varekamp, Verbeek, & Dijk, 2006).

CYSTIC FIBROSIS

Etiology, Pathogenesis, and Clinical Characteristics

CF is a genetic deficiency disease characterized by recurrent respiratory tract infections and progressive respiratory insufficiency. A specific gene responsible for CF was first discovered in 1989, although scientists have recently discovered that there are numerous gene mutations associated with CF (O'Sullivan & Freedman, 2009). Because of these varied gene mutations, the severity of CF may vary from person to person. It has been estimated that one out of every 20 people is a carrier of a defective gene associated with CF. It occurs more often in Caucasians (1 in 2,500 births) than in other racial groups (Tsui & Buchwald, 1991). Because of advances in treatment, median survival now exceeds 37.4 years (Cystic Fibrosis Foundation, 2007). However, even more prolonged survival is increasingly common with better medical management and lung transplantation. Increased survival has created a need for increased social and psychological support for these patients.

The primary genetic defect in CF affects the mechanism by which sodium and chloride pass out of cells. In CF, the epithelial cells that line the surface passageways of many organs such as the lung and pancreas retain increased amounts of sodium and chloride. The high concentration of these electrolytes draws water from the airways of the lung, pancreatic ducts, and the secretory ducts of other organs producing thicker, dehydrated mucus secretions. This highly viscous mucus obstructs and plugs the passageways leading to infection and destruction of tissue. Although pulmonary involvement is the most striking manifestation of CF, multiple organs may be affected including the pancreas, liver, intestines, and reproductive organs.

Functional Disability

Recurrent respiratory tract infection is characteristic of CF. The patient has a chronic cough with wheezing, dyspnea, recurrent bronchitis, pneumonia, and sinusitis. Hemoptysis (coughing up blood or bloody sputum) and bronchiectasis also occur. Pancreatic and intestinal involvement leads to nutrition malabsorption, poor growth, and abdominal discomfort. Liver involvement can lead to jaundice and cirrhosis while sodium loss in sweat may lead to circulatory compromise. Genitourinary tract abnormalities often cause reproductive failure and renal difficulties. There is considerable variation in the time of presentation of these symptoms. Although approximately 75% of patients with CF are diagnosed before age 6, some individuals may not exhibit serious symptoms until adolescence or later in life (Fitzsimmons, 1998).

Medical Evaluation

The diagnosis of CF is usually made clinically by the presence of pancreatic insufficiency and recurrent respiratory tract infections. The sweat test, demonstrating an elevated sodium concentration in sweat, continues to be the most readily available and clinically useful way of making the diagnosis for CF. In general, a diagnosis of CF can be made in an individual with clinical features of the disease if the concentration of chloride in sweat is greater than 60 mmol/L and two disease-causing CF transmembrane conductance regulator (CFTR) mutations are identified (O'Sullivan & Freedman, 2009). Chest x-ray findings depend on the stage of CF and show varying degrees of bronchiectasis, fibrosis, mucus plugging, and hyperinflation. PFTs are useful in documenting the progress and severity of the disease. As in patients with COPD and asthma, there is evidence of airway obstruction and ultimately "air trapping," which results in hyperinflation. Blood gases often reveal a decrease in oxygen levels early in the disease with elevation of carbon dioxide being noted later on. Progressive pulmonary disease may ultimately lead to cardiac failure as well.

Treatment

Advances in antibiotic therapy, nutritional support, airway clearance techniques, and having treatments coordinated at centers specializing in the care of individuals with CF have markedly increased survival into adulthood (O'Sullivan & Freedman, 2009). Heart–lung transplants are also being more commonly used with increasing success (Yankaskas & Mallory, 1998). Patients with CF usually require frequent chest physiotherapy to loosen secretions and prevent stagnation of mucus and subsequent infection. Chest wall percussion including with pressurized vest devices as well as vibratory airway clearance devices are used. Inhaled hypertonic saline (Elkins et al., 2006) and DNAse enzyme therapy (Fuchs et al., 1999) decrease sputum viscosity, and improve lung function. Antibiotics are essential in treating infections and usually must be given intravenously for prolonged periods. Inhalational antibiotic therapy has also been successfully used and inhaled tobramycin or aztreonam in patients colonized with *Pseudomonas aeruginosa* is frequently provided (Ramsey et al., 1999). Azithromycin can decrease lung inflammation in CF patients colonized with *Pseudomonas* (Saiman et al., 2003). Often intravenous and inhalational antibiotic therapy can be used at home, thereby decreasing hospitalization time. Because of the malabsorption problems inherent in this illness, nutritional support is critical in managing these patients.

Advances in the understanding of the molecular pathogenesis of CF have led to the development of drugs that can improve the function of some mutant CFTR proteins. Ivacaftor, a "CFTR potentiator" was associated with sustained improvement in lung function, weight, and sweat chloride concentration in patients with CF due to an infrequently occurring mutation (Ramsey et al., 2011). There is hope that personalized medicine may significantly improve the treatment and outcome for a greater proportion of patients with CF in the future.

Regular aerobic exercise has been shown to attenuate the decline in pulmonary function over a 3-year period in a randomized clinical trial (Schneiderman-Walker et al., 2000). In addition, appropriate vigorous physical activity enhances cardiovascular fitness, increases functional capacity, and improves quality of life. For these reasons, all adults with CF should be encouraged to exercise, unless their clinical condition prevents it (Yankaskas, Marshall, Sufian, Simon, & Rodman, 2004).

Vocational Implications

Patients with CF often have excellent educational abilities and can be very productive individuals. The patient's vocational counselor has to work with employers to provide needed support mechanisms that will allow the patient to remain in his or her workplace for as long as possible. This might include time for airway clearance techniques or antibiotic therapy during the workday. Also, the work environment must be reviewed to ensure the absence of inhaled irritants that might exacerbate the pulmonary aspect of this disease. Supplemental oxygen may sometimes be necessary to allow the patient to remain productive and ambulatory. Psychological problems often revolve around factors involving the patient's altered physical appearance, chronic cough, chronic dyspnea, loneliness, and family issues that normally arise in the course of any chronic illness. Faced with these numerous problems and additional concerns over sexual function, individuals with CF may develop anxiety and/or depression. Therefore, psychological evaluation and treatment will often be necessary. The counselor may also have to work with the patient's family to improve support at home that will allow the patient to increase his or her social and vocational activities.

INTERSTITIAL LUNG DISEASES

Etiology, Pathophysiology, and Clinical Features

Interstitial lung diseases (ILDs) are a group of pulmonary disorders that involve inflammation, scarring, and fibrosis of the alveoli, the gas exchanging units of the lung, and the supporting structure or interstitium of the lung in which the alveoli are located. Although ILD represents a heterogeneous group of diseases in which there is inflammation, fibrosis, and scarring of the alveolar walls (alveolitis), blood vessels, and small airways, there are many features common to this group of disorders. One major characteristic of ILD in general is the loss of lung volume, which causes what is described as a restrictive pattern on pulmonary function testing. In other words, the lungs are restricted in terms of their ability to expand on inhalation. This is in contrast to the obstructive pattern of COPD, asthma, and other similar diseases that are primarily airway diseases that result in obstruction to expiratory airflow.

The etiologies of the ILDs and ensuing pulmonary fibrosis are often unknown. However, inhalation of certain organic or inorganic dusts and chemicals may result in a hypersensitivity pneumonitis. This is an inflammatory disease of the lung in which inflammatory cells infiltrate into the lung tissue as a response to this exposure, causing the lung tissue to become thickened and fibrotic. These inhaled organic and inorganic particles, dusts, and chemicals may originate from a variety of sources including animal proteins, agricultural, and industrial by-products. These illnesses are often named after the occupation with which they are associated. For example, *farmer's lung* results from exposure to fungal particles found in moldy hay. *Bird breeder's lung* results from the inhalation of avian proteins such as those found in pigeon coops and birdcages. Sometimes the ILD caused by the inhalation of inorganic dusts and chemicals is termed "pneumoconiosis." Silica and asbestos are examples of inorganic dusts that may produce ILD and pulmonary fibrosis. Other potential causes of industrial dust pneumoconiosis are aluminum, beryllium, and cobalt. In pneumoconiosis, the duration and intensity of exposure to the offending material as well as the smoking history are important factors in determining etiology and severity. It should also be noted that the development of pulmonary fibrosis in pneumoconiosis can often occur years after the initial exposure and that symptoms frequently occur after the patient has left the occupation in which he or she was initially exposed (Muir et al., 1989).

Idiopathic pulmonary fibrosis (IPF) is a type of ILD in which the cause of the fibrosis is unknown. At times, pulmonary fibrosis will exist in conjunction with systemic diseases such as rheumatoid arthritis (rheumatoid lung). Sarcoidosis is another illness of unknown etiology, which can result in ILD and ultimately pulmonary fibrosis. Although sarcoidosis is often a benign disease of young adults that may present with eye or skin lesions, pulmonary involvement may result in severe fibrosis and disability.

A common clinical feature of patients with ILD is dyspnea or shortness of breath, particularly on exertion. With mild disease, the patient may be relatively asymptomatic. Difficulty in stair climbing may be noted first, but as the disease progresses, the patient may become quite symptomatic with marked shortness of breath and cough on minimal activity. Simple daily activities such as eating, dressing, and bathing may become progressively more difficult. Patients with severe disease demonstrate striking air hunger with rapid respiratory rates and obvious respiratory distress. Cough can also be a predominant feature. Patients with ILD, particularly those caused by hypersensitivity pneumonitis, may present with other constitutional symptoms such as fever. Patients with rheumatoid arthritis and pulmonary fibrosis will typically have severe joint disease, and patients with other connective tissue diseases such as systemic lupus erythematosus may have ILD associated with the typical symptoms of systemic lupus. Likewise, patients with pulmonary sarcoidosis may have extrapulmonary manifestations of their disease with involvement of skin, eyes, bones, and internal organs. The pulmonary fibrosis associated with progressive ILD can lead not only to the destruction of alveoli but also to the obliteration of the pulmonary capillary bed, resulting in pulmonary hypertension, right ventricular enlargement, and ultimately right ventricular failure.

Medical Evaluation

The medical evaluation of the patient with ILD will resemble that of the COPD and asthma patient as detailed earlier. A thorough and detailed occupational history will be necessary and is essential to the diagnosis of hypersensitivity pneumonitis and pneumoconiosis. Diagnosis will also depend on chest x-ray findings in many of these disease entities. In pneumoconiosis, the chest x-ray is often used as a means to grade severity and intensity of exposure. X-ray findings are particularly useful in establishing the diagnosis and severity of disease in silicosis and asbestosis. Often, the x-ray findings of pulmonary fibrosis may be nonspecific in terms of etiology, but they may be useful in helping to evaluate the severity of disease. High-resolution CT scanning is a necessary step and reveals a more detailed picture of the anatomical abnormalities of ILD (AMA, 2008). In view of the large number of disease entities that comprise the category of ILD, a lung biopsy is often necessary to establish a more definitive diagnosis.

As with COPD and asthma patients, pulmonary function testing is essential in determining disability in patients with pulmonary fibrosis or ILD. The characteristic pulmonary function pattern in patients with ILD is restrictive, with loss of vital capacity (the maximum amount of air that can be expelled from the lungs by a forceful effort following a maximal inspiration), functional residual capacity (the amount of air remaining in the lung following a normal exhalation), residual volume (the amount of air remaining in the lung following a maximal exhalation), and total lung capacity (the total amount of air in the lungs at maximal inspiration; see Figure 21.1).

In the early stages of inflammation and fibrosis, and occasionally in patients with more advanced disease, little change in lung volume may be noted, but more significant reduction will be seen in diffusion

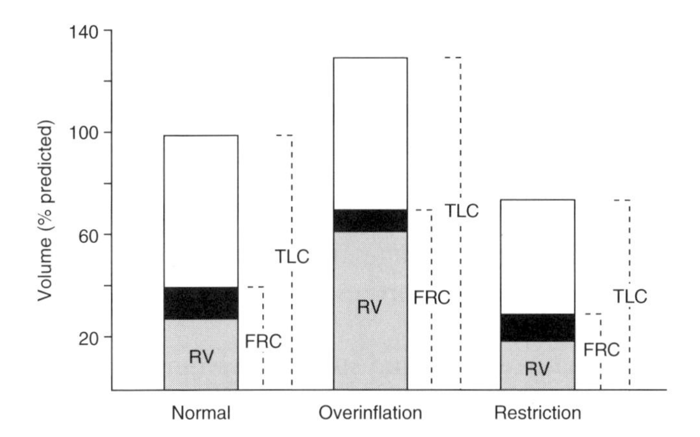

FIGURE 21.1 Lung volumes and capacities.
Source: Baum (1983). Copyright 1983 by Little Brown. Reprinted with permission from Lippincott Williams & Wilkins.

capacity and blood gases. Measurement of diffusion capacity for carbon monoxide may also be useful in detecting significant abnormalities in oxygen absorption across the alveolar–capillary membrane of the lung due to ILD. However, abnormalities in oxygenation and gas exchange at rest may not accurately predict the magnitude of the abnormality that may be seen during exercise (ATS, 2000). Therefore, exercise studies may be very useful in demonstrating deterioration in gas exchange during physical activity (Epler, Saber, & Gaensler, 1980), playing a greater role in the evaluation of impairment in ILD than in COPD or asthma (Balmes & Barnhart, 2005). Individuals with IPF demonstrate a marked decline in arterial oxygen saturation during mild-to-moderate exercise (Hsai, 1999). To increase their minute ventilation (volume of air breathed in and out in 1 minute) during exercise, individuals with IPF, unlike normal individuals, must increase their respiratory rate rather than tidal volume breath size because of the restricted expansion capability of the lung (ATS, 2000). Therefore, individuals with restrictive lung disease develop a higher ventilatory requirement, a greater work of breathing, and a greater respiratory muscle oxygen requirement compared with normal individuals because of decreased lung compliance (Hsai, 1999).

Pulmonary impairment due to ILD is marked by reduction in lung volume and gas exchange, as well as by hypoxemia. For disability compensation related to ILD, specific agencies have rating scales for the determination of disability in ILD. These include Social Security, Workers' Compensation Insurance, Department of Veterans Affairs U.S. Department of Labor, and the Department of Energy.

Treatment

Knowledge of the natural history of each type of ILD is essential in regard to management. In this heterogeneous group of diseases, the ability to reverse the disease process will vary considerably according to the nature of the illness and the stage at which the disease is first detected. In hypersensitivity pneumonitis, for example, withdrawal of the offending material from the patient's environment is necessary and may have dramatic results in terms of improvement. In pneumoconiosis, reduction of intensity and duration of exposure will help to reduce the severity of the disease. For a disease that may be reversible, introduction of drug therapy during the earliest stages of disease is essential. Because immunologically mediated inflammation is characteristic of many ILDs, corticosteroids are often the first drug of choice. Other immunosuppressive agents are also used in combination with corticosteroids or alone. Two antifibrotic drugs, perfenidone and nintedanib, have been shown to limit the progression of restrictive lung disease in IPF (King et al., 2014; Richeldi et al., 2014).

Vocational Implications

In regard to occupational lung diseases, the counselor should work with the physician and employer in determining the offending substances that must be avoided. Retraining, relocation, and extension of education may be necessary for those with occupationally induced diseases. A counselor may have to work with employers to make adjustments in the workplace to achieve an environment that will allow the patient continued employment. Supplemental oxygen and rehabilitation programs may increase a patient's functional abilities. As in COPD, significant psychosocial disabilities may result from severe breathlessness in patients with ILDs. Anxiety and depression are very common not only as a result of the air hunger but also from a drastic change in lifestyle activities associated with respiratory compromise. Family members are also often affected by the patient's deteriorating health and concerns regarding the social and financial issues relating to the patient's inability to function normally. Social service evaluation in connection with the patient's family status may be helpful in determining the extent of the patient's support mechanisms at home.

ROLE OF PULMONARY REHABILITATION IN CHRONIC LUNG DISEASE

Definition

As defined by the ATS, PR is a comprehensive intervention based on a thorough patient assessment followed by patient-tailored therapies that include, but are not limited to, exercise training, education, and behavior change, designed to improve the physical and psychological condition of people with chronic respiratory disease and to promote long-term adherence to health-enhancing behaviors. PR has become an important part of the standard of care for individuals with lung disease and benefits those with COPD and many other chronic lung diseases (Spruit et al., 2013).

Goals and Rationale

PR attempts to reverse the systemic consequences of lung disease, not to improve lung function (Casaburi & Zu Wallach, 2009; Troosters et al., 2008). Systemic consequences contributing to exercise intolerance in pulmonary disorders include limitations in ventilation and gas exchange, as well as cardiac, skeletal muscle, and respiratory muscle dysfunction (Nici et al., 2006).

The goal of PR is to improve the functional abilities of those with chronic lung disease by addressing muscle weakness, exercise intolerance, exertional dyspnea, fatigue, nutritional deprivation, and psychological issues (Nici et al., 2006; Troosters et al., 2008). Target areas for improvement through PR include desensitization to dyspnea, decreased anxiety/depression, reduction in dynamic hyperinflation (air trapping during exercise), and improved skeletal muscle function (Casaburi & Zu Wallach, 2009).

PR Team Members and Areas of Focus

A comprehensive PR program is multidisciplinary and may include physicians, physical therapists, occupational therapists, nurses, exercise physiologists, psychologists, nutritionists, respiratory therapists, pharmacists, and social workers (British Thoracic Society, 2001). The multidisciplinary team will address the following areas to help optimize the individual's clinical status:

- Smoking cessation
- Disease education
- Proper use of handheld nebulizers and inhalers for medication administration
- Secretion clearance techniques
- Controlled breathing techniques—pursed-lip, paced, and diaphragmatic breathing
- Recovery from shortness of breath positions and coping strategies
- Exercise training and strength training
- Nutritional counseling
- Energy conservation during activities of daily living
- Social support and psychological counseling

Exercise Training

The exercise portion is considered the cornerstone of a PR program and has the potential to reverse the effects of deconditioning (Troosters et al., 2008). Deconditioning occurs when individuals with lung disease experience dyspnea on exertion and gradually limit their activity over time, which result in further muscle weakness. Pulmonary status should be maximized prior to initiating an exercise program. Optimal bronchodilator therapy is recommended for individuals with airflow limitations (Nici et al., 2006; Ries et al., 2007). Oxygen supplementation during PR, regardless of whether or not oxygen desaturation occurs, often allows higher training intensities and/or reduced symptoms in the research setting; however, oxygen supplementation in this setting has not been definitively shown to improve clinical outcomes when studied in small randomized trials, but may be used on a tailored individual basis (Spruit et al., 2013).

Measures of baseline functional status are usually documented prior to initiation of an exercise program. The functional measure may be an established treadmill exercise testing protocol, a 6-minute walk test (ATS, 2002), or a bicycle ergometer test protocol. Following completion of the exercise program, the functional measure is repeated to determine whether improvement in functional status has been achieved.

Physiological monitoring to ensure patient safety during exercise training includes continuous heart rate and oxygen saturation monitoring, with blood pressure monitored at frequent intervals. Visual scales for rating level of exertion or dyspnea are also utilized to record symptoms, such as the Borg Scale of Perceived Exertion, which asks patients to rate their level of exertion by examining a number scale with word descriptions of exercise intensities. The numbers on the Borg Scale correlate roughly to the patient's pulse rate (Borg, 1982).

Principles of exercise training used in the healthy elderly population are utilized for those with COPD. Exercise is preceded by a warm-up session of stretching and warm-up exercises, a core exercise program, 30 minutes of continuous or intermittent active exercise, followed by a cool-down period (Troosters et al., 2008). Improvement in muscle function will be seen in the muscles that have actively participated in exercise training. Therefore, programs that emphasize endurance activities (treadmill walking and cycling) yield muscle changes that improve endurance, whereas training programs that emphasize tasks requiring strength (machine weights, free weight, elastic resistance, and lifting the body against gravity) yield muscle changes improving strength (Ries et al., 2007).

PR programs have traditionally focused on lower extremity training to improve ambulation (Ries et al., 2007; Spruit et al., 2013). Currently, greater emphasis is being placed on the inclusion of upper extremity exercise as well, since the upper extremities, used in unsupported positions, are crucial to the performance of many activities of daily living (Ries et al., 2007). When continuous exercise is difficult for those with severe lung disease, severe symptoms, or those just beginning to exercise, interval training, which involves short exercise periods alternating with rest periods, can be helpful (Spruit et al., 2013).

Exercise Training Interventions Included in PR

Endurance exercise involves using large muscle groups in continuous repetitive motions, with emphasis on the muscles of ambulation (Ries et al., 2007). This includes cycling, walking/treadmill walking, and exercise stepping machines. The smaller muscles of the upper extremities are necessary for activities of daily living and there is benefit to training involving those muscle groups (Spruit et al., 2013), including the use of upper body ergometry, ball tossing, and rowing machines. Cross-country ski machines, stationary bicycles with arm resistance, or swimming can exercise arms and legs simultaneously. Strength training can increase muscle strength and muscle mass (Ries et al., 2007). Strength training is particularly indicated for individuals with significant muscle atrophy, and may have benefit in maintenance of bone mineral density (Spruit et al., 2013). Exercise modalities used in strength training include machine or free weights, elastic resistance, and lifting the body against gravity (Ries et al., 2007). Recent emphasis has been placed on leisure walking as a functional training modality. Respiratory muscle training provides resistance to the inspiratory muscles through the use of inspiratory muscle trainers (IMTs) and is included in many PR programs. However, current evidence does not support the routine use of IMT as a standard component of PR programs (Spruit et al., 2013).

Length of PR Programs and Outcome Measures

PR programs differ in duration and number of sessions per week, and programs lasting 6 to 12 weeks have been recommended by the American College of Chest Physicians and the American Association of Cardiovascular and Pulmonary Rehabilitation to achieve physiological benefits. Programs lasting longer than 12 weeks are noted to produce greater sustained benefits than shorter programs (Spruit et al., 2013). PR programs are an important component in the management programs for individuals with chronic lung disease, particularly COPD, with statistically and clinically significant improvements seen in four important quality-of-life issues: dyspnea, fatigue, emotional state, and sense of control over the disease (Lacasse, Goldstein, Lasserson, & Martin, 2009). Significant improvements for the exercise measures of maximum exercise capacity, endurance time, and walking distance following PR for COPD were reported in a meta-analysis of outcome measures, with maximum exercise capacity and walking distance improvements sustained for up to 9 months after PR (Cambach, Wagenaar, Koelman, Ton van Keimpema, & Kemper, 1999).

Individuals with ILD may also achieve gains in functional status following PR by virtue of improved skills for coping with symptoms of their illness and better energy conservation with activity.

Future research is needed to clarify the benefits and outcome measures for individuals with other chronic lung diseases following PR programs.

CONCLUSION

Chronic pulmonary diseases encompass a wide variety of disorders including COPD, asthma, CF, ILD, and others. The economic impact of these disorders is enormous and can only be estimated in terms of the cost of treatment, reduced work productivity, morbidity, and mortality. Understanding the etiology, pathogenesis, and pathophysiology of these diseases is crucial to the development of methods to prevent and treat these disorders. With proper medical treatment programs including PR, many individuals with pulmonary disease may achieve enough improvement in their physical capability to be able to return to useful work, thereby lessening the financial burden on society and improving their quality of life.

REFERENCES

Abbey, D. E., Burchette, R. J., Knutson, S. F., McDonnell, W. F., Lebowitz, M. D., & Enright, P. L. (1998). Long term particulate and other air pollutants and lung function in nonsmokers. *American Journal of Respiratory and Critical Care Medicine, 158*, 289–298.

Albert, R. K., Connett, J., Bailey, W. C., Casaburi, R., Cooper, J. A, Criner, G. J., . . . COPD Clinical Research Network. (2011). Azithromycin for prevention of exacerbations of COPD. *New England Journal of Medicine*, 365, 689–698.

American Lung Association Fact Sheet, May 2014.

American Medical Association. (2008). The pulmonary system. In R. D. Rondinelli (Ed.), *Guides to the evaluation of permanent impairment* (6th ed., pp. 77–99). Chicago, IL: American Medical Association.

American Thoracic Society. (1986). Evaluation of impairment/disability secondary to respiratory disorders. *American Review of Respiratory Disease, 133*, 1205–1209.

American Thoracic Society. (1993). Guidelines for the evaluation of impairment/disability in patients with asthma. *American Review of Respiratory Disease, 147*, 1056–1061.

American Thoracic Society. (2000). Idiopathic pulmonary fibrosis: Diagnosis and treatment: International consensus statement. *American Journal of Respiratory and Critical Care Medicine, 161*, 646–664.

American Thoracic Society. (2004). Guidelines for assessing and managing asthma risk at work, school and recreation. *American Journal of Respiratory and Critical Care Medicine, 169*, 873–887.

American Thoracic Society Statement. (2002). Guidelines for the six-minute walk test. *American Journal of Respiratory and Critical Care Medicine, 166*, 111–117.

Anthonisen, N. R., Connett, J. E., Kiley, J. P., Altose, M. D., Bailey, W. C., Buist, A. S., . . . O'Hara, P. (1994). Effects of smoking intervention and use of an inhaled anticholinergic bronchodilator on the rate of decline of FEV_1. The Lung Health Study. *Journal of the American Medical Association*, 272, 1497–1505.

Balmes, J. R., & Barnhart, S. (2005). Evaluation of respiratory impairment/disability. In R. J. Mason, V. C. Broaddus, J. F. Murray, & J. A. Nadel (Eds.), *Textbook of respiratory medicine* (4th ed., pp. 795–812). Philadelphia, PA: Elsevier Saunders.

Barnes, P. J. (2004). Macrophages as orchestrators of COPD. *Journal of Chronic Obstructive Pulmonary Disease, 1*, 59–70.

Barnes, P. J., & Celli, B. R. (2009). Systemic manifestations and comorbidities of COPD. *European Respiratory Journal, 33*, 1165–1185

Baum E. L. (Ed.). (1983). *Textbook of pulmonary diseases*. Boston, MA: Little, Brown.

Borg, G. A. (1982). Psychophysical bases of perceived exertion. *Medicine and Science in Sports and Exercise, 14*, 337–381.

British Thoracic Society. Standards of Care Subcommittee on Pulmonary Rehabilitation. (2001). Pulmonary rehabilitation. *Thorax, 56*, 827–834.

Brooks, S. M., Hammad, Y., Richards, I., Giovinco-Barbas, J., & Jenkins, K. (1998). The spectrum of irritant-induced asthma: Sudden and not-so-sudden onset and the role of allergy. *Chest, 113*, 42–49.

Brooks, S. M., Weiss, M. A., & Bernstein, I. L. (1985). Reactive airways dysfunction syndrome (RADS) after high level irritant exposures. *Chest, 88*, 376–384.

Burgel, P. R., & Nadel, J. A. (2004). Roles of epidermal growth factor receptor activation in epithelial cell repair and mucin production in airway epithelium. *Thorax, 59*, 992–996.

Cambach, W., Wagenaar, R. C., Koelman, T. W., Ton van Keimpema, A. R., & Kemper, H. C. (1999). The long-term effects of pulmonary rehabilitation in patients with asthma and chronic obstructive pulmonary disease: A research synthesis. *Archives of Physical Medicine and Rehabilitation, 80*, 103–111.

Casaburi, R., & ZuWallach, R. (2009). Pulmonary rehabilitation for management of chronic obstructive pulmonary disease. *The New England Journal of Medicine, 360*, 1329–1335.

Centers for Disease Control and Prevention. (2012, November). Chronic Obstructive Pulmonary Disease Among Adults—United States, 2011. *Morbidity and Mortality Weekly Report*, *61*(46), 938–943.

Centers for Disease Control and Prevention. (2013a, June). 2011 national health survey interview data. Retrieved from http://www.cdc.gov/asthma/nhis/2011/data.htm

Centers for Disease Control and Prevention. (2013b). *National Vital Statistics Reports*, 61(4).

Claverly, P. M. A., Anderson, J. A., Celli, B., Ferguson, G. T., Jenkins, C., Jones, P. W., . . . TORCH investigators. (2007). Salmeterol and fluticasone proprionate and survival in chronic obstructive pulmonary disease. *New England Journal of Medicine*, *356*, 775–789.

Cystic Fibrosis Foundation. (2007). *Patient registry, 2007 annual data report*. Retrieved from www.cff.org

Eisner, M. D., Yelin, E. H., Trupin, L., & Blanc, P. D. (2002). The influence of chronic respiratory conditions on health status and work disability. *American Journal of Public Heath*, *92*, 1506–1513.

Elkins M. R., Robinson, M., Rose, B. R., Harbour, C., Moriarty, C. P., & Marks, G. B., . . . National Hypertonic Saline in Cystic Fibrosis (NHSCF) Study Group. (2006). A controlled trial of long-term inhaled hypertonic saline in patients with cystic fibrosis. *New England Journal of Medicine*, *354*, 229–240.

Epler, G., Saber, F., & Gaensler, E. (1980). Determination of severe impairment (disability) in interstitial lung disease. *American Review of Respiratory Disease, 121*, 647–659.

Fabbri, L. M., Calverley, P. M., Izquierdo-Alonso, J. L., Bundschuh, D. S., Brose, M., Martinez, F. J., . . . M2-127 and M2-128 study groups. (2009). Roflumilast in moderate-to-severe chronic obstructive lung disease treated with longacting bronchodilators: Two randomised clinical trials. *The Lancet*, *347*, 695–703.

Fitzsimmons, S. C. (1998). *CFF patient registry, 1997 annual data report*, Bethesda, MD.

Gallagher, C. G. (1994). Exercise limitations and clinical exercise testing in chronic obstructive lung disease. *Clinics in Chest Medicine, 15*, 305–326.

Garcia-Rio, F., Rojo, B., Casita, R., Lores, V., Madero, R., & Romero, D., . . . Villasante, C. (2012). Prognostic value of the objective measurement of daily physical activity in patients with COPD. *Chest*, *142*, 338–346.

GOLD Report, Global Initiative for Chronic Obstructive Lung Disease. (2008). *Global strategy for the diagnosis, management, and prevention of chronic obstructive pulmonary disease*. Retrieved from www .goldcopd.org

GOLD Report, Global Initiative for Chronic Obstructive Lung Disease. (2016). *Global strategy for the diagnosis, management, and prevention of chronic obstructive pulmonary disease* [Updated]. Retrieved from www.goldcopd.org

Halbert, R. J., Isonaka, S., George, D., & Iqbal, A. (2003). Interpreting COPD prevalence estimates: What is the true burden of disease? *Chest, 123*, 1684–1692.

Halbert, R. J., Natoli, J. L., Gano, A., Badamgarav, E., Buist, A. S., & Mannino, D. M. (2006). Global burden of COPD: Systematic review and meta-analysis. *European Respiratory Journal, 28*, 523–532.

Hsai, C. C. W. (1999). Cardiopulmonary limitations to exercise in restrictive lung disease. *Medicine and Science in Sports and Exercise, 31*, S28–S32.

Isawa, T., Techima, T., Hirano, T., Ebina, A., & Kono, K. (1984). Mucociliary clearance in smoking and non-smoking subjects. *Journal of Nuclear Medicine, 25*, 352–359.

Jemal, A., Ward, E., Hao, Y., & Thun, M. (2005). Trends in the leading causes of death in the United States. 1970–2002. *Journal of the American Medical Association, 294*, 1255–1259.

King, T. E., Bradford, W. Z., Castro-Bernardini, S., Fagan, E. A., Glaspole, I., & Glassberg, M. K., . . . ASCEND Study Group. (2014). A phase 3 trial of pirfenidone in patients with idiopathic pulmonary fibrosis. *New England Journal of Medicine, 370*, 2083–2092.

Kremer, A. M., Pal, T. M., & van Keimpema, A. R. J. (2006). Employment and disability for work in patients with COPD: A cross-sectional study among Dutch patients. *Internal Archives of Occupational and Environmental Health, 80*, 78–86.

Lacasse, Y., Goldstein, R., Lasserson, T. J., & Martin, S. (2009). Pulmonary rehabilitation for chronic obstructive pulmonary disease (Review). *Cochrane Database of Systematic Reviews*. Retrieved from http://www.thecochranelibrary.com

Lane, D. J., & Howell, J. B. L. (1970). Relationship between sensitivity to carbon dioxide and clinical features in patients with chronic airways obstruction. *Thorax, 25*, 150 159.

Mannino, D. M., & Kiriz, V. A. (2006). The changing burden of COPD mortality. *International Journal of Chronic Obstructive Pulmonary Disease, 1*(3), 219–233.

Mannino, D. M., Homa, D. M., Akinbami, L. J., Ford, E. S., & Redd, S. C. (2002). Chronic obstructive pulmonary disease surveillance-United States, 1971–2000. *Morbidity and Mortality Weekly Reports, 51*(6), 1–16

McArdle, W. D., Katch, V. L., & Katch, F. I. (Eds.). (1994). Energy expenditure at rest and during exercise. In *Essentials of exercise physiology* (pp. 78–113). Philadelphia, PA: Lea & Febinger.

Minino, A., Xu, J., & Kochanek, K. (2010). Deaths: Preliminary data for 2008. *National Vital Statistics Reports, 59*(22), 1–52.

Muir, D. C., Julian, J. A., Shannon, H. S., Verma, D. K., Sebestyen, A., & Bernholz, C. D. (1989). Silica exposure and silicosis among Ontario hardrock miners: III. Analysis and risk estimates. *The American Journal of Industrial Medicine, 16*, 29–43.

Nici, L., Donner, C., Wouters, E., Wallack, R., Ambrosin, N., Bourbeau, J., . . . ATS/ERS Pulmonary Rehabilitation Writing Committee. (2006). American Thoracic Society/European Respiratory Society Statement on Pulmonary Rehabilitation. *Americal Journal of Respiratory and Critical Care Medicine, 173*, 1390–1413.

O'Sullivan, B. P., & Freedman, S. D. (2009). Cystic fibrosis. *The Lancet, 373*, 1891–1904.

Orbon, K. H., Schermer, T. R., van der Gulden, J. W., Chavannes, N. H., Akkermans, R. P., van & Schayck, O. P., . . . Folgering, H. T. (2005). Employment status and quality of life in patients with chronic obstructive pulmonary disease. *International Archives of Occupational and Environmental Health, 78*, 467–474.

Ramsey B. W., Davies, J., McElvaney, N. G., Tullis, E., Bell, S. C., & Dřevínek, P., . . . VX08-770-102 Study Group. (2011). A CFTR potentiator in patients with cystic fibrosis and the G551D mutation. *New England Journal of Medicine, 365*, 1663–1672.

Ramsey B. W., Pepe, M. S., Quan, J. M., Otto, K. L., Montgomery, A. B., & Williams-Warren, J., . . . Smith, A. L. (1999). Intermittent administration of inhaled tobramycin in patients with cystic fibrosis. *New England Journal of Medicine, 340*, 23–30.

Riccioni, G., Dillio, C., Theoharides, T., & D'Orazio, N. (2004). Advances in therapy with antileukotriene drugs. *Annals of Clinical Laboratory Science, 34*, 379–387.

Richeldi, L., du Bois, RM., Raghu, G., Azuma, A., Brown, K. K., & Costabel, U., . . . INPULSIS Trial Investigators. (2014). Efficacy and safety of nintedanib in idiopathic pulmonary fibrosis. *New England Journal of Medicine, 370*, 2071–2082.

Ries, A. L., Bauldoff, G. S., Carlin, B. W., Casaburi, R., Emery, C. F., & Mahler, D., . . . Herrerias, C. (2007). Pulmonary rehabilitation: Joint ACCP/AACVPR evidenced based clinical practice guidelines. *Chest, 131*, 4S–42S.

Saiman, L. Marshall, B. C., Mayer-Hamblett, N., Burns, J. L., Quittner, A. L., Cibene, D. A., . . . Macrolide Study Group. (2003). Azithromycin in patients with cystic fibrosis chronically infected with pseudomonas aeruginosa. *New England Journal of Medicine, 290*, 1749–1756.

Schneiderman-Walker, J., Pollack, S. L., Corey, M., Wilkes, D. D., Canny, G. J., Pedder, L., . . . Reisman, J. J. (2000). A randomized controlled trial of a 3-year home exercise program in cystic fibrosis. *Journal of Pediatrics, 136*, 304–310.

Sethi, S., Maloney, J., Grove, L., Wrona, C., & Berenson, C. S. (2001). Airway inflammation and bronchial bacterial colonization in chronic obstructive pulmonary disease. *American Journal of Respiratory and Critical Care Medicine, 164*, 469–473.

Sin, D. D., Stafinsk, T., Ng, Y. C., Bell, N. R., & Jacobs, P. (2002). The impact of chronic obstructive pulmonary disease on work loss in the United States. *American Journal of Respiratory and Critical Care Medicine, 165*, 704–707.

Spruit, M. A., Singh, S. J., Garvey, C., ZuWallack, R., Nici, L., Rochester, C., . . . ATS/ERS Task Force on Pulmonary Rehabilitation. (2013). An official American thoracic society/European respiratory society statement: Key concepts and advances in pulmonary rehabilitation. *American Journal of Respiratory and Critical Care Medicine, 188*, e13–e64.

Stockley, R. A. (2002). Neutrophils and the pathogenesis of COPD. *Chest, 121*(Suppl. 5), 151S–155S.

Stoller, J. K., & Aboussouan, L. S. (2005). Alpha 1-antitrypsin deficiency. *The Lancet, 365*, 2225–2236.

Stoller, J. K., Panos, R. J., Krachman, S., Doherty, D. E., Make, B., & Long-term Oxygen Treatment Trial Research Group. (2010). Oxygen therapy for patients with COPD. Current evidence and the long-term oxygen treatment trial. *Chest, 138*, 179–187.

Sullivan, S. D., Strassels, S., & Smith, D. H. (1996). Characterization of the incidence and cost of COPD in the U.S. *European Respiratory Journal, 9*(Suppl. 23), S421.

Tashkin, D. P., Celli, B., Senn, S., Burkhart, D., Kesten, S., Menjoge, S., . . . UPLIFT Study Investigators. (2008). A 4-year trial of tiotropium in chronic obstructive pulmonary disease. *New England Journal of Medicine, 359*, 1543–1554.

Troosters, T., Gosselink, R., Burtin, C., & DeCramer, M. (2008). Exercise training in COPD in clinical management of chronic obstructive pulmonary disease. In S. I. Rennard, R. Rodriguez-Rosin, G. Huchon, & N. Roche (Eds.), *Lung biology in health and disease* (2nd ed., pp. 371–384). New York, NY: Informa Health Care.

Tsui, L. C., & Buchwald, M. (1991). Biochemical and molecular genetics of cystic fibrosis. *Advanced Human Genetics, 20*, 153–266, 311–312.

Varekamp, I., Verbeek, J. H. A. M., & Dijk, F. J. H. (2006). How can we help employees with chronic diseases to stay at work? A review of interventions aimed at job retention and based on an empowerment perspective. *International Archives of Occupational and Environmental Health, 80*, 87–97.

Venables, K. M., & Chan-Yeung, M. (1997). Occupational asthma. *The Lancet, 349*, 1465–1469.
World Health Organization. (2008). *The global burden of disease 2004 (update 2008)*. Retrieved from http://www.who.int/topics/global_burden_of_disease/en
World Health Organization. (2012, December). *The global burden of disease study 2010*. Retrieved from http://www.thelancet.com/global-burden-of-disease
World Health Organization. (2014, May). *The top 10 causes of death 2000 and 2014*. Retrieved from www.who.int/mediacentre/factssheets/fs310/en
Yankaskas, J. R., & Mallory, G. B. (1998). Lung transplantation in cystic fibrosis: Consensus Conference Statement. *Chest, 113*, 217–226.
Yankaskas, J. R., Marshall, B. C., Sufian, B., Simon, R. H., & Rodman, D. (2004). Cystic fibrosis adult care consensus conference report. *Chest, 125*(Suppl. 1), 1S–39S.

CHAPTER

Chronic Kidney Disease

Sushma Bhusal, Kotresha Neelakantappa, and Jerome Lowenstein

Chronic renal failure poses a singular challenge for health professionals who deal with illness-related disability and rehabilitation. The course of progressive chronic kidney disease (CKD) leading to renal failure often spans many years; during the period before dialysis or renal transplantation is undertaken, the patient may experience disabilities related to cardiovascular disease, anemia, malnutrition, metabolic bone disease, neuropathy, muscle wasting, and acid–base and electrolyte disturbances. Dialysis treatment and transplantation significantly prolong the lives of patients with renal failure, but often allow some of the most disabling features of renal disease to persist or progress. A better understanding of the pathophysiological basis for many of the disabling aspects of chronic renal failure has led to therapies that may reduce the frequency and/or severity of these aspects of the disease. Prevention of disability and rehabilitation has become increasingly important as the number of patients treated with dialysis therapy and renal transplantation has become more common. U.S. Renal Data System's (USRDS, 2015) Annual Data Report (ADR) shows that the prevalence rate of end-stage renal disease (ESRD) was 661,648 as of December 31, 2013, affecting 2,034 per million of the U.S. population. This number has increased more than seven times since 1980. The annual incidence rate (the number of new patients entering the program) was 117,162 cases in 2013. The incidence had been increasing in the 1980s and 1990s, plateaued in 2000, and has declined since the peak in 2006.

ANATOMY AND PHYSIOLOGY OF THE NEPHRON

Each functioning unit of the kidney is called a nephron, and there are a million nephrons in each kidney. The nephron is composed of the glomerulus, which is a tuft of capillaries invaginated in the Bowman's capsule. The glomerular tuft arises from the afferent arteriole. The glomerular capillaries reunite to form the efferent arteriole, which divides a second time to form peritubular capillaries, which ultimately drain into the renal vein. The Bowman's capsule, which forms the urinary space, opens into the renal tubule.

Glomerulus

The glomerular tuft contains the capillary network, an epithelial cell layer that arises from the Bowman's capsule and surrounds each of the capillaries and the mesangial cellular matrix forming the stalk. The filtration of water and small water soluble solutes across the capillary endothelium is governed by the balance of hydrostatic and oncotic pressures across the glomerular capillary. Reduced glomerular filtration in CKD is almost always attributable to reduced surface area for filtration (glomerular sclerosis).

The barrier to filtration of macromolecules is formed by the fenestrated capillary endothelium, the visceral epithelial layer of the Bowman's capsule, and the common basement membrane between these two. The visceral epithelial cell is a large specialized cell called a podocyte, which forms long interdigitating foot processes that rest on the basement membrane, completely covering the outside of the basement membrane. The adjacent foot processes are separated by the slit diaphragm. The podocyte, with its foot processes, and the slit diaphragm serve as a barrier to protein filtration during health and alterations in their structure and function during disease. The ultrastructure of the filtration barrier is shown in Figure 22.1. Disorders of the podocyte and slit diaphragm are manifested by proteinuria.

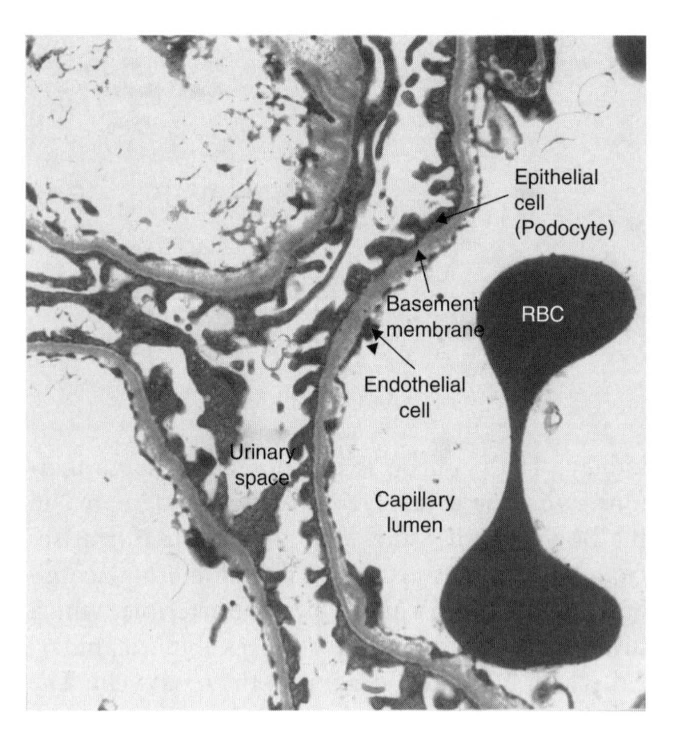

FIGURE 22.1 Electron micrograph of glomerular filtration barrier.

Source: Copyright © by Dr. Barisoni. All rights reserved.

Renal Tubule

The renal tubule consists of several segments—proximal tubule (PT), loop of Henle, distal tubule, and collecting tubule. The renal tubule serves to reabsorb most of the glomerular filtrate and to secrete a number of solutes that are too large to be filtered at the glomerulus or are poorly filtered as a consequence of protein binding. The epithelium in each segment is equipped with a number of transporters—transmembrane proteins that serve to facilitate the movement of solutes and water into or out of the tubular lumen across the lipid bilayer plasma membrane of renal tubular epithelial cells or through the "tight junctions" between tubular epithelial cells. These transport activities are carried out by membrane proteins characterized as exchangers, pumps, transporters, channels, and claudins (Figure 22.2).

This tubular transport is energy-dependent. The energy for these transporters is derived, in most cases, from the hydrolysis of adenosine triphosphate (ATP) by Na+/K+ATPase or H+ATPase. A second class of transport proteins, claudins, line the spaces between epithelial cells (Yu, 2015). Transport through these "tight junctions" permits the selective passage of many small molecules across the renal tubule in a manner that is regulated but independent of energy expenditure as it is driven by concentration gradients.

Disorders of renal tubular transport in chronic renal disease are manifested by abnormalities of acid–base, electrolyte, and fluid balance. In addition to the well-recognized acidosis, hyperkalemia, and hyperphosphatemia, failure to transport (secrete) protein-bound solutes in chronic disease may play an important role in the accumulation of protein-bound uremic retention solutes ("uremic toxins") in chronic renal disease (Sirich, Funk, Plummer, Hostetter, & Meyer, 2014).

CHRONIC KIDNEY DISEASE

Although the kidney serves multiple functions, including regulation of red blood cell production, through the secretion of erythropoietin (EPO), and the hydroxylation of vitamin D to its active form, 1,25 Vit D, its main function is to excrete the daily accumulation of nitrogenous waste products, acid, and ingested water and electrolytes. To excrete the metabolic waste products, such as urea, in a reasonably small volume of fluid, at a concentration much higher than in the plasma, the kidney filters 180 liters of plasma water a day (with all the dissolved solutes at the same concentration as that in the plasma) at the glomerulus and reabsorbs virtually all of the filtered essential components, such as glucose, water, and electrolytes, excreting only 1 to 2 liters of urine with a high concentration of waste products. Renal function is traditionally expressed in terms of glomerular filtration rate (GFR) per minute. However, GFR, measured as the clearance of inulin, is not often measured in clinical medicine. An estimate of glomerular filtration rate (estimated GFR [eGFR]) is derived from application of data derived from estimation of GFR from the blood clearance of injected radiolabeled iothalamate in the Modification of Diet in Renal Disease (MDRD) study (Levey et al., 2009)

The National Kidney Foundation (NKF; Table 22.1) has proposed to consider CKD as a continuum, based largely on impaired eGFR (NKF Kidney Disease Outcomes Quality Initiative [NKF-KDOQI], NKF, 2002), and more recently the presence of persistently increased protein excretion in the urine (proteinuria; Hallan et al., 2009).

The prevalence of CKD of stages 1 to 4 defined as in Table 22.1 was estimated to have increased

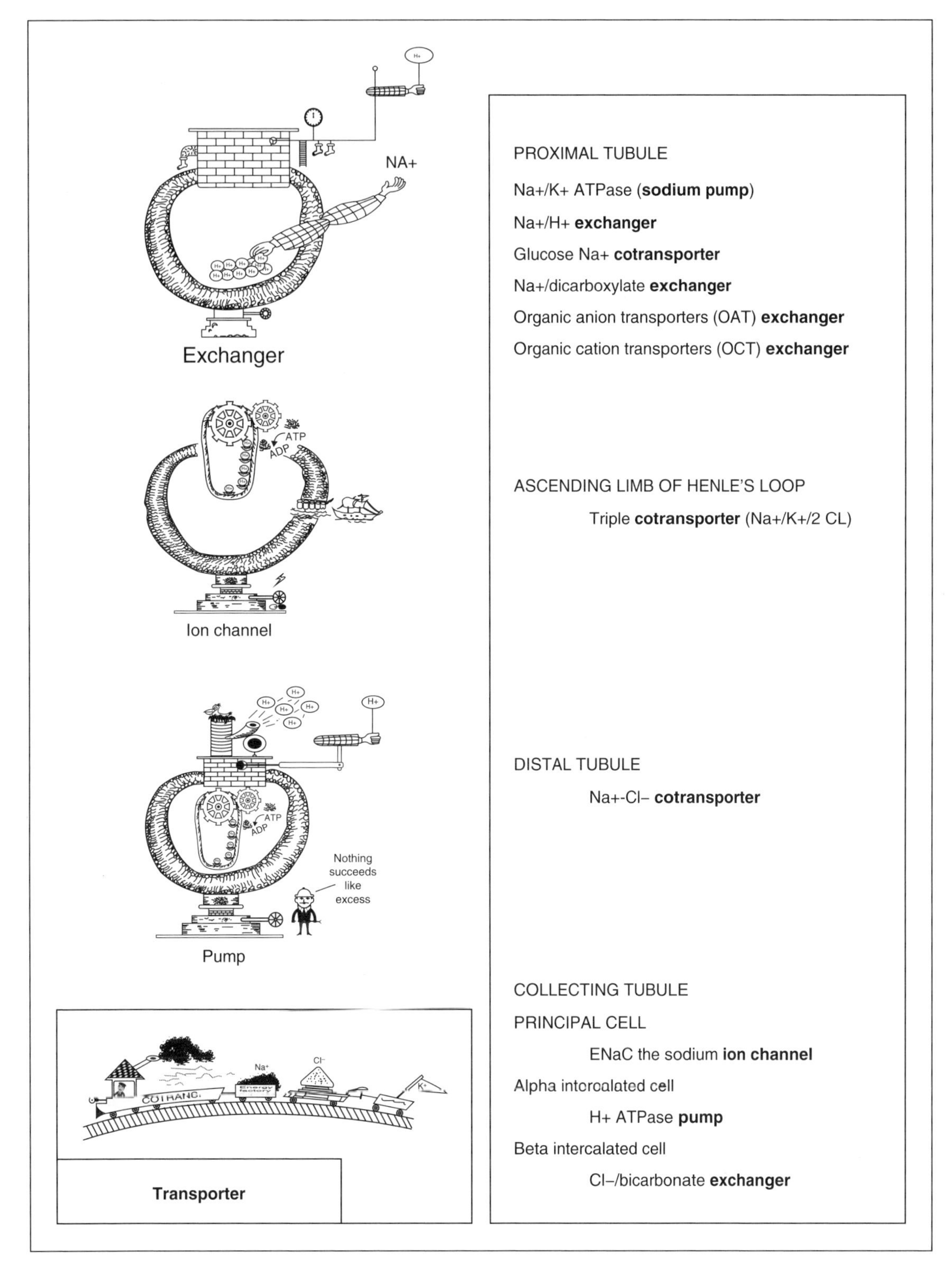

FIGURE 22.2 Renal tubular transporters. These can be viewed as proteins that move substances across the membranes of renal tubular cells to achieve secretion or reabsorption.
Claudins, not shown here, line the paracellular pathways, are activated or inactivated by specific stimuli, and participate in the movement of substances into or out of the renal tubule through paracellular pathways.

from 14% to 16.8% between National Health and Nutrition Examination Surveys (NHANESs) of 1988 to 1994 and 1999 to 2004. This may in part be secondary to increased identification. CKD classification carries the implicit message that renal disease (defined simply as reduced GFR) may be expected to progress, albeit at a variable rate, to renal failure and the need for either dialysis or

TABLE 22.1

NATIONAL KIDNEY FOUNDATION KIDNEY DISEASE OUTCOMES QUALITY INITIATIVE (NKF-KDOQI) CLASSIFICATION OF CHRONIC KIDNEY DISEASE			
Stage	**Description**	**GFR (mL/min/1.73 m^2)**	**Prevalence in the United States (NHANES 2007–2012)**
1	Kidney damage with normal or ↑ in GFR	>90	5.7%
2	Kidney damage with mild ↓ in GFR	60–89	5.4%
3	Moderate ↓ in GFR	30–59	5.4%
4	Severe ↓ in GFR	15–29	0.4%
5	Kidney failure	<15 (or dialysis)	

Note: Chronic kidney disease is defined as either evidence of kidney damage or impaired glomerular filtration rate (GFR) of <60 mL/min/1.73 m^2 for ≥3 months.

Source: Coresh et al. (2007).

renal transplantation. This may not be the case. It is now well recognized that many patients classed as CKD 2 or 3 may not have intrinsic renal disease. Couser (Couser, 2007) stated:

> Identification of stages of CKD implies, perhaps unintentionally, that CKD is a progressive process with those afflicted moving eventually from earlier to more advanced stages of disease. Although this clearly happens in many patients with *defined* [italics added] forms of kidney disease like diabetes and glomerulonephritis, there is a paucity of data documenting such progression in patients with CKD defined *only* as GFR <60 mL/min or GFR <60 mL/min with microalbuminuria. Indeed, it is clear from several studies that many such patients do not progress over several years of follow-up. (Couser, 2007)

More recently, Hallan et al. (2009) have shown that combining GFR and albuminuria to classify CKD improves prediction of progression to ESRD. In a study of 65,589 adults, these authors showed that adding presence of albuminuria to impaired GFR would reduce the identified individuals who are predicted to progress to ESRD from 4.7% to 1.4% of the population and still identify 65.6% versus 69.4% of all individuals progressing to ESRD.

CKD and Cardiovascular Disease

While reduced GFR in CKD classes 2, 3, and even 4 does not often progress to ESRD and the need for dialysis or renal transplantation there is abundant evidence that impaired GFR is associated with increased risk of cardiovascular morbidity and mortality usually defined as sudden cardiac death, cardiac arrhythmia, coronary calcification, or myocardial infarction (Hage et al., 2009; Go, 1974; Lindner, Charra, Sherrard, & Scribner, 1974). Several large multicenter studies (Khan et al., 2006; Tokmakova et al., 2004) reported that even mild reductions in GFR in patients with coronary artery disease and impaired left ventricular function is associated with higher mortality and morbidity. The relationship between impaired glomerular filtration and outcomes in cardiovascular disease is confounded by the fact that many important risk factors are common to both conditions. Diabetes mellitus, hypertension, and hyperlipidemia are risk factors common to both renal disease and coronary artery disease. Risk factor assessment using the scores developed in the Framingham studies appears to underestimate cardiovascular outcomes in the presence of reduced GFR (Henry et al., 2002). Analysis of cardiovascular and renal outcomes in the VALIANT study (Anavekar et al., 2004) composed of more than 14,000 patients with acute myocardial infarction and heart failure or left ventricular dysfunction demonstrated a significant and graded increase in mortality and cardiovascular events over a range of GFR that spanned the CKD categories 2 through 4. Patients presenting with greater reduction in GFR (CKD 5) were excluded from the study. Although the rate of renal events (e.g., hyperkalemia) increased with declining eGFRs, the adverse outcomes were predominantly cardiovascular. Below 81.0 mL/min/1.73 m^2, each reduction of the eGFR by 10 mL/min/1.73 m^2 was associated with a hazard ratio for death and nonfatal cardiovascular outcomes of 1.10.

Although there is strong evidence of an association between renal disease with reduced GFR and accelerated atherosclerosis, the relative contributions of traditional cardiovascular risk factors (e.g., hypertension, diabetes, hyperlipidemia), factors unique to renal disease (e.g., profibrotic or proinflammatory mediators), and the adverse effect of cardiac performance on renal function are not clearly defined.

CKD and Its Progression

Most renal parenchymal diseases, regardless of the etiology of the underlying disease, exhibit progressive scarring and loss of function over a period of many years (see Table 22.1). In some instances, progression occurs because of persistent disease or repeated recurrences of the primary disease, but more frequently progression occurs without evidence of residual activity of the primary disease. Studies of the mechanisms underlying "nonimmunological" progression have provided therapeutic strategies for delaying the onset of renal failure.

The proposed mechanisms for progression fall into two categories—hemodynamic and signal-mediated fibrosis. Many of the studies directed at understanding the hemodynamic mechanisms have been carried out in the "remnant kidney" model in rats subjected to five-sixths nephrectomy. The animals go on to develop progressive scarring and renal failure. Studies have shown that after ablation of a critical mass of renal tissue, single nephron plasma flow and glomerular capillary hydrostatic pressure are increased in the remaining nephrons. The factors responsible for glomerular hemodynamic alterations and glomerular hypertrophy are not well understood. Increased levels of growth hormone, certain dietary amino acids, vasodilator renal prostaglandins, increased local concentrations of angiotensin II, endothelins (vasoconstrictor proteins produced by the endothelial cells), and autoregulation of glomerular blood flow leading to glomerular hypertension have all been implicated. The increase in glomerular hydrostatic pressure may occur in the absence of systemic hypertension. Increased surface area of the glomerular filtering bed and glomerular hypertension in the remnant nephron, while maintaining overall GFR close to normal, appear to lead to accelerated glomerular injury and fibrosis of the remaining nephrons. Treatment with antihypertensive agents is beneficial in slowing the rate of progression in various renal diseases in both experimental animals and humans. Angiotensin converting enzyme inhibitors (ACEIs) and angiotensin II receptor blockers (ARBs) independently appear to exert a protective effect in CKD, which may be independent of the reduction in systemic blood pressure (BP).

Studies directed at identifying specific cellular mechanisms responsible for glomerular or interstitial fibrosis have usually been performed in experimental models of renal disease such as the unilateral obstructive nephropathy and forms of glomerular injury in which inflammation is absent (puromycin nephrotoxicity or experimental models characterized by the nephrotic syndrome). Attention has been focused on the role of transforming growth factor beta (TGF-β; Böttinger & Bitzer, 2002) and other profibrotic or proinflammatory molecules such as endothelin-1, monocyte attractant protein-1, and RANTES (Benigni & Remuzzi, 2001) in the progression of glomerular and tubulointerstitial renal diseases. More recently, attention has been focused on the role of uremic retention solutes as responsible for progression of renal scarring (Jhawar et al., 2015; VanHolder et al., 2008). While it is attractive to seek profibrotic factors in progressive renal diseases characterized by tissue fibrosis, other cellular mechanisms including apoptosis, proliferation, and endothelial–mesangial transdifferentiation may be important components in slowly progressive renal diseases.

FUNCTIONAL ADAPTATION TO NEPHRON LOSS

At birth, there are approximately 1 million nephrons in each kidney; with considerable interindividual variability, the number is proportional to birth weight (Luyckx & Brenner, 2010). During the course of progressive renal diseases, many of the functions of the kidney appear to decline in parallel. This has been termed the "whole nephron hypothesis." It is not known whether whole nephrons drop out or this is a statistical artifact. In virtually all forms of parenchymal renal disease, as nephrons are lost, adaptive changes in residual nephrons permit the kidney to retain much of its function despite marked reduction in the total number of intact nephrons. Systemic and intrarenal hemodynamic changes, hormonal stimuli, and possibly structural changes along the nephron lead to increase in single nephron GFR and to changes in tubular reabsorption and tubular secretion of various metabolites in the surviving nephrons. With further nephron loss, compensatory changes in the residual nephrons fail to maintain normal total renal function, and abnormalities in blood composition become evident.

Minute changes in body composition resulting from retention of some substances (e.g., phosphate retention) trigger mechanisms, which result in compensatory increase in their excretion with little change in the internal milieu. These mechanisms themselves are associated with varying degrees of untoward effects, but these are considered to be less harmful effects than those of retention of the substance in question. This is referred to as the *trade-off hypothesis*. It is well illustrated by the compensatory responses that maintain external balance of sodium, potassium, hydrogen ion, calcium, and phosphate (Figure 22.3).

Sodium

Under normal circumstances, approximately 25,000 mEq of sodium (Na^+) are filtered daily. All except about 150 mEq (average daily intake) are reabsorbed. As the GFR and the filtered load of sodium decline with progressive renal disease, there is a reciprocal increase in the fraction of filtered sodium that escapes reabsorption. Despite marked reduction in filtered sodium in advanced renal failure, overt sodium retention and edema are not seen until the most advanced stage with decreased urine output, unless complicated by other problems such as heart failure or the nephrotic syndrome.

Potassium

Filtered potassium is completely reabsorbed before the glomerular filtrate reaches the distal convoluted tubule (DCT). Potassium balance is maintained mainly by secretion of potassium by the principal cells in the late DCT and cortical-collecting duct. Hyperkalemia (increased blood level of potassium) is usually not observed until GFR declines to less than 10% to 15% of the normal value.

Hydrogen Ion

Daily metabolism leads to generation of fixed acids (predominantly sulfuric acid), which dissociate into their respective anions (e.g., sulfate) and the cation H^+ (proton). Daily metabolic acid production averages about 1 mEq/kg/day. Renal acid excretion is reduced only modestly despite marked reduction in nephron number as renal disease progresses. This is the result of an increase in titratable acid excretion per nephron facilitated by decreased tubular reabsorption of phosphate and by enhanced ammonia production per residual nephron.

Calcium and Phosphorus

Calcium and phosphorus metabolism are markedly altered in progressive renal disease. The concentration of 1,25-D3, the active form of vitamin D, is governed by the enzymatic hydroxylation of 25-D3 by the kidneys. As 1,25-D3 is reduced in renal failure and calcium absorption by the intestine decreases, hypocalcemia (reduced blood level of calcium) develops.

Normally 80% to 90% of the filtered phosphorus is reabsorbed. In renal failure, even though the filtered load of phosphorus declines steadily, the serum phosphorus level does not rise, since the daily load can be excreted by reduction in reabsorption down to nearly 50%. Beyond this point, steady state is achieved by a combination of further reduction in reabsorption and a relative increase in the filtered load achieved by a rise in the plasma level. In large part this is attributable to increased parathyroid hormone (PTH) secretion. PTH not only reduces tubular reabsorption of phosphate, but also mobilizes calcium from the skeletal system. The "trade-off" for maintenance of calcium and phosphorus concentrations is the development of bone disease secondary to hyperparathyroidism characterized by osteomalacia and osteitis fibrosa cystica.

Uremic Retention Solutes

After almost 50 years during which the number of patients treated by dialysis has risen to more than half a million in the United States, it is only within the past 10 years that studies have addressed the question of what toxins are removed by dialysis and, more importantly, what toxins might not be

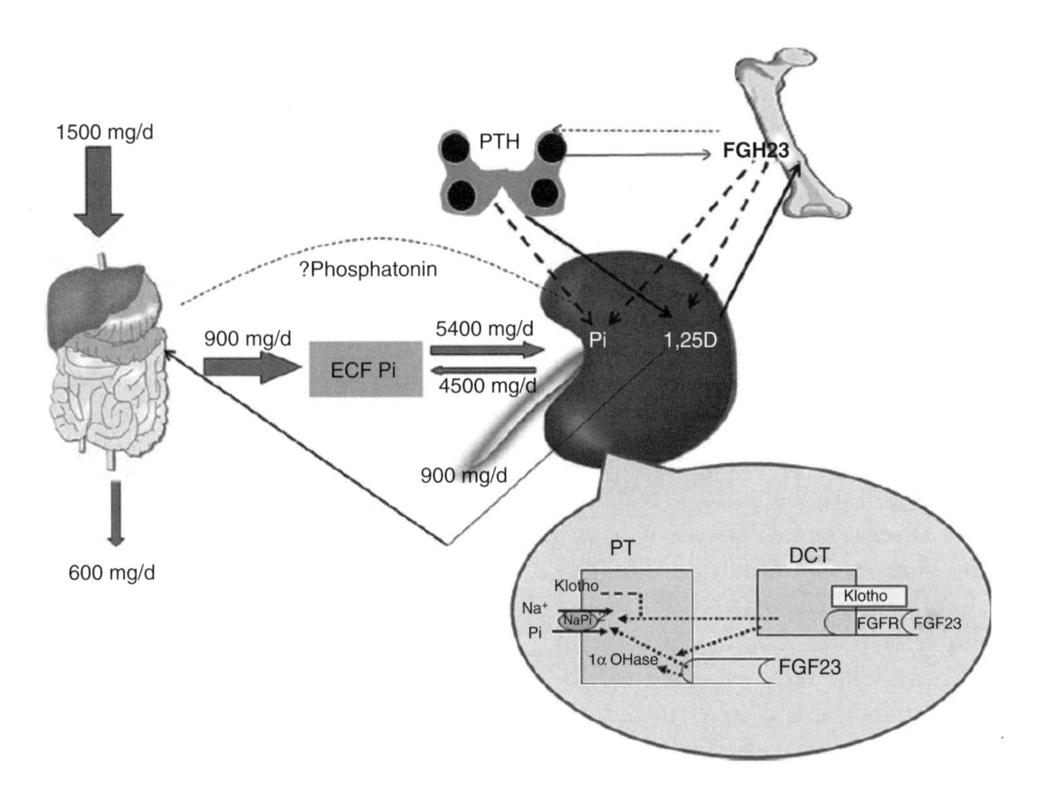

FIGURE 22.3 Normal phosphate balance. Normal dietary phosphate intake is 1,000 to 1,500 mg/day of which 60% to 80% is absorbed. Calcitriol (1,25D) stimulates intestinal phosphate absorption while fibroblast growth factor 23 (FGF23) indirectly decreases intestinal phosphate absorption by lowering 1,25D values. The gut may also regulate phosphate homeostasis by producing an unknown phosphatonin in response to dietary phosphate loading. Bone regulates internal phosphate balance by serving as a reservoir for phosphate. PTH and 1,25D regulate bone deposition and release of phosphate. Bone also is the site of FGF23 production. The primary regulator of phosphate homeostasis is the kidney, which adjusts the excretory load to the dietary load of phosphate. The proximal tubule (PT) is the primary site for phosphate reabsorption. Phosphate transporters, NaPi-2a, and 2c, responsible for transepithelial transport, are primarily regulated by phosphate load, PTH, and FGF23/klotho. Both PTH and FGF23 inhibit PT phosphate reabsorption. FGF23 acts through the FGF receptor (FGFR) system using the protein klotho as a cofactor. The majority of renal klotho expression is in the distal convoluted tubule (DCT), but the mechanism of transmission of the FGF23 signal to the PT remains unidentified. One possibility is that secreted klotho may be the messenger between the DCT and PT and another is that small amounts of klotho expressed in the PT may be sufficient for FGF23 to act directly on the PT. The production and action of FGF23 is modified by several factors including 1,25D, phosphate load, calcium intake, and PTH. FGF23 in turn inhibits PTH production, parathyroid gland expression of the CaSR and VDR, and 1,25D production forming a closed loop. Solid lines indicate a positive effect and broken/dotted lines an inhibitory effect.

effectively removed by hemodialysis or peritoneal dialysis. The EUTOX group (Van Holder et al., 2003) identified a wide range of solutes that were found to be significantly increased in concentration in patients recognized as having renal disease with decreased glomerular filtration. Since it has not been established whether these solutes are toxic, the term "uremic retention solutes" seems more appropriate than "uremic toxins." About one-half of these are small water soluble substances, such as urea and creatinine, normally removed by glomerular filtration, roughly a quarter are "middle molecules" (such as beta-2-microglobulin or complement) too large to be filtered across the glomerulus, and one quarter are small molecules (approximately 250 D) bound to protein, mainly albumin. As a consequence of protein binding, reportedly 95%, these solutes are poorly filtered at the glomerulus. These uremic retention solutes are secreted by renal tubules, the majority via one of several organic anion transporters (OATs) in proximal renal tubular cells (Masereeuw et al., 2014; Sekine, Miyazaki, & Endou, 2006). Several of these protein-bound uremic solutes, indoxyl sulfate and p-cresyl sulfate, are derived from the metabolism of dietary amino acids by gut bacteria (Evenpoel, Meijers, Bammens, & Verbeke, 2009; Poesen, 2013). The excretion of such protein-bound molecules is reduced as the nephron number declines. Studies in rats with partial nephrectomy suggest that retention of several protein-bound solutes, most notably indoxyl sulfate, may be responsible for progressive renal scarring (fibrosis). These protein-bound uremic retention solutes require OATs for their transport and are not effectively removed by hemodialysis or peritoneal dialysis.

TREATMENT OF CHRONIC RENAL FAILURE

Preservation of Residual Renal Function

Most patients still excrete urine when dialysis is initiated but anuria, defined as urine production of less than 200 mL/day, developed during 13-month follow-up in 130 of the 542 patients treated with peritoneal dialysis (Moist et al., 2000). Analysis of large data sets suggests that patients with residual renal function (RRF), that is, continued urine production while undergoing hemodialysis or peritoneal dialysis, have better survival and less cardiovascular disease than patients who are anuric (Bargman, Thorpe, Churchill, & Canada–USA [CANUSA] Peritoneal Dialysis Study Group, 2001; Termorshuizen et al., 2004). Patients in the NECOSAD Study who retained RRF exhibited better survival than those who were anuric. Survival in the latter group was closely correlated with parameters of dialysis efficiency while survival of patients with RRF was almost independent of the efficacy of dialysis Kt/V_{creat}. It has been estimated that RRF provides clearance of the conventional surrogate uremic markers, urea and creatinine, roughly equivalent to prolonging each hemodialysis by only 33 minutes The findings of less severe cardiovascular disease and the observation that survival is virtually independent of the dialyzer clearance of creatinine in patients with RRF suggest the possibility that RRF confers a cardiovascular benefit to patients with ESRD and suggests a unique mechanism for continued urine production when glomerular filtration is markedly reduced.

Marquez et al. (2011) measured the renal clearance of indoxyl sulfate in a small group of patients with RRF undergoing chronic hemodialysis and concluded that the clearance of indoxyl sulfate relative to the clearance of urea or creatinine was evidence of an important contribution of renal tubular secretion of indoxyl sulfate.

These findings highlight the importance of RRF and suggest a paradigm shift in the treatment of patients with chronic renal failure. This would include avoidance, when possible of the administration of nephrotoxic radiographic contrast agents, initiating treatment with peritoneal dialysis rather than hemodialysis, and the use of ACEIs and calcium channel blockers to preserve RRF (Lowenstein, 2012).

Delaying Progression of Renal Disease

The course of chronic renal failure may extend over many years and presents a great number of disabilities that require careful management.

Hypertension

Although hypertension is almost always a result rather than a cause of renal disease, it leads to accelerated progression of the underlying disease, creating a vicious circle. Control of hypertension in renal disease is directed at both a reduction in cardiovascular morbidity and the slowing of progression of the underlying renal disease. Antihypertensive drugs have selective actions on afferent or efferent arterioles and differ in their ability to reduce glomerular hypertension. ACEIs (Lewis, Hunsicker, Bain, & Rohde, 1993) and ARBs (Brenner et al., 2001; Lewis et al., 2001), which lower glomerular capillary pressure (P_{GC}), have been shown to reduce proteinuria and delay progression in both diabetic and nondiabetic renal diseases (The GISEN Group, 1997). Although some studies have shown beneficial effect of the combination of ACEI and ARB in reducing proteinuria and delaying progression of renal disease, a randomized controlled trial (RCT; Mann et al., 2008) of combination therapy of the ACEI ramipril and the ARB telmisartan showed that there was no improvement in proteinuria or reduction in the rate of decline in renal function with either therapy alone or in combination. However, the increase in proteinuria during the study period was the least with combination therapy with ACEI and ARB. A meta-analysis of RCTs of combination therapy with ACEI and ARB reported significant decrease in proteinuria, without clinically significant hyperkalemia or decline in GFR. The jury is still out regarding the use of this combination (MacKinnon et al., 2006). Calcium channel blockers differ in their effect on the kidney. Dihydropyridines, which are potent vasodilators, lead to an increase in proteinuria, perhaps because afferent arteriolar dilatation leaves P_{GC} unchanged or increased. Nondihydropyridines have been shown to reduce proteinuria, which is additive to that brought about by ACEI.

The goal BP in patients with CKD has been variable but mostly based upon the presence or absence of proteinuria, race, and other risk factors such as diabetes. An RCT in Black patients did not find any difference in the progression of CKD in patients with and without intensive BP control, defined as BP less than 130/80, but did find a potential benefit in patients with proteinuria (urine protein/creatinine ratio >0.22; Appel et al., 2010). The Kidney Disease: Improving Global Outcomes (KDIGO) guidelines (2012) recommend BP of ≤140/90 in diabetics and nondiabetics with CKD without proteinuria and BP goal of ≤130/80 in diabetics and nondiabetics with CKD with microalbuminuria or proteinuria. It also recommends the use of ACEI/ARBs in patients with microalbuminuria.

Antifibrotic Agents

Recently, considerable evidence has shown that the accumulation of extracellular matrix proteins characterizes most forms of progressive CKD. Support for this comes from studies wherein inhibition of factors that promote fibrosis, mainly TGF-β and connective tissue growth factor (CTGF) and enhancement of mediators that inhibit fibrosis like bone morphogenetic protein 7 (BMP7) and hepatocyte growth factor (HGF), delay progression of CKD. Antibodies to TGF-β and CTGF are being studied in clinical trials and have shown promising early response (Declèves & Sharma, 2014; Lee, Kim, & Choi, 2015).

Other strategies to delay the progression have included antifibrotic agents such as tranilast, supplementation of glycosaminoglycans to restore glomerular integrity and function, counteracting advanced glycation end products (AGEs) in diabetics with agents such as aminoguanidine, antagonists for the receptor for AGE, inhibitors of protein kinase C, preventing its oxidant injury, and so on. Pleiotropic effects of statins, erythropoiesis-stimulating agents, and vitamin D in delaying progression of renal disease have also been observed and are being explored. But, so far, either the benefit of these therapies has been marginal or the side effects have been significant, and therefore none of these has been advised.

Metabolic Abnormalities

With declining GFR, serum bicarbonate declines. Daily excretion of titratable acid is not much changed, but the excretion of NH4+ is reduced. This is attributed to decreased ammoniagenesis. Metabolic acidosis in chronic renal disease is generally well tolerated and is usually not treated unless it is severe. The arguments against treatment have included the risk of sodium overload associated with sodium bicarbonate therapy, reduction in ionized calcium concentration resulting in tetany (sustained painful contraction of a group of muscles), and seizures and perhaps diminished oxygen (O_2) delivery to tissues due to reversal of an adaptive change in the O_2 dissociation curve. More recent evidence suggests that the benefits of treatment outweigh these objections. Epidemiological studies (Dobre, Rahman, & Hostetter, 2015) have shown independent association between low serum bicarbonate levels and adverse renal outcomes. Banerjee et al. (2015) examined the association between dietary acid load (DAL) and the risk of ESRD in 1,486 adults enrolled in NHANES and found that higher DAL conferred increased risk of ESRD. Small alkali interventional trials and an unblinded RCT in late-stage CKD patients with acidosis, showed that correction of acidosis slowed progression of CKD to ESRD (de Brito-Ashurst, Varagunam, Raftery, & Yaqoob, 2009). Treatment of metabolic acidosis with bicarbonate or with a metabolizable anion, which can act as a substitute for bicarbonate (e.g., citrate or lactate), has been shown to prevent growth retardation in children with renal tubular acidosis. It has been shown that correction of metabolic acidosis, by increasing dialysate bicarbonate concentration in patients with ESRD, improves bone mineralization, diminishes bone resorption, and reduces the severity of secondary hyperparathyroidism.

Chronic metabolic acidosis is associated with muscle weakness and decreased lean body mass. Forearm muscle studies in patients with chronic renal disease have demonstrated that the rate of protein degradation is directly related to the degree of acidosis and to plasma cortisol levels; plasma cortisol levels, in turn, are directly related to the degree of acidosis. Further, albumin synthesis is diminished and negative nitrogen balance increased in patients with chronic renal disease made acidotic by the administration of ammonium chloride. The downregulation of protein degradation seen in patients with chronic renal disease placed on a protein-restricted diet is impaired in those who also have metabolic acidosis; this can be corrected by treatment of acidosis with bicarbonate.

Anemia

Among several factors, such as nutritional deficiency, infection, inflammation, occult blood loss, inadequate dialysis, and so on, that cause anemia in chronic renal disease, reduced EPO production by the kidney seems to be the most important factor. Reduced oxygen delivery to the kidney, acting through hypoxia inducible factor (HIF-1), normally results in increased production of EPO, which increases the production of red blood cells (Semenza, 2000). EPO levels are markedly reduced in patients with anemia of chronic renal disease. The introduction of erythropoietin-stimulating agents (ESAs) in the late 1980s, has revolutionized the treatment of anemia in CKD. Administration of recombinant human EPO (rHuEPO) corrects the anemia of renal disease in a dose-dependent manner. Ninety percent of patients on dialysis in the United States and many patients with chronic renal disease who are not yet on dialysis receive rHuEPO therapy. A longer acting preparation, darbepoetin alfa (Aranesp), has made administration and compliance more convenient for patients not yet receiving dialysis. The most common cause of resistance to rHuEPO is iron deficiency. Lack of response to oral iron administration is common among patients with ESRD and is attributed to the effects of hepcidin, which is produced by the liver, on the iron channel, ferroportin, preventing intestinal iron absorption (Ganz, 2007). Patients with superimposed iron deficiency are treated with IV iron preparations quite safely. Several RCTs have compared the efficacy and safety of oral versus IV iron in nondialysis patients with CKD 3 to 5. The FIND-CKD study by Macdougall et al. (2014) found significant difference between high ferritin-target IV iron versus oral iron groups in the initiation of additional anemia treatment strategies (blood transfusion, ESAs) without the occurrence of renal toxicity or difference in cardiovascular and infectious complications between the groups. In contrast, the REVOKE trial comparing oral iron to IV iron sucrose was terminated early on the chance of detecting no difference in the slope of decline of GFR but higher risk of serious adverse effects in the IV iron group (Agarwal, Kusek, & Pappas, 2015). Other causes of resistance to EPO include bone marrow fibrosis, inflammatory conditions, poor nutrition, and underdialysis.

Anemia has been found to be an independent predictor of the de novo occurrence of congestive heart failure and increased mortality in ESRD. Left ventricular hypertrophy (LVH) has also been found to be associated with increased mortality in ESRD. Successful treatment of anemia with rHuEPO has been shown to reverse cardiovascular and hemodynamic abnormalities such as LVH, increased cardiac output, and decreased peripheral vascular resistance. Patients report improved vitality and exercise tolerance. Amelioration of angina, congestive heart failure, and fatigue has been observed. Other beneficial effects of EPO therapy include improvement in platelet dysfunction of uremia, uremic pruritus (itching), impaired carbohydrate and cortisol metabolism, and sexual function in male patients.

Despite such positive effects of treatment of anemia, attempts at complete correction of anemia with higher doses of epoetin are associated with increased cardiovascular risk and mortality (Drüeke et al., 2006; Singh et al., 2006). The 2007 update by KDOQI (2007) suggests hemoglobin levels be maintained between 11 and 12 g/dL and not exceed 13 g/dL. KDIGO guidelines (2012) recommend that ESAs not be started in patients whose Hb levels are >10 g/dL. They also recommend Hb should not be maintained at ≥11.5 g/dL, individualizing treatment if quality of life is improved at levels ≥11.5 g/dL, but not to exceed 13 g/dL. A recent placebo-controlled study (Pfeffer et al., 2009) showed that treatment of type 2 diabetes and CKD with darbepoetin alfa did not show a significant difference in death or cardiovascular events and death or ESRD, but that there was a significantly higher rate of fatal and nonfatal strokes in the darbepoetin group. There was only a modest improvement in the patient-reported fatigue in the darbepoetin group. Target hemoglobin was 13 g/dL and rescue darbepoetin was used even in the placebo group for hemoglobin of less than 9 g/dL. Subset analysis and finer details of the trial are still being studied. Treatment of patients with systolic heart failure and anemia with darbepoetin did not improve clinical outcomes in a double-blind RCT (Agarwal et al., 2015). In addition, the RED-HF cohort with heart failure, anemia, diabetes, and CKD observed double the risk of stroke, which provided confirmation of the increased stroke risk associated with darbepoetin use (Bello et al., 2015) identified in TREAT patients studied by Pfeffer et al. (2009).

Hepcidin is an inflammatory mediator produced by the liver as an acute phase reactant. The levels of hepcidin are elevated in CKD and ESRD as well as chronic inflammatory states. Elevated levels of hepcidin are associated with increased cardiovascular risk as well as decreased intestinal iron absorption and release from certain types of white cells (macrophages) and liver cells that store iron (Ganz, 2007). HIF-1 normally inhibits hepcidin. It has been suggested that higher doses of rHuEPO rather than the higher hemoglobin levels are responsible for the increased cardiovascular risk. It is thought that rHuEPO might lead to decreased HIF-1 levels in a feedback fashion, thus releasing the inhibitory effect on hepcidin. Newer classes of agents that stabilize HIF-1 and hence stimulate endogenous EPO production and at the same time have a suppressive effect on hepcidin are under investigation, some of which are in the clinical development phase. Agents targeting the EPO receptor such as EPO mimetic peptides, EPO fusion proteins, antibody against EPO receptors, and EPO gene therapy are under investigation (Bonomini, Del Vecchio, Sirolli, & Locatelli, 2016).

CKD Mineral and Bone Disorder

This is the clinical syndrome that develops as a systemic disorder of mineral and bone metabolism due to CKD, manifested by abnormalities in bone and mineral metabolism and/or extraskeletal calcification. It begins early in CKD and initially consists of vascular smooth muscle calcification, osteodystrophy, FGF23 secretion, and decrease in klotho all of which lead to progressive worsening of bone metabolism. Factors that help repair the kidney disease such as Wnt inhibitors and Activin are released in the circulation and contribute to the pathogenesis of CKD-mineral and bone disorder (CKD-MBD; Hruska, Seifert, & Sugatani, 2015).

Although symptomatic renal osteodystrophy, for example, bone pain and fractures, seldom occurs before the onset of ESRD, altered mineral metabolism is present early in the course of renal failure. The two classic forms of renal osteodystrophy are secondary hyperparathyroidism with osteitis fibrosa, characterized by an increased rate of a high bone turnover rate secondary to hyperparathyroidism, and osteomalacia in which bone turnover is diminished and there is an increased volume of unmineralized bone (osteoid). Osteomalacia may result from vitamin D deficiency and aluminum toxicity in patients with ESRD. The incidence of aluminum toxicity has markedly diminished since the use of aluminum-containing phosphate binders has been discontinued and the aluminum content of the water used for dialysate is regularly monitored and kept below the recommended level. More recently, a third entity called adynamic bone disease or aplastic bone disease is well described. Low levels of PTH, diminished skeletal turnover, and reduced rate of osteoid formation characterize this condition. In some cases, it may result from excessive suppression of PTH or with parathyroidectomy.

The management of renal osteodystrophy involves both suppression of hyperparathyroidism and control of hyperphosphatemia. Dysregulated calcium and phosphorus homeostasis is the major driving force for vascular smooth muscle calcification and cardiovascular mortality (Shanahan, Crouthamel, Kapustin, & Giachelli, 2011) in addition to the increased calcium and phosphate product, which has been shown to increase the relative risk of dying in the dialysis population (Block et al., 2004). Dysregulated mineral homeostasis directly acts on the vascular smooth muscle and activates pathways that lead to vascular calcification. Although the administration of 1–25 (OH)2 vitamin D3 has been extremely useful in the suppression of hyperparathyroidism, hypercalcemia (elevated calcium level) has been a limiting factor. This has led to the development of other vitamin D analogs, such as doxercalciferol and paricalcitol, which preferentially stimulate vitamin D receptors on the parathyroid gland and have less of an effect on intestinal calcium and phosphate absorption. These agents have better ability to suppress PTH for a given calcium level. In recent years, a new generation of products referred to as calcimimetic agents, has been investigated. Cinacalcet HCl (Sensipar) is the only approved drug of this class and is widely used in the United States. These drugs increase the sensitivity of the calcium-sensing receptor to calcium and are devoid of the potential for hypercalcemia or hyperphosphatemia. The level of the calcium phosphorus product, which increases the risk of soft tissue calcification including vascular calcification and coronary artery disease, is not elevated with the use of cinacalcet. The key clinical event rates from the post hoc analysis of phase 3 studies show that parathyroidectomies were 0.3 per 100 patient years in the cinacalcet group versus 4.1 in the control group. Fractures were half as frequent, but mortality was not significantly different (NKF, 2003). However, the Evaluation of Cinacalcet Therapy to Lower Cardiovascular

Events (EVOLVE) study, a global, phase 3, double-blind, randomized, placebo-controlled trial evaluating the effects of cinacalcet on mortality and cardiovascular events in hemodialysis patients with secondary hyperparathyroidism did not show any significant difference between the cinacalcet and placebo groups (Chertow et al., 2012). In addition, an intention-to-treat analysis done on the EVOLVE trial patients did not show reduction in the rate of clinical fracture compared to placebo. However, when differences in baseline characteristics, multiple fractures, and/or events prompting discontinuation of study drug were accounted for, cinacalcet reduced the rate of clinical fracture by 16% to 29% (Moe et al., 2011).

Most patients with stages 4 and 5 CKD need phosphate binders, even if they are on dialysis. Aluminum-containing antacids have been replaced by calcium carbonate and calcium acetate as dietary phosphate binders, to avoid the risk of aluminum toxicity. Even calcium-containing compounds have come under scrutiny because of the positive calcium balance and soft tissue calcification such as coronary and other vascular calcification in dialysis patients. Examples of calcium-free phosphate binders available in the United States include sevelamer chloride (Renagel), recently replaced by sevelamer carbonate (Renvela) to avoid metabolic acidosis, and lanthanum carbonate (Fosrenol). Most recently, iron-based phosphate binders have found their way into the clinical field, two of which are ferric citrate and sucroferric oxyhydroxide (Nastou et al., 2014; Negri & Ureña Torres, 2015). The ability to control hyperparathyroidism and hyperphosphatemia has resulted in a marked reduction in the incidence of renal osteodystrophy.

In certain instances, the nodular parathyroid hyperplasia is so severe that it is not possible to suppress it medically, a condition referred to as tertiary hyperparathyroidism in the past; this may necessitate surgical parathyroidectomy.

■ Vitamin D

Vitamin D deficiency is common in patients with CKD and treatment with vitamin D analogs has been associated with better survival and lower cardiovascular risk. Vitamin D plays a major role in bone metabolism and intestinal absorption of calcium and phosphorus. Sources of vitamin D include the following: (a) endogenous production by the skin from 7-dehydrocholesterol when exposed to ultraviolet (UV) radiation from the sun, (b) ingestion of preformed vitamin D from animal sources, and (c) from plants. Vitamin D derived from animals, including endogenously produced product, is named cholecalciferol or vitamin D3 and the one derived from plants is named ergocalciferol or vitamin D2.

Vitamin D, once produced or ingested, needs to be hydroxylated by the liver and the kidney before it is biologically active. Hydroxylation at the 25th carbon position occurs in the liver by one or more cytochrome P450 vitamin D 25 hydroxylases resulting in the formation of 25-hydroxyvitamin D3 (25(OH)D3), which is then transported by vitamin D binding protein (DBP) to the PT of the kidney. It is then internalized by megalin (a member of the low-density lipoprotein [LDL] receptor superfamily) and hydroxylated at the 1st or 24th position by 1α-hydroxylase (biologically active form) or 24-hydroxylase respectively (Christakos, Ajibade, Dhawan, Fechner, & Mady, 2010). Vitamin D deficiency (<20–25 ng/mL) is defined by 25-hydroxy vitamin D levels. Patients with liver disease require supplementation of 25-hydroxy vitamin D (1–25 OH vitamin D is used in the United States since 25 OH vitamin D is not available) and those with kidney disease need either 1α-hydroxy vitamin D or 1–25 dihydroxy vitamin D. The role of 24–25 dihydroxy D is less well understood and is being investigated. It decreases the available pool of 1,25-hydroxy vitamin D. Since hydroxylation at the 1 and 24 position occurs in the kidney, it is not surprising that the levels of 1–25 and 24–25 OH D are diminished in patients with kidney disease. Several mechanisms have been postulated to cause vitamin D dysregulation during the course of CKD. Decreased GFR and proteinuria limit 25(OH) D-DBP in the circulation and hence formation of the biologically active 1,25-hydroxy D. FGF23 levels rise early in CKD, which suppresses the activity of 1,25(OH)2D by inhibiting 1-α-hydroxylase and degrades 1,25(OH)2D via the stimulation of 24-hydroxylase (Zhu, Wang, Gu, Wang, & Yuan, 2015). The levels of 24–25 OH D are decreased early in the course of CKD and those of 1–25 OH D later in the course. However, 25 OH D deficiency is also known to exist in CKD and ESRD throughout the United States (LaClair et al., 2005). Based on NHANES III, the prevalence of 25(OH) D levels <20 ng/mL among adults with stages 1 to 3 CKD is 9% to 14%. Among adults with eGFR

<30 mL/min/1.73 m^2, more than 27% had 25(OH) D deficiency. Furthermore, nearly 80% of dialysis patients had vitamin D deficiency or insufficiency (<30 ng/mL).

Vitamin D deficiency has been associated with decreased bone mineral density and increase in the risk of fractures (Elder & Mackun, 2006). However there have been several studies with conflicting results regarding vitamin D supplementation and prevention of falls. A recent RCT examining the vitamin D supplementation and targeted exercise on women between 70 and 80 years did not affect the rate of falls, while exercise decreased the rate of injurious falls and injured fallers (Uusi-Rasi et al., 2015). However a meta-analysis of 26 trials on the use of vitamin D and falls found a combination of vitamin D and calcium reduced the risk of falls; the reduction of falls with vitamin D alone did not reach statistical significance (Murad et al., 2011).

A recent interesting finding has been the discovery that higher vitamin D levels and treatment with vitamin D analogs are associated with a survival advantage and lower cardiovascular mortality (Duranton et al., 2013; Shoji et al., 2004; Wolf et al., 2007). The pathophysiological basis for this is not clear and thought to be due to favorable influence on other physiological functions like BP regulation due to inhibition of renin–angiotensin system, modulation of immune system, anti-inflammatory effects, and insulin and lipid metabolism, which need to be studied further. Receptors for vitamin D have been identified in more than 30 tissues in the body. Vitamin D may favorably influence the renin–angiotensin system, vascular smooth muscle cells, and cardiomyocytes. Ultrasound Doppler studies of brachial artery pulse, aortic pulse wave velocity, and brachial artery distensibility indicate a correlation between low vitamin D levels and increased atherosclerosis. However randomized trial data in CKD suggest no effect on LVH in predialysis CKD patients.

Uremic Neuropathy

Uremic neuropathy can present as either a polyneuropathy or a mononeuropathy involving both sensory and motor fibers. It generally occurs in advanced renal failure and is an indication to start dialysis for ESRD. When it occurs in patients who are already on dialysis, one needs to consider inadequate dialysis as a cause. Though quite common, the prevalence is underestimated in patients with dialysis. In a cross-sectional study done in two Italian centers (225 patients), 16.4% patients were found to have uremic neuropathy using a questionnaire scoring system, which correlated well with nerve conduction velocity studies (Mambelli et al., 2012). Surprisingly 9% could not be picked up by the scoring system despite having positive neuropathic symptoms. The neurological symptoms increase with the degree of renal failure in predialysis patients (Aggarwal, Sood, Jain, Kaverappa, & Yadav, 2013).

Pathologically, uremic polyneuropathy is associated with demyelination (loss of insulation surrounding nerve fibers) and axonal degeneration, and the involvement is directly proportional to the length of the nerve, affecting longer axons first. It is usually symmetrical. The metabolic and chemical defects leading to these changes are not well understood. Clinically, it first presents as paresthesias (numbness), burning sensation, and pain in distal areas such as feet. Sensory symptoms usually precede motor symptoms. The onset of motor symptoms reflects advanced disease, which unlike the sensory neuropathy may not reverse with the institution of dialysis. Electrophysiological studies are very useful in detecting subclinical neuropathy. Uremic mononeuropathy usually involves median and ulnar nerves. Other nerves involved include seventh and eighth cranial nerves and peroneal nerves. Carpal tunnel syndrome is common in ESRD. It results from compression of the median nerve at the wrist between carpal bones and transverse carpal ligament. Deposition of beta-2-microglobulin-related amyloid fibrils in the carpal tunnel plays an important role in the pathogenesis of the syndrome. Early initiation of dialysis, the use of better dialysis membranes with higher clearance for beta-2-microglobulin, and close attention to the adequacy of dialysis have reduced the incidence of uremic neuropathy. The extent of recovery is inversely related to the degree of dysfunction before initiation of dialysis. In recent years, high-tone external muscle stimulation (HTEMS) has shown improvement in objective electrophysiologic parameters in dialysis patients with severe uremic neuropathy whose symptoms have been refractory to medical management. Restoration of renal function with renal transplantation results in remarkable recovery from even the most severe sensory and motor neuropathy (Strempska et al., 2013).

Sexual Dysfunction

Infertility and sexual dysfunction are common but poorly studied in both men and women on dialysis. Erectile dysfunction (ED) and a decrease in both libido and frequency of intercourse are present in more than half the men with uremia; almost 70% of men with CKD report ED. This is organic in nature as evidenced by a decline in nocturnal penile tumescence. The decline in nocturnal penile tumescence is more marked as compared with normal controls and in patients with other chronic illness, suggesting that it is the effect of uremia and yet does not improve with hemodialysis. ED is multifactorial in etiology and is contributed by psychological, neurological, endocrine, vascular, and iatrogenic factors apart from uremia (Papadopoulou, Varouktsi, Lazaridis, Boutari, & Doumas, 2015). Factors other than uremia that contribute to ED include peripheral neuropathy, autonomic nervous system dysfunction, and peripheral vascular disease. Men on dialysis have impaired spermatogenesis and well as decreased free testosterone levels (Holley & Schmidt, 2013). Treatment with phosphodiesterase 5 (PDE5) inhibitors such as sildenafil and vardenafil remains first-line therapy for ED and has shown benefit. Psychological and physical stress may also play a role.

Lack of estradiol-stimulated cyclic luteinizing hormone secretion in women on dialysis is thought to lead to ovarian failure (anovulation), which is presumed to be the primary cause of infertility. Lack of ovulation and scant menstruation are common in women with chronic renal failure. Some women may have menorrhagia (excessive menstrual bleeding) leading to worsening of anemia. Pregnancy can rarely occur with chronic renal failure but fetal loss is almost universal. Elevated prolactin levels are also seen in women with chronic renal disease. Although suppression of very high prolactin levels with bromocriptine in women with normal renal function improves the clinical syndrome of amenorrhea (loss of menstruation) and galactorrhea (abnormal milky discharge from the nipple), it fails to restore normal menstruation or correct galactorrhea in uremic women. A few studies have demonstrated improvement in fertility and better pregnancy rates in a small number of women on nocturnal home hemodialysis perhaps by restoration of a more normal hormonal milieu. Successful renal transplantation, however, leads to restoration of fertility and sexual function in most patients (Holley & Schmidt, 2013).

Drug Treatment in Patients With Chronic Renal Failure

In light of the evidence that OATs play a major role in the excretion of indoxyl sulfate and/or similar protein-bound uremic retention solutes, and the knowledge that very many substances compete for OATs, choice of therapeutic agents should focus not only on adjustment for the rate of removal, but also on consideration of possible competition for organic anion transport (Lowenstein, 2012). The modification of drug dosage in patients with reduced renal function is typically based on the value of eGFR. This is subject to two important limitations. Drugs that are secreted by one of the OATs in the PT may require very different dosage modification than those excreted by glomerular filtration. The list of drugs that compete for transport is very long (Burckhardt & Burckhardt, 2011).

It seems reasonable that competition between excreted solutes should be considered in prescribing drugs just as consideration is given to propensity for hemorrhage or thrombosis, G-6-PD deficiency, or cytochrome P-450 status (Dresser, Spence, & Bailey, 2000). Further, glomerular filtration may change dramatically, before there is a measurable increase in serum creatinine (and decline in eGFR) at the onset of acute renal failure, and adjusting drug dosing based on serum creatinine or eGFR might result in overdosing of drugs that are known to be removed by glomerular filtration.

TREATMENT OF END-STAGE RENAL FAILURE

Treating the Symptoms of Renal Failure

Traditionally, treatment of patients with chronic renal disease has been directed at reducing uremic symptoms such as nausea, vomiting, pruritus, seizures, coma, and death. Most of these symptoms are effectively ameliorated by hemodialysis or peritoneal dialysis but other metabolic abnormalities and symptoms persist during renal replacement therapy.

When Willem Johan Kolff introduced his rotating drum artificial kidney in 1943, it was described as an effective treatment of patients with acute reversible renal failure. Today, hemodialysis and peritoneal dialysis serve to support and rehabilitate a growing number of patients with end-stage irreversible renal failure. The incident hemodialysis population is now nearly eight times larger than what it was in 1978, and in 2006 it topped 100,000 patients for the first time. The number of new peritoneal dialysis patients peaked at 9,407 in 1995, and has since fallen to 6,725; this population now accounts for 6.2% of new dialysis patients, a ratio that continues to decline from its peak of 15% during 1982 to 1985.

As of December 31, 2011, the last year for which such data are available, 396,656 patients were receiving hemodialysis therapy, 31,684 were on peritoneal dialysis (8% of the dialysis population), and 185,626 had a functioning renal transplant. The number of new patients starting hemodialysis decreased by 1.5%, the first decrease in the past 30 years, whereas new patients starting peritoneal dialysis increased for the third year in a row to 6.6%, reflecting the clear incentives for peritoneal dialysis in the new bundled payment system. The greatest growth has occurred in the renal transplant population, which has increased 5.5% to 6.0% each year since 2001. The number of patients who receive a kidney transplant as their first ESRD therapy reached 2,855 in in 2011. In 2011, 90,474 patients were waiting to receive a transplant. The total cost of ESRD to Medicare was $32.9 billion for 2010.

The NKF-KDOQI has provided evidence-based clinical practice guidelines for all stages of CKD and related complications (NKF, 1997) since 1997. Recognized throughout the world for improving the diagnosis and treatment of kidney disease, the NKF-KDOQI guidelines have changed the practices of numerous specialties and disciplines and improved the lives of thousands of kidney patients.

Hemodialysis

Hemodialysis is typically performed three times a week. The procedure involves diffusion of solutes between the plasma and the dialysis bath (dialysate) across the semipermeable dialyzer membrane down a concentration gradient. Fluid (usually equal to the volume retained from one dialysis to the next) is removed by ultrafiltration by regulating the dialyzer transmembrane hydrostatic pressure. Blood flow rates through the dialyzers in the range of 350 to 450 mL/min are necessary to obtain sufficient clearance of solutes over a reasonably short period of time. Since the normal blood flow rates in peripheral veins are insufficient for this purpose, it is necessary to have some form of access to circulation where the blood flow rate is well in excess of this range. Simple catheters placed in a central vein and an arteriovenous (AV) fistula/shunt, with or without the interposition of a synthetic vascular graft, serve as the most common forms of hemodialysis access. Although tunneled central vein catheters are very useful to provide dialysis when a vascular access such as an AV fistula or AV graft is not available, continued use of these catheters is associated with the risk of serious infections, including bacterial endocarditis and decreased survival on dialysis and is greatly discouraged. Among all types of vascular access for dialysis, AV fistulas have the best outcome and are preferred the most. Since 6 to 8 weeks are required for full maturation of an AV fistula, preemptive AV fistula creation in patients who anticipate going on hemodialysis is strongly advised.

Peritoneal Dialysis

In this technique, the patient's peritoneum substitutes for the dialyzer membrane. When the peritoneal cavity is filled with dialysate solution, diffusion of solutes occurs between the plasma flowing in the capillaries supplying the peritoneum and the dialysate until concentration equilibrium is reached. In 1976 (Papovich, Moncrief, Decherd, Bomar, & Pyle, 1976), the basic concept of continuous ambulatory peritoneal dialysis (CAPD) was described. The authors made use of the fact that although the diffusion of solutes into the peritoneal fluid started to slow down after about 30 minutes, some solute transfer continued to occur for as long as 4 to 5 hours and one could achieve sufficient solute clearance with four to five 2-liter exchanges of dialysis fluid on a daily basis. This led the way to the use of peritoneal dialysis as a treatment option for patients with ESRD. The incidence of peritonitis as a complication of this procedure has been markedly reduced by improvements in techniques and the design of catheters, connections, and automated cyclers, which can be used at night when the patients are asleep.

Despite advances in medical care, mortality in the ESRD population has remained relatively high (20% annually) and a substantial component of this mortality is attributable to cardiovascular disease This has been the major factor that has led to increased dialysis intensity, but the cardiovascular mortality has been little effected (Go, Chertow, Fan, McCulloch, & Hsu, 2004; Hage, 2009; Lindner et al., 1974).

It has become increasingly apparent that hemodialysis fails to remove protein-bound uremic retention solutes as dialyzer clearance is dependent on the concentration of free (unbound) solute (Figure 22.4; Jhawar et al., 2015).

These data suggest that indoxyl sulfate is a major uremic retention solute. The ability of indoxyl sulfate to cause the dysregulation of almost 1,500 genes can be related to the action of indoxyl sulfate as a transcription factor. Indoxyl sulfate is transported across the renal tubular cell membrane by OAT1 and OAT3. Within the cytoplasm, indoxyl sulfate combines with the aryl hydrocarbon receptor (AHR), which is then transported across the nuclear membrane where it binds to the aryl hydrocarbon receptor nuclear transporter (ARNT). The AHR–ARNT heterodimer interacts with several histone acetyltransferases and chromatin remodeling factors in the nucleus. This promotes the transcription of genes containing xenobiotic response elements (XRE) in their promoters (Noakes, 2015). This is believed to result in the activation of inflammatory mediators and the formation of cholesterol laden foam cells (Wu et al., 2011).

Plasma concentrations of indoxyl sulfate in patients undergoing thrice weekly hemodialysis are elevated much more than the increase in creatinine as protein binding renders indoxyl sulfate poorly dialyzable. Alternate methods of dialyzing protein-bound solutes, altering the gut microbiome to reduce the production of uremic retention solutes, or altering the binding of indoxyl sulfate to

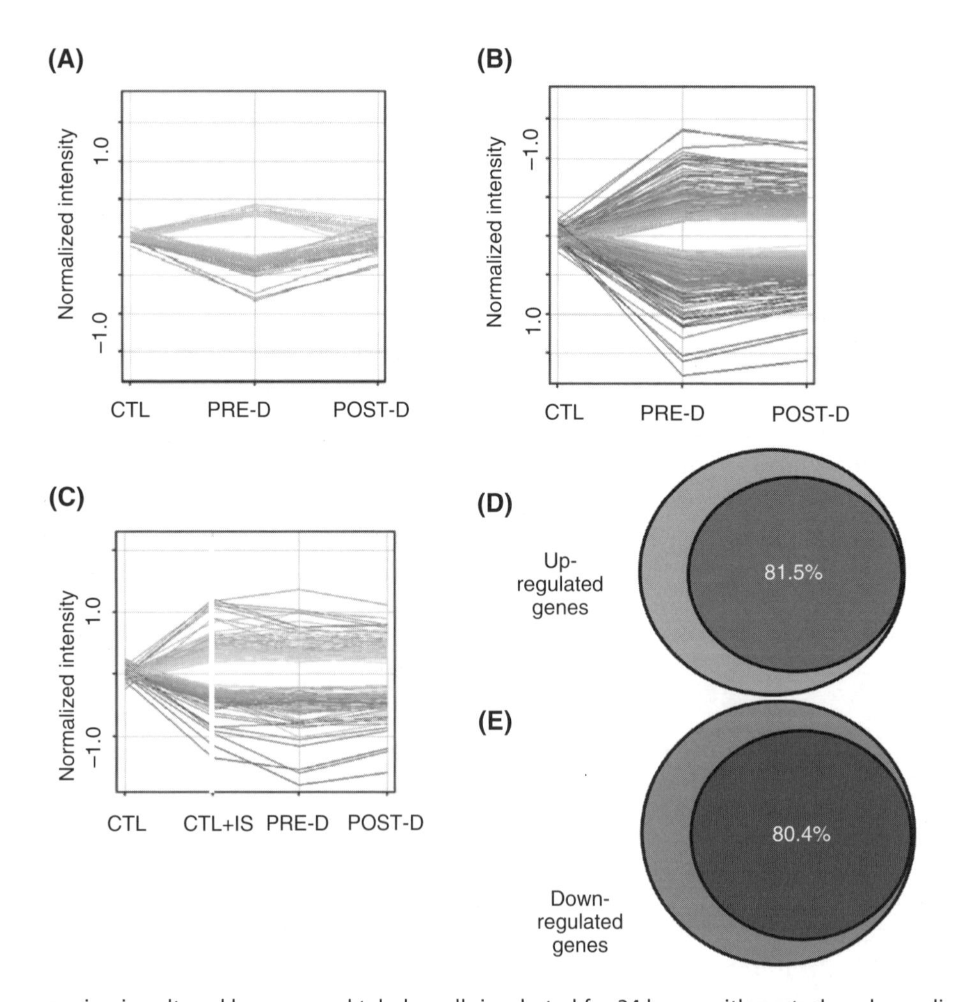

FIGURE 22.4 Gene expression in cultured human renal tubular cells incubated for 24 hours with control, prehemodialysis, and post-hemodialysis plasma. The expression of over 2,000 genes was "dysregulated" either increased or decreased.

(A) The expression of roughly 500 genes was normalized by a 3.5-hours hemodialysis.

(B) The expression of more than 1,500 genes remained dysregulated following hemodialysis.

(C) Indoxyl sulfate added to control plasma simulated more than 80% of the gene dysregulation observed when cells were incubated with uremic plasma (the inner circle of Venn diagrams D and E).

protein Chun (2014) may allow for more effective reduction in the plasma concentration of uremic retention solutes.

Survival of ESRD Patients

Although maintenance dialysis prevents death from uremia, patient survival is still limited. The USRDS 2013 ADR data show a mean expected remaining life span of 9.7 years for patients beginning dialysis between the ages of 40 and 44 and 5.1 years for those beginning between the ages of 60 and 64 years, for the year 2011. These are roughly one fourth the expected life span for the general U.S. population of comparable age groups. In comparison, the remaining life span for patients with successful renal transplantation was 26.4 years for the 40 to 44 years age group and 14.0 years for those between 60 and 64 years. Understandably, survival depends on comorbid conditions. The probability of survival for 5 years after starting dialysis for incident diabetic patients during 2008 was 38%.

Although all-cause mortality has declined steadily since 1988, cardiovascular events (strokes and heart attack) account for about 50% of deaths in ESRD. The other important causes of death in ESRD are infections, most often stemming from hemodialysis access sites or peritonitis in those on peritoneal dialysis. The number of patients withdrawing from dialysis has increased from 21% in 2000–2001 to 24% in 2005–2006. Most of this increase has been in patients 75 years and older.

Adequacy of Dialysis

The National Cooperative Dialysis Study, a prospectively randomized and controlled study, demonstrated that the *dose of dialysis* as measured by urea clearance correlated with morbidity (Lowrie, Laird, Parker, & Sargent, 1981). Although it is recognized that urea and creatinine are not uremic toxins, they have been seen as surrogate markers for dialyzable uremic toxins. No data are available that might evaluate the adequacy of dialysis from measurements of the removal of poorly dialyzed protein-bound uremic retention solutes (Eloot et al., 2013).

The dose of dialysis can be expressed as the virtual volume of plasma completely cleared of urea during dialysis, relative to the volume of distribution. The formula K*t*/V expresses this, where K is urea clearance, *t* is duration of dialysis, and V is volume of distribution. The urea reduction ratio (URR) is also a correlate of K*t*/V. Several studies (Hakim, Breyer, Ismail, & Schulman, 1994; Held et al., 1996; Parker, Husni, Huang, Lew, & Lowrie, 1994) have shown that increasing the dose of dialysis reduces mortality, which in one study (Held et al., 1996) was 7% for each 0.1 unit increment in K*t*/V. However, increasing URR and K*t*/V to higher levels (75% and 1.7) does not seem to be associated with further reduction in morbidity and mortality (Eknoyan et al., 2002). A target URR of more than 65% set by NKF-KDOQI was met by 96% of patients on hemodialysis in 2007.

Similar observations have been made regarding adequacy of dialysis and mortality and morbidity for patients on maintenance peritoneal dialysis. The CANUSA Peritoneal Dialysis Study Group (1996), in a prospective cohort study, found that a decrease in 0.1 unit K*t*/V was associated with a 5% increase in the relative risk of death. Randomized-controlled studies have supported lowering the minimum dose of weekly K*t*/V to 1.7 (Moran & Correa-Rotter, 2006). As per USRDS data, 92.2% of patients in the United States met this goal as of 2006.

Survival on hemodialysis has been lower in the United States than in Japan and Europe. The reasons for regional variations in survival may be multiple, such as genetics, underlying comorbid conditions, different etiologies of ESRD, and relative prevalence of diabetes and atherosclerosis, as well as differences in criteria for accepting a patient for maintenance hemodialysis. One particular group from Tassin, France, has reported particularly excellent outcome in the control of BP and anemia as well as survival and has drawn attention to their practice pattern (Charra et al., 1992). Patients are dialyzed for longer periods (24 hours compared to 9 to 12 hours per week) than any other dialysis unit. A study of 22,000 patients from seven countries participating in the Dialysis Outcomes and Practice Patterns Study (DOPPS) found that longer treatment times and slower ultrafiltration rates are associated with better survival even after adjusting for comorbidities, dose of dialysis as determined by K*t*/V, and body size (Saran et al., 2006).

Nutrition

Malnutrition is common in chronic renal disease. It results not only from protein restriction in an attempt to slow the progression of renal disease, but also as a function of advancing renal disease. Mild-to-moderate protein–calorie malnutrition is present in one-third of the patients on maintenance dialysis. Factors contributing to malnutrition in the dialysis population include poor nutrient intake, intercurrent illness, and dialysis itself.

Protein energy wasting (PEW), a complex umbrella term used to describe the end result of poor nutrient intake and catabolic wasting, has been linked to poor outcomes in CKD and ESRD. PEW can be ascertained by a combination of biochemical abnormalities and changes in nutrient intake, body weight, and muscle mass, which have been individually associated with poor outcomes in observational studies. Lower body mass index (BMI) and higher mortality have been shown repeatedly in various studies of dialysis patients. Since BMI is not a proper measure of body composition, direct assessment of muscle and fat mass with measures such as mid-arm circumference or more sophisticated methods such as bioimpedance or dual-energy x-ray absorptiometry (DEXA) are used. Both higher muscle mass and higher fat mass are associated with lower mortality in ESRD patients. Various biochemical measures of PEW such as low albumin, prealbumin, transferrin, insulin-like growth factor-1 (IGF-1), cholesterol, and creatinine have been linked to higher mortality, increased hospitalization rates, and poor quality of life. Of these, low serum albumin concentration seems to be the strongest predictor of mortality (Kovesdy, 2016).

The odds ratio for the risk of death is inversely related, exponentially, to serum albumin concentration in patients maintained on either hemo- or peritoneal dialysis. Nearly half the patients with ESRD starting dialysis have serum albumin concentration below the normal range. Even though peritoneal losses contribute to hypoalbuminemia in CAPD patients (Lowrie, Huang, & Lew, 1995), the relative risk of death was the same for hemodialysis and CAPD patients with hypoalbuminemia, suggesting that regardless of the mechanism, hypoalbuminemia carried the same risk.

Evidence suggests that various interventions ranging from simple nutritional supplements to administration of intradialytic parenteral nutrition may be of value in improving the nutritional status in patients with ESRD. In addition to dietary interventions, several nondietary therapies have been shown to improve markers of PEW such as albumin or lean body mass. These include among others appetite stimulants (e.g., megestrol acetate, L-carnitine, growth factors including recombinant human growth hormone, IGF-1, and anabolic steroids). High-quality observational studies have linked nutritional supplementation in dialyzed patients with PEW to significant improvement in mortality and hospitalization rates. A post hoc analysis of a RCT, which compared the impact on mortality of intradialytic parenteral nutrition plus oral nutritional supplementation to oral intervention alone in 186 malnourished hemodialysis patients, showed that an increase in prealbumin level of >30 mg/L within 3 months of either intervention predicted a 54% decrease in mortality, reduced hospitalizations, and improved general well-being (Cheu et al., 2013).

PHYSICAL REHABILITATION

CKD is associated with an increased risk of functional impairment, independent of age, gender, comorbidities, and cardiovascular events. As in any other chronic illness, rehabilitation is extremely important if patients with ESRD are to live as normal a life as possible. Even though hemodialysis and peritoneal dialysis provide means to sustain life in the absence of kidney function, patients are generally weak and disabled to a variable extent. The trend in favor of institution of dialysis before severe debility is incurred has made rehabilitation more effective.

Frailty is common among dialysis patients as the median age and comorbid conditions of these patients have increased in recent years. A study of more than 2,000 patients in the Dialysis Morbidity and Mortality Wave 2 study (Johansen, Chertow, Jin, & Kutner, 2007) revealed that two thirds met the definition of frailty, which comprised self-reported poor physical functioning, exhaustion/fatigue, low physical activity, and undernutrition. Older age, female gender, and hemodialysis, rather than peritoneal dialysis, were independently associated with frailty. The hazard ratio for death was 2.24 among patients with frailty.

The 2008 ADR from USRDS shows that the prevalence of walking disability in the CKD population is about twice that of the non-CKD population, and is much more likely to lead to death.

Early identification of CKD patients with walking disabilities, and recognition that they are at high risk for falls, could lead to increased use of exercise interventions and rehabilitation to maintain or restore balance and function.

One of the most serious problems that patients with advanced renal disease experience is falling. Patients with renal disease have multiple risk factors for falls and "fragility fractures." This is especially true of elderly dialysis patients. Muscle weakness, low BP, particularly when upright (orthostatic hypotension) either caused by fluid removal during hemodialysis or antihypertensive medications, peripheral neuropathy, and vitamin D deficiency all contribute to the risk of serious falls in patients with renal disease. Desmet, Beguin, Swine, Jadoul, and Université Catholique de Louvain Collaborative Group (2005) identified older age, diabetes, increased number of prescription drugs, use of antidepressants, and inability to walk more than 10 m without assistance as risk factors associated with falls. A third of the falls required medical attention and 3.9% of patients with a history of falling during an 8-week period of the study sustained a fall fracture during that year. Falls have been shown to be an independent risk factor of increased mortality, even after adjusting for age, dialysis vintage, comorbidity, and laboratory variables in the dialysis population (Li, Tomlinson, Naglie, Cook, & Jassal, 2008). Falls may also lead to decreased mobility, hospitalization, depressive symptoms, functional decline, decreased social activity, and poor quality of life. Sterky et al. observed that elderly patients on dialysis had 50% less functional capacity than gender- and age-matched healthy subjects. Only 13% of subjects after 1 year of hemodialysis maintain stable functionality (Intiso, 2014).

Physical therapy aimed at improving flexibility, balance, and range of movement will help improve patients' abilities to perform activities of daily living, such as stooping, bending, and reaching. During the past 30 years, there have been a significantly increasing number of published studies concerning the effect of regular exercise training in adults with CKD. There is evidence for significant beneficial effects of regular exercise on physical fitness, walking capacity, cardiovascular dimensions (e.g., BP and heart rate), health-related quality of life, and some nutritional parameters in adults with CKD. Physical activity has the potential to positively impact upon aerobic and functional ability, and the quality of life of all CKD patients independent of the stage of the disease process (Intiso, 2014).

Preliminary studies in patients with CKD indicate that resistance training reduces markers of inflammation such as C-reactive protein and interleukin-6 as well as leads to skeletal muscle hypertrophy (Castaneda et al., 2004).

Maximal aerobic capacity as measured by peak oxygen uptake (VO_2 max) is reduced in patients with ESRD to roughly half of what is seen in normal sedentary individuals. Correction of anemia with rHuEPO results in an increase in the arterial oxygen content and improves VO_2 max by an average of 28%, but the change in VO_2 max is much smaller than that expected for the change in hemoglobin and arterial oxygen content. Painter and Moore (1994) have determined that normal subjects get nearly twice the VO_2 change per change in hemoglobin as compared to dialysis patients. Exercise training alone has been shown to improve VO_2 max by 25%. Patients with peak VO_2 values (<17.5 mL kg^{-1} min^{-1}) may obtain the largest survival benefit from exercise training.

As is well appreciated in the general population, exercise training offers other health benefits in dialysis patients. Endurance exercise training in hemodialysis patients offers cardiovascular risk benefits, including lowering of both systolic and diastolic BP sufficient to decrease or withdraw antihypertensive therapy in a number of patients, and a decline in plasma triglycerides and very-low-density lipoprotein (VLDL) levels while increasing high-lipoprotein level (Hagberg et al., 1983; Harter & Goldberg, 1985; Miller, Cress, Johnson, Nichols, & Schnitzler, 2002). Benefits associated with exercise training are improved peak VO_2, cardiac function, quality of life, and sympatho-adrenal activity. Significant improvements in lean body mass, quadriceps muscle area, knee extension, hip abduction, and flexion strength have been also reported.

Exercise training may be delivered in nondialysis time, either as outpatients or at home, and also during dialysis, termed intradialytic exercise. Although the best time for exercise in relation to hemodialysis is not clear, exercise training during dialysis sessions has the advantages of supervision and encouragement by the staff as well as a productive use of dialysis time. One can expect an improved compliance to the exercise program. Flexibility, strengthening, and aerobic exercises can all be performed effectively during dialysis.

Because of the likelihood of hypotension and muscle cramps during the latter part of dialysis, exercise is best performed in the first hour of dialysis. It has been suggested that exercise during dialysis might improve efficiency of the latter. Although there are some risks of musculoskeletal injury associated with participation in an exercise program for a patient with ESRD, proper patient selection makes this risk negligible.

Although traditionally vitamin D has been viewed in relation to its effects on bone and mineral metabolism and much emphasis has been placed on the bioactive form, 1–25 dihydroxy D3 (1–25 OH D3), there has been renewed interest in its precursor 25-hydroxy D3 (25 OH D3) and its effects on muscle strength, pain, cognitive function, autoimmune disease, heart disease, cancer, and mortality (Kovesdy & Kalantar-Zadeh, 2008; Stechschulte, Kirsner, & Federman, 2009; Taskapan, Wei, & Oreopoulos, 2006; Wolf et al., 2007). 25 OH D3 levels are found to be low in most patients with CKD and are associated with muscle weakness and musculoskeletal pain. Supplementation with 25 OH D3 has been shown to result in improvement in muscle strength and decrease the incidence of falls (Prince et al., 2008). The need for supplementation of 25 OH D3 in addition to optimum management of secondary hyperparathyroidism with active form of vitamin D (1–25 OH D3) or its analogs in patients with kidney disease has not been well studied.

PSYCHOLOGICAL AND VOCATIONAL REHABILITATION

Cognitive impairment is another aspect of disability in patients undergoing hemodialysis. Twenty-two percent have mild cognitive impairment and 8% have moderate-to-severe impairment. More importantly there is a high burden of unrecognized cognitive impairment in this population. Adults undergoing hemodialysis who have cognitive dementia are at a high risk of mortality. Poor cognitive function may be one pathway linking frailty to adverse outcomes on hemodialysis. McAdams-DeMarco et al. (2015) studied 324 incident hemodialysis patients in a longitudinal cohort (Predictors of Arrhythmic and Cardiovascular Risk in ESRD) who were classified into three groups (frail, intermediately frail, and nonfrail) based on the Fried frailty phenotype. Global cognitive function (3MS) and speed/attention (Trail Making Tests A and B [TMTA and TMTB]) were assessed at cohort entry and 1-year follow-up. They found that the prevalences of frailty and intermediate frailty were 34.0% and 37.7%, respectively, and frailty was independently associated with lower cognitive function at cohort entry. They concluded that in adult incident hemodialysis patients, frailty is associated with worse cognitive function, particularly global cognitive function. Interventions to recognize cognitive impairment in frail adults initiating hemodialysis should therefore be identified (McAdams-DeMarco et al., 2015).

In addition to the appropriate management of the gamut of abnormalities resulting from chronic renal failure outlined earlier, one must also address the issue of the patient returning to living a full life. For some, this may not mean returning to work, but feeling well enough to enjoy one's family and surroundings. The goal should be to help the patient to resume all the duties, responsibilities, and benefits he or she enjoyed before the illness. Psychological problems stemming from chronic illness, dependence on dialysis, sexual dysfunction, and change in status from an earning and supporting member of the family to a dependent person need to be identified and addressed. Gainful employment is extremely important for an adult in the earning period of his or her life to regain self-esteem and to interact with the society he or she lives in with confidence. However, the fear of losing financial benefits such as Social Security disability insurance and Social Security income may deter some patients from seeking employment, even if they are able to return to work. In several states, there are work-incentive programs whereby the state agencies waive the termination of financial benefits to persons with disabilities if they seek employment (Renal Rehabilitation Report, 1997). Assistance by a knowledgeable social worker in the field is extremely helpful in this regard. The USRDS Dialysis Morbidity and Mortality Study: Wave 2 conducted in 1996 (USRDS 2003 ADR) found that 37% of younger (18–54 years) and 16% of older (55+ years) patients reported that they were able to work at the start of therapy for ESRD. Of these, only 60% of the younger and 40% of the older group were actually employed. Patients' educational levels correlated with reported ability to work and with employment status. Consistent with the association of lower educational level and increased risk of chronic disease in the general population, dialysis patients with lower educational status were more likely to be diabetic. Rasgon et al. (1993, 1996) have shown that multidisciplinary predialysis intervention leads to maintenance of employment in a larger number of patients starting dialysis, both in the in-center setting as well as in the home hemodialysis and ambulatory peritoneal dialysis population. The quality of life is significantly better after a successful transplantation. A long-term study (Matas et al., 1996) showed that more than 40% of transplant recipients were employed part time or full time 8 years after transplantation.

The Life Options Rehabilitation Advisory Council, which was formed in 1993 by a group of patients, health care providers, researchers, government representatives, and private business persons, has played a major role in bringing the rehabilitation and quality-of-life issues into focus. Through its website (www.lifeoptions.org), it acts as a resource guide for important issues related to encouragement, education, exercise, employment, and evaluation—the five Es—described as the bridges to rehabilitation for people with kidney failure. There are free publications on these issues directed not only toward patients, but also for health care professionals and social workers.

REFERENCES

Agarwal, R., Kusek, J. W., & Pappas, M. K. (2015). A randomized trial of intravenous and oral iron in chronic kidney disease. *Kidney International*, *88*(4), 905–914.

Aggarwal, H. K., Sood, S., Jain, D., Kaverappa, V., & Yadav, S. (2013). Evaluation of spectrum of peripheral neuropathy in predialysis patients with chronic kidney disease. *Renal Failure*, *35*(10), 1323–1329.

Anavekar, N. S., McMurray, J. J. V., Velazquez, E. J., Solomon, S. D., Kober, L., Rouleau, J.-L., . . . Pfeffer, M. A. (2004). Relation between renal dysfunction and cardiovascular outcomes after myocardial infarction. *The New England Journal of Medicine*, *351*(13), 1285–1295.

Appel, L. J., Wright, J. T., Greene, T., Agodoa, L. Y., Astor, B. C., Bakris, G. L., . . . AASK Collaborative Research Group. (2010). Intensive blood-pressure control in hypertensive chronic kidney disease. *The New England Journal of Medicine*, *363*(10), 918–929.

Banerjee, T., Crews, D. C., Wesson, D. E., Tilea, A. M., Saran, R., Ríos-Burrows, N., . . . Centers for Disease Control and Prevention Chronic Kidney Disease Surveillance Team. (2015). High dietary acid load predicts ESRD among adults with CKD. *Journal of the American Society of Nephrology*, *26*(7), 1693–1700.

Bargman, J. M., Thorpe, K. E., Churchill, D. N., & CANUSA Peritoneal Dialysis Study Group. (2001). Relative contribution of residual renal function and peritoneal clearance to adequacy of dialysis: a reanalysis of the CANUSA study. *Journal of the American Society of Nephrology*, *12*(10), 2158–2162.

Bello, N. A., Lewis, E. F., Desai, A. S., Anand, I. S., Krum, H., McMurray, J. J. V, . . . Pfeffer, M. A. (2015). Increased risk of stroke with darbepoetin alfa in anaemic heart failure patients with diabetes and chronic kidney disease. *European Journal of Heart Failure*, *17*(11), 1201–1207.

Benigni, A., & Remuzzi, G. (2001). How renal cytokines and growth factors contribute to renal disease progression. *American Journal of Kidney Diseases: The Official Journal of the National Kidney Foundation*, *37*(1, Suppl. 2), S21–S24.

Block, G. A., Klassen, P. S., Lazarus, J. M., Ofsthun, N., Lowrie, E. G., & Chertow, G. M. (2004). Mineral metabolism, mortality, and morbidity in maintenance hemodialysis. *Journal of the American Society of Nephrology*, *15*(8), 2208–2218.

Bonomini, M., Del Vecchio, L., Sirolli, V., & Locatelli, F. (2016). New treatment approaches for the anemia of CKD. *American Journal of Kidney Diseases: The Official Journal of the National Kidney Foundation*, *67*(1), 133–142.

Böttinger, E. P., & Bitzer, M. (2002). TGF-beta signaling in renal disease. *Journal of the American Society of Nephrology*, *13*(10), 2600–2610.

Brenner, B. M., Cooper, M. E., de Zeeuw, D., Keane, W. F., Mitch, W. E., Parving, H. H., . . . RENAAL Study Investigators. (2001). Effects of losartan on renal and cardiovascular outcomes in patients with type 2 diabetes and nephropathy. *The New England Journal of Medicine*, *345*(12), 861–869.

Burckhardt, G., & Burckhardt, B. C. (2011). In vitro and in vivo evidence of the importance of organic anion transporters (OATs) in drug therapy. *Handbook of Experimental Pharmacology*, *201*, 29–104.

Canada-USA (CANUSA) Peritoneal Dialysis Study Group. (1996). Adequacy of dialysis and nutrition in continuous peritoneal dialysis: association with clinical outcomes. Canada-usa (canusa) peritoneal dialysis study group. *Journal of the American Society of Nephrology*, *7*(2), 198–207.

Castaneda, C., Gordon, P. L., Parker, R. C., Uhlin, K. L., Roubenoff, R., & Levey, A. S. (2004). Resistance training to reduce the malnutrition-inflammation complex syndrome of chronic kidney disease. *American Journal of Kidney Diseases: The Official Journal of the National Kidney Foundation*, *43*(4), 607–616.

Charra, B., Calemard, E., Ruffet, M., Chazot, C., Terrat, J. C., Vanel, T., . . . Laurent, G. (1992). Survival as an index of adequacy of dialysis. *Kidney International*, *41*(5), 1286–91.

Chertow, G. M., Block, G. A., Correa-Rotter, R., Drüeke, T. B., Floege, J., Goodman, W. G., . . . Parfrey, P. S. (2012). Effect of cinacalcet on cardiovascular disease in patients undergoing dialysis. *The New England Journal of Medicine*, *367*(26), 2482–2494.

Cheu, C., Pearson, J., Dahlerus, C., Lantz, B., Chowdhury, T., Sauer, P. F., & Ramirez, S. P. B. (2013). Association between oral nutritional supplementation and clinical outcomes among patients with ESRD. *Clinical Journal of the American Society of Nephrology*, *8*(1), 100–107.

Christakos, S., Ajibade, D. V., Dhawan, P., Fechner, A. J., & Mady, L. J. (2010). Vitamin D: Metabolism. *Endocrinology and Metabolism Clinics of North America*, *39*(2), 243–253.

Chun, K. S., Singh, P., Jhawar, S., & Lowenstein, J. (2014). Changes in pH during hemodialysis determine indoxyl sulfate binding and limit its removal. *American Society of Nephrology*.

Coresh, J., Selvin, E., Stevens, L. A., Manzi, J., Kusek, J. W., Eggers, P., . . . Levey, A. S. (2007). Prevalence of chronic kidney disease in the United States. *The Journal of the American Medical Association*, *298*(17), 2038–2047.

Couser, W. G. (2007). Chronic kidney disease the promise and the perils. *Journal of the American Society of Nephrology*, *18*(11), 2803–2805.

de Brito-Ashurst, I., Varagunam, M., Raftery, M. J., & Yaqoob, M. M. (2009). Bicarbonate supplementation slows progression of CKD and improves nutritional status. *Journal of the American Society of Nephrology*, *20*(9), 2075–2084.

Declèves, A.-E., & Sharma, K. (2014). Novel targets of antifibrotic and anti-inflammatory treatment in CKD. *Nature Reviews. Nephrology*, *10*(5), 257–267.

Desmet, C., Beguin, C., Swine, C., Jadoul, M., & Université Catholique de Louvain Collaborative Group. (2005). Falls in hemodialysis patients: Prospective study of incidence, risk factors, and complications. *American Journal of Kidney Diseases: The Official Journal of the National Kidney Foundation*, *45*(1), 148–153.

Dobre, M., Rahman, M., & Hostetter, T. H. (2015). Current status of bicarbonate in CKD. *Journal of the American Society of Nephrology*, *26*(3), 515–523.

Dresser, G. K., Spence, J. D., & Bailey, D. G. (2000). Pharmacokinetic-pharmacodynamic consequences and clinical relevance of cytochrome P450 3A4 inhibition. *Clinical Pharmacokinetics*, *38*(1), 41–57.

Drüeke, T. B., Locatelli, F., Clyne, N., Eckardt, K.-U., Macdougall, I. C., Tsakiris, D., . . . Create Investigators. (2006). Normalization of hemoglobin level in patients with chronic kidney disease and anemia. *The New England Journal of Medicine*, *355*(20), 2071–2084.

Duranton, F., Rodriguez-Ortiz, M. E., Duny, Y., Rodriguez, M., Daurès, J.-P., & Argilés, A. (2013). Vitamin D treatment and mortality in chronic kidney disease: a systematic review and meta-analysis. *American Journal of Nephrology*, *37*(3), 239–248.

Eknoyan, G., Beck, G. J., Cheung, A. K., Daugirdas, J. T., Greene, T., Kusek, J. W., . . . Hemodialysis (HEMO) Study Group. (2002). Effect of dialysis dose and membrane flux in maintenance hemodialysis. *The New England Journal of Medicine*, *347*(25), 2010–2019.

Elder, G. J., & Mackun, K. (2006). 25-Hydroxyvitamin D deficiency and diabetes predict reduced BMD in patients with chronic kidney disease. *Journal of Bone and Mineral Research: The Official Journal of the American Society for Bone and Mineral Research*, *21*(11), 1778–1784.

Eloot, S., Van Biesen, W., Glorieux, G., Neirynck, N., Dhondt, A., & Vanholder, R. (2013). Does the adequacy parameter Kt/V(urea) reflect uremic toxin concentrations in hemodialysis patients? *PLOS ONE*, *8*(11), e76838.

Evenepoel, P., Meijers, B. K. I., Bammens, B. R. M., & Verbeke, K. (2009). Uremic toxins originating from colonic microbial metabolism. *Kidney International. Supplement*, (114), S12–S19.

Ganz, T. (2007). Molecular control of iron transport. *Journal of the American Society of Nephrology*, *18*(2), 394–400.

The GISEN Group. (1997). Randomised placebo-controlled trial of effect of ramipril on decline in glomerular filtration rate and risk of terminal renal failure in proteinuric, non-diabetic nephropathy. The GISEN group (Gruppo Italiano di Studi Epidemiologici in Nefrologia). *The Lancet*, *349*(9069), 1857–1863.

Go, A. S., Chertow, G. M., Fan, D., McCulloch, C. E., & Hsu, C. (2004). Chronic kidney disease and the risks of death, cardiovascular events, and hospitalization. *The New England Journal of Medicine*, *351*(13), 1296–1305.

Hagberg, J. M., Goldberg, A. P., Ehsani, A. A., Heath, G. W., Delmez, J. A., & Harter, H. R. (1983). Exercise training improves hypertension in hemodialysis patients. *American Journal of Nephrology*, *3*(4), 209–212.

Hage, F. G., Venkataraman, R., Zoghbi, G. J., Perry, G. J., DeMattos, A. M., & Iskandrian, A. E. (2009). The scope of coronary heart disease in patients with chronic kidney disease. *Journal of the American College of Cardiology*, *53*(23), 2129–2140.

Hakim, R. M., Breyer, J., Ismail, N., & Schulman, G. (1994). Effects of dose of dialysis on morbidity and mortality. *American Journal of Kidney Diseases: The Official Journal of the National Kidney Foundation*, *23*(5), 661–669.

Hallan, S. I., Ritz, E., Lydersen, S., Romundstad, S., Kvenild, K., & Orth, S. R. (2009). Combining GFR and albuminuria to classify CKD improves prediction of ESRD. *Journal of the American Society of Nephrology*, *20*(5), 1069–1077.

Harter, H. R., & Goldberg, A. P. (1985). Endurance exercise training. An effective therapeutic modality for hemodialysis patients. *The Medical Clinics of North America*, *69*(1), 159–175.

Held, P. J., Port, F. K., Wolfe, R. A., Stannard, D. C., Carroll, C. E., Daugirdas, J. T., . . . Hakim, R. M. (1996). The dose of hemodialysis and patient mortality. *Kidney International*, *50*(2), 550–556.

Henry, R. M. A., Kostense, P. J., Bos, G., Dekker, J. M., Nijpels, G., Heine, R. J., . . . Stehouwer, C. D. A. (2002). Mild renal insufficiency is associated with increased cardiovascular mortality: The Hoorn study. *Kidney International*, *62*(4), 1402–1407.

Holley, J. L., & Schmidt, R. J. (2013). Changes in fertility and hormone replacement therapy in kidney disease. *Advances in Chronic Kidney Disease*, *20*(3), 240–245.

Hruska, K. A., Seifert, M., & Sugatani, T. (2015). Pathophysiology of the chronic kidney disease-mineral bone disorder. *Current Opinion in Nephrology and Hypertension*, *24*(4), 303–309.

Ikizler, T. A., Greene, J. H., Wingard, R. L., Parker, R. A., & Hakim, R. M. (1995). Spontaneous dietary protein intake during progression of chronic renal failure. *Journal of the American Society of Nephrology*, *6*(5), 1386–1391.

Intiso, D. (2014). The rehabilitation role in chronic kidney and end stage renal disease. *Kidney & Blood Pressure Research*, *39*(2–3), 180–188.

Jhawar, S., Singh, P., Torres, D., Ramirez-Valle, F., Kassem, H., Banerjee, T., . . . Lowenstein, J. (2015). Functional genomic analysis identifies indoxyl sulfate as a major, poorly dialyzable uremic toxin in end-stage renal disease. *PLOS ONE*, *10*(3), e0118703.

Johansen, K. L., Chertow, G. M., Jin, C., & Kutner, N. G. (2007). Significance of frailty among dialysis patients. *Journal of the American Society of Nephrology*, *18*(11), 2960–2967.

KDOQI. (2007). KDOQI clinical practice guideline and clinical practice recommendations for anemia in chronic kidney disease: 2007 update of hemoglobin target. *American Journal of Kidney Diseases: The Official Journal of the National Kidney Foundation*, *50*(3), 471–530.

Khan, N. A., Ma, I., Thompson, C. R., Humphries, K., Salem, D. N., Sarnak, M. J., & Levin, A. (2006). Kidney function and mortality among patients with left ventricular systolic dysfunction. *Journal of the American Society of Nephrology*, *17*(1), 244–253.

Kovesdy, C. P., & Kalantar-Zadeh, K. (2008). Vitamin D receptor activation and survival in chronic kidney disease. *Kidney International*, *73*(12), 1355–1363.

LaClair, R. E., Hellman, R. N., Karp, S. L., Kraus, M., Ofner, S., Li, Q., . . . Moe, S. M. (2005). Prevalence of calcidiol deficiency in CKD: A cross-sectional study across latitudes in the United States. *American Journal of Kidney Diseases: The Official Journal of the National Kidney Foundation*, *45*(6), 1026–1033.

Lee, S.-Y., Kim, S. I., & Choi, M. E. (2015). Therapeutic targets for treating fibrotic kidney diseases. *Translational Research: The Journal of Laboratory and Clinical Medicine*, *165*(4), 512–530.

Levey, A. S., Stevens, L. A., Schmid, C. H., Zhang, Y. L., Castro, A. F., Feldman, H. I., . . . Chronic Kidney Disease Epidemiology Collaboration. (2009). A new equation to estimate glomerular filtration rate. *Annals of Internal Medicine*, *150*(9), 604–612.

Lewis, E. J., Hunsicker, L. G., Bain, R. P., & Rohde, R. D. (1993). The effect of angiotensin-converting-enzyme inhibition on diabetic nephropathy. The Collaborative Study Group. *The New England Journal of Medicine*, *329*(20), 1456–1462.

Lewis, E. J., Hunsicker, L. G., Clarke, W. R., Berl, T., Pohl, M. A., Lewis, J. B., . . . Collaborative Study Group. (2001). Renoprotective effect of the angiotensin-receptor antagonist irbesartan in patients with nephropathy due to type 2 diabetes. *The New England Journal of Medicine*, *345*(12), 851–860.

Li, M., Tomlinson, G., Naglie, G., Cook, W. L., & Jassal, S. V. (2008). Geriatric comorbidities, such as falls, confer an independent mortality risk to elderly dialysis patients. *Nephrology, Dialysis, Transplantation: Official Publication of the European Dialysis and Transplant Association-European Renal Association*, *23*(4), 1396–1400.

Lindner, A., Charra, B., Sherrard, D. J., & Scribner, B. H. (1974). Accelerated atherosclerosis in prolonged maintenance hemodialysis. *The New England Journal of Medicine*, *290*(13), 697–701.

Lowenstein, J. (2012). Competition for organic anion transporters in chronic renal disease. *Kidney International*, *82*(9), 1033.

Lowrie, E. G., Huang, W. H., & Lew, N. L. (1995). Death risk predictors among peritoneal dialysis and hemodialysis patients: A preliminary comparison. *American Journal of Kidney Diseases: The Official Journal of the National Kidney Foundation*, *26*(1), 220–228.

Lowrie, E. G., Laird, N. M., Parker, T. F., & Sargent, J. A. (1981). Effect of the hemodialysis prescription of patient morbidity: Report from the National cooperative dialysis study. *The New England Journal of Medicine*, *305*(20), 1176–1181.

Luyckx, V. A., & Brenner, B. M. (2010). The clinical importance of nephron mass. *Journal of the American Society of Nephrology*, *21*(6), 898–910.

Macdougall, I. C., Bock, A. H., Carrera, F., Eckardt, K.-U., Gaillard, C., Van Wyck, D., . . . FIND-CKD Study Investigators. (2014). FIND-CKD: A randomized trial of intravenous ferric carboxymaltose versus oral iron in patients with chronic kidney disease and iron deficiency anaemia. *Nephrology, Dialysis, Transplantation: Official Publication of the European Dialysis and Transplant Association-European Renal Association*, *29*(11), 2075–2084.

MacKinnon, M., Shurraw, S., Akbari, A., Knoll, G. A., Jaffey, J., & Clark, H. D. (2006). Combination therapy with an angiotensin receptor blocker and an ACE inhibitor in proteinuric renal disease: A systematic review of the efficacy and safety data. *American Journal of Kidney Diseases: The Official Journal of the National Kidney Foundation*, *48*(1), 8–20.

Mambelli, E., Barrella, M., Facchini, M. G., Mancini, E., Sicuso, C., Bainotti, S., . . . Santoro, A. (2012). The prevalence of peripheral neuropathy in hemodialysis patients. *Clinical Nephrology*, *77*(6), 468–475.

Mann, J. F. E., Schmieder, R. E., McQueen, M., Dyal, L., Schumacher, H., Pogue, J., . . . ONTARGET investigators. (2008). Renal outcomes with telmisartan, ramipril, or both, in people at high vascular risk (the ONTARGET study): A multicentre, randomised, double-blind, controlled trial. *The Lancet*, *372*(9638), 547–553.

Marquez, I. O., Tambra, S., Luo, F. Y., Li, Y., Plummer, N. S., Hostetter, T. H., & Meyer, T. W. (2011). Contribution of residual function to removal of protein-bound solutes in hemodialysis. *Clinical Journal of the American Society of Nephrology*, *6*(2), 290–296.

Masereeuw, R., Mutsaers, H. A. M., Toyohara, T., Abe, T., Jhawar, S., Sweet, D. H., & Lowenstein, J. (2014). The kidney and uremic toxin removal: glomerulus or tubule? *Seminars in Nephrology*, *34*(2), 191–208.

Matas, A. J., Lawson, W., McHugh, L., Gillingham, K., Payne, W. D., Dunn, D. L., . . . Najarian, J. S. (1996). Employment patterns after successful kidney transplantation. *Transplantation*, *61*(5), 729–733.

McAdams-DeMarco, M. A., Tan, J., Salter, M. L., Gross, A., Meoni, L. A., Jaar, B. G., . . . Sozio, S. M. (2015). Frailty and cognitive function in incident hemodialysis patients. *Clinical Journal of the American Society of Nephrology*, *10*(12), 2181–2189.

Miller, B. W., Cress, C. L., Johnson, M. E., Nichols, D. H., & Schnitzler, M. A. (2002). Exercise during hemodialysis decreases the use of antihypertensive medications. *American Journal of Kidney Diseases: The Official Journal of the National Kidney Foundation*, *39*(4), 828–833.

Moe, S. M., Abdalla, S., Chertow, G. M., Parfrey, P. S., Block, G. A., Correa-Rotter, R., . . . Evaluation of Cinacalcet HCl Therapy to Lower Cardiovascular Events (EVOLVE) Trial Investigators. (2015). Effects of cinacalcet on fracture events in patients receiving hemodialysis: The EVOLVE Trial. *Journal of the American Society of Nephrology*, *26*(6), 1466–1475.

Moist, L. M., Port, F. K., Orzol, S. M., Young, E. W., Ostbye, T., Wolfe, R. A., . . . Bloembergen, W. E. (2000). Predictors of loss of residual renal function among new dialysis patients. *Journal of the American Society of Nephrology*, *11*(3), 556–564.

Moran, J., & Correa-Rotter, R. (2006). Revisiting the peritoneal dialysis dose. *Seminars in Dialysis*, *19*(2), 102–104.

Murad, M. H., Elamin, K. B., Abu Elnour, N. O., Elamin, M. B., Alkatib, A. A., Fatourechi, M. M., . . . Montori, V. M. (2011). Clinical review: The effect of vitamin D on falls: a systematic review and meta-analysis. *The Journal of Clinical Endocrinology and Metabolism*, *96*(10), 2997–3006.

Nastou, D., Fernández-Fernández, B., Elewa, U., González-Espinoza, L., González-Parra, E., Sanchez-Niño, M. D., . . . Ortiz, A. (2014). Next-generation phosphate binders: focus on iron-based binders. *Drugs*, *74*(8), 863–877.

National Kidney Foundation. (1997). NKF-DOQI clinical practice guidelines for hemodialysis adequacy. National Kidney Foundation. *American Journal of Kidney Diseases: The Official Journal of the National Kidney Foundation*, *30*(3, Suppl. 2), S15–S66.

National Kidney Foundation. (2002). K/DOQI clinical practice guidelines for chronic kidney disease: evaluation, classification, and stratification. *American Journal of Kidney Diseases: The Official Journal of the National Kidney Foundation*, *39*(2 Suppl. 1), S1–S266.

National Kidney Foundation. (2003). K/DOQI clinical practice guidelines for bone metabolism and disease in chronic kidney disease. *American Journal of Kidney Diseases: The Official Journal of the National Kidney Foundation*, *42*(4, Suppl. 3), S1–S201.

Negri, A. L., & Ureña Torres, P. A. (2015). Iron-based phosphate binders: Do they offer advantages over currently available phosphate binders? *Clinical Kidney Journal*, *8*(2), 161–167.

Noakes, R. (2015). The aryl hydrocarbon receptor: A review of its role in the physiology and pathology of the integument and its relationship to the tryptophan metabolism. *International Journal of Tryptophan Research*, *8*, 7–18.

Painter, P., & Moore, G. E. (1994). The impact of recombinant human erythropoietin on exercise capacity in hemodialysis patients. *Advances in Renal Replacement Therapy*, *1*(1), 55–65.

Papadopoulou, E., Varouktsi, A., Lazaridis, A., Boutari, C., & Doumas, M. (2015). Erectile dysfunction in chronic kidney disease: From pathophysiology to management. *World Journal of Nephrology*, *4*(3), 379–387.

Papovich, R. P., Moncrief, J. W., Decherd, J. F., Bomar, J. B., & Pyle, W. K. (1976). The definition of a novel portable-wearable equilibrium peritoneal dialysis technique [Abstract]. *Transactions of the American Society of Artificial Internal Organs*, *5*, 64.

Parker, T. F., Husni, L., Huang, W., Lew, N., & Lowrie, E. G. (1994). Survival of hemodialysis patients in the United States is improved with a greater quantity of dialysis. *American Journal of Kidney Diseases: The Official Journal of the National Kidney Foundation, 23*(5), 670–680.

Pfeffer, M. A., Burdmann, E. A., Chen, C.-Y., Cooper, M. E., de Zeeuw, D., Eckardt, K.-U., . . . TREAT Investigators. (2009). A trial of darbepoetin alfa in type 2 diabetes and chronic kidney disease. *The New England Journal of Medicine, 361*(21), 2019–2032.

Poesen, R., Viaene, L., Verbeke, K., Claes, K., Bammens, B., Sprangers, B., . . . Meijers, B. (2013). Renal clearance and intestinal generation of p-cresyl sulfate and indoxyl sulfate in CKD. *Clinical Journal of the American Society of Nephrology, 8*(9), 1508–1514.

Prince, R. L., Austin, N., Devine, A., Dick, I. M., Bruce, D., & Zhu, K. (2008). Effects of ergocalciferol added to calcium on the risk of falls in elderly high-risk women. *Archives of Internal Medicine, 168*(1), 103–108.

Rasgon, S. A., Chemleski, B. L., Ho, S., Widrow, L., Yeoh, H. H., Schwankovsky, L., . . . Butts, E. (1996). Benefits of a multidisciplinary predialysis program in maintaining employment among patients on home dialysis. *Advances in Peritoneal Dialysis. Conference on Peritoneal Dialysis, 12*, 132–135.

Rasgon, S., Schwankovsky, L., James-Rogers, A., Widrow, L., Glick, J., & Butts, E. (1993). An intervention for employment maintenance among blue-collar workers with end-stage renal disease. *American Journal of Kidney Diseases: The Official Journal of the National Kidney Foundation, 22*(3), 403–412.

Saran, R., Bragg-Gresham, J. L., Levin, N. W., Twardowski, Z. J., Wizemann, V., Saito, A., . . . Port, F. K. (2006). Longer treatment time and slower ultrafiltration in hemodialysis: Associations with reduced mortality in the DOPPS. *Kidney International, 69*(7), 1222–1228.

Sekine, T., Miyazaki, H., & Endou, H. (2006). Molecular physiology of renal organic anion transporters. *American Journal of Physiology Renal Physiology, 290*(2), F251–F261.

Semenza, G. L. (2000). Surviving ischemia: Adaptive responses mediated by hypoxia-inducible factor 1. *The Journal of Clinical Investigation, 106*(7), 809–812.

Shanahan, C. M., Crouthamel, M. H., Kapustin, A., & Giachelli, C. M. (2011). Arterial calcification in chronic kidney disease: Key roles for calcium and phosphate. *Circulation Research, 109*(6), 697–711.

Shoji, T., Shinohara, K., Kimoto, E., Emoto, M., Tahara, H., Koyama, H., . . . Nishizawa, Y. (2004). Lower risk for cardiovascular mortality in oral 1alpha-hydroxy vitamin D3 users in a haemodialysis population. *Nephrology, Dialysis, Transplantation: Official Publication of the European Dialysis and Transplant Association - European Renal Association, 19*(1), 179–184.

Singh, A. K., Szczech, L., Tang, K. L., Barnhart, H., Sapp, S., Wolfson, M., . . . CHOIR Investigators. (2006). Correction of anemia with epoetin alfa in chronic kidney disease. *The New England Journal of Medicine, 355*(20), 2085–2098.

Sirich, T. L., Funk, B. A., Plummer, N. S., Hostetter, T. H., & Meyer, T. W. (2014). Prominent accumulation in hemodialysis patients of solutes normally cleared by tubular secretion. *Journal of the American Society of Nephrology, 25*(3), 615–622.

Stechschulte, S. A., Kirsner, R. S., & Federman, D. G. (2009). Vitamin D: Bone and beyond, rationale and recommendations for supplementation. *The American Journal of Medicine, 122*(9), 793–802.

Strempska, B., Bilinska, M., Weyde, W., Koszewicz, M., Madziarska, K., Golebiowski, T., & Klinger, M. (2013). The effect of high-tone external muscle stimulation on symptoms and electrophysiological parameters of uremic peripheral neuropathy. *Clinical Nephrology, 79*(Suppl. 1), S24–S27.

Taskapan, H., Wei, M., & Oreopoulos, D. G. (2006). 25(OH) vitamin D3 in patients with chronic kidney disease and those on dialysis: Rediscovering its importance. *International Urology and Nephrology, 38*(2), 323–329.

Termorshuizen, F., Dekker, F. W., van Manen, J. G., Korevaar, J. C., Boeschoten, E. W., Krediet, R. T., & NECOSAD Study Group. (2004). Relative contribution of residual renal function and different measures of adequacy to survival in hemodialysis patients: An analysis of the Netherlands cooperative study on the adequacy of dialysis (NECOSAD)-2. *Journal of the American Society of Nephrology, 15*(4), 1061–1070.

Tokmakova, M. P., Skali, H., Kenchaiah, S., Braunwald, E., Rouleau, J. L., Packer, M., . . . Solomon, S. D. (2004). Chronic kidney disease, cardiovascular risk, and response to angiotensin-converting enzyme inhibition after myocardial infarction: The survival and ventricular enlargement (SAVE) study. *Circulation, 110*(24), 3667–3673.

Uusi-Rasi, K., Patil, R., Karinkanta, S., Kannus, P., Tokola, K., Lamberg-Allardt, C., & Sievänen, H. (2015). Exercise and vitamin D in fall prevention among older women: A randomized clinical trial. *JAMA Internal Medicine, 175*(5), 703–711.

Vanholder, R., Baurmeister, U., Brunet, P., Cohen, G., Glorieux, G., Jankowski, J., & European Uremic Toxin Work Group. (2008). A bench to bedside view of uremic toxins. *Journal of the American Society of Nephrology, 19*(5), 863–870.

Vanholder, R., De Smet, R., Glorieux, G., Argilés, A., Baurmeister, U., Brunet, P., . . . European Uremic Toxin Work Group (EUTox). (2003). Review on uremic toxins: Classification, concentration, and interindividual variability. *Kidney International, 63*(5), 1934–1943.

Wolf, M., Shah, A., Gutierrez, O., Ankers, E., Monroy, M., Tamez, H., . . . Thadhani, R. (2007). Vitamin D levels and early mortality among incident hemodialysis patients. *Kidney International*, *72*(8), 1004–1013.

Work incentives: Thoughts from an expert. (1997). *Renal Rehabilitation Report, 5,* 3.

Wu, D., Nishimura, N., Kuo, V., Fiehn, O., Shahbaz, S., Van Winkle, L., . . . Vogel, C. F. A. (2011). Activation of aryl hydrocarbon receptor induces vascular inflammation and promotes atherosclerosis in apolipoprotein E-/- mice. *Arteriosclerosis, Thrombosis, and Vascular Biology,* 31(6), 1260–1267.

Yu, A. S. L. (2015). Claudins and the kidney. *Journal of the American Society of Nephrology*, *26*(1), 11–9.

Zhu, N., Wang, J., Gu, L., Wang, L., & Yuan, W. (2015). Vitamin D supplements in chronic kidney disease. *Renal Failure*, *37*(6), 917–924.

23

CHAPTER

Rheumatic Diseases

Sicy H. Lee, Pamela B. Rosenthal, and Steven B. Abramson

Rheumatic diseases encompass all disorders in which some portion of the musculoskeletal system, including synovial joints, periarticular structures, or muscle, is involved. Arthritis is the general term used when joint disease predominates in the patient's illness. Examples of some inflammatory arthritides include rheumatoid arthritis, reactive arthritis, and psoriatic arthritis. In other conditions, the periarticular soft tissue or muscle disease is the primary concern, and the joint complaints are only a minor component. Some examples of these diseases include fibromyalgia, polymyositis, polymyalgia rheumatica, and scleroderma.

The classification of rheumatic diseases established by the American College of Rheumatology (ACR), the professional medical organization of the subspecialty of rheumatology, lists 116 rheumatic diseases under 10 major general classes of disorders. The current classification is based on known pathological changes induced in affected tissues, clinical patterns, and/or causative agents of each disease. The classification of the rheumatic diseases is a dynamic process that undergoes periodic review as important new information and concepts concerning pathophysiological mechanisms of these diseases are discovered.

According to the latest estimates derived from numerous surveys, there are over 52.5 million persons suffering from some form of arthritis or related diseases in the United States (Barbour et al., 2013). This number will reach 67 million by year 2030 (Hootman & Helmick, 2006). Among these individuals at least 26% are partially disabled and about 10% are totally disabled. Arthritis and related diseases resulted in at least 45 million lost workdays yearly. These figures underscore the magnitude and the problems in diagnosis and management of these diseases. Furthermore, because most rheumatic diseases are chronic disabling conditions, these diseases as a group have significant social and economic ramifications. The rheumatic diseases detailed in this chapter, rheumatoid arthritis, spondyloarthropathies, and particularly degenerative joint disease, are chronic disabling forms of arthritis that afflict otherwise healthy working adults.

RHEUMATOID ARTHRITIS

The prevalence of rheumatoid arthritis in most Caucasian populations approaches 1% among adults aged 18 and older and increases with age, approaching 2% and 5% in men and women, respectively, by 65. The incidence also increases with age, peaking between the fourth and sixth decades. The annual incidence for all adults has been estimated at 67/100,000. Both prevalence and incidence are two and three times greater in women than in men (Hochberg, 1981).

Racial factors appear to be important in rheumatoid arthritis. African Americans, native Japanese, and Chinese may have a lower prevalence of rheumatoid arthritis than do Whites, whereas several North American Indian tribes (the Yakima of central Washington State and the Mille-Lac Band of Chippewa in Minnesota) have a high prevalence of rheumatoid arthritis (Cunningham & Kelsey, 1984). Reasons for these differences are unknown but may relate to both genetic and environmental factors.

Genetic factors play an important role in the susceptibility to rheumatoid arthritis. The concordance among monozygotic twins is 25% to 50%, whereas the concordance among dizygotic twins is only 10%. One of the most significant genetic risk factors for rheumatoid arthritis is the presence of a common amino acid sequence on the DR beta-1 chain of the human leukocyte antigen (HLA) genes

(Gregersen, Lee, Silver, & Winchester, 1987). The proteins produced from HLA genes are important in allowing the immune system to distinguish self-antigens from foreign proteins made by invaders such as viruses and bacteria. Changes in the protein tyrosine phosphatase 22 (PTPN22) gene, which is considered an autoimmune gene, are also associated with increased risk of developing rheumatoid arthritis.

Long-term smoking is a well-established environmental risk factor for developing rheumatoid arthritis; it is also associated with more severe signs and symptoms and worse treatment outcome in people who have rheumatoid arthritis. Other environmental factors, particularly infectious agents, as a causal factor in rheumatoid arthritis remain under active investigation.

Etiology and Pathogenesis

Rheumatoid arthritis is an autoimmune disease in which the normal immune response is directed against an individual's own tissue, including the joints, tendons, and bones, resulting in inflammation and destruction of these tissues. The cause of rheumatoid arthritis is not known, but current evidence suggests that the initiating event is an immune reaction to a foreign antigen such as a virus or bacteria. In an individual with the genetic susceptibility for rheumatoid arthritis, this normal immune response is unchecked, perpetuating the inflammatory response. This theory is supported by the presence of rheumatoid factor (RF) and anticitrullinated protein antibodies, which can appear 10 years prior to the symptomatic onset of rheumatoid arthritis. An experimental arthritis in animals similar to rheumatoid arthritis can be induced following inoculation of protein substances similar to these antibodies, supporting this hypothesis in part (Holmdahl, Nordling, Rubin, Tarkowski, & Klareskog, 1986).

During this process of inflammation, cells of the immune system, including monocytes, T lymphocytes, B lymphocytes, and neutrophils, are activated to secrete a variety of chemical substances. These chemical messengers, cytokines and chemokines, among others, further stimulate proliferation of the synovial cells that normally line the joints, causing fluid accumulation in the joints (effusion), destruction of cartilage, and erosion of bone. The erosions in the bone can be observed radiographically and are characteristic of rheumatoid arthritis. Pathologically, the typical feature is the invasion of the cartilage and bone by the pannus, a vascular granulation tissue composed of various numbers of inflammatory cells, synovial cells, and new blood vessels. The tendons and ligaments can be similarly affected.

Clinical Manifestations

Rheumatoid arthritis is a systemic disease manifested primarily as polyarthritis. Although the diagnosis is made on clinical grounds, the most recent criteria, established by the ACR in 2010, aim to identify rheumatoid arthritis much earlier than the previous 1987 set of criteria with the goal of initiating treatment as early as possible (Arnett et al., 1988; Aletaha et al., 2010). Patients with at least one joint with definite clinical synovitis not explained by another disease will be considered to have definite rheumatoid arthritis if the cumulative score is greater than 6/10 based on: (a) joint involvement: 2 to 10 large joints scores 1 point, 1 to 3 small joints 2 points, 4 to 10 small joints 3 points, >10 joints 5 points, (b) presence of RF or anticitrullinated protein antibodies: low positivity (less than three times upper limit of normal) scores 2 points, high positivity (greater than three times upper limit of normal) scores 3 points, (c) abnormal C-reactive protein (CRP) or erythrocyte sedimentation rate (ESR) scores 1 point, and (d) duration of symptoms greater than 6 weeks scores 1 point (Smolen et al., 2010).

Rheumatoid arthritis usually has an insidious, slow onset over weeks to months. About 15% to 20% of individuals have a more rapid onset that develops over days to weeks. About 8% to 15% actually have acute onset of symptoms that develop over days. The initial symptoms may be systemic or articular. In some patients, fatigue, malaise, low-grade fever, or diffuse musculoskeletal pain may be the first nonspecific complaints. Morning stiffness is frequently the first presenting symptom prior to onset of joint pain. Although symmetric pattern is common, asymmetric presentation is not unusual. The usual involvement is oligoarthritis progressing to polyarthritis in an additive but not migratory pattern. The most common joints involved in rheumatoid arthritis are metacarpophalangeals (MCPs) (87%), proximal interphalangeals (PIPs) (82%), and wrists (63%). Among larger joints, knees are most commonly involved (56%), followed by the shoulders (47%) and the hips. Medium-size joints are the least commonly involved, with the ankles (53%) affected more frequently than the elbows (21%; Harris, 1997).

The natural history of rheumatoid arthritis is varied. In a minority of patients the intermittent course is marked by partial to complete remission without need for continuous therapy. This pattern of disease is usually mild. Initially, only a few joints are involved. Insidious return of the disease is often marked by progressive joint involvement. The majority of patients develop persistent disease requiring chronic therapy. At least 50% will develop erosive disease of cartilage in bone, which in a significant minority of patients is progressive and debilitating. In a seminal 1992 study, Pincus and Callahan (1992) and others underscored the increased all-cause mortality and morbidity among patients with rheumatoid arthritis. More recently, the risk of premature cardiovascular disease is an area of interest and research focus (Solomon et al., 2015).

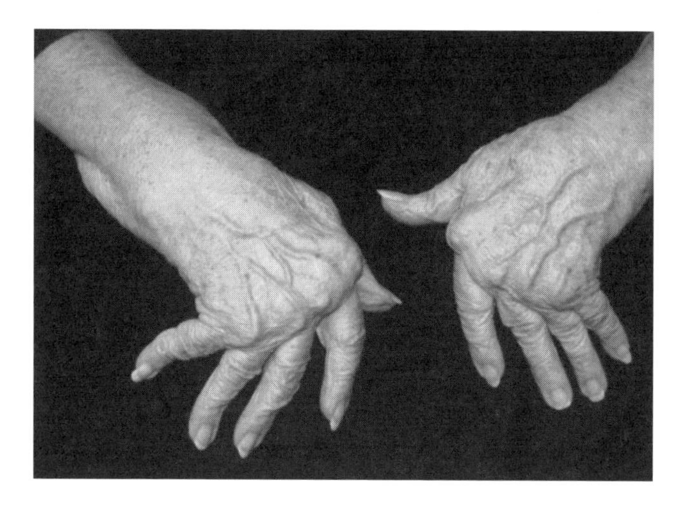

FIGURE 23.1 Rheumatoid arthritis: ulnar deviation with subluxation of the metacarpophalangeal joints. The joints are swollen. Muscle atrophy has developed in the dorsal musculature of both hands.

Source: Chung and Pushman (2011). Copyright 2011. Published by Elsevier.

Functional Presentation and Disability

In the initial stages of each joint involvement, there is warmth, pain, and redness, with corresponding decrease of range of motion of the affected joint. In the hand, soft tissue swelling occurs as an early finding in rheumatoid arthritis and usually appears as fusiform enlargement of the PIPs. Patients describe difficulty in activity requiring motion of these joints, particularly in the morning. Progression of the disease results in reducible and later fixed deformities, including ulnar deviation, swan-neck, or boutonniere deformities (Figures 23.1–23.3). The distal interphalangeal joints (DIPs) are seldom involved in rheumatoid arthritis. Many patients are able to continue performing activities of daily living as well as various nondexterous vocational tasks. The most severe form is arthritis mutilans, in which there is complete bone and joint destruction and all movement is severely limited. At the wrist, there is decreased ability to extend or flex, with progression toward eventual fusion. An exaggerated flexion with near dislocation (subluxation) can occur in severe disease.

Deformities also occur at other joints. At the neck, there can be limitation in extension/flexion as well as rotation. The more serious deformities are those that result in neurological problems such as weakness and paralysis. The transverse ligaments that stabilize C-1 and C-2 vertebrae can become eroded. This results in C-1–C-2 (atlantoaxial) subluxation and can cause instability, with possible compression of the spinal cord or upward migration of the cervical spine and impingement of the medulla (brain). Such neurological involvement requires surgical intervention. The knees can decrease in flexion and can also develop flexion contracture. The hip may become limited in rotation or flexion extension. The ankle can be affected,

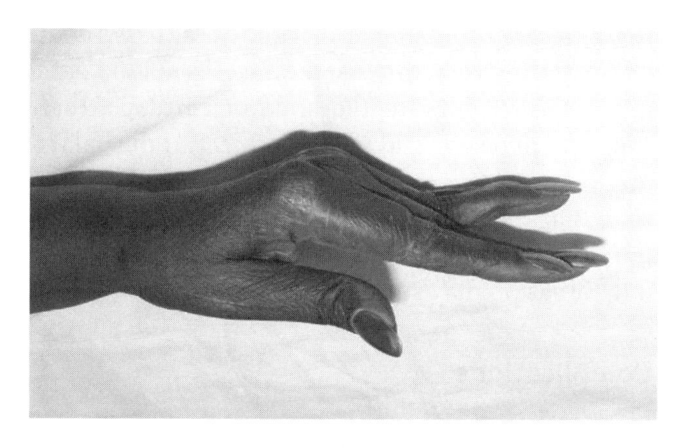

FIGURE 23.2 Rheumatoid arthritis: swan-neck deformity is seen in the fourth digit of a patient with chronic rheumatoid arthritis.

Source: Chung and Pushman (2011). Copyright 2011. Published by Elsevier.

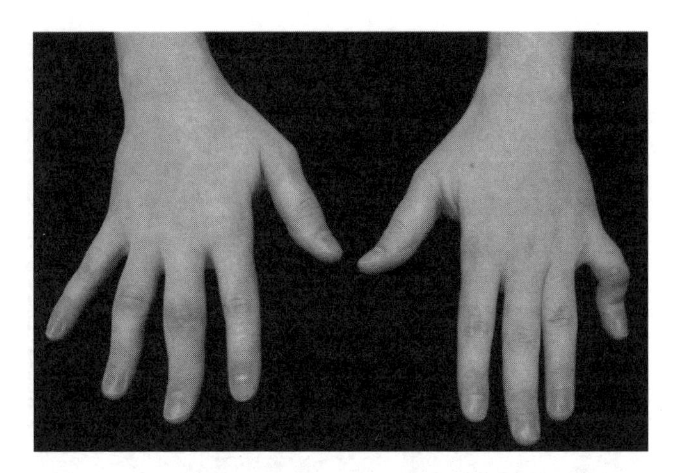

FIGURE 23.3 Rheumatoid arthritis: A boutonnière deformity of the fifth digit is present.

Source: Chung and Pushman (2011). Copyright 2011. Published by Elsevier.

with decreased ability to invert/evert or flex/extend. With inflammation or rupture of certain tendons, pes planus or flat foot can develop. The toes mirror what occurs in the hands with involvement of the metatarsal phalangeal joints (MTPs) and PIPs. The most common deformities are hammer or cockup toes with MTP subluxation and callus formation of the planter surface.

Muscle weakness and atrophy develop early in the course of the disease in many patients. The exact cause of these problems is not clear. One observation is that perhaps patients are unable to move because of pain, and this lack of movement can cause further muscle atrophy and weakness. The combination of pain and muscle atrophy further diminishes the patient's ability to perform activities requiring both strength and dexterity. Therefore, the vocational and functional skills of the patient may be impaired early by pain, inflammation, and weakness. If the inflammation clears after several weeks and no damage has been done to the bone or cartilage, there usually will be no residual impairment. If the inflammation persists, permanent deformities can develop such that the mechanics of the joint are altered and the joint cannot function well, even though pain and inflammation may subside eventually.

Complications

There are a number of complications in rheumatoid arthritis. These include carpal tunnel syndrome, Baker's cyst, vasculitis, subcutaneous nodules, Sjogren's syndrome, peripheral neuropathy, cardiac and pulmonary involvement, Felty's syndrome, and anemia (Hurd, 1984). With the exception of carpal tunnel syndrome and Baker's cyst, these complications usually occur in the presence of seropositive, progressive, and destructive disease.

Carpal tunnel syndrome occurs when the proliferating synovial tissue compresses on the median nerve as it travels through the narrow space in the flexor surface of the wrist. It is characterized by numbness, tingling, and eventual loss of feeling in the thumb, second, and third fingers. The small muscles of the thumb may weaken and atrophy when the compression is not relieved.

Baker's cyst occurs when the synovial fluid escapes from the knee and collects in the space behind the knee, with extension into the calf. Rupture of the Baker's cyst can occur abruptly and cause sudden pain and swelling in the calf. These symptoms must be distinguished from venous thrombophlebitis by ultrasound studies.

Vasculitis is the inflammation of blood vessels, affecting capillaries and small and medium-size blood vessels. It can lead to skin lesions such as ulcers and subcutaneous nodules and to more severe problems, such as mononeuritis multiplex.

Subcutaneous nodules may develop in approximately 20% to 25% of seropositive patients. They typically occur in areas subject to pressure, such as the elbows, occiput, or sacrum. They may occasionally break down or become infected but generally are asymptomatic.

In Sjogren's syndrome, lymphocytes invade the glandular tissue of the mouth, nose, eyes, throat, and lungs, resulting in dry eyes (keratoconjunctivitis sicca) and dry mouth (xerostomia). The loss of glandular function may cause ulcers of the eye tissue, dental caries, and an inability to chew food normally. When dry eyes and dry mouth occur alone, the sicca syndrome is said to be present. When sicca syndrome is accompanied by rheumatoid arthritis, the condition is termed Sjogren's syndrome. The lymphocytes can also invade the kidneys, liver, lungs, and other internal organs, resulting in their dysfunction.

Many patients with rheumatoid arthritis can develop peripheral neuropathy and complain of mild numbness and tingling in their fingers and toes. Rarely, they can develop mononeuritis and lose complete function of a major nerve. This loss of nerve function is due to inflammation of the blood vessels that supply the nerve. When more than one nerve is involved, it is termed mononeuritis multiplex.

The most common cardiac involvement in rheumatoid arthritis is pericardial effusion or accumulation of fluid around the heart, which is reported in about 40% of patients at autopsy but is usually clinically asymptomatic. When symptomatic pericarditis occurs, it will rarely proceed to pericardial tamponade where emergency surgical intervention to relieve the pressure around the heart is necessary. Sometimes a focal myocarditis may be recognized. Lesions similar to rheumatoid nodules may be found involving the myocardium and the valves. Valvular insufficiency and conduction abnormalities secondary to these inflammatory lesions may occasionally be seen as clinical manifestations of rheumatoid heart disease.

There is an increased risk of premature death in patients with rheumatoid arthritis. Recently, it has become clear that this is largely due to cardiovascular disease, particularly coronary artery disease (CAD). A meta-analysis of 24 observational studies comprising 111,758 patients concluded that the risk of CAD mortality was higher by 59% in patients with rheumatoid arthritis (Avina-Zubieta et al., 2008).

Several forms of pulmonary disease can occur in patients with rheumatoid arthritis. Rheumatoid pleural disease, though frequently found at autopsy, is most commonly asymptomatic. Pleural effusions or fluid in the pleural cavity can develop, but rarely will they accumulate to a significant size and cause respiratory distress. Multiple pulmonary nodules may occur bilaterally. Another, more serious pulmonary manifestation of rheumatoid arthritis is interstitial fibrosis with pneumonitis. This may progress to a honeycomb appearance on x-rays, with bronchiectasis, chronic cough, and progressive dyspnea. Lung biopsy can show chronic inflammatory cell infiltration accompanied by neutrophils and eosinophils. Laryngeal obstruction can also be caused by arthritis of the cricoarytenoid joint.

Felty's syndrome is characterized by splenomegaly, lymphadenopathy, anemia, thrombocytopenia, and neutropenia in association with chronic active rheumatoid arthritis. Systemic manifestations such as fever, fatigue, anorexia, and weight loss are common. Hyperpigmentation and leg ulcers may accompany Felty's syndrome.

The anemia of rheumatoid arthritis can be due either to chronic inflammation that primarily affects the production of red blood cells in the bone marrow or to iron deficiency secondary to occult blood loss among individuals treated with medications that can cause gastritis or peptic ulcer disease. Frequently, a combination of both factors can be present.

Laboratory Diagnosis

RF, antibodies to cyclic citrullinated peptides (CCPs), increased levels of the ESR and CRP are associated with rheumatoid arthritis. RFs and anti-CCP antibodies are useful in diagnosis and may be helpful in monitoring the activity of disease (Visser, le Cessie, Vos, Breedveld, & Hazes, 2002). RFs, which are antibodies to the constant region of immunoglobulins, occur in 70% to 80% of patients with rheumatoid arthritis. They are not specific for rheumatoid arthritis, as they are also found in patients with mixed cryoglobulinemia, Sjögren's syndrome, 20% to 30% of those with systemic lupus erythematosus (SLE), and 5% to 10% of healthy individuals. In contrast, anti-CCP antibodies are found in 60% to 70% of patients with rheumatoid arthritis but less often in other diseases. The presence of RF yields 85% specificity and 69% sensitivity while anticitrullinated antibodies yields 95% specificity and 67% sensitivity in the diagnosis of rheumatoid arthritis. Both RF and anti-CCP antibodies predict erosive disease among patients with rheumatoid arthritis.

Treatment and Prognosis

A variety of medications are available in the treatment of rheumatoid arthritis (Harris, 1997). The approach to the individual patient with rheumatoid arthritis is determined by a careful analysis of the severity of the patient's disease and rate of progression of the disease as well as an assessment of the patient's other comorbid conditions. Clinical assessment is supplemented by laboratory and radiographic assessment. Because articular cartilage or bone in humans cannot be replaced, the goal of the therapy must be to arrest the synovitis prior to any irreversible damage. In 2015, the ACR established guidelines for treatment of rheumatoid arthritis (Singh et al., 2015). The primary goal of treat-to-target is to achieve the clinical state of remission or low disease activity in established long-standing disease. This treatment target should be maintained throughout the course of disease and drug therapy should be adjusted every 3 months using validated composite measures to guide treatment decisions and should be influenced by comorbidities, patient factors, and drug-related risks. The drugs available to treat rheumatoid arthritis can be divided into several broad categories (Table 23.1).

Analgesics

These drugs include topical (e.g., capsaicin or diclofenac) and oral agents such as acetaminophen (paracetamol), propoxyphene, tramadol, and more potent opioids (e.g., oxycodone, hydrocodone).

Nonsteroidal anti-inflammatory drugs (NSAIDs), which include cyclooxygenase 2 (COX-2) selective agents, have both analgesic and anti-inflammatory properties, but do not alter disease outcomes. Selective inhibitors are preferred for patients at higher risk for adverse gastroduodenal effects, although the well-publicized concern for an association with vascular events should be factored into agent selection as well (Desai et al., 2008).

Glucocorticoids

In patients with extensive synovitis who do not obtain relief from NSAIDs, low-dose steroids can be given for temporary relief. Prednisone in doses up to 7.5 mg daily is used in rheumatoid arthritis for symptomatic control. Even at low doses oral corticosteroids may promote osteoporosis and therefore concomitant treatment with antiresorptive agents should be considered. Moreover, patients who require treatment with corticosteroids should be considered for disease-modifying antirheumatic drug (DMARD) treatment, and once the disease is controlled or improved on DMARDs, steroid therapy should be tapered and discontinued. Steroids alone should never be the mainstay of medical therapy because they do not appear to prevent cartilage damage and because of their side effects. Long-term steroid use can result in early cataract formation, osteoporosis, peptic ulcer disease, augmentation or initiation of hypertension and diabetes, increased skin and vascular fragility, delayed wound healing, muscle weakness, unsightly weight gain and fat accumulation on the face and the trunk, and poor resistance to bacterial and other opportunistic (e.g., fungal) infections.

Disease-Modifying Antirheumatic Drugs

DMARDs may be either traditional drugs or biologics, which are produced by recombinant DNA technology. DMARDs have the potential to reduce or prevent joint damage, preserve joint integrity and function. In individuals who have persistent disease, DMARDs should be initiated as soon as possible.

There is now an increasing tendency to begin DMARDs earlier and more aggressively in the course of the patient's illness. This tendency resulted from the emerging view that there is a brief window of opportunity early in the patient's illness to halt the inflammatory process. Once articular damage occurs, the destructive process appears to self-perpetuate and cannot be reversed with medications. There is evidence that for many patients radiographic damage can occur soon after the onset of disease. Therefore, individuals who have evidence of disease activity as measured by swollen and tender joints, elevated CRP or sedimentation rate, elevated RF and/or anti-CCP, constitutional symptoms including morning stiffness, fever, and weight loss should be aggressively treated with DMARDs so that remission is achieved as soon as possible. The traditional DMARDs include hydroxychloroquine, sulfasalazine, methotrexate, leflunomide, and minocycline. Among traditional DMARDs, methotrexate and leflunomide are preferred to sulfasalazine in patients with high disease activity and features associated with a poor prognosis (Saag et al., 2008)

D-penicillamine is rarely used and has potential major side effects, including nephrosis (protein in the urine), anemia, leukopenia, thrombocytopenia, stomatitis, skin rash, and interstitial pulmonary fibrosis. Therefore, close laboratory and clinical monitoring is required while patients are on these medications. In order for the patient to accept these potentially toxic medications, the physician must adequately explain the necessity for their use. Oral gold and antimalarials have less toxic side effects but are also less likely to be effective. Because of the potential damage to the retina, regular ophthalmological examination is necessary while the patient is on antimalarials. Methotrexate has gained widespread use and is relatively easy to administer as it is given once a week. The drug is effective, but there are concerns about long-term toxicity, particularly

TABLE 23.1

AGENTS USED TO TREAT RHEUMATOID ARTHRITIS	
Agent	**Dose**
ANALGESICS/ANTI-INFLAMMATORIES	
Salicylates Aspirin Sodium salicylate Salicylic acid (Trilisate) Diflunisal (Dolobid)	1,000–5,000 mg/day (adjusted based on serum salicylate levels)
NSAIDs *COX-2 Inhibition* Celecoxib (Celebrex) Ibuprofen (Motrin/Advil) Sulindac (Clinoril) Piroxicam (Feldene) Indomethacin (Indocin) Meclofenamate (Meclomen) Naproxen (Naprosyn/Aleve) Ketoprofen (Orudis/Oruvail) Oxaprozin (Daypro) Tolmetin (Tolectin) Diclofenac (Voltaren/Arthrotec) Flurbiprofen (Ansaid)	 200 mg daily 400–800 mg t.i.d.-q.i.d. 150–200 mg b.i.d. 10–20 mg q.d. 25–50 mg b.i.d.-q.i.d., 75 mg SR 50–100 mg b.i.d.-q.i.d. 250–500 mg b.i.d. 50–75 mg b.i.d.-q.i.d., 200 mg q.d. 1,200–1,800 mg q.d. 200–400 mg b.i.d.-q.i.d. 25–75 mg b.i.d. 50–100 mg b.i.d.
Corticosteroids Oral prednisone Intra-articular	5.0–15 mg q.d. for arthritis Higher doses for extra-articular disease Varies with joint size
Disease-modifying agents (slow-acting agents) D-penicillamine (Depen) Hydroxychloroquine (Plaquenil) Sulfasalazine (Entab)	 125–1000 mg q.d. 200–600 mg q.d. 1000–1500 mg b.i.d.
Immunosuppressive agents Methotrexate (PO, IM, IV) Azathioprine (Imuran) Leflunomide (Arava) Cyclophosphamide (Cytoxan) Mycophenolate acid (Cellcept) Cyclosporin (Neoral)	 5.0–30 mg/week 25–150 mg q.d. 10–20 mg q.d. 25–150 mg q.d. 1 gm b.i.d. 2 4 mg/kg/day
BIOLOGIC AGENTS	
TNF receptor antagonist Etanercept (Enbrel) Adalimumab (Humira) Infliximab (Remicade) Golimumab (Simponi) Certolizumab (Cimzia)	 SQ 50 mg q week SQ 40 mg q 2 weeks IV 3–10 mg/kg q 2 months SQ 50 mg q month or IV 2 mg/kg q 8 weeks SQ 200 mg q 2 weeks
Interleukin-6 antibody Tocilizumab (Actemra)	 IV 8 mg/kg q month or SQ 162 mg q 2 weeks
Anti-CTLA-4 monoclonal antibody Abatacept (Orencia)	 IV 500–1000 mg q month or SQ 125 mg weekly

(*continued*)

TABLE 23.1 (*continued*)

AGENTS USED TO TREAT RHEUMATOID ARTHRITIS	
Agent	**Dose**
JAK inhibitor	
Tofacitinib (Xeljanz)	5 mg b.i.d.
Anti-CD20 monoclonal antibody	
Rituximab (Rituxan)	IV 500–1,000 mg days 1 and 15 every 6 months

COX-2, cyclooxygenase 2; IM, intramuscular; IV, intravenous; JAK, Janus kinase; NSAIDs, nonsteroidal anti-inflammatory drugs; PO, per oral; TNF, tumor necrosis factor.

pulmonary and hepatic fibrosis (Tugwell, Bennett, & Gent, 1987). Sulfasalazine had gained popularity in Europe as an effective DMARD (Pinals, Kaplan, Lawson, & Hepburn, 1986). The adverse effects associated with the use of this drug include blood dyscrasias, drug fever, hepatitis, allergic pneumonitis, drug-induced lupus, vasculitis, and significant cutaneous reaction including exfoliative dermatitis. Very few serious reactions have been reported in rheumatoid arthritis patients, and the adverse events appear to occur more commonly among slow acetylators. Leflunomide (Arava) is a reversible pyrimidine inhibitor and appears similar to methotrexate in efficacy; the major potential adverse effect is hepatotoxicity, and monitoring is required monthly (Smolen, Kalden, & Scott, 1999; Strand, Cohen, & Schiff, 1999). Other cytotoxic drugs (azathioprine, cyclophosphamide) appear effective but also have many potential side effects, particularly hepatic and hematologic toxicities, and require careful monitoring.

Biologicals

The newest group of DMARDs in the treatment of rheumatoid arthritis is the biological agents (Siddiqui, 2007). These agents are unique in that they target a specific arm or subpopulation of cells within the immune system so that the inflammatory response in rheumatoid arthritis is abrogated. The majority of the approved agents target tumor necrosis factor (TNF). Etanercept (Enbrel) is a soluble TNF receptor antagonist and is a recombinant receptor fusion protein (Bathon, Martin, & Fleishmann, 2000). Infliximab (Remicade) is a chimeric anti-TNF monoclonal antibody (approximately 25% mouse protein) and approved for the treatment of rheumatoid arthritis in combination with methotrexate (Maini, Clair, & Breedveld, 1999). Adalimumab (Humira) and golimumab (Simponi) are fully humanized anti-TNF monoclonal antibodies (Weinblatt, Keystone, & Furt, 2003). Certolizumab (Cimzia) is a recombinant humanized Fab' anti-TNF antibody conjugated to polyethylene glycol. Other non-anti-TNF approved biologic therapies for rheumatoid arthritis include rituximab (Rituxan), an anti-CD20 monoclonal antibody; abatacept (Orencia), a cytotoxic T-lymphocyte antigen 4 immunoglobulin monoclonal antibody; and tocilizumab (Actemra), an anti-interleukin-6 receptor monoclonal antibody. Tofacitinib (Xeljanz) is the member of a new class of oral targeted synthetic compounds. Tofacitinib is a moderately selective inhibitor of Janus kinase 3.

Another growing trend in the medical management of rheumatoid arthritis is the early use of combination drug therapy in aggressive disease. Smaller doses of multiple drugs with synergistic effects are used, in effect lowering the level of toxicity of individual drugs and enhancing the efficacy of treatment. Multiple studies have demonstrated that giving a biologic agent in combination with methotrexate is more effective in preventing radiographic progression than when methotrexate or any of the biologic agents is given as monotherapy. The ultimate challenge for the future is to devise safe and effective therapies that can be administered in early stages of the disease.

Surgical treatment in rheumatoid arthritis should be used in combination with medical therapy. In patients with severe synovitis and in whom the slow-acting agents have not yet taken effect, early synovectomy (removal of the synovial tissue to as great a degree as possible) can be considered for the elbows and knees. When permanent deformities have developed despite medical therapy, surgery can be performed to correct these deformities to decrease pain and improve the patient's functional status. These procedures include joint fusions (e.g., wrist fusion to provide a stable and painless wrist), resections (e.g., resection of the distal ends of the metatarsal heads to reduce foot pain and improve comfort and walking), and joint prosthesis. The most successful total joint replacements are the hips and knees; joint replacement for the shoulder, elbow, and ankle are available but less successful.

Rehabilitation therapy is an integral part of treatment in rheumatoid arthritis. In early disease, the goal is to reduce pain and inflammation and to prevent deformities and muscle atrophy. As the disease progresses, it is an important modality to correct deformities and increase strength. The major goal at each stage is to improve functional skills in the patient. Modalities that are used to reduce pain and inflammation include moist heat, paraffin baths, and cold packs, which allow more activities to be performed with less discomfort. Acupuncture sometimes can be used as an adjunct to decrease swelling or pain. The choice of treatment depends largely on the patient's preference because there are few data upon which one can base the choice. The pain relief is temporary, lasting perhaps 2 hours. It is important, therefore, that the patient be taught how to perform these treatments at home. Placing a joint in plastic, fiberglass, or plaster splints will protect the joint and diminish the inflammation. There must be a balance between exercise and rest, however, to prevent deterioration of motion and muscle atrophy. Splints are most conveniently placed on the wrists or hands. For some, night use alone may be sufficient.

Exercise is important to help prevent contractures as well as preserve and improve muscle strength. Non-weight-bearing and isometric exercises will allow improvement in strength without joint inflammation. Passive range-of-motion exercises will help preserve motion without stress on the joints. Physical and occupational therapists should also evaluate the patient's functional limitations in activities of daily living and ambulation. Patients should be taught ambulation and transfer techniques. Devices such as reachers, hooks, and built-up utensil handles can be provided. The occupational therapist may also make energy or labor-saving recommendations for the home, such as the raising or lowering of table tops or changing to more easily activated faucet handles. All of these measures aim to allow the patient to be more functional and independent.

With the advent of biologics and implementation of early diagnosis and treatment, attaining clinical remission is a realistic goal for many patients with rheumatoid arthritis, defined as absence of radiographic progression and clinical symptoms. Even in patients who do not achieve clinical remission where there is gradual diminution of inflammation but progression of deformities, the speed of progression to deformities can be significantly slowed. Poor prognostic factors include persistent inflammation despite aggressive medical therapy of more than 1 year's duration; onset of disease below age 30; presence of extra-articular manifestation of rheumatoid arthritis, including subcutaneous nodules, vasculitis, Sjogren's syndrome, and neuropathy; anticitrulline protein antibody and persistent high-titer RF.

PSYCHOLOGICAL AND VOCATIONAL IMPLICATIONS

Patients with rheumatoid arthritis undergo several stages of psychological adjustments. In the early stages of disease, it is common for patients with rheumatoid arthritis to be frightened because of the uncertainty of the prognosis of the disease and the degree of disability. Many patients also tend to blame themselves or a particular incident for the onset of the disease. Along with this feeling of guilt, there is also denial. Many patients do not give up hope that one day the disease and pain will miraculously vanish. This type of denial may lead to unrealistic expectations and resistance to medical treatment. As the disease progresses, the patient may express various degrees of anger, frustration, resentment, and depression. Some patients adapt to their disease and disability and function well with limited abilities, whereas other patients seem incapacitated by fairly minimal involvement. Adaptation to rheumatoid arthritis requires the patient to have self-confidence and willingness to adjust certain aspects of lifestyle without sacrificing independence. This adaptation is difficult and may be thwarted by pain denial, anger, and depression. Another reaction to the disease is hopelessness and increased dependency. Faced with the prospect of progressive deformities and apparent deterioration, the patient may give up trying to remain active by increasingly depending on others for care.

Not all individuals with rheumatoid arthritis progress unremittingly to disability. In the minority of patients with mild disease, fewer adjustments are required and vocational goals can be easily met. However, in individuals in whom the disease is an evolving and dynamic process, the vocational counselor should make frequent assessment of the patient's functional ability as the disease progresses and provide realistic goals and support through the more difficult periods so that employment can be sustained.

In general, motor coordination, finger and hand dexterity, and eye–hand–foot coordination are adversely affected by rheumatoid arthritis. Vocational goals dependent upon fine, dexterous, or coordinated movements of the hand are therefore not ideal for patients with rheumatoid arthritis. Loss of motion and pain on motion slow the patient's movements and diminish coordination. Therefore, the operation of machines requiring repetitive, dexterous, and rapid movements is also not a desirable choice. However, if the force required is quite low, dexterous tasks such as typing on a computer keyboard, are possible.

Most jobs requiring medium-to-heavy physical activity are also not desirable. Although most patients may be able to perform moderate manual labor (i.e., lift 25–30 lb), such level of activity will not be sustainable as the disease progresses. In addition, such a workload may be harmful to the joints. Activities such as climbing, balancing, stooping, kneeling, standing, or walking are all hampered by pain on weight bearing or with motion. Although these activities can be accomplished by most individuals with milder forms of rheumatoid arthritis, jobs requiring such activities repetitively and without periods of rest cannot be sustained and indeed may damage joints.

It is usual for patients with rheumatoid arthritis to detect changes in humidity, temperature, or barometric pressure. Therefore, extremes of weather or abrupt changes in temperature should be avoided, and an indoor climate in which the environment is relatively controlled is recommended. Excessive noise, vibration, fumes, gases, dust, and poor ventilation have no specific effects on patients with rheumatoid arthritis except for those individuals with appreciable pulmonary involvement.

Advanced or additional educational goals such as vocational training and/or college courses of 2 to 4 years should be strongly considered for individuals with recent-onset rheumatoid arthritis and those with long-standing disease despite increased mortality and morbidity among the latter. Educational goals should be guided by the patient's interest and aptitude. It is important to realize that the individual with rheumatoid arthritis does not have a permanent invariant disability but rather a changing disability with chronic pain (which can vary from day to day) that generally results in a progressive and unfavorable outcome. Such individuals require ongoing coordinated counseling that provides a combination of empathy, encouragement, and adequate evaluation and treatment.

SERONEGATIVE SPONDYLOARTHROPATHIES

The seronegative spondyloarthropathies consist of a group of related disorders that include reactive arthritis syndrome, ankylosing spondylitis, psoriatic arthritis, and arthritis in association with inflammatory bowel disease. This group of diseases occurs more commonly among young men, with a mean age at diagnosis in the third decade and a peak incidence between ages 25 and 34. The prevalence appears to be approximately 1%. The male-to-female ratio approaches 4 to 1 among adult Caucasians (Hochberg, 1992).

Genetic factors play an important role in the susceptibility to each disease. Among Caucasians, over 90% of patients with ankylosing spondylitis are HLA-B27, and approximately 20% of individuals with the HLA-B27 antigen will develop some form of spondyloarthritis. In addition, disease concordance for ankylosing spondylitis among monozygotic twins exceeds 50%. Linkage to other major histocompatibility complex (MHC) class I antigens that are cross-reactive with B27 (B7, B22, B40, B42) also has been observed, particularly among people of African descent, in whom the association between ankylosing spondylitis and HLA-B27 (40%–50%) is not as striking as that in Caucasians (Arnett, 1984).

Etiology and Pathogenesis

The cause of spondyloarthritis is unclear, but there is strong evidence that the initial event involves interaction between genetic factors determined by class I MHC genes and environmental factors, particularly bacterial infections. The onset of musculoskeletal symptoms following exposure to infections suggests an immunologically mediated process, as does the finding of lymphocytes at the sites of inflammation. In addition, there is mounting interest in the role of the intestinal microbiome in the pathoetiology of spondyloarthropathies. An intestinal microbiome dysbiosis, whereby skewed bacterial populations may result in priming and activation of the innate immune response, which results in the activation of inflammatory pathways, such as those mediated by TH17 cells, ultimately resulting in enthesitis and synovitis, is a hypothesis under active investigation. In psoriatic arthritis the dysbiosis is characterized by a decreased intestinal species diversity compared to healthy controls, suggesting that in this instance the dysbiosis is characterized by the relative absence of beneficial intestinal bacterial species (Scher et al., 2015). In the past several years the role of the TH17 pathway as typified by the production of the cytokines, IL17 and IL22, is increasingly recognized as central to the inflammatory drive in the spondyloarthropathies. Of interest, the TH17 pathway functions as part of the innate immune response, supporting host defense against extracellular infections and fungi (Mease, 2015).

Reactive arthritis may follow a wide range of gastrointestinal infections, including species of *Salmonella, Shigella, Yersinia, Campylobacter,* and *Escherichia coli* (Arnett, 1984). Work by Schumacher has identified chlamydial organisms in the synovial tissue. *Giardia, Brucella,* and *Streptococcus* organisms have also been implicated, as well as amoebas, and episodes of diarrhea in which no specific pathogen can be identified have been reported (Callin & Fries, 1976; Voltonen, Leirisalo, & Pentikainen, 1985). Arthritis also occurs in association with inflammatory bowel disease in patients who have undergone intestinal bypass operations for obesity and in Whipple's disease. Bowel inflammation has been implicated in the pathogenesis of endemic reactive arthritis, psoriatic arthritis, and ankylosing spondylitis. A putative link between these diverse conditions is the ability of enteric organisms to gain access to the systemic circulation and initiate an immune response in a genetically susceptible individual. The observation that some bacterial antigens share certain amino acid sequences with the HLA-B27 molecule suggests molecular mimicry as a possible mechanism to explain the link between infection and arthritis in the presence of HLA-B27 (Inman, Chiu, Johnston, & Falk, 1992). This association, however, does not explain why only 20% of HLA-B27 individuals develop arthritis in the face of appropriate enteric infection, suggesting that additional genetic or environmental factors influence the development of disease.

Clinical Manifestations

Spondyloarthropathies share certain common features, including the absence of serum RF, an oligoarthritis commonly involving large joints in the lower extremities, frequent involvement of the axial skeleton, familial clustering, and linkage to HLA-B27. Unlike rheumatoid arthritis, in which the predominant site of inflammation is the synovium, these disorders are characterized by inflammation at sites of attachment of ligament, tendon, fascia, or joint capsule to bone (enthesopathy).

Because the musculoskeletal presentation in each of the seronegative disorders is indistinguishable, current classification schemes are based on the presence of extra-articular features that include dermal, ophthalmologic, gastrointestinal and/or urological inflammation. For example, the diagnosis of psoriatic arthritis is supported by the typical cutaneous psoriasis rash, and/or nail bed changes, and perhaps inflammatory eye disease. However, reactive arthritis is often associated with urethral inflammation (urethritis), colitis, inflammatory eye disease, and/or a scaly rash of the palmar surface of the hands and feet (keratoderma blenorrhagicum). However, unfortunately, none of these features is unique to any particular disease. Psoriasis may occur in the setting of inflammatory bowel disease, aphthous stomatitis may occur in any of the seronegative disorders, keratoderma may be indistinguishable from pustular psoriasis, and axial changes in psoriatic or colitic arthritis can be indistinguishable from primary ankylosing spondylitis. Overlap syndromes are common. Finally, there are patients with oligoarthritis and enthesopathy who lack sufficient extra-articular features to allow a specific diagnosis by existing criteria. HLA typing may provide a means of establishing that these patients have a disorder that falls within the spectrum of spondyloarthropathy. Given these pitfalls, the most accurate way of classifying a given patient may be to delineate fully the clinical features of the disease as well as the immunogenetic background in which it occurs.

Ankylosing spondylitis is the prototype disease among this group of disorders. The diagnosis is confirmed by clinical and radiographic findings. Existing criteria include the Rome and the New York criteria (Table 23.2; Bennett & Burch, 1967). Ankylosing spondylitis is considered primary if no other rheumatological disorder is present and secondary if the patient has evidence of reactive arthritis, psoriasis, or colitis.

Reactive arthritis was first described by Hans Conrad Julius Reiter in 1916, in reference to a World War I soldier's arthritis and associated symptoms. For many years the syndrome was known by the eponym "Reiter's syndrome," but the usage of the eponym has been dropped because of Dr. Reiter's conviction as a Nazi war criminal. Reactive arthritis consists of the triad of arthritis, urethritis, and conjunctivitis. Paronen (1948) subsequently pointed out the association of antecedent infectious urethritis or dysentery with the clinical trial. Arnett introduced the concept of incomplete "Reiter's syndrome" to describe those individuals who had only two of the features of the triad and underscored the association of the incomplete syndrome with HLA-B27 (Arnett, McClusky, & Schacter, 1976). The most current ACR criteria are much broader; they define reactive arthritis as a seronegative arthritis that follows urethritis, cervicitis, or dysentery. Possible associated features include balanitis, inflammatory eye disease, oral ulcers, and keratoderma. Callin has proposed a broader definition (Table 23.3) that gives added weight to these extra-articular features (Fox, Callin, Gerber, & Gibson, 1979).

Psoriatic arthritis is not a single disease entity but consists of many different patterns of musculoskeletal disorders occurring in individuals with psoriasis. Patients may present with disease that is clinically indistinguishable from rheumatoid arthritis, ankylosing spondylitis, or reactive arthritis. The most widely used criteria are those of Moil and Wright (Table 23.4; Bennett & Burch, 1967). Complicating this classification scheme is the observation that in up to 20% of patients the musculoskeletal disease antedates the onset of psoriasis. Therefore, an individual with dactylitis and radiographic evidence of pencil-in-cup deformities may be considered to have psoriatic arthritis even if the patient lacks skin disease. A family history of psoriasis or the presence of psoriasis-associated HLA alleles would further support this diagnosis (Mielants, Veys, & Cuvelier, 1985).

There are no distinct criteria for the enteropathic arthritis accompanying ulcerative colitis or Crohn's disease. A clinical spectrum of diseases similar to those seen in association with psoriasis may be observed. In an individual patient, axial disease, peripheral arthritis, or enthesopathy may

TABLE 23.2

CLINICAL CRITERIA FOR ANKYLOSING SPONDYLITIS: NEW YORK CRITERIA (1966)
Diagnosis
1. Limitation of the lumbar spine in all three planes—anterior flexion, lateral flexion, and extension
2. History of or presence of pain in the dorsolumbar junction or in the lumbar spine
3. Limitation of chest expansion to 1 inch (2.5 cm) or less measured at the level of the fourth intercostal space
Grading (requires radiographs of sacroiliac joints)
Definite AS
Grade 3–4 bilateral sacroiliitis with at least one clinical criterion
Grade 3–4 unilateral or grade 2 bilateral sacroiliitis with clinical criterion 1 or with clinical criteria 2 and 3
Probable AS
Grade 3–4 bilateral sacroiliitis with no clinical criteria

AS, ankylosing spondylitis.

Source: Adapted from Bennett and Burch (1967). Reprinted by permission.

TABLE 23.3

CLINICAL CRITERIA FOR REACTIVE ARTHRITIS
Seronegative asymmetric arthropathy (predominately lower extremity) plus one or more of the following: Urethritis Cervicitis Inflammatory eye disease Mucocutaneous disease: balanitis, oral ulceration, or keratoderma
Exclusions Primary ankylosing spondylitis Psoriatic arthropathy Other rheumatic diseases

Source: Adapted from Fox et al. (1979). Reprinted by permission.

predominate. Peripheral arthritis tends to parallel activity of bowel disease, whereas axial disease may progress independent of bowel activity. Complicating the concept of enteropathic arthritis as a distinct disease is the observation that low-grade bowel inflammation may be found on colonic or ileal biopsy in all of the seronegative disorders.

Patients with spondyloarthropathy may also develop inflammation of the aorta (aortitis) and the aortic valve, resulting in aortic insufficiency. Pulmonary fibrosis may also occur, resulting in diminished diffusion capacity and restrictive lung disease.

Functional Presentation and Disability

When the axial skeleton is involved, the initial symptom is morning stiffness and lower-back pain. As the disease worsens, there is progressive diminution of motion of the spine. Eventually, the sacroiliac joints, lumbar, thoracic, and cervical spine become fused, although the process may skip over parts. At this stage, the spine is no longer painful, but the patient has lost all ability to flex or rotate the spine and generally develops a hunched-over posture with fused flexion of the cervical spine and flexion contracture of the hips to compensate for the loss of the lordosis curvature in the lumbar spine. The joints where the ribs attach to the vertebrae are also affected, and chest expansion and lung volume are decreased. Frequently, peripheral joints are involved, and the pattern is usually asymmetric oligoarthritis involving primarily the large or medium joints, including the hips, knees, and ankles. Rarely are smaller joints or the joints in the upper extremities involved. Enthesopathy can occur at multiple sites but more commonly presents as planter fasciitis, Achilles tendonitis, and medial or lateral epicondylitis.

Loss of motion of the spine or pain in the spine with motion generally affects a patient's mobility, making certain chores difficult. Walking, however, remains unimpaired unless the hips and knees are affected. Frequent stooping and bending become

TABLE 23.4

DIAGNOSIS OF PSORIATIC ARTHRITIS		
Established inflammatory musculoskeletal disease (joint, spine, or entheseal) with three or more of the following		
1. Psoriasis	(a) Current	Psoriatic skin or scalp disease present today as judged by a qualified health professional
	(b) History	A history of psoriasis that may be obtained from patient or qualified health professional
	(c) Family history	A history of psoriasis in a first- or second-degree relative according to patient report
2. Nail changes		Typical psoriatic nail dystrophy including onycholysis, pitting, and hyperkeratosis observed on current physical examination
3. A negative test for rheumatoid factor		By any method except latex but preferably by ELISA or nephelometry, according to the local laboratory reference range
4. Dactylitis	(a) Current	Swelling of an entire digit
	(b) History	A history of dactylitis recorded by a qualified health professional
5. Radiological evidence of juxta-articular new bone formation		Ill-defined ossification near joint margins (but excluding osteophyte formation) on plain x-rays of hand or foot

Source: Taylor et al. (2006). Reprinted with permission.

impossible. Toilet activities and dressing may be difficult, but rarely does the patient become dependent. In fact, a patient with ankylosing spondylitis typically is able to continue vocational activity despite progressive stiffness, unless it requires significant back mobility or physical labor.

Treatment and Prognosis

Although the spondyloarthropathies share many features in common they form a diverse and distinctive group of syndromes with their own rapidly evolving targeted therapeutic options. And because they share the hallmark lesion of inflammatory synovitis with rheumatoid arthritis, both conventional DMARDs and anti-TNF agents are efficacious, but recently an anti-IL12/IL23, an anti-IL17A, and a phosphodiesterase 4 (PDE4) inhibitor have been approved for the treatment of psoriatic arthritis (Ramiro, Smolen, & Landewé, 2015).

Historically, NSAIDs are the initial choice for the treatment of seronegative spondyloarthritis. The 2015 American College of Rheumatology ankylosing spondylitis treatment recommendations continue to recommend NSAIDs as first-line therapy for ankylosing spondylitis (Ward et al., 2015). Although the ankylosing spondylitis treatment group does not favor any particular NSAID, indomethacin is commonly regarded as being the most effective. Other NSAIDs, including naproxen, piroxicam, meclofenamate, and flurbiprofen, are also efficacious. Salicylates generally are not effective treatment. Although the benefit of corticosteroids varies by syndrome, in some instances corticosteroids, when given at significantly higher doses than that used in rheumatoid arthritis, can also be quite effective. If the inflammation does not completely resolve with NSAIDs alone or erosive disease is present at the initial evaluation, DMARDs should be given to prevent joint destruction and fusion. Just as in rheumatoid arthritis, the initiation of DMARDs in early disease is recommended to prevent progression of disease. The more common DMARDs used in the treatment of spondyloarthritis include sulfasalazine and methotrexate (Nissila, Lehtinen, & Leirisalo-Repo, 1988). Anti-TNF biologic agents are currently FDA approved in the treatment of psoriatic arthritis and ankylosing spondylitis. The current ankylosing spondylitis treatment guidelines do not distinguish between anti-TNF therapies, except in the instance where there is concomitant inflammatory bowel disease, in which case one of the several anticytokine monoclonal antibodies is preferred. Surgical intervention includes either early synovectomy or total joint replacement in the later stages of disease. In particular, there is strong recommendation for total hip arthroplasty in ankylosing spondylitis patients with advanced hip arthritis. Physical therapy is also an integral part of treatment in this disease and is strongly recommended. Exercises should be done daily and should include those that enable the patient to maintain maximum chest expansion and erect posture as well as maximal axial flexibility.

Three novel therapies have recently been approved for the treatment of psoriasis and psoriatic arthritis. In 2013, ustekinumab (Stelara) was approved; in 2014, apremilast (Otezla); and in 2015 secukinumab (Cosentyx). Ustekinumab is a monoclonal antibody directed against the pro-inflammatory cytokines IL12/IL23 and is in the biologic DMARD (bDMARD) class of therapeutics. Secukinumab (Cosentyx) is another bDMARD. Following from the growing understanding of the role of the TH17 mediated pathways in the pathogenesis of the spondyloarthropathies, secukinumab is targeted against the cytokine IL17A. Taking a different approach, apremilast is an oral synthetic PDE4 inhibitor. PDE4 inhibition limits TNF production. All three drugs have side effect profiles that are considered to be comparable to existing therapies, although there is an increase in *Candida* infections with the IL17A inhibitor. All three have been shown to improve clinical and structural outcomes both for patients who are treated with methotrexate, but not previously treated with anti-TNF therapies and for patients who have previously failed anti-TNF therapy. There are other compounds targeting these and other pathways currently in development. Of note, another IL17A targeted compound, brodalumab was suspended from further clinical development because of a concern for increased suicidal ideation among study patients receiving the compound (Lebwohl et al., 2015).

Spondyloarthritis follows at least three different courses. The majority of the patients experience recurrent episodes of arthritis. A minority have only one self-limiting episode of the disease. A smaller minority of patients suffer a continuous and unremitting aggressive course. Although most patients can continue to work, most are affected and become disabled as the disease progresses (Fox et al., 1979).

Vocational Implications

The patient with spondylitis should be considered for vocational or professional education as resources and interests dictate. Although motor coordination, eye–hand coordination, and eye–hand–foot coordination will not be impaired among individuals with minimum peripheral arthritis, a stiff back will limit the patient's rotation and flexion so that overall dexterity may be affected. Tasks that require reaching or bending will be difficult. Work requiring lifting of over 10 to 15 lb may cause increased back pain. Climbing and balancing skills, stooping, and kneeling may be tolerated initially but become difficult as the disease worsens. Even with sedentary tasks, the patient must be allowed the opportunity to stretch the spine frequently. Although many individuals describe joint pain in relation to weather changes, patients with spondylitis should not necessarily require an indoor environment. Some noise, vibration, fumes, gas, dust, and poor ventilation should not be more intolerable than they are to an individual without spondyloarthritis unless significant pulmonary involvement is present. In general, patients with advanced education or clerical skills will frequently be able to continue meaningful employment, whereas those with only manual skills will become disabled.

OSTEOARTHRITIS

Osteoarthritis, which is also known as degenerative joint disease, is the most common of all joint derangements. It is characterized by progressive loss of cartilage and reactive changes at the margins of the joint, the subchondral bone, and the often mild inflammation of the synovium (Attur, Samuels, Krasnokutsky, & Abramson, 2010). The disease usually begins in the fourth decade; prevalence increases with age, and the disease becomes almost universal in individuals aged 65 and older (Scott & Hochberg, 1984). It primarily affects weight-bearing joints such as the knees, hips, and lumbosacral spine. Frequently, the DIPs and PIPs are involved. Rarely, the shoulder can also be affected.

Etiology and Pathogenesis

Osteoarthritis involves three tissues: bone, articular cartilage, and the synovium. Mechanical stress, trauma, joint misalignment, meniscal surgery, and genetic predisposition can all contribute to the development of osteoarthritis. Obesity is frequently associated with degenerative joint disease in the weight-bearing joints (Hartz, Fischer, & Bril, 1986). Genetic factors play a role in the development of osteoarthritis of the PIPs and DIPs and appear to involve a single autosomal gene that is sex-influenced and dominant in females, resulting in an incidence 10 times greater than in men.

Degenerative changes begin as focal erosion of cartilage at various points of stress. There follows an increase in water content of the cartilage and quantitative and qualitative changes in the cartilage proteoglycans. Enzymes capable of degrading proteoglycans and collagen are increased in the osteoarthritis cartilage. As the disease progresses, cartilage erosions become confluent and lead to large areas of denuded surface. The final outcome is full-thickness loss of cartilage down to bone. In contrast with this structural ulcerative breakdown, there is a proliferative cartilage and bone response leading to thickening of the subchondral bone and increased bony formation (osteophyte). Low-grade synovitis is common, particularly in advanced disease, and is due to release of inflammatory mediators or humoral and cell-mediated immune responses to damaged joint components (Samuels, Krasnokutsky, & Abramson, 2008).

Abnormal mechanical stress can result in production of inflammatory cytokines including TNF-α and interleukins (IL) -1β, -6, and -8 and proteases (e.g., matrix metalloproteinase) that can degrade cartilage (Samuels et al., 2008). It is important to note that inflammatory events also contribute to the pain characteristic of osteoarthritis. Inflammatory molecules, including prostaglandin E_1 and leukotriene B_4, can sensitize nerve fibers in joints so that their responses are increased to both painful and nonpainful stimuli. Other inflammatory molecules (e.g., bradykinin, histamine, serotonin, prostacyclin) released in joints can cause fibers to signal pain even when the joint is still (Bonnet & Walsh, 2005).

Clinical Manifestations

In early disease, pain occurs only after joint use and is relieved by rest. As the disease progresses, pain occurs with minimal motion or even at rest. Nocturnal pain is commonly associated with severe disease. Acute inflammatory flares may be precipitated by trauma or, in some patients, by crystal-induced synovitis in response to crystals of calcium pyrophosphate or apatite. Stiffness usually occurs only in affected joints. Local tenderness, pain on passive motion, and crepitus are prominent findings. Joint enlargement results from synovitis, synovial effusion, or proliferative changes in cartilage and bone (osteophyte formation). Clinical symptoms usually show positive correlation with radiological abnormalities. In a given patient, however, the lack of correlation between joint symptoms and plain radiographic findings may be striking. However, there is mounting interest in the correlation between bone marrow lesions, and synovitis as documented by MRI and pain, as well as progression of joint deterioration (Roemer et al., 2015).

Osteophytes formed at the DIPs are termed Heberden's nodes, and similar changes at the PIPs are called Bouchard's nodes. Flexor and lateral deviations of the DIPs are common. In most patients, Heberden's nodes develop slowly over months or years. These deformities are generally asymptomatic and primarily concern the patient for cosmetic reasons. In other patients, onset is rapid and associated with moderately severe inflammatory changes. This pattern of osteoarthritis is termed erosive osteoarthritis and frequently occurs during the fourth decade in women with a strong familial history. The first metacarpal (MP) joints are frequently involved, leading to tenderness at the base of the first MP bone and a squared appearance of the hand.

Osteoarthritis of the knee is characterized by localized tenderness over various components of the joint and pain on passive or active motion. Crepitus is usually present, and muscle atrophy is seen secondary to disuse. Disproportionate losses of cartilage localized to the medial or lateral compartments of the knee lead to secondary genu varum or valgum deformity. Chondromalacia patellae is commonly detected and is associated with softening and erosion of the patellar articular cartilage. Pain, localized around the patella, is aggravated by activity such as climbing stairs.

Osteoarthritic changes in the hip present with an insidious onset of pain. Pain is usually localized to the groin or along the inner aspect of the thigh, although patients often complain of pain in the buttocks, sciatic region, or the knee due to pain referral along contiguous nerves. Physical examination shows loss of hip motion, initially most marked on internal rotation or extension.

Osteoarthritis of the MTPs can lead to MTP subluxation with corresponding hammer toe deformities. In the first MTP, the most common change is hallux valgus deformities. The severity of these deformities is usually aggravated by inappropriate footwear such as high heels and narrow, pointed, tight shoes.

Osteoarthritis of the spine results from involvement of the intervertebral discs, vertebral bodies, or posterior apophyseal articulations. Associated symptoms include local pain and stiffness and radicular pain due to compression of contiguous nerve roots. Lumbar spinal stenosis is the term used when the middle or the sides of the spinal canal are narrowed and may compress or irritate spinal cord or spinal nerves. The presenting symptom can be pain on walking (claudication) and must be differentiated from claudication secondary to vascular incompetence. The presence of nocturnal pain can be a differentiating symptom for lumbar disease. In severe cases, myelopathy can develop, leading to weakness, sensory loss, loss of bowel and bladder control, muscle atrophy, and disability, which at times can be severe or catastrophic. Surgical intervention is recommended when there are signs of myelopathy.

Functional Disabilities

Osteoarthritis affects the patient's performance by impeding use of the involved joint. Because the hips, knees, and lower back are common sites of degenerative joint disease, walking and transfer activities may be impaired. At first the patient will be able to function well in a limited area, but as the disease progresses, the patient's functional capability decreases. Generally, however, activities of daily living, including dressing and eating, will not be significantly impaired.

Treatment and Prognosis

Major guidelines for the treatment of osteoarthritis are all quite similar in that all of them recommend a combination of nonpharmacologic and pharmacologic treatments (Zhang et al., 2008). All guidelines also recommend a stepped approach to pharmacotherapy for pain management in osteoarthritis patients. The primary goal in the treatment of osteoarthritis is pain control and improvement of function in the affected joint. NSAIDs should only be used intermittently in patients who show signs of inflammation in the affected joint. Analgesic agents such as acetaminophen can be used with low dose on a continuous basis, rather than NSAIDs, for pain control. Oral or parenteral therapy with corticosteroids is contraindicated in the treatment of osteoarthritis. Intra-articular injections of corticosteroids, however, may be beneficial when used judiciously in the management of acute flares, when inflammatory response appears to be a major component. Injections should be infrequent because joint deterioration may be accelerated by masking of pain and subsequent joint overuse or by a direct deleterious effect of these drugs on cartilage (Hochberg et al., 2012).

Newer therapies are in the horizon aimed at preserving the joint function and preventing further damage. These potential treatments can be divided into disease- or structural-modifying drugs and those that improve functional status only. The disease-modifying agents include tetracyclines, gene therapy, and use of growth factors and cytokines (Howell & Altman, 1993). The mode of action is either through inhibition of collagenase activity, increase in the level of tissue inhibitor of metalloproteinases (TIMP), or manipulation of these factors via cytokines or gene therapy. Increased understanding of molecular events involved in the pathobiology of osteoarthritis has prompted development of disease-modifying osteoarthritis drugs, although there is no FDA approved DMARD to date. Many of these agents (e.g., matrix metalloproteinase inhibitors, TNF-α inhibitors, IL-1β inhibitors) are aimed at blocking the actions of the inflammatory cytokines and degradative enzymes described in the preceding paragraphs and they may also decrease the pain experienced by osteoarthritis patients (Hunter & Hellio Le Graverand-Gastineau, 2009). However, pain should also be a primary focus in the overall management of osteoarthritis patients because it has been repeatedly shown that the achievement of significant pain relief is associated with significant improvements in quality of life for this population (Rabenda et al., 2005). Potential agents that are used only for symptomatic treatment of osteoarthritis include glucosamine sulfate, chondroitin sulfate, and intra-articular administration of hyaluronic acid derivatives. Glucosamine sulfate and chondroitin sulfate are available in the United States as nutritional supplements. Some evidence exists from Europe that these drugs may modify symptoms in selected patients, but controlled trial has failed to establish its effect in structural modification. Although hyaluronic acid derivatives are often mentioned as potential structure-modifying drugs, these products are currently considered to be long-acting symptom-modifying drugs only (Peyron, 1993).

The goal in early rehabilitation is to improve the functional status and prevent further deterioration of the affected joint. Patients should be instructed in daily non-weight-bearing exercise to strengthen muscles and thus protect joints from overuse. In addition, they should be taught weight-bearing techniques. Appliances such as canes are also beneficial.

Surgical procedures in the treatment of osteoarthritis include arthroplasty, osteotomy, and total prosthetic replacement. Hip and knee replacement procedures produce striking symptomatic relief and improved range of motion. Advances in arthroscopic techniques have led to increased surgical management such as debridement to remove loose bodies and abrasion chondroplasty earlier in the disease.

Osteoarthritis is a slowly progressive disease. Although medical and rehabilitative treatment can lead to improvement of function and diminution of pain in most patients, the effect is generally temporary. There is currently no established disease-modifying drug in the treatment of osteoarthritis. The eventual outcome is complete destruction of the joint, and ultimately surgical intervention is required.

Vocational Implications

Because osteoarthritis is not always a systemic disease, successful treatment of a single involved joint may result in continued employment in the patient's current job unless it requires dexterous or heavy use of the involved joint. Even if surgical or medical treatment results in an increased range of motion, diminished pain, and increased functional ability of the affected joint, the use of that joint should be limited. Heavy lifting, which places repetitive stress on the hips, knees, or lumbosacral spine, should be avoided by those who have osteoarthritis in these areas. Light-to-medium work should be possible.

Climbing, balancing skills, stooping, and kneeling will be impaired in many patients with osteoarthritis. The environment has no significant effect on patients with osteoarthritis even though changes in relative humidity and barometric pressures may cause transient joint discomfort.

Returning to work after undergoing successful surgery requires intensive postoperative rehabilitation and continued exercise to maintain muscle strength. As the patient's endurance and tolerance for activity normalize, work can be resumed. However, heavy manual work should be avoided, as the durability of the prosthetic implants is still limited. Stooping and kneeling may be accomplished without pain following surgery but should be limited. Certain motions involved with stooping and kneeling may cause dislocation of a prosthetic hip. Climbing and balancing can be accomplished, but such repetitive motions are hazardous and should also be limited. Most individuals with osteoarthritis are able to sustain gainful employment and a normal level of activity following successful medical and surgical therapy.

REFERENCES

Aletaha, D., Neogi, T., Silman, A. J., Funovits, J., Felson, D. T., Bingham, C. O., . . . Hawker, G. (2010). 2010 rheumatoid arthritis classification criteria: An American College of Rheumatology/European League Against Rheumatism collaborative initiative. *Arthritis & Rheumatism, 62*(9), 2569–2581.

Arnett, F. C. (1984). HLA and the spondyloarthropathies. In A. Callin (Ed.), *Spondyloarthropathies* (pp. 297–321). Orlando, FL: Grune & Stratton.

Arnett, F. C., Edworthy, S. M., Bloch, D. A., McShane, D. J., Fries, J. F., Cooper, N. S., . . . Luthra, H. S. (1988). The American rheumatism association 1987 revised criteria for the classification of rheumatoid arthritis. *Arthritis & Rheumatism, 31*, 315–324.

Arnett, F., McClusky, O. E., & Schacter, B. Z. (1976). Incomplete reiter's syndrome: Discriminating features and HLAB w27 in diagnosis. *Annals of Internal Medicine, 84*, 8–13.

Attur, M., Samuels, J., Krasnokutsky, S., & Abramson, S. (2010). Targeting the synovial tissue for treating osteoarthritis (OA): Where is the evidence? *Best Practice & Research Clinical Rheumatology, 24*(1), 71–79.

Avina-Zubieta, J. A., Choi, H. K., Sadatsafavi, M., Etminan, M., Esdaile, J. M., & Lacaille, D. (2008). Risk of cardiovascular mortality in patients with rheumatoid arthritis: A meta-analysis of observational studies. *Arthritis & Rheumatism, 59*, 1690–1697.

Barbour, K. E., Helmick, C. G., Theis, K. A., Murphy, L. B., Hootman, J. M., & Brady T. J. (2013). Prevalence of doctor-diagnosed arthritis and arthritis-attributable activity limitation—United States, 2010–2012. *Morbidity and Mortality Weekly Report, 62*(44), 869–873.

Bathon, J. M., Martin, R. W., & Fleishmann R. M. (2000). A comparison of etanercept and methotrexate in patients with early rheumatoid arthritis. *New England Journal of Medicine, 343*, 1586–1593.

Bennett, P. H., & Burch, T. A. (1967). New York symposium on population studies in the rheumatic diseases: New diagnostic criteria. *Bulletin on the Rheumatic Diseases, 17*, 453–469.

Bonnet, C. S., & Walsh, D. A. (2005). Osteoarthritis, angiogenesis and inflammation. *Rheumatology, 44*(1), 7–16.

Callin, A., & Fries, J. F. (1976). An "experimental" epidemic of Reiter's syndrome, revisited: Follow-up evidence on genetic and environmental factors. *Annals of Internal Medicine, 84*, 564–574.

Chung, K. C., & Pushman, A. G. (2011). Current Concepts in the Management of the Rheumatoid Hand. *The Journal of Hand Surgery, 36*(4), 736–747.

Cunningham, L. S., & Kelsey, J. L. (1984). Epidemiology of musculoskeletal impairments and associated disability. *American Journal of Public Health, 74*, 574–579.

Desai, S. P., Solomon, D. H., Abramson, S. B., Buckley, L., Crofford, L. J., Cush, J. C., . . . Saag, K. G. (2008). American college of rheumatology ad hoc group on use of selective and nonselective nonsteroidal antiinflammatory drugs. *Arthritis & Rheumatism, 59*(8), 1058–1073.

Fox, R., Callin, A., Gerber, R. C., & Gibson, D. (1979). The chronicity of symptoms and disability in Reiter's syndrome: An analysis of 131 consecutive patients. *Annals of Internal Medicine, 91*, 190–207.

Gregersen, P. K., Lee, S., Silver, J., & Winchester, R. (1987). The shared epitope hypothesis: An approach to understanding the molecular genetics of rheumatoid arthritis susceptibility. *Arthritis & Rheumatism, 30*, 1205–1213.

Harris, H. D., Jr. (1997). The clinical features of rheumatoid arthritis & treatment of rheumatoid arthritis. In W. N. Kelly, E. D. Harris, S. Ruddy, & C. Sledge (Eds.), *Textbook of rheumatology* (pp. 898–950). Philadelphia, PA: W. B. Saunders.

Hartz, A. J., Fischer, M. E., & Bril, G. (1986). The association of obesity with joint pain and osteoarthritis. *Journal of Chronic Diseases, 39*, 311–319.

Hochberg, M. C. (1981). Adult and juvenile rheumatoid arthritis: Current epidemiologic concepts. *Epidemiology Review, 3*, 27–41.

Hochberg, M., Altman, R. D., April, K. T., Benkhalti, M., Guyatt, G., McGowan, J., . . . American College of Rheumatology. (2012). American college of rheumatology 2012 recommendations for the use of nonpharmacologic and pharmacologic therapies in osteoarthritis of the hand, hip, and knee. *Arthritis Care & Research, 64*, 465–474.

Hochberg, M. C. (1992). Epidemiology. In A. Callin (Ed.), *Spondyloarthropathies*. Orlando, FL: Grune & Walton.

Holmdahl, R., Nordling, C., Rubin, K., Tarkowski, A., & Klareskog, L. (1986). Generation of monoclonal rheumatoid factors after immunization with collagen II-anti-collagen II immune complexes: An anti-idiotype antibody to anti-collagen II is also a rheumatoid factor. *Scandinavian Journal of Immunology, 24*, 197–212.

Hootman, J. L., & Helmick, C. G. (2006). Projections of US prevalence of arthritis and associated activity limitations. *Arthritis & Rheumatism, 54*(1), 226–229.

Howell, D. S., & Altman, R. D. (1993). Cartilage repair and conservaion in osteoarthritis. *Rheumatic Diseases Clinics of North America, 19*, 713–724.

Hunter, D. J., & Hellio Le Graverand-Gastineau, M. P. (2009). How close are we to having structure-modifying drugs available? *Medical Clinics of North America, 93*(1), 223–234, xiii.

Hurd, E. R. (1984). Extra-articular manifestations of rheumatoid arthritis. *Seminars in Rheumatic Diseases, 8*, 151–163.

Inman, R. D., Chiu, B., Johnston, M. E. A., & Falk, J. (1992). Molecular mimicry in reiter's syndrome: Cytotoxicity and ELISA studies of HLA-microbial relationships. *Immunology, 58*, 501–512.

Lebwohl, M., Strober, B., Menter, A., Gordon, K., Weglowska, J., Puig, L., . . . Nirula, A. (2015). Phase 3 studies comparing brodalumab with ustekinumab in psoriasis. *New England Journal of Medicine, 373*(14), 1318–1328.

Mease, P. (2015). Inhibition of interleukin-17, interleukin-23 and the TH17 cell pathway in the treatment of psoriatic arthritis and psoriasis. *Current Opinion in Rheumatology, 27*(2), 127.

Maini, R., St., Clair, E. W., & Breedveld, F. (1999). Infliximab versus placebo in rheumatoid arthritis patients receiving concomitant methotrexate, a randomized phase III trial. ATTRACT study group. *The Lancet, 354*, 1932–1939.

Mielants, H., Veys, E. M., & Cuvelier, C. (1985). HLA B27 related arthritis and bowel inflammation: Part 2. Ileocolonoscopy and bowel histology in patients with HLA B27 related arthritis. *Journal of Rheumatology, 12*, 294–299.

Nissila, M., Lehtinen, K., & Leirisalo-Repo, M. (1988). Sulfasalazine in the treatment of ankylosing spondylitis: A 26-week placebo-controlled clinical trial. *Arthritis and Rheumatism, 31*, 1111–1117.

Paronen, A. (1948). Reiter's disease: A study of 344 cases observed in Finland. *Acta Medica Scandinavica, 131*, 1–143.

Peyron, J. G. (1993). Intraarticular hyaluronan injection in the treatment of osteoarthritis: State-of-the-art review. *Journal of Rheumatology, 20*(39), 10–15.

Pinals, R. S., Kaplan, S. B., Lawson, J. G., & Hepburn, B. (1986). Sulfasalazine in rheumatoid arthritis. *Arthritis & Rheumatism, 29*(12), 1427–1434.

Pincus, T., & Callahan, L. F. (1992). Taking mortality in rheumatoid arthritis seriously: Predictive markers, socio-economic status and co-morbidity. *Journal of Rheumatology, 13*, 841–845.

Rabenda, V., Burlet, N., Ethgen, O., Raeman, F., Belaiche, J., & Reginster, J. Y. (2005). A naturalistic study of the determinants of health related quality of life improvement in osteoarthritic patients treated with non-specific non-steroidal anti-inflammatory drugs. *Annals of the Rheumatic Diseases, 64*(5), 688–693.

Ramiro, S., Smolen, J. S., & Landewé, R. (2015). Pharmacological treatment of psoriatic arthritis: a systematic literature review for the 2015 update of the EULAR recommendations for the management of psoriatic arthritis. *Annals of the Rheumatic Diseases, 75*, 490–498. doi:10.1136/annrheumdis-2015-208466

Reiter, H. (1916). Über eine bisher unbekannte spirochaeten infektion (Spirochaetosis arthritica). *Deutsche Medicin Wochenschrift, 42*, 1535–1536.

Roemer, F., Kwoh, K., Hannon, M., Hunter, D., Eckstein, F., Fujii, T., . . . Guermazi, A. (2015). What comes first? multitissue involvement leading to radiographic osteoarthritis: magnetic resonance imaging–based trajectory analysis over four years in the osteoarthritis Initiative. *Arthritis & Rheumatology, 67*(8), 2085–2096.

Saag, K. G., Teng, G. G., Patkar, N. M., Anuntiyo, J., Finney, C., Curtis, J. R., . . . American College of Rheumatology. (2008). American College of Rheumatology 2008 recommendations for the use of nonbiologic and biologic disease-modifying antirheumatic drugs in rheumatoid arthritis. *Arthritis & Rheumatism, 59*, 762–784.

Samuels, J., Krasnokutsky, S., & Abramson, S. B. (2008). Osteoarthritis: A tale of three tissues. *Bulletin of the NYU Hospital for Joint Diseases, 66*(3), 244–250.

Scher, J., Ubeda, C., Artacho, A., Attur, M., Isaac, S., Reddy, S., . . . Abramson, S. (2015). Decreased bacterial diversity characterizes the altered gut microbiota in patients with psoriatic arthritis, resembling dysbiosis in inflammatory bowel Disease. *Arthritis & Rheumatology, 67*(1), 128–139.

Scott, J. C., & Hochberg, M. C. (1984). Osteoarthritis. *Maryland Medical Journal, 33*, 712–716.

Siddiqui, M. A. (2007). The efficacy and tolerability of newer biologics in rheumatoid arthritis: Best current evidence. *Current Opinion in Rheumatology*, *19*(3), 308–313.

Singh, J., Saag, K., Bridges, S., Akl, E., Bannuru, R., Sullivan, M., . . . McAlindon, T. (2016). 2015 American College of Rheumatology guideline for the treatment of rheumatoid arthritis. *Arthritis Care & Research, 68*(1), 1–25.

Smolen, J. S., Aletaha, D., Bijlsma, J. W. J., Breedveld, F. C., Boumpas, D., Burmester, G., . . . van der Heijde, D. (2010). Treating rheumatoid arthritis to target: Recommendations of an international task force. *Annals of the Rheumatic Diseases, 69*(4), 631–637.

Smolen, J. S., Kalden, J. R., & Scott, D. L. (1999). Efficacy and safety of leflunomide compared with placebo and sulphasalazine in active rheumatoid arthritis: A double-blind, randomized, multicentre trial. European leflunomide study group. *The Lancet*, *353*, 259–266.

Solomon, D. H., Reed, G., Kremer, J. M., Curtis, J. R., Farkouh, M. E., Harrold, L. R., . . . Greenberg, J. D. (2015). Disease activity in rheumatoid arthritis and the risk of cardiovascular events. *Arthritis & Rheumatology,* *67*(6), 1449–1455 doi:10.1002/art.39098

Strand, V., Cohen, S., & Schiff, M. (1999). Treatment of active rheumatoid arthritis with leflunomide compared with placebo and methotrexate. European leflunomide Study Group. *Archives of Internal Medicine*, *159*, 2542–2550.

Taylor, W. J., Gladman, D., Helliwell, P., Marchesoni, A., Mease, P., Mielants, H., . . . CASPAR Study Group. (2006). Classification criteria for psoriatic arthritis: Development of new criteria from a large international study. *Arthritis & Rheumatism, 54*, 2665–2673.

Tugwell, P., Bennett, K., & Gent, M. (1987). Methotrexate in rheumatoid arthritis: Indications, contraindications, efficacy, and safety. *Annals of Internal Medicine*, *107*, 358–366.

Visser, H., le Cessie, S., Vos, K., Breedveld, F. C., & Hazes, J. M. (2002). How to diagnose rheumatoid arthritis early: A prediction model for persistent (erosive) arthritis. *Arthritis & Rheumatism, 46*, 357–365.

Voltonen, V. V., Leirisalo, M., & Pentikainen, P. J. (1985). Triggering infections in reactive arthritis. *Annals of Rheumatic Diseases*, *44*, 399–412.

Ward, M., Deodhar, A., Akl, E., Lui, A., Ermann, J., Gensler, L., . . . Caplan, L. (2015). American College of Rheumatology/Spondylitis Association of America/ spondyloarthritis research and treatment network 2015 recommendations for the treatment of ankylosing spondylitis and nonradiographic axial Spondyloarthritis. *Arthritis & Rheumatology*, *68*, 282–298.

Weinblatt, M. E., Keystone, E. C., & Furt, D. E. (2003). Adalimumab, a fully human anti-tumor necrosis factor a monoclonal antibody, for the treatment of rheumatoid arthritis in patients taking concomitant methotrexate: The ARMADA trial. *Arthritis & Rheumatism*, *48*, 35–45.

Zhang, W., Moskowitz, R. W., Nuki, G., Abramson, S., Altman, R. D., Arden, N., . . . Tugwell, P. (2008). OARSI recommendations for the management of hip and knee osteoarthritis, Part II: OARSI evidence-based, expert consensus guidelines. *Osteoarthritis & Cartilage*, *16*(2), 137–162.

Spinal Cord Injury

Christopher Boudakian, Jeffrey Berliner, and Jung Ahn

Sir Ludwig Guttmann, a physician who was a pioneer in the care and treatment of patients with spinal cord injury (SCI), put it succinctly when he said, "Of the many forms of disability which can beset mankind, a severe injury or disease of the spinal cord undoubtedly constitutes one of the most devastating calamities in human life." Given that we do not have a cure as of now, the best treatment continues to be prevention.

Since World War I, great strides have been made in understanding the pathophysiology of SCI. Physicians who work with patients with SCI deal not only with spinal stability and physical disability but also with secondary medical complications. These secondary medical complications involve the dysregulation of the nerve supply to the cardiopulmonary, digestive, integumentary, and urological systems.

Over the past three decades we have witnessed great progress in the management of SCI-related complications, significant changes in SCI epidemiology, new diagnostic modalities used to assess the status of spinal trauma, and tremendous advances in research aimed at alleviating secondary functional deficits resulting from SCI. The complexity of the spinal cord leaves many unknown variables that play key roles in its function. When an injury occurs, a cascade of events are triggered, which lead to further damage of tissues. We are just beginning to understand the role of these mediators of damage and their effects. Research is now focused on interrupting the pathological processes at different points and on helping foster an environment to regrow healthy nerve tissue. The ultimate goal in SCI treatment is the repair of altered neural function and restoration of normal physiology. A cure remains to be a hope for the future.

This chapter addresses the medical, physical, neurological, psychological, social, and vocational aspects of SCI medicine.

HISTORY

The first recorded account describing SCI was discovered in the Edwin Smith papyrus and dates back to 3000 BCE (Donovan, 2007). It was described as an "ailment not to be treated." Centuries later in Greece, treatment for SCIs had changed little. According to the Greek physician Hippocrates (460–377 BCE), "there were no treatment options for spinal cord injuries that resulted in paralysis; unfortunately, those patients were destined to die" (Hughes, 1988). Hippocrates did, however, create a traction machine to help realign the spinal column. Revolutionary gains in treatment of SCI were not made until centuries later when Paul of Aegina (625–690 CE) recommended surgical intervention for vertebral fractures. Surgical treatments were discussed in further detail and refined in India in the Sushruta Samhita during the sixth century and the Royal Book written in Baghdad during the tenth century (Belen & Aciduman, 2006; Delisa & Hammond, 2002; Donovan, 2007; Eltorai, 2002; Hughes, 1988).

Advances in the care of persons with SCI have come through prevention of injury and secondary complications. Today, there is hope that with better understanding of the inner workings of the spinal cord and the neuronal damage caused by SCI, in conjunction with new technology, future treatments and therapies will help reverse injury and restore function.

TERMINOLOGY

SCI is defined as an insult to the spinal cord resulting in a change, either temporary or permanent, in normal motor, sensory, or autonomic function. The term paraplegia refers to the lower extremities, whereas tetraplegia (formally referred to as quadriplegia) refers to all extremities. SCI does not only affect the ability to walk or the use of the hands, but also alters interaction with people and the environment. The injury can affect any or all of the following: the ability to earn income and to obtain or hold a job, relationships with loved ones and friends, sexuality, bowel and bladder functioning, dynamics of marriages, health, and emotion. Although the initial injury often provides a bleak picture, persons with SCI can enjoy fruitful and fulfilling lives.

FACTS AND FIGURES

The National Spinal Cord Injury Statistical Center has been in existence since 1973 and is a culmination of the efforts of Model Spinal Cord Injury Systems. In 2015, there were 14 model system centers across the United States, which worked in a collaborative effort, with the goal of improving care for persons affected by SCI. The model systems are sponsored by the National Institute on Disability and Rehabilitation Research (National SCI Statistical Center, 2014).

The incidence of SCI in the United States is approximately 12,500 new cases per year and the prevalence or number of people alive with SCI in the United States is estimated to be approximately 276,000. The majority of SCIs, 38%, occur from motor vehicle accidents, whereas falls account for 30% and violence 14%. The average age of onset of injury is 42 with a bimodal peak. The highest incidence of SCI occurs during the teenage years through the mid-20s and then another increase is seen after the age of 65. Motor vehicle accidents and sport-related injuries predominate the younger age bracket whereas falls and degenerative spinal stenosis (a narrowing of the spinal canal due to ligamentous and bony overgrowth) affect the latter population. SCI affects males roughly four to one over females with a causal relationship to high-risk behaviors (DeVivo, Krause, & Lammertse, 1999; Jain et al., 2015; National SCI Statistical Center, 2014). The cost of care for a patient with SCI is colossal. The average cost in the first year of injury exceeds $300,000 for all levels of injury and can surpass $1 million for a person with ventilator-dependent tetraplegia. The lifetime-associated medical cost for an injury occurring at the age of 25 for a person with paraplegia is greater than $2.2 million and the estimated lifetime cost for a person with tetraplegia is more than $ 4.6 million. The cost of the injury is augmented by the fact that only half of the patients are covered by insurance at the time of injury and that income is generally lost during hospitalization and recovery. Unemployment among those with SCI is extremely high and estimated to be approximately 47% at 10 years after injury (National SCI Statistical Center, 2014).

Life expectancy for a person with SCI has dramatically risen over the past 50 years. A person with paraplegia injured at the age of 20 can be expected to live for 45 years after the injury. Life expectancy for the uninjured population is 78.8 years. A person with tetraplegia and ventilator-dependent at the age of 20 has an average life expectancy of 25 years after injury, although if the patient has a C1–C4 injury and is able to be weaned from the ventilator, the life expectancy rises to 37 years. This underscores the importance of ventilator weaning (National SCI Statistical Center, 2014). People with SCI undergo a dramatic change in lifestyle. This change in lifestyle not only affects the injured person but also the family members, friends, and loved ones. This may put a strain on relationships as persons now attempt to redefine their roles as caregiver and patient. Among those married at the time of injury (52%), there is a slightly increased divorce rate when compared with the general population (EI Ghatit & Hanson, 1975; National SCI Statistical Center, 2014). Among those who remain married, a limited number of studies showed a better quality of marriage and life-satisfaction rating for both the injured person and his or her spouse.

SCI is often associated with risk-taking behavior. The prevalence of alcohol abuse is high when compared with that of the general population. Mckinley, Kolakowsky, and Kreutzer (1999) found that at the time of initial injury, 53% of patients had positive toxicology screens and among those, 75% were over the state legal limit for intoxication. About 25% of positive toxicology screens were positive for both drugs and alcohol (Allen & Darlene, 1998). Heinemann and colleagues also found that "persons with spinal cord injury have a greater lifetime exposure to and use of substances" as compared to their able-bodied counterparts in the age group of 18 to 25 years (Charles & Carl, 1998).

ANATOMY AND PHYSIOLOGY OF THE SPINAL CORD

Armed with a basic understanding of spinal cord anatomy and physiology, location of the injury, and extent of the spinal cord insult, it becomes possible to predict and anticipate the functions that may be lost, impaired, and regained.

The Spinal Cord

The spinal cord is composed of a bundle of tracts and neurons that are responsible for modulating and transmitting information between the outside environment and the brain and vice versa. The brain and the spinal cord comprise the central nervous system; the spinal cord contains lower motor neurons (LMNs) as well. Upper motor neurons (UMNs) have their origins in the brain or brain stem and transmit information to the spinal cord level, whereas LMNs connect the information from the UMNs to the muscle. Both UMNs and LMNs aid in the movement of muscles. The peripheral nervous system has its origin outside the central nervous system and connects the central nervous system to various muscles and organs.

An adult spinal cord contains more than 1 billion neurons, some of which extend roughly 45 cm in length. These neurons form two specific regions of the spinal cord referred to as gray and white matter. To understand this concept better, it helps to think of the brain and the spinal cord as two computers gathering information and sharing it with one another. The white matter functions to connect the two computers. The gray matter, located in the center of the spinal cord, is made of neuronal cell bodies and processes information. After the information is processed, it is then passed to connector neurons, termed interneurons, and then to the white matter. The white matter is composed of axons and is organized into long tracts. Separate tracts relay sensory, motor, and autonomic information to and from the brain.

To gain a better understanding of how the spinal cord works, let us follow the pathway of the sensation of vibration. The feeling of vibration is sensed by receptors underneath the skin termed Pacinian corpuscles. The information is transmitted to the back of the spinal cord via peripheral nerves. This information is relayed to the posterior gray matter in the back of the spinal cord, processed and transferred to the ascending long tracts (fasciculus gracilis and fasciculus cuneatus) of the white matter, and then transferred to the brain. These ascending tracts are situated in the back of the spinal cord, and are known as the posterior column. The information is processed within the brain and delivered to the sen sory cortex of the parietal lobe (Figure 24.1).

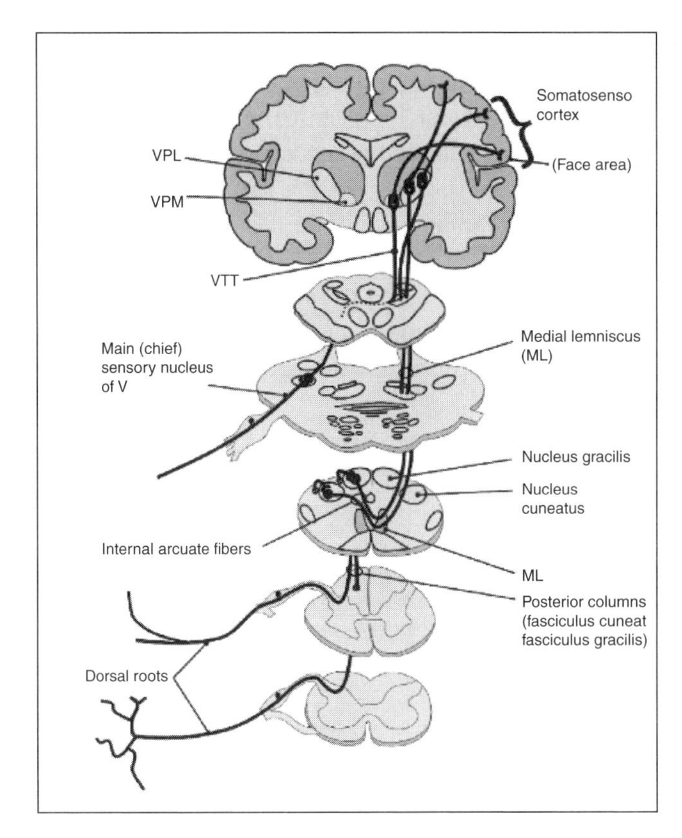

FIGURE 24.1 The fibers making up the posterior column system, critical for proprioception and fine tactual discrimination, enter ipsilateral dorsal cord without synapsing until they reach the nucleus cuneatus and nucleus gracilis in the lower medulla. Second-order neurons then cross the midline and ascend as the medical lemniscus to the ventral posterolateral nuclei of the thalamus, there giving rise to third-order thalamocortical fibers.

Vertebrae

The spinal cord is encased and protected by the vertebrae, numbering about 33 at birth. Taken together, the 33 vertebrae make up the vertebral (spinal) column. This column is typically divided into four levels, referred from top to bottom as the cervical, thoracic, lumbar, and sacral spine. The cervical spine contains seven bones located in the neck region. The thoracic spine contains twelve vertebrae. The next three levels, caudal to the thoracic spine, are the lumbar spine, sacrum, and coccyx containing five, five, and three to four segments respectively. The spinal cord terminates around the inferior border of the first lumbar vertebra, forming the conus medullaris (Figure 24.2).

Sequelae of SCI

SCIs are classified using the ASIA Impairment Scale (AIS). Using a standard classification scale allows clinicians to communicate the location and the extent of injury accurately. The scale also allows clinicians to predict the potential for recovery and monitor the effects of particular interventions on outcome more accurately.

The International Standards for Neurological Classification of Spinal Cord Injury (ISNCSCI) examination involves 10 key muscle groups (myotomes) and 28 key sensory levels (dermatomes) on each side of the body (Figure 24.3). After testing all myotomes and dermatomes, a score of A through

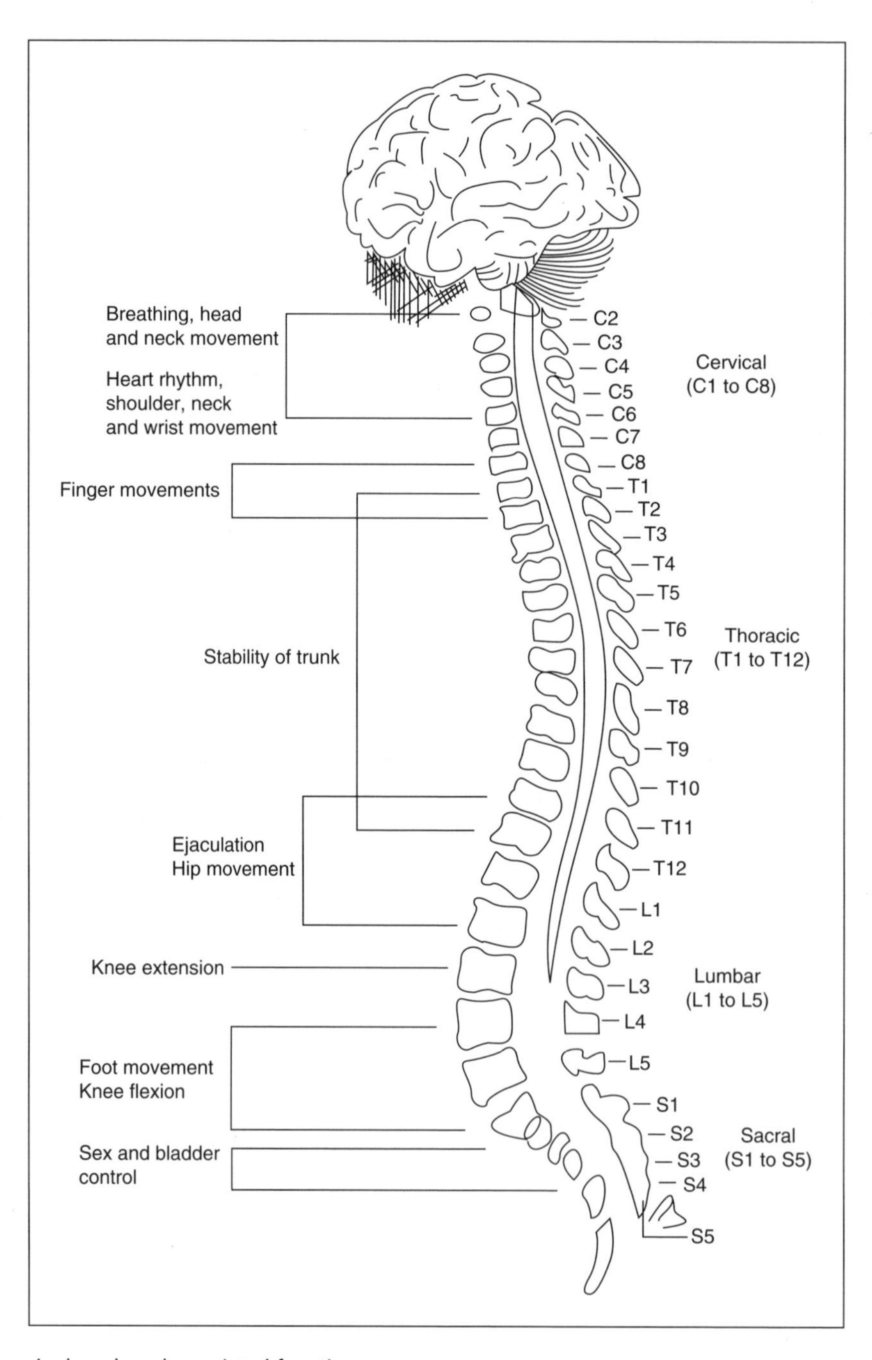

FIGURE 24.2 The spine, spinal cord, and associated functions.

Source: American Spinal Injury Association: International Standards for Neurological Classification of Spinal Cord Injury, revised 2011; Atlanta, GA, Revised 2011, Updated 2015 and International Spinal Cord Society (ISCOS)

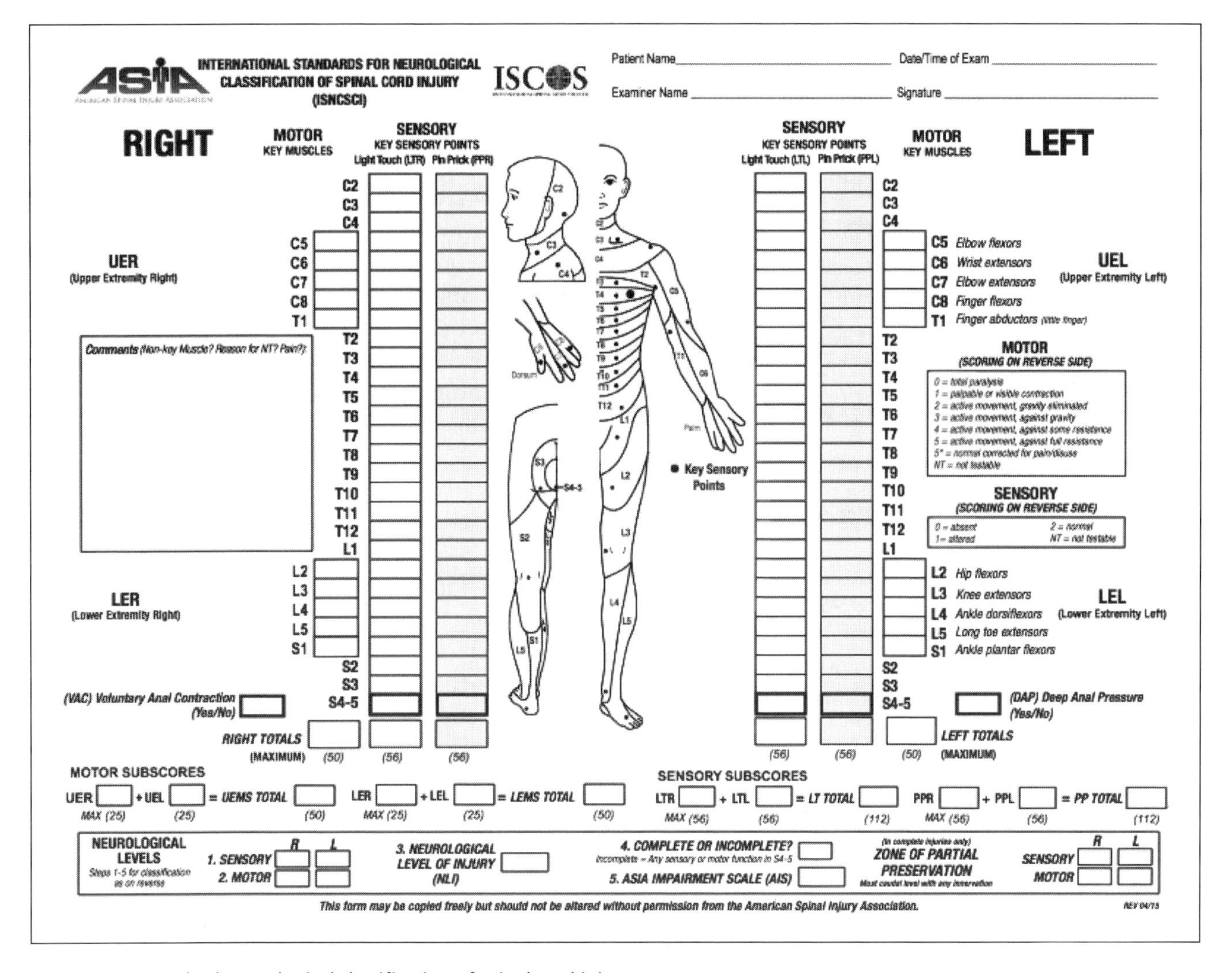

INTERNATIONAL STANDARDS FOR NEUROLOGICAL CLASSIFICATION OF SPINAL CORD INJURY (ISNCSCI)

Patient Name ______ Date/Time of Exam ______

Examiner Name ______ Signature ______

RIGHT — MOTOR KEY MUSCLES — SENSORY KEY SENSORY POINTS Light Touch (LTR) Pin Prick (PPR)

LEFT — SENSORY KEY SENSORY POINTS Light Touch (LTL) Pin Prick (PPL) — MOTOR KEY MUSCLES

C2, C3, C4

UER (Upper Extremity Right) / UEL (Upper Extremity Left)

- C5 Elbow flexors
- C6 Wrist extensors
- C7 Elbow extensors
- C8 Finger flexors
- T1 Finger abductors (little finger)

T2, T3, T4, T5, T6, T7, T8, T9, T10, T11, T12, L1

Comments (Non-key Muscle? Reason for NT? Pain?):

MOTOR (SCORING ON REVERSE SIDE)

0 = total paralysis
1 = palpable or visible contraction
2 = active movement, gravity eliminated
3 = active movement, against gravity
4 = active movement, against some resistance
5 = active movement, against full resistance
5* = normal corrected for pain/disuse
NT = not testable

SENSORY (SCORING ON REVERSE SIDE)

0 = absent 2 = normal
1 = altered NT = not testable

• Key Sensory Points

LER (Lower Extremity Right) / LEL (Lower Extremity Left)

- L2 Hip flexors
- L3 Knee extensors
- L4 Ankle dorsiflexors
- L5 Long toe extensors
- S1 Ankle plantar flexors

S2, S3, S4-5

(VAC) Voluntary Anal Contraction (Yes/No)

(DAP) Deep Anal Pressure (Yes/No)

RIGHT TOTALS (MAXIMUM) (50) (56) (56)

LEFT TOTALS (MAXIMUM) (56) (56) (50)

MOTOR SUBSCORES

UER ☐ + UEL ☐ = UEMS TOTAL ☐ MAX (25) (25) (50)

LER ☐ + LEL ☐ = LEMS TOTAL ☐ MAX (25) (25) (50)

SENSORY SUBSCORES

LTR ☐ + LTL ☐ = LT TOTAL ☐ MAX (56) (56) (112)

PPR ☐ + PPL ☐ = PP TOTAL ☐ MAX (56) (56) (112)

NEUROLOGICAL LEVELS (Steps 1-5 for classification as on reverse)

1. SENSORY R ☐ L ☐
2. MOTOR R ☐ L ☐
3. NEUROLOGICAL LEVEL OF INJURY (NLI) ☐
4. COMPLETE OR INCOMPLETE? ☐ (Incomplete = Any sensory or motor function in S4-5)
5. ASIA IMPAIRMENT SCALE (AIS) ☐

ZONE OF PARTIAL PRESERVATION (In complete injuries only) — Most caudal level with any innervation: SENSORY R ☐ L ☐; MOTOR R ☐ L ☐

This form may be copied freely but should not be altered without permission from the American Spinal Injury Association. REV 04/15

FIGURE 24.3 Standard neurological classification of spinal cord injury.

Source: American Spinal Injury Association: International Standards for Neurological Classification of Spinal Cord Injury, revised 2011; Atlanta, GA, Revised 2011, Updated 2015 and International Spinal Cord Society (ISCOS).

E is given. The scale in Figure 24.4 is truncated for improved ease of understanding (Oleson, Burns, Ditunno, Geisler, & Coleman, 2005).

A complete injury is the most severe injury and is graded as an AIS A. This infers that there is no sensory perception or motor strength in the sacral segments. An injury that has sensation in the most caudal sacral dermatome is termed incomplete and confers a better prognosis for recovery.

Prognosis

"Will I walk again?" This is one of the first questions asked by those with severe SCI and the answer is very complicated. Different mechanisms of injury are known to have different prognoses. Tumors convey a different prognosis as compared to traumatic SCI, and falls have a different prognosis for return of function than bullet injuries. This section focuses on the return of function in traumatic SCI. Even with accurate research, however, there is still a dearth of literature on return of function and many questions remain unanswered.

It is the goal of every patient with an SCI to "walk again." Walking after SCI is often divided into three different categories: walking for exercise only, walking for household distances, and walking in the community. As of now it is possible for persons with paraplegia with injury as high as the second thoracic level to ambulate short distances using a walking aid with bilateral long leg braces. Most patients without motor strength in their legs walk for exercise only as the energy requirement for walking is too great, and the quality of the gait is poor and inefficient. Walking for exercise is not without merit as walking and standing even for short periods of time has been

A = Complete. No sensory or motor function is preserved in the sacral segments S4-S5.

B = Sensory Incomplete. Sensory but not motor function is preserved below the neurological level and includes the sacral segments S4-S5 (light touch or pin prick at S4-S5 or deep anal pressure) AND no motor function is preserved more than three levels below the motor level on either side of the body.

C = Motor Incomplete. Motor function is preserved at the most caudal sacral segments for voluntary anal contraction (VAC) OR the patient meets the criteria for sensory incomplete status (sensory function preserved at the most caudal sacral segments [S4-S5] by light touch [LT], pin prick [PP] or deep anal pressure [DAP]), and has some sparing of motor function more than three levels below the ipsilateral motor level on either side of the body.
(This includes key or non-key muscle functions to determine motor incomplete status). For AIS C – less than half of key muscle functions below the single neurological level of injury [NLI] have a muscle grade ≥ 3.

D = Motor Incomplete. Motor incomplete status as defined above, with at least half (half or more) of key muscle functions below the single NLI having a muscle grade ≥ 3.

E = Normal. If sensation and motor function as tested with the International Standards for Neurological Classification of Spinal Cord Injury (ISNCSCI) are graded as normal in all segments, and the patient had prior deficits, then the AIS grade is E. Someone without an initial SCI does not receive an AIS grade.

Using ND: To document the sensory, motor and NLI levels, the ASIA Impairment Scale grade, and/or the zone of partial preservation (ZPP) when they are unable to be determined based on the examination results

FIGURE 24.4 American Spinal Injury Association impairment scale (AIS).
Source: American Spinal Injury Association (ASIA).

shown to be beneficial for the psychosocial aspect of the patient. Walking is also good for cardiovascular health. However, it is true that the lower the level of injury and the greater the strength in the lower extremities, the higher the predictive value for functional gait (Chen, 2000; Freund et al., 2007; Kwon et al., 2008).

Functional recovery is predicted using the AIS (Figure 24.4). Improvements in predicting functional recovery have been demonstrated by Curt, Keck, and Dietz (1999) when combining the AIS with electrodiagnostic testing. In persons with tetraplegia, most of the recovery of arm function is believed to occur within the first 6 months after injury. Studies by Ditunno, Flanders, Kirshblum, and Graziani (1994) found that if subjects had a complete injury with no motor function at the level of injury by 1 week, only 45% of patients demonstrated antigravity strength in that same muscle by 9 to 12 months. However, if subjects had some motor power, more than 90% gained antigravity strength over the same period (Kirshblum & O'Connor, 1998). This is important because antigravity strength helps make muscles functional on their own. The quicker the recovery begins, the quicker the progress is made, and often the recovery is more complete. For patients who have incomplete injuries, recovery is often faster and more complete.

Walking in persons with tetraplegia and paraplegia is accomplished through return of lower extremity motor strength (Crozier et al., 1992; Waters, Adkins, Yakura, & Sie, 1993). Prediction of walking in complete and incomplete SCI, studied by Burns, Golding, Rolle, Graziani, and Ditunno (1997) and most recently by Scivoletto, Donna, Kim, Eng, and Whittaker (2004), has yielded interesting results. A person with a complete SCI (AIS A) has a 5% chance of recovering to an AIS C and a 3% chance of recovering to an AIS D by 1 year's time. How this correlates into walking with or without an assistive device remains largely unknown. With the development of new technology, such as tractography, an MRI technology that is able to look at individual tracts of the spinal cord, and advances in electrodiagnostic testing, it may be possible that in the future physicians will be better able to predict recovery for the individual patient.

Secondary Complications

When asked to visualize a patient with an SCI, people typically envision a person in a wheelchair. The inability to walk is only one of many alterations of function that affects the quality of life for a person living with an SCI. Understanding the repercussions that an SCI has on daily life offers a window into the injury's psychosocial ramifications.

■ Respiratory System

Injuries involving the cervical and thoracic spinal cord have a deleterious effect on the respiratory system. Nerves exiting the spine at cervical levels 3, 4, and 5 are of particular importance as they join to form the phrenic nerve, which innervates the primary muscle of quiet respiration known as the diaphragm. Weakness or paralysis of the diaphragm may result in temporary or permanent respiratory failure, requiring the assistance of mechanical ventilation. As ventilatory demand increases with activity, accessory muscles, innervated by segments of the thoracic and cervical cord, are recruited to aid in inhalation and exhalation. Quiet exhalation is primarily a passive process requiring little muscle activation. Actions such a cough, however, require significant force generation by the internal intercostals and abdominal musculature. Thoracic cord injury may result in weakness of these muscles with profound effects on pulmonary toileting (Daniel et al., 2011).

Physicians specializing in SCI medicine and pulmonology are gaining a better understanding of how to help people with SCI gain independence from ventilators. When medically feasible, avoiding mechanical ventilation improves quality of life and extends the life span. Although lifelong ventilator support may appear to paint a bleak picture, studies have demonstrated that patients on a ventilator can enjoy a high quality of life (Charlifue et al., 2011).

Prevention of respiratory complications is of the utmost importance. In general, tetraplegics with the loss of diaphragm and accessory respiratory muscle function are unable to remove phlegm by themselves because of their inability to cough effectively. This can cause pneumonia, the leading cause of death in both the acute and chronic phases of SCI. Other complications include atelectasis, mucus plugging, pleural effusion, empyema, pneumothorax, and pulmonary embolism.

Measures to prevent respiratory complications in the acute phase of high-level SCI require a team approach. Secretion management, cough assist techniques, proper pulmonary toileting, chest physical therapy, in-line ventilator equipment, and proper oral hygiene are just a few of the many techniques that help reduce pulmonary complications. Long-term pulmonary management includes yearly influenza vaccination and pneumococcal vaccination every 5 years.

Phrenic nerve pacing provides an exciting alternative to long-term ventilator support. This involves pulsatile electrical stimulation applied to the phrenic nerves, provided by a diaphragmatic pacemaker, resulting in stimulation of the diaphragm and thus ventilator-free breathing. To qualify for the procedure, the patient must have at least partially preserved function of the phrenic nerve in addition to an intact diaphragm. The procedure is not without complications, such as electrical failure and electrode migration (Berliner & Ahn, 2006; Onders et al., 2007). The diaphragmatic pacemaker is a device in which the electrodes are implanted directly into and provide stimulation to the diaphragm. Research on the practicality and efficacy of the diaphragmatic pacemaker is ongoing. In a multicenter review including a total of 29 patients, 72% of pacemaker eligible patients ($n = 22$) were completely free of ventilator support within 2 weeks of implantation (Posluszny et al., 2014). With advances in technology and respiratory care for persons with high-level tetraplegia comes the hope for improved quality of life.

Cardiovascular System

Historically, the pulmonary and renal systems were related to mortality following an SCI. The function of the cardiovascular system, particularly with injuries above the level of the sixth thoracic vertebra, becomes compromised after an injury. The cardiovascular system not only includes the heart, but the massive network of blood vessels that supply all of the body's organs with oxygen and nutrients in addition to carrying away waste materials. The heart receives input from the sympathetic and parasympathetic nervous systems. These signals allow the heart rate to speed up or slow down in response to the body's needs. Blood vessel constriction and dilation respond to sympathetic signals only. These sympathetic signals predominantly come from the thoracic spinal cord. Therefore, any injury that blocks the pathway from the brain to the heart and blood vessels causes disturbance with the function of these organs. In SCI, this can present with at least three distinct complications: orthostatic hypotension, autonomic dysreflexia, and venous thrombus formation (blood clots).

Orthostatic hypotension occurs when the body is unable to maintain adequate blood pressure to perfuse the brain with positional changes. Since the vessels are under the control of the sympathetic system, most injuries that involve the thoracic segments will experience this disturbance to some degree. Symptoms resulting from hypotension include dizziness, visual disturbance, blurry vision, confusion, weakness, fatigue, and nausea. These momentary drops in blood pressure can be especially problematic when standing from a sitting or lying position or during transfers and can result in loss of balance and falls. These symptoms tend to improve with time. Rehabilitation focuses on minimizing these effects with the use of a tilt table, assistive devices, and medications to ensure safety and preserve quality of life.

Autonomic dysreflexia, a potentially fatal complication, is a sharp rise in blood pressure resulting from a noxious (usually interpreted as painful) stimulus below the level of injury. These events may be triggered by bladder distention (most common), fecal impaction, wounds, or tight clothing. Signals from receptors in these regions relay to the spinal cord, in turn, causing excitation of the nerves in those segments of cord resulting in increased sympathetic activity. Without communication with the brain, these stimuli lead to constriction of blood vessels with a spike in blood pressure. Treatment includes placing the patient in an upright position to minimize cerebral pressure, removing all constrictive clothing, along with identification and removal of the noxious stimulus. Antihypertensive medications can be used to control excessively high pressures.

Persons with SCI are at higher than normal risk of blood clot formation in the veins. While the exact cause is unknown, it is thought decreased mobility and decreased muscle function coupled with impaired blood vessel tone can result in pooling and ultimately clotting of blood. These clots can subsequently dislodge and travel to the lungs with potentially fatal consequences. Prophylactic treatment early in the course of injury (within 72 hours), including mechanical and pharmacological prevention, is critical to prevent these complications. While there are differing schools of thought regarding the method and length of treatment, it is accepted that treatment should be instituted as soon as possible after injury (Dhall et al., 2013).

Genitourinary System

The importance of proper urinary management for persons with SCI cannot be overstated. Before World War II, the leading cause of death among patients with SCI was related to urinary complications (Boone, 2000). Over the past three decades we have learned to reduce urinary tract complications including infection, stone formation, and hydronephrosis.

The urinary system is made up of the kidneys, ureters, urinary bladder, bladder neck (internal sphincter), external urethral sphincter, and urethra. Storage and excretion of urine work in a coordinated manner that is under the control of the brain, brainstem, spinal cord, and peripheral nervous system. Following SCI, there is a disruption in the signals being sent between the brain and the genitourinary system. The effects seen on the bladder depend on whether UMNs or LMNs have been affected.

UMN injuries cause a reflexogenic bladder; as the bladder fills, an uncontrollable contraction of the detrusor occurs forcing urine against a closed outlet. This can result in one of two problems: incontinence or a backflow of urine to the kidneys. Long-standing backflow of urine to the kidneys may lead to hydronephrosis. LMN lesions cause flaccidity of the detrusor, resulting in areflexia of the bladder with urinary retention. Increased urinary volumes result in elevated bladder pressure leading to overflow incontinence with eventual hydronephrosis.

Treatment of a neurogenic bladder is tailored to individual needs and may consist of catheter care, pharmacological intervention, and surgery. Two common forms of initial management for the neurogenic bladder are intermittent catheterization or indwelling urinary catheterization. These two approaches are performed in an effort to eliminate residual urine from the bladder and to protect the kidneys from backflow. To perform intermittent catheterization, a catheter is inserted through the urethra and into the urinary bladder to drain the urine. This is usually performed every 4 to 6 hours depending on daily fluid intake and urine production. This means that every 4 to 6 hours a person will need to find an appropriate place to perform catheterization. An indwelling catheterization is an alternative procedure where catheter is placed in the bladder to drain the urine constantly into a bag. Both of these methods have advantages and disadvantages.

Pharmacological treatment has also provided an increased quality of life for persons with SCI by increasing urine flow, preventing incontinence, and decreasing urinary tract infections (Berliner & Ahn, 2006; Raghavan & Shenot, 2009).

Surgical intervention may be considered to increase the size of the urinary bladder, reduce the tone of the external sphincter, and increase independence with self-care with bladder management. For example, the Mitrofanoff procedure allows a patient with poor hand function to catheterize through a small opening, usually placed in the umbilicus, which is connected to the bladder by utilizing the appendix. In persons without an appendix, a piece of ileum may be substituted and this is known as the Monti procedure. Other procedures include suprapubic tube placement, external sphincterotomy, bladder augmentation, and artificial sphincter placement.

The use of botulinum toxin has also evolved for the management of a spastic bladder. In this procedure, botulinum toxin is injected directly into the bladder wall by use of cystoscopy allowing for increased storage capacity and decreased incontinence episodes. This procedure is usually effective for 3 to 6 months, and needs to be repeated to maintain efficacy (Darouiche, 2001; Raghavan & Shenot, 2009).

Bladder care research offers hope for improved quality of life for patients with neurogenic bladder. Hyperreflexic (overactive) bladders lead to loss of compliance requiring augmentation surgery to increase the size of the bladder. A new augmentation surgery is currently being investigated using an autologous neo-bladder construct. In this study, a patient's own bladder cells are isolated and grown in a medium and placed in a scaffold in the shape of the bladder. The neo-bladder is then surgically placed to augment the patient's own bladder (Raghavan & Shenot, 2009).

Advances in care and an improved understanding of the physiological changes resulting from SCI have led to decreased mortality from renal failure. The evolution of neurogenic bladder management lies in the restoration of function by reinnervation utilizing stem cell based therapies. Elimination of catheterization will result in decreased bacterial colonization and, subsequently, urinary tract infections (Cho et al., 2014).

Gastrointestinal System

In SCI, the normal physiology of defecation is impaired. The gastrointestinal system relies on coordinated neural function between the central nervous system and the autonomic nervous system to function properly. When interrupted, there is a disruption of normal stool transit time and defecation. In general, "if the spinal cord injury is above the twelfth thoracic vertebrae, the ability to feel when the rectum is full may be lost. The anal sphincter muscle may remain tight, and bowel movements will occur on a reflex basis" (Rosito, Nino-Murcia, Wolfe, Kiratli, & Perkash, 2002). The injury to the bowel is termed an UMN-type bowel. A spinal cord injury below the twelfth thoracic vertebrae may damage the defecation reflex and cause paralysis of the anal sphincter muscle. Fluid absorption in the transverse colon is also partially impaired. This is known as a LMN or "flaccid bowel." These two conditions require different approaches to management of bowel care (Rosito et al., 2002).

The UMN reflexogenic bowel may be treated with diet modification, gentle digital stretching to the anal sphincter, digital disimpaction, and medications in the form of stool softeners, bulking agents, colonic stimulants, suppositories, and enemas. Taken together, the bowel regimen is termed a "bowel care program," which is typically performed daily or every other day. In preparation of bowel movements, the patient or care provider checks the rectal vault for stool. If no stool is present in the rectum, an enema or suppository may be inserted. If no result is noted within 15 minutes of insertion, digital anal stretching or digital rectal stimulation may be necessary. Digital stimulation is performed by inserting a lubricated, gloved finger inside the anus maintaining contact with the rectal mucosa. The patient or care provider then rotates the finger in a circular motion until the wall relaxes. This usually takes 15 to 60 seconds. Digital stimulation takes advantage of an intact reflex, which causes peristalsis (reflex contraction of the intestines) to occur, which in turn pushes the stool along (Kalat, 1998).

The LMN bowel routine is different from that of the UMN bowel program because there are no reflexes. This renders digital stimulation and many medications such as suppositories and laxatives useless. There is also a flaccid anal sphincter, which allows stool to pass uninhibited. The LMN bowel treatment program may consist of a high-fiber diet and bulking agents such as fiber-based medicines. It may also require high colonic enemas to empty the distal colon and rectum for prevention of fecal incontinence.

In some cases, the bowel care program may take more than 3 hours, greatly compromising quality of life. One alternative is the Malone procedure (appendicostomy). The Malone procedure involves connecting the appendix to the abdominal wall creating a stoma with a one-way valve. The person can then place an enema into the intestines through this opening using a catheter. The one-way valve when working properly ensures that no fecal matter passes to the abdomen. Another alternative to the bowel treatment programmed is a colostomy. This procedure involves connecting the colon to the anterior abdominal wall, creating a stoma. The feces then evacuate through the stoma and into a collecting bag. High satisfaction with this procedure for both the caregiver and patient has been reported. A recently introduced transanal irrigation system shows promise as a less invasive method of facilitating stool evacuation as compared to the Malone or colostomy procedures. Early studies demonstrate improved quality of life with decreased symptoms of neurogenic bowel (Christensen, Andreasen, & Ehlers, 2008).

Integumentary System

Patients with SCI are at high risk of developing pressure ulcers over the bony prominences below the level of injury due to loss of sensation. The skin is truly one of the areas where "an ounce of prevention is worth a pound of cure" (Benjamin Franklin). "Now let us look at a means of preventing bedsores. Daily care must be devoted to keep integrity of the skin for once they appear, it is often difficult to get rid of them."

Normal skin is resistant to the development of a pressure sore by means of sensory feedback to the brain from the peripheral nervous system. This feedback alerts our body that it is time to move. Changing positions or performing "weight shifts" will allow the arterial blood supply to reach the skin and underlying soft tissue to provide oxygen as well as to wash out noxious waste (Regan et al., 2007). It is estimated that 50% to 80% of all persons with SCI experience pressure ulcers within their lifetime. The cost of pressure ulcers remains high and a single pressure ulcer can cost between $2,000 and $7,000 per year (Regan et al., 2007). This cost is enormous, but the emotional cost to the affected person may be even higher. A patient with an ischial pressure ulcer will need to avoid sitting for prolonged periods of time. Since sitting in and pushing a wheelchair is the primary means of locomotion, stopping this activity may cause time missed at work and school, in addition to social isolation and financial hardship.

A pressure ulcer is defined by the National Pressure Ulcer Advisory Panel (NPUAP) as a "localized injury to the skin and/or underlying tissue usually over a bony prominence, as a result of pressure, or pressure in combination with shear, moisture and/or friction. A number of contributing or confounding factors are associated with pressure ulcers" (Figure 24.5).

Proper lying and sitting surfaces reduce pressure on vulnerable areas. Cushioned mattresses and wheelchair seating systems effectively disperse pressure over the entire region rather than over a

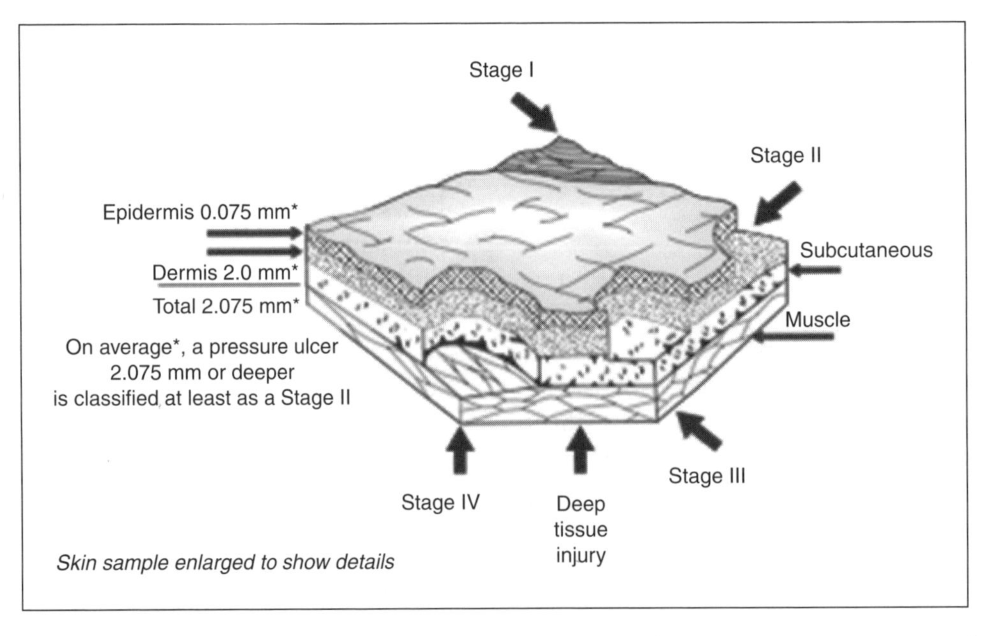

FIGURE 24.5 Stages of a pressure ulcer according to the National Pressure Ulcer Advisory Panel (NPUAP) guidelines. If the wound base is covered by slough and/or eschar, it is considered "unstageable."

bony prominence (Regan et al., 2007). Educating patients and families on ways to relieve pressure and to perform daily skin inspection is an imperative means of preventing pressure ulcers (Brown, Hill, & Baker, 2006; O'Connor & Salcido, 2002). Pressure relief while lying in bed entails changing position every 2 hours. To perform pressure relief when sitting, persons with active triceps function (C7) and strength can lift the upper body from the wheelchair for either 15 seconds every 15 minutes or 30 seconds every 30 minutes, termed the 15/15 or 30/30 rule (Kalat, 1998; Sipski & Arenas, 2006). Patients who do not possess enough upper limb strength to lift themselves can modify local pressure using an electric wheelchair that tilts or reclines the upper body posteriorly. This will take pressure off the sitting surface. Pressure mapping is a way to evaluate the safety of a seating surface further. It involves using sensors to quantify the pressure between the person and the seat cushion. Other means of improving skin care include good nutritional support, maintaining proper body weight, smoking cessation, and avoiding moist and caustic substances, such as urine or stool to remain on the skin for prolonged periods of time (Brown et al., 2006).

The treatment of a pressure ulcer depends on many variables including its appearance, cleanliness, degree of penetration through the skin and underlying structures, location, and drainage. The general principles of pressure ulcer treatment are to eliminate predisposing conditions, avoid friction, shear stress and tissue maceration, and debride devitalized tissue (Sipski & Arenas, 2006). There are multiple pharmacological agents that aid in pressure ulcer healing. Treatments that may be used in conjunction with pharmacological management include whirlpool therapy, electrical stimulation, hyperbaric oxygen, and vacuum-assisted dressings. Eating a nutritious diet high in protein and cessation of smoking are encouraged to provide a proper medium for wound healing.

If a wound is large, deep, and complex, a surgical closure may be a viable alternative. Surgical techniques include sharp debridement and rotational myocutaneous flap closure. After the operation, an air-fluidized bed is frequently used for surgical site care. Typically, a patient is kept on bed rest for 6 weeks. Subsequently, a progressive sitting program is implemented under close observation by a treating physician and rehabilitation nurse as long as the surgical site remains intact (Consortium for Spinal Cord Medicine, 2000; Priebe, Martin, Wuermser, Castillo, & McFarlin, 2002).

Sexuality and Fertility

Sexuality and intimacy are important components of psychological health and emotional well-being. Sexuality encompasses much more than just the act of sex but involves closeness and interpersonal relationship between people. Persons with SCI may continue to express sexual desire and remain sexually active but often face many barriers to a return to intimacy. Often these embarrassing topics remain largely unaddressed by health care providers, leaving persons with SCI and their partners in the dark. They are left without answers to questions regarding sexuality and childbearing.

SCI affects sexuality in both males and females and may affect interest, arousal, ejaculation, and orgasm. Interest in performing sexual activity remains high in the SCI community but there are logistical considerations and hurdles. Before sexual activity, bowel and bladder care may need to be performed to prevent incontinence during the sexual act (Kalat, 1998). Males may need to premedicate to achieve erection, and females may need added lubrication. Sexual positioning may also need to be planned. In the right environment and with open dialogue, many of the aforementioned obstacles are incorporated into, as opposed to being a deterrent from, the sexual act.

The effect of SCI on sexual response is generally discussed based upon the degree of completeness or incompleteness of the patient's injury, and whether the neurological damage caused an upper or LMN injury. In males, SCI may affect the ability to achieve or maintain an erection. Erections, if achieved, are often incomplete or unsustainable for the purpose of intercourse (Westgren & Levi, 1995). A multitude of treatment options are available for men with erectile dysfunction. These include vacuum tumescence devices (vacuum-assisted erections), oral medications, placement of medication into the urethral opening, injection of medication into the penile shaft (intracavernous injections), and penile implantation surgery.

The effects of SCI on sexuality and fertility of females are less evident and have been less well studied. The arousal stage for females is affected, manifested by a decrease in vaginal lubrication.

Ejaculation is defined as the expulsion of seminal fluid from the urethra. This is greatly diminished in the male with SCI and may occur in only 4% of persons. If the goal of ejaculation is for siring a child, then assistive reproductive technology may be tried. Methods of semen retrieval include vibroejaculation, electroejaculation, and removal of semen directly from the testicles or seminal tract (Bors & Commar, 1960; Kirshblum et al., 2002; Kreuter, Siösteen, & Biering-Sørensen, 2008; Linsenmeyer, 2002; Consortium for Spinal Cord Medicine, 1999; Ricciardi, Szabo, & Poullos, 2007; Westgren & Levi, 1995; Wirz, van Hedel, Rupp, Curt, & Dietz, 2006).

Female reproductive capability does not appear to be affected by SCI. It is important for an obstetrician to be familiar with SCI as secondary complications during pregnancy occur at a substantially higher rate than in able-bodied females. Persons with a tendency for autonomic dysreflexia, those with injuries higher than the sixth thoracic level, should have spinal epidural anesthesia to reduce dysreflexic episodes during labor regardless of whether they have sensation (American College of Obstetricians and Gynecologists, 2002). Parenting after SCI has been studied by Westgren and Levi (1995), and there appears to be no negative consequences for the child or parents. Children stated that mothers with SCI were no different than other mothers, and the partner did not feel that extra burden of care shifted toward them.

> We found an overall favorable outcome as regards to the parameters evaluated. The families seem to live a rich and complete family life with very little demand for external help. They report a well functioning social network and seem socially integrated both as individuals and as families (Crozier et al., 1992).

REHABILITATION

Rehabilitation begins in the early acute phase of SCI and continues as a lifelong process. The rehabilitation team may consist of many or all of the following disciplines: a physiatrist (physicians specializing in physical medicine and rehabilitation), rehabilitation nurse, physical therapist, occupational therapist, speech pathologist, swallow therapist, psychologist, nutritionist, recreational therapist, respiratory therapist, vocational counselor, and social worker.

The team, led by the physiatrist, provides medical care, therapies, and psychosocial support to foster medical stability, improve function, and assist with community return. The acute period is always an intense and rough period for the person with a newly acquired SCI. They often feel that a piece of them has been taken away, and that they are not whole anymore. The goal of the team is to support and encourage the patient to overcome many difficulties the patient will face in activities of daily living and to come out as a strong, independent, and confident individual. The interdisciplinary team members communicate with one another to ensure that the patient, patient's family, and caregivers receive the support they need.

The ultimate goal of rehabilitation after SCI is to maximize function, minimize dysfunction, and facilitate a smooth return to life activities. The rehabilitation process begins once the patient enters the emergency department and is a lifelong process thereafter. Because no two patients are the same, no two rehabilitation programs can be the same and must be tailored to each patient. In the acute phase of SCI, rehabilitation focuses on patient and family/caregiver education and prevention of secondary complications.

Such initial rehabilitation program includes prevention of joint contractures, pneumonia, pressure ulcers, urinary tract infections, ileus, autonomic dysreflexia, orthostatic hypotension, and thromboembolic disease. This helps provide optimal patient care and alleviates physical suffering (Waters, Adkins, Yakura, & Vigil, 1994). The information provided in the acute phase will be reinforced throughout the entire rehabilitation process. Once the patient with SCI is medically and surgically stabilized, he or she is transferred to an inpatient rehabilitation hospital for acute SCI inpatient rehabilitation.

Attainable goals for patients with SCI are based on level of injury, AIS, comorbidities, previous function, precautions, and psychosocial status. These interdisciplinary goals are reassessed weekly, as function, endurance, and task achievement may change over the inpatient stay.

Injury levels have been correlated with functional outcome, and individuals may attain or often exceed expectations. Adaptive technology can also allow the injured to become more independent in activities of daily living. Patients with high complete injury at cervical levels 1 through 4 have no hand function but can obtain independence in wheelchair mobility, weight shifts, and directing transfers. Environmental control units allow persons to open and close doors, turn on and off lights, use computers, and control the television. Persons with high SCIs have learned to hunt and fish with mouth units termed sip and puff even without arm or hand movement. The more caudal (toward the feet) the injury and the more key muscles a patient recovers for use, the more functional and independent an individual can become (Albin, White, Yashon, & Harris, 1969).

TRENDS IN SCI RESEARCH

The cure for SCI has been elusive, but current research is paving the way for a future cure.

Acute Injury

In an ideal world, clinicians would be able to stop the cascade of damaging events triggered by an SCI. One attempt at stopping the cascade is spinal cord hypothermia. This procedure was originally invented by Dr. Alfred Reginald Allen in 1911 and was used to treat SCI by Dr. Maurice Albin, but in 1969 it was deemed to have no medical value (Belen & Aciduman, 2006). Spinal cooling has recently been repopularized after use on a professional football player who was injured during a game. Although a cogent biological rationale may exist for the use of local or systemic hypothermia in acute traumatic SCI, little scientific literature is currently available to substantiate the clinical use of either in human patients (Festoff et al., 2006). Experiments are currently under way using different methods of cooling in an attempt to prove efficacy. Other attempts to stop neural tissue inflammation have included activated macrophage trials, antibodies against NOGO-A, a molecule that destroys the protective covering of nerve cells, and inhibitors of nitrous oxide synthetase. No single agent has yet been successful to alter the outcome of SCI (Yick, So, Cheung, & Wu, 2004). Use of hyperbaric oxygen in animal models has shown promise in reducing secondary cord injury by downregulating harmful mediators in the inflammatory cascade and improving the local microenvironment for neural regeneration (Li, Wang, Zhang, & Luo, 2014).

Immunosuppressive therapy has recently gained ground in SCI research as a means of blocking the entire inflammatory cascade. Tacrolimus and cyclosporine are primarily used to inhibit autoimmune reactions in transplanted organs or tissue. It has been hypothesized that, through the same mechanism, the body would be unable to mount an immune and inflammatory response after SCI (Sayer, Kronvall, & Nilsson, 2006).

Other attempts have also been made to stop programmed cell death (apoptosis) after injury in the form of inhibitors of caspase and calpain, and with the use of minocycline (Hurlbert, 2001). Lithium, a drug long known to alter sodium transport and inhibit the body's immune reaction, is currently being trialed as well (Consortium for Spinal Cord Medicine, 2008).

Neuroprotection After SCI

The use of steroids for treating SCI is noted as early as the 1970s; during this time, steroids were thought to have no efficacy in treating cervical SCI sustained from trauma. After results of the second National Acute Spinal Cord Injury Study were reported in 1990, administration of high-dose steroids within 8 hours of SCI appeared to be the standard of care. The 2013 guidelines set forth by the American Association of Neurological Surgeons and Congress of Neurological Surgeons recommended against the routine administration of steroids for acute SCIs. A recent Cochrane review performed in 2015 confirmed benefit was shown for early high-dose steroid administration in motor neurologic function and functional status. The use of steroids is still a debated topic, and only time and additional research will determine its usefulness (Evaniew & Marcel, 2015; Fouad et al., 2005; Keirstead, 2005; Nistor, 2004).

Neural Regeneration

Cajal and Golgi, two neuroscientists in the late 1800s, laid the framework for the modern view of neuroanatomy and are believed to be the founders of modern neuroscience. Since that time, many efforts have been made to assess and promote neural reconnections in the spinal cord. As early as 1980, it was shown that neural regrowth is possible after SCI in a rodent model (Fawcett, 2009). Attempts to translate that experiment and many subsequent experiments have not been able to provide a functional recovery in humans.

Cell Transplantation and Replacement

Stem cell research offers hope for recovery of SCI and has provided evidence of efficacy in animal models. Stem cells have been isolated from the bone marrow, olfactory cells, umbilical cord blood, placenta, and embryo. When placed in an appropriate medium, these cells undergo division and regenerate a line of cells, which produce a desired function.

In the case of SCI, the goal of stem cell research is to generate viable neurons within a damaged lesion. One successful experiment produced oligodendrocytes, cells that produce a sheath covering over the nerve, called myelin. An experiment by McDonald et al. (1999) provided evidence that transplanted mouse embryonic stem cells into the damaged spinal cord could not only survive up to 5 weeks but could also differentiate into oligodendrocytes. Improvement in motor function was also reported. Keirstead (2005) showed that embryonic cells taken from human fetal tissue, when transplanted into a rat, could also grow, survive, and produce cells that helped replace the myelin. Current stem cell research offers hope for a cure for paralysis (Eltorai, 2002). Recent studies have shown remarkable promise including neural recovery and restoration of function (El-Kheir et al., 2014). However, great care needs to be taken with the development of new stem cell sources ensuring genetic stability and screening for potential tumor formation or other adverse events.

Functional Recovery

Restoration of function is a prime consideration for persons with SCI. A multitude of research studies are being conducted to evaluate the effects of interventions on walking and return of function in patients with SCI. Some equipment and therapies currently under investigation are examining the effects of functional electrical stimulation on muscle recovery and body-weight-supported treadmill training on functional recovery.

Electrical stimulation has been shown to have numerous benefits including muscle hypertrophy and recover of lost bone mass in the SCI population (Martin, Sadowsky, Obst, Brooke, & McDonald, 2012). However, this gain rarely translates to functional improvement. Epidural spinal cord stimulation is widely used for neuromodulation of chronic pain with a minimally invasive technique. This idea has been adapted to initiate voluntary muscle movement in the lower limbs with the hopes of independent ambulation. Animal models have demonstrated successful locomotion by stimulation of a central pattern generator found in mammalian spinal cords (Guertin, 2009). Recent trials have demonstrated the possibility of locomotor training with voluntary muscle control in persons with complete motor and sensory paralysis (Sayenko et al., 2015, Shah et al., 2016).

In recent years, the use of exoskeleton robots has become more common in the rehabilitation setting. A variety of designs are currently available for professional use with one model available for use in the home. These devices have a training mode where the action is controlled by the therapist; however, as the user advances they are able to imitate steps by shifting body weight or activating a trigger mechanism. Most users require an assistive device in the form of crutches or a walker. These devices show promise in preventing bone demineralization, and may possibly serve to maintain or improve bone strength. As the technology progresses, lighter weight, quieter, more cost-effective, and increased ease of use are expected. Neurologically controlled devices are currently in the experimental phase.

CONCLUSION

SCI is a devastating disease, which affects almost all aspects of a person's life. Through proper medical management, psychosocial support, and rehabilitation therapies as well as the patient's motivation and family/caregiver's participation, it is possible for a person with SCI to pursue a productive and satisfying life.

REFERENCES

American College of Obstetricians and Gynecologists. (2002). ACOG Committee opinion Number 275, September 2002: Obstetric management of patients with spinal cord injuries. *Obstetrics & Gynecology, 100,* 625–627.

Albin, M. S., White, R. J., Yashon, D., & Harris, L. S. (1969). Effects of localized cooling on spinal cord trauma. *The Journal of Trauma, 9*, 1000–1008.

Allen, W. H., & Darlene, H. (1998). Substance abuse and medical complication following spinal cord injury. *Rehabilitation Psychology, 43*, 219–231.

Belen, D., & Aciduman, A. (2006). A pioneer from the islamic golden age: Haly Abbas and spinal traumas in his principal work, The royal book. *Journal of Neurosurgery, Spine, 5*, 381–383.

Berliner, J. C., & Ahn, J. H. (2006). Pharmacological management of urological dysfunction. *Journal of Korean American Medical Association, 12*, 85–93.

Boone, T. B. (2000). Recent advances in the management of neurogenic bladder. *Urology, 56*, 76–81.

Bors, E., & Commar, A. E. (1960). Neurological disturbances of sexual function with special reference to 529 patients with spinal cord injury. *Urological Survey, 10*, 191–222.

Brown, D. J., Hill, S. T., & Baker, H. W. (2006). Male fertility and sexual function after spinal cord injury. *Progress in Brain Research, 152*, 427–439.

Burns, S. P., Golding, D. G., Rolle, W. A., Jr., Graziani, V., & Ditunno, J. F. (1997). Recovery of ambulation in motor incomplete tetraplegia. *Archives of Physical Medicine and Rehabilitation, 78*, 1169–1172.

Charlifue, S., Apple, D., Burns, S. P., Chen, D., Cuthbert, J. P., Donovan, W. H., . . . Pretz, C. R. (2011). Mechanical ventilation, health, and quality of life following spinal cord injury. *Archives of Physical Medicine and Rehabilitation*, *92*, 457–463.

Charles, H. B., & Carl, T. R. (1998). Alcohol use and readiness to change after spinal cord injury. *Archives of Physical Medicine and Rehabilitation, 79*, 1110–1115.

Chen, M. S. (2000). Nogo-A is a myelin-associated neurite outgrowth inhibitor and an antigen for monoclonal antibody IN-1. *Nature, 403*, 434–439.

Cho, Y. S., Ko, I. G., Kim, S. E., Lee, S. M., Shin, M. S., Kim, C. J., . . . Kim, K. H. (2014). Oral mucosa stem cells alleviates spinal cord injury-induced neurogenic bladder symptoms in rats. *Journal of Biomedical Science, 21*, 1–43.

Christensen, P., Andreasen J., & Ehlers, L. (2008). Cost-effectiveness of transanal irrigation versus conservative bowel management for spinal cord injury patients. *Spinal Cord*, *47*, 138–143.

Consortium for Spinal Cord Medicine. (1999). Outcomes Following Traumatic Spinal Cord Injury: Clinical practice guideline for health care professionals. Retrieved from http://www.kintera.org/AccountTempFiles/Account403152/ECSoft/OutcomesCPG.pdf

Consortium for Spinal Cord Medicine. (2000). Pressure ulcer prevention and treatment following spinal cord injury: A clinical practice guideline for health care professionals. Retrieved from http://www.pva.org/atf/cf/%7BCA2A0FFB-6859-4BC1-BC96-6B57F57F0391%7D/cpg_pressure%20ulcers.pdf

Consortium for Spinal Cord Medicine. (2008). Early acute management in adults with spinal cord injury: A clinical practice guideline for health-care professionals. *Journal of Spinal Cord Medicine, 31*(4), 403–479.

Crozier, K. S., Cheng, L. L., Graziani, V., Zorn, G., Herbison, G., & Ditunno, J. F., Jr. (1992). Spinal cord injury: Prognosis for ambulation based on quadriceps recovery. *Paraplegia, 30*, 762–767.

Curt, A., Keck, M. E., & Dietz, V. (1999). Functional outcome following spinal cord injury: Significance of motor-evoked potentials and ASIA scores. *Archives of Physical Medicine and Rehabilitation, 79*, 81–86.

Daniela, G. L., Terson, D. P., William, B. M., Rodney, J. F., & Alexander, V. O. (2011). Respiratory motor control disrupted by spinal cord injury: Mechanisms, evaluation, and restoration. *Translational Stroke Research, 2*, 463–473.

Darouiche, R. (2001). Pilot trial of bacterial interference for preventing urinary tract infection. *Urology, 58*, 339–344.

Delisa, J., & Hammond, M. (2002). The history of the subspecialty of spinal cord injury medicine. In S. Kirshblum, D. Campagnolo, & J. Delisa (Eds.), *Spinal cord medicine* (pp. 1–4). Philadelphia, PA: Lippincott Williams and Wilkins.

DeVivo, M. J., Krause, J. S., & Lammertse, D. P. (1999). Recent trends in mortality and causes of death among persons with spinal cord injury. *Archives of Physical Medicine and Rehabilitation, 80*, 1411–1419.

Dhall, S. S., Hadley, M. N., Aarabi, B., Gelb, D. E., Hurlbert, R. J., . . . Walters BC. (2013). Deep venous thrombosis and thromboembolism in patients with cervical spinal cord injuries. *Neurosurgery, 72*, 244–254.

Ditunno, J., Flanders, A., Kirshblum, S., Graziani, V., & Tessler, A. (1994). Predicting outcomes in traumatic spinal cord injuries. In S. Kirshblum, D. Campagnolo, & J. Delisa (Eds.), *Spinal cord medicine* (pp. 108–120). Philadelphia, PA: Lippincott Williams and Wilkins.

Donovan, W. H. (2007). Spinal cord injury: Past, present, and future. *Journal of Spinal Cord Medicine, 30*, 85–100.

El Ghatit, A. Z., & Hanson, R. W. (1975). Outcome of marriages existing at the time of a male's spinal cord injury. *Journal of Chronic Diseases, 28*, 383–388.

El-Kheir, W. A., Gabr, H., Awad, M. R., Ghannam, O., Barakat, Y., Farghali, H. A., . . . Sabaawy, H. E. (2014). Autologous bone marrow-derived cell therapy combined with physical therapy induces functional improvement in chronic spinal cord injury patients. *Cell Transplantation Cell Transplant*, *23*(6), 729–745.

Eltorai, I. M. (2002). History of spinal cord medicine. In V. Lin (Ed.), *Spinal cord medicine, principles and practice* (pp. 3–14). New York, NY: Demos Medical Publishing.

Evaniew, N., & Marcel, D. (2015). Cochrane in CORR®: Steroids for acute spinal cord injury (Review). *Clinical Orthopaedics and Related Research®, 474*, 19–24.

Fawcett, J. W. (2009). Recovery from spinal cord injury: Regeneration, plasticity and rehabilitation. *Brain, 132*, 1417–1418.

Festoff, B. W., Ameenuddin, S., Arnold, P. M., Wong, A., Santacruz, K. S., & Citron, B. A. (2006). Minocycline neuroprotects, reduces microgliosis, and inhibits caspase protease expression early after spinal cord injury. *Journal of Neurochemistry, 97*, 1314–1326.

Fouad, K., Schnell, L., Bunge, M. B., Schwab, M. E., Liebscher, T., & Pearse, D. D. (2005). Combining Schwann cell bridges and olfactory-ensheathing glia grafts with chondroitinase promotes locomotor recovery after complete transection of the spinal cord. *Journal of Neuroscience, 25*, 1169–1178.

Freund, P., Wannier, T., Schmidlin, E., Bloch, J., Mir, A., Schwab, M. E., & Rouiller, E. M. (2007). Anti-Nogo-A antibody treatment enhances sprouting of corticospinal axons rostral to a unilateral cervical spinal cord lesion in adult macaque monkey. *Journal of Comparative Neurology, 502*, 644–659.

Guertin, P. A. (2009). The mammalian central pattern generator for locomotion. *Brain Research Reviews, 62*(1), 45–56.

Hughes, J. T. (1988). The Edwin Smith papyrus: An analysis of the first case reports of spinal cord injuries. *Paraplegia, 26*, 71–82.

Hurlbert, R. J. (2001). Methylprednisolone for acute spinal cord injury. An inappropriate standard of care. *Journal of Spinal Disorders, 13*, 185–199.

Jain, N. B., Ayers, G. D., Peterson, E. N., Harris, M. B., Morse, L., O'Connor, K. C., . . . Garshickm, E. (2015). Traumatic spinal cord injury in the United States, 1993–2012. *Journal of the American Medical Association, 33*, 2236.

Kalat, J. W. (1998). *Biological psychology* (6th ed., p. 24). Pacific Grove, CA: Brooks/Cole.

Keirstead, H. S. (2005). Human embryonic stem cell-derived oligodendrocyte progenitor cell transplants remyelinate and restore locomotion after spinal cord injury. *Journal of Neuroscience, 25*, 4694–4705.

Kirshblum, S., Ho, C. H., House, J. G., Druin, E., Nead, C., & Drastal, S. (2002). Rehabilitation of spinal cord injury. In S. Kirshblum, D. Campagnolo, & J. Delisa (Eds.), *Spinal cord medicine* (pp. 275–298). Philadelphia, PA: Lippincott Williams and Wilkins.

Kirshblum, S. C., Burns, S. P., Biering–Sorensen, F., Donovan, W., Graves, D. E., Jha, A., . . . Waring, W. (2011). International standards for neurological classification of spinal cord injury (revised 2011). *Journal of Spinal Cord Medicine, 34*, 535–546.

Kirshblum, S. C., & O'Connor, K. C. (1998). Bowel care practices in chronic spinal cord injury. *Archives of Physical Medicine and Rehabilitation, 79*, 1456–1466.

Kreuter, M., Siösteen, A., & Biering-Sørensen, F. (2008). Sexuality and sexual life in women with spinal cord injury: A controlled study. *Journal of Rehabilitation Medicine, 40*, 61–69.

Kwon, B. K., Mann, C., Sohn, H. M., Hilibrand, A. S., Phillips, F. M., Wang, J. C., . . . NASS Section on Biologics. (2008). Hypothermia for spinal cord injury. *The Spine Journal, 8*, 859–874.

Li, Y., Wang, Y., Zhang, S., & Luo, M. (2014). Hyperbaric oxygen therapy improves local microenvironment after spinal cord injury. *Neural Regeneration Research, 9*(24), 2182.

Linsenmeyer, T. (2002). Sexual function and fertility following spinal cord injury. In S. Kirshblum, D. Campagnolo, & J. Delisa (Eds.), *Spinal cord medicine* (pp. 322–328). Philadelphia, PA: Lippincott Williams and Wilkins.

Martin, R., Sadowsky, C., Obst, K., Brooke, M., & McDonald, J. (2012). Functional electrical stimulation in spinal cord injury: From theory to practice. *Topics in Spinal Cord Injury Rehabilitation, 18*(1), 28–33.

McDonald, J. W., Liu, X. Z., Qu, Y., Liu, S., Mickey, S. K., Turetsky, D., . . . Choi, D. W. (1999). Transplanted embryonic stem cells, survive, differentiate and promote recovery in injured rat spinal cord. *Nature Medicine, 5*, 1410–1412.

McKinley, W. O., Kolakowsky, S. A., & Kreutzer, J. S. (1999). Substance abuse, violence, and outcome after traumatic spinal cord injury. *American Journal of Physical Medicine & Rehabilitation, 78*, 306–312.

National SCI Statistical Center. (2014). *Spinal cord injury: Facts and figures at a glance*. Birmingham, AL: University of Alabama at Birmingham National Spinal Cord Injury Center.

Nistor, G. I. (2004). Human embryonic stem cells differentiate into oligodendrocytes in high purity and myelinate after spinal cord transplantation. *Glia, 49*, 385–396.

O'Connor, K., & Salcido, R. (2002). Pressure ulcer management and spinal cord injury. In S. Kirshblum, D. Campagnolo, & J. Delisa (Eds.), *Spinal cord medicine* (pp. 207–220). Philadelphia, PA: Lippincott Williams and Wilkins.

Oleson, C. V., Burns, A. S., Ditunno, J. F., Geisler, F. H., & Coleman, W. P. (2005). Prognostic value of pin-prick preservation in motor complete, sensory incomplete spinal cord injury. *Archives of Physical Medicine and Rehabilitation, 86*, 988–992.

Onders, R., McGee, M. F., Marks, J., Chak, A., Schilz, R., Rosen, M. J., . . . Ponsky, J. (2007). Diaphragm pacing with natural orifice transluminal endoscopic surgery: Potential for difficult-to-wean intensive care unit patients. *Surgical Endoscopy, 21*, 471–479.

Posluszny, J. A., Raymond, O., Andrew, J. K., Michael, S. W., Deborah, M. S., Jennifer, K., . . . Diebel, L. (2014). Multicenter review of diaphragm pacing in spinal cord injury. *Journal of Trauma and Acute Care Surgery, 76*, 303–310.

Priebe, M. M., Martin, M., Wuermser, L. A., Castillo, T., & McFarlin, J. (2002). The medical management of pressure ulcers. In V. Lin (Ed.), *Spinal cord medicine, principles and practice* (pp. 567–587). New York, NY: Demos Medical Publishing.

Raghavan, A. M., & Shenot, P. J. (2009). Bladder augmentation using an autologous neo-bladder construct. *Kidney International, 76*, 236.

Regan, M., et al. (2007). Pressure ulcers following spinal cord injury, spinal cord injury rehabilitation evidence, ICORD. Retrieved from http://www.icord.org/scire

Ricciardi, R., Szabo, C., & Poullos, A. (2007). Sexuality and spinal cord injury. *Nursing Clinics of North America, 42*, 675–684.

Rosito, O., Nino-Murcia, M., Wolfe, V. A., Kiratli, B. J., & Perkash, I. (2002). The effects of colostomy on the quality of life in patients with spinal cord injury: A retrospective analysis. *Journal of Spinal Cord Medicine, 25*, 174–183.

Sayenko, D. G., Atkinson, D. A., Floyd, T. C., Gorodnichev, R. M., Moshonkina, T. R., Harkema, S. J., . . . Gerasimenko, Y. P. (2015). Effects of paired transcutaneous electrical stimulation delivered at single and dual sites over lumbosacral spinal cord. *Neuroscience Letters, 609*, 229–234.

Sayer, F., Kronvall, E., & Nilsson, O. (2006). Methylprednisolone treatment in acute spinal cord injury: The myth challenged through a structured analysis of published literature. *The Spine Journal, 6*, 335–343.

Scivoletto, G., Di Donna, V., Kim, C. M., Eng, J. J., & Whittaker, M. W. (2004). Level walking and ambulatory capacity in persons with incomplete spinal cord injury: Relationship with muscle strength. *Spinal Cord, 42*, 156–162.

Shah, P., Sureddi, S., Alam, M., Zhong, H., Roy, R. R., Edgerton, V. R., . . . Gerasimenko, Y. (2016). Unique spatiotemporal neuromodulation of the lumbosacral circuitry shapes locomotor success after spinal cord injury. *Journal of Neurotrauma, 33*(18), 1709–1723.

Sipski, M. L., & Arenas, A. (2006). Female sexual function after spinal cord injury. *Progress in Brain Research, 152*, 441–447.

Spinal cord injury bowel management. (2009). Retrieved from http://www.sci-info-pages.com/bowel.html

Waters, R. L., Adkins, R. H., Yakura, J. S., & Sie, I. (1993). Motor and sensory recovery following complete tetraplegia. *Archives of Physical Medicine and Rehabilitation, 74*(3), 242–247.

Waters, R. L., Adkins, R., Yakura, J., & Vigil, D. (1994). Prediction of ambulatory performance based on motor scores, derived from standards of the American spinal injury association. *Archives of Physical Medicine and Rehabilitation, 75*, 756–760.

Westgren, N., & Levi, R. (1995). Motherhood after traumatic spinal cord injury. *Obstetrics and Gynecology, 50*, 260–261.

Wirz, M., van Hedel, H. J., Rupp, R., Curt, A., & Dietz, V. (2006). Muscle force and gait performance: Relationships after spinal cord injury. *Archives of Physical Medicine and Rehabilitation, 87*, 1218–1222.

Yick, L. W., So, K. F., Cheung, P. T., & Wu, W. T. (2004). Lithium chloride reinforces the regeneration-promoting effect of chondroitinase ABC on rubrospinal neurons after spinal cord injury. *Journal of Neurotrauma, 21*, 932–943.

CHAPTER 25

Stroke

Heidi N. Fusco, Koto Ishida, Jaime M. Levine, and Jose Torres

INTRODUCTION

Stroke is a common and prevalent disease. It is the second leading cause of death and the third leading cause of disability in the world. In 2010, there were 33 million strokes worldwide, with 16.9 million people having their first stroke (Lozano et al., 2012). In the United States, large campaigns promoting early stroke symptom recognition and treatment have led to a 30% reduction in the stroke death rate in the past 10 years. Despite this success, stroke remains the fifth leading cause of death and a leading cause of disability. Every year almost 800,000 people have a stroke in the United States with 600,000 experiencing a stroke for the first time in their lives. Stroke kills 130,000 Americans each year, causes almost 1 out of every 20 deaths, and costs over $34 billion a year in health care services, medications, and missed work (Mozaffarian et al., 2015).

Stroke presents a greater burden of disease to minority populations and older patients. The incidence of first time stroke ranges from 88/100,000 in Caucasians to 149/100,000 in Hispanics and 191/100,000 in African Americans (White et al., 2005). Although stroke affects people over the age of 65 disproportionately, 34% of stroke patients are younger than 65 years (Mozaffarian et al., 2015). Stroke also affects certain regions within the United States more than others. The southeastern part of the country has the highest stroke rates and is often referred to as the Stroke Belt (Glymour, Kosheleva, & Boden-Albala, 2009). Despite these racial, regional, and age disparities, stroke can affect any person of any race, gender, or age in any part of the country. Because of this, knowledge of stroke is key in continuing efforts to decrease the burden of this devastating disease. In this chapter, we discuss the major subtypes of stroke, ischemic and hemorrhagic, as well as their symptoms, causes, risk factors, medical complications, and treatments.

ISCHEMIC STROKE/TRANSIENT ISCHEMIC ATTACK

Ischemic strokes comprise 85% of all strokes in the United States (Mozaffarian et al., 2015). They occur when brain tissue does not receive sufficient blood flow and, therefore, sufficient nutrition, causing irreversible damage. This decrease in blood flow usually occurs when there is either systemic hypoperfusion decreasing blood flow to the entire brain or local hypoperfusion from clot formation inside the arteries of the brain or movement of a clot to the brain from other parts of the body. Some patients can experience temporary stroke-like symptoms that resolve within 24 hours and do not cause permanent injury to brain tissue, called transient ischemic attacks (TIAs). Patients who experience TIAs are at increased risk for stroke. In some cases, stroke risk is as high as 8% in the first 30 days after a TIA (Johnston, 2002, 2005). Therefore, even though these patients return to normal, they are taken as seriously as patients who have persisting symptoms and undergo rapid assessment and risk factor modification in order to prevent future strokes.

Etiology and Risk Factors

Ischemic strokes can be caused by a variety of disease processes including small vessel disease, large vessel disease, and cardioembolism. Small vessel strokes are present in 25% of ischemic stroke patients. They result from damage that occurs to the small, nonmuscular, perforating arteries that branch from the middle cerebral and basilar arteries. This damage occurs from sustained damage to the vessels from chronic diseases such as hypertension, diabetes, and hyperlipidemia. Over time, these vessels can become occluded through a process called lipohyalinosis, causing strokes. These strokes tend to be small in size, usually less than 1.5 cm in largest diameter and usually occur in the thalamus, basal ganglia, and brainstem. While many of these strokes are silent and without any clear clinical correlates, some can result in severe acute neurologic symptoms such as unilateral weakness and unilateral numbness.

Twenty percent of stroke patients have cardioembolic strokes, where blood clots travel, or embolize, from the heart to the brain and occlude the intracranial arteries. Cardioembolism can result from abnormal cardiac rhythms such as atrial fibrillation, abnormal cardiac function such as severely low ejection fraction, abnormal valves such as infected or mechanical valves, or even as a result of tumors in the heart. Patients who present with cardioembolic strokes often have strokes in multiple vascular territories and symptoms tend to be maximal at onset but can improve as the clot breaks up and travels more distally.

Twenty percent of ischemic stroke patients have large vessel disease, which is due to the formation of cholesterol plaque in the main arteries of the brain. This plaque usually forms at arterial bifurcations where turbulent flow can cause damage to the inner lining of the vessels causing local inflammation. This inflammation in patients with hypertension, diabetes, and hyperlipidemia causes abnormal buildup of cholesterol plaque, which over time can cause severe stenosis of the arteries and even completely occlude them. In some cases, this plaque can rupture, exposing blood to the very thrombogenic material underlying the plaque and allow for clot formation that can either occlude the artery locally or embolize into the brain, causing stroke. These patients often present with watershed strokes, that is, strokes in locations that are not served by dedicated arterial blood supplies but instead, receive overflow circulation from other arteries.

Finally, 5% of patients have ischemic strokes from a variety of other reasons such as tearing of the inner lining of the arteries, a condition called arterial dissection, genetic disorders that predispose patients to clot formation such as antiphospholipid syndrome, and even infections such as syphilis, which can cause inflammatory damage of the arteries. Given this wide array of causative conditions, treatment of stroke depends greatly on identifying the underlying cause. Consequently, assessment of the potential causes of stroke in these patients usually consists of blood tests that look for vascular risk factors, such as diabetes and high cholesterol, imaging of the blood vessels to look for atherosclerosis, imaging of the heart to look at the heart walls and valves, and continuous cardiac rhythm monitoring to look for arrhythmias such as atrial fibrillation. Despite this workup, however, in 30% of patients no clear cause is found in the immediate period after stroke (Albers, Amarenco, Easton, Sacco, & Teal, 2004). The etiology of these strokes is termed cryptogenic, meaning they occurred without an identified cause. Up to 30% of patients with cryptogenic strokes are later diagnosed with intermittent atrial fibrillation, which is thought to be the likely cause of their strokes. Identifying atrial fibrillation in these patients often requires monitoring over a period of years (Sanna et al., 2014).

Stroke risk factors vary as widely as stroke causes. Age is the most important nonmodifiable risk factor in stroke patients. Stroke risk doubles every decade after the age of 55 years in both men and women. High blood pressure is the single most important modifiable risk factor. Patients with blood pressures greater than 160/90 are 10 times more likely to have a stroke than those with blood pressures under 120/80, with studies showing a linear increase in risk with increasing blood pressures (Rapsomaniki et al., 2014). Patients who have atrial fibrillation, a common heart rhythm abnormality in older adults, are up to five times more likely to have a stroke than those without atrial fibrillation, independent of age and other risk factors. Smokers have two to three times the stroke risk of nonsmokers with risk noted to be dose-dependent (Kawachi et al., 1993). Diabetes has been shown to almost triple the risk of stroke with poorly controlled patients having the most risk (Emerging Risk Factors Collaboration, 2010). Finally, while the role of cholesterol in heart disease and the formation of arterial plaque is without question, its role in ischemic stroke is not yet completely clear.

Some studies have shown increased risk for stroke in patients with high cholesterol while others have not. What has been consistent in all studies is that decreasing cholesterol can lead to up to 50% reduction in stroke in patients with hyperlipidemia (Adams, 1999; Kernan, 2014).

Signs and Symptoms

Stroke symptoms can vary depending on the area of the brain affected, ranging from sudden onset hearing loss, imbalance, or neglect of one side of space. However, the most common symptoms are covered by the FAST acronym, which is currently being used by the American Heart and Stroke Associations in their stroke awareness campaign. FAST stands for Facial droop, Arm weakness, Speech difficulty (both understanding and production of speech), and Time, indicating the importance of early recognition and treatment in patient outcomes. Eighty percent of patients present with these symptoms (Goldstein & Simel, 2005). The other 20% of patients present with symptoms such as dizziness, imbalance, nausea/vomiting, and blurry/double vision (Jauch, 2013).

ACUTE ISCHEMIC STROKE MANAGEMENT

Initial Assessment

When patients present with stroke symptoms to an emergency department, rapid and efficient triage, assessment, and treatment are crucial because it has been shown that the human brain loses approximately 2 million neurons for every minute an area of brain receives insufficient blood flow (Saver, 2006). The initial assessment includes looking for airway, respiratory, or circulatory compromise that may put the patient's life in immediate danger. An EKG, blood glucose level, and vital signs are also obtained immediately after going into the emergency department. A brief history is then obtained. The history focuses on the time of onset of symptoms or when the patient was last seen normal, if no clear onset time is known, any pertinent past medical history, and what medications the patient is taking. After the history, a brief neurologic exam is performed. The most commonly accepted method in the United States is to assess the patient's National Institutes of Health Stroke Scale (NIHSS) score. The scale tests 15 items and provides a score from 0 to 42 (Jauch, 2013). In general, the NIHSS is not a strict measurement of disability but rather a measure of how large the stroke will be if not treated. For instance, a patient with a small stroke in the hand area of the brain can have an NIHSS of 0 despite having no movement in his or her fingers because the NIHSS tests the movement of the whole arm and not the hand. Conversely, a patient with a large stroke affecting the motor, sensory, and language areas of the brain will likely have an NIHSS of over 15. Both patients would suffer disability, but the latter would have a much larger stroke as reflected in his or her NIHSS score. Nevertheless, while not perfect, the NIHSS is widely used and remains one of the best validated stroke scales with excellent inter-rater reliability (Goldstein & Samsa, 1997). It has also been shown to correlate well with patient outcomes (Adams, 1999).

After this, all ischemic stroke patients undergo emergent noncontrast CT head scans. These scans only show evidence of stroke a fraction of the time and their primary purpose is to rule out a brain hemorrhage, which, as we discuss later on, requires very different management than ischemic stroke. CT scans may also show brain tumors, infections, vascular malformations, or other lesions that may explain patients' symptoms (Jauch, 2013).

Treatment

After head CT, neurologic examination, and history are obtained, the next and most important step is in deciding whether the patient is a candidate for any acute treatment. The only medication approved by the Food and Drug Administration in the United States for this purpose is intravenous tissue plasminogen activator (IV tPA), which is a thrombolytic or clot busting medication. IV tPA has been shown to improve outcomes when given within 4.5 hours of symptom onset. Overall, when compared to patients who are not treated with tPA, 30% more patients who receive tPA return to normal or are functionally independent (Emberson et al., 2014). The effects and risks of tPA are extremely time-dependent. For every 15 minutes tPA administration is delayed, the likelihood of impairment increases by 4% and the risk of adverse effects of tPA increases by 4% (Saver et al., 2013).

Bleeding is the most significant complication associated with IV tPA. Systemic bleeding has been seen in 1% to 2% of patients and brain hemorrhage has been seen in 6% of patients (Emberson et al., 2014). The greatest risk factors for intracerebral hemorrhage are elevated blood pressure and large stroke size. Because of this, tPA is contraindicated in patients who are at high risk of systemic bleeding, have severely elevated blood pressure, or have large strokes on head imaging. If tPA is given, the blood pressures of patients are closely followed and maintained under 180/105 (Jauch, 2013). One to eight percent of patients can have tongue swelling with tPA. However, this is not associated with increased death rate in patients who receive tPA (Hill et al., 2003).

In some cases, the patients who present with stroke-like symptoms are diagnosed with a "stroke mimic," which includes seizure, migraine, metabolic abnormalities, and psychiatric disease. It is very difficult to distinguish real strokes from mimics and even when it has been determined that the patient is having a mimic, he or she could also be having a stroke. Moreover, tPA has been shown to be much safer in mimics than in patients with actual strokes. Overall, 4.3% of patients who receive tPA are ultimately found to have a stroke mimic and of those, 0.5% have intracranial bleeding and 0.3% have tongue swelling (Chernyshev et al., 2010; Winkler et al., 2009). Therefore, tPA should not be withheld from patients even when there is suspicion of a stroke mimic.

In select patients whose symptoms do not resolve immediately with IV tPA, mechanical clot retrieval is now considered the standard of care. Several studies have demonstrated the overwhelming efficacy of this procedure in patients who present within 6 hours of symptom onset, who are shown to have a large clot in the intracranial vessels (like the distal internal carotid and proximal middle cerebral arteries), and who do not already have a large stroke on head CT when treatment is initiated (Powers et al., 2015). The imaging modality most commonly used to demonstrate the presence of intracranial clot is a CT angiogram. In this study, iodinated contrast is injected into the veins and then makes its way into the arteries of the brain. If a thrombus is present in an artery of the brain, the contrast will not travel past the clot or may not fill the artery completely. If this is the case and the patient meets the other criteria discussed previously, he or she is taken for the clot retrieval procedure, which involves passage of a catheter from the femoral artery in the groin to the arteries of the brain, deployment of a stent inside the thrombus, which causes it to adhere to the stent, and retrieval of the stent with the adherent thrombus. Suctioning of the clot is also possible. When compared to patients who are not candidates for the procedure, those who undergo clot retrieval are almost twice as likely to be without impairment or be functionally independent (Berkhemer et al., 2015; Goyal et al., 2015; Jovin et al., 2015; Saver et al., 2015; Campbell et al., 2014).

Course and Prognosis

After treatment with IV tPA, clot retrieval, or both, patients are usually admitted to a stroke unit where they are managed carefully prior to their placement in a rehabilitation facility if needed. The most important part of this management is the preservation of at-risk brain tissue called penumbra that will be irreversibly damaged if sufficient blood flow does not reach the brain. This is because despite our best treatments, the interventions noted do not completely open all of the arteries that have clot in them. In patients with evidence of continued blockage of blood flow, blood pressure is augmented with intravenous fluids and reduction in the doses of blood pressure medications so that sufficient blood flow can make it beyond the blockage, through collateral circulation. However, care must be taken to not allow severe blood pressure elevations, as blood pressures above 200 systolic can lead to intracerebral hemorrhage (Jauch, 2013). Great care is also taken to prevent fevers and hyperglycemia as both have been shown to lead to worse outcomes (Azzimondi, 1995; Capes et al., 2001). As noted, a detailed assessment is undertaken to determine the cause of the stroke and to determine whether the patient should be started on antiplatelets such as aspirin and clopidogrel, which prevent platelet aggregation or anticoagulants like warfarin, which is a potent blood thinner. In general, high risk causes of stroke such as atrial fibrillation or intracardiac thrombus are treated with stronger medications such as warfarin while most other conditions are treated with aspirin or clopidogrel or a combination of both. Risk factors are also treated. Despite initial blood pressure augmentation, the long-term blood pressure goal in stroke patients is normotension and hypertension is treated aggressively 1 to 2 weeks after the stroke with angiotensin converting enzyme inhibitors (ACEIs) and calcium channel blockers. Elevated cholesterol is treated with high-dose statin medications and diabetes is treated with oral hypoglycemics and insulin. In cases where the stroke is due to severe carotid artery plaque, carotid endarterectomy may be pursued to physically remove the plaque from the diseased artery. Finally, in patients with infectious causes of stroke such as infections of the heart valves, or endocarditis, the most effective treatment is antibiotic therapy (Kernan et al., 2014). Patients are assessed by speech, physical and occupational therapists, and, if needed, are referred to inpatient acute and subacute facilities for further management.

Most recovery after an ischemic stroke occurs in the first 3 to 6 months after the event (Nakayama et al., 1994; Veerbeek et al., 2011). Prognosis after stroke depends on a variety of factors including the patient's age, the severity of the stroke, and the stroke size. Studies have demonstrated that larger stroke sizes and higher NIHSS at presentation predict worst outcomes (Adams et al., 1999; Vogt, Laage, Shuaib, Schneider, & Collaboration, 2012). For instance, one study demonstrated that patients with an NIHSS of 7 to 10 have a 46% chance of being independent at 3 months whereas those with an NIHSS of 11 to 23 have a 23% chance (Adams et al., 1999). Patients over the age of 65 have higher mortality after stroke and are more likely to require long-term nursing care (Steiner et al., 1997).

HEMORRHAGIC STROKE

Hemorrhagic strokes occur when there is seepage of blood out of intracranial vessels into the brain or into the subarachnoid space. Hemorrhagic strokes comprise 15% of all strokes in the United States and have an incidence of 12 to 31 per 100,000 people with the rate doubling every 10 years after the age of 35 (Stein et al., 2012). Unlike ischemic stroke, Asian and Caucasian Americans are affected disproportionately over African Americans and Hispanics with rates ranging from 51.8/100,000 person-years in Asians to 24.2/100,000 person-years in Caucasians, 22.9/100,000 person-years in African Americans, and 19.6/100 000 person-years in Hispanics (van Asch et al., 2010). However, as with ischemic strokes, patients of any age and gender may be affected and early treatment and management are crucial for ensuring favorable patient outcomes.

Etiology and Risk Factors

Hemorrhagic strokes can be subdivided into subarachnoid hemorrhage and intraparenchymal hemorrhage. Subarachnoid hemorrhage occurs when there is seepage of blood into the subarachnoid space. It affects 10–15/100,000 people and usually occurs after rupture of an aneurysm, allowing blood to fill the subarachnoid space under arterial pressure (Labovitz et al., 2006). Aneurysms affect 2% to 3% of the population with 20% to 30% of these patients having multiple aneurysms. Approximately 10% of patients with ruptured intracranial aneurysms die before they reach the hospital (Vlak, Algra, Brandenburg, & Rinkel, 2011). Parenchymal hemorrhages occur when there is direct damage or rupture of vessels in the brain itself allowing blood to seep out into the brain tissue. As blood seeps out, it creates a hematoma that can cause increased intracranial pressure, which eventually causes blood to stop flowing out of the affected artery.

Parenchymal hemorrhages are usually the result of high blood pressure. However, other causes include vascular malformations, trauma, drugs, and amyloid angiopathy. Severe elevations of blood pressure can damage the small arteries of the brain over time, causing the vessel to become occluded via lipohyalinosis. However, these nonmuscular walls can also rupture from the mechanical pressure, causing intracranial hemorrhage. Vascular malformations tend to have abnormal vessel walls that are weak and can spontaneously rupture. They affect 0.1% of the population and underlie 3% of strokes in young patients and 9% of intraparenchymal hemorrhages (Al-Shahi & Warlow, 2001). Amyloid angiopathy is due to the abnormal deposition of amyloid beta protein in intracranial vessel walls causing them to crack and rupture. It affects 12% of people over the age of 85 (Viswanathan & Greenberg, 2011). The greatest risk factors associated with intracerebral hemorrhage are elevated blood pressure, age, and the use of blood thinners. Hypertension increases the risk for hemorrhage fourfold (Woo, 2004). Older age is another important risk factor, with risk doubling every 10 years after the age of 35 (Broderick, 2007). Finally, the use of blood thinners such as warfarin increases hemorrhagic risk by two to five times and also confers poorer prognosis (Cucchiara, 2008; Flibotte, Hagan, O'Donnell, Greenberg, & Rosand; Rosand, Eckman, Knudsen, Singer, & Greenberg, 2004).

Signs and Symptoms

Common symptoms after a hemorrhagic stroke are headache, vomiting, decreased level of consciousness, and seizures. "The worst headache of my life" complaint occurs in up to 97% of patients who present with subarachnoid hemorrhage (Gorelick, Hier, Caplan, & Langenberg, 1986). Overall, headaches occur in 90% of all intracerebral hemorrhage patients and are due to elevated intracranial pressure from hematomas or increased blood in the subarachnoid space, as mentioned earlier, as well as irritation of pain fibers that supply the meningeal covering of the brain. Vomiting occurs in 50% of patients and is also the result of elevated intracranial pressure. Seizures have been noted to occur in up to 29% of patients and are due to irritation of brain tissue by blood in the brain. Finally, decreased level of consciousness is also seen in these patients and is also due to increased intracranial pressure preventing blood from flowing into the brain. These symptoms are less common with ischemic strokes, where less than 20% of patients have headache and less than 10% have nausea and vomiting. Like ischemic stroke patients, hemorrhagic stroke patients will also present with focal neurologic symptoms that will depend on the location of the hemorrhage. The most frequent locations for hemorrhage are the thalamus, basal ganglia, and brainstem causing symptoms such as unilateral weakness and sensory loss, eye movement abnormalities, and imbalance (Broderick, 2007).

ACUTE HEMORRHAGIC STROKE MANAGEMENT

Initial Assessment

As with ischemic stroke patients, initial management includes assessment of airway, breathing and circulation and ensuring the patient's hemodynamic stability. After this is done, vital signs, EKG, and blood glucose are obtained. A quick history and neurologic examination, again with an NIHSS, is also performed. Most importantly, after these assessments, the patient is emergently taken for a noncontrast head CT, which has 95% sensitivity in detecting intracerebral hemorrhages. In some instances, particularly with patients presenting with the worst headache of their lives with suspicion of subarachnoid hemorrhage, a head CT may not show intracranial hemorrhage and a lumbar puncture is then required. The combined sensitivity of head CT and lumbar puncture for detecting subarachnoid hemorrhage is 99% (Morgenstern et al., 2010).

Treatment

Careful blood pressure control is the initial treatment in patients with hemorrhagic stroke. Cerebral blood flow is dependent on systemic blood pressure and intracranial pressure and must be maintained. Current recommendations suggest lowering the patient's blood pressure to 140–160/90 (Morgenstern et al., 2010). This has been shown to improve outcomes when done carefully (Anderson et al., 2013). Reversal of any blood thinners should occur promptly and if the patient is taking medications such as aspirin or clopidogrel, which affect how platelets adhere to one another to form clots, platelet transfusions may be necessary. The head of bed is usually elevated to 30 degrees to reduce intracranial pressure and hypertonic and hyperosmotic therapies can be used.

One of the most feared complications of hemorrhage is herniation of brain tissue and compression of the brainstem where crucial life sustaining centers reside. Herniation occurs because the hemorrhage takes up space in an already crowded cranial cavity. Brain tissue cannot move anywhere to compensate for the hematoma or the subarachnoid hemorrhage because the brain is encased in bone, so it shifts down into the brainstem. In cases where herniation occurs despite maximal medical management, surgical decompression is a possible intervention. During this procedure a piece of skull is removed to allow the brain to shift outward, thus decreasing intracranial pressure and preventing herniation. In cases where patients are found to have aneurysms or vascular malformations, surgery and/or endovascular therapies can be used to treat these underlying lesions (Morgenstern et al., 2010).

Long-term blood pressure control is the first-line treatment modality in preventing future hemorrhagic stroke. This, along with treatment of underlying causative lesions such as aneurysms and vascular malformations, confers the greatest risk reduction in hemorrhagic stroke patients. Unfortunately, there is no specific treatment for patients with amyloid angiopathy except for lifelong avoidance of blood thinners and antiplatelets as well as maintaining good blood pressure control (Morgenstern et al., 2010).

Course and Prognosis

The prognosis of patients with hemorrhagic stroke is poorer than that of patients with ischemic stroke. The 30-day mortality ranges from 30% to 50% with half of the deaths occurring in the first 48 hours (van Asch et al., 2010). These deaths occur as a result of complications from the hemorrhage such as respiratory compromise or herniation. A major predictor of mortality is the Intracerebral Hemorrhage (ICH) score. This score is a 6-point scale looking at factors such as level of consciousness, age, volume of hemorrhage, and location of hemorrhage. It is validated in hemorrhagic stroke patients and is widely used in the United States. In patients with a score of 5 or more, the risk of death in 30 days approaches 100% (Hemphill, Bonovich, Besmertis, Manley, & Johnston, 2001; Hemphill, Farrant, & Neill, 2009).

Long-term prognosis in those who survive the acute hemorrhage period depends on the location and size of the hemorrhage, the age of the patient, and the use of blood thinners. Larger hemorrhages that occur in or around the brainstem (thus increasing the risk of herniation) in older patients are all associated with poor outcomes (van Asch, 2010). Growth of hemorrhage within the first 24 hours is also associated with poor prognosis. Patients experiencing early hematoma growth had a 20% increase in 30-day mortality. Finally, patients who use blood thinners have also been shown to have larger hemorrhages and worse outcomes (Cucchiara et al., 2008).

As with ischemic strokes, those patients who survive the initial period are assessed for possible placement in inpatient acute and subacute rehabilitation facilities. Most of the recovery will occur in the first 3 to 6 months. Depending on the amount of intracranial hemorrhage, reabsorption of blood products occurs over weeks to months. Studies have found up to 40% of patients are functionally independent at 3 months (Morgenstern et al., 2010). Although the overall prognosis is poorer for hemorrhage patients, as with ischemic stroke, early recognition is key to improved outcomes.

MEDICAL COMPLICATIONS OF STROKE

Medical complications are frequent after stroke and are known to increase hospital length of stay as well as worsen functional outcome (Johnston et al., 1998). Such complications may include cardiac abnormalities, dysphagia, venous thrombosis, falls, bowel dysfunction, genitourinary abnormalities, seizures, systemic infections, pressure ulcers, pain, spasticity, and mood disorders. Those with more severe, disabling strokes are at particularly high risk for complications in addition to older patients and those with preexisting comorbid medical conditions. Most occur within the first few weeks after stroke onset although late complications may also occur (Langhorne et al., 2000).

Dysphagia

Dysphagia, or impairment of swallowing function, is a common complication of stroke. When severe, it can involve aspiration of food, medications, and oral secretions that can lead to aspiration pneumonia. Age greater than 70, male gender, and disabling stroke are independent predictors of dysphagia as well as specific characteristics of swallowing function including incomplete oral clearance, impaired pharyngeal response, and palatal asymmetry or weakness (Mann & Hankey, 2001). A systematic review of 24 studies of aspiration in stroke patients demonstrated that both dysphagia (RR 3.17; 95% CIs [2.07, 4.87]) and aspiration (RR 11.56; 95% CIs [3.36, 39.77]) were associated with a significant increase in the risk of pneumonia as compared with control patients with normal swallowing function (Martino et al., 2005). Furthermore, severe dysphagia was associated with an 11-fold increase in risk of developing pneumonia (Martino et al., 2005; Smithard, O'Neill, Parks, & Morris, 1996).

Bedside tests for dysphagia are less sensitive than more comprehensive testing by speech pathologists, but are important screening tools to prevent aspiration after stroke prior to oral intake of food or medications. One review of 16 studies found that the water swallow test was the most commonly performed bedside screening test. This test is feasible and safe but abnormal response (cough or voice change) was only found to have low-to-moderate sensitivity and moderate-to-high specificity for predicting aspiration (Daniels, Anderson, & Willson, 2012). Dysphagia incidence is lowest for this kind of bedside screening test (37%–45%), moderate for testing by trained speech therapists (51%–55%), and highest with imaging studies such as video fluoroscopy (64%–78%; Martino et al., 2005). Despite the lower sensitivity for bedside testing, however, dysphagia screening prior to oral administration of medications or food is important for prevention of aspiration pneumonia. One prospective multicenter study found significantly decreased risk of aspiration pneumonia in centers that employed a formal dysphagia screening protocol such as the water swallow test for all stroke patients (adjusted odds ratio [OR] 0.10; 95% confidence interval [CI] [0.03, 0.45]; Hinchey et al., 2005).

Systemic Infection

Infection remains one of the most common medical complications after stroke, with an estimated incidence ranging from 25% to 65% (Aslanyan, Weir, Diener, Kaste, & Lees, 2004; Kwan, & Hand, 2007; Langhorne et al., 2000). Most commonly, this involves pneumonia and urinary tract infections (UTI).

Pneumonia is common after stroke with incidence ranging from 5% to 9% overall and much higher for those admitted to the neurologic intensive care unit (ICU) or who require nasogastric tube feeding (Ingeman, Andersen, Hundborg, Svendsen, & Johnsen, 2011). Pneumonia is the most common cause of fever within the first 48 hours after stroke and is the most frequent complication within the first 2 to 4 weeks after supratentorial ischemic stroke. In this population, roughly 60% is attributed to aspiration (Grau et al., 1999). Retrospective Medicare data suggest that poststroke pneumonia is one of the leading causes of hospital readmission in the first 5 years after stroke (Bravata, Ho, Meehan, Brass, & Concato, 2007).

Aspiration of oropharyngeal contents colonized by oral bacterial flora may cause pneumonia requiring antimicrobial treatment for gram-negative bacilli and gram-positive cocci while aspiration of acidic gastric contents may only lead to aspiration pneumonitis, a self-limited sterile lung injury (Kumar, Selim, & Caplan, 2010). Timing of radiographic abnormalities can be helpful in differentiating between pneumonia and pneumonitis as rapid resolution is more consistent with aspiration pneumonitis and delayed but longer lasting (weeks) opacities more suggestive of frank pneumonia. Risk factors for developing pneumonia after stroke include older age (>65 years), symptomatic speech impairment, poststroke disability, cognitive impairment, and dysphagia (Sellars et al., 2007) as well as depressed level of consciousness, significant facial weakness, mechanical ventilation, and brainstem or multiple infarcts (Hilker et al., 2003). Nursing care including frequent suctioning, elevation of the head of the bed, assisted feeding, and regular oral care may decrease risk for pneumonia (Yoneyama, Yoshida, Matsui, & Sasaki, 1999). In mechanically ventilated patients, oral antiseptic treatment may further lower risk. Current data do not support the use of prophylactic antibiotics in this population. Some studies have reported increased incidence of pneumonia associated with the use of proton pump inhibitors or histamine receptor antagonists for gastric acid suppression (Herzig, Howell, Ngo, & Marcantonio, 2009).

UTIs are also very common after stroke with estimates of incidence ranging from 11% to 15% by 3 months (Ingeman et al., 2011; Langhorne et al., 2000). Independent predictors of UTI include older age, female gender, stroke severity, and urinary catheterization (Aslanyan et al., 2004). Most are uncomplicated and related to primary *Escherichia coli* infection; however, 1% of stroke patients will suffer serious or prolonged complication as a result of UTI. Avoidance of unnecessary indwelling catheterization is important, given direct association with development of UTI; however, data supporting decreased incidence of infection with external catheter alternatives are limited. Because patients with catheter-associated UTI are often asymptomatic or minimally symptomatic and can have relatively normal peripheral white blood cell (WBC) counts, urine cultures can be useful to confirm diagnosis and guide antibiotic selection.

Cardiac Complications

Preexisting cardiac disease is common in patients with stroke, particularly given the significant overlap in risk factors between cardiovascular and cerebrovascular disease. This link is so strong that stroke has been established as a coronary heart disease risk equivalent. Furthermore, because cardiac abnormalities can be both the cause and effect of stroke and often present concurrently, differentiation can be challenging. Cardiac complications after stroke include myocardial infarction (MI), cardiac arrhythmias, and congestive heart failure (CHF) or cardiomyopathy. These tend to occur early after stroke onset. High-risk patients include those with established CHF or prior MI, diabetes, renal insufficiency, severe or debilitating strokes, peripheral vascular disease, and prolonged QTc on EKG (Liao et al., 2009; Prosser et al., 2007).

Cardiac ischemia including angina and MI may complicate nearly 6% of acute strokes and are serious or life-threatening in 1% (Hinchey et al., 2008). The risk is highest in the acute poststroke time period and one study of consecutive stroke patients reported 2.3% incidence of in-hospital MI. These patients were at significantly higher risk for severe disability or death at hospital discharge (OR 2.51; 95% CIs [1.42, 2.10]) and higher rates of mortality at 1 year (Liao et al., 2009). Cardiac enzymes may also be elevated in the setting of acute ischemic stroke. These elevations are often minor and although patients may not meet full criteria for MI, any elevation of troponin may result in significantly increased in-hospital mortality (RR 3.2; 95% CIs [1.7, 5.8]; James et al., 2000).

Cardiac arrhythmias, including atrial fibrillation, supraventricular tachycardia, ventricular tachycardia, and ventricular ectopic beats are frequently observed after stroke. One prospective study reported 25% incidence of serious cardiac arrhythmia within the first 72 hours after stroke, highest in the first 24 hours (Kallmünzer et al., 2012). The most common of these serious arrhythmias remains atrial fibrillation, which accounts for more than half of all cases. Diagnosis of atrial fibrillation in particular is important since it may be the causative mechanism for the initial presenting stroke and impacts management decisions. Many of these patients who develop cardiac arrhythmias have otherwise normal cardiac function, which suggests an underlying neurogenic etiology. Moreover, stroke location may influence arrhythmia type, including tachycardia, bradycardia, or heart block.

Right insular strokes in particular may be associated with increased cardiac enzyme concentrations as well as repolarization abnormalities, cardiac arrhythmias, heart failure, and sudden death (Ay et al., 2006; Lane, Wallace, Petrosky, Schwartz, & Gradman, 1992; Oppenheimer, Wilson, Guiraudon, & Cechetto, 1991). The exact mechanism remains unclear but is likely related to disturbance of normal cardiovascular autonomic regulation. Some data suggest that right insular strokes are more likely to result in both brady- as well as tachyarrhythmias (Daniele, Caravaglios, Fierro, & Natalè, 2002; Dütsch, Burger, Dörfler, Schwab, & Hilz, 2007; Lane et al., 1992).

Less is known about the incidence of heart failure after acute stroke; however, concurrent CHF does significantly increase mortality in this population. One subset of often reversible cardiomyopathy after stroke, including subarachnoid hemorrhage, is stress cardiomyopathy or Takotsubo syndrome. The characteristic apical ballooning has been described after stroke with reported incidence in one consecutive cohort as high as 1.2% within the first 2 weeks (Yoshimura et al., 2008).

Venous Thromboembolism

Both deep vein thrombosis (DVT) and pulmonary embolism (PE) are potentially life-threatening examples of venous thromboembolism (VTE) complicating acute stroke. Clinically evident DVT after acute stroke ranges in incidence from 1% to 10% (Amin, Lin, Thompson, & Wiederkehr, 2013; Dennis et al., 2009; Sandercock, 1997) depending upon the method of detection including Doppler ultrasound as well as blood markers. Not surprisingly, prevalence of asymptomatic DVT is even higher. Incidence of MRI diagnosed DVT as high as 40% has been reported in patients 3 weeks after stroke, on aspirin, who were wearing graded compression stockings (Kelly et al., 2004). Similar to cardiac complications, venous thromboembolic events tend to occur early after stroke with the highest incidence in days 2 to 7 (Kelly, Rudd, Lewis, & Hunt, 2001).

Patients with advanced age, dehydration, severe strokes, and who are immobile or hemiparetic are at highest risk for DVT (Kelly et al., 2004). Consistent with these data, thrombosis is significantly more common in the ipsilateral rather than contralateral leg (73% vs. 11%) and degree of weakness and immobility appears to correlate with DVT risk (Dennis, Mordi, Graham, & Sandercock, 2011; Warlow, Ogston, & Douglas, 1976).

Prevention of VTE is varied and includes pharmacologic as well as nonpharmacologic options. For immobile acute ischemic stroke patients, intermittent pneumatic compression (IPC) devices have been shown to significantly reduce the incidence of proximal DVT at 30 days (8.5 vs. 12.1%, ARR 3.6%; CIs [1.4, 5.8]). This reduction was not associated with any major adverse events although there was a significant increase in skin breaks from 1.4% to 3.1% (Dennis et al., 2013). IPC is contraindicated in those with leg ischemia from peripheral vascular disease, severe leg edema, skin lesions including ulcerations or dermatitis, and those who have already been immobilized for more than 72 hours after stroke onset. The latter recommendation is related to the theoretical risk of embolization of a recently formed venous clot. In contrast to IPC, graduated compression stockings have not been shown to effectively prevent VTE and may in fact be harmful in acute stroke patients, given similar cutaneous side effects as IPC devices (Dennis et al., 2011, 2013; Lederle, Zylla, MacDonald, & Wilt, 2011).

Pharmacologic VTE prophylaxis with subcutaneous anticoagulation has also been proven effective. Both unfractionated heparin (UFH) and low molecular weight heparin (LMWH) in varying doses have been prospectively studied in patients after acute ischemic stroke (Kamphuisen & Agnelli, 2007; Sandercock, 1997). UFH at low-dose (≤15,000 units/day) significantly decreased the risk of DVT (OR 0.17; 95% CIs [0.11, 0.26]) but not PE. There was also no difference in risk of major hemorrhage, either intra- or extracranial. High-dose UFH (>15,000 units/day) did significantly reduce risk of PE (OR 0.49; 95% CIs [0.29, 0.83]) but at the cost of higher rates of major intracranial (OR 3.86; 95% CIs [2.41, 6.19]) and extracranial (OR 4.74; 95% CIs [2.88, 7.78]) hemorrhage. Low-dose LMWH (≤6000 IU/day) was associated with the optimal benefit–risk ratio with significantly decreased incidence of both DVT (OR 0.34; 95% CIs [0.19, 0.59]) and PE (OR 0.36; 95% CIs [0.15, 0.87]) without concurrent increase in major intracranial or extracranial hemorrhage. Higher dose LMWH was also associated with lower rates of DVT and PE but did result in significant increase in intracranial hemorrhage with a trend toward increased extracranial hemorrhage also. In another meta-analysis, prophylaxis with LMWH was superior to UFH for prevention of any VTE (OR 0.54; 95% CIs [0.41, 0.95]) without associated difference in major bleeding including intracranial, or overall mortality (Shorr, Jackson, Sherner, & Moores, 2008). Aspirin may also decrease VTE frequency in high-risk patients, but to a lesser degree. Newer generation oral anticoagulants have not yet been evaluated for VTE prophylaxis in acute stroke patients but there is growing evidence for possible efficacy in the post-surgical and high-risk medical populations.

The most dangerous complication of DVT is PE. Fatal PE can occur in up to 15% of patients with untreated proximal DVT and is the most common cause of death between 2 and 4 weeks after stroke (Kelly et al., 2001). The mortality rate of acute, untreated PE nears 30%. The mainstay of treatment for PE is anticoagulation and many of these patients will require stabilization in an ICU. The risks of hemorrhagic transformation (especially symptomatic) must be weighed against the degree of clinical suspicion and severity of PE.

Seizures

Acute stroke is the most common cause of clinical seizures in older adults (>60 years old), accounting for nearly 50% of all seizures in this population (Loiseau et al., 1990). Most of these will occur within the first 48 hours of stroke onset. Similarly, incidence of seizure after acute cerebrovascular events including TIA is also common, ranging from 4% to 15% with about 55% of these occurring early, within the first month (Bladin et al., 2000; Conrad et al., 2013).

Inconsistent method of seizure determination, duration of follow-up, retrospective versus prospective design, and recruitment criteria may account for some of this variability across studies. The risk of early symptomatic seizure (within the first week) is as high as 4% in ischemic stroke although this risk triples with hemorrhagic conversion and quadruples for those with primary intracerebral hemorrhage (Beghi et al., 2011). These early seizures are thought to be triggered by the metabolic and physiologic imbalances associated with acute ischemia or hemorrhage. In contrast, late seizures (weeks to years) may be more related to long-standing alterations in neuronal networks resulting in ongoing hyperexcitability. Risk factors for seizure include younger age at stroke, hemorrhagic stroke, coagulopathy, larger stroke volume, higher severity, and cortical location. Most are secondary generalized seizures. The overall risk of epilepsy after stroke is 5% to 9%; however, this rate surges to nearly 35% in those with acute stroke related seizure (So, Annegers, Hauser, O'Brien, & Whisnant, 1996). Early 30-day mortality increases significantly in patients with early seizure compared to those without seizures (12.5% vs. 6.3%, risk ratio [RR] 2.6; Beghi et al., 2011).

Bowel Dysfunction

After stroke, bowel dysfunction is increased sevenfold and includes but is not limited to constipation and fecal incontinence (Engler et al., 2014). Both problems have demonstrated negative influences on quality of life, functional outcomes, and disposition destination (Camara-Lemarroy, Ibarra-Yruegas, & Gongora-Rivera, 2014; Krogh, Christensen, & Laurberg, 2001).

The prevalence of constipation is reported to be 74% acutely after stroke (Engler et al., 2014; Su et al., 2009) and can result in pain and discomfort, decreased nutritional intake, and have urgent life-threatening outcomes if not treated. Constipation after stroke is thought to be due to decreased mobility, dysphagia (resulting in decreased fiber and fluid intake), dysfunctional intestinal contractility, and deficits in cognition, consciousness, and communication (Lim et al., 2015).

The prevalence of bowel incontinence after stroke is as high as 40% (Brittain, Peet, & Castleden, 1998; Camara-Lemarroy, Ibarra-Yruegas, & Gongora-Rivera, 2014) and is an even greater barrier for a patient to return home or to assimilate into the community. Fecal incontinence has been shown to be more prevalent in stroke patients who were older, had greater stroke severity, and other disabling comorbidities such as diabetes (Harari, Coshall, Rudd, & Wolfe, 2003).

In the evaluation and treatment of bowel dysfunction after stroke, the clinician must first evaluate the pattern of patient's bowel movements, and perform an adequate clinical exam. A rectal exam and radiograph should be performed if there is suspicion for impaction or obstruction. When managing bowel dysfunction after stroke, the clinician should first focus on a bowel schedule (usually after breakfast or dinner) and then can use dietary adjustments to increase fiber and fluid. Several agents can be used to treat constipation and bowel dysfunction. Psyllium husk is a bulk producing laxative and fiber supplement that increases stool bulk, resulting in firming or solidifying very loose stools, or softening very hard small stools. Docusate sodium and polyethylene glycol are stool softeners that increase the amount of water in the stool making the stool softer and easier to pass. Senakot and bisacodyl are stimulant laxatives that irritate bowel tissues. Care should be taken to wean off use of stimulant laxatives, as overuse can result in dependence. Enemas are useful when there is an impaction. Finally, simethicone is useful in treating pain from discomfort from gas by decreasing stomach and intestinal gas bubble surface tension and aiding gas elimination.

Urinary Incontinence and Urinary Retention

Urinary incontinence and urinary retention unfortunately are common disorders after stroke with incidences as high as 80% for incontinence and 30% for retention (McKenzie & Badlani; Williams, 2012). In understanding bladder dysfunction, it is first useful to understand the normal bladder physiology. In low volumes, the bladder accommodates by relaxing the detrusor muscle, or the smooth muscle found in the bladder. As the bladder fills, there is automatic stimulation of internal urethral sphincter to contract, thus further maintaining continence. The external urethral sphincter and levator ani muscles can also be consciously contracted to further maintain continence. After the bladder volume reaches between 300 and 600 mL urine, there is a strong signal to void voluntarily by relaxing the external and levator ani muscles, which then involuntarily cause coordinated contraction of the detrusor muscle, and relaxation of the internal urethral sphincter.

Urinary incontinence has been associated with impaired cognition, aphasia, and motor deficits (Gelber, Good, Laven, & Verhulst, 1993) and is associated with decreased quality of life, skin breakdown, discomfort, decreased social interaction and community living as well as has been associated with higher mortality rates (McKenzie & Badlani, 2012). Urinary incontinence can be due to retention and subsequent overflow, loss of bladder control, and most commonly, detrusor overactivity.

Contrary to previous belief, incontinence has not been associated with specific hemispheric lesions (McKenzie & Badlani, 2012).

When evaluating urinary dysfunction, one first needs to review a detailed recording of the volume and frequency of urination. Laboratories and clinical exam can assess if the patent is adequately hydrated or has a UTI. Nurses can perform bedside bladder scans (ultrasound measurement of bladder urine volume) or postvoid residuals (PVR), which is ultrasound measurement of bladder urine volume after voiding. If a bladder scanner is not available, sometimes a nurse can perform intermittent catheterization if there has been no void for several hours to not only empty the bladder but also determine the volume in the bladder.

A urodynamic study (UDS) is performed by a skilled clinician where a special catheter is inserted into the urethra and bladder and measures the filling pressure of the bladder and sphincter activity. UDS is helpful if micturition history, physical exam, and PVRs do not declare the cause of incontinence or retention.

In detrusor overactivity, a patient demonstrates frequent low volume incontinence episodes, where the detrusor muscle contracts at lower than normal bladder volumes. The patient may feel frequent and urgent needs to void, with loss of bladder control. In treating detrusor overactivity, timed voiding is deemed the gold standard, with documentation of decreased incontinence episodes from 80% to 20% (McKenzie & Badlani, 2012; Ostaszkiewicz, Johnston, & Roe, 2004). In timed voiding, the patient is assisted in voiding at short intervals (every 2–3 hours). Length of time between voids is only increased once continence is maintained between these intervals. Time voiding may also be used in conjunction with an anticholinergic medication such as oxybutynin. Still, timed voiding alone, or timed voiding with oxybutynin has been demonstrated to be more effective than oxybutynin alone (Gelber et al., 1993; Ostaszkiewicz et al., 2004). In addition, anticholinergic medications should be prescribed with caution in the stroke population as these medications can exacerbate constipation, dry mouth, drowsiness, and cognitive impairment.

Although not as common after stroke, urinary retention poses immediate danger to the patient as it can quickly lead to bladder infection, bladder overdistension, ureter reflux, hydronephrosis, and renal failure. Causes of urinary retention after stroke include outflow obstruction due to an enlarged prostate or urethral stricture and detrusor–sphincter dyssynergia (DSD). DSD occurs when there is loss of coordinated contraction of the detrusor muscle and relaxation of the internal and external urethral sphincters. A patient may still have incontinence when he or she has retention due to overflow from an overdistended bladder and detrusor overactivity. Clean intermittent catheterization is preferred over indwelling catheters for the treatment of urinary retention. The patient will need to be catheterized on a schedule to avoid overfilling. Finally, if there is bladder outlet obstruction, such as an enlarged prostate, alpha-blockers such as doxazosin and tamsulosin have been demonstrated to improve urinary flow and PVR (McKenzie & Badlani, 2012), but care should be taken as these medications can cause orthostasis.

Pressure Ulcers

Pressure ulcers are areas of damaged skin and underlying tissue that form over bony prominences or weight-bearing surfaces. Patients with stroke are at risk for pressure ulcers due to impaired mobility, decreased nutrition, altered level of consciousness and sensation, and bowel and bladder incontinence (Tânia, 2013). The most common areas of pressure ulcer in patients who have suffered cerebrovascular accident include occiput, scapula, sacrum, buttocks, and heels. Pressure ulcer development after stroke has demonstrated increased poststroke mortality (Lee, 2016).

Treatment of pressure ulcers requires multidisciplinary management with modification of support surfaces, optimization of nutrition, wound dressing and applications, positioning, and surgical repair if required (Tânia, 2013). Wound care clinicians are specialized in prescribing the proper dressing and seating/bedding type for the patient, which in part is determined by the type of ulcer (necrotic, dry, moist, etc.) Despite the advances in dressings, it is imperative to first focus on correcting the underlying issues identified earlier.

Falls

The fall prevalence of patients hospitalized for stroke is as high as 65% (Batchelor, Mackintosh, Said, & Hill, 2012; Callaly et al., 2015). There is increased risk of fall in patients with nondominant-hemispheric stroke, possibly related to decreased awareness and attention to physical deficits. Fall during rehabilitation hospitalization has been associated with an increased mean length of stay compared to patients who did not fall; reported mean is 11 days longer (Wong, Brooks, & Mansfield, 2015). Fall after stroke is associated with a fracture rate of 5% to 23% (Callaly et al., 2015). Those with mobility impairment are more likely to fall than patients who are mobility-dependent (Callaly et al., 2015).

Fall prevention in the home includes environmental modifications (removing clutter, coffee tables and throw rugs, improving lighting, and use of bedside commodes or urinals), and treatment of orthostasis, dizziness, and weakness. In the inpatient setting, a patient is assessed for impulsivity and insight into deficits and can be placed on continuous or intermittent monitoring, and also have bed and chair alarms placed. Physical restraints are not recommended for fall prevention.

After a fall, a patient should be evaluated thoroughly by a skilled clinician. Detailed documentation should include mechanism of the fall, how the patient was found, if the fall was witnessed, and if the patient reports any pain or symptom. The patient should be examined fully, making special note of skin injury or joint deformity. The clinician should consider radiographic imaging if there is any deformity, change in range of motion, neurological status change, or if there is a chance the patient hit his or her head.

Pain

Pain after stroke is sometimes not adequately assessed due to communication difficulties or cognitive impairments. Pain sources poststroke that the clinician should consider include headache, central pain, shoulder subluxation, spasticity-related pain, and contracture. In addition, a patient's preexisting pain generators such as arthritis and neuropathies should also be taken into consideration (Nesbitt, Moxham, Ramadurai, & Williams, 2015).

Central poststroke pain (CPSP) arises from a central nervous system (CNS) lesion and has prevalence as high as 35 % (Oh & Seo, 2015). It was first named in 1906 and initially called Dejerine–Roussy syndrome. CPSP usually develops weeks to months after the CNS injury and is both insidious and progressive (Szczudlik et al., 2014). CPSP has a variety of descriptions, and has been described as a sensation of numbness, tingling, lancinating, burning, sharp, prickling, shooting, pulling, and swelling. It is most likely to be constant, but can be intermittent and has been thought to be due to alterations of excitatory and inhibitory mechanisms of pain receptors (Oh & Seo, 2015). CPSP is associated with depression, anxiety, sleep disturbance, and decreased quality of life (Oh & Seo, 2015; Szczudlik et al., 2014).

The pharmacological treatment of CPSP includes the first-line agent, amitriptyline, but side effects of dry mouth, urinary retention, and sedation can limit its use. Other tricyclic antidepressants can also be tried for better tolerance. Selective serotonin–norepinephrine reuptake inhibitors, such as venlafaxine or duloxetine, have some reports of efficacy. Anticonvulsants have been used, which include carbamazepine, lamotrigine, gabapentin, pregabalin, and levetiracetam, but also have varying reports of efficacy. Morphine, ketamine, lidocaine, and propofol have been shown to relieve CPSP but obviously require close monitoring of use and can be difficult to manage in the outpatient setting. There is ongoing evaluation for the use of transcutaneous electrical nerve stimulation (TENS), motor cortex stimulation, caloric stimulation, deep brain stimulation (DBS), and repetitive transcranial magnetic stimulation (rTMS; Harrison & Field, 2015; Oh & Seo, 2015; Szczudlik et al., 2014).

Musculoskeletal shoulder pain can occur from shoulder subluxation and joint contracture and has reported occurrence in over half of patients with stroke (Dromerick, Edwards, & Kumar, 2008). Shoulder subluxation is likely to occur in patients with hemiplegia, as it is a unique joint with decreased bony constraints and relies on muscles for stability. In contracture, there is shortening of the soft tissues in the joint resulting in decreased range. When subluxation is present, external supports such as pillows, lap trays and external slings are useful in preventing joint injury and pain. TENS has proposed efficacy in treating shoulder pain, and functional electrical stimulation (FES) targeting the supraspinatus, trapezius, and posterior deltoid muscle for muscle stability (Ping Gu, Juan-juan Ran, & Lei Yu, 2016). Finally, if there is spasticity in the shoulder, treatment of spasticity would be required (and is discussed in the following section).

Spasticity

Spasticity is defined as velocity-dependent increased resistance to passive stretch. Common after stroke, it has an incidence of 25% of patients after 1 week from stroke (Harrison & Field, 2015). Spasticity is an upper motor neuron sign that occurs when there is a lesion to the CNS with other upper motor neuron signs including clonus, pronator drift, dystonia, muscle stiffness, and joint contracture (Harrison & Field, 2015; Lance, 1980). Spasticity is thought to be due to signal mishandling at the spinal cord level and lack of inhibition of the stretch reflex from the supraspinal cord level (Lance, 1980). Spasticity is problematic in stroke recovery as it is painful, causes deformities of the limb and joint, hinders function and mobility, and can affect proper positioning and hygiene (Sunnerhagen, Olver, & Francisco, 2013).

When evaluating spasticity, it is important to measure muscle tone, joint range of motion, muscle stretch reflexes, strength, and motor coordination. The Tardieu Scale and Modified Ashworth Scale are commonly used scales to objectively measure and document spasticity (Bethoux, 2015; Sunnerhagen et al., 2013). They also set goals of treatment with patients and their caregivers (Sunnerhagen et al., 2013). Treatment is multidisciplinary and involves nonpharmacologic and pharmacologic interventions. Muscle stretching therapies are the first-line therapies for spasticity and can be directed by a skilled rehabilitation therapist. These include prolonged positioning and passive, active, isokinetic, and isotonic stretching, which all promote length of muscle tendon unit and decreased motor unit excitability (Nakao et al., 2010; Sunnerhagen et al., 2013). Currently under study are other modalities, which include FES and transcutaneous electrical stimulation (Sunnerhagen et al., 2013).

Pharmacologic treatment includes central and peripheral acting antispasmodics. Central acting antispasmodics include benzodiazepines that act on gamma-aminobutyric acid (GABA) suppression of spinal reflexes; the most commonly used agent is diazepam. Side effects of benzodiazepines include sedation and muscle weakness. Tizanidine depresses the spasticity pathway via alpha-agonist properties and side effects are also sedation, weakness, and transaminitis (Nakao et al., 2010; Sunnerhagen et al., 2013). Gabapentin has documented use in treating spasticity at high doses (2,400–3,600 mg per day) but this is likely limited to side effects of fainting, somnolence, nystagmus, headache, and tremor. Baclofen is a GABA agonist and pre- and postsynaptically inhibits spinal reflexes. Dantrolene sodium inhibits muscle contractility but can cause liver toxicity at doses greater than 200 to 300 mg per day (Nesbitt et al., 2015).

Botulinum toxin is valuable in the treatment of poststroke spasticity, as it does not cause sedation or confusion. Botulinum toxin is injected directly into the spastic muscle and inhibits the release of acetylcholine at the neuromuscular junction, thus preventing the firing of the muscle contraction. It comes in different formulations and has been demonstrated in multiple randomized controlled trials to improve spasticity and a patient's achievement of personal goals (McCrory et al., 2009; Sunnerhagen et al., 2013). Also injected peripherally, phenol has been used for chemodenervation; however, side effects include dysesthesia and soft tissue fibrosis (Sunnerhagen et al., 2013).

For treatment of more severe widespread spasticity, intrathecal baclofen (ITB) can be used. Lower doses of baclofen are used when administered intrathecally, which causes decreased side effects compared with oral baclofen (McCormick et al., 2015). In ITB, baclofen is administered to the intrathecal space continuously through a catheter attached to a small pump implanted into the abdominal wall. The pump requires maintenance with setting adjustments, percutaneous refills at least every 6 months, and battery changes every 5 to 7 years (McCormick et al., 2015), which can be difficult for a patient with a decreased support system or impaired mobility.

Joint contractures can occur after stroke and are thought to be due to shortening of the muscle tendon ligaments and joint capsules (Ada, Goddard, McCully, Stavrinos, & Bampton, 2005; Goldspink & Williams, 1990). After stroke, common patterns of contracture are shoulder abduction and internal rotation, hip and knee flexion, and ankle plantar flexion. Prevention of contractures is most important, with passive range of motion through the functional range of motion several times a day (Ada et al., 2005; Wright et al., 2012). Contractures are treated with prolonged static stretch, serial casting with a skilled therapy team, and with adequate spasticity management (Ada et al., 2005). If contractures are severe and minimally responsive to conservative measures, and are limiting functional gains, a patient may be referred for surgical release (Tafti, Cramer, & Gupta, 2008).

Depression and Anxiety

Depression and anxiety are common after stroke, both with a reported prevalence of roughly one fourth to one third of patients after a stroke (Guajardo et al., 2015; Hackett & Pickles, 2014; Menlove, 2015). Depression and anxiety are associated with worse prognosis, increased mortality, decreased quality of life, and decreased function (Bethoux, 2015). Treatment includes comprehensive psychosocial and pharmacologic interventions. A neuropsychologist or specialized psychologist can provide skilled evaluation and therapy for a patient with stroke, even in the presence of a cognitive and linguistic disorder.

Pharmacological treatment of mood disorder after stroke first includes treatment of pain, and physiological disturbances such as nutrition, infection, constipation, and urinary dysfunction. In addition, patients require addressing of mobility, community entry, and support systems. Referral to social work is helpful. Finally, adjustment of medications with mood-altering side effects can be useful. For instance, some beta-blockers, beta-agonists, antibiotics, antiepileptic drugs, and anti-spasticity agents have documented side effects of depression, anxiety, and irritability.

Selective serotonin reuptake inhibitors (SSRIs) are useful in treating both depression and anxiety after stroke and have been demonstrated to improve neurological outcomes (Chollet et al., 2011; Mead et al., 2012). In a double-blind, placebo-controlled trial, early use of fluoxetine 20 mg resulted in significant motor gains after 90 days (Chollet et al., 2011). Use of SSRIs should be discussed with a patient's neurologist after hemorrhagic stroke, given effects on platelet function. Finally, exercise should not be overlooked as a treatment of depression and anxiety after stroke, given its multiple documented beneficial effects in the literature (Adamson, Ensari, & Motl, 2015).

STAGES OF STROKE RECOVERY

The classical pattern of recovery from stroke has been described by several people. Among the most widely known descriptions are by Twitchell and Brunnstrom (Figure 25.1). Twitchell began publishing descriptions of motor recovery in the 1950s (Twitchell, 1951). He observed that patients who demonstrated some recovery of hand function by 4 weeks had a 70% chance of making a full or good recovery. He observed that most motor recovery occurs in the first 3 months poststroke, and that recovery tends to plateau beyond 6 months. We now know that in many instances motor recovery poststroke can occur well beyond that time frame.

Stage	
1	Flaccidity. No voluntary movement.
2	Spasticity appears. Minimal voluntary movement within synergistic pattern.
3	Increase in spasticity. Patient gains voluntary control over synergy.
4	Decrease in spasticity. Some movement outside of synergy appears, but synergy dominates.
5	Further decrease in spasticity. More complex movement combinations are learned. Synergies lose their dominance.
6	Disappearance of spasticity. Individual joint movements possible. Coordination approaches normal.
7	Normal function.

FIGURE 25.1 Brunnstrom stages of motor recovery.
Source: Lozano et al. (2012) and Mozaffarian et al. (2015).

The Brunnstrom stages were first described by a Swedish physical therapist in the 1960s to describe the synergistic pattern of recovery noted in recovery from flaccid hemiplegia, to normal motor function (Brunnstrom, 1966; Perry, 1967). The term "synergy" refers to recruitment of a whole chain of muscles to perform a given motion, when only a small number of muscles would normally be needed to perform that task. An example of the synergy referred to by Brunnstrom is the whole-arm flexion pattern seen when a patient with a paretic upper extremity tries to flex at their elbow. While all patients do not follow these stages, they serve as a starting point for conversations on prognosis with patients and their families. Also of note is the fact that patterns of poststroke deficits in some cases are becoming less predictable, given the advent of interventions such as administration of thrombolytic therapies during stroke, as well as mechanical thrombectomies.

REHABILITATION THERAPIES

Various rehabilitation specialists partner with stroke survivors throughout their recovery, and under the leadership of a physiatrist, provide therapeutic interventions needed to promote recovery and improve functional independence. Among these professionals are: occupational therapists, physical therapists, speech and language pathologists (SLPs), recreational therapists, vocational rehabilitation specialists, and neuropsychologists.

One common role shared by all therapy disciplines is caregiver education and training. Caregivers are called upon to reinforce strategies learned in rehabilitation, maintain a safe home environment for the patient, and be a source of information for the rehabilitation team should the patient have a cognitive or communicative impairment. In essence, the caregiver becomes an essential part of the rehabilitation team.

Occupational Therapy

The field of occupational therapy emphasizes retraining patients to perform activities of daily living (ADL), as well as upper extremity function in general, while dealing with new neurological deficits (American Occupational Therapy Association, 2016). After stroke, many patients have hemiparesis or hemiplegia, making it necessary for them to relearn techniques for performing their most basic self-care tasks, such as dressing and bathing. Additionally, some occupational therapists have specialized training in vision rehabilitation and driving rehabilitation. As patients return to the community, the role of an occupational therapist may also involve an individualized home assessment through a Barrier Free Design program, which strives to make the home uniquely accessible, given the patient's individual pattern of deficits.

Physical Therapy

The field of physical therapy focuses on enhancing and retraining all aspects of gross functional mobility. With a special focus on gait and transferring, physical therapists employ a range of therapeutic techniques aimed at strengthening muscle groups, improving muscle control, and retraining balance (American Physical Therapy Association, 2011). Physical therapists evaluate patients for assistive devices when appropriate, such as a rolling walker or cane, to improve a patient's functional capacity and overall safety.

The fields of occupational therapy and physical therapy utilize many new technologies to enhance rehabilitation training, several of which are described later in this chapter, including robot-assisted therapy and constraint-induced movement therapy (CIMT).

Speech and Language Pathology

The SLP focuses on improving the impairments of speech (dysarthria), language (aphasia), and swallowing (dysphagia) through specialized rehabilitation interventions. The SLP also addresses the cognitive aspects of communication (e.g., attention, memory, problem solving, executive functioning).

The SLP works closely with the medical and nursing teams to ensure that a patient is administered medications, fluids, and solid foods in the safest way possible. Some patients with dysphagia, or a decrease in arousal or responsiveness, may require a specialized type of diet to ensure their risk of aspiration is minimized. The risk of aspiration, or passage of foreign substance into the lungs, may be increased following stroke should dysphagia be present, or arousal compromised. SLPs are highly trained to use both bedside and radiographic measures to assess for aspiration risk and to determine at what stage of the swallow mechanism the problem exists. They devise strategies the patient can use to maximize safety and minimize aspiration risk while eating or drinking, and train nurses and caregivers in how to promote compliance. Dysphagia responds to rehabilitation techniques and these are overseen by the SLP in parallel to speech and language rehabilitation as needed.

Recreational Therapy

The recreational therapist uses novel activities to promote recovery and well-being during the rehabilitation phase. Recreational therapy can come in many forms, among them horticulture, art, music, and pet-assisted therapy. While a patient may be distracted with what feels to them like a leisure activity, the recreational therapist is sure to reinforce strategies learned in other rehabilitation sessions such as fine motor skills, use of affected extremity, concentration, receptive language skills, and memory.

Vocational Therapy

The role of the vocational therapist becomes most salient once it is appropriate to begin discussions and planning around a stroke survivor's return to either work or school. For many patients, a return to precisely the same job description is not feasible, and plans need to be made for some alternative. Some patients are able to return to the same organization, but their job description may be different, to match their current functional status. Patients with cognitive or communicative impairments are less likely to return to any form of employment poststroke when compared to their counterparts with only physical impairments.

Vocational rehabilitation serves as a liaison between the patient, place of employment or school, and the rehabilitation team, including the physiatrist. In some cases, specific training is recommended to redirect someone's employment course, and the vocational rehabilitation counselor helps to introduce and coordinate this.

Neuropsychology

The field of neuropsychology studies the structure and function of the brain as they relate to specific behaviors and psychological processes. A neuropsychologist delves deeply into the areas of behavior and cognition, and studies how they are affected by neurological disorders such as stroke. A neuropsychologist may become involved early on in the stroke rehabilitation process, to identify areas of cognition, mood, or behavior that require immediate attention, or pose a safety concern; they are also likely to remain involved well into the recovery process to address areas of adjustment and cognitive deficits that have meaningful impact on a person's life.

Some patients benefit from undergoing neuropsychological testing during their recovery from stroke. This assessment closely analyzes all aspects of cognition, and identifies areas of strength and weakness. Following neuropsychological testing, some patients may undergo cognitive remediation, administered by a neuropsychologist, designed to teach new strategies to overcome or circumvent areas of cognitive weakness. This therapy most often occurs in a one-on-one format with a neuropsychologist, but sometimes may occur in a group setting. Individual patient characteristics, chronicity, and prognosis determine which setting is most appropriate for a given patient.

EMERGING TREATMENTS

Transcranial Direct Current Stimulation and Transcranial Magnetic Stimulation

Transcranial direct current stimulation (tDCS) is a form of neuromodulation that uses constant, low electrical current delivered to a chosen area of the brain using electrodes on the scalp. It was originally developed to help patients with brain injuries such as strokes. Tests on healthy adults demonstrated that tDCS can increase cognitive performance on a variety of tasks, depending on the area of the brain being stimulated. tDCS has been theorized to enhance language and mathematical ability, attention span, problem solving, memory, and coordination. Because tDCS is still in early phases of clinical research, it is not yet widely available in the various stroke rehabilitation settings, but it does remain a promising tool for continued study and future use.

While the tDCS method is gaining interest, the most commonly used method of brain neuromodulation is transcranial magnetic stimulation (TMS; Brown, Lutsep, Cramer, & Weinand, 2003; Hummel & Cohen, 2005). This technique of brain stimulation utilizes an electric coil held above the area of interest on the scalp that uses rapidly changing magnetic fields to induce small electrical currents in the brain. There are two types of TMS: repetitive TMS and single-pulse TMS. So far, repetitive TMS has been shown to have longer lasting results. Several studies have looked at TMS in the diagnosis, prognosis, and therapy for poststroke motor deficits.

Both TMS and tDCS are painless and considered safe; however, TMS is more expensive, and more technically difficult to utilize, while tDCS is relatively easy to use. TMS causes the neuron's action potentials to fire, resulting in a stronger effect. Since tDCS only causes increased spontaneous cell firing, it does not have as big of an effect. One benefit of tDCS when compared to TMS is that, due to the smaller effect, there is a much smaller chance of causing harm.

Neuromuscular Electrical Stimulation

Neuromuscular electrical stimulation, commonly referred to as e-stim, can be an effective adjunct treatment following stroke. E-stim artificially bypasses the communication loop from the brain to the muscle, and instead sends a signal directly to the muscle prompting it to contract. When cortical tissue is injured from a stroke, commonly leading to motor weakness in the extremities, the brain is unable to send this signal itself. The clinical uses of e-stim are broad and include spasticity reduction, slowing the development of disuse atrophy, reduction in joint pain, and decreasing the size of shoulder subluxations. E-stim has even been shown to improve swallow function if used to stimulate the muscles involved in the swallow mechanism.

E-stim can also be used as neuroprostheses (Bioness, 2016; Innovative Neurotronics, 2016). Several products are available for patient use, one of which is essentially an ankle–foot orthosis designed for a patient with foot drop, which is wired for use as e-stim, and is designed to trigger dorsiflexion during the appropriate stage of gait. A similar device is available for promotion of wrist extension.

Deep Brain Stimulation

DBS involves neurosurgical implantation of a neurostimulator, which sends electrical impulses through implanted electrodes to chosen parts of the brain (Kringelbach, Jenkinson, Owen, & Aziz, 2007). DBS use in the context of stroke recovery and rehabilitation has been most often studied for its pain reducing properties. Some stroke survivors suffer from a variety of painful syndromes resulting from their brain injury, and DBS is a proposed method of treatment for the severe, intractable cases. DBS for the purpose of stroke recovery or improvement of symptoms is not FDA approved, but it continues to be the subject of ongoing clinical research.

Constraint-Induced Movement Therapy

Many patients suffer from hemiparesis or hemiplegia following stroke, and to compensate often will primarily use their unaffected side to perform tasks. Survivors may initially try to use their affected extremity, especially if it is their dominant side, but their initial failure may discourage them from future efforts. This phenomenon has been described by Dr. Edward Taub and is termed "learned nonuse." Dr. Taub developed CIMT to combat this (Reiss, Wolf, Hammel, McLeod, & Williams, 2012). CIMT involves forced use of the affected side by restraining the unaffected side. With CIMT, the therapist constrains the survivor's unaffected arm in a sling, and the survivor then uses his or her affected arm intensively and repetitively for 2 weeks. The most compelling evidence in favor of CIMT comes from the EXCITE trial (Wolf et al., 2008).

Robotics

There have been numerous recent studies highlighting the use of robotic devices or robot-assisted therapies in the process of stroke recovery (Mehrholz & Pohl, 2012; Mehrholz, Werner, Kugler, & Pohl, 2007; Norouzi-Gheidari, Archambault, & Fung, 2012). To summarize available research, the role of robot-assisted therapy in stroke rehabilitation is currently an adjunct rather than a replacement for traditional rehabilitation therapies. Whole body vibration is used in some clinical settings with the goal of improving motor recovery and neuromuscular control poststroke; however, whole body vibration has recently been shown to have no effect on improving outcomes beyond leg exercises alone (Lau, Yip, & Pang, 2012).

Neuropharmacology in Stroke Recovery

Stroke recovery is the result of multiple simultaneous processes. Intrinsic processes include neuroplasticity and other spontaneous healing mechanisms the brain will undergo on its own. Additionally, avoidance of medical setbacks and complications can eliminate symptoms, which may mask neurological recovery. Extrinsic processes include rehabilitation techniques and other novel treatments mentioned earlier. There is now growing support for the addition of pharmacological agents to promote neurological recovery from stroke. There exists literature to support the use of pharmacologic agents to aid motor recovery (Chollet et al., 2011; Marquez-Romero, Arauz, & Ruiz-Sandoval, 2013) and aphasia recovery (Allen, Mehta, & McClure, 2012; Berthier, Green, & Higueras, 2006). However, there is also evidence that medications can play a positive role in improving memory, mood, and behavior following stroke. The idea is that the addition of these agents creates a synergy with the other recovery mechanisms, as well as promote the recovery process.

CONCLUSION

As stroke still remains the second leading cause of death and third leading cause of disability in the world, it will likely remain a focus in the health care world. Each year we strive to develop improved management strategies, improved survival rates, and decreased impairments in survivors. Still, for patients who have suffered stroke, they have to face ongoing challenges from the first evaluation in the emergency department, through their days in ICU rehabilitation, and upon reentering the community. As they face these challenges, it is paramount that their medical team be attentive to their proper management needs, thus facilitating survival, quality of life, overall function, and return to the community.

REFERENCES

Ada, L., Goddard, E., McCully, J., Stavrinos, T., & Bampton, J. (2005). Thirty minutes of positioning reduces the development of shoulder external rotation contracture after stroke: A randomized controlled trial. *Archives of Physical Medicine and Rehabilitation, 86*(2), 230–234.

Adams, H. P., Jr., Davis, P. H., Leira, E. C., Chang, K. C., Bendixen, B. H., Clarke, W. R., . . . Hansen, M. D. (1999). Baseline NIH stroke scale score strongly predicts outcome after stroke: A report of the trial of org 10172 in acute stroke treatment (TOAST). *Neurology, 53*(1), 126–131.

Adamson, B. C., Ensari, I., & Motl, R. W. (2015). Effect of exercise on depressive symptoms in adults with neurologic disorders: A systematic review and meta-analysis. *Archives of Physical Medicine and Rehabilitation, 96*(7), 1329–1338.

Albers, G. W., Amarenco, P., Easton, J. D., Sacco, R. L., & Teal, P. (2004). Antithrombotic and thrombolytic therapy for ischemic stroke: The seventh ACCP conference on antithrombotic and thrombolytic therapy. *Chest, 126*(Suppl. 3), 483S–512S. doi:10.1378/chest.126.3_suppl.483S

Allen, L., Mehta, S., & McClure, J. A. (2012). Therapeutic interventions for aphasia initiated more than six months post stroke: A review of the evidence. *Topics in Stroke Rehabilitation, 6*, 523–535.

Al-Shahi, R., & Warlow, C. (2001). A systematic review of the frequency and prognosis of arteriovenous malformations of the brain in adults. *Brain, 124*(Pt. 10), 1900–1926.

American Occupational Therapy Association. (2016). Retrieved from http://www.aota.org

American Physical Therapy Association. (2011). Today's physical therapist. Retrieved from http://www.apta.org

Amin, A. N., Lin, J., Thompson, S., & Wiederkehr, D. (2013). Rate of deep-vein thrombosis and pulmonary embolism during the care continuum in patients with acute ischemic stroke in the United States. *BMC Neurology, 13*, 17. doi:10.1186/1471-2377-13-17

Anderson, C. S., Heeley, E., Huang, Y., Wang, J., Stapf, C., Delcourt, C., . . . Investigators, I. (2013). Rapid blood-pressure lowering in patients with acute intracerebral hemorrhage. *New England Journal of Medicine*, 368(25), 2355–2365. doi:10.1056/NEJMoa1214609

Aslanyan, S., Weir, C. J., Diener, H. C., Kaste, M., & Lees, K. R. (2004). Pneumonia and urinary tract infection after acute ischaemic stroke: A tertiary analysis of the GAIN International trial. *European Journal of Neurology, 11*(1), 49–53. doi:10.1046/j.1468-1331.2003.00749.x

Ay, H., Koroshetz, W. J., Benner, T., Vangel, M. G., Melinosky, C., Arsava, E. M., . . . Sorensen, A. G. (2006). Neuroanatomic correlates of stroke-related myocardial injury. *Neurology, 66*, 1325–1329. doi:10.1212/01.wnl.0000206077.13705.6d

Azzimondi, G., Bassein, L., Nonino, F., Fiorani, L., Vignatelli, L., Re, G., . . . D'Alessandro, R. (1995). Fever in acute stroke worsens prognosis. A prospective study. *Stroke, 26*(11), 2040–2043.

Batchelor, F. A., Mackintosh, S. F., Said, C. M., & Hill, K. D. (2012). Falls after stroke. *International Journal of Stroke*, 7, 482–490.

Beghi, E., D'Alessandro, R., Beretta, S., Consoli, D., Crespi, V., Delaj, L., . . . Zaccara, G. (2011). Incidence and predictors of acute symptomatic seizures after stroke. *Neurology, 77*, 1785–1793. doi:10.1212/WNL.0b013e3182364878

Berkhemer, O. A., Fransen, P. S., Beumer, D., van den Berg, L. A., Lingsma, H. F., Yoo, A. J., . . . Investigators, M. C. (2015). A randomized trial of intraarterial treatment for acute ischemic stroke. *The Journal of Emergency Medicine, 372*(1), 11–20. doi:10.1056/NEJMoa1411587

Berthier M. L., Green, C., & Higueras, C. (2006). A randomized, placebo-controlled study of donepezil in poststroke aphasia. *Neurology, 9*, 1687–1689.

Bethoux, F. (2015). Spasticity management after stroke. *Physical Medicine and Rehabilitation Clinics of North America, 4*, 625–639. doi:10.1016/j.pmr.2015.07.003

Bioness. (2016). Retrieved from http://www.bioness.com/Healthcare_Professionals/Exoskeletal_Products/L300_for_Foot_Drop.php

Bladin, C. F., Alexandrov, A. V., Bellavance, A., Bornstein, N., Chambers, B., Coté, R., . . . Norris, J. W. (2000). Seizures after stroke: A prospective multicenter study. *Archives of Neurology, 57*, 1617–1622. doi:10.1001/archneur.57.11.1617

Bravata, D. M., Ho, S. Y., Meehan, T. P., Brass, L. M., & Concato, J. (2007). Readmission and death after hospitalization for acute ischemic stroke: 5-year follow-up in the medicare population. *Stroke, 38*, 1899–1904. doi:10.1161/STROKEAHA.106.481465

Brittain, P. S., & Castleden, C., (1998). Stroke and incontinence. *Stroke, 29*, 524–528.

Broderick, J., Connolly, S., Feldmann, E., Hanley, D., Kase, C., Krieger, D., . . . Outcomes in Research Interdisciplinary Working Group. (2007). Guidelines for the management of spontaneous intracerebral hemorrhage in adults: 2007 update: A guideline from the American Heart Association/American Stroke Association Stroke Council, High Blood Pressure Research Council, and the quality of care and outcomes in research interdisciplinary working group. *Stroke, 38*(6), 2001–2023. doi:10.1161/STROKEAHA.107.183689

Brown, J. A., Lutsep, H., Cramer, S. C., & Weinand, M. (2003). Motor cortex stimulation for enhancement of recovery after stroke: Case report. *Neurological Research, 25*(8), 815–818.

Brunnstrom, S. (1966). Motor testing procedures in hemiplegia: Based on sequential recovery stages. *Physical Therapy, 46*(4), 357–375.

Callaly, E. L., Chroinin, D., Hannon, N., Sheehan, O., Marnane, M., Merwick, A., . . . Kyne, L. (2015). Falls and fractures 2 years after acute stroke: The North Dublin population stroke study. *Age and Ageing, 5*, 882–886. doi:10.1093/ageing/afv093

Camara-Lemarroy, C. R., Ibarra-Yruegas, B. E., & Gongora-Rivera, F. (2014). Gastrointestinal complications after ischemic stroke. *Journal of the Neurological Sciences, 15*, 20–25. doi:10.1016/j.jns.2014.08.027

Campbell, B. C., Mitchell, P. J., Yan, B., Parsons, M. W., Christensen, S., Churilov, L., . . . EXTEND-IA investigators. (2014). A multicenter, randomized, controlled study to investigate Extending the time for thrombolysis in emergency neurological deficits with intra-arterial therapy (EXTEND-IA). *International Journal of Stroke, 9*(1), 126–132. doi:10.1111/ijs.12206

Capes, S. E., Hunt, D., Malmberg, K., Pathak, P., & Gerstein, H. C. (2001). Stress hyperglycemia and prognosis of stroke in nondiabetic and diabetic patients: A systematic overview. *Stroke, 32*(10), 2426–2432.

Chernyshev, O. Y., Martin-Schild, S., Albright, K. C., Barreto, A., Misra, V., Acosta, I., . . . Savitz, S. I. (2010). Safety of tPA in stroke mimics and neuroimaging-negative cerebral ischemia. *Neurology, 74*(17), 1340–1345. doi:10.1212/WNL.0b013e3181dad5a6

Chollet, F., Tardy, J., Albucher, J. F., Thalamas, C., Berard, E., Lamy, C., . . . Loubinoux, I. (2011). Fluoxetine for motor recovery after acute ischaemic stroke (FLAME): A randomised placebo-controlled trial. *The Lancet Neurology, 10*(2), 123–130. doi:10.1016/S1474-4422(10)70314-8

Conrad, J., Pawlowski, M., Dogan, M., Kovac, S., Ritter, M. A., & Evers, S. (2013). Seizures after cerebrovascular events: Risk factors and clinical features. *Seizure: The Journal of the British Epilepsy Association, 22*, 275–282. doi:10.1016/j.seizure.2013.01.014

Cucchiara, B., Messe, S., Sansing, L., Kasner, S., Lyden, P., & CHANT Investigators. (2008). Hematoma growth in oral anticoagulant related intracerebral hemorrhage. *Stroke, 39*(11), 2993–2996. doi:10.1161/STROKEAHA.108.520668

Daniele, O., Caravaglios, G., Fierro, B., & Natalè, E. (2002). Stroke and cardiac arrhythmias. *Journal of Stroke and Cerebrovascular Diseases, 11*, 28–33. doi:10.1053/jscd.2002.123972

Daniels, S. K., Anderson, J. A., & Willson, P. C. (2012). Valid items for screening dysphagia risk in patients with stroke: A systematic review. *Stroke, 43*, 892–897. doi:10.1161/STROKEAHA.111.640946

Dennis, M., Mordi, N., Graham, C., & Sandercock, P. (2011). The timing, extent, progression and regression of deep vein thrombosis in immobile stroke patients: Observational data from the CLOTS multicenter randomized trials. *Journal of Thrombosis and Haemostasis, 9*, 2193–2200. doi:10.1111/j.1538-7836.2011.04486.x

Dennis, M., Sandercock, P. A. G., Reid, J., Graham, C., Murray, G., Venables, G., . . . CLOTS Trials Collaboration. (2009). Effectiveness of thigh-length graduated compression stockings to reduce the risk of deep vein thrombosis after stroke (CLOTS trial 1): A multicentre, randomised controlled trial. *The Lancet, 373*, 1958–1965. doi:10.1016/S0140-6736(09)60941-7

Dennis, M., Sandercock, P., Reid, J., Graham, C., Forbes, J., & Murray, G. (2013). Effectiveness of intermittent pneumatic compression in reduction of risk of deep vein thrombosis in patients who have had a stroke (CLOTS 3): A multicentre randomised controlled trial. *The Lancet, 382*(9891), 516–524. doi:10.1016/S0140-6736(13)61050-8

Dromerick, A. W., Edwards, D. F., & Kumar, A. (2008). Hemiplegic shoulder pain syndrome: Frequency and characteristics during inpatient stroke rehabilitation. *Archives of Physical Medicine and Rehabilitation, 89*, 1589–1593.

Dütsch, M., Burger, M., Dörfler, C., Schwab, S., & Hilz, M. J. (2007). Cardiovascular autonomic function in poststroke patients. *Neurology, 69*, 2249–2255. doi:10.1212/01.wnl.0000286946.06639.a7

Emberson, J., Lees, K. R., Lyden, P., Blackwell, L., Albers, G., Bluhmki, E., . . . Stroke Thrombolysis Trialists' Collaborative Group. (2014). Effect of treatment delay, age, and stroke severity on the effects of intravenous thrombolysis with alteplase for acute ischaemic stroke: A meta-analysis of individual patient data from randomised trials. *The Lancet, 384*(9958), 1929–1935. doi:10.1016/S0140-6736(14)60584-5

Emerging Risk Factors Collaboration., Sarwar, N., Gao, P., Seshasai, S. R., Gobin, R., Kaptoge, S., . . . Danesh, J. (2010). Diabetes mellitus, fasting blood glucose concentration, and risk of vascular disease: A collaborative meta-analysis of 102 prospective studies. *The Lancet, 375*(9733), 2215–2222. doi:10.1016/S0140-6736(10)60484-9

Engler, T. M., Dourado, C. C., Amâncio. T. G., Farage, L., de Mello, P. A., & Padula. M. P. (2014). Stroke: bowel dysfunction in patients admitted for rehabilitation. *The Open Nursing Journal*, 8, 43–47. doi:10.2174/1874434601408010043

Flibotte, J. J., Hagan, N., O'Donnell, J., Greenberg, S. M., & Rosand, J. (2004). Warfarin, hematoma expansion, and outcome of intracerebral hemorrhage. *Neurology, 63*(6), 1059–1064.

Gelber, D. A., Good, D. C., Laven, L. J., & Verhulst, S. J. (1993). Causes of urinary incontinence after acute hemispheric stroke. *Stroke, 3*, 378–382.

Glymour, M. M., Kosheleva, A., & Boden-Albala, B. (2009). Birth and adult residence in the Stroke Belt independently predict stroke mortality. *Neurology, 73*(22), 1858–1865. doi:10.1212/WNL.0b013e3181c47cad

Goldspink, G., & Williams, P. E. (1990). Muscle fibre and connective tissue changes associated with use and disuse. In L. Ada & C. Canning (Eds.), *Key issues in neurological physiotherapy* (pp. 197–218). Oxford, England: Butterworth-Heinemann.

Goldstein, L. B., & Samsa, G. P. (1997). Reliability of the National institutes of health stroke scale. Extension to non-neurologists in the context of a clinical trial. *Stroke, 28*(2), 307–310.

Goldstein, L. B., & Simel, D. L. (2005). Is this patient having a stroke? *Journal of the American Medical Association, 293*(19), 2391–2402. doi:10.1001/jama.293.19.2391

Gorelick, P. B., Hier, D. B., Caplan, L. R., & Langenberg, P. (1986). Headache in acute cerebrovascular disease. *Neurology, 36*, 1445–1450.

Goyal, M., Demchuk, A. M., Menon, B. K., Eesa, M., Rempel, J. L., Thornton, J., . . . ESCAPE Trial Investigators. (2015). Randomized assessment of rapid endovascular treatment of ischemic stroke. *New England Journal of Medicine, 372*(11), 1019–1030. doi:10.1056/NEJMoa1414905

Grau, A. J., Buggle, F., Schnitzler, P., Spiel, M., Lichy, C., & Hacke, W. (1999). Fever and infection early after ischemic stroke. *Journal of the Neurological Sciences, 171*, 115–120. doi:10.1016/S0022-510X(99)00261-0

Guajardo, V. D., Terroni, L., Sobreiro, M. deF., Zerbini, M. I., Tinone, G., Scaff, M., . . . Fráguas, R. (2015). The influence of depressive symptoms on quality of life after stroke: A prospective study. *Journal of Stroke and Cerebrovascular Diseases, 24*(1), 201–209. doi:10.1016/j.jstrokecerebrovasdis.2014.08.020

Hackett, M. L., & Pickles, K. (2014). Part I: Frequency of depression after stroke: An updated systematic review and meta-analysis of observational studies. *International Journal of Stroke, 9*(8), 1017–1025. doi:10.1111/ijs.12357

Harari, D., Coshall, C., Rudd, A. G., & Wolfe, C. D. (2003). New-onset fecal incontinence after stroke: Prevalence, natural history, risk factors, and impact. *Stroke, 34*, 144–150.

Harrison, R. A., & Field, T. S. (2015). Post stroke pain: Identification, assessment, and therapy. *Cerebrovascular Diseases, 39*, 190–201. doi:10.1159/000375397

Hemphill, J. C., 3rd., Bonovich, D. C., Besmertis, L., Manley, G. T., & Johnston, S. C. (2001). The ICH score: A simple, reliable grading scale for intracerebral hemorrhage. *Stroke, 32*(4), 891–897.

Hemphill, J. C., 3rd., Farrant, M., & Neill, T. A., Jr. (2009). Prospective validation of the ICH Score for 12-month functional outcome. *Neurology, 73*(14), 1088–1094. doi:10.1212/WNL.0b013e3181b8b332

Herzig, S. J., Howell, M. D., Ngo, L. H., & Marcantonio, E. R. (2009). Acid-suppressive medication use and the risk for hospital-acquired pneumonia. *Journal of the American Medical Association, 301*, 2120–2128. doi:10.1001/jama.2009.722

Hilker, R., Poetter, C., Findeisen, N., Sobesky, J., Jacobs, A., Neveling, M., & Heiss, W. D. (2003). Nosocomial pneumonia after acute stroke: Implications for neurological intensive care medicine. *Stroke, 34*, 975–981. doi:10.1161/01.STR.0000063373.70993.CD

Hill, M. D., Lye, T., Moss, H., Barber, P. A., Demchuk, A. M., Newcommon, N. J., . . . Buchan, A. M. (2003). Hemi-orolingual angioedema and ACE inhibition after alteplase treatment of stroke. *Neurology, 60*(9), 1525–1527.

Hinchey, J. A., Shephard, T., Furie, K., Smith, D., Wang, D., & Tonn, S. (2005). Formal dysphagia screening protocols prevent pneumonia. *Stroke, 36*, 1972–1976. doi:10.1161/01.STR.0000177529.86868.8d

Hummel, F., & Cohen, L. G. (2005). Improvement of motor function with noninvasive cortical stimulation in a patient with chronic stroke. *Neurorehabilitation and Neural Repair, 19*(1), 14–19.

Ingeman, A., Andersen, G., Hundborg, H. H., Svendsen, M. L., & Johnsen, S. P. (2011). In-hospital medical complications, length of stay, and mortality among stroke unit patients. *Stroke, 42*, 3214–3218. doi:10.1161/STROKEAHA.110.610881

Innovative Neurotronics. (2016). Retrieved from http://walkaide.com/patients/Pages/default.aspx

James, P., Ellis, C. J., Whitlock, R. M., McNeil, A. R., Henley, J., & Anderson, N. E. (2000). Relation between troponin T concentration and mortality in patients presenting with an acute stroke: Observational study. *British Medical Journal (Clinical Research ed.), 320*, 1502–1504.

Jauch, E. C., Saver, J. L., Adams, H. P., Jr., Bruno, A., Connors, J. J., Demaerschalk, B. M., . . . Council on Clinical. (2013). Guidelines for the early management of patients with acute ischemic stroke: A guideline for healthcare professionals from the American Heart Association/American Stroke Association. *Stroke, 44*(3), 870–947. doi:10.1161/STR.0b013e318284056a

Johnston, K. C., Li, J. Y., Lyden, P. D., Hanson, S. K., Feasby, T. E., Adams, R. J., . . . Haley, E. C. (1998). Medical and neurological complications of ischemic stroke: Experience from the RANTTAS trial. RANTTAS Investigators. *Stroke: A Journal of Cerebral Circulation, 29*, 447–453. doi:10.1161/01.STR.29.2.447

Johnston, S. C. (2002). Clinical practice. Transient ischemic attack. *New England Journal of Medicine, 347*(21), 1687–1692. doi:10.1056/NEJMcp020891

Johnston, S. C. (2005). Transient ischemic attack: A dangerous Harbinger and an opportunity to intervene. *Seminars in Neurology, 25*(4), 362–370. doi:10.1055/s-2005-923530

Jovin, T. G., Chamorro, A., Cobo, E., de Miquel, M. A., Molina, C. A., Rovira, A., . . . Investigators, R. T. (2015). Thrombectomy within 8 hours after symptom onset in ischemic stroke. *New England Journal of Medicine, 372*(24), 2296–2306. doi:10.1056/NEJMoa1503780

Kallmünzer, B., Breuer, L., Kahl, N., Bobinger, T., Raaz-Schrauder, D., Huttner, H. B., . . . Köhrmann, M. (2012). Serious cardiac arrhythmias after stroke: Incidence, time course, and predictors-a systematic, prospective analysis. *Stroke, 43*, 2892–2897. doi:10.1161/STROKEAHA.112.664318

Kamphuisen, P. W., & Agnelli, G. (2007). What is the optimal pharmacological prophylaxis for the prevention of deep-vein thrombosis and pulmonary embolism in patients with acute ischemic stroke? *Thrombosis Research, 119*, 265–274. doi:10.1016/j.thromres.2006.03.010

Kawachi, I., Colditz, G. A., Stampfer, M. J., Willett, W. C., Manson, J. E., Rosner, B., . . . Hennekens, C. H. (1993). Smoking cessation and decreased risk of stroke in women. *Journal of the American Medical Association, 269*(2), 232–236.

Kelly, J., Rudd, A., Lewis, R. R., Coshall, C., Moody, A., & Hunt, B. J. (2004). Venous thromboembolism after acute ischemic stroke: A prospective study using magnetic resonance direct thrombus imaging. *Stroke; A Journal of Cerebral Circulation, 35*, 2320–2325. doi:10.1161/01.STR.0000140741.13279.4f

Kelly, J., Rudd, A., Lewis, R., & Hunt, B. J. (2001). Venous thromboembolism after acute stroke. *Stroke, 32*(1), 262–267. doi:10.1161/01.STR.32.1.262

Kernan, W. N., Ovbiagele, B., Black, H. R., Bravata, D. M., Chimowitz, M. I., Ezekowitz, M. D., . . . Council on Peripheral Vascular. (2014). Guidelines for the prevention of stroke in patients with stroke and transient ischemic attack: A guideline for healthcare professionals from the American heart association/American stroke association. *Stroke, 45*(7), 2160–2236. doi:10.1161/STR.0000000000000024

Kong, K. H., & Young, S. (2000). Incidence and outcome of poststroke urinary retention: A prospective study. *Archives of Physical Medicine and Rehabilitation, 11*, 1464–1467.

Kringelbach, M. L., Jenkinson, N., Owen, S. L. F., & Aziz, T. Z. (2007). Translational principles of deep brain stimulation. *Nature Reviews Neuroscience, 8*(8), 623–635. doi:10.1038/nrn2196

Krogh, K., Christensen, P., & Laurberg, S. (2001). Colorectal symptoms in patients with neurological diseases. *Acta Neurologica Scandinavica, 103*, 335–343.

Kumar, S., Selim, M. H., & Caplan, L. R. (2010). Medical complications after stroke. *The Lancet Neurology, 9*(1), 105–118. doi:10.1016/S1474-4422(09)70266-2

Kwan, J., & Hand, P. (2007). Infection after acute stroke is associated with poor short-term outcome. *Acta Neurologica Scandinavica, 115*, 331–338. doi:10.1111/j.1600-0404.2006.00783.x

Labovitz, D. L., Halim, A. X., Brent, B., Boden-Albala, B., Hauser, W. A., & Sacco, R. L. (2006). Subarachnoid hemorrhage incidence among whites, blacks and caribbean hispanics: The northern manhattan study. *Neuroepidemiology, 26*(3), 147–150. doi:10.1159/000091655

Lance, J. W. (1980). Spasticity: Disordered motor control. In R. G. Feldman, R. R. Young, W. P. Koella (Ed.), *Symposium synopsis* (pp. 485–494). Chicago, IL: Year Book Medical Publishers.

Lane, R. D., Wallace, J. D., Petrosky, P. P., Schwartz, G. E., & Gradman, A. H. (1992). Supraventricular tachycardia in patients with right hemisphere strokes. *Stroke: A Journal of Cerebral Circulation, 23*, 362–366. doi:10.1161/01.STR.23.3.362

Langhorne, P., Stott, D. J., Robertson, L., MacDonald, J., Jones, L., McAlpine, C., . . . Murray, G. (2000). Medical complications after stroke: A multicenter study. *Stroke: A Journal of Cerebral Circulation, 31*, 1223–1229. doi:10.1161/01.STR.31.6.1223

Lapeyre, E., Kuks, J., & Meijler, W. J. (2010). Spasticity: Revisiting the role and the individual value of several pharmacological treatments. *NeuroRehabilitation, 27*(2), 193–200. doi:10.3233/NRE-2010-0596

Lau, R. W., Yip, S. P., & Pang, M. Y. (2012). Whole-body vibration has no effect on neuromotor function and falls in chronic stroke. *Medicine & Science in Sports & Exercise, 44*(8), 1409–1418.

Lederle, F. A., Zylla, D., MacDonald, R., & Wilt, T. J. (2011). Venous thromboembolism prophylaxis in hospitalized medical patients and those with stroke: A background review for an American college of physicians clinical practice guideline. *Annals of Internal Medicine, 155*(9), 602–615. doi:10.7326/0003-4819-155-9-201111010-00008

Lee, S. Y., Chou, C. L., Hsu, S. P., Yeh, C. C., Hung, C. J., Chen, T. L., & Liao, C. C. (2016). Outcomes after stroke in patients with previous pressure ulcer: A nationwide matched retrospective cohort study. *Journal of Stroke and Cerebrovascular Diseases*, 1, 220–227. doi:10.1016/j.jstrokecerebrovasdis.2015.09.022

Liao, J., O'Donnell, M. J., Silver, F. L., Thiruchelvam, D., Saposnik, G., Fang, J., . . . Kapral, M. K. (2009). In-hospital myocardial infarction following acute ischaemic stroke: An observational study. *European Journal of Neurology, 16*, 1035–1040. doi:10.1111/j.1468-1331.2009.02647

Lim, S. F., Ong, S. Y., Tan, Y. L., Ng, Y. S., Chan, Y. H., & Childs, C. (2015). Incidence and predictors of new-onset constipation during acute hospitalisation after stroke. *International Journal of Clinical Practice*, *4*, 422–428. doi:10.1111/ijcp.12528

Loiseau, J., Loiseau, P., Duché, B., Guyot, M., Dartigues, J. F., & Aublet, B. (1990). A survey of epileptic disorders in southwest France: Seizures in elderly patients. *Annals of Neurology, 27*, 232–237. doi:10.1002/ana.410270304

Lozano, R., Naghavi, M., Foreman, K., Lim, S., Shibuya, K., Aboyans, V., . . . Memish, Z. A. (2012). Global and regional mortality from 235 causes of death for 20 age groups in 1990 and 2010: A systematic analysis for the global burden of disease study 2010. *The Lancet, 380*(9859), 2095–2128. doi:10.1016/S0140-6736(12)61728-0

Mann, G., & Hankey, G. J. (2001). Initial clinical and demographic predictors of swallowing impairment following acute stroke. *Dysphagia, 16*, 208–215.

Marquez-Romero, J. M., Arauz, A., & Ruiz-Sandoval, J. L. (2013). Fluoxetine for motor recovery after acute intracerebral hemorrhage (FMRICH): Study protocol for a randomized, double-blind, placebo-controlled, multicenter trial. *Trials*, *14*, 77.

Martino, R., Foley, N., Bhogal, S., Diamant, N., Speechley, M., & Teasell, R. (2005). Dysphagia after stroke: Incidence, diagnosis, and pulmonary complications. *Stroke: A Journal of Cerebral Circulation, 36*, 2756–2763. doi:10.1161/01.STR.0000190056.76543.eb

McCormick, Z. L., Chu, S. K., Binler, D., Neudorf, D., Mathur, S. N., Lee, J., & Marciniak, C. (2015). Intrathecal versus oral baclofen: A matched cohort study of spasticity, pain, sleep, fatigue, and quality of life. *PM&R: The Journal of Injury, Function and Rehabilitation, 7*(9), S1934–S1482. doi:10.1016/j.pmrj.2015.10.005

McCrory, P., Turner-Stokes, L., Baguley, I. J., De Graaff, S., Katrak, P., Sandanam, J., . . . Hughes, A. (2009). Botulinum toxin A for treatment of upper limb spasticity following stroke: A multi-centre randomized placebo-controlled study of the effects on quality of life and other person-centred outcomes. *Journal of Rehabilitation Medicine, 41*(7), 536–544. doi:10.2340/16501977-0366

McKenzie, P., & Badlani, G. H. (2012). The incidence and etiology of overactive bladder in patients after cerebrovascular accident. *Current Urology Reports, 5*, 402–406. doi:10.1007/s11934-012-0269-6

Mead, G. E., Hsieh, C. F., Lee, R., Kutlubaev, M. A., Claxton, A., Hankey, G. J., . . . Hackett, M. L. (2012). Selective serotonin reuptake inhibitors (SSRIs) for stroke recovery. *Cochrane Database of Systematic Reviews, 14*, 11, CD009286. doi:0.1002/14651858

Mehrholz, J., & Pohl, M. (2012). Electromechanical-assisted gait training after stroke: A systematic review comparing end-effector and exoskeleton devices. *Journal of Rehabilitation Medicine, 44*, 193–199.

Mehrholz, J., Werner, C., Kugler, J., & Pohl, M. (2007). Electromechanical-assisted training for walking after stroke. *Cochrane Database of Systematic Reviews*, 4, CD006185.

Menlove, L., Crayton, E., Kneebone, I., Allen-Crooks, R., Otto, E., & Harder, H. (2015). Predictors of anxiety after stroke: A systematic review of observational studies. *Journal of Stroke and Cerebrovascular Diseases, 24*(6), 1107–1117. doi:10.1016/j.jstrokecerebrovasdis.2014.12.036

Morgenstern, L. B., Hemphill, J. C., 3rd., Anderson, C., Becker, K., Broderick, J. P., Connolly, E. S., Jr., . . . Council on Cardiovascular. (2010). Guidelines for the management of spontaneous intracerebral hemorrhage: A guideline for healthcare professionals from the American heart association/American stroke association. *Stroke, 41*(9), 2108–2129. doi:10.1161/STR.0b013e3181ec611b

Mozaffarian, D., Benjamin, E. J., Go, A. S., Arnett, D. K., Blaha, M. J., Cushman, M., . . . Stroke Statistics. (2015). Heart disease and stroke statistics--2015 update: A report from the American Heart Association. *Circulation, 131*(4), e29–322. doi:10.1161/CIR.0000000000000152

Nakao, S., Takata, S., Uemura, H., Kashihara, M., Osawa, T., Komatsu, K., . . . Yasui, N. (2010). Relationship between barthel index scores during the acute phase of rehabilitation and subsequent ADL in stroke patients. *The Journal of Medical Investigation, 57*(1–2), 81–88.

Nakayama, H., Jorgensen, H. S., Raaschou, H. O., & Olsen, T. S. (1994). Recovery of upper extremity function in stroke patients: The copenhagen stroke study. *Archives of Physical Medicine and Rehabilitation, 75*(4), 394–398.

Nesbitt, J., Moxham, S., Ramadurai, G., & Williams, L. (2015). Improving pain assessment and managment in stroke patients. *BMJ Quality Improvement Reports, 4*(1). doi:10.1136/bmjquality.u203375.w3105

Norouzi-Gheidari, N., Archambault, P. S., & Fung, J. (2012). Effects of robot-assisted therapy on stroke rehabilitation in upper limbs: Systematic review and meta-analysis of the literature. *The Journal of Rehabilitation Research and Development, 49*, 479–496.

Oh, H., & Seo, W. A. (2015). Comprehensive review of central post-stroke pain. *Pain Management Nursing, 5*, 804–818. doi:10.1016/j.pmn.2015.03.002

Oppenheimer, S. M., Wilson, J. X., Guiraudon, C., & Cechetto, D. F. (1991). Insular cortex stimulation produces lethal cardiac arrhythmias: A mechanism of sudden death? *Brain Research, 550*, 115–121. doi:10.1016/0006-8993(91)90412-O

Ostaszkiewicz, J., Johnston, L., & Roe, B. (2004). Habit retraining for the management of urinary incontinence in adults. *Cochrane Database of Systematic Reviews*, (2), CD002801.

Perry, C. E. (1967). Principles and techniques of the Brunnstrom approach to the treatment of hemiplegia. *Australian Occupational Therapy Journal, 46*(1), 789–815.

Ping Gu, M. M., Juan-juan Ran, M. M., & Lei Yu, M. M. (2016). Electrical stimulation for hemiplegic shoulder function: A systematic review and metaanalysis of 15 randomized controlled trials. *Archives of Physical Medicine and Rehabilitation, 16*, 30147-30152. doi:10.1016/j.apmr.2016.04.011

Powers, W. J., Derdeyn, C. P., Biller, J., Coffey, C. S., Hoh, B. L., Jauch, E. C., . . . American Heart Association Stroke. (2015). 2015 American Heart Association/American Stroke Association focused update of the 2013 guidelines for the early management of patients with acute ischemic stroke regarding endovascular treatment: A guideline for healthcare professionals from the American heart Association/American Stroke Association. *Stroke, 46*(10), 3020–3035. doi:10.1161/STR.0000000000000074

Prosser, J., MacGregor, L., Lees, K. R., Diener, H.-C., Hacke, W., & Davis, S. (2007). Predictors of early cardiac morbidity and mortality after ischemic stroke. *Stroke: A Journal of Cerebral Circulation, 38*, 2295–2302. doi:10.1161/STROKEAHA.106.471813

Rapsomaniki, E., Timmis, A., George, J., Pujades-Rodriguez, M., Shah, A. D., Denaxas, S., . . . Hemingway, H. (2014). Blood pressure and incidence of twelve cardiovascular diseases: Lifetime risks, healthy life-years lost, and age-specific associations in 1.25 million people. *The Lancet, 383*(9932), 1899–1911. doi:10.1016/S0140-6736(14)60685-1

Reiss, A. P., Wolf, S. L., Hammel, E. A., McLeod, E. L., & Williams, E. A. (2012). Constraint-induced movement therapy (CIMT): Current perspectives and future directions. *Stroke Research and Treatment, 2012*, 159391. doi:10.1155/2012/159391

Rosand, J., Eckman, M. H., Knudsen, K. A., Singer, D. E., & Greenberg, S. M. (2004). The effect of warfarin and intensity of anticoagulation on outcome of intracerebral hemorrhage. *Archives of Internal Medicine, 164*(8), 880–884. doi:10.1001/archinte.164.8.880

Rovira, A., Grive, E., Rovira, A., & Alvarez-Sabin, J. (2005). Distribution territories and causative mechanisms of ischemic stroke. *European Radiology, 15*(3), 416–426. doi:10.1007/s00330-004-2633-5

Sandercock, P. A. G. (1997). The International Stroke Trial (IST): A randomised trial of aspirin, subcutaneous heparin, both, or neither among 19,435 patients with acute ischaemic stroke. *The Lancet, 349*, 1569–1581. doi:10.1016/S0140-6736(97)04011-7

Sanna, T., Diener, H. C., Passman, R. S., Di Lazzaro, V., Bernstein, R. A., Morillo, C. A., . . . Investigators, C. A. (2014). Cryptogenic stroke and underlying atrial fibrillation. *New England Journal of Medicine, 370*(26), 2478–2486. doi:10.1056/NEJMoa1313600

Saver, J. L. (2006). Time is brain--quantified. *Stroke, 37*(1), 263–266. doi:10.1161/01.STR.0000196957.55928.ab

Saver, J. L., Fonarow, G. C., Smith, E. E., Reeves, M. J., Grau-Sepulveda, M. V., Pan, W., . . . Schwamm, L. H. (2013). Time to treatment with intravenous tissue plasminogen activator and outcome from acute ischemic stroke. *Journal of the American Medical Association, 309*(23), 2480–2488. doi:10.1001/jama.2013.6959

Saver, J. L., Goyal, M., Bonafe, A., Diener, H. C., Levy, E. I., Pereira, V. M., . . . SWIFT PRIME Investigators. (2015). Solitaire with the intention for thrombectomy as primary endovascular treatment for acute ischemic stroke (SWIFT PRIME) trial: Protocol for a randomized, controlled, multicenter study comparing the Solitaire revascularization device with IV tPA with IV tPA alone in acute ischemic stroke. *International Journal of Stroke, 10*(3), 439–448. doi:10.1111/ijs.12459

Sellars, C., Bowie, L., Bagg, J., Sweeney, M. P., Miller, H., Tilston, J., . . . Stott, D. J. (2007). Risk factors for chest infection in acute stroke: A prospective cohort study. *Stroke: A Journal of Cerebral Circulation, 38*, 2284–2291. doi:10.1161/STROKEAHA.106.478156

Shorr, A. F., Jackson, W. L., Sherner, J. H., & Moores, L. K. (2008). Differences between low-molecular-weight and unfractionated heparin for venous thromboembolism prevention following ischemic stroke: A metaanalysis. *Chest, 133*, 149–155. doi:10.1378/chest.07-1826

Smithard, D. G., O'Neill, P. A., Parks, C., & Morris, J. (1996). Complications and outcome after acute stroke. Does dysphagia matter? *Stroke: A Journal of Cerebral Circulation, 27*, 1200–1204. doi:10.1161/01.STR.27.7.1200

So, E. L., Annegers, J. F., Hauser, W. A., O'Brien, P. C., & Whisnant, J. P. (1996). Population-based study of seizure disorders after cerebral infarction. *Neurology, 46*, 350–5. doi:10.1212/WNL.46.2.350

Stein, M., Misselwitz, B., Hamann, G. F., Scharbrodt, W., Schummer, D. I., & Oertel, M. F. (2012). Intracerebral hemorrhage in the very old: Future demographic trends of an aging population. *Stroke, 43*(4), 1126–1128. doi:10.1161/STROKEAHA.111.644716

Steiner, T., Mendoza, G., De Georgia, M., Schellinger, P., Holle, R., & Hacke, W. (1997). Prognosis of stroke patients requiring mechanical ventilation in a neurological critical care unit. *Stroke, 28*(4), 711–715.

Su, Y., Zhang, X., Zeng, J., Pei Z., Cheung, R., & Zhou, Q. (2009). New-onset constipation at acute stage after first stroke: Incidence, risk factors, and impact on the stroke outcome. *Stroke, 40*, 1304–1309.

Sunnerhagen, K. S., Olver, J., & Francisco, G. E. (2013). Assessing and treating functional impairment in poststroke spasticity. *Neurology, 80*, 35–44. doi:10.1212/WNL.0b013e3182764aa2

Szczudlik, A., Dobrogowski, J., Wordliczek, J., Stępień, A., Krajnik, M., Leppert, W., . . . Malec-Milewska, M. (2014). Diagnosis and management of neuropathic pain: Review of literature and recommendations of the Polish Association for the study of pain and the Polish Neurological Society-part one. *Neurologia i Neurochirurgia Polska, 4*, 262–271. doi:10.1016/j.pjnns.2014.07.011

Tafti, M. A., Cramer, S. C., & Gupta, R. (2008). Orthopaedic management of the upper extremity of stroke patients. *Journal of the American Academy of Orthopaedic Surgeons, 16*(8), 462–470.

Tânia, M. N., de Engler, C., Thais, G. D., Amâncio, L., Farage, P., de Mello, A., & Marcele, P. C. Padula. (2013). *Dressing materials for the treatment of pressure ulcers in patients in long-term care facilities: A review of the comparative clinical effectiveness and guidelines* [Internet]. Ottawa, ON: Canadian Agency for Drugs and Technologies in Health.

Twitchell, T. E. (1951). The restoration of motor function following hemiplegia in man. *Brain, 74*(4), 443–480. doi:10.1093/brain/74.4.443

van Asch, C. J., Luitse, M. J., Rinkel, G. J., van der Tweel, I., Algra, A., & Klijn, C. J. (2010). Incidence, case fatality, and functional outcome of intracerebral haemorrhage over time, according to age, sex, and ethnic origin: A systematic review and meta-analysis. *The Lancet Neurology, 9*(2), 167–176. doi:10.1016/S1474-4422(09)70340-0

Veerbeek, J. M., Van Wegen, E. E., Harmeling-Van der Wel, B. C., Kwakkel, G., & EPOS Investigators. (2011). Is accurate prediction of gait in nonambulatory stroke patients possible within 72 hours poststroke? The EPOS study. *Neurorehabilitation and Neural Repair, 25*(3), 268–274. doi:10.1177/1545968310384271

Viswanathan, A., & Greenberg, S. M. (2011). Cerebral amyloid angiopathy in the elderly. *Annals of Neurology, 70*(6), 871–880. doi:10.1002/ana.22516

Vlak, M. H., Algra, A., Brandenburg, R., & Rinkel, G. J. (2011). Prevalence of unruptured intracranial aneurysms, with emphasis on sex, age, comorbidity, country, and time period: A systematic review and meta-analysis. *The Lancet Neurology, 10*(7), 626–636. doi:10.1016/S1474-4422(11)70109-0

Vogt, G., Laage, R., Shuaib, A., Schneider, A., & VISTA Collaboration. (2012). Initial lesion volume is an independent predictor of clinical stroke outcome at day 90: An analysis of the virtual international stroke trials archive (VISTA) database. *Stroke, 43*(5), 1266–1272. doi:10.1161/STROKEAHA.111.646570

Warlow, C., Ogston, D., & Douglas, A. S. (1976). Deep venous thrombosis of the legs after strokes. Part I—incidence and predisposing factors. *British Medical Journal, 1*, 1178–1181. doi:10.1136/bmj.1.6019.1178

White, H., Boden-Albala, B., Wang, C., Elkind, M. S., Rundek, T., Wright, C. B., & Sacco, R. L. (2005). Ischemic stroke subtype incidence among whites, blacks, and Hispanics: The northern manhattan study. *Circulation, 111*(10), 1327–1331. doi:10.1161/01.CIR.0000157736.19739.D0

Williams, M. P. (2012). Urinary symptoms and natural history of urinary continence after first-ever stroke--a longitudinal population-based study. *Age and Ageing, 3*, 371–6.

Winkler, D. T., Fluri, F., Fuhr, P., Wetzel, S. G., Lyrer, P. A., Ruegg, S., & Engelter, S. T. (2009). Thrombolysis in stroke mimics: Frequency, clinical characteristics, and outcome. *Stroke, 40*(4), 1522–1525. doi:10.1161/STROKEAHA.108.530352

Wolf, S. L., Winstein, C. J., Miller, J. P., Thompson, P. A., Taub, E., Uswatte, G., . . . Clark, P. C. (2008). The EXCITE trial: Retention of improved upper extremity function among stroke survivors receiving CI movement therapy. *The Lancet Neurology, 7*(1), 33–40. doi:10.1016/S1474-4422(07)70294-6

Wong, J. S., Brooks, D., & Mansfield, A. (2015). Do falls experienced during in-patient stroke rehabilitation affect length of stay, functional status, and discharge destination? *Archives of Physical Medicine and Rehabilitation, 15*, 1501–1054. doi:10.1016/j.apmr.2015.12.005

Woo, D., Haverbusch, M., Sekar, P., Kissela, B., Khoury, J., Schneider, A., . . . Broderick, J. (2004). Effect of untreated hypertension on hemorrhagic stroke. *Stroke, 35*(7), 1703–1708. doi:10.1161/01.STR.0000130855.70683.c8

Wright, L., Hill, K. M., Bernhardt, J., Lindley, R., Ada, L., Bajorek, B. V., . . . National Stroke Foundation Stroke Guidelines Expert Working Group. Stroke management: Updated recommendations for treatment along the care continuum. *Internal Medicine Journal, 42*(5), 562–569.

Yoneyama, T., Yoshida, M., Matsui, T., & Sasaki, H. (1999). Oral care and pneumonia. *The Lancet, 354*(9177), 515. doi:10.1016/S0140-6736(05)75550-1

Yoshimura, S., Toyoda, K., Ohara, T., Nagasawa, H., Ohtani, N., Kuwashiro, T., . . . Minematsu, K. (2008). Takotsubo cardiomyopathy in acute ischemic stroke. *Annals of Neurology, 64*, 547–554. doi:10.1002/ana.21459

26 CHAPTER

Visual Impairments

Bruce P. Rosenthal, Roy Gordon Cole, and Elsa Escalera

The world population clock stood at 7,301,964,110 on January 29, 2016 and will add 2 billion plus people by the year 2040 (U.S. Census Bureau, n.d.-b). The world and United States population pyramids (U.S. Census Bureau, n.d.-a) continue to expand toward the apex confirming a significant increase in the 65 to 100+ age population. The marked growth in the numbers of older persons is already translating into an increased prevalence of ocular disease, resulting in an upsurge in visual impairment worldwide. The increase is especially significant, as Congdon, O'Colmain, et al. (2004) have noted, because Americans aged 80 and older have the highest rates of blindness, as well as being in the fastest growing segment of the population.

The progression is most common in the escalation of age-related eye diseases such as cataract, diabetic retinopathy, glaucoma, and age-related macular degeneration (AMD). Complications resulting from systemic conditions, including diabetes, stroke, ischemic disease, multiple sclerosis, and tumors, may also result in severe disabling vision loss. These individuals will in turn require access to vision rehabilitation and particularly low-vision services. Figure 26.1 illustrates that the trend between the years 2010 and 2050 estimates that the number of people affected by the most common eye diseases will double.

It was also noted that although those aged 80 and older make up only 8% of the population, they accounted for 69% of the cases of blindness. There will also be a concomitant increase in the life expectancy in the United States from 75.8 in males and 80.9 in females in 2010 to 80.8 in males and 85.3 in females in 2050 (Figure 26.1; U.S. Census Bureau, n.d.-b).

DEFINITIONS AND STATISTICS

Visual Acuity

There are more than 38 million Americans aged 40 and older who are classified as either "blind," have low vision, or an age-related eye disease (Eye Disease Prevalence Research Group, 2004). These estimates are based on only two parameters in the United States: visual acuity or visual field loss.

Visual acuity charts that are currently in use were developed in the 1860s. They can be based on either the foot or the metric system (e.g., 20/20 or 6/6). The numerator in 20/20 relates to a test distance of 20 feet while the numerator in 6/18 (equivalent to 20/60 in feet notation) is the Metric distance (6 meters) used in the second fraction. Eye doctors in the United States, other than low-vision specialists, continue to use feet notation, whereas most of the rest of the world uses the metric system (Figure 26.2).

Measured visual acuity gives us an indication of the patient's sharpness of vision, that is, the ability to resolve detail. "Normal" acuity (i.e., 20/20) is based on the assumption that an individual should be able to separate objects that are 1′ apart in visual angle. People can have even better vision (20/15 and even 20/10). The limitation on acuity is generally determined by the spacing of the retinal cells.

There are many definitions used worldwide to define vision loss.

Vision Impairment

"Vision impairment" is perhaps the most used definition. It can be described as irreversible reduced vision that interferes with an individual's ability

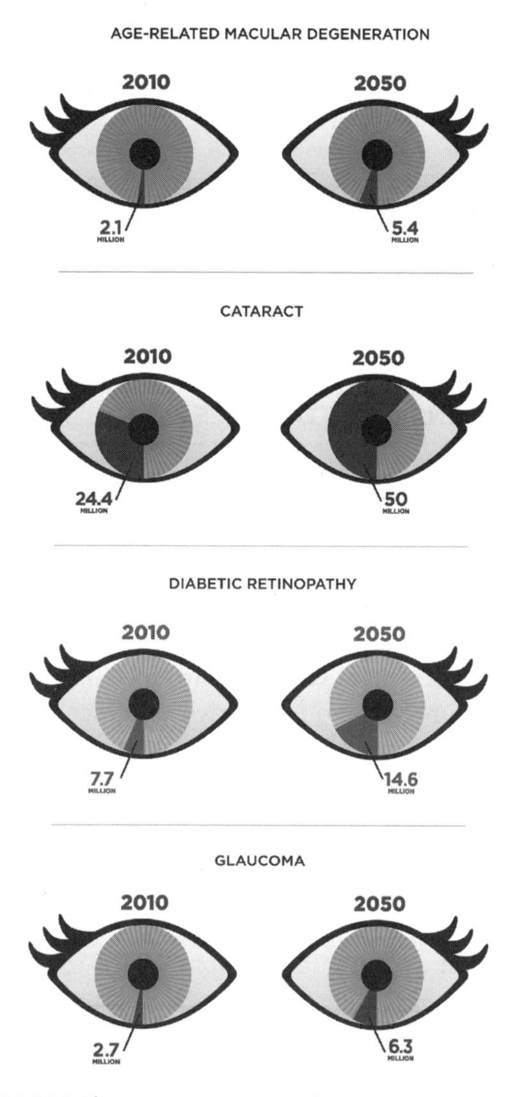

FIGURE 26.1 The most common eye diseases. Each eye represents a total of 80 million people, the estimated number of Americans who will be 65 and older in 2050, the population most affected by these diseases.

Source: National Eye Institute (2015).

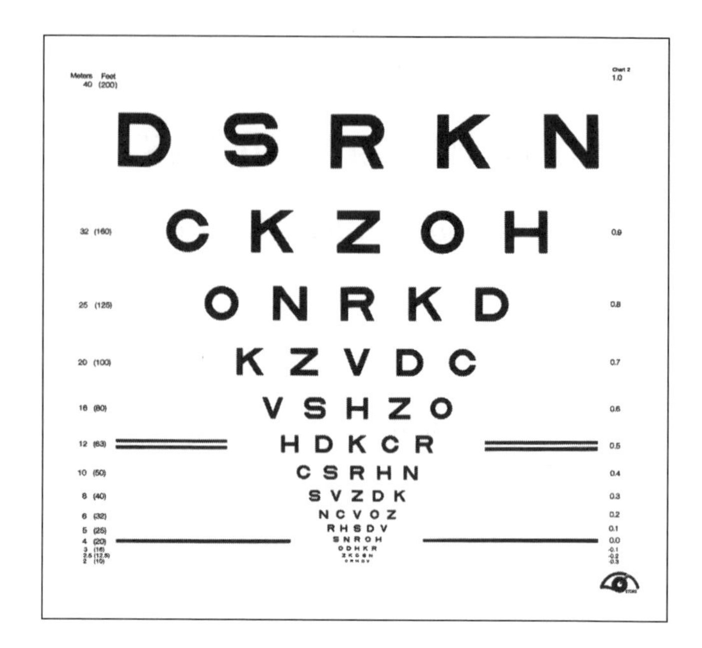

FIGURE 26.2 Visual acuity chart.

Source: National Eye Institute, National Institutes of Health (n.d.-c).

to do their normal daily activities. It can also be defined as having a visual acuity of 20/70 or worse in the better eye, even with eyeglasses, or in the presence of a significant visual field loss (International Statistical Classification of Diseases and Related Health Problems, 10th Revision [ICD-10], 2016). A broader definition of vision impairment, according to Prevent Blindness America (2008), is having a visual acuity of 20/40 or worse in the better eye even with eyeglasses. Visual impairment was categorized as moderate, severe, profound, near-total, or total vision loss depending on the degree of loss of visual acuity or visual field (Pearson Education, 2009); there are also categories of vision called "normal" and "near normal" that are not considered to be impaired vision).

Another categorization is "moderate," "severe," and blindness (which would include profound, near-total, and total vision loss, as used in Pearson Education, 2009). This categorization of visual impairment, currently in use worldwide, is based on the ICD-10-World Health Organization (WHO) Version for 2016 (WHO, n.d.).

A person with low vision is one who has impairment of visual functioning even after treatment and/or standard refractive correction, and has a visual acuity of less than 6/18 (20/60) to light perception, or a visual field of less than 10° from the point of fixation (20° width in the horizontal meridian), but who uses, or is potentially able to use, vision for planning and/or execution of a task.

With the implementation of the ICD-10-CM American version on October 1, 2015, blindness and low vision have five subheadings: H54.0 blindness, both eyes; H54.2 low vision, both eyes; H54.3 unqualified visual loss, both eyes; H54.7, unspecified visual loss; and H54.8, legal blindness, as defined in the the United States (ICD-10, American Version).

Americans across racial and ethnic groups describe losing eyesight as potentially having the greatest impact on their day-to-day life—more so than other coconditions, including loss of memory, hearing, and speech. A higher percentage of African Americans (57%) cite this concern compared to non-Hispanic Whites (49%), Asians (43%), and

Hispanics (38%; The Association for Research in Vision and Ophthalmology, 2014).

Fortunately, the blindness that people often think of (cannot see light, needs a guide dog, and has to learn Braille) rarely occurs. However, it is not uncommon to have a loss of vision to the point that one has a significant problem in maintaining a satisfactory quality of life. What this means can vary from individual to individual; therefore, a careful evaluation of the patient's abilities and needs is required before attempting to implement a rehabilitation program.

Legal Blindness

According to the National Eye Institute, the leading causes of new cases of legal blindness are macular degeneration, glaucoma, and diabetic retinopathy. The most common definition of blindness is most likely that used by the Social Security Department to determine disability. It states that an individual is legally (statutorily) blind if either the best-corrected visual acuity (with standard lenses) is 20/200 (6/60) or worse in the better eye, or if the remaining central visual field is restricted to 20° or less in the widest meridian of the better eye. To take into account the visual acuity charts that are often used in clinical low-vision care (e.g., the Early Treatment of Diabetic Retinopathy Study chart) the visual acuity criteria were recently clarified by the Social Security Department to be a visual acuity of less than 20/100 (Social Security Online, n.d.).

The acuity part of this definition dates back to 1935, when the Social Security Act, with its benefits to the blind, was passed. The visual field part was added as an amendment the following year (Simons, 1991). This definition has been adopted widely by federal, state, and local agencies throughout the United States to determine eligibility and benefits. It is even used by the Internal Revenue Service to determine tax benefits.

The problem with this definition of legal blindness is that it has little or no validated experimental basis. Anyone working in the field has had patients with relatively poor visual acuity or visual field (considered legally blind) who functioned well, and other patients with relatively good visual acuity and fields (not legally blind) who could barely do anything for themselves. It also does not address reduced contrast sensitivity, field loss as result of stroke (e.g., hemianopia), and central scotomas that interfere with functional capability but do not necessarily impact acuity significantly. Thus, from a rehabilitation point of view, it makes more sense to talk in terms of visual disability.

FACTORS AFFECTING VISUAL FUNCTION AND ITS TREATMENT

The main impairments affecting visual function are reduced visual acuity, visual field loss (central or peripheral), poor contrast sensitivity, lighting and glare problems, and visual skills and binocularity problems. Although not commonly encountered, and not on this list, when color vision problems are found, they are compensated for with adaptive techniques and devices, although they cannot be cured.

Visual acuity is usually written as a fraction, the numerator represents the test distance, and the denominator represents the letter size.

$$\text{Visual acuity} = \frac{\text{Testing distance}}{\text{Letter size}}$$

The letter size is actually a distance measurement: the distance at which the letter must be held to subtend a visual angle of 5′ at the eye, that is, the same as a 20/20 letter. When test distances in feet are used, we see acuities such as 20/20 or 20/200. When metric distances are used, these acuities become 6/6 or 6/60. All acuities can be represented as decimal acuities, and this is done by "dividing out the fraction"; that is, 20/20 becomes 1.0 and 20/200 becomes 0.1.

Another way of writing this definition is

$$\text{Visual acuity} = \frac{\text{Distance at which letter was used}}{\text{Distance at which letter subtends } 5' \text{ of arc}}$$

For example, a 20-feet letter size read at 10 feet would be equivalent to 10/20 or 20/40 acuity. The conversion is done by simply converting the fraction so that it has a "20" on top, in this case multiplying both the top and the bottom numbers by 2.

When working with people whose vision is significantly reduced, the acuity can still be measured accurately. One technique simply involves walking the patient up to the test chart, thus reducing the test distance and increasing the sensitivity of the chart. Another technique is to use a test chart with larger letters or numbers and a larger selection of intermediate sizes. In this case, low levels of vision can still be measured, even worse than 20/2000. Legal (statutory) blindness in the United States is based on a best-corrected (with standard glasses or contact lenses) visual acuity of 20/200 or less. The WHO definition, which most of the rest of the world uses, based on visual acuity has legal blindness starting at 20/400. ICD-10, which was implemented in the United States in 2015, actually uses this definition, but does have a separate code for legal blindness, as defined in United States (20/200 or worse, or a central field of 20 degrees or less): H54.8.

One other system that is used is the log MAR system. MAR = minimum angle of resolution. The formula is

$$VA = \log MAR$$

The MAR of a 20/20 letter is 1′ of arc. The log (base 10) of 1 is 0, so in this case, logMAR = 0. The MAR of 20/200 would be 10 degrees, and the logMAR of this would be 1.0.

In some cases, all that is needed to allow a patient with reduced visual acuity to resolve detail is an up-to-date refraction, resulting in a new pair of glasses or contact lenses for general wear. When glasses by themselves are not adequate, additional interventions must be initiated. This is generally accomplished by making the image on the retina larger. This magnification can be provided in one of three ways: making the object larger (e.g., large-print books), moving the object closer (e.g., sitting closer to the television or bringing the reading material closer to the eyes when using stronger reading glasses), or using some optical device to make the object look bigger (e.g., a telescope to see distant objects better or a magnifier for reading). One of the goals of the low-vision examination is to determine and prescribe the appropriate level and type of magnification for the desired tasks.

Visual Field

Primary care physicians should be especially aware that "vision loss is a leading cause of falls in the elderly. One study found that visual field loss was associated with a 6-fold risk of frequent falls" (Ramrattan et al., 2001).

The visual field gives us information regarding the patency of the whole retina (the central and peripheral areas of the retina). When we test the visual field, we are generally, but not exclusively, evaluating peripheral field (side vision). This is important for the patient to be able to detect objects around them. Once the individual detects an object, the individual can look at it and identify it (using visual acuity and central field). The peripheral visual field becomes an especially important factor when discussing and considering training for mobility problems.

Peripheral visual field loss is the other way someone can be certified as legally blind. The criteria used in the United States is that the peripheral field is constricted resulting in a central field of vision subtending an overall angle of 20° or less at the eye. This is also WHO's definition of legal blindness based on peripheral field loss.

Perimetry, which is the measurement of the visual field, uses a variety of techniques. These may include manual and automated evaluation of the entire visual field with kinetic or static stimuli. The automated perimeter has paved the way for more standardized and accurate visual field testing in all types of patients, including those with low vision (Bass & Sherman, 1996).

There are different ways that the visual field can be affected. A loss of vision in a specific area is referred to as a scotoma (scotomas can range from "black holes" in vision to areas that are distorted or hazy to see through). It should be noted that scotomas in the visual field can have almost any size, shape, and number. They can be located in the center of the macula (referred to as a central scotoma), affecting straight-ahead vision with a concurrent reduction in visual acuity. The magnification principles discussed would apply in these cases. Scotomas can also be located adjacent to the central area (paracentral scotoma). In this case, acuity is usually not affected; interference comes from the closeness of scotoma to what is being viewed. Central and paracentral scotomas can be plotted using a microperimetry technique such as scanning laser ophthalmoscopy or with a handheld laser (the Fletcher central field test) as described by Cole (Cole, 2008). Sometimes, central scotomas or distortions can be identified with a diagnostic test known as the Amsler grid (a grid of 20 × 20 squares that is equivalent to 20° of the visual field when held 13 inches from the eye). Unfortunately, "the sensitivity of Amsler charts in detecting macular disease can be less than 50%, implying that presentation may be delayed in over half of patients with advancing disease relying on the Amsler chart to detect progression" (Crossland, & Rubin, 2007).

An overall peripheral field defect, which may be caused by glaucoma or retinitis pigmentosa (RP), can interfere with mobility. This is the situation when only a small central part of the visual field remains. Significant mobility problems generally occur when the overall remaining central field subtends an angle of about 5° or less (the normal field of vision with both eyes open is 180° and with one eye is 140°), but some patients are bothered even earlier. Scotomas usually caused by stroke or head trauma can be limited to one side of the visual field (hemianopia), or to one sector. These can be detrimental to patient function because the patient cannot see objects to that side. This can interfere significantly with general mobility and with near tasks such as reading and writing. Laser photocoagulation for diabetic retinopathy results in scotomas as well.

The treatment of a visual field defect will vary depending on the size, location, number, and severity of the scotomas. Generally, there is no good optical treatment available for significant loss of the peripheral visual field. However, optical remediation with prisms, mirrors, or reversed telescopes has been used in training and maximizing the residual visual field. Usually, the patient must learn to live with and compensate for the defect. Orientation and mobility training (especially cane travel), and visual scanning training, will often be helpful in the case of peripheral field loss and sometimes in the case of severe central field loss. For patients who have central field loss (central and paracentral scotomas), eccentric viewing training, which teaches the patient to look off-center, that is, away from the fovea (the area of the retina that gives us the greatest detail when looking at an object), can sometimes help with tasks such as reading and even with seeing in general. Eccentric viewing training is usually only done for central scotomas accompanied with a loss of visual acuity. Also, basic visual skills training (fixation, pursuits, saccades, etc.) can also be helpful with some of these patients.

Contrast

Visual acuity charts measure high-contrast vision (the ability to resolve very black letters on a very light, usually white, background). Most of the world, however, is not high contrast, and this can explain some situations in which patients feel that their vision has worsened, although the measured visual acuity on the eye chart is the same. Contrast sensitivity charts are specially designed charts that can measure any decrement in this visual function and would account for the patient's perception of a decrease in their vision. An example can be seen in Figure 26.3.

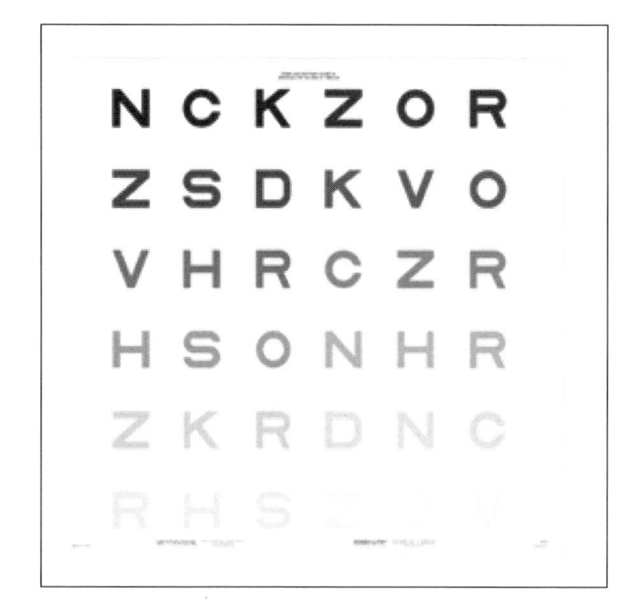

FIGURE 26.3 Evans Contrast Sensitivity Chart.
Source: Reprinted with permission of the Good-Lite Company

Visual acuity, the main measure of visual capability for the last 142 years, has not correlated well to functional vision. In particular, low-vision practitioners have noted the discrepancy between the "quantity" and "quality" of vision and patient performance as measured by acuity. Contrast sensitivity has emerged as a more complete performance-related measure of the "quality" of functional vision. Differences in individual contrast sensitivity, but not visual acuity, of normal observers have been shown to be related to differences in complex visual tasks. The results from normal observers suggest that contrast sensitivity may also help in the evaluation of functional vision of low-vision patients (Ginsburg et al., 1987).

Contrast sensitivity is increasingly recognized as an important factor influencing navigation in the visual environment. Many patients having a worsening loss in contrast sensitivity and complaints that objects are hard to see cannot be identified using standard clinical acuity testing (Kupersmith, Karen, & Seiple, 1989).

There is an increased risk for accidents when there is a decrease in the contrast sensitivity function. Reduced contrast sensitivity may also affect the ability to walk down steps, recognize faces, drive at night or in the rain, find a telephone number in a directory, read instructions on a medicine container, or navigate safely through unfamiliar environments. Unfortunately, contrast sensitivity testing is still not a part of the routine eye medical evaluation. Low-vision doctors do, however, routinely use this test.

The benefit of contrast sensitivity testing is that it often gives us an indication of who will respond poorly to standard (or predicted) magnification levels, sometimes needing significantly higher magnification, or who will need higher levels of lighting or glare control to perform desired tasks. In fact, it is not unusual to see patients with contrast sensitivity problems function with significantly weaker lenses when bright lighting is incorporated into the task, along with appropriate glare-control techniques.

Lighting and Glare

It is often impossible to predict how much light a patient needs. Too much can be as detrimental as not enough. The best way to determine the appropriate level is to see how the patient responds to different intensities and types of lighting (fluorescent, light emitting diode [LED], etc.) and note the effect of the lighting on patient performance. The easiest way to change the intensity of light on a page is to either change the brightness (lumens) of the bulb, or the distance of the light from the page. Intensity approximately follows the inverse-square law: If you move the light, the intensity (I) changes by an amount inversely proportional to the square of the change in the distance (Δd) from the page: $I = I_o/(\Delta d)^2$. For example, if you move a light to one half the original distance from the page, the intensity on the page increases by four times:

$$I = I_o/(0.5)^2 = 4I_o$$

Patients also complain about glare. One broad definition of glare is "light that does not contribute to retinal imagery but has an adverse effect on visual efficiency, visual comfort, or resolution" (Waiss & Cohen, 1991). Intraocular glare problems can sometimes be solved by removing the source of glare (e.g., cataracts). If the glare source is external, one can either modify the environment or filter out the distracting wavelengths causing the glare problem by using special filters, such as yellow or amber lenses, or visors. One very handy device is a typoscope (also called a reading guide). This is simply a matte-black card with a slot cut in it that, when placed on printed material, exposes two to three lines of print. The surrounding black material reduces the reflected light from the page, thus reducing the total amount of light entering the eye. Concurrently, the intensity of light on the exposed printed material can be increased, thus increasing the perceived contrast of the print.

Visual Skills and Binocularity Problems

Some people have problems moving their eyes (scanning), locating objects, aiming the eyes at the object (fixating), and maintaining this fixation when following the object (tracking). They might have trouble using the two eyes together (binocularity) easily and comfortably. They might also have trouble moving the eyes accurately across a printed line or jumping from the end of one line to the next when reading. When this happens, skills training can be done. This consists of a series of exercises that are designed to improve these skills and are generally done over a period of some weeks. Optometrists, occupational therapists, and vision rehabilitation therapists generally provide this type of training, when indicated.

THE ROLE OF PATHOLOGY IN VISUAL IMPAIRMENT

One of the ways to understand the various pathologies that cause a visual impairment is to understand how light travels through the eye (Figure 26.4).

The cornea (the transparent window in the front) and the lens are the primary refracting structures of the eye that focus images onto the retina, which is located at the back of the eye. After passing through the lens, the light must travel through the vitreous, which is a clear, jelly-like material that fills the interior of the eye. Problems such as cataracts and corneal disease affect these systems and generally result in the person experiencing an overall blurred image (reduced visual acuity), decreased contrast, and glare.

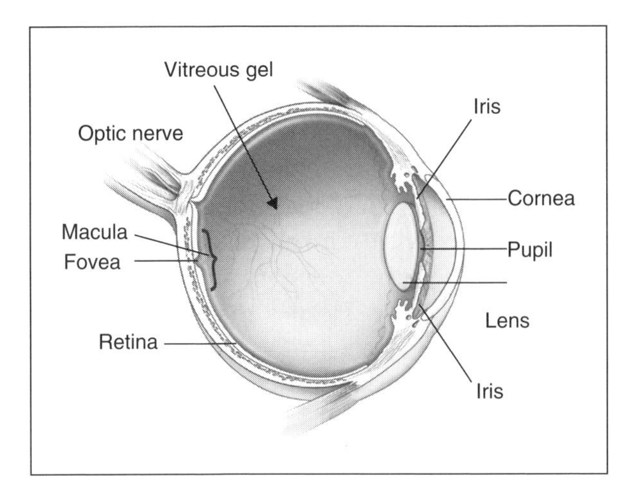

FIGURE 26.4 The eye.
Source: National Eye Institute (n.d.-a).

Eventually, the light will fall on the retina, a structure that is, in effect, a dual image-processing system. The central portion of the retina (macular area) is associated with straight-ahead vision, including detail discrimination and color. The macular area plays a major role in reading, facial discrimination, and object identification. Problems in the macular area can cause a reduction in visual acuity or a loss of central visual field (a central scotoma or blind spot). Some of the common conditions in which the macular region is affected include macular degeneration, diabetic retinopathy, and albinism.

The second portion of the retina, the peripheral retina, is associated with object awareness and motion detection. Its function is to allow one to become aware of objects to the side (peripherally; i.e., up, down, right, left), and it plays a major role in mobility (one's ability to navigate around objects and people without bumping into them). Conditions that affect the peripheral retina result in a loss of side vision, with or without a concurrent reduction in visual acuity. Some of these conditions are glaucoma, RP, strokes, and tumors.

The retina converts light energy into electrical impulses that leave the eye through the optic nerve. The fibers carrying the information travel through the visual pathways to the occipital region, and other areas in the brain, where the interpretation and interaction with other body systems take place.

The following are the most common pathological eye conditions that may result in severe vision loss.

Cataract

Description of Medical Condition

Primary care physicians should be aware that many visual complaints may be related to the development of a cataract. Cataracts, in fact, become significantly more prevalent after the age of 40, with nearly 20.5 million Americans having some type of change in the lens of the eye. This number is expected to markedly increase to 30.1 million by 2020. It has also been found in the United States that women have a higher prevalence of cataracts than men (Congdon, Vingerling, et al., 2004) and that Caucasians are three times as likely as Blacks to develop cataracts. Women smoking at least 35 cigarettes a day increased the risk by about 50% (Lindblad, Håkansson, Svensson, Philipson, & Wolk, 2005). And the most recent study reveals that one in two Americans aged 85 years or older stated that their cataracts have been removed (Centers for Disease Control and Prevention, 2011).

The lens is composed of three layers: the nucleus (center), the cortex, and the capsule. It is clear at birth, but throughout life, the lens continues to produce cells that become increasingly yellow with age. Cataracts develop as a result of aging, trauma, hereditary factors, birth defects, or a systemic condition such as diabetes. Cataracts (opacity or clouding of the lens) may appear in all parts of the lens and are classified into four main anatomical types: the nuclear, cortical, posterior subcapsular, and mixed.

Treatment and Prognosis

Cataracts are one of the four major eye diseases in the United States (cataracts, macular degeneration, glaucoma, and diabetic retinopathy), and surgery is considered to be a routine outpatient procedure. The most common procedure involves a "stitchless" incision and replacement of the cataractous lens with an intraocular lens. Cataract extraction is considered to be one of the safest and cost-effective surgical procedures. Assuming a healthy retina, the prognosis for functional cure and restoration of normal vision is high.

Patients should be referred for a low-vision examination if cataract surgery is deferred due to risk factors such as a complication that occured during or following the surgery on the fellow eye.

Although magnification itself might not be as successful as in other eye conditions, approaches using lighting, glare control, and contrast enhancement can often go a long way in helping the patient.

Corneal Disease

The cornea functions to protect the eye from dust and germs and, as noted, is the primary refracting surface (65%–70% of the eye's total focusing power for light entering the eye) (National Eye Institute [NEI], 2013).

Description of Medical Condition

The cornea is composed of the anterior corneal epithelium, Bowman's membrane, the corneal stroma, Descemet's membrane, and the endothelium as well as a possible thin sixth layer that is just anterior to Descemet's membrane (Dua et al., 2013). The cornea is a structure that is prone to degenerations, dystrophies, inflammation, abrasion, neovascularization, ulcers, deposition, edema, scarring, pigmentation, cysts, noninflammatory progressive degenerative diseases, thinning (e.g., keratoconus), infection, viral diseases, and trauma. Changes in any of the corneal layers or membranes from any of these conditions may result in blurred, distorted, or even total loss of vision in the affected eye.

Functional Presentation of Medical Condition

Interference with corneal integrity can result in a blurred or distorted image on the retina. A totally opaque cornea from trauma or late onset disease can prevent light from reaching the retina altogether. Patients with corneal disease may experience severe glare, cloudy vision, and problems with reduced visual acuity. Herpes zoster is a condition that may involve the cornea. The incidence and severity increases with advancing age, with persons over the age of 60 are at the highest risk (Chapman, Cross, & Fleming, 2003).

Visual function, however, may be restored with medical treatment, including laser, a corneal transplant, or a keratoprosthesis. If the treatment is not totally successful in restoring vision, the patient should be referred for a low-vision examination. Although magnification itself might not be as successful as in other eye conditions, approaches using lighting, glare control, and contrast enhancement can often go a long way in helping the patient.

Macular Degeneration

Description of Medical Condition

AMD is the most common cause of irreversible visual impairment in older populations in industrialized nations (Figure 26.5; Yonekawa, Miller, & Kim, 2015).

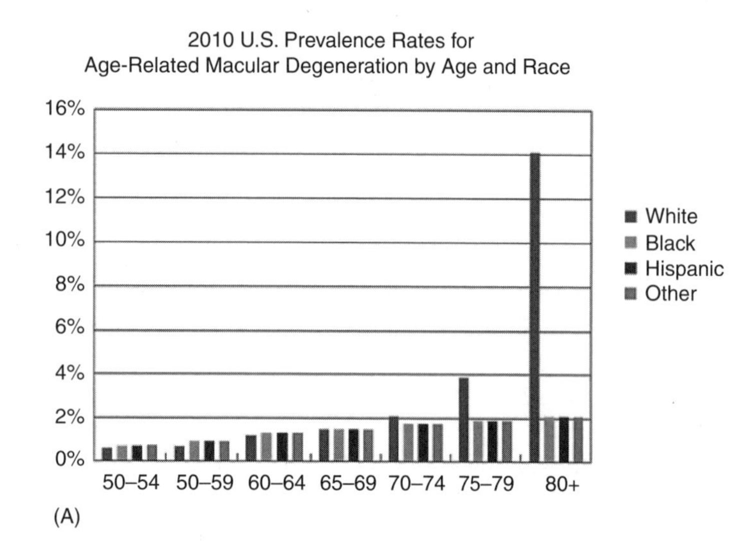

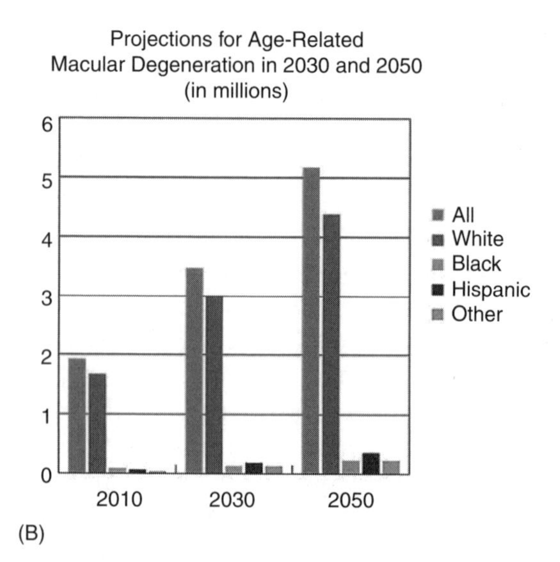

FIGURE 26.5 U.S. Age-specific prevalence rates for age-related macular degeneration (AMD) by age and race/ethnicity for 2010.
Source: National Eye Institute (n.d.-b).

By 2050, the estimated number of people with AMD is expected to more than double from 2.07 million to 5.44 million. White Americans will continue to account for the majority of cases. However, Hispanics will see the greatest rate of increase, with a nearly sixfold rise in the number of expected cases from 2010 to 2050.

There are many risk factors (Clemons, Milton, Klein, Seddon, & Ferris, 2005) associated with macular degeneration, which include increasing age, ethnicity (Caucasian), family history, high blood pressure, obesity (Seddon, Cote, Davis, & Rosner, 2003), a history of hypertension (Klein, Klein, Tomany, & Cruickshanks, 2005), and light iris color (Maguire, 1997). Another risk factor associated with macular degeneration is smoking. The incidence of macular degeneration in smokers (Congdon, O'Colmain, et al., 2004) seems to be two to four times higher than that in nonsmokers, and genes also play an ever-increasing role in the development of AMD. Previous cataract surgery and a family history of AMD showed strong and consistent associations with late AMD. Risk factors with moderate and consistent associations were higher body mass index, history of cardiovascular disease (Tan, Mitchell, Smith, & Wang, 2007), hypertension, and higher plasma fibrinogen.

Early AMD is characterized by the presence of drusen and pigmentary abnormalities. Drusen are yellow deposits that are made up of lipids (a fatty protein) and deposit under the retina. The presence of drusen in the retina may also be a risk factor in developing AMD.

A new era has begun with clinical trials underway for nonexudative complications of AMD (Zarbin, Casaroli-Marano, & Rosenfeld, 2014). Research has revealed new pathways that may be amenable to treatment. Individuals having the CFH gene variant, for example, were found to have an increased risk for developing macular degeneration by about 2.5 to 5.5 times (Haines et al., 2005)

The Age-Related Eye Disease Study (AREDS; Chew, Lindblad, Clemons, & The Age-Related Eye Disease Study Research Group, 2009) showed that supplementing the diet with antioxidant vitamins, including C and E, zinc, and copper, along with the betacarotenoid has been effective in reducing the severity of AMD. In 2013, the NEI completed the Age-Related Eye Disease Study 2, which tested several changes to orginal AREDS by including omega-3 fatty acids, as well as the antioxidants lutein and zeaxanthin. Lutein and zeaxanthin together appeared to be as safe and effective alternative to beta-carotene (NEI, 2013).

Treatment and Prognosis

Optical coherence tomography (OCT) is a noninvasive imaging technique that provides high-resolution, cross-sectional images of the retina, retinal nerve fiber layer, and the optic nerve head (Adhi & Duker, 2013). It has not only become the gold standard in imaging and treating retinal and other disorders of the eye, but revolutionized the clinical practice of ophthalmology and optometry. Fluorescein angiography (FA) and indocyanine green angiography (ICG; Yannuzzi, Slakter, Sorenson, Guyer, & Orlock, 1992) are two other diagnostic procedures used, along with OCT, to evaluate the permeable blood vessels that form in response to vascular endothelial growth factor (VEGF) in macular degeneration. Numerous clinical studies have confirmed the efficacy and benefits from the use of anti-VEGF treatments (Patel et al., 2011).

Patients are also able to monitor the course of the disease with the Amsler grid to determine whether there is a change in the macular function from disease processes (Figure 26.6). Any sudden change of

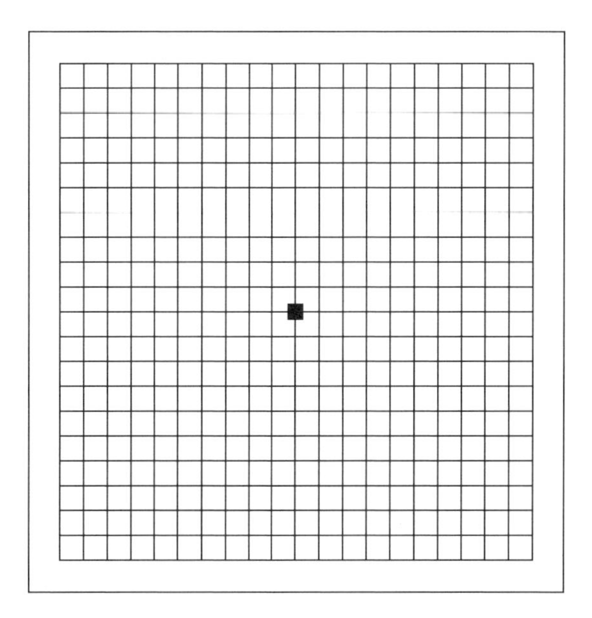

FIGURE 26.6 Amsler grid.
Source: National Eye Institute, National Institutes of Health (n.d.-a).

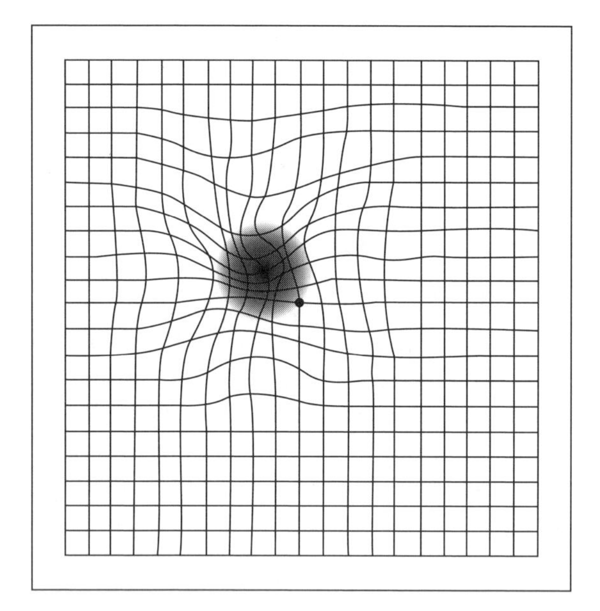

FIGURE 26.7 Amsler grid as it might appear to someone with age-related macular degeneration (AMD).

Source: National Eye Institute, National Institutes of Health (n.d.-b).

the grid (such as waviness, black areas [scotomas], or distortion) may be indicative of a leaking retina that might be amenable to anti-VEGF treatment, especially if done early. Additional treatments that have been under investigation are combination therapies, including anti-VEGF treatment (ranibizumab) with photodynamic therapy (cold laser) and dexamethasone. The rationale for the combination therapies is the targeting of different processes in the development of new blood vessels. The Amsler grid will often reflect the benefits of the treatments with a decrease in the waviness in the grid (Figure 26.7)

Diabetic Retinopathy

Description of Medical Condition

Most clinicians are not aware that "diabetic eye disease comprises a group of eye conditions that affect people with diabetes. These conditions include diabetic retinopathy, diabetic macular edema (DME), cataract, and glaucoma." It is also important for all clinicians to recognize that "all forms of diabetic eye disease have the potential to cause severe vision loss and blindness" (NEI diabetic eye disease, n.d.).

More than 7.6 million Americans aged 40 and older have diabetic retinopathy (Prevent Blindness America, 2008). Nearly, all persons with type 1 diabetes will develop diabetic retinopathy, and 60% of patients with type 2 will develop retinopathy within two decades of the disease diagnosis (Fong et al., 2004). In the National Eye Institute Los Angeles Latino Eye Study, the Latino population was shown to have a significant prevalence of diabetic retinopathy. It was found that approximately 50% of the participants who had diabetes had diabetic retinopathy (Varma, Torres, Peña, Klein, & Azen, 2004). In the United States, diabetic retinopathy causes vision loss during the working years, translating into more disability and person-years of vision lost than any other eye disease (Kempen et al., 2004).

The early or background stage of diabetic retinopathy manifests itself with small hemorrhages in the eye. This eventually may lead to the more serious proliferative type, which can cause retinal scarring, hemorrhaging into the vitreous, and even retinal detachment.

Treatment and Prognosis

The Diabetes Control and Complications Trial (DCCT) study showed that strict control of blood sugar is required to reduce the incidence of complications once considered an inevitable result of diabetes (Fuchs, 1996). Intensive blood glucose control was shown to reduce the risk for eye disease by 76%, kidney disease by 50%, and nerve disease by 60%. Study results also showed that intensive therapy reduced the risk for developing retinopathy by 76%.

Despite regulation of the condition with diet, oral medication, or insulin, many individuals still continue to have progressive visual loss. Photocoagulation may be indicated when there is leaking of the blood vessels. In addition, panretinal photocoagulation of the peripheral retina may be indicated to preserve remaining vision, as well as the possibility of having cataracts removed.

Despite continued vision loss, low-vision devices, including prisms for transitory diplopia, will often be of value in enabling an individual to maintain everyday activities.

Exciting research in reducing the devastating effects of diabetes are in clinical trials. A gene transfer process, for example, that produces a VEGF receptor prevents retinal vascular permeability (RVP) associated with diabetes that could have value in treating diabetic retinopathy (Ramirez et al., 2011).

Glaucoma

Description and Demographics of Medical Condition

An estimated 2.2 million Americans aged 40 and older have glaucoma. Of these, 711,000 Americans aged 80 and older (7.7% of the population) have the condition (Friedman, 2004). Glaucoma is more prevalent in the Hispanic and Black population and accounts for 28.6% cases of blindness (Congdon, O'Colmain, et al., 2004).

Glaucoma is a disease in which the optic nerve is damaged when the intraocular pressure (IOP) of the eye increases. Generally, "normal" eye pressure ranges between 10 and 20 mmHg, but it has been found that thin corneas may be a significant risk factor in damaging the optic nerve. If left untreated, glaucoma will result in the loss of the cells in the eye, the rods that are located primarily in the peripheral retina. A continuing loss of the rods (and their function) will impact a patient's ability to travel independently and result in nightblindness.

The causes of glaucoma are varied and generally result from a blockage in the drainage canal of Schlemm, which drains the aqueous fluid in the eye. The blockage takes place in an area known as the trabecular meshwork (filter-like tissue) located in the anterior segment of the eye (see Figure 26.8). The causes may be congenital, hereditary, systemic, traumatic, drug induced, neoplastic, or surgically induced.

There are primarily three types of glaucoma that affect the eye: (a) chronic (open-angle) glaucoma, in which increased pressure over time eventually affects the optic nerve and visual field; (b) acute (closed-angle) glaucoma, in which there is a rapid increase or spiking of the IOP that may be accompanied by intense pain and even nausea or vomiting; and (c) low-tension glaucoma, which may be caused by a decrease in blood flow to the optic nerve.

Risk factors have been found to include thin corneas (Gordon et al., 2002) and optineurin (defect in the gene directing the production of the protein found in the trabecular meshwork; Sarfarazi & Rezaie, 2004).

Treatment and Prognosis

Medications that decrease production of aqueous humor or facilitate outflow of fluid through the trabecular meshwork are generally the first treatments instituted for the patient with glaucoma (Figure 26.7). Some of the drugs used to reduce the IOP are the anticholinergic drugs, beta-adrenergic receptor antagonists, alpha-2 adrenergic agonists, sympathomimetics (Epifrin), carbonic anhydrase inhibitors, prostaglandin analogs, and miotic agents (parasympathomimetics, such as pilocarpine).

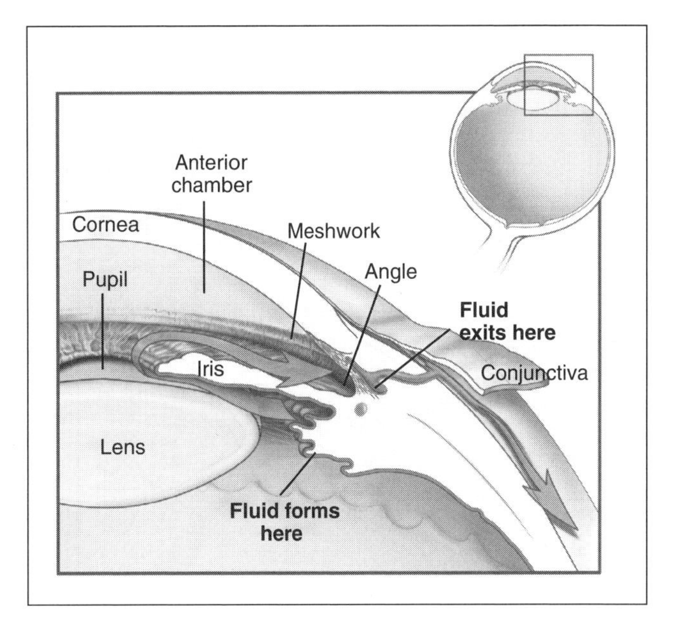

FIGURE 26.8 The aqueous fluid. A clear fluid flows continuously in and out of the anterior chamber and nourishes nearby tissues. The fluid leaves the chamber at the open angle where the cornea and iris meet. When the fluid reaches the angle, it flows through a spongy meshwork and leaves the eye.

Source: National Eye Institute, National Institutes of Health (n.d.-d).

Argon laser trabeculoplasty, in use since 1979, relieves buildup of pressure by creating drainage holes. Another procedure is a trabeculectomy, which is designed to lower pressure by cutting out a small section of the drainage system (Parc, Johnson, Oliver, Hattenhauer, & Hodge, 2001; see Figure 26.9).

Albinism

Description of Medical Condition/Disability Condition

Albinism differs from the other conditions discussed. Albinism is a trait that is inherited through autosomal recessive, or sex-linked, transmission and results in characteristics that affect the pigmentation of the skin and hair, as well as the iris and retina.

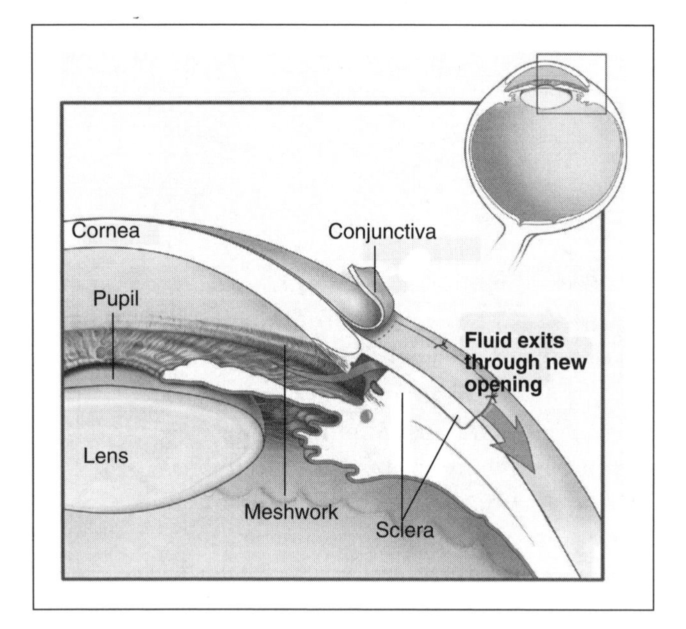

FIGURE 26.9 Conventional surgery to treat glaucoma makes a new opening in the meshwork. This new opening helps fluid to leave the eye and lowers intraocular pressure.

Source: National Eye Institute, National Institutes of Health (n.d.-e)

In addition, nystagmus (involuntary pendular movement of the eyes) and a significant refractive error are also generally associated with albinism. There is a lack of the pigment in the body and the eye in the tyrosinase-negative (ty-neg oculocutaneous) form of albinism. The "typical" individual with albinism has white or platinum hair and irises that appear to be pink. In the tyrosinase-positive (ty-positive oculocutaneous) type of albinism, there is some degree of pigmentation in the eye and skin. The ocular albino, however, is distinctive in that the lack of pigmentation is restricted to the eyes only. This person has a normal (and often dark) skin and hair coloring.

Functional Presentation of Medical Condition/Disability Condition

Photophobia varies with the type of albinism. For example, the ty-negative albino is characteristically more sensitive to light than the ty-positive or ocular albino. Nystagmus is also more noticeable in the ty-negative albino than in the ocular albino.

Persons with albinism have a decrease in visual acuity because of macular aplasia, but, as mentioned, the severity of the loss of vision varies with the type of albinism. With regard to visual acuity, the ty-negative albino has the most severe visual impairment, and the ocular albino has the least.

Treatment and Prognosis

Because refractive errors are generally significant, persons with albinism should be evaluated for corrective spectacle lenses, as well as for absorptive lenses, as early as possible to reduce light sensitivity. The individual with albinism also responds favorably to low-vision devices, including strong microscopic reading lenses, magnifiers, absorptive lenses, and telescopic lenses, and should be referred to a low-vision specialist before entry into school. The presence of nystagmus is in no way a contraindication to the use of low-vision devices, and people with albinism are often our best low-vision patients.

Retinitis Pigmentosa

Description of Medical Condition/Disability Condition

RP, which is a progressive eye disease that affects the pigmentary layer of the retina, is the most common cause of inherited blindness (NEI, 1993). In addition, approximately 30% of people with RP report some degree of hearing loss (National Retinitis Pigmentosa Foundation, 1995). Although there are many variants of RP, it most commonly affects the periphery or midperiphery of the retina. The speed of the progression of visual field loss varies with each individual; some progress to a significant loss of functional visual field. Multiple genes, when mutated, can cause the RP phenotype.

The electroretinogram is essential in the differential diagnosis of RP. The electroretinogram will typically reveal a decreased or absent scotopic response and a reduction in the photopic response as the condition progresses. The visual field is also diagnostically significant in recording the progression of the visual field loss. It is impossible, however, to predict whether an individual diagnosed in the early stages will rapidly progress to a loss of functional vision.

Functional Presentation of Medical Condition/Disability Condition

Night vision and peripheral vision loss go hand in hand. The more advanced the RP, the greater the loss of peripheral vision, and the more difficult it is to travel. Legal blindness, as previously noted, is a field restricted to 20° or less in the better eye.

Mobility, however, does not generally become a significant problem until the remaining visual field is 5° or less. Reading also becomes progressively more difficult as the visual field becomes small.

Glare or light sensitivity is frequently associated with RP, especially when a small posterior subcapsular cataract is associated with the condition. The need for good lighting, however, is an important factor in providing optimal visual function.

Treatment and Prognosis

Currently, no medical or surgical treatments are known to stop or decrease the progression of RP. Periodic eye examinations are essential in monitoring the progression of the condition. Refractive corrections are necessary, along with absorptive lenses, to cut down on glare or light sensitivity. In addition, contrast-enhancing lenses such as the NOIR or Corning CPF series may be beneficial in enhancing performance and reducing adaptation times between outdoors and indoors.

The closed-circuit television (CCTV) is also indicated when reading becomes too difficult with optical devices. The CCTV provides the ability to reverse polarity so that white letters can be seen on a black background, and it enables one to regulate the brightness and contrast of the image viewed. Special prism lenses have been used in the later stages of RP to increase the awareness of the periphery. The Nightscope, which was intended to be used for mobility under dim illumination by individuals with RP, has been found to have limited use.

As the progression of the RP continues, so will the loss in mobility. A traveling cane, long cane, sensory device, or seeing-eye dog may be indicated to assist in independent travel.

Peripheral Visual Field Loss From Strokes or Tumors

Description of Medical Condition

Peripheral visual field loss can be the result of inflammatory, vascular, congenital, toxic, or degenerative changes that can occur anywhere in the visual pathway as well as the eye itself. A person who has a stroke or tumor can be left with a resultant visual field loss that may be partial, bilateral, unilateral, homonymous, eccentric, bitemporal, superior, inferior, or nasal. See Figure 26.10 for a representation of a right homonymous hemianopia (loss of half the field to the right in both eyes). This problem may be compounded by the cognitive, motor, and language disorders that may result from the initial neurological injury that caused the field loss, such as stroke or brain trauma (Cohen & Waiss, 1994). In addition, there are more complex aspects of the visual process that can be affected. These include perception of visual form, color, object meaning, recognition, and attention. There may also be disorders of the visual system such as hallucinations (Brown & Murphy, 1992).

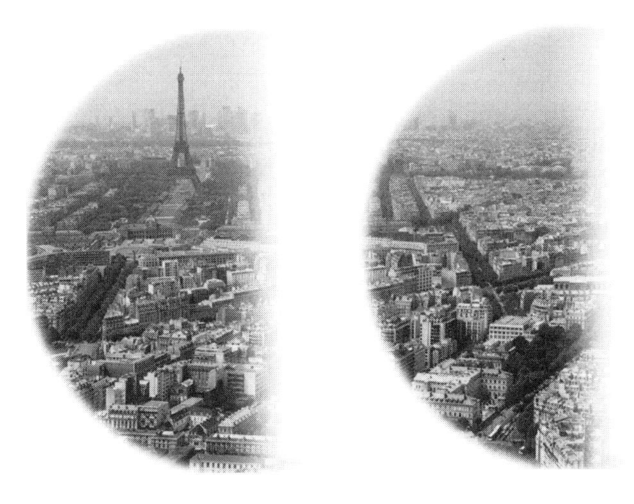

FIGURE 26.10 Simulation of right homonymous hemianopia visual field loss.
Source: Wikipedia. Homonymous hemianopia (n.d.).

Treatment and Prognosis

Generally, visual field loss is accompanied by "spatial neglect" in the area of the field loss. Prisms have been used to enhance rather than expand spatial awareness when there is a loss in the peripheral visual field. Furthermore, mirrors have been placed on glasses, with less success than prisms, to facilitate peripheral field awareness. Low-vision devices, including the CCTV, have also been of value in reading and vocational pursuits.

Functional Presentation of Medical Condition

The pathological condition may result in very different functional presentations. For example, the greater the progression of the cataract, the greater the visual impairment from the effects of decreased visual acuity, loss of contrast, and glare. The primary care physician should be aware of the consequences that may be impacted by cataract formation such as driving, especially at night, as well as the increase in falls with the progression of a cataract.

The changes in the macula may be manifested by decreased visual acuity, decreased color recognition, loss of contrast, or as a "black hole" (area of no vision [scotoma]). Reading may become progressively more difficult as the disease progresses, driving may have to be discontinued, and employment may be impossible without special low-vision intervention. In addition, macular degeneration has been linked with depression.

Individuals with diabetes often experience fluctuating or severely decreased visual acuity, which in turn may cause difficulty in reading and seeing the markings on a syringe. They are at a higher risk for cataracts, which may be manifested by glare and reduced contrast sensitivity (e.g., how black a letter needs to be seen).

Irreversible optic nerve and visual field damage may result in impaired night vision, decreased visual acuity or traveling independently. Stroke may also affect the ability for independent travel with a loss of side vision and not being able to see the ground.

OVERVIEW OF VISION REHABILITATION

Vision rehabilitation addresses functional deficits resulting from a medical condition (congenital or acquired). Before any type of visual rehabilitation is contemplated, it is preferable that the patient have a thorough medical eye evaluation, along with the initiation of any medical and/or surgical interventions. The patient should also have received standard refractive eye care to be certain that the cause of reduced vision is not uncorrected or undercorrected refractive error or presbyopia, and to be sure the patient is seeing the best they can with standard spectacle correction. The ultimate goal in the rehabilitation of a person with visual impairment is to maximize the use of any residual vision and compensate for vision loss by using either vision enhancement or vision substitution techniques and devices. Vision rehabilitation can be thought of as having two components:

1. Clinical low-vision care results in the prescription of and training with vision-assistive devices and the development of a treatment plan for vision rehabilitation training. These services are provided by optometrists or ophthalmologists.
2. Vision rehabilitation training instructs and trains the patient in the use of techniques and devices to allow for greater independence and the achievement of the patient's goals and objectives to the greatest extent possible. These services are provided by occupational therapists and other nonmedical professionals, such as vision rehabilitation trainers, orientation and mobility specialists, and low-vision instructors.

The ultimate goal of vision rehabilitation is to have the person lead a life of independence and safety to the greatest degree possible.

Maximizing the Use of Residual Vision With Clinical Low-Vision Care

Before vision rehabilitation training is recommended and implemented, it is important to perform a low-vision examination. The low-vision examination will identify the patient's functional goals, assess the patient's current level of visual functioning, and determine whether any modifications can be made to attain these goals. These modifications (or interventions) can include the provision of magnification, lighting, glare control, visual field loss compensation, and visual skills training.

As mentioned, the objective of the low-vision examination is to maximize the use of the residual vision. On the basis of the results of this examination, the patient will be categorized as either "sighted" or "blind" and will be guided into the rehabilitation model with the appropriate emphasis. Thus, the low-vision examination is the key component that ties together medical care and rehabilitative care, making certain that patients are channeled into the correct programs. It is this service that mostly responds to the chief complaint of older persons with vision loss. The chief complaint of a majority of older persons was previously identified as "I want to see well."

Compensating for Vision Loss With Vision Rehabilitation Training

Once the clinical low-vision care has been completed or has progressed to the point that current functional levels and desired goals have been determined, the vision rehabilitation training of the patient can be initiated. Sometimes the entry point for the patient into rehabilitation services occurs in the settings providing vision rehabilitation training. A low-vision examination must be an essential and early component of any rehabilitation services. Rehabilitation can include, but is not necessarily limited to, the following:

Activities of daily living (ADL) and instrumental activities of daily living (IADL) training are activities providing instruction in the use of special devices or techniques to compensate for visual impairment.

ADLs are basic but important general tasks required for day-to-day living. IADLs consist of activities that are less basic than ADLs, and need to be done but on a less time-sensitive schedule.

While ADLs apply to all degrees of disability, IADLs become more relevant as the individual wants to become more independent. Sometimes these activities are grouped together and loosely referred to as ADL training.

Orientation and mobility training is designed to enable the person to navigate safely both indoors and outdoors. This training stresses safe travel and teaches techniques that can be used when traveling alone or with someone else (guide technique).

Communications skills training is designed to develop the ability of the patient to handle common interactions with other individuals. This includes verbal communication between individuals, writing, using the telephone and other technologies, and special hearing-amplifying devices.

Educational and vocational training is designed to provide the patient with the education and training needed to achieve a specific goal. This should include the training required to become as independent as possible. Any special optical or adaptive devices needed should be provided.

Psychological and social counseling is designed to help the patient deal with the loss of vision and interact with other people. Support groups and family and peer counseling may also provide help in adjusting to vision loss. Depression is a major problem, and Javitt, Zhou, and Wilke (2007) found that a progression of vision loss from normal to blind is associated with more than 1.5-fold increased odds of depression and injury and 2.5- to 3-fold increased odds of utilization of skilled nursing facilities and long-term care. Horowitz, Reinhardt, and Kennedy (2005) note in a study of new applicants for rehabilitative services who had recent vision loss that 7% had current major depression and 26.9% met the criteria for subthreshold depression.

Other needed services are required by some patients with specific and/or unusual needs, and it is important that these are identified and addressed. One example is diabetes education, which teaches self-management of diabetes, including but not limited to blood sugar level monitoring and the preparation and injection of insulin. Also included is instruction in proper nutrition and exercise. This service is generally provided by a team consisting of a nurse and a dietician, both certified diabetes educators.

LOW-VISION INTERVENTION

Fortunately, patients with macular degeneration and other age-related and early onset eye diseases can often be helped with low-vision interventions recommended during a low-vision evaluation. The power and type of magnification is determined by the extent of the visual loss. Except in a minority of cases, functional ability is generally retained throughout an affected person's life with the use of low-vision devices such as microscopic and telescopic lens systems and absorptive lenses. Electronic CCTVs allow the ability to magnify as well as enhance the contrast of the letters from black letter on a white background to white letters on a black background. A new generation of portable CCTVs allows for greater freedom, such as reading menus under poor lighting conditions.

Perhaps the greatest change in this century has been the introduction of hi-tech devices that can increase font size and boldness, and reverse polarity of reading material from white on black to black on white. But voice input and speech output devices can also read documents, identifiy colors, currency denominations, make automatic telephone calls, give locations, or provide access to e-mail.

Talking books are available, free of charge, from the local library system through the Library of Congress. Bold felt-tip pens, talking clocks, and checkbook stencils are some other nonoptical devices that are available for the person with macular disease and low vision. Through the use of low-vision devices, individuals are often able to function with visual acuity as low as 20/1000. However, a new generation of portable optical character recognition devices enables individuals with little or no vision to access newspapers, magazines, or books. Other types of rehabilitation, as discussed in this chapter, are also generally beneficial to the patient.

Low-vision devices, including spectacles, hand and stand magnifiers, CCTV, lighting, and nonoptical devices, are used to return an individual with glaucoma to normal, or at least improved, visual function. Absorptive lenses, especially those that transmit in the yellow visible portion of the spectrum, seem to enhance the contrast and seem to be especially beneficial for outdoor and indoor wear. These lenses also may enhance the apparent brightness of the scene and often aid in mobility.

Psychological and Vocational Implications

Each pathological condition may have psychological or vocational implications.

A cosmetic contact lens or prosthetic shell following corneal surgery, for example, may improve the cosmetic appearance and enhance professional or personal goals. But macular degeneration or glaucoma may require that the individual, even with the best optical intervention, no longer operate a motor vehicle.

Individuals are often depressed and should be directed to a social worker, psychiatrist, psychologist, or discussion group for support. For conditions such as RP and glaucoma, the fear of total blindness and loss of independence are uppermost in their minds. Psychological and family counseling, as well as genetic counseling, are indicated for persons contemplating having children.

Loss in the areas of the visual field (e.g., hemianopia) will benefit from optical intervention including the use of prisms and mirrors. Mobility and night vision may be impaired, as well as difficulty in reading, if there is a loss in either the left or the right visual field.

WHERE WE HAVE COME FROM AND WHERE WE ARE

Vision rehabilitation got its start after World War II (as did medical rehabilitation) when blinded veterans came back from the war and recovered from their wounds but were still blind. Attention was paid more to psychosocial and vocational issues, and care was provided by an interdisciplinary team. The two rehabilitation programs (vision and medical) split apart, and the first civilian Low Vision Rehabilitation Center was opened at the VA Hospital in Hines, Illinois, in 1948. Initially, this system (vision rehabilitation) worked mainly with healthy, blind veterans, but in 1978, there was an amendment to the Rehabilitation Act of 1973 designating funds for independent living skills training for older adults. Because older adults develop many other health problems, it would make sense for these two systems to come back together, and that continues today (Wainapel, 2001).

Currently, these two systems in the United States, the Blindness System (sometimes referred to as an educational model) and the Health Care System (sometimes referred to as a medical model), are starting to integrate. There is also a third system, the Aging System, which works with aging and sick adults but not primarily with the visually impaired or blind. Aging and visually impaired people sometimes fall through the cracks, with each group (vision and aging) feeling that the other should be taking care of these individuals. Again, this is beginning to be addressed somewhat at present (Warren, 2000), especially with occupational therapists getting more involved in providing vision rehabilitation care, thus bringing together the health and vision issues of the patient. In addition, there have been changes in Medicare and also legislative attempts to provide more care and coverage for visually impaired or blind adults, discussed at the end of this chapter.

THE MODEL OF DISABILITY

There is no single descriptor for the type of functional vision loss an individual is experiencing. Three major categories are currenly used in ICD-10 (ICD-10, American version) to describe the continuum in the classification of visual performance:

- Normal vision: visual acuities down to greater than 20/70
- Low vision: visual acuities from 20/70 to greater than 20/400

- Blindness: visual acuities of 20/400 or worse, including counting fingers (CF) at about 3 m or less, hand motion (HM), some light perception (LP), and no light perception (NLP), or a central visual field of 20° or less in the greatest diameter.

See Table 26.1 for the various impairment categories and the ICD-10 codes.

Colenbrander (1977) described how an organ's structural disorder can lead to an impairment, which is "a disorder interfering with an organ function" (e.g., reduced visual acuity, reduced visual

TABLE 26.1

ICD-10 CODES FOR IMPAIRMENT CATEGORIES AND VISUAL FIELD LOSS, PLUS OTHER USEFUL CODES

		VISION IMPAIRMENT OF **RIGHT** EYE		**RIGHT** EYE
		BLINDNESS 20/400 → NLP 20° or Less Field	**LOW VISION** 20/70 → >20/400	**NORMAL VISION** 20/10 → >20/70
VISUAL IMPARIMENT OF LEFT EYE	**BLINDNESS** 20/400→NLP 20° or Less Field	H54.0	H54.12	H54.42
	LOW VISION 20/70→>20/400	H54.11	H54.2	H54.52
LEFT EYE	**NORMAL VISION** 20/10 → > 20/70	H54.41	H54.51	

VISUAL FIELD LOSS CODES

Homonymous hemianop(s)ia, Quadrant anop(s)ia

Homonymous bilateral field defects right side: H53.461
Homonymous bilateral field defects left side: H53.462
Homonymous bilateral field defects unspecified side: H53.469

Heteronymous bilateral field defects, hemianop(s)ia

Heteronymous bilateral field defects: H53.47
Heteronymous hemianop(s)ia: H53.47

Central scotoma

right eye: H53.411
left eye: H53.412
bilateral: H53.413
unspecified eye: H53.419

Generalized contraction of visual field

right eye: H53.481
left eye: H53.482
bilateral: H53.483
unspecified eye: H53.489

SOME OTHER USEFUL CODES

H54.8: Legal Blindness, as defined in the United States.
H53.71: Glare Sensitivity
H53.72: Decreased Contrast
H53.8: Other Visual Disturbance
H53.9: Unspecified Visual Disturbance

NLP, No light perception.

Source: Impairment Code Table designed by Roy Cole, OD. Lighthouse Guild, New York, NY. 2015. Based on ICD-10 (American Version).

field). An impairment can lead an individual's inability to adequately do an activity (disability), such as not being able to read a newspaper.

An inability to do an activity can lead to a limitation in the ability to participate in a role that is normal for that individual (handicap). An example of a problem with participation would be if reading the newspaper is an activity that is important in a person's life and the activity cannot be done. Individuals who do not need or want to read the newspaper should not be considered handicapped by this disability.

This model is based on the "social model of disability," emphasizing functioning (impairments at the organ level, and doing activities at the person level) and participation in a social context, instead of a diagnosis due to an individual medical condition (A. Colenbrander, personal communication, July 22, 2008). Although these classification systems would be helpful in sharing information, defining function, and doing research, they have not been universally adopted for use in the United States. Doctors and rehabilitation professionals generally code with a medical diagnosis code (ICD-10, 2016) combined with a procedure code. It should be noted that there are some vision impairment codes in the ICD-10 that are used by rehabilitation professionals (particularly occupational therapists) as their primary codes and some low-vision doctors as secondary codes (see Table 26.1), but most doctors still use only the medical diagnosis codes.

Arditi and Rosenthal (1996) included contrast sensitivity and defined visual impairment as a significant limitation of visual capability (vision function) resulting from disease, trauma, or congenital condition that cannot be fully ameliorated by standard refractive correction, medication, or surgery. Impairment is manifested by one or more of the following:

1. Insufficient visual resolution (worse than 20/60 in the better eye with best correction of ametropia);
2. Inadequate field of vision (worse than 20° along the widest meridian in the eye, with the more intact central field, or homonymous hemianopia);
3. Reduced peak contrast sensitivity (less than 1.7 log CS binocularly).

Unfortunately, this definition has not been adopted for use, the main problem being a lack of accepted criteria for reduced contrast sensitivity.

In addition to reduced contrast sensitivity, two other problems can cause functional performance issues in individuals: lighting and glare problems, and visual skills and binocularity problems. Although recognized and addressed in low-vision rehabilitation care, these have not been defined to an extent that will allow them to be included in a classification system.

MEDICARE, THIRD-PARTY COVERAGE, AND LEGISLATION

The problem with Medicare coverage in the past was that there was no distinct national policy on coverage of vision rehabilitation services. Local medical review policies were inconsistent and/or nonexistent. Vision-impaired patients were denied full and consistent access to rehabilitation services. This started to change with statements in two appropriations bills in two consecutive years. The Appropriations Committee urged the Health Care Financing Administration (HCFA) to study the impact of vision loss on beneficiary health status and health care costs and urged the Center for Medicare and Medicaid Services (CMS) to direct its carriers to inform physicians and other providers about the availability of medically necessary rehabilitation services for these beneficiaries.

Program Memorandum—2002

These statements resulted in the issuing of a Program Memorandum by Medicare (AB-02-78) on May 29, 2002. It clarified equal access and coverage of necessary rehabilitation services, stating that Medicare-covered therapeutic services could include mobility, ADLs, and other rehabilitation goals that are medically necessary. One major change that this memorandum brought was the fact that visually impaired people who are *not* legally blind can get coverage. It raised the acuity level requirement from 20/200 (severely impaired—legally blind) to 20/70 (moderately impaired), and added a number of visual field conditions that could also now be covered (Program Memorandum, 2002).

Medicare Vision Rehabilitation Services Act of 2003

In 2003, Congress put language in the Appropriation Bill to encourage CMS to direct carriers and intermediaries to recognize the delivery of additional vision rehabilitation in the home that are included in a clinical care plan.

Medicare Prescription Drug, Improvement, and Modernization Act of 2003

There had been legislative attempts to implement coverage since 1999, but none had passed either house of Congress as of the beginning of 2016. The latest language coming out of Congress was in the Medicare Drug Bill, Section 645, which was signed into law in December 2003. When the compromise bill finally came out, it directed the Secretary of Health and Human Services to study the feasibility and advisability of Medicare payment for services of vision rehabilitation professionals (orientation and mobility specialists, rehabilitation teachers, or low-vision therapists; Medicare Drug Act, 2003)

Two other provider proposals came out in 2003 in the Conference Report on H.R. 2673, Consolidated Appropriations Act, 2004—(House of Representatives—November 25, 2003). One directed the Secretary to report on the provision of services by vision rehabilitation professionals (including in the home) under "general" supervision. The other requested a nationwide outpatient vision rehabilitation services demonstration project to examine the impact of "standardized" national vision rehabilitation provided in the home by physicians, occupational therapists, and vision rehabilitation teachers (Consolidated Appropriations Act, 2004).

Because other third-party coverage generally follows Medicare, it is expected that other policies will ultimately cover vision rehabilitation, if they are not already doing so. It should be noted that Medicare does not cover the low-vision examination done by optometrists and ophthalmologists. The medical part of the exam would be covered, but there is generally a charge to the patient for the noncovered part ("refractive" or "optical"). Medicare also does not currently cover the provision of low-vision devices that are so beneficial to most of these patients. The American Academy of Ophthalmology and the American Optometric Association are currently trying to address these issues. In the current climate of downsizing and budget limitations, this is not an easy task.

Demonstration Project Gets Underway—2003

The Demonstration Project, described in the Medicare Prescription Drug, Improvement, and Modernization Act of 2003 (Medicare Drug Act, 2003), began on April 1, 2006, and was planned to run through March 31, 2011 in six demonstration sites. It extended the provider list for rehabilitation training to include certified low-vision therapists, orientation and mobility specialists, and rehabilitation teachers, and allowed these individuals to provide services under general supervision.

At the conclusion, a report was to be produced to determine whether low-vision rehabilitation services should be covered for the additional providers for all Medicare recipients across the country. Unfortunately, the project did not run as long as planned. There was very little participation, and nothing was really demonstrated. Two shortcomings in the way the care system served the beneficiaries were identified:

> First, some medical providers were reported to lack knowledge of and referral relationships with low vision (LV) providers. Second, the lack of coverage of devices and other adaptive items in the Low Vision Rehabilitation Demonstration benefit was a barrier to receiving help for some beneficiaries, and the barrier would have been greater had the Center for Visual Impairment not covered devices through charitable funds. (Bishop, 2010)

It should be noted that concerns about the Demonstration Project had been expressed: "There are intrinsic flaws in the scope and design of the project that preclude its successful implementation and may even undermine the services that have been expended by Medicare to beneficiaries with visual impairments in the last decade" (Mogk, Watson, & Williams, 2008). The article concluded that the Demonstration Project should be either completely restructured or terminated.

Americans with Disabilities Amendments Act of 2008

The Americans with Disabilities Amendments Act of 2008 (ADA; 110 325 [S3406]) was passed by

Congress and signed by the President on September 25, 2008. Its purpose is to restore the intent and protections of the Americans with Disabilities Act of 1990. It includes two important features of particular interest:

- If an individual has a visual disability that impacts a major life activity, such as reading, and is using low-vision devices to compensate for that disability, their disability status is evaluated based on the person's normal visual abilities with ordinary eye glasses or contact lenses, but not with low-vision devices.
- It makes the important distinction between glasses/contact lenses and low-vision devices:
  - (I) the term "ordinary eyeglasses or contact lenses" means lenses that are intended to fully correct visual acuity or eliminate refractive error; and
  - (II) the term "low-vision devices" means devices that magnify, enhance, or otherwise augment a visual image.
  (ADA Amendments Act of 2008)

Demonstration Project Rejuvinated—2013

On December 12, 2013, H.R.3749, the Medicare Demonstration of Coverage for Low Vision Devices Act of 2013 was introduced to the House Energy and Commerce and Ways and Means committees. It was referred to the Subcommittee on Health. The American Council for the Blind initiated this bill. The bill

> directs the Secretary of Health and Human Services (HHS) to commence a project to demonstrate and evaluate the impact of covering low vision devices under part B (Supplementary Medical Insurance) of title XVIII (Medicare) of the Social Security Act in the same or similar manner as coverage is provided for durable medical equipment under such part (H.R.3749, 2013).

The demonstration project is to run for 5 years. Participants receiving services would have to complete a low-vision examination performed by a physician (Medical Doctor or Doctor of Optometry), and the recommended low-vision device would have to be deemed as medically necessary. The bill would "allow reimbursement for certain low vision devices that are the most function-rich, most powerful, and most expensive" (Roberts, 2015). What exactly would be covered was not described in the bill. There is a general description in the bill of the term "low vision device" as meaning "a device, prescribed by a physician that magnifies, enhances, or otherwise augments or interprets visual images irrespective of the size, form, or technological features of such device and does not include ordinary eye-glasses or contact lenses" (H.R.729, 2015). No action has been taken as of November 20, 2015.

A Major Stumbling Block for Medicare Coverage of Low-Vision Devices

A major problem with any bill trying to get coverage of low vision devices (optical and/or electro-optical) is that Medicare does not cover them because they are included under the eyeglasses exclusion. It defines them as "all devices irrespective of their size, form, or technological features that use one or more lenses to aid vision or *provide magnification of images for impaired vision*" (italicized by the authors; Center for Medicare Advocacy, Inc., 2013).

This problem should have been remedied with the passage of the ADA Amendments Act of 2008, described earlier. Unfortunately, this does not seem to be the case. The Center for Medicare Advocacy continues to use the same argument against coverage. It has been noted that "Medicare's limited coverage for eyeglasses and vision assistance is a significant gap that poses a problem for many beneficiaries" (Center for Medicare Advocacy, Inc., 2013). It appears that it may be successfully challenged in litigation, based on the three federal court decisions that have interpreted the Medicare statute as allowing coverage of low-vision devices, but only those pertaining to the cases.

For additional information about Medicare coverage of vision assistive equipment (low-vision devices), see (Morse, 2010; Whitson, 2014).

CONCLUSION

The prevalence of vision loss is markedly increasing with the aging U.S. and worldwide populations. The leading conditions resulting in this vision loss will continue to be AMD, glaucoma, diabetic retinopathy, and cataracts.

Advances in the treatment and understanding of the mechanisms in the "dry" and "wet" forms of

AMD, as well as new treatments for diabetic retinopathy, glaucoma, and many other ocular conditions will ultimately have long-term effects in preserving visual function. These treatments now include both genetic and stem cell therapies, as well as new nutritional and pharmaceutical approaches. This is of great importance, especially because the annual cost of adult vision problems in the United States was around $51.4 billion in 2007 (Prevent Blindness America, 2008). A significantly larger cost was calculated for 2011, coming to $139 billion based on the 2011 U.S. population (including children and adults under age 40) in 2013 dollars. It was also estimated that uncorrectable vision loss resulted in a social burden of 283 disability-adjusted life years (DALYs) lost. If this was included in the monetary cost of vision loss (assuming $50,000 per DALY), the total economic burden would increase by $14 billion to a total of $153 billion (Rein & Wittenborn, 2013).

A study published in 2013 gave a value for lost productivity due to lower wages and reduced workforce participation of $48.4 billion for the visually impaired and blind ages 18 and over, of which $24.6 billion was attributed to ages 65 and over. On top of this, there is also productivity losses resulting from informal care, which refers to care provided by someone for visually impaired family members. The total for ages 18 and over is $2.1 billion, with $1.3 billion attributed to those 65 and over (Rein & Wittenborn, 2013).

Screening and early detection, along with new therapies and treatments, will result not only in great cost savings to society but also in increased quality of life for persons affected with age-related eye disease. Unfortunately, as the older population in the United States is increasing, and in particular the leading age of the baby boomers who are now moving into their 70+ years of age, we are not sure how much the total cost curve can be brought down, if at all.

REFERENCES

ADA Amendments Act of 2008. Retrieved from http://www.eeoc.gov/laws/statutes/adaaa.cfm

Adhi, M., Duker, J. S. (2013). Optical coherence tomography–current and future applications. *Current Opinion in Ophthalmology, 24*(3), 213–221.

Arditi, A., & Rosenthal, B. (1996, July). *Developing an objective definition of visual impairment*. Paper presented at the VISION 96 International Conference on Low-Vision Proceedings (Book 1), Madrid, Spain.

The Association for Research in Vision and Ophthalmology. (2014). New poll: Americans fear blindness more than loss of other senses, strongly support more funding for research. Retrieved from http://www.arvo.org/About_ARVO/Press_Room/New_poll__Americans_fear_blindness_more_than_loss_of_other_senses,_strongly_support_more_funding_for_research

Bass, S. J., & Sherman, J. (1996). Visual field testing in the low vision patient. In B. P. Rosenthal & R. G. Cole (Eds.), *Functional assessment of low vision* (pp. 89–100). St. Louis, MO: C. V. Mosby.

Bishop, C. (2010). *Evaluation of the medicare low vision rehabilitation demonstration-beneficiary case study—Final report* (p. vi). Schneider Institutes for Health Policy, The Heller School for Social Policy and Management, Brandeis University.

Brown, G. C., & Murphy, R. P. (1992). Visual symptoms associated with choroidal neovascularization: Photopsias and the Charles bonnet syndrome. *Archives of Ophthalmology, 110*, 1251.

Center for Medicare Advocacy, Inc. (2013). Medicare coverage of eyeglasses and low vision devices. Retrieved from http://www.medicareadvocacy.org/old-site/News/Archives/PartB_07.09.20.eyeglasses.htm#_ednref15

Centers for Disease Control and Prevention. (2011). *The state of vision, aging, and public health in America*. Washington, DC: U.S. Department of Health and Human Services. Retrieved from http://www.cdc.gov/aging/data/stateofaging.htm

Chapman, R. S., Cross, K. W., & Fleming, D. M. (2003). The incidence of shingles and its implications for vaccination policy. *Vaccine, 21*, 2541–2547.

Chew, E. Y., Lindblad, A. S., Clemons, T., & The Age-Related Eye Disease Study Research Group. (2009). Summary results and recommendations from the age-related eye disease study. *Archives of Ophthalmology, 127*(12), 1678–1679.

Clemons, T. E., Milton, R. C., Klein, R., Seddon, J. M., & Ferris, F. L., 3rd. (2005). Age-related eye disease study research group: Risk factors for the incidence of advanced age-related macular degeneration in the age-related eye disease study (AREDS) AREDS report No. 19. *Ophthalmology, 112*, 533–539.

Cohen, J. M., & Waiss, B. M. (1994). An overview of visual rehabilitation for stroke and head trauma patients. *Aging and Vision News, 6*, 3, 11.

Cole, R. J. (2008). Modifications to the Fletcher central field test for patients with low vision. *Journal of Visual Impairment & Blindness, 102*, 659.

Colenbrander, A. (1977). Dimensions of visual performance. *Transactions of the American Academy of Ophthalmology and Otolaryngology, 83*, 322.

Congdon, N., Vingerling, J. R., Klein, B. E., West, S., Friedman, D. S., Kempen, J., . . . Eye Diseases Prevalence Research Group. (2004). Prevalence of cataract and pseudophakia/aphakia among adults in the United States. *Archives of Ophthalmology, 122*, 487–494.

Consolidated Appropriations Act, Pub. L. 108–199. (2004). Retrieved from http://thomas.loc.gov/cgi-bin/query/z?c108:H.R.2673 (Select Version 6).

Crossland, M., & Rubin, G. (2007). The amsler chart: Absence of evidence is not evidence of absence. *The British Journal of Ophthalmology, 91*(3), 391–393. doi:10.1136/bjo.2006.095315

Dua, H. S., Faraj, L. A., Said, D. G., Gray, T., & Lowe, J. (2013). Human corneal anatomy redefined. *Ophthalmology, 120*(9), 1778–1785. doi:10.1016/j.ophtha.2013.01.018

Eye Disease Prevalence Research Group. (2004). Blindness. *Archives of Ophthalmology, 122*, 437–676.

Fong, D. S., Aiello, L., Gardner, T. W., King, G. L., Blankenship, F., Cavallereno, J. D., . . . American Diabetes Association. (2004). Retinopathy in diabetes. *Diabetes Care, 27*, S99–S102.

Friedman, D. S., O'Colmain, B. J., Munoz, B., Tomany, S. C., McCarty, C., de Jong, P. T., . . . For the Eye Disease Prevalence Research Group. (2004). Prevalence of age-related macular degeneration in the United States. *Archives of Ophthalmology, 122*, 564–573.

Friedman, D. S., Wolfs, R. C., O'Colmain, B. J., Klein, B. E., Taylor, H. R., West, S., . . . Eye Disease Prevalence Research Group. (2004). Prevalence of open-angle glaucoma among adults in the United States. *Archives of Ophthalmology, 122*, 532–538.

Fuchs, W. (1996). Preventing diabetic vision loss. *Aging and Vision News, 8*, 6–7.

Ginsburg, A. P., Rosenthal, B., & Cohen, J. (1987). The evaluation of the reading capability of low vision patients using the Vision Contrast Test System (VCTS). In G. C. Woo (Ed.), *Low vision: Principles and applications* (pp. 17–28). New York, NY: Springer-Verlag.

Gordon, M. O., Beiser, J. A., Brandt, J. D., Heuer, D. K., Higginbotham, E. J., Johnson, C. A., . . . Kass, M. A. (2002). The ocular hypertension treatment study: Baselines factors that predict the onset of primary open-angle glaucoma. *Archives of Ophthalmology, 120*, 714–720.

H.R.3749–Medicare Demonstration of Coverage for Low Vision Devices Act of 2013. (2013). Retrieved from https://www.congress.gov/bill/113th-congress/house-bill/3749

H.R.729–Medicare Demonstration of Coverage for Low Vision Devices Act of 2015. (2015). Retrieved from https://www.congress.gov/bill/114th-congress/house-bill/729

Haines, J. L., Hauser, M. A., Schmidt, S., Scott, W. K., Olson, L. M., Gallins, P., . . . Pericak-Vance, M. A. (2005). Complement factor H variant increases the risk of age-related macular degeneration. *Science, 308*, 419–421.

Homonymous hemianopsia. (n.d.). Retrieved from https://en.wikipedia.org/wiki/Homonymous_hemianopsia#/media/File:Rhvf.png

Horowitz, A., Reinhardt, J. P., & Kennedy, G. J. (2005). Major and subthreshold depression among older adults seeking vision rehabilitation services. *American Journal of Geriatric Psychiatry, 13*, 180–187.

ICD-10 (American Version). Retrieved from http://www.icd10data.com

ICD-10. World Health Organization-ICD-10 Version. (2016). Retrieved from http://apps.who.int/classifications/icd10/browse/2016/en

Javitt, J. C., Zhou, Z., & Wilke, R. J. (2007). Association between vision loss and higher medical care costs in medicare beneficiaries: Costs are greater for those with progressive vision loss. *Ophthalmology, 114*, 238–245.

Kempen, J. H., O'Colmain, B. J., Leske, M. C., Haffner, S. M., Klein, R., Moss, S. E., . . . Eye Disease Prevalence Research Group. (2004). The prevalence of diabetic retinopathy among adults in the United States. *Archives of Ophthalmology, 122*, 552–563.

Klein, R., Klein, B. E. K., Tomany, S. C., & Cruickshanks, K. J. (2003). The association of cardiovascular disease with the long-term incidence of age-related maculopathy: The Beaver Dam eye study. *Ophthalmology, 110*, 636–643.

Kupersmith, M. J., Karen, H., & Seiple, W. H. (1989). Contrast sensitivity testing. In M. Wall & A. A. Sadun (Eds.), *New methods of sensory visual testing* (pp. 53–67). New York, NY: Springer-Verlag.

Lindblad, B., Håkansson, N., Svensson, H., Philipson, B., & Wolk, A. (2005). Intensity of smoking and smoking cessation in relation to risk of cataract extraction: A prospective study of women. *American Journal of Epidemiology, 162*, 73–79.

Maguire, M. (1997). Who is at risk? *Aging and Vision News, 9*, 5.

Medicare Drug Act. (2003). Overview of the medicare prescription drug, improvement, and modernization Act of 2003. Retrieved from http://royce.house.gov/uploadedfiles/overview%20of%20medicare.pdf

Mogk, L., Watson, G., & Williams, M. (2008). A commentary on the medicare low vision rehabilitation demonstration project. *Journal of Visual Impairment & Blindness, 102*, 69–75.

Morse, A., Massof, R., Cole, R., Mogk, L., O'Hearn, A., Hsu, Y., . . . Jackson, M. (2010). Medicare coverage for vision assistive equipment. *Archives of Ophthalmology*, 128(10), 1350.

National Eye Institute. (1993). *Vision research: A National plan 1994–1998* (NIH Publication No. 95-3186). Bethesda, MD: Author.

National Eye Institute. (2013). *Age-related eye disease study 2 (AREDS2)*. Retrieved from https://nei.nih.gov/areds2

National Eye Institute. (2015). The most common eye diseases: NEI looks ahead. Retrieved from https://www.flickr.com/photos/nationaleyeinstitute/21997059516/in/album-72157646733299877

National Eye Institute. (n.d.-a.). Drawing of the eye. Retrieved from http://www.nationaleyeinstitute.net/photo/keyword.asp?conditions=Normal+Eye+Images&match=all

National Eye Institute. (n.d.-b.). Age-related macular degeneration (AMD). Retrieve from https://nei.nih.gov/eyedata/amd#5

National Eye Institute diabetic eye disease. (n.d.). Facts about diabetic eye disease. Retrieved from https://nei.nih.gov/health/diabetic/retinopathy

National Eye Institute, National Institutes of Health. (n.d.-a.). Amsler grid. Retrieved from https://www.flickr.com/search/?text=amsler%20grid

National Eye Institute, National Institutes of Health. (n.d.-b.). Distorted Amsler grid. Retrieved from https://www.flickr.com/photos/nationaleyeinstitute/7544605480

National Eye Institute, National Institutes of Health. (n.d.-c.). Visual acuity chart. Retrieved from https://www.flickr.com/photos/nationaleyeinstitute/7544604904/in/album-72157646870593861

National Eye Institute, National Institutes of Health. (n.d.-d.). Drawing of the eye. Retrieved from https://www.flickr.com/photos/nationaleyeinstitute/7544457582/in/album-72157646829197286

National Eye Institute, National Institutes of Health. (n.d.-e.). Surgery to treat glaucoma. Retrieved from https://www.flickr.com/photos/nationaleyeinstitute/7544457494/in/album-72157646829197286

National Retinitis Pigmentosa Foundation. (1995). *Fact sheets: Information about retinitis pigmentosa.* Retrieved from http://www.fightblindness.org/site/PageServer?pagename=VisionNation_Fact_Sheet

Parc, C. E., Johnson, D. H., Oliver, J. E., Hattenhauer, M. G., & Hodge, D. O. (2001). The long-term outcome of glaucoma filtration surgery. *American Journal of Ophthalmology, 132*, 27–35.

Patel, P. J., Chen, F. K., Da Cruz, L., Rubin G. S., Rufail, A., & the ABC Trial Study Group. (2011). Contrast sensitivity outcomes in the ABC trial: A randomized trial of bevacizumab for neovascular age-related macular degeneration. *Investigative Opthalmology & Visual Science*, *52*(6), 3089–3093. Retrieved from http://iovs.arvojournals.org/article.aspx?articleid=2165605

Pearson Education. (2009). *ICD-9-CM 2009 Hospital/Payer Edition* (Vol. 1, 2, 1st ed.). Retrieved from https://www.amazon.com/ICD-9-CM-2009-Hospital-Payer-Volumes/dp/0135099374.

Prevent Blindness America. (2012). *Vision problems in the U.S.: Prevalence of adult vision impairment and age-related eye disease in America.* Chicago, IL: Prevent Blindness America. Retrieved from http://www.visionproblemsus.org/index.html

Program Memorandum. (2002). Program memorandum intermediaries/carriers. Retrieved from https://www.cms.gov/Regulations-and-Guidance/Guidance/Transmittals/downloads/AB02078.pdf

Ramirez, M., Wu, Z., Moreno-Carranza, B., Jeziorski, M. C., Arnold, E., Díaz-Lezama, N., . . . Clapp, C. (2011). Vasoinhibin gene transfer by adenoassociated virus type 2 products against VEGF-and diabetes-induced retinal vasopermeability. *Investigative Opthalmology & Visual Science*, *52*(12), 8944–8950.

Ramrattan, R. S., Wolfs, R. C., Panda-Jones, S., Jonas, J. B., Bakker, D., Pols, H. A., Hofman, A., & de Jong, P. T. (2001). Prevalence and causes of visual field loss in the elderly and associations with impairment in daily functioning. *Archives of Ophthalmology*, *119*(12), 1788–1794. Retrieved from http://archopht.ama-assn.org/cgi/content/abstract/119/12/1788?ck=nck

Rein, D. B., & Wittenborn, J. S. (2013). *Cost of vision problems: The economic burden of vision loss and eye disorders in the United States. ResearchGate. NORC (National Opinion Research Center) at the University of Chicago.* Retrieved from http://www.researchgate.net/publication/249960785_Cost_of_Vision_Problems_The_Economic_Burden_of_Vision_Loss_and_Eye_Disorders_in_the_United_States

Roberts. (2015). Retrieved from http://lowvision.preventblindness.org/latest-news/legislation-re-introduced-to-cover-medicare-payment-for-low-vision-devices

Sarfarazi, M., & Rezaie, T. (2004). Optineurin in primary open angle glaucoma. *Ophthalmology Clinics of North America, 16*, 529–541.

Seddon, J. M., Cote, J., Davis, N., & Rosner, B. (2003). Progression of age-related macular degeneration: Association with body mass index, waist circumference, and waist-hip ratio. *Archives of Ophthalmology, 121*, 785–792.

Simons, K. (1991). Visual acuity and the functional definition of blindness. In W. Tasman & E. A. Jaeger (Eds.), *Duane's clinical ophthalmology* (Vol. 5, pp. 1–21). Philadelphia, PA: J. B. Lippincott.

Social Security Online. (n.d.). Retrieved from https://www.ssa.gov/disability/professionals/bluebook/2.00-SpecialSensesandSpeech-Adult.htm

Tan, J. S., Mitchell, P., Smith, W., & Wang, J. J. (2007). Cardiovascular risk factors and the long-term incidence of age-related macular degeneration: The blue mountains eye study. *Ophthalmology*, *114*(6), 1143–1150.

U.S. Census Bureau. (n.d.-a.). Retrieved from http://www.census.gov/popest/estimates.php

U.S. Census Bureau. (n.d.-b.). Retrieved from http://www.census.gov/popclock

Varma, R., Torres, M., Peña, F., Klein, R., & Azen, S. P. (2004). Prevalence of diabetic retinopathy in adult Latinos: The Los Angeles Latino eye study. *Ophthalmology, 111*, 1298–1306.

Wainapel, S. F. (2001). Low vision rehabilitation and rehabilitation medicine: A parable of parallels. In R. W. Massof & L. Lidoff (Eds.), *Issues in low vision rehabilitation—Service delivery, policy, and funding* (pp. 55–59). New York, NY: AFB Press.

Waiss, B., & Cohen, J. (1991). Glare and contrast sensitivity for low vision practitioners. *Problems in Optometry, 3*, 436.

Warren, M. (2000). An overview of low vision rehabilitation and the role of occupational therapy. In M. Warren (Ed.), *Low vision: Occupational therapy with the older adult* (pp. 11–14). Bethesda, MD: American Occupational Therapy Association.

Whitson, H. E. (2014). Hearing and vision care for older adults: Sensing a need to update medicare policy. *Journal of the American Medical Association, 312*(17), 1739–1740.

World Health Organization. (n.d.). International statistical classification of diseases and related health problems 10th revision of ICD-10-WHO version for 2016. Retrieved from http://www.who.int/classifications/icf/en

Yannuzzi, L. A., Slakter, J. S., Sorenson, J. A., Guyer, D. R., & Orlock, D. A. (1992). Digital indocyanine green videoangiography and choroidal neovascularization. *Retina, 12*, 191–223.

Yonekawa, Y., Miller, J. W., Kim I. K. (2015). Age-Related Macular Degeneration: Advances in Management and Diagnosis. *Journal of Clinical Medicine*, 4(2), 343–59. doi:10.3390/jcm4020343

Zarbin, M. A., Casaroli-Marano, R. P., & Rosenfeld, P. J. (2014). Age-related macular degeneration: Clinical findings, histopathology and imaging techniques. *Developments in Ophthalmology, 53*, 1–32. doi:10.1159/000358536

27

CHAPTER

Integrative Medicine

Charles Kim

Absence of evidence is not evidence of absence.
—Sagan (2006)

The term "integrative medicine" has been an evolving growth of semantics that arose from historical trends over several decades attempting to describe a wide body of practices, many of which trace back thousands of years. What has been and is still termed as "fringe" or "pseudo" medicine has evolved into a wide-ranging body of knowledge and practices that has been classified into systematic and formal groupings for clinical and research purposes. We have seen the terms change over the decades—description of these practices as "alternative" morph into "complementary," then to "complementary–alternative," to its present day descriptor as "integrative." It is no surprise to those in the modern medical field that integrative medicine is indeed an enmeshed part of the fabric of health care approaches, whether we choose to accept them or not. It is also no surprise in the scientific communities that integrative medicine needs to continue being studied and researched to validate its integration into "mainstream medicine."

In 1991, the U.S. government allocated funding to establish the Office of Alternative Medicine (OAM), charged to objectively test and research alternative medicine treatments. As the public interest and use of complementary alternative medicine (CAM) therapies increased, the OAM was elevated, with increased funding, to the National Center for Complementary and Alternative Medicine (NCCAM) in 1998. In 2014, the NCCAM changed its name to the National Center for Complementary and Integrative Health (NCCIH). The NCCIH is one of the 27 institutes of the National Institutes of Health (NIH).

In July 1999, representatives from eight academic medical centers (Duke University, Harvard University, Stanford University, University of California-San Francisco, University of Arizona, University of Maryland, University of Massachusetts, and the University of Minnesota) met in Kalamazoo, Michigan, to further develop and expand the field of integrative medicine (Academic Consortium for Integrative Medicine and Health, 2015). This meeting was termed the "Consortium of Integrative Medicine." Since its inception, this organization has grown and currently includes over 60 academic center members spread over the United States, Canada, and Mexico. The current name of this organization is the Consortium of Academic Health Centers for Integrative Medicine & Health (Consortium).

Integrative medicine has been most simply defined by *Merriam-Webster* as "medicine that integrates the therapies of alternative medicine with those practiced by mainstream medical practitioners."[1] With the help of the scientific method and studies, the term has meant to further validate and bring to "mainstream" medicine those "nonconventional" therapies that have been shown to hold scientific merit.

The National Health Interview Survey (NHIS; Centers for Disease Control and Prevention [CDC] and NCCIH) examined the trends of complementary health approaches among adults in the United States between 2002–2012 (Clark, Black, Stussman, Barnes, & Nahin, 2015). This study examined survey data from 88,962 adults over the age of 18 years. Overall, 34% of American adults utilized some form of CAM in 2012. They found that nonvitamin, nonmineral dietary supplements were the most popular CAM modality utilized. They also found that the use of body-based therapies (yoga, t'ai chi, and qi gong) increased linearly over this time period (Barnes, Bloom, & Nahin, 2008).

[1]From Merriam-Webster's Collegiate® Dictionary, 11th Edition © 2016 by Merriam-Webster, Inc. (www.Merriam-Webster.com).

In 2007, the NHIS found that Americans spent $33.9 billion in out-of-pocket costs for CAM therapies within a 12-month period. This figure comprised 11.2% of all total out-of-pocket expenditures on health care in the United States. Although no absolute figures are readily available, the coverage of these services by third-party payers has been showing steadily increasing acceptance, particularly for acupuncture services.

The NCCIH has adopted a classification system that organizes the wide-ranging and almost infinite amount of nonconventionally based medical practices and treatments into five primary areas. These include:

1. Whole medical systems
2. Mind–body medicine
3. Biologically based practices
4. Manipulative and body-based practices
5. Energy therapies

This chapter briefly discusses integrative medicine utilizing the classification approaches devised by the NCCIH, and provides selected research findings regarding some of their most popular examples.

WHOLE-MEDICAL SYSTEMS

Alternative can be best used to describe this class of CAM therapies. One of the most well-known whole medical systems is traditional Chinese medicine (TCM), which dates back in origin to 200 BCE, and has spread to other Asian cultures (e.g., Korea, Japan, India, Vietnam). Other examples of whole medical systems include Ayurveda, homeopathy, naturopathy, osteopathy, and chiropracty. The basic tenet of these medical systems is that they are "standalone" systems of health care utilizing their own unique "complete systems with explanation of disease, diagnosis, and therapy," as defined by the *Merck Manual* (Novella, 2015).

Example: Traditional Chinese Medicine

TCM focuses on the basic theory that all living beings (animals, plants) have a life energy flow. This life energy flow is called "Qi" (pronounced "chee") that flows throughout the body. When this flow of Qi is slowed, stagnant, or blocked, it is believed that illness, pain, and sickness occur. It is though interventions in TCM that the proper flow of Qi is manipulated and encouraged to promote health and well-being. Interventions in TCM that are utilized for this purpose include diet, medicinal patent herbs, exercise (Qi Gong), and acupuncture.

In one of the most comprehensive systematic reviews of TCM studies to date, Manheimer Wieland, Kimborough, Cheng, and Berman (2009) reviewed the *Cochrane Database of Systematic Reviews*. The group identified 70 studies of TCM: acupuncture (n = 26), Chinese herbal medicine (n = 42), moxibustion (n = 1), and t'ai chi (n = 1). Their conclusion was that most studies of TCM were inconclusive, due to poor methodology and heterogeneity.

Example: Acupuncture

Acupuncture has been one of the most well-known, researched, and used of the CAM therapies that have been integrated into modern medicine. With acupuncture, insertion of thin needles at focal points of the body impart therapeutic effects to the flow of Qi in the body. Acupuncture was one of the earliest therapies that brought attention to CAM, when the mainstream media first lauded its effectiveness in July 1971. It was a *New York Times* reporter, James Reston, who developed acute appendicitis in Peking, while covering President Richard Nixon's China visit. He underwent a conventional appendectomy at the Anti-Imperialist Hospital in Peking, but his postoperative pain was reportedly treated effectively with acupuncture (Reston, 1971). Reston's reported experiences with acupuncture, which appeared in the *Times* on July 26, 1971, was a pivotal event in CAM history, placing acupuncture on the world's center stage (Prensky, 1995).

Besides being one of the most popular of the CAM therapies, acupuncture has also been one of the most researched utilizing "Western" methodologies. Pomeranz and Cheng (1979) have been one of the pioneering Western researchers studying acupuncture. He showed that the analgesic effects of acupuncture could be blocked utilizing opiate antagonists, such as naloxone, as well as steroids.

As medical technologies advanced, so did the studies that examined acupuncture. Around the new millennium, several researches examined the effects of acupuncture on the body, utilizing technologies, such as functional MRI (fMRI) and single-photon emission CT (SPECT). Hui et al. (2000) found that acupuncture manipulations on normal subjects significantly reduced fMRI signals in the nucleus accumbens, amygdala, hippocampus, parahippocampus, hypothalamus, ventral tegmental area, anterior cingulate gyrus, caudate, putamen, temporal lobe, and insula. Newberg, Lariccia, Lee, Farrar, Lee, and Alavi (2005) looked at a pool of patients with chronic pain compared to controls after having acupuncture treatments. Utilizing SPECT imaging, they found that asymmetric uptake of radioisotope in the thalami of chronic pain subjects at baseline, compared to controls, normalized after having acupuncture. These functional imaging studies were able to show that acupuncture imparts observable attenuations in complex and key regions that are activated in the pain response.

In a more recent study, Torres-Rosas and his group at Rutgers looked at acupuncture's effects on immune response. They used a mouse model for sepsis and examined the effects of electro-acupuncture on systemic inflammation. They found that the acupuncture modulated the inflammatory response and reduced the sequelae of clinical sepsis, similar to dopamine-agonist effects (Torres-Rosas et al., 2014).

Berman, Powell-Griner, McFann, and Nahin (2004) examined acupuncture therapies for the treatment of osteoarthritis of the knee utilizing a randomized controlled trial (RCT). His group studied 570 subjects with osteoarthritis of the knee. The subjects were randomized into three groups: treatment, sham, and control (conventional therapy). After a treatment period of 26 weeks, they measured outcomes based on the Western Ontario and McMaster Universities Osteoarthritis Index (WOMAC) pain and function scores. They found significant improvements in pain relief and function in the acupuncture group versus the sham and control groups.

In one of the largest RCTs to date examining acupuncture, Haake et al. (2007) examined the effectiveness of acupuncture for the treatment of chronic low back pain. They studied 1,162 subjects, randomized into three groups: verum (true acupuncture points), sham (fake acupuncture points), and control (physical therapy, conventional medication, and exercise). After 6 months of intervention, they measured pain-related items on the Von Korff Chronic Pain Grade Scale questionnaire. They found that both verum and the sham acupuncture groups had significantly improved measures of pain compared to the control group. The difference between the verum and sham groups was not found to be significant.

The safety of acupuncture in clinical practice has also been reviewed. White, Hayoe, Hart, and Ernst (2001) conducted a prospective survey of 32,000 treatment consultations in Britain. They found that the rate of adverse events from acupuncture interventions numbered at a rate of 14 per 10,000 treatments. All these events cleared within 1 week, except one case that lasted 2 weeks, and another that lasted several weeks. The most commonly reported events found were bleeding (310 per 10,000) and needling pain (110 per 10,000). Wu et al. (2015) examined data from acupuncture-related complications from 1980 to 2013 in China. Over these 33 years, they found 182 incidents. Pneumothorax (n = 30), internal organ puncture (n = 22), syncope (n = 18), infections (n = 17), hemorrhage (n = 10), central nervous system injury (n = 37), peripheral nerve injury (n = 8), broken needles (n = 7), and others (n = 15) were determined to be the most serious adverse events. Although acupuncture is considered a very safe treatment modality, this large review highlights the wide range of potential adverse events.

MIND–BODY MEDICINE

The NCCIH defines mind–body interventions as those practices that "employ a variety of techniques designed to facilitate the mind's capacity to affect bodily function and symptoms." Some therapies included in this domain are guided imagery, hypnosis, meditation, prayer, mental healing, art therapy, music therapy, and dance therapy.

Example: Fibromyalgia

In a systematic review and meta-analysis study, Theadom, Cropley, Smith, Feigin, and McPherson (2015) looked at various mind–body therapies for the treatment of fibromyalgia pain, function, and mood. Fibromyalgia is categorized as a chronic disorder characterized by diffuse, widespread body pain, often accompanied by fatigue, sleep problems, anxiety, and depression. This group examined 62 RCTs to date, which included 4,234 adults. They found that there was low-quality evidence that psychological therapies helped patients with fibromyalgia. They also found that that subjects receiving mindfulness and relaxation training, showed little or no difference in physical functioning, pain, and mood.

Acupuncture for the treatment of fibromyalgia, has been more widely studied. Martin, Sletten, Williams, and Berger (2006) conducted a prospective, partially blinded, controlled, randomized clinical trial to examine acupuncture for the treatment of fibromyalgia. Fifty patients were randomized to an acupuncture group ($n = 25$) and a control group ($n = 25$) that received "sham" acupuncture. The symptoms of fibromyalgia were measured using the Fibromyalgia Impact Questionnaire (FIQ) and the Multidimensional Pain Inventory (MPI) at baseline, immediately after treatment, and at 1 and 7 months posttreatment. They found that acupuncture significantly improved pain symptoms of fibromyalgia, as well as decreasing fatigue and anxiety. In a more recent meta-analysis of acupuncture and fibromyalgia, Deare et al. (2013) found that there was low- to moderate-level evidence that acupuncture improved pain and stiffness in patients with fibromyalgia more effectively than with either no treatments or standard therapy. They also acknowledged the weak level of evidence and the problem of providing an ideal sham acupuncture in control subjects.

Example: Mindfulness Meditation

Mindfulness meditation is defined by *Mosby's Medical Dictionary* as "a technique of meditation in which distracting thoughts and feeling are not ignored but rather acknowledged and observed nonjudgmentally as they arise to create detachment from them and gain insight and awareness."[2]

Zeidan et al. (2015) examined mindfulness meditation for pain relief. They randomly assigned 75 healthy volunteers into four groups: (a) mindfulness mediation, (b) placebo conditioning, (c) sham mindfulness meditation, or (d) book-listening control intervention. The subjects were then assessed with psychophysical and functional neuroimaging to experimentally induced pain. They found that mindfulness-related pain relief was distinct from placebo analgesia. Specifically, they found that mindfulness-meditation related relief was associated with greater activation in brain regions associated with the cognitive modulation of pain (orbitofrontal, subgenual anterior cingulate, and anterior insular cortex).

Example: Music Therapy

Hole, Hirsch, Ball, and Meads (2015) reviewed the role of music as an adjunct for the postoperative recovery in adults. In a meta-analysis of 4,261 titles and abstracts, including 73 randomized control studies, they found that music significantly reduced postoperative pain, anxiety, and analgesia use, but no changes in length of stay. Other key points they found was that the choice of music by the patient, timing of the music being played, and when the patients were under general anesthesia, made no significant difference in outcomes.

BIOLOGICALLY BASED THERAPIES

As defined by the *Merck Manual*, "biologically based therapies are naturally occurring substances and include individual biologic therapies (such as using shark cartilage to treat cancer and glucosamine to treat osteoarthritis), diet therapy, herbal medicine, orthomolecular medicine, and chelation therapy."

Example: Shark Cartilage

In Chinese culture and TCM, shark cartilage has been used for centuries to treat various ailments, as well as a tonic to vivify health and well-being. Shark fin has been prepared in powdered form to easily mix with other ingredients for patent traditional Chinese medicines. It has also been ingested in food, as in the traditional "shark fin soup" that is often served at special events, such as weddings and banquets.

The use of shark fin for cancer treatments has been controversial (Pollack, 2007). Opponents note that it contains significant levels of neurotoxins, such as mercury and beta-N-methylamino-l-alanine (BMAA), potentially causing harm without proven cancer fighting benefits (Mondo et al., 2014).

[2] Mosby's Medical Dictionary, 9th edition. © 2009, Elsevier.

Lu et al. (2010) added a shark cartilage extract (*AE-941*) to traditional chemoradiotherapy for roughly one half of a total subject pool of 379 patients with unresectable Stage III non-small cell lung cancer. The randomized experiment group received the standard chemoradiotherapy with the *AE-941*, while the control group received only the traditional chemoradiotherapy. They found that there was no statistically significant difference in overall survival between these two groups.

Example: Ginseng

Ginseng is a group of slow-growing plants with fleshy roots typically found in cooler climates in North America and eastern Asia. Ginseng has been used for thousands of years as a medicinal herb and tonic and can be found in small doses in various energy drinks, herbal teas, and cosmetic preparations.

Barton et al. (2010) looked at using American ginseng (*Panax quinquefolius*) in treating cancer-related fatigue. Two hundred ninety cancer patients were randomized to receive American ginseng in doses of 750, 1,000, or 2,000 mg/day, or placebo given twice daily over 8 weeks. Their outcome measures included the Brief Fatigue Inventory, the vitality subscale of the Medical Outcome Scale Short Form-36 (SF-36), and the Global Impression of Benefit Scale, at 4 and 8 weeks. They found that over twice as many patients on ginseng perceived a benefit, and were satisfied with treatment over the placebo group with no significant toxicity measured between the dose arms. Although they did not find definite dose response, they concluded that there appeared to be some activity and tolerable toxicity at the 1,000 to 2,000 mg/day doses of the American ginseng with regard to cancer-related fatigue.

Example: Glucosamine

The popularity of glucosamine supplement use for patients with osteoarthritis has become one of the most commonly utilized of the CAM therapies. Glucosamine is a sugar that is the precursor in the production of glycosaminoglycans, proteoglycans, and glycolipids, which are substances required for normal joint function. Glucosamine is readily available in different chemical forms, including glucosamine sulfate, glucosamine hydrochloride, and N-acetylglucosamine. It is also available in combination with chondroitin sulfate, a structural component of cartilage.

The use of glucosamine products has been steadily rising over the past several decades. The global market for glucosamine products is expected to grow to $1.25 billion from 2014 to 2020, up from a $528.8 million market in 2013 (Grand View Research, 2016).

Bruyere et al. (2004) looked at glucosamine sulfate on disease progression in two 3-year, randomized, placebo-controlled, prospective, independent studies specifically focusing on post-menopausal women with knee osteoarthritis ($n = 414$). They examined joint space narrowing, as well as functional WOMAC scores, at baseline and after 3 years. They found that glucosamine use resulted in significantly less joint space narrowing and improvements in physical function scales (WOMAC) over time. These studies demonstrated for the first time that pharmacologic intervention for osteoarthritis has a disease-modifying effect.

Hochberg et al. (2016) studies led the Multicentre Osteoarthritis interVEntion trial (MOVES) that examined the efficacy and safety of chondroitin sulfate and glucosamine hydrochloride (GH+CS) compared to celecoxib, a nonsteroidal anti-inflammatory drug in patients with knee osteoarthritis. Six hundred six subjects with moderate to severe pain were randomized into groups: GH 500 mg + CS 400 mg, three times a day versus 200 mg celecoxib for 6 months. They found that the GH+CS group had similar efficacy to celecoxib with significant reduction in pain, stiffness, functional limitations, and joint swelling/effusion, with a good safety profile.

MANIPULATIVE AND BODY-BASED THERAPIES

Manipulative and body-based practices focus primarily on the structures and systems of the body, including the bones and joints, soft tissues, and the circulatory and lymphatic systems (Brainline.org).

Some examples of this group of integrative therapies include, chiropractic, osteopathic manipulation, massage therapy, cupping, Tui Na, reflexology, rolfing, Alexander technique, and Feldenkrais method.

Example: Cupping

Cupping therapy utilizes a sustained and controlled local suction over the skin, often creating bruises and ecchymosis. The cup is usually made of ceramic, glass, or plastic. The suction is produced with either heat or a pump mechanism. Cupping therapy dates back to as early as 3000 BCE and has been historically documented as a health intervention in ancient Egypt, China, Greece, and Persia, among others. When the skin is pierced to produce bleeding prior to the application of the cups, this is called "wet cupping." "Dry cupping" is provided without bleeding. Cupping has been used for a broad range of medical conditions, such as pain, bleeding disorders, skin diseases, respiratory diseases, rheumatic diseases, and fertility.

Kim et al. (2012) assessed cupping therapy in the treatment of neck pain in video display terminal (VDT) users. They randomized 40 VDT workers with moderate to severe neck pain into a treatment group receiving six sessions of wet and dry cupping, and a heating pad application control group. They measured response to the interventions during and after a 7-week period with a 0 to 100 numeric pain scale for neck pain numeric rating scale (NRS), Measure Yourself Medical Outcome Profile 2 score (MYMOP2), cervical spine range of motion, neck disability index (NDI), the EuroQoL health index (EQ-5D), short form stress response inventory, and fatigue severity scale (FSS). They found that compared with heating pad control, the cupping group reported significant improvements across all measured responses.

Example: Alexander Technique

The Alexander technique is named after Frederick Matthias Alexander (1869–1955) who was a Shakespearean orator. He found that awareness of postural activities led to decreased physical problems, such as vocal hoarseness and pain. The Alexander technique focuses on helping people recognize and unlearn maladaptive physical motions and imbalances in favor of a more balanced state of alignment.

The Alexander technique and acupuncture were used to treat patients with chronic neck pain in a randomized trial. In this study, MacPherson et al. (2015) randomized 517 patients with neck pain, which lasted for a median duration of 6 years, into three groups: (a) acupuncture, (b) Alexander lessons, and (c) usual care control (prescribed medications and physical therapy). They then measured the subjects' response to the interventions with the Northwick Park Questionnaire (NPQ) for neck pain and Chronic Pain Self-Efficacy Scale. Over a study period of 1 year, they assessed interventions at 0, 3, 6, and 12 months. They found significant reductions in neck pain and associated disability in the acupuncture and Alexander groups, compared to usual care, at study completion.

In another study, Lauche et al. (2016) conducted a RCT evaluating the efficacy of the Alexander technique in treating chronic nonspecific neck pain. They randomized 72 patients into three parallel groups: (a) Alexander group, (b) local heat application, and (c) guided imagery. They measured response to treatments at Week 5 with a 100-mm visual analog scale. They did not find any significant superiority of Alexander technique to local heat application but did show significant superiority of Alexander technique to guided imagery.

Example: Feldenkrais Method

The Feldenkrais method was developed by Moshe Feldenkrais (1904–1984), an Israeli physicist. He theorized that increasing a person's kinesthetic and proprioceptive self-awareness of functional movement improved function and decreased pain (Thomas, 1985).

Lundqvist, Zetterlund, and Richter (2014) studied the efficacy of the Feldenkrais method in chronic neck/scapular pain in people with visual impairment. Sixty-one subjects were randomized into either the Feldenkrais method or an untreated control group. The treatment group received one 2-hour Feldenkrais method session per week for 12 consecutive weeks. They measured pain with the Medical Outcomes Study 36-item Short-Form Health Survey bodily pain scale. They found that the Feldenkrais group reported significantly less pain than the control group at 12 weeks, and at 1-year follow-up.

Hiller and Worley (2015) performed a systematic review of randomized controlled studies to date examining the evidence for the benefits of the Feldenkrais method. Their review included 20 RCTs, which they found were highly heterogeneous in population, outcome, and findings.

Of these 20 RCTs, they were able to perform a meta-analysis on seven studies, finding that the Feldenkrais method improved balance in aging populations and functional reach test. However, they concluded that further research was required to draw conclusions as the effects of Feldenkrais method appear to be generic, supporting the idea that it works on a learning paradigm instead of disease-based mechanisms.

Example: Massage Therapy

Massage is defined by *Merriam-Webster* as the "manipulation of tissues (as by rubbing, stroking, kneading, or tapping) with the hand or an instrument especially for therapeutic purposes."[3] Massage therapy is one of the oldest therapeutic modalities, with historical evidence found in many ancient civilizations from Asia (China, Japan, India, Korea), Europe (Greek, Roman), and Persia. There are numerous types of massage therapies such as acupressure, Shiatsu, Bowen technique, craniosacral therapy, Kum Nye, lymphatic drainage, medical massage, myofascial release, Namaste massage, Reflexology, sports massage, Swedish massage, Traditional Chinese massage, Thai massage, Tui na, trigger point therapy, and many others.

Massage therapy is among the most commonly provided CAM treatments in both inpatient and ambulatory settings. According to a survey conducted by the American Hospital Association and Samueli Institute in 2010, the top CAM services offered at hospital outpatient sites were massage therapy, acupuncture, and guided imagery. The survey found that the top CAM services offered at hospital inpatient sites were: pet therapy, massage, and music/art therapies. The survey also found that these services were associated with 85% patient satisfaction.

Furlan et al. (2015) performed a meta-analysis of 25 trials involving 3,096 subjects examining massage therapy for lower back pain in a Cochrane Database Systematic Review. They found significant bias effects in these studies due to difficulty in subject and therapist blinding, as well as measuring outcomes due to a lack of standardized tools. They found that massage was associated with only a short-term decrease in pain in subjects with chronic, acute, and subacute lower back pain when compared with inactive controls. The confidence of these findings, due to the inherent study biases, was minimal, thus no definitive conclusion on its effectiveness was made by the investigators.

ENERGY THERAPIES

In a variety of health systems and practices, there is belief that there is an invisible energy force that flows through the body. For example, in TCM, this is *qi*. In Ayurvedic medicine, this is called *prana*. In this energy force view, it is thought that the proper flow of energy in our bodies is essential for good health. An imbalance or blockage of flow is thought to cause illness or pain. The goal of these energy therapies is to promote "health" by ensuring balanced flow of the energy force. Biofield and bioelectric–magnetic based therapies, such as Reiki, therapeutic touch, magnetic therapies, are also based on theories that purport to rebalance energy flow through manipulation treatments geared to treat illness and pain (Tabish, 2008).

In a Cochrane review by So, Jiang, and Qin (2008), several touch therapies (healing touch, therapeutic touch, and Reiki) were examined via research database search. Twenty-four randomized controlled studies with a total of 1,153 participants were included in the analysis. They found that participants having touch therapy had an average of 0.83 units (on a 0–10 pain scale) lower pain intensity compared to control groups. The authors found greater effects with Reiki studies and from trials by more experienced practitioners. They concluded a "modest effect" in pain relief with touch therapies, noting that more studies were needed.

In a systematic review and meta-analysis of randomized trials, Pittler Brown, and Ernst (2007) examined static magnets for the reduction of pain. They identified nine RCTs with placebos with visual analog scale measures. They did not find significant evidence to support the use of static magnets for pain relief.

Example: Qigong

According to the National Qigong Association, Qigong is "an integration of physical postures,

[3] From Merriam-Webster's Collegiate® Dictionary, 11th Edition © 2016 by Merriam-Webster, Inc. (www.Merriam-Webster.com).

breathing techniques, and focused intentions." The goal of Qigong is to help manipulate and improve the circulation of *Qi*, a life energy force based in TCM philosophies. According to the National Health Interview Survey (NHIS) on CAM by the CDC, between 2002 and 2007, the number of Americans practicing Qigong rose from 527,000 in 2002, to 625,000 in 2007 (Barnes et al., 2004, 2008).

Lynch, Sawynok, Hiew, and Marcon (2012) examined the effectiveness of Qigong for fibromyalgia. They randomized 100 subjects with fibromyalgia into immediate treatment, delayed treatment, and control care (waitlist, "usual care") groups for Chaoyi Fanhuan Qigong. They measured pain using the 11-point pain intensity numerical rating scale (PI-NRS), FIQ, sleep (Pittsburgh Sleep Quality Index), physical and mental function at baseline (SF-36 Health Survey), at 8 weeks, 4 months, and 6 months. They found that Qigong provided significant posttreatment benefits in several of the core domains in fibromyalgia (pain, sleep, and physical and mental function).

In another study, by von Trott et al. (2009), Qigong was studied versus traditional exercise therapy for elderly patient with chronic neck pain. They randomized 117 elderly patients with chronic neck pain (>6 months) to a Qigong group, exercise group, and a waitlist control group. Utilizing standard questionnaires, they measured neck pain using a visual analog scale, neck pain and disability (NPAD) scale, and quality of life (SF-36), at baseline, and after 3 and 6 months. They found that there was no significant difference between the Qigong and traditional exercise group. However, they did find that Qigong was more effective than no treatment (waitlist) group. The authors concluded that a larger sample should be utilized without a wait-list control group to better clarify the value of Qigong compared to exercise therapy.

CONCLUSION

The term "integrative medicine" has been borne out of the scientific need to translate "non-conventional" health therapies and systems, to better serve modern society's health care needs. It is no surprise that the main driver of increased use of CAM derives from the demand of consumers of health care. To meet this demand, health systems have significantly increased their resources to the consumers. In a 2011 follow-up survey by the American Hospital Association, 42% of responding hospitals indicated they offer one or more CAM therapies; up from 37% reported in their survey in 2007. Most importantly, the study found that 85% of responding hospitals indicated patient demand as the primary rationale in offering CAM services and 70% of survey respondents stated clinical effectiveness as their top reason (American Hospital Association and Samueli Institute, 2011; Ananth, 2009, 2011).

Perhaps as a sign that we "practice what we preach," a study examining therapeutics used by U.S. health care workers in 2012, a subject pool of 14,329 subjects indicated that they were more likely than the general population to utilize CAM services (Johnson, Ward, Knutson, & Sendelbach, 2012).

As can be seen by the increasing demand by the consumers of health care services, as well as a desire for further understanding by those in "mainstream" medicine, the future of integrative medicine will be determined by the successful marriage of the art, history, and science of medicine.

REFERENCES

Academic Consortium for Integrative Medicine and Health. (2015). *Member listing*.

American Hospital Association and Samueli Institute. (2011). *2010 complementary and alternative medicine survey*.

Ananth, S. (2009, March 31). A steady growth in CAM services. *Hospitals & Health Networks Magazine*.

Ananth, S. (2011). 2010 complementary and alternative medicine survey of hospitals. Retrieved from http://samueliinstitute.org

Barnes, P. M., Bloom, B., & Nahin, R. L. (2008, December 10). Complementary and alternative medicine use among adults and children: United States, 2007. *National Health Statistics Reports*, (12), 1–23.

Barnes, P. M., Powell-Griner, E., McFann, K., & Nahin, R. L. (2004, May 27). Complementary and alternative medicine use among adults: United States, 2002. *Advance Data*, (343), 1–19.

Barton, D. L., Soori, G. S., Bauer, B. A., Sloan, J. A., Johnson, P. A., Figueras, C., . . . Loprinzi, C. L. (2010, February). Pilot study of *Panax quinquefolius* (American ginseng) to improve cancer-related fatigue: A randomized, double-blind, dose-finding evaluation: NCCTG trial N03CA. *Support Care Cancer*, *18*(2), 179–187.

Berman, B. M., Lao, L., Langenberg, P., Lee, W. L., Gilpin, A. M., & Hochberg, M. C. (2004, December). Effectiveness of acupuncture as adjunctive therapy in osteoarthritis of the knee: A randomized, controlled trial. *Annals of Internal Medicine, 141*(12), 901–910.

Bruyere, O., Pavelka, K., Rovati, L. C., Deroisy, R., Olejaorva, M., Gatterova, J., . . . Reginster, J. Y. (2004). Glucosamine sulfate reduces osteoarthritis progression in postmenopausal women with knee osteoarthritis: Evidence for two 3-year studies. *Menopause, 11*(2), 138–143.

Clark, T. C., Black, L. I., Stussman, B. J., Barnes, P. M., & Nahin, R. L. (2015). *Trends in the use of complementary health approaches among adults: United States, 2002–2012* (National health statistics reports; No. 79). Hyattsville, MD: National Center for Health Statistics.

Deare, J. C., Zheng, Z., Xue, C. C., Liu, J. P., Shang, J., Scott, S. W., & Littlejohn, G. (2013, May 31). Acupuncture for treating fibromyalgia. *Cochrane Database of Systematic Reviews,* (5), CDC007070.

Furlan, A. D., Giraldo, M., Baswill, A., Irvin, E., & Imamura, M. (2015, September 1). Massage for low-back pain. *Cochrane Database of Systematic Reviews,* (9), CD001929.

Grand View Research. (2016). Glucosamine market analysis by application (nutritional supplements, food & beverages, dairy products) and segment forecasts to 2022. Retrieved from http://www.grandviewresearch.com/industry-analysis/glucosamine-market

Haake, M., Müller, H. H., Schade-Brittinger, C., Basler, H. D., Schäfer, H., Maier, C., . . . Molsberger, A. (2007). German Acupuncture Trials (GERAC) for chronic low back pain: Randomized, multicenter, blinded, parallel-group trial with 3 groups. *Archives of Internal Medicine, 167*(17), 1892–1898.

Hiller, S., & Worley, A. (2015). The effectiveness of the Feldenkrais method: A systematic review of the evidence. *Evidence-Based Complementary and Alternative Medicine, 2015,* 752160. doi:10.1155/2015/752160

Hochberg, M. C., Martel-Pelletier, J., Monfort, J., Moller, I., Castillo, J. R., Arden, N., . . . Pelletier, J. P. (2016). Combined chondroitin sulfate and glucosamine for painful knee osteoarthritis: A multicentre, randomised, double-blind, non-inferiority trial versus celecoxib. *Annals of the Rheumatic Diseases, 75*(1), 37–44.

Hole, J., Hirsch, M., Ball, E., & Meads, C. (2015, October 24). Music as an aid for postoperative recovery in adults: A systematic review and meta-analysis. *The Lancet, 386*(10004), 1659–1671.

Hui, K. K., Liu, J., Makris, N., Gollub, R. L., Chen, A. J., Moore, C. L., . . . Kwong, K. K. (2000). Acupuncture modulates the limbic system and subcortical gray structures of the human brain: Evidence from fMRI studies in normal subjects. *Human Brain Mapping, 9*(1), 13–25.

Johnson, P. J., Ward, A., Knutson, L., & Sendelbach, S. (2012). Personal use of complementary and alternative medicine (CAM) by U.S. health care workers. *Health Services Research, 47*(1, Pt. 1), 211–227.

Kim, T. H., Kang, J. W., Kim, K. H., Lee, M. H., Kim, J. E., Kim, J. H., . . . Hong, K. E. (2012). Cupping for treating neck pain in video display terminal (VDT) users: A randomized controlled pilot trial. *Journal of Occupational Health, 54*(6), 416–426.

Lauche, R., Schuth, M., Schwickert, M., Ludtke, R., Musial, F., Michalsen, A., . . . Choi, K. E. (2016). Efficacy of the Alexander technique in treating chronic non-specific neck pain: A randomized controlled trial. *Clinical Rehabilitation, 30*(3), 247–258.

Lu, C., Lee, J. J., Komaki, R., Herbst, R. S., Feng, L., Evans, W. K., . . . Fisch, M. J. (2010, June 16). Chemoradiotherapy with or without AE-941 in stage III non-small lung cancer: A randomized phase III trial. *Journal of the National Cancer Institute, 102*(12), 859–865.

Lundqvist, L. O., Zetterlund, C., & Richter, H. O. (2014, September). Effects of Feldenkrais method on chronic neck/scapular pain in people with visual impairment: A randomized controlled trial with one-year follow-up. *Archives of Physical Medicine and Rehabilitation, 95*(9), 1656–1661.

Lynch, M., Sawynok, J., Hiew, C., & Marcon, D. (2012, August 3). A randomized controlled-trial of Qigong for fibromyalgia. *Arthritis Research & Therapy, 14*(4), R178.

MacPherson, H., Tilbrook, H., Richmond, S., Woodman, J., Ballard, K., Atkin, K., . . . Watt, I. (2015, November 3). Alexander technique lessons or acupuncture sessions with persons with chronic neck pain: A randomized trial. *Annals of Internal Medicine, 163*(9), 653–662.

Manheimer, E., Wieland, S., Kimborough, E., Cheng, K., & Berman, B. M. (2009, September). Evidence from the Cochrane Collaboration for traditional Chinese Medicine therapies. *The Journal of Alternative and Complementary Medicine, 15*(9), 1001–1014.

Martin, D. P., Sletten, C. D., Williams, B. A., & Berger, I. H. (2006, June 8). Improvement in fibromyalgia symptoms with acupuncture: Results of a randomized controlled trial. *Mayo Clinic Proceedings, 81*(6), 749–757.

Mondo, K., Broc Glover, W., Murch, S. J., Liu, G., Cai, Y., Davis, D. A., & Mash, D. C. (2014, August). Environmental neurotoxins Beta-N-methylamino-l-alanine (BMAA) and mercury in shark cartilage dietary supplements. *Food and Chemical Toxicology, 70,* 26–32.

National Center for Complementary and Integrative Health – Organization – The NIH Almanac – National Institutes of Health. (n.d.). Retrieved from https://www.nih.gov/about-nih/what-we-do/nih-almanac/national-center-complementary-integrative-health-nccih

Newberg, A. B., Lariccia, P. J., Lee, B. Y., Farrar, J. T., Lee, L., & Alavi, A. (2005, January). Cerebral blood flow effects of pain and acupuncture: A preliminary single-photon emission computed tomography imaging study. *Journal of Neuroimaging, 15*(1), 43–49.

Novella, S. (2015). Alternative whole medical systems. *Merck Manual Professional Version.* Retrieved from https://www.merckmanuals.com/professional/special-subjects/complementary-and-alternative-medicine/alternative-whole-medical-systems

Pittler, M. H., Brown, E. M., & Ernst, E. (2008, September 25). Static magnets for reducing pain: A systematic review and meta-analysis of randomized trials. *Canadian Medical Association Journal, 177*(7), 736–742.

Pollack, A. (2007, June 3). Shark cartilage, not a cancer therapy. *The New York Times*, A32.

Pomeranz, B., & Cheng, R. (1979). Suppression of noxious responses in single neurons of cat spinal cord by electroacupuncture and its reveral by the opiate anatagosist naloxone. *Experimental Neurology, 64*(2), 327–341.

Prensky, W. L. (1995, December 14). Reston helped open a door to acupuncture. *The New York Times.* Retrieved from http://www.nytimes.com/1995/12/14/opinion/l-reston-helped-open-a-door-to-acupuncture-011282.html

Reston, J. (1971, July 26). Now about my operation in Peking. *The New York Times*, 1.

Sagan, C. (2006, November 2). *The varieties of scientific experience: A personal view of the search for god.* New York, NY: Penguin Press.

So, P. S., Jiang, Y., & Qin, Y. (2008, October 8). Touch therapies for pain relief in adults. *Cochrane Database of Systematic Reviews,* (4).

Tabish, S. A. (2008). Complementary and alternative healthcare: is it evidence-based? *International Journal of Health Sciences, 2*(1), V–IX.

Theadom, A., Cropley, M., Smith, H. E., Feigin, V. L., & McPherson, K. (2015, April 9). Mind and body therapy for fibromyalgia. *Cochrane Database of Systematic Reviews,* (4), CD001980.

Thomas, C. (1995). *Bodywork: What type of massage to get and how to make the most of it* (pp. 75–88). New York, NY: William Morrow and Co.

Torres-Rosas, R., Yehia, G., Pena, G., Mishra, P., del Rocio Thompson-Bonilla, M., Moreno-Eutimio, M. A., . . . Ulloa, L. (2014, March). Dopamine mediates vagal modulates vagal modulation of the immune system by electroacupuncture. *Nature Medicine, 20*(3), 291–295.

von Trott, P., Widermann, A. M., Ludtke, R., Reishauer, A., Willich, S. N., & Witt, C. M. (2009, May). Qigong and exercise therapy for elderly patients with chronic neck pain (QIBANE): A randomized controlled study. *The Journal of Pain, 10*(5), 501–508.

White, A., Hayoe, S., Hart, A., & Ernst, E. (2001, September 1). Adverse events following acupuncture: prospective survey of 32,000 consultations with doctors and physiotherapists. *BMJ: British Medical Journal*, *323*(7311), 485.

Wu, J., Hu, Y., Zhu, Y., Yin, P., Litscher, G., & Xu, S. (2015). Systematic review of adverse effects: a further step towards modernization of acupuncture in China. *Evidence-Based Complementary and Alternative Medicine, 2015*, 432–467.

Zeidan, F., Emerson, N. M., Farris, S. R., Ray, J. N., Jung, Y., McHaffie, J. G., & Coghill, R. C. (2015, November 18). Mindfulness meditation-based pain relief employs different neural mechanisms than placebo and sham mindfulness meditation-induced analgesia. *Journal of Neuroscience, 35*(46), 15307–15325.

28

CHAPTER

Rehabilitation Nursing

Mary Anne Loftus and Ana Mola

OVERVIEW

In this chapter, the decisions to highlight the selected nursing care topics were based on themes that span various disabilities and are essential to the patient's rehabilitation process. The scope of rehabilitation nursing care is broad; hence, the topics selected are core elements related to basic human needs with an overarching perspective of psychosocial health, which is vital to the patients' recovery.

INTRODUCTION

Based on the pioneering work of Dr. Frank Krusen and Dr. Howard Rusk, in 1947 the American Board of Physical Medicine and Rehabilitation was established. As the medical specialty of rehabilitation advanced, the need for the nursing community to expand its knowledge in this specialty grew as well. The Association of Rehabilitation Nursing (ARN) was founded in 1974 and, in 1976, the American Nurses Association (ANA) formally recognized ARN as a specialty nursing organization (Williams, 2011).

The ANA describes nursing as the "protection, promotion, and optimization of health and abilities, prevention of illness and injury, alleviation of suffering through the diagnosis and treatment of human response, and advocacy in the care of individuals, families, communities, and populations" (ANA, 2010, p. 66). The ARN, in collaboration with the ANA, further defines rehabilitation nursing as "a specialty practice area within the domain of professional nursing. It involves the diagnosis and treatment of individual and group human responses to actual or potential health problems related to altered functional ability and lifestyle" (Association of Rehabilitation Nurses, 2014, p. 7).

The rehabilitation nurse's practice is guided by both standards of practice and standards of professional performance to which the nurse is held accountable. The standards of practice refer to a "competent level of nursing care as demonstrated by critical thinking model known as the nursing process" (ANA, 2010, p. 9). These practices include assessing, diagnosing, planning, and implementing aspects of patient care, educating patients and their families, identifying patient outcomes, and coordinating care. The standards of professional performance "describe a competent level of behavior in the professional role" (ANA, 2010, p. 10), that includes working in an ethical, collaborative manner with patients, families, and other members of the health care team while utilizing research to maintain knowledge of the most current evidence-based practices in order to provide quality patient care.

The goal of the rehabilitation nurse as defined by ARN is "to assist the individual who has a disability or chronic illness in restoring, maintaining, and promoting maximal health" (2014, p. 7). The rehabilitation nurse works with the emotional, as well as the physical, aspects of the patient's condition. As patients and their families face these life-changing challenges, emphasis is placed on their abilities—what they are able to do versus what they are not able to do. Rehabilitation nurses understand that patients must learn to adapt to their situation and encourage patients to maximize their function. The rehabilitation nurse should be able to address the needs of the patient by anticipating what community resources patients, their families, and caregivers will need after discharge.

As with any nursing specialty, the rehabilitation nurse must possess a distinct knowledge and set of skills in order to assist all patients to achieve positive outcomes. Nursing has always focused on knowledge about people and their environment (Roy & Andrews, 1999). The nursing theoretical models are used as professional practice guidelines for organizing nursing knowledge, research, clinical practice, educational programs, and administrative systems (Fawcett, 2000). In caring for patients in rehabilitation clinical practice, these nursing models provide a framework to examine and interpret human health experiences by which nurses can interpret, plan, intervene, and evaluate the human behavior responses to an illness, disease trajectory, or disability (Fawcett, 2000). The goal of nursing, through its professional knowledge, is to empower patients to understand and embrace the rehabilitation self-care management practices.

Nurses in the rehabilitation setting have an opportunity to engage both the patients and caregivers within a model of shared decision making (SDM). This model has been mandated in the recent federal legislation of health care redesign within the Patient Protection and Affordable Care Act, Public Law 111-148, (March 23, 2010), as modified by the Health Care and Education Reconciliation Act of 2010, Public Law 111-152 (March 30, 2010), Title III, Subtitle F, Section 3506 (Frosch et al., 2011). The model of SDM is a collaborative process in which patients are supported by their health care professional to select from the available options with the goal being to protect and improve the health of populations and individual patients, while also helping control health care costs (Frosch et al., 2011).

An SDM dialogue is formed between the nurse and patient that includes a combination of a rehabilitation consultation, or conversations of the best scientific evidence, and the patient's value system and preferences. The patient's value system, which is a factor in SDM, is formed by the patient's beliefs, attitudes, and personal constructs, including contextual factors related to age, family, and social relationships. These factors are addressed by the process of both mutual information and interactive discussion among the patient, nurse, and other members of the health care team. It replaces the former approach of a traditional clinician-centered practice, where patients were dependent on their health care professional in a paternalistic manner to make decisions about their care (The Health Foundation, 2012). The SDM model is a positive development for patients' well-being in their path to recovery. Engaging patients, caregivers, and the health care team in the SDM process will allow all stakeholders to benefit from the health care system through increased patient experience, increased quality of care, and lower costs (Frosch et al., 2011).

SKIN INTEGRITY

The skin, which is the largest organ of the body, is responsible for providing a variety of major functions, including thermoregulation, sensation, metabolism, prevention of fluid loss, prevention of infection, and assisting in the elimination of waste products. It is of paramount importance that the patient's skin be assessed on a daily basis to ensure its integrity is maintained in order to prevent pressure ulcers. "A pressure ulcer is a localized injury to the skin and/or underlying tissue usually over a bony prominence, as a result of pressure or pressure in combination with shear" (National Pressure Ulcer Advisory Panel [NPUAP], the European Pressure Ulcer Advisory Panel [EPUAP], and Pan Pacific Pressure Injury Alliance [PPPIA], 2014).

Along with the elderly, the rehabilitation patient population includes those with spinal cord injuries (SCIs), burns, multiple sclerosis, Parkinsonism, strokes, and amputations that are at high risk to develop skin breakdown and pressure ulcers. The reasons that contribute to this complication are decreased mobility, lack of sensation, cognitive deficits, depression, vascular compromise, incontinence, and underlying acute or chronic medical conditions (Anton, 2012).

The NPUAP (2015) estimated that in the United States, the annual cost of pressure ulcer care approached $11 billion. The cost of treating an individual pressure ulcer ranges from $500 to $70,000. In addition to the high economic impact that comes with treating pressure ulcers, the psychological and social impact it has on the patients' quality of life can be devastating. During treatment, patients may require bed rest, which results in missed work or school, decreased social interaction, decreased functional status, increased cost for home care, depression, and secondary complications related to immobilization. A crucial goal for rehabilitation nursing is to maintain the patient's skin integrity and continually assess for the risk factors that contribute to skin breakdown in this vulnerable patient population. The nursing staff, in collaboration with the interdisciplinary team, works to minimize the potential for skin breakdown through implementing preventive strategies and assessing the effectiveness of those strategies based on the patient's individualized plan of care. Education provided to patients and their caregivers should focus on the causes and risk factors related to pressure ulcers and the strategies to use to minimize these risk factors. Patients should be encouraged to increase their activity as rapidly as tolerated in order to optimize maintenance of their skin integrity.

To identify patients who are at risk for developing pressure ulcers, a structured skin assessment should be completed upon admission to the hospital, as well as on a daily basis or more frequently if it is warranted by the patient's condition. The recommendation from the NPUAP, EPUAP, and the PPPIA (2014) is that a valid and reliable risk assessment tool be used to conduct a structured assessment with the following elements: patient's activity and mobility status, oxygenation, nutritional status, age, sensory perception, skin moisture, and general health status. This assessment should focus on the skin temperature, blanching response, and changes in tissue consistency and discoloration over bony prominences such as the sacrum, hips, and heels.

General Care Strategies

Pressure ulcer prevention is one of the most important proactive strategies employed by the rehabilitation nurse. Preventive interventions should be individualized to each patient and focused on the patient's identified risk factors, underlying condition, and diseases process. Interventions should address strategies for skin care, nutrition, repositioning and pressure redistribution, and support surfaces.

■ Skin Care

To maintain the integrity of the skin, the skin should be kept clean and dry. Avoid using water that is too hot or soaps that will dry out the skin. Moisturizers can be used to hydrate dry skin. If patients become incontinent, they should promptly be cleaned up. If there is difficultly maintaining dry skin owing to incontinence, drainage, or sweat, a skin barrier product can be utilized to protect the skin (Yap & Kennerly, 2011). In addition, the use of protective pads on beds and chairs can wick moisture away from the skin. The establishment of a bladder and/or bowel program for patients who are incontinent should be implemented to minimize or eliminate contact of urine and stool with the skin that would otherwise increase the risk of friction and shear (Wound, Ostomy and Continence Nurses Society [WOCN], 2010).

The patient's skin should be continuously assessed for potential breakdown related to impaired circulation caused by pressure. Pressure is defined by force divided by the total area that force is acting on. Thus, pressure will be higher for any given force when it is applied over a smaller surface. When the body is in certain positions, its weight (or force) can be unevenly distributed, causing excessive pressure in certain areas. For example, when sitting, the weight of the body (force) is concentrated over a small area (the ischium of the pelvis) resulting in high pressure. When pressure on the skin is high enough, it restricts capillary blood flow, causing localized areas of ischemia that may result in the development of pressure sores (Consortium for Spinal Cord Medicine, 2014). Therefore, the most common sites for the development of pressure ulcers are over bony prominences where body weight is concentrated, and include the sacrum, greater trochanter, ischium, and scapula. Massaging the skin over bony prominences is not recommended as this could lead to tissue damage (NPUAP, EPUAP, & PPPIA, 2014; Yap & Kennerly, 2011). Soft tissue such as the ear lobes, back of the head, elbows, and heels are also at risk for developing pressure ulcers if left in contact with various surfaces, such as beds and wheelchair components for prolonged periods of time (NPUAP, EPUAP, & PPPIA, 2014; WOCN, 2010). Nursing staff must be cognizant that pressure from positioning of medical devices including endotracheal tubes, nasal cannulas, tracheostomy ties, braces, and splints can also result in excessive pressure and possible skin breakdown. Strategies to reduce risks include repositioning of the devices and ensuring that devices are correctly sized, fit appropriately, and are sufficiently secured to avoid excessive pressure (NPUAP, EPUAP, & PPPIA, 2014).

Nutrition

Adequate nutrition and hydration are also vital components to maintaining skin integrity and healing pressure sores once they develop. All patients should have a nutritional screening completed on admission, which will assist the rehabilitation staff to understand what the patient's caloric, protein, and fluid intake should be each day. Malnutrition will result if the patient is not ingesting the required caloric and protein requirements needed by the body. Oral nutritional supplements can be provided to patients between meals if they are not consuming an adequate diet. Alternative options to consider if a patient's oral intake is not adequate to maintain appropriate nutrition include enteral or parenteral tube feeding if this is the patient's preference or the family's if the patient cannot express his or her wishes. Patients should be monitored for weight loss and signs of dehydration throughout the rehabilitation process (NPUAP, EPUAP, & PPPIA, 2014).

Repositioning

For patients who are immobile or require staff to reposition them, it is imperative to provide pressure relief on a regularly scheduled basis. This can be best accomplished by establishing repositioning schedules that are individualized to the patient's needs. To ensure appropriate pressure relief, patients who are bed bound should be turned and repositioned every 2 hours whether or not they are on a pressure relief mattress (NPUAP, EPUAP, & PPPIA, 2014; WOCN, 2010). Based on the patient's clinical condition, more frequent repositioning may be required. The head of the bed should not be raised more than 30° unless there is a clear medical rationale in order to more evenly distribute force over a larger surface area and prevent shear-related injuries from the patient sliding down in the bed (Yap & Kennerly, 2011). As well, the head of the bed should not be raised higher that 30° when positions are rotated (left side, back, right side). The prone position could also be used if it can be tolerated by the patient. When repositioning patients in bed or transferring them, utilizing lifting devices such as a lift sheet allows the patients to be moved rather being dragged, thereby reducing the possibility of exposing the patient to friction and shear. Positioning pillows or wedges can be used to provide protection over bony prominences to cushion them against surfaces. Pressure to the heel can be reduced by "floating" the patient's heels off the bed by using a pillow or heel protectors (NPUAP, EPUAP, & PPPIA, 2014; WOCN, 2010). Whenever possible, overhead trapezes and slide boards should be utilized to allow for patients to assist with mobility (WOCN, 2010).

For dependent patients who are chair bound, pressure redistribution should occur every hour or more often, as needed. Patients who are chair bound who are independent can be trained to provide pressure relief by shifting their weigh every 15 to 30 minutes. Patients with impairments of the spinal cord should maintain an offload position for at least 1 to 2 minutes every 30 minutes (Consortium for Spinal Cord Medicine, 2014). When in chairs, patients should be positioned comfortably ensuring support is provided to their arms and feet in order to minimize pressure and maintain a supported comfortable position. Rings or donut-shaped devices should not be used because they can create areas of high pressure (NPUAP, EPUAP, & PPPIA, 2014; WOCN, 2010).

Support Surfaces

Support surfaces are defined as "specialized devices for pressure redistribution designed for management of tissue loads, microclimate and/or other therapeutic function" (NPUAP, EPUAP, & PPPIA, 2014, p. 27). Selection of an appropriate support surface (utilized for both beds and chairs) is based on the individual needs of each patient. As the patient's condition changes, the support surfaces should also be reassessed for their effectiveness. Mattresses and support surfaces for beds are designed to either increase the body surface that comes into contact with the surface in order to reduce interface pressure, or reduce pressure at a given anatomical site by sequentially altering the part of the body that is bearing pressure (NPUAP, EPUAP, & PPPIA, 2014). It is important to assess all support surfaces for proper size and signs of daily wear. Ensuring that surfaces are providing effective pressure relief can be assessed by placing a hand under the mattress or cushion below the area at risk for skin breakdown, and if there is less than 1 inch between the patient and support material, the support surface is not providing adequate pressure relief (WOCN, 2010). Even when pressure redistributing support surfaces are being utilized, the importance of repositioning patients to provide comfort and pressure relief cannot be overemphasized.

Treatment

If a pressure ulcer exists, it is important to document if it was present on admission or developed after admission. A standardized measurement system is used to classify or stage the pressure ulcers based on the depth of the wound and the tissue layers involved. The treatment plan established is based on both patient and wound-related factors. Daily wound reassessment, pain management, and many of the previously mentioned strategies for prevention will need to be continued and incorporated into treatment plans. Nonsurgical treatment plans can involve wound cleansing, management of wound drainage, debridement, application of specialized wound dressings, and infection management. Surgical management might be necessary to close wounds that are not responding to conservative nonsurgical interventions (Preston, Tebben, & Johnson, 2008). The literature described several alternative treatment modalities that have been studied to promote healing of pressure ulcers, including electrical stimulation, ultraviolet and laser phototherapy, negative pressure wound therapy, hydrotherapy, and hyperbaric oxygen therapy. At this time, only electrical stimulation has scientific evidence to support its use in treating pressure ulcers (Garber, 2012).

BLADDER AND BOWEL MANAGEMENT

Patients in rehabilitation settings often experience bladder and bowel dysfunction as a result of their disease process. Based on the patient's diagnosis, there can be associated impairments with mobility, dexterity, cognitive functioning, pain, communication, and behavioral deficits, which will affect the patient's level of participation in carrying out successful bladder and bowel management. Consequently, this can lead to a variety of complications including incontinence, urinary retention, kidney stones, urinary tract infections (UTI), constipation, and fecal impaction. These can present major barriers to successful community integration, employment, and social activities for patients, and can adversely impact the quality of life of the patient and their caregivers. Rehabilitation nurses must be able to assess and recognize bowel and bladder disruptions and implement appropriate interventions that will result in effective elimination patterns. Nurses collaborate with the patient, caregiver, and other members of the rehabilitation team in the establishment of a realistic, achievable program to best meet the patient's needs, foster an increasing level of independence, and encourage compliance with the program. The elements of the program must be individualized to meet the needs of the patient's disease process, functional status, preferences, and safety issues, as well as whether or not a caregiver will be involved in assisting with the patient's management program.

As with all aspects of caring for patients in a rehabilitation setting, the interdisciplinary team develops a partnership and SDM with patients and their caregivers to develop an effective plan of care. Nurses are the members of the health care team who work most closely with the patient when it comes to bladder and bowel management. Rehabilitation nurses must provide an environment of encouragement, support, and privacy that will promote a sense of independence and confidence during this difficult time. Patients are encouraged to raise issues and fears they may have related to management of their bladder and bowel routine in order to assist with learning acceptance of their new "norm."

Education for both the patient and caregiver is essential for the bladder and bowel management program. Nurses ensure the patient and caregiver have adequate knowledge on the importance of maintaining a regular elimination schedule both inside and outside the home. They educate patients to recognize the signs and symptoms related to bladder and bowel impairment and strategies to prevent complications. Training is provided to the patient and caregiver on the techniques that will be used to perform the patient's bladder and/or bowel program, as well as the management and cleaning of equipment and supplies. Providing opportunities for return demonstrations of the psychomotor skills of the required techniques will assist the nursing staff in evaluating the effectiveness of the training. Nurses facilitate discussions on problem-solving strategies that can be utilized if the bladder and/or bowel program requires adjustment.

The patient and family are taught that after the patient has returned to the home setting, the program needs to be reevaluated on a regular basis and any required modifications to the program should be discussed with the physician.

Bladder Management

The urinary tract is composed of kidneys, ureters, bladder, and urethra. When the neurological system is intact, there is coordination between the bladder and the nervous system to allow for voluntary voiding. In patients with neurological impairment, there is often disruption of nerve impulses to the bladder that may cause them to experience incontinence (leaking of urine), have voiding difficulty and not be able to empty the bladder. Urinary incontinence is caused by a variety of factors including physiological, pathological, and psychological factors. Incontinence can be transient and is often reversible; however, when associated with a neurogenic bladder, dysfunction is more chronic in nature. The types of incontinence as described by Rye and Mauk (2012) and Anderson, Kautz, Bryant, and Clanin (2011) are:

- Stress incontinence: sudden, uncontrollable loss of small amounts of urine associated with activities such as coughing, laughing, sneezing, lifting, or exercising
- Urge incontinence: sudden, strong, frequent urges to void without the ability to delay urination
- Mixed incontinence: combination of both stress and urge incontinence
- Total incontinence: continuous uninhibited loss of urine
- Overflow incontinence: frequent dribbling of urine due to the inability to empty the bladder completely because of overdistension or retention
- Functional incontinence: loss of urine at inappropriate times and locations, without physiological cause.

The term "neurogenic bladder" refers to a variety of disorders that affect the bladder owing to disruption of the central nervous system through disease or trauma. As described by Rye and Mauk (2012), there are three classifications of neurogenic bladder disorders:

- Uninhibited bladder: This is associated with disorders of the brain and typically occurs in patients with stroke, brain injury, multiple sclerosis (MS), Parkinson's disease, and Alzheimer's disease. Patients experience the sensation to void but lack sufficient voluntary control to delay it, which results in incontinence, urgency, frequency, and nocturia.
- Reflexic or spastic bladder: Patients with this this type of neurogenic bladder, which is also known as bladder sphincter dyssynergia, most commonly have a SCI. The contractions of the bladder and urinary sphincter are poorly coordinated, which can result in high bladder pressure and back flow of urine to the kidney (Consortium for Spinal Cord Medicine, 2006). If not addressed properly, it can result in urinary tract infection, kidney stones, and kidney damage.
- Areflexic or flaccid bladder: Patients fail to empty their bladders because they have no sensation or voluntary voiding capacity. These patients, including those with lower motor neuron (LMN) SCIs and inflammation of the spinal cord, can experience urinary retention, reflux of urine into the kidneys, and overflow incontinence.

General Care Strategies

The desired outcome for bladder management is for the patient "to remain continent, empty the bladder completely, and avoid recurrent urinary tract infections and other complication of the bladder dysfunction" (Anderson et al., 2011, p. 118). There are a variety of techniques, interventions, and medications that can be combined to achieve a successful bladder management program based on the type of bladder dysfunction the patient experiences. Before any bladder management program is initiated, a comprehensive patient assessment needs to take place including the patient's voiding history and patterns as well as the patient's ability and willingness to perform necessary tasks. The assessment could include urine analysis, urine cultures, post void residual (PVR) volume measurements, and urodynamic studies.

General strategies that can be used by staff, patients, and caregivers include monitoring the patient's fluid intake and output and developing a fluid intake schedule. If patients are having difficulty with nighttime frequency, or nocturia, they should be instructed to stop drinking fluids 2 hours before bedtime. Initially, diapers can be used during both day and nighttime with the goal to only use absorbent underpads on the beds at night. Urinals should not be propped and patients should not be left on the bedpan for long periods of time as this can lead to skin breakdown. Routinely assess the patient's skin for signs of breakdown. Clean the patient's skin immediately after an episode of incontinence and apply barrier protection as warranted. As the patient's condition improves, discontinue the use of urinals and bedpans and assist the patient to a commode or to the bathroom (Anderson et al., 2011).

Bladder Training

The goals of a bladder training program are to reduce the number of episodes of incontinence and to assist the patient to regain control over bladder function. These programs can include fluid restrictions, scheduled voiding, prompted voiding, and medication. A flexible approach needs to be taken when collaborating with patients and caregivers to establish a program that will best meet the physical, cognitive, and lifestyle needs of the patient. Whether on a patient-initiated schedule or staff-prompted voiding schedule for those cognitively impaired, patients are placed on the bedpan, commode, or toilet every 2 hours for at least 5 minutes. As the patient's level of continence improves, the time intervals can be increased (Anderson et al., 2011; Stevens, 2008). Patients who have an uninhibited bladder, or experience transient incontinence, can be trained to perform pelvic floor muscle trainings (Kegel exercises), which strengthen the muscles used to prevent leakage of urine (Cournan, 2012).

Intermittent Catheterization

For patients who have difficultly emptying their bladder, intermittent catheterization is preferred to indwelling catheters (Healthcare Infection Control Practice Advisory Committee [HICPAC], 2009). Intermittent catheterization is recommended for patients who have the manual dexterity to execute this procedure, or have a caregiver who is willing to perform the catheterization. Intermittent catheterization is a method of removing urine from a neurogenic bladder that the patient is not able to voluntarily empty on his or her own. A flexible catheter is inserted into the bladder and removed once the urine has been drained. The normal bladder capacity for an adult is between 400 to 500 mL. In order to prevent overdistention of the bladder, the volume of urine should be maintained at less than 500 mL. The patient and/or caregiver is instructed to catheterize the bladder every 4 to 6 hours, noting that the frequency can be adjusted based on the volume of urine obtained. For example, if more than 500 mL is frequently retrieved, the frequency of catheterization should increase or the patient's fluid intake should be evaluated (Consortium for Spinal Cord Medicine, 2006; Goldmark, Niver & Ginsberg, 2014). In the home setting, a clean (nonsterile) technique is used verses the sterile techniques that is used in hospitals (HICPAC, 2009).

Indwelling Catheters

This type of catheter is inserted into the bladder for an extended period of time and continuously drains urine into a closed collection system. This can be done by using either a urethral or suprapubic catheter (inserted into bladder through the lower abdomen). Ideally, indwelling catheters should be removed as soon as possible to help facilitate bladder sphincter control and decrease the risk of infection (Cournan, 2012). However, the benefit of using an indwelling catheter may outweigh the risk in those patients who have poor hand skills, have high fluid intake, have not had success with other methods of bladder management, or do not have the availability of a caregiver (Consortium for Spinal Cord Medicine, 2006). Sterile equipment and technique should be used when inserting an indwelling catheter. If there is a break in technique, the catheter becomes disconnected from the drainage bag or there is leakage of urine, replace the catheter and closed drainage system (HICPAC, 2009). As recommended by the Consortium for Spinal Cord Medicine (2006), an indwelling urethral catheter should be replaced every 2 to 4 weeks or every 1 to 2 weeks if the patient is prone to catheter crustation or bladder stones. Patients with suprapubic catheters should change catheters every 4 weeks or more frequently if the patient has catheter crustation or bladder stones. Catheters and the collection tubing should be kept free from kinks and the collection bag should always be kept below the level of the bladder.

Educating patients and their caregivers regarding the signs and symptoms of all complications of bladder dysfunction is an essential component of being able to manage care as they transition to home. One of the most important conditions for patients, caregivers, and health care providers to quickly recognize is autonomic dysreflexia, which is a life-threatening emergency that requires immediate attention. It occurs in patients who have sustained an injury at or above spinal cord level T6 (see Chapter 24). Autonomic dysreflexia is initiated by a noxious stimulus below the level of the patient's neurological injury level, with the most common source being bladder distension followed by bowel distension. A common cause is restricted or blocked urine flow within an indwelling catheter, causing the bladder to become overdistended. The stimulus causes unopposed sympathetic nervous system activity below the level of injury resulting in blood vessel constriction and potentially dangerous hypertension. Corresponding parasympathetic activity above the injury level results in bradycardia, flushing, perspiration, and pounding headache. Other initiating stimuli can be from decubitus ulcers, urological procedures, pregnancy and delivery, restrictive clothing, and ingrown toe nails. Immediate treatment is focused on removing the offending stimulus and reducing the patient's blood pressure. The head of the bed should be raised, tight clothing should be loosened, and the bladder or rectal vault should be emptied. If left untreated, it can result in stroke, coma, or death (Martinkewiz, Furr, Farnan, & Martinez, 2011).

■ Credé and Valsalva Techniques

These are two techniques that can be used by patients with LMN injuries with low outlet resistance to assist with emptying the bladder. The bladder is typically flaccid following an injury to the most caudal portion of the spinal cord, thus lacking the ability to contract and empty normally. The Credé technique involves application of gentle pressure with the blade of the hand to the lower abdomen above the pubic area. The Valsalva maneuver utilizes the abdominal muscles and the diaphragm to push down on the bladder (Rye & Mauk, 2012), both of which can aid in evacuation of urine.

Bowel Management

Neurogenic bowel dysfunction occurs when there is a disruption in the central nervous system, either through disease or injury, that results in alterations in bowel function and impaired elimination. Patients can experience severe constipation, diarrhea, fecal urgency, and incontinence (Coggrave & Norton, 2013). The classifications of neurogenic bowel disorders are:

- Uninhibited bowel: This is seen in patients with lesions in the brain or above level C1 in the spinal cord and includes patients who have suffered strokes, brain injury, Parkinson's disease, MS, and dementia. Although the bowel sensation and reflex activity are intact, the brain does not have the same control over inhibitory processes so urgency and incontinence can occur. Patients experiencing this type of bowel dysfunction may regain adequate control by utilizing interventions such as scheduled toileting, medications and managing diet, physical activity, and fluid intake (Rye & Mauk, 2012).
- Reflexic bowel: This upper motor neuron (UMN) bowel disorder occurs in patients with SCIs above level T12 resulting from trauma or disease, such as MS and tumors. Patients lack sensation and are unaware of when the rectum is full, but as the defecation reflex remains intact, emptying can occur on a reflex basis resulting in episodes of incontinence. The anal sphincter remains tight so this can also cause patients to experience constipation (Coggrave & Norton, 2013; Rye & Mauk, 2012).
- Areflexic or flaccid bowel: A SCI below level T12 is considered to be an LMN disorder resulting in damage to the defecation reflex arc, relaxed anal sphincter, and a prolonged transit time (Coggrave & Norton, 2013). Patients experience frequent incontinent episodes, constipation, impaction, and stool leakage.

■ General Care Strategies

The goals of a bowel management program are for the patient "to remain continent, have formed bowel movements on a regular schedule, prevent diarrhea and constipation, and prevent complications such as hemorrhoids, abdominal distention, autonomic dysreflexia, and fecal impaction" (Anderson et al., 2011, p.118). Similar to a bladder management program, a comprehensive patient assessment needs to be taken focusing on the patient's premorbid bowel function, bowel habits (including time of day, stool characteristics, and medication use), and difficulties the patient might have experienced with evacuation. The assessment should include the patient's medical condition and the type of bowel dysfunction the patient is currently experiencing. A successful individualized bowel program must also address the patient's life style, personal preferences, and whether or not the patient's physical and cognitive ability will allow him or her to manage and maintain the program independently. The population with SCI will have a more complex regimen in comparison to those that have experienced a stroke or traumatic brain injury (Rye & Mauk, 2012).

Before oral medications are introduced into the bowel regimen, all natural methods should be utilized first. Monitoring the patient's daily fluid and fiber intake is essential to normalize stool consistency. The appropriate amount of fluid and fiber should be based on the patient's bowel dysfunction, but as a general guideline it is recommended that patients have an intake of 2 L of fluid a day with 20 to 35 g of dietary fiber (Rye & Mauk, 2012). Encouraging patients to engage in physical exercise and activities promotes gastrointestinal motility and assists in the prevention and treatment of constipation. Whenever possible, patients should be toileted and/or perform their bowel program in an upright position on a toilet or commode. This allows for gravity to assist in stool evacuation. If this is not feasible, it is recommended that patients lie on their left side to receive an enema or suppository (this supports absorption) and lay on their right side to facilitate elimination (Anderson et al., 2011).

The importance of determining a consistently timed toileting schedule to establish a predictable elimination response cannot be overemphasized. This not only assists in reducing the possibility of having incontinent episodes, but also allows patients to have some control over their daily schedules. In order to have the patient benefit from the gastrocolic reflex, encourage toileting to take place 15 to 30 minutes after a meal (Coggrave & Norton, 2013; Consortium for Spinal Cord Medicine, 1998). This reflex may also be stimulated by ingesting hot liquids.

Bowel Programs

The rehabilitation nursing staff needs to assist patients and families to understand that establishing an effective bowel program may take several months (especially for the population with SCI) and will involve periods of "trial and error." If patient outcomes are not being achieved, modification to the bowel program will need to occur. Unless the patient is experiencing serious complications, only one aspect (e.g., diet, frequency of care, medication) of the bowel program should be changed at a time. This allows the evaluation of the change in intervention to be assessed for effectiveness (Consortium for Spinal Cord Medicine, 1998). As with patients with bladder dysfunctions, the patients with bowel dysfunction may experience autonomic dysreflexia. Patients and caregivers need to be educated that this complication can be triggered though fecal impaction and rectal stimulation.

Reflexic (UMN) Bowel Program

In order to evacuate the bowel more effectively, the goal for patients with a reflexic bowel is to have a soft-formed stool consistency. In conjunction with monitoring the patient's diet to ensure the patient is taking in an adequate amount of fiber and fluid, bulking agents and stool softeners can be given to improve general bowel function and ensure the appropriate stool consistency. Suppositories and enemas are chemical stimulants that are used to stimulate a bowel movement and relieve constipation.

It has been described that the use of chemical stimulants alone will not do an adequate job of completely evacuating the rectum and most patients require digital stimulation or digital evacuation (Coggrave et al., 2009). Digital stimulation is a mechanical technique that involves gently stretching the anal sphincter muscle so that it relaxes. It is performed by inserting a gloved lubricated finger into the rectum and slowly rotating the finger in a circular motion so that it remains in contact with the rectum wall. The stimulation is continued until the relaxation of the anal wall is felt, the patient expels flatus or stool or the internal sphincter contracts. It should occur within 15 to 20 seconds and is seldom required for more than 1 minute (Coggrave & Norton, 2013; Consortium for Spinal Cord Medicine, 1998). This should be repeated every 5 to 10 minutes until evacuation occurs (Consortium for Spinal Cord Medicine, 1998). Bowel care should be scheduled on a daily basis until an effective program has been established and then can move to an every-other-day basis.

Areflexic (LMN) Bowel Program

The goal for patients with an areflexic bowel is for patients to have firm stool consistency through the use of high fiber and bulking agents. Maintaining this consistency assists in preventing diarrhea and facilitates the ease of removing stool though the mechanical process of manual evacuation. This type of evacuation involves inserting one or two lubricated fingers into the rectum to break up the stool and remove it from the rectum. To assist with propelling the stool further down into the rectum, the Valsalva maneuver should be performed before and after each manual evacuation. Patients with a LMN bowel dysfunction are at higher risk for fecal incontinence, so this bowel program may have to be performed twice daily (Coggrave & Norton 2013; Consortium for Spinal Cord Medicine, 1998).

Alternate Strategies

There are a variety of strategies that have been utilized with patients that have bowel dysfunctions. Biofeedback has been used for fecal incontinence and constipation with patients who are able to voluntarily contract their anal sphincter. Several surgical procedures have been used to create a stoma to facilitate the elimination of stool. This option has been utilized in patients who have persistent problems with pressure ulcers, or those who have been unsuccessful in establishing an effective bowel management program. Evidence has shown that many patients feel that utilizing a colostomy as their method of bowel management has added to their quality of life by reducing bowel-related complications and time spent preforming their bowel routine (Coggrave & Norton, 2013; Consortium for Spinal Cord Medicine, 1998; Pardee, Bricker, Rundquist, MacRae, & Tebben, 2012).

SLEEP DISTURBANCES

Sleep is essential to maintaining health, strength, and cognitive functioning. One of the most common consequences of a TBI and stroke are disturbances or alteration in the patient's normal sleep pattern, or circadian rhythm. The circadian rhythm is the internal 24-hour clock that controls the body's natural sleep and wake hours (Mollayeva, Colantonio, Mollayeva, & Shapiro, 2013). It is estimated that 50% of patients who have had brain injury experienced some form of sleep disturbance (Mathias & Alvaro, 2012; Ouellet, Beaulieu-Bonneau, & Morin, 2015). These disturbances are seen in patients who have had brain injury in whom the severity of their injuries ranges from mild to severe, and they can occur early after the injury is sustained and continue for many years (Mathias & Alvaro, 2012; Ponsford & Sinclair, 2013). It has been found that 20% to 40% of patients who have had a stroke experience some form of sleeping disturbance (Duraski, Denby, Danzy, & Sullivan, 2012).

These sleep disturbances includes hypersomnia, insomnia, excessive daytime sleepiness (EDS), delayed sleep onset, early wakening, and poor sleep quality (Ponsford & Sinclair, 2013). The effects of interrupted sleep can exacerbate symptoms such as fatigue, depression, anxiety, pain, and cognitive deficits, and negatively impact the patient's ability to participate in a rehabilitation program and impede healing. The goal of a multifaceted approach, including treating the patient's underlying medical conditions along with nonpharmacological management and pharmacological management of the patient's sleep disturbance, will lead to optimizing the patient's recovery and improve functional outcomes.

Nonpharmacological Management

The implementation of a sleep hygiene program to manage the individual needs of patients may assist in improving nighttime sleep quality. There are a variety of components described in the literature that can be implemented by the nursing staff, patients, and caregivers to create an effective sleep hygiene program for patients. Cognitive behavioral therapy utilizes cognitive restructuring to learn healthier ways to cope with the patient's thoughts, beliefs, and attitudes that might contribute to negative or unrealistic expectations about sleep (Ouellet et al., 2015). Sleep restriction consolidates sleep to a specific period of time to "improve sleep continuity and enhance sleep drive" (De La Rue-Evans, Nesbitt, & Oka, 2013), while stimulus control reinforces positive associations between the bed, bedroom, and sleep in order to establish a regular sleep–wake schedule.

General Care Strategies

The following are strategies that can be utilized to establish an effective sleep hygiene program by the nursing staff, patients, and caregivers while the patient is in the rehabilitation setting with the goal that the strategies could be modified by patients and their caregivers when they return home. Establish a constant time the patient should go to bed each night and awake each day. Patients should be discouraged to take naps during the day (Ouellet et al., 2015). Caffeine and other stimulates should be avoided 4 to 6 hours before bedtime. A relaxing bedtime routine should be carried out in an unrushed manner. If needed, assistance should be provided to the patient with changing into sleep wear, ensure toileting has taken place before the lights are turned out, and providing oral and personal hygiene. Allow the patient to participate in relaxation activities that will promote sleep, such as reading, guided imagery, listening to soft music, or prayer (Anderson et al., 2011; De La Rue-Evans et al., 2013).

Establish an environment conducive to sleep by turning off the television at a predetermined time and ensuring there are low levels of light and noise around the patient's room. Maintain the room at an appropriate temperature (cooler is preferable to warmer) and ensure that the patient is in a comfortable position and has all items he or she will require to keep warm during the night such as blankets or socks (Anderson et al., 2011).

Enforce the concept that the bed is only used for sleep (Ouellet et al., 2015). Patients should be seated in a chair for all meals. Many people believe that if they cannot sleep, they should stay in bed to rest. Patients and their caregivers should be instructed that if the patient cannot fall asleep after a predetermined amount of time, they should get out of bed and read or perform a relaxing activity until the patient gets sleepy then return to bed (De La Rue-Evans et al., 2013). Assure the patient that he or she can fall asleep without the use of medication through the use of comfort techniques, such as relaxation (Anderson et al., 2011).

After discharge, it may be necessary for patients and their caregivers to modify the sleep hygiene program that was established in rehabilitation. Nursing staff can educate patient and caregiver to assist them in identifying barriers in the home that may disrupt sleep. Daily routines and household activities need to be monitored and modified to provide appropriate timed rest periods along with energy conservation strategies in order to minimize fatigue.

Other Nonpharmacological Treatments

A recent study using acupuncture to treat brain-injured patients with insomnia reported improvement in cognitive functioning and "improvement in the perception of sleep was sustained for at least a month after the cessation of acupuncture (Zollman, Larson, Wasek-Throm, Cyborski, & Bode, 2012). Blue light therapy has been shown to be effectively used with traumatic brain injury patients experiencing fatigue and daytime sleepiness (Sinclair, Ponsford, Taffe, Lockley, & Rajaratnam, 2014).

Pharmacological Management

The goal should be to reduce the amount of sleep medication the patient receives because it not only results in an artificial sleep but also puts the patient at a higher risk for falls (Anderson et al., 2011). In addition, medication prescribed to treat sleep disorders in the rehabilitation patient population can have adverse effects that include exacerbating cognitive deficits, reducing daytime alertness, increasing hallucinatory behaviors, fatigue, and dizziness (Ouellet et al., 2015; Ponsford & Sinclair, 2013). Nonpharmacological management of patient's sleep disorders should be the first line of treatment, but if these interventions are not effective, physicians will prescribe medications for short-term use. Nurses must carefully monitor patients as well as educate them on the side effects of these medications.

PSYCHOLOGICAL HEALTH

Rehabilitation nurses practice with the knowledge and understanding of all aspects of psychosocial development. The psychosocial attributes of patients' self-concept, self-esteem, grief process, coping and stress tolerance, and depression are impacted by disability or injury and are addressed by rehabilitation nurses in the patient's plan of care (Sims, 2012). The patient recovering from an injury or disability is continually assessed by the nurse in a holistic manner, and a collaborative decision of care among nurse, patient, and caregiver needs to be formulated.

Self-Concept and Self-Esteem

Self-concept is a person's perception of himself or herself, influenced by social interactions that lead the individual to exhibit behaviors that impact self-worth, self-respect, and status. Studies highlight that a person with a healthy self-concept handles life's realities and challenges with appropriate coping behaviors, while an individual with a poor self-concept has worse outcomes (Craven & Hirnle, 2009; Jacelon, 2011).

Self-concept, or an individual's beliefs about himself or herself, may have a key role in the psychological adjustment process for people with SCI (Kaiser & Kennedy, 2011). In particular, post-traumatic stress symptoms have been noted among people with SCI who report a negative perception of themselves (Hatcher, Whitaker, & Karl, 2009). With improved self-concept, people with SCI may cope better with their injuries. Proactive cognitive and behavioral coping skills may enhance self-esteem and self-efficacy for individuals with SCI (Chen, Lai, & Wu, 2011; Geyh et al., 2012).

Self-esteem refers to overall feelings about the self and is relatively resistant to change. Specific aspects of self-image and self-esteem are more easily influenced by situational events that disrupt a particular substructure of the self, such as one's role, appearance, or function. The literature in nursing and other health fields supports the concept of situational alteration in self-esteem based on factors, such as altered body image or function, that can be caused by a disability or injury. Several studies report an association between negatively perceived body image changes and lowered self-esteem. Conversely, the literature points to the influence of self-esteem on healing and general adaptation to body image changes (Peter, Muller, Cieza, & Geyh, 2012).

Stroke survivors inevitably go through a period of confusion and struggle while trying to discover their new self as their values undergo a transformation. Studies have investigated self-esteem in stroke survivors and have concluded that self-esteem is an important element of mental health and quality of life, and is lowered by traumatic experiences and long-term stress. The ultimate goal of providing assistance to patients is to help recovering patients transform their values, and to help them recognize and find value in their self-esteem (Shida, Sugawara, Goto, & Sekito, 2014).

Norris, Kunes-Connell, and Stockard-Spelic (1998) performed a grounded theory study to explore physical alterations in appearance or function that influence self-esteem. What emerged from their study was a grounded theory of reimaging. The themes that emerged from this exploration process are that reimaging is highly subjective, unique to the person, and occurs simultaneously with the process of grieving the loss of the person's former appearance or function. Three phases of reimaging occurred: body image disruption, wishing for restoration, and reimaging the self. In phase one, patients may experience a significant alteration in their body image due to either their appearance or ability to function and a call for reimaging. In phase two, which is wishing for restoration, participants may have maintained the hope that surgery, prosthetics, or other medical technologies and therapies would restore them to the way they were prior to the disruption. Phase three emerged as participants experienced the exploration of continued accommodation efforts such as physical therapy, reconstructive surgery, or prosthetics use against the cost in energy, time, and effort of recovery from the disability. This phase was the turning point in which many participants begin to embrace a more realistic view of the self and self-capabilities and transform the focus from one of restoring the body to reimaging the self.

■ General Care Strategies

The goal of rehabilitation is to assist the patient in recovering from an injury or disability by maintaining the patient's self-concept and self-esteem. This can be accomplished by providing patients opportunities to set their own goals, practice the skills they have learned, and direct their own self-care. Encouraging activities in community-based social integration programs will reinforce social skills. By fostering relationships with people with similar disabilities, the patient can form a network of support. Encouraging the patient's spirituality as a basis for self-concept has been related to positive rehabilitation outcomes (Jacelon, 2011).

The families and caregivers should be educated to observe for disruptions in the patients' self-concept and self-esteem as evidenced by feelings of defeat, failure, worthlessness, hopelessness, vulnerability, fragility, and inadequacy (Sims, 2012). Families and caregivers should support patients with disabilities in the promotion and maintenance of their self-concept through positive thinking, satisfaction with small successes, and valuing their contributions to the family unit. Encouraging honest and open dialogue among the patient, family, and friends allows everyone the opportunity to express their concerns, frustrations, fears, and anxiety about the patient's recovery. This communication will also reassure patients that they are loved for themselves and not for their appearance, physical abilities, or work capacity (Sims, 2012).

Coping and Stress Tolerance

There are stressors that impact coping when patients and caregivers confront an illness, injury, or disability. Some of the factors include age, severity of impairment, visibility of the impairment, sense of control, prior coping abilities, values (spiritual, cultural, philosophical, and religious), and perceived social support. Adaptation to illness and injury demands resilience of various coping strategies especially when enduring changes in functioning (Sims, 2012). Lazarus and Folkman (1984) suggested two categories of coping behaviors. Emotion-focused behavior uses avoidance efforts to divert away from thoughts and feelings caused by stress. These behaviors are maladaptive and result in poor outcomes. The other is problem-focused behavior, which utilizes adaptation and results in improved outcome. The emotion-focused behavior can be destructive and is related to increased levels of depression. Maladaptive behavior is critical to identify and manage early for prevention of complications in selected rehabilitation outcomes.

Livneh and Martz (2014) investigated whether SCI survivors' use of coping resources (e.g., hope, sense of coherence) and coping strategies (e.g., engagement coping, seeking social support) influenced their psychosocial adaptation, and whether their use of coping strategies moderated the effect of coping resources, after controlling for the influence of depression and anxiety, on psychosocial adaptation. Results indicated that coping resources and coping strategies were significantly associated with psychosocial adaptation. Findings indicated that both coping resources and strategies (especially engagement coping) were reliably linked to adaptation to SCI.

■ General Care Strategies

Encourage patients to participate in integrative health modalities, such as guided imagery and relaxation techniques to manage stress, anxiety, and mood state (Freeman et al., 2008). Patients may also find comfort in journaling or expressing feelings in writing, meditation, prayer, or yoga (Crowe & Lutz, 2005). Provide community integration resources to allow the opportunity for people with disabilities to expand their leisure activities, and opportunities to engage in academic and/or vocational endeavors that will enhance their coping strategies (Jacelon, 2011).

Depression

Major depressive disorder (MDD) is a primary mood disorder that is a common condition impacting the recovery of rehabilitation patients. Rehabilitation nurses are critical in assessing and caring for depressed patients who are admitted to postacute care services. It has been described that patients with MDD are less adherent to their rehabilitation programs, have longer inpatient stays, do not engage in recreational activities, do not use adaptive equipment, and engage in less social contacts. Other mental health disorders such as dysthymia, reactive adjustment disorder, and bipolar depression, that have similar classical presentations as MDD, should be considered when evaluating patients (Gunderson & Tomwokiak, 2005).

The diagnosis of MDD appears to be the most prevalent psychiatric disorder after traumatic brain injury (TBI) with a prevalence rate over 52% within the first year after injury (Fann et al., 2003). The increased risk of depression is seen in patients with mild, moderate, and severe TBI (Hoge et al., 2008). It is essential for all members of the rehabilitation team to assess and monitor for symptoms of depression in patients with TBI.

Depressive symptoms are common among patients with heart failure (HF), and prevalence ranges from 9% to 60% (Rutledge, Reis, Linke, Greenberg, & Mills, 2006). A meta-analysis study by Fan et al. (2014) revealed that depressive mood after HF diagnosis increased the risk of future cardiovascular and all-cause mortality. Sherwood et al. (2011) demonstrated that worsening symptoms of depression are associated with a poorer prognosis in HF patients. Routine assessment of symptoms of depression in HF patients may help to guide appropriate medical management of these patients who are at increased risk for adverse clinical outcomes.

Patients with HF due to coronary heart disease initially classified as depressed who remained depressed after exercise training (ET) had nearly a fourfold higher mortality than patients whose depression resolved after ET. Patients with depression who completed ET had a 59% lower mortality compared to depressed dropout subjects not undergoing ET. Survival benefits after ET were concentrated to those patients with depression who improved exercise capacity. Structured ET is effective in decreasing depressive symptoms, a factor that correlates with improved long-term survival (Milani, Lavie, Mehra, & Ventura, 2011).

General Care Strategies

Nurses should encourage patient and caregiver to engage in family therapy with a focus on the entire family, which should include counseling about injury, disability, and illness with strategies for handling emotional distress and with assistive coping services (Deutsch, Allison, & Cimino-Ferguson, 2005). Based on the level of disability there may be a change in the role of the patient within the family. This will require supportive discussions about protective measures of coping regarding role changes, and the impact this will have on the family unit (Dacey & Margolis, 2006; Jacelon, 2011). Strong family, caregiver, and social support are various forms of social interventions that may improve a patient's adjustment to disability and level of participation in social activities (Tsouna-Hadjis, Vemmos, Zakopoulos, & Stamatelopoulos, 2000).

Nurses can refer patients with TBI for cognitive behavioral therapy (CBT), which has shown efficacy comparable to that of antidepressant medication (DeRubeis et al., 2005). According to one meta-analysis, therapies focusing on behavioral activation, even in simple forms such as activity scheduling, problem-solving therapy, and social problem-solving therapy used in multidisciplinary programs for TBI are at least as effective for depression as CBT (Cuijpers, van Straten, & Wamerdam, 2007). Nurses can engage patients in all forms of behavioral activation that can have an impact on the treatment of their MDD.

Nurses should regularly evaluate symptoms of depression in patients with diagnosed HF (Fan et al., 2014). Various forms of depression can present as fatigue (National Institute of Health, 2013). The rehabilitation team can encourage patients with HF and caregivers to demonstrate understanding of activity intolerance by modifying activity, encouraging rest periods in order to prevent fatigue as a presenting symptom of depression. Nurses can promote the referral of patients with HF to cardiac rehabilitation. The patients will be evaluated for depression and be provided with information about support groups and social services to enhance their well-being.

In relation to psychosocial health, therapeutic emotion work has been used to insightfully examine relations among health care providers as they manage their own feelings as well as those of colleagues and patients as part of efforts to improve the physical and psychosocial health outcomes of patients (Miller et al., 2008). Nurses should explore therapeutic emotion work to enhance the care they provide to their patients in rehabilitation in their journey to recovery.

SEXUAL HEALTH

World Health Organization (WHO) defines sexual health as "a state of physical, emotional, mental and social well-being in relation to sexuality; it is not merely the absence of disease, dysfunction or infirmity" (Centers for Disease Control and Prevention [CDC], 2014). Furthermore, WHO advocates that "sexual health can also be influenced by mental health, acute and chronic illnesses, and violence. Addressing sexual health at the individual, family, community or health system level requires integrated interventions by trained health providers and a functioning referral system" (WHO, 2002).

Research that has explored the experiences of people with disabilities and chronic illness suggests that body changes and function confound the individual's psychosocial and sexual life, and impacts negatively on the individual's self-esteem, sense of attractiveness, relationships, and sexual functioning (Higgins et al., 2012). Sexuality is a multidimensional concept with biological, psychological, social, cultural, and spiritual dimensions. These dimensions should be espoused by the health care team, including the nurse, to provide holistic care to patients. The rehabilitation nurse in collaboration with patients and their partners, have the opportunity to address sexual health both as an educator and advocate through the promotion of enhanced relationship intimacy and sexual function in adults with traumatic injury, chronic illness, and disability (Moore, Kautz, & Cournan, 2012).

General Care Strategies

A conceptual model for nurses to employ when addressing sexual concerns of patients and their partners is the PLISSIT model (permission, limited information, specific suggestions, and intensive therapy) developed by Annon (1976). The model describes four different levels of sexual counseling and interventions. The elements of the PLISSIT are permission, which engages and encourages patients and their partners to raise sexual concerns; limited information highlights that information for overcoming sexual problems by providing education and information on sexual activity is necessary; specific suggestions can include treatments for erectile dysfunction and/or vaginal dryness, adopting comfortable positions for intercourse, methods of managing spasticity during intercourse, and instructing patients on bed and wheelchair mobility during sexual activities. The last element of the PLISSIT is intensive therapy that advocates for marital couple or sex therapy and cognitive remediation therapy; the latter focuses on patient or partner counseling for maintaining intimacy in relationships with chronic illness and disability to enhance overall sexual function (Anderson et al., 2011; Moore et al., 2012).

Rehabilitation nurses can emphasize further sexual health education and practices on general concepts that highlight methods to enhance sensuality by using all available senses and provide information on sexual assistive devices (sex toys) that are sometimes used to enhance sexual experiences (Consortium for Spinal Cord Medicine, 2011). The nurse can review with patients and/or partners the common classes of medications and the effects these medications may have on sexual functioning (e.g., antidepressants, antihypertensive, anticholinergics, anticonvulsants, and opioids; Kennedy & Rizvi, 2009). Nursing interventions for sexual functional problems related to sensory and/or perceptions include counseling the patient and partner on tactile sensitivity, and stimulation to defined body areas after an injury or disability. The patient's partner can use pillows for alternate positioning strategies for comfort and to produce less stress on muscles that tend to spasm (Anderson et al., 2011).

The patient and partner can use the following reminders for addressing bowel and bladder needs before initiating foreplay: Restrict fluids before sexual activity, complete bowel regimen before sexual activity, tape Foley catheters to the side (for women to the thigh and for men on the abdomen or place a condom over the shaft of the penis); and avoid positions that increases pressure to the bladder and bowel (Anderson et al., 2011; Ricciardi, Szabo, & Poullos, 2007). Ensure that patients with disabilities and their partners understand that they remain at risk for transmitting or acquiring sexually transmitted infections.

Evidence-based practices for healthy lifestyles for therapeutic management of erectile dysfunction and vaginal dryness include smoking cessation, drinking no more than moderate amounts of alcohol, increasing physical activity, and reducing obesity (Kautz, Van Horn, & Moore, 2009; Moore et al., 2012).

CONCLUSION

It is crucial for the rehabilitation nurses to collaborate with patients and families in understanding that rehabilitation is a process. It is not only the patient, but the family and those who care for the patient that have experienced a loss. The loss can have a direct impact on these individuals and disrupt their way of life. The role of the rehabilitation nurse is essential in guiding these individuals to adapt to their new "norm." Patients and families need to be aware that everyone moves through this process at varying speeds and the importance of allowing time to cope with this transition is a critical step. This rehabilitation process will continue long after the patient leaves the rehabilitation facility and assimilates back into the community.

REFERENCES

American Nurses Association. (2010). *Nursing: Scope and standards of practice* (2nd ed.). Silver Spring, MD: Author.

Anderson, C. D., Kautz, D. D., Bryant, S., & Clanin, N. (2011). Physical healthcare patterns and nursing interventions. In C. S. Jacelon (Ed.), *The specialty practice of rehabilitation nursing: A core curriculum* (6th ed., pp. 103–144). Glenview, IL: Association of Rehabilitation Nurses.

Anton, P. A. (2012). Maintaining skin integrity. In K. L. Mauk (Ed.), *Rehabilitation nursing: A contemporary approach to practice* (pp. 100–120). Sudbury, MA: Jones & Bartlett Learning.

Association of Rehabilitation Nurses. (2014). *Standards and scope of rehabilitation nursing practice*. Glenview, IL: Author.

Annon, J. (1976). The PLISSIT model: A proposed conceptual scheme for the behavioral treatment of sexual problems. *Journal of Sex Education Therapists, 2*, 1–15.

Center for Disease Control and Prevention. (2014). Sexual health. Retrieved from http://www.cdc.gov/sexualhealth

Chen, H. Y., Lai, C. H., & Wu, T. J. (2011). A study of factors affecting moving-forward behavior among people with spinal cord injury. *Rehabilitation Nursing, 36*, 91–97.

Coggrave, M., & Norton, C. (2013). Neurogenic bowel. In M. P. Barnes & D. C. Good (Eds.), *Neurological rehabilitation: Handbook of clinical neurology* (3rd Series, Vol. 110, pp. 221–228). Retrieved from http://www.sciencedirect.com/science/handbooks/00729752/110

Coggrave, M., Norton, C., & Wilson-Barnett, J., (2009). Management of neurogenic bowel dysfunction in the community after a spinal cord injury: A postal survey in the United Kingdom. *Spinal Cord, 47*, 323–333. doi:10.1038/sc.2008.137

Consortium for Spinal Cord Medicine. (1998). *Neurogenic bowel management in adults with spinal cord injury: A clinical practice guideline for healthcare providers*. Washington, DC: Paralyzed Veterans of America.

Consortium for Spinal Cord Medicine. (2006). *Bladder management for adults with spinal cord injury: A clinical practice guideline for healthcare providers*. Washington, DC: Paralyzed Veterans of America.

Consortium for Spinal Cord Medicine. (2011). *Sexuality and reproductive health in adults with spinal cord injury: What you should know*. Washington, DC: Paralyzed Veterans of America.

Consortium for Spinal Cord Medicine. (2014). *Pressure ulcer prevention and treatment following spinal cord injury: A clinical practice guideline for healthcare providers*. Washington, DC: Paralyzed Veterans of America.

Cournan, M. (2012). Bladder management in female stroke survivors: Translating research into practice. *Rehabilitation Nursing, 37*, 220–230.

Craven, R. F., & Hirnle, C. J. (2009). *Fundamentals of nursing: Human health and function* (6th ed.). Philadelphia, PA: Lippincott Williams & Wilkins.

Crowe, M., & Lutz, S. (2005). Nonpharmacologic treatments for older adults with depression. *Geriatrics & Aging, 8*(8), 30–33.

Cuijpers, P., van Straten, A., & Wamerdam, L. (2007). Behavioral activation treatments of depression: A meta-analysis. *Clinical Psychology Review, 27*, 318–326.

Dacey, J., & Margolis, D. (2006). Psychological developmental: Adolescence and sexuality. In K. Thies & J. Travers (Eds.), *Handbook of human development for health care professionals* (pp. 191–218). Boston, MA: Jones & Bartlett.

De La Rue-Evans, L., Nesbitt, K., & Oka, R. K. (2013). Sleep hygiene program implementation in patients with traumatic brain injury. *Rehabilitation Nursing, 38*, 2–10.

DeRubeis, R. J., Hollon, S. D., Amsterdam, J. D., Shelton, R. C., Young, P. R., & Salomon, R. M. (2005). Cognitive therapy vs. medications in the treatment of moderate to severe depression. *Archives of General Psychiatry, 62*(4), 409–416.

Deutsch, P. M., Allison, L., & Cimino-Ferguson, S. (2005). Life care planning assessments and their impact on life in spinal cord injury. *Topics in Spinal Cord Rehabilitation, 10*(4), 135–145.

Duraski, S. A., Denby, F. A., Danzy, L. V., & Sullivan, S. (2012). Stroke. In K. L. Mauk (Ed.), *Rehabilitation nursing: A contemporary approach to practice* (pp. 215–254). Sudbury, MA: Jones & Bartlett Learning.

Fan, H., Yu, W., Zhang, Q., Cao, H., Li, J., Wang, J., . . . Hu, X. (2014). Depression after heart failure and risk of cardiovascular and all-cause mortality: A meta-analysis. *Preventive Medicine, 63*, 36–42.

Fann, J. R., Bombardier, C. H., Temkin, N. R., Esselman, P., Pelzer, E., Keough, M., . . . Dikmen, S. (2003). Incidence, severity, and phenomenology of depression and anxiety in patients with moderate to severe traumatic brain injury. *Psychosomatics, 44*, 161.

Fawcett, J. (2000). *Analysis and evaluation of contemporary nursing knowledge: Nursing models and theories*. Philadelphia, PA: F. A. Davis.

Freeman, L., Cohen, L., Stewart, M., White, R., Link, J., Palmer, J. L., . . . Hild, C. M. (2008). The experience of imagery as a post-treatment intervention in patients with breast cancer: program, process, and patient recommendations. *Oncology Nursing Forum, 35*(6), E116–E121.

Frosch, D. L., Moulton, B. W., Wexler, R. M., Holmes-Rovner, M., Volk, R. J., & Levin, C. A. (2011). Shared decision making in the United States: Policy and implementation activity on multiple fronts. *Zeitschrift für Evidenz, Fortbildung und Qualität im Gesundheitswesen, 105*(4), 305–312.

Garber, S. L. (2012). Wounds in special populations: Spinal cord injury population. In S. Baranoski & E. A. Ayello (Eds.), *Wound care essentials: Practice principles* (3rd ed., pp. 520–529). Ambler, PA: Lippincott Williams & Wilkins.

Geyh, S., Nick, E., Stirnimann, D., Ehrat, S., Michel, F., Peter, C., & Lude, P. (2012). Self-efficacy and self-esteem as predictors of participation in spinal cord injury–an ICF-based study. *Spinal Cord, 50*, 699–706.

Goldmark, E., Niver, N., & Ginsberg, D. A. (2014). Neurogenic bladder: From diagnosis to management. *Current Urology Reports, 15*(448), 1–8. Retrieved from http://link.springer.com/article/10.1007%2Fs11934-014-0448-8#

Gunderson, A., & Tomwokiak, J. (2005). Major depression in rehabilitation care. *Rehabilitation Nursing, 30*(6), 219–220.

Hatcher, M. B., Whitaker, C., & Karl, A. (2009). What predicts post-traumatic stress following spinal cord injury? *British Journal Health Psychology, 14*, 541–561.

The Health Foundation. (2012). Evidence: Helping people shared decision making. Retrieved from http://personcentredcare.health.org.uk/person-centred-care/shared-decision-making

Healthcare Infection Control Practice Advisory Committee. (2009). *Guideline for the prevention of catheter associated urinary tract infections.* Washington, DC: U.S. Department of Health and Human Services and Centers for Disease Control and Prevention.

Higgins, A., Sharek, D., Nolan, M., Sheerin, B., Flanagan, P., & Slaicuinaite, S. (2012). Mixed methods evaluation of an interdisciplinary sexuality education programme for staff working with people who have an acquired physical disability. *Journal of Advanced Nursing, 68*(11), 2559–2569.

Hoge, C. W., McGurk, D., Thomas, J. L., Cox, A. L., Engel, C. C., & Castro, C. A. (2008). Mild traumatic brain injury in U.S. soldiers returning from Iraq. *New England Journal of Medicine, 358*, 453–463.

Jacelon, C. S. (2011). Psychosocial healthcare patterns and nursing interventions. In C. S. Jacelon (Ed.), *The specialty practice of rehabilitation nursing: A core curriculum* (6th ed., pp. 145–168). Glenview, IL: Association of Rehabilitation Nurses.

Kaiser, S., & Kennedy, P. (2011). An exploration of cognitive appraisals following spinal cord injury. *Psychology Health Medicine, 16*, 708–718

Kautz, D., Van Horn, E., & Moore, C. (2009). Promoting family integrity to inspire hope in rehabilitation. *Rehabilitation Nursing, 34*(4), 168–172.

Kennedy, S. H., & Rizvi, S. (2009). Sexual dysfunction, depression and the impact of anitdepressants. *Journal of Clinical Pharmacology*, 29, 157–164.

Lazarus, R. S., & Folkman, S. (1984). *Stress, appraisal, and coping*. New York, NY: Springer Publishing.

Livneh, H., & Martz, E. (2014). Coping strategies and resources as predictors of psychosocial adaptation among people with spinal cord injury. *Rehabilitation Psychology, 59*(3), 329–339.

Martinkewiz, P., Furr, B. J., Farnan, C., & Martinez, P. G. (2011). Traumatic injuries: Traumatic brain injury and spinal cord injury. In C. S. Jacelon (Ed.), *The specialty practice of rehabilitation nursing: A core curriculum* (6th ed., pp. 251–287). Glenview, IL: Association of Rehabilitation Nurses.

Mathias, J. L., & Alvaro, P. K. (2012). Prevalence of sleep disturbances, disorders, and problems following traumatic brain injury: A meta-analysis. *Sleep Medicine, 13*, 898–905.

Milani, R. V., Lavie, C. J., Mehra, M. D., & Ventura, H. O. (2011). Impact of exercise training and depression on Survival in heart failure due to coronary heart disease. *American Journal of Cardiology, 107*, 64–68.

Miller, K. L., Reeves, S., Zwarenstein, M., Beales, J. D., Kenaszchuk, C., & Conn, L. G. (2008). Nursing emotion work and Interprofessional collaboration in general internal medicine wards: A qualitative study. *Journal of Advanced Nursing, 64*, 332–343.

Mollayeva, T., Colantonio, A., Mollayeva, S., & Shapiro, C. M. (2013). Screening for sleep dysfunction after traumatic brain injury. *Sleep Medicine, 14*, 1235–1246.

Moore, C., Kautz, D. D., & Cournan, M. (2012). Sexuality and disability. In K. L. Mauk (Ed.), *Rehabilitation nursing: A contemporary approach to practice* (pp. 161–175). Sudbury, MA: Jones & Bartlett Learning.

National Institute of Health. (2013). *Depression.* Washington, DC: U.S. Department of Health and Human Services. Retrieved from http://www.nimh.nih.gov/health/publications/depression-easy-to-read/depression-trifold-new_150043.pdf

National Pressure Ulcer Advisory Panel. (2015). World wide pressure ulcer prevention day 2015. Retrieved from http://www.npuap.org/world-wide-pressure-ulcer-prevention-day

National Pressure Ulcer Advisory Panel, European Pressure Ulcer Advisory Panel, and Pan Pacific Pressure Injury Alliance. (2014). *Prevention and treatment of pressure ulcers: Quick reference guide*. E. Haesler (Ed.). Retrieved from http://www.npuap.org/resources/educational-and-clinical-resources/prevention-and-treatment-of-pressure-ulcers-clinical-practice-guideline

Norris, J., Kunes-Connell, M., & Stockard Spelic, S. (1998). A grounded theory of reimaging. *Advances in Nursing Science, 20*(3), 1–12.

Ouellet, M.-C., Beaulieu-Bonneau, S., & Morin, C. M. (2015). Sleep-wake disturbances after traumatic brain injury. *The Lancet Neurology, 14*, 746–757.

Pardee, C., Bricker, D., Rundquist, J., MacRae, C., & Tebben, C. (2012). Characteristics of neurogenic bowel in spinal cord injury and perceived quality of life. *Rehabilitation Nursing, 37*, 128–135.

Peter, C., Muller, R., Cieza, A., & Geyh, S. (2012). Psychological resources in spinal cord injury: A systematic literature review. *Spinal Cord, 50*, 188–201.

Ponsford, J. L., & Sinclair, K. L. (2013). Sleep and fatigue following traumatic brain injury. *Psychiatric Clinics of North America, 37*, 77–89.

Preston, M., Tebben, C., & Johnson, K. M. M. (2008). Skin integrity. In S. P. Hoeman (Ed.), *Rehabilitation nursing: Prevention, intervention and outcomes* (4th ed., pp. 258–280). St. Louis, MO: Mosby/Elsevier.

Ricciardi, R., Szabo, M., & Poullos, A. Y. (2007). Sexuality and spinal cord injury. *Nursing Clinics of North America, 42*(4), 675–684.

Roy, C., & Andrews, H. A. (1999). *The Roy adaptation model* (2nd ed.). Upper Saddle River, NJ: Pearson.

Rutledge, T., Reis, V. A., Linke, S. E., Greenberg, B. H., & Mills, P. J. (2006). Depression in heart failure: Prelevance, intervention effects, and associations with clinical outcomes. *Journal of American College of Cardiology, 48*, 1527–1537.

Rye, J., & Mauk, K. L. (2012). Bowel and bladder management. In K. L. Mauk (Ed.), *Rehabilitation nursing: A contemporary approach to practice* (pp. 121–135). Sudbury, MA: Jones & Bartlett Learning.

Sherwood, A., Blumenthal, J. A., Hinderliter, A. L., Koch, G. G., Adams, K. F., Jr, Dupree, C. S., . . . O'Connor, C. M. (2011). Worsening depressive symptoms are associated with adverse clinical outcomes in patients with heart failure. *Journal of the American College of Cardiology, 57*(4), 418–423.

Shida, J., Sugawara, K., Goto, J., & Sekito, Y. (2014). Relationship between self-esteem and living conditions among stroke survivors at home. *Japan Journal of Nursing Science, 11*, 229–240.

Sims, G. L. (2012). The art of caring: Addressing psychosocial and spiritual issues: Spirituality, coping, depression, grieving, adjustment, and adaptation. In K. L. Mauk (Ed.), R*ehabilitation nursing: A contemporary approach to practice* (pp. 200–214). Sudbury, MA: Jones & Bartlett Learning.

Sinclair, K. L., Ponsford, J. L., Taffe, J., Lockley, S. W., & Rajaratnam, S. M. W. (2014). Randomized controlled trial of light therapy for fatigue following traumatic brain injury. *Neurorehabilitation and Neural Repair, 28*, 303–313.

Stevens, K. A. (2008). Urinary elimination and continence. In S. P. Hoeman (Ed.), *Rehabilitation nursing: Prevention, intervention and outcomes* (4th ed., pp. 334–368). St. Louis, MO: Mosby/Elsevier.

Tsouna-Hadjis, E., Vemmos, K. N., Zakopoulos, N., & Stamatelopoulos, S. (2000). First-stroke recovery process: The role of family social support. *Archives of Physical Medicine Rehabilitation, 81*(7), 881–887.

Williams, D. (2011). Rehabilitation nursing: Past, present, and future. In C. S. Jacelon (Ed.), *The specialty practice of rehabilitation nursing: A core curriculum* (6th ed., pp. 15–29). Glenview, IL: Association of Rehabilitation Nurses.

World Health Organization. (2002). Defining sexual health. Retrieved from http://www.who.int/reproductivehealth/topics/sexual_health/sh_definitions/en

Wound, Ostomy and Continence Nurses Society. (2010). Prevention of pressure ulcers. Retrieved from www.guideline.gov/synthesis/synthesis.aspx?id=47794

Yap, T. L., & Kennerly, S. M. (2011). A nurse-led approach to preventing pressure ulcers. *Rehabilitation Nursing, 36*, 106–110.

Zollman, F. S., Larson, E. B., Wasek-Throm, L. K., Cyborski, C. M., & Bode, R. K. (2012). Acupuncture for treatment of insomnia in patients with traumatic brain injury: A pilot intervention study. *Journal of Head Trauma Rehabilitation, 27*, 135–142.

CHAPTER 29

Adult Medical Speech–Language Pathology

Mary Regina Reilly and Matina Balou

> *Words are singularly the most powerful force available to humanity. We can choose to use this force constructively with words of encouragement, or destructively using words of despair. Words have energy and power with the ability to help, to heal, to hinder, to hurt, to harm, to humiliate and to humble.*
>
> —Yehda Berg

As defined by *Merriam-Webster*, communication is the act or process of using words, sounds, signs, or behaviors to express or exchange information (Merriam-Webster: Dictionary and Thesaurus, n.d.).[1] From our earliest days on this Earth, humans have devised ways to relate their thoughts and needs to others. Some communication is verbal, while other forms, though profound, are silent. Our voice frequently provides a reflection of our emotional state. During our recent past, strides that have made in the scientific community to enhance, restore, and to initiate verbal communication have been remarkable.

Speech–language pathologists are professionals who specialize in understanding the science behind the process of human communication. As a member of the interdisciplinary team in a medical setting, speech–language pathologists diagnose and treat disorders of speech sound production, resonance, voice, fluency, language, cognition, feeding, and swallowing. At times, the therapists encourage development of untapped potential and skill. In working with those with chronic disabilities, the speech–language pathologist may focus on the appreciation and development of the patients' preserved abilities. In the acute hospital arena, the speech–language pathologist serves to identify cognitive communication or swallowing deficits, to educate patients and families regarding areas of concern, and to suggest appropriate discharge treatment options aimed to enhance self-sufficiency. The goal of intervention is not geared to "cure" a disability, but rather to foster an optimal level of independence and function.

MOTOR SPEECH PRODUCTION

Speech is a means of communicating verbally. Speech sounds are produced by speech movements. The four subsystems of speech production include respiration, phonation, resonance, and articulation. The process involves the generation of airflow and the creation of air pressure by the displacement of bodily structures, which, taken together, cause the disturbances of air that constitute phonemes, the smallest meaningful units of sound (Behrman, 2013). The speech system is modulated by central and peripheral innervation, including cranial nerves V, X, XI, and XII, as well as with the phrenic and intercostal nerves (Melfi et al., 2015). Speech features are defined by the rate of production, rhythm, pitch, prosody, timing, and volume modulation for production. Partially overlapping brain regions, including the left frontal operculum and anterior insula, have been identified in both singular and group case studies (Nestor et al., 2013) that implicate these dominant anterior regions in the motor programming of speech.

Motor speech disorders result from neurological impairment affecting the motor programming or neuromuscular execution of speech. They encompass the dysarthrias and apraxia of speech (Duffy, 2013). The objective in assessment of motor speech disorders is to detect or confirm a suspected

[1]From Merriam-Webster's Collegiate® Dictionary, 11th Edition © 2016 by Merriam-Webster, Inc. (www.Merriam-Webster.com).

problem, establish a differential diagnosis, define the severity of the problem and its impact on function and, when appropriate, to outline a therapeutic care plan. Darley, Aronson, and Brown (1975) outlined six salient neuromuscular features that influence speech production, including strength, speed of movement, range of movement, accuracy, steadiness, and tone. The evaluation may include both perceptual and instrumental measurement of the subsystems involved in production of speech. Both clinical perception and instrumental measurement are frequently employed to interpret overall intelligibility.

The Dysarthrias

Dysarthia is a term that comes from the Greek *dys arthroun*, referring to an inability to verbalize clearly. Dysarthria encompasses a group of related motor speech disorders resulting from disturbed muscular control over the mechanisms of speech (Table 29.1; Rosenbeck & LaPointe, 1985). Dysarthria may have either a congenital or an acquired etiology. Overall intelligibility of speech production with patients with dysarthria varies based on the extent of damage. Some or all of the motor structures that support speech may be impaired. As such, vocalizations may appear audibly ill coordinated, weak, harsh, labored, hypernasal, or hyponasal. Dysarthria is most commonly secondary to a peripheral disorder, although it can occasionally be produced by cerebral damage (Broussolle et al., 1996). Possible etiologies attributable for the various forms of dysarthria include progressive neurological disease or trauma and can include stroke, facial palsy, tumor, encephalitis, myasthenia gravis, Parkinson's disease, toxic effects of substances such as alcohol and drugs, cerebral palsy, multiple sclerosis, amyotrophic lateral sclerosis, Shy–Drager syndrome, Wilson's disease, and Huntington's disease. If not accompanied by a concomitant language/cognitive disorder, language processing remains intact in patients with dysarthria.

Primary remediation techniques for dysarthria include the focus on the distinct impaired subsystems of speech and are based on the individual's presentation and preserved abilities. Compensatory strategies are stressed to maximize function.

Acquired Apraxia of Speech

Apraxia of speech (AOS) is a motor speech disorder caused by a disturbance in programming the sequential movement for volitional speech production. Knollman-Porter describes apraxia of speech as "a disturbed ability to produce purposeful learned movements despite intact mobility,

TABLE 29.1

CHARACTERISTICS OF DYSARTHRIA

Type	Location	Perceptual Deficits
Flaccid dysarthria	Lower motor neuron	Variation depending on the specific cranial nerve involved. Specific compensation depending on site of weakness; may include hypernasality, compromised articulatory precision, breathy vocal quality, and nasal emissions
Spastic dysarthria	Upper motor neuron	Slower speaking rate, effortful speech, fatigue when vocalizing, harsh vocal quality, hypernasality
Ataxic dysarthria	Cerebellar system	"Drunk" sounding speech, poor coordination of breath support for vocalization, stumbling over words, irregular articulatory breakdowns, prolongations of phonemes and intervals
Hypokinetic dysarthria	Extrapyramidal system	Monotone, mono-loudness, rapid rate, difficulty initiating speech
Hyperkinetic dysarthria	Extrapyramidal system	Chorea: effortful speech, involuntary oral movements
Mixed dysarthia	Upper and lower motor neurons	Varies depending on whether the upper motor neuron or lower motor neuron remain mostly intact

Source: Adapted from Duffy (2013).

secondary to brain damage." Clinical presentation can range from an inability to produce speech, to fluent output with labored speech, accompanied with minor sound distortions. The clinical features of AOS convey the impression that muscles are capable of normal function and that the appropriate message has been formulated, but that there is either difficulty enacting the planned message or that the perceptual characteristics of the sounds that emerge are not what is intended (Duffy, 2013). Speech behaviors associated with AOS include articulatory groping, perseverative errors, increased errors with increased word length, and initiation difficulties with speech (McNeil, Robin, & Schmidt, 2009). The perceptual characteristics of AOS include disturbances in articulation, rate, and prosody, or in the rhythm of the spoken utterance (Croot, Ballard, Leyton, & Hodges. 2012; Wambaugh, 2006).

McNeil reports that the primary clinical characteristics of AOS include:

- a slow rate of speech resulting in lengthened sound segments and intersegment duration
- sound distortions and or sound substitutions
- variability in error production
- dysprosody or abnormal intonation, rhythm, and stress

Controversy exists in the literature regarding the correlation of AOS to a singular brain region. Presentation of the disorder is highly associated with lesions to Broca's area (Hillis et al., 2007); the left frontal and temporoparietal cortex (Square, Roy, & Martin, 1997; McNeil, Doyle, & Wambaugh, 2000); the left, superior anterior region of the insula (Dronkers, 1996); as well as the left subcortical structures, particularly within the basal ganglia (Duffy, 2013; Square, Martin, & Bose, 2001; Peach & Tonkovich, 2004).

Therapeutic intervention for acquired AOS is focused on improvement of overall communicative function. A review of the AOS treatment literature was conducted by the Apraxia of Speech Treatment Guidelines Committee of the Academy of Neurological Communication Disorders and Sciences (Wambaugh, 2006) and revealed that treatments for this motor speech disorder are generally associated with four general areas including:

- Articulatory–kinematic treatments: Focus on maximizing the temporal and spatial aspects of speech production via use of modeling repetition, integral stimulations, and articulatory cueing.
- Rate/rhythm control treatments: Involve the manipulation of rate and/or rhythm to maximize overall speech intelligibility. Metronomic pacing and metrical pacing maybe introduced.
- Intersystemic facilitation/reorganization treatments: Make use of the more intact system to encourage speech productions. Iconic gestures, rhythmic gestures, vibrotactile stimulations, or singing maybe utilized.
- Alternative and augmentative communication approaches: Supplemental gestures, or use of communication boards/notebooks, spoken computer output, or an electrolarynx may be employed as alternative strategies.

Stuttering

Stuttering is a chronic communication disorder that involves a disruption to fluent speech output. It is characterized by an abnormally high frequency and/or duration of stoppages in the forward flow of speech. Stoppages generally take the form of repetitions of sound, syllables, or one-syllable words, prolongations of sounds, or "blocks" of airflow and/or voicing in speech (Guitar, 2013). Stuttering can have profound influences on daily function. People who stutter have reported negative reactions to stuttering, difficulty communicating in key situations, diminished satisfaction with life, and a reduced ability to achieve their goals (Yaruss, 2010). Stuttering can be neurogenic in nature as a result from an acute brain injury. With prevalence greater in males than in females, the precipitating factors for persistent stuttering remain speculative. Recent studies appear to indicate a genetic predisposition to disfluent production in certain individuals. Emotional trauma is now considered a rare risk factor for stuttering onset.

Stuttering signs and symptoms may include:

- Difficulty with initiation of verbal production at a word, sentence, or phrase level
- Prolongations, or involuntary extension of certain letters or sounds
- Unpredictable speech blocks

- Part word repetitions
- Uneven speech rate
- Addition of fillers "um," "like" in spontaneous production
- Tension, tightness, or concomitant movement during vocalization attempt

People who stutter may develop secondary behaviors in reaction to the fear of stuttering. Interchanging words might be utilized to divert a word that might be considered formidable. Starter techniques, such as eye blinking or facial grimaces, maybe observed during vocal production.

Treatment for stuttering employs various approaches to best provide care for the patient's individual areas of difficulty. Skilled intervention may focus on controlling speech patterns by utilization of slower rates of speech and shorter sentence or phrase length. Delayed auditory feedback and other electrical devices might be utilized in the treatment process. Therapeutic interventions concentrate on stuttering modification, and focused attention to feelings and attitudes of the patient to his or her stuttering throughout the therapeutic process.

Voice

Voice is the sound that is the product of the passage of air through the laryngeal mechanism. The generation of air flow sets the vocal folds into vibration creating a series of pressure waves in the air that we perceive as sound. Colton (2000) explains that the quality of the voice is determined by physiological and acoustic characteristics of the sound source, the vocal folds, and the resonating system above the vocal folds. The properties of pitch, loudness, and quality help to define vocal production. Variations in the rhythm, loudness, pitch, and rate of speech establish the overall tone of the communicative message.

Voice disorders can result from a variety of causes and are generally multifactorial. Organic voice disorders are biological, psychological, and sociocultural (Brown, Vinson, & Crary, 2000). Dysphonias can be debilitating and can significantly impact an individual's ability to function in personal and professional contexts. A voice disorder is characterized by the abnormal production and/or absences of vocal quality, pitch, loudness, resonance, and or duration, which is inappropriate for an individual's age, culture, and/or gender. Optimal diagnosis and treatment of voice disorders generally involve team coordination and may include a specialty trained otolaryngologist, speech–language pathologist, neurologists, gastroenterologist, singing teacher, or vocal coach. Deficits can range in severity from mild hoarseness to complete aphonia. Bless and Hick (1996) report that a plethora of assessment methods exist, including laryngeal imaging, acoustics, aerodynamic movement, and neurophysiologic direct and indirect measures of the laryngeal structure and its function. The specific tools utilized depend on the patient's clinical symptomatology and medical diagnosis.

Misuse of the vocal instrument may result in vocal nodules or contact ulcers. Vocal cord nodules are benign growths that develop on the vocal cords, generally at the anterior two thirds of the glottal opening. The general etiology of vocal nodules is thought to be vocal abuse or misuse. Triggers for vocal abuse/misuse are multifactorial and are defined during the assessment and treatment process. Perceptually, voice characteristics with nodules include a "rough," or "raspy," "breathy" quality and decreased pitch range. The main factors involved in producing these perceptible characteristics are breathiness, overpressure (medical compression) of the vocal folds and perceived as voice tension and asymmetrical vocal fold vibration (Case, 1984). Variable perceptual voice characteristics include weak, breathy vocalizations, and vocal fry, frequently described as a "froglike" or "gravely" vocal quality observed when productions are made in a lower register.

A vocal polyp is a soft, benign growth, which appears as a "blister like" lesion on the vocal cords. Causes for vocal polyps igclude long-term cigarette smoking, thyroid imbalance, gastroesophageal reflux disease (GERD), and continued overuse of the voice in a suboptimal manner. Behaviors including excessive throat clearing, screaming, and the presence of excessive tension in the muscles in the perilaryngeal area are additional triggers for the development of a polyp. Treatment for vocal polyps may include voice therapy and surgical intervention.

Paradoxical vocal cord dysfunction or movement (PVCM) is a disorder characterized by unintentional paradoxical adduction of the vocal cords, resulting in episodic shortness of breath, wheezing, and stridor (Campainha, Ribeiro, & Guimaraes, 2012). PVCM is characterized by an abnormal closing of the vocal cords during inspiration, therefore, producing airflow obstruction. The vocal cords typically function well; however, when episodes are triggered in an unpredictable manner, the cords adduct when they should abduct. Direct visualization of the vocal cords via laryngoscopy is the "gold standard" for making this diagnosis. The foundation for management of PVCM includes both voice therapy by a trained speech-language pathologist and behavioral management.

Head and Neck Cancer

Laryngeal tumors are frequently classified by their origin (Figure 29.1), and are divided as supraglottic, glottic, or subglottic. The supraglottic zone involves the epiglottic regions, including the valleculae, the aryepiglottic folds, the aryntenoid cartilages, the ventricular folds, and the ventricular cavity. Glottic tumors emerge on the vocal folds and on the anterior or posterior commissure. Subglottic tumors are rare and arise more commonly from the lower margins of the vocal folds (Case, 1984).

Signs and symptoms of laryngeal cancer include hoarseness, difficulty swallowing, cough or chest infection, halitosis, weight loss, and prolonged earache. Most laryngeal cancers are squamous cell cancer are determined based the size, location, and stage of the cancer's progression. Larynx preservation programs offer a combination of radiation and chemotherapy delivered together, reserving surgical intervention for a recurrence. A total laryngectomy results in a complete loss of voice known as aphonia. Speech–language pathologists play a critical role in facilitating the overall communication competence of patients with speech involvement. Presurgical counseling is of most importance in explaining how surgical intervention will affect voice. Augmentative communications are provided immediately after surgery. Treatment regimens for speech restoration for those with a total laryngectomy might include:

- Esophageal speech: vocalization that is produced on controlled air that has been ingested via forced inhalation.
- Training and instruction with an artificial larynx: a device that can be utilized via placement in the mouth or on the neck to produce words from a vibratory tone.
- Tracheoesophageal puncture: surgical placement of a voice prosthesis that allows for vocalization. Air is directed from the lungs into the esophagus where it vibrates in the pharyngoesophageal segment to produce a vocalization.

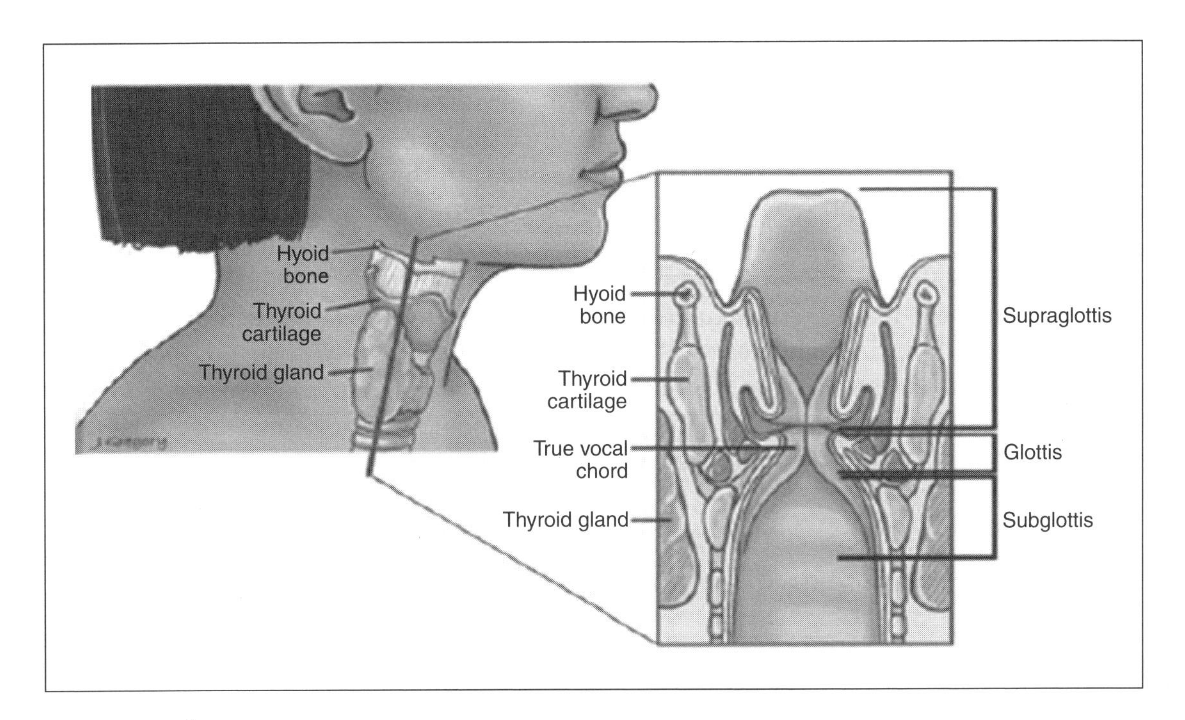

FIGURE 29.1 Laryngeal Tumors.

Source: Reprinted with permission. This image was created by Jill Gregory on behalf of the THANC Foundation as an educational tool for the Head and Neck Cancer Guide www.headandneckcancerguide.com

Artificial Airways

Placement of a tracheostomy tube hinders the ability of an individual to communicate verbally. Tracheotomy is the procedure of making an incision over the trachea. The term tracheostomy is used to indicate the procedure involving the incision on the trachea followed by insertion of a tube that maintains the patency of the opening in the trachea either temporarily or permanently (Muralidhar, 2008). Varying in size and type, tracheostomy tubes are either cuffed, cuffless, fenestrated, or communication tubes. A tracheostomy team is generally compromised of the primary physician, otolaryngologist, pulmonologist, respiratory therapist, nurse, and speech–language pathologist. Patients requiring mechanical ventilation often require either an endotracheal tube or a tracheostomy tube placement. When a patient is intubated, communication is often accomplished through facial expressions, gestures, and/or writing, depending on the person's neurological status and sedation level (Batty, 2009). However, these primary modes of communication are not consistently effective and often result in heightened frustration for the patient (Patak et al., 2006). Patients must be stable enough to tolerate cuff deflation prior to verbalization attempts. In mechanically ventilated patients, speech can be provided by the use of a talking tracheostomy tube, using a cuff-down technique, via use of a speaking valve, or using a cuff-down technique with a speaking valve (Hess, 2005). Patients breathing spontaneously with a tracheostomy tube placement may be trained to use digital occlusion to produce speech. A variety of speaking valves are available that can be attached to the hub of the tracheostomy tube prior to capping. Fenestrated tracheostomy tubes can be used to direct airflow through the vocal cords to produce vocalization. Tracheostomy and ventilator use is life sustaining. Speech for patients with tracheostomies or ventilators is life enriching (ASHA, 2007).

Language and Higher-Level Cognitive Linguistic Function

Language is made up of socially shared rules. The conversion of thoughts into meaningful symbols occurs through the use of language. The effective use of language is a multitiered process involving semantics, morphology, and pragmatic functioning. For the majority of the population, the left hemisphere is dominant for language. However, a review of the literature reveals some evidence of lateralization of language to the right hemisphere. Dominant handedness has been linked with hemispheric language dominance in healthy humans.

Aphasia

Aphasia is an acquired neurological communication disorder that affects a person's ability to process and use language efficiently. Aphasia originates from the Greek word *aphatos* meaning speechless. It is most commonly the result of damage to the cerebral cortex of brain's left hemisphere, although injury to subcortical structures may also result in aphasia. Aphasia is characterized by a reduction in and dysfunction of language content or meaning, language form or structure, language *use* or function, and the cognitive processes that underlie language, such as memory and thinking (Chapey, 1981). The National Institute on Neurological Disorders and Stroke estimates that approximately 1 million individuals suffer from aphasia in the United States. Despite its noted prevalence, aphasia is poorly recognized in the general community. Dependent on lesion size and location, aphasia can vary significantly in severity and may affect a single or multiple aspects of communication. Aphasia may impair expressive language including speaking and writing, auditory comprehension, and reading and writing skills.

Owing to the unique and variable presentation of symptoms in aphasia, it is most challenging to subscribe to a single classification system of aphasia. Traditionally, aphasia is described as expressive or receptive. Patients with expressive aphasia typically have challenges in producing fluent output and are believed to have a lesion in Broca's area in the dominant frontal lobe. Damage to the anterior speech areas result in slow, labored speech with limited output and prosody, and difficulty in producing grammatical sentences (Hopper & Holland, 2005). Nonfluency may be due to a number of different factors, including decreased phrase length, agrammatism, poor articulation, or slower speech rate (Hillis et al., 2007). Speech production in patients with nonfluent aphasia is largely noted as "halting," utilizing nouns and verbs with higher frequency than articles and prepositions. Auditory comprehension is generally better preserved than expression, leading to frustration in communication attempts. Examples of nonfluent aphasia include Broca's aphasia, transcortical motor aphasia, transcortical mixed aphasia, and global aphasia. Deficits in comprehending language are thought to be associated with a lesion in the Wernicke's area of the dominant temporal lobe, and are frequently referred to as a receptive or sensory aphasia. Lesions anterior to the fissure of Rolando generally result in nonfluent aphasias, while posterior lesions to this fissure have a higher correspondence to a fluent aphasia. Fluent aphasias occur when damage occurs in the posterior language areas of the brain, where sensory stimuli from hearing, sight, and bodily sensation converge (Hopper & Holland, 2005). The same author explains that prosody and flow of speech is maintained and one typically must listen closely to recognize that speech is not normal. Examples of fluent aphasia include Wernicke's aphasia, anomic aphasia, conduction aphasia, and transcortical sensory aphasia (Figure 29.2).

As patients rarely fit into a defined structure, it is often more clinically relevant to describe and summarize the actual cognitive–linguistic (content and form) and communicative abilities and impairments of each individual (Chapey, 1981). Generally, aphasia is classified on integration of data based on the location of the brain lesion, observation of a spontaneous language sample, and an analysis of specific language tasks across modalities of auditory/visual comprehension, expression, higher-level language processing, reading, and writing.

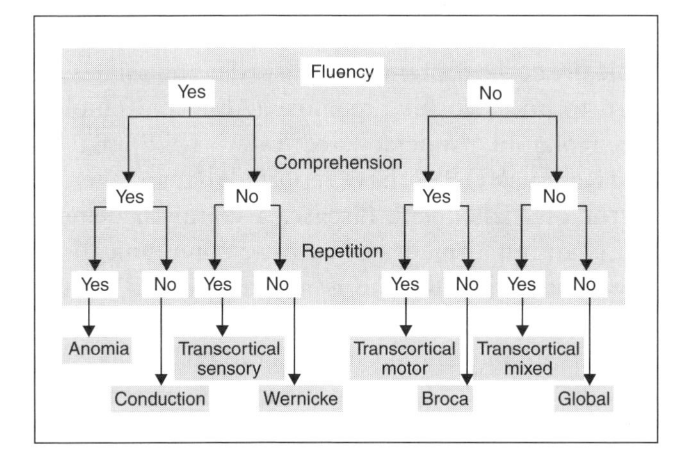

FIGURE 29.2 Classification of the aphasias.

Source: Reprinted with permission from Medscape Drugs & Diseases

Validated and reliable screening tools and comprehensive assessment batteries are available to assist speech–language pathologists in the measurement process.

Individuals with aphasia have difficulty in finding the "right" words to effectively communicate. Impaired content at the level of individual words is evident as a marred vocabulary. Various forms of naming errors can have a profound impact on the patient's functional communication. Anomia affects some categories of words more than others. Nouns appear to be especially difficult for aphasic patients to retrieve from memory while the labels for numbers and letters are often recalled with relative ease (Goodglass & Kaplan, 1983). With primary involvement of the verbal knowledge store, there are typically high consistent deficits that affect naming both to confrontation and from description, but which affect unusual low frequency items (e.g., hippopotamus) more than common, high frequency items (e.g., cat; Rohrer et al., 2008). The patient may use approximate or imprecise expressions, circumlocutions that substitute a vague term for an explicit label. Paraphasias refers to the production of unintended syllables, words, or phrases during the effort to speak (Goodglass & Kaplan, 1983) and indicate word-finding difficulty. The classification of paraphasias include literal/phonological, neologistic and semantic/verbal. More than half of the intended word is produced correctly in literal or phonological paraphasias. For example, a patient may say /pun/ instead of /fun/. Neologistic paraphasias occur when a "nonsense" word is utilized to replace a target word, "arfty" for "chair." Semantic or verbal paraphasias replace a target word with a word from a similar semantic category, such as "mother" for "daughter." Repetition tasks are assessed to better differentiate clinical presentation.

Reading deficits in aphasia can have profound implications on functional communicative tasks. Deficits can include a lack of recognition of printed words, dysfluent reading, word omission/substitutions and poor comprehension of material that was read. A challenge with writing in the context of language processing is known as agraphia. Deficits in the written modality of language can include mislabeling objects, omission of grammatical forms, syntactic deficiencies, disorganization in writing, difficulties with recall as to what letters mean, and inefficient copying of letters, words, and sentences. Some aphasic patients may encounter noted difficulty in writing to dictation.

The goal of therapeutic intervention is both restorative and compensatory in nature. Various forms of aphasia therapy include cognitive linguistic therapy to support adaptation of the deviant communication deficits, education regarding optimal use of residual language abilities, programmed simulation, forced use aphasia therapy, community and group participation, transcranial magnetic stimulation, melodic intonation therapy, promoting aphasic communicative effectiveness (PACE), and utilization of augmentative communication devices. Family counseling in regard to expectations and management of deficits is of prime importance.

Cognitive Communication Deficits

Advances in imaging techniques have demonstrated the contributions of right hemispheric (nondominant) structures in the linguistic process. The diagnosis of cognitive disorders is made by an interdisciplinary team of professionals. Speech–language pathologists have competency in understanding brain–behavior relationships as they relate to linguistic functioning. Cognitive–communicative disorders may affect the ability to communicate by impairing pragmatic language use, or the social rules of language (Tompkins, 2012). Areas for assessment and intervention in cognitive communication include orientation, latent processing of novel stimuli, attention, judgement, memory problems, and the linguistic elements of executive function. Executive functions include initiation, goal maintenance, task persistence, awareness, organization, problem solving, and cognitive flexibility (Norman & Shallice, 1986). Patients with frontal lesions are more likely to have impaired executive function. An appreciation of concomitant factors such as hearing loss, visual impairment, depression, effects of chemical agents, and management of the parameters of sugar levels and hydration are of key importance in this assessment process.

Right Hemisphere Dysfunction

Most individuals are left hemisphere dominant for language function. Although the left hemisphere of the brain houses the dominant functions of speech and language in most individuals, the right hemisphere contributes to the effectiveness of communication. Right hemisphere dysfunction may result in perceptual, attentional, and other behavioral deficits. However, the right hemisphere is a major contributor to nonverbal, emotional aspects of communication (Borod et al., 1983), and complex aspect of linguistic processing (Gardner, Brownell, & Wapner, 1983). Injury to the prefrontal cortex disrupts the regulation and initiation of behavior, including language, vocational behavior, learning/studying behavior, and social behavior, all of which have profound impact on communication. Challenges in patients with right hemisphere dysfunction (RHD) may include prosodic problems, use of anomalous speech and inappropriate or subtle changes in social language exchanges. Difficulty can be seen in integrating information in stories and implying meanings across the modalities of language. Speech language intervention for patients with RHD attempts to build on preserved communicative strengths and are developed on an individual basis. Emphasis may focus on improving a patient's self-awareness of deficits. Empowerment of caregivers via education of the nuances of RHD communicative impairment is essential.

Dementia

Dementia is an acquired neurological syndrome associated with a gradual and permanent decline in intellectual and communicative functions and general behavior that is sustained over a period of months or years. Communication challenges affecting an individual's ability to comprehend and produce linguistic information are present in most types of dementia. Poor comprehension skills are typically at the center of this disorder and relates, in part, to poor working memory (Almore, Kempler, MacDonanld, Anderson, & Tyler, 1999). Bayles and Kaszniak (1987) have reported that an inherent factor of Alzheimer's disease, a common dementia, is an impairment in linguistic communication. Communication decline is also influenced by the common presence of repetitiousness and anxiety. Cognitive linguistic decline is gradual and permanent in nature. The assessment of a person with dementia requires the collaboration of a medical team. Speech–language pathologists assist individuals with dementia in maintaining the highest level of linguistic independence throughout the course of the disease. Based on the severity of impaired linguistic skills, deficits may range from inefficient language comprehension and calculations, spontaneous compulsive repetition of words/phrases, and naming difficulties. Therapeutic intervention for patients with dementia may be restorative or compensatory in nature. Family orientation treatment is of noted importance owing to the progressive nature of the communicative decline.

Communication Challenges in Typical Aging

Stedman's Medical Dictionary defines aging as the gradual deterioration of a mature organism resulting from time-dependent, irreversible changes in structure that is intrinsic to the particular species. Owing to the rapid growth of the older population, attention has been allocated to age-related health issues in the elderly. Suppression of sensory input with dulled hearing and vison changes impact overall processing of the communicative message. Aging is responsible for changes in hearing, voice, and speech processes (Caruso, Muellar, & Shadden, 1995). There is a correlate between aging and increased frequency of word-finding challenges. Vocabulary, grammatical judgment, and repetition ability are relatively stable with age; comprehension of complex utterances may decline (Lubinski, 1995). Older adults exhibit retrieval difficulties in spelling, suggestive of challenges with word phonology and orthography (Burke & Shafto, 2004). The role of speech–language pathologists in this population is best served in assisting in differentiating between normal aging and disordered communication or swallowing function (ASHA, 2007).

Dysphagia as a Disorder

The primary purpose of swallowing is to transport the food or liquid from the lips to the stomach. Flow of the bolus (food or liquid) through the oropharyngeal mechanism can be either stopped, as in oropharyngeal residue, or misdirected, as in penetration or aspiration of material into the airway. Dysphagia is not a primary medical diagnosis but a symptom of an underlying disease or medical diagnosis. Although the true incidence of dysphagia may be unknown, it seems that this disorder is widespread with severe consequences. The diagnosis is often not easily recognized, requiring an accurate and complete medical history and clinical examination in addition to various diagnostic tests. Numerous treatments and interventions have been developed to prevent aspiration with greater awareness of the disorder's importance among various health care providers being an important component of care.

Normal Swallow Physiology

Normal swallow is a coordinated mechanism involving several anatomical chambers divided by muscular sphincters (Leonard & Kendall, 2014). The propulsion pressures are generated by muscles that retract and expand within the chambers in a coordinated manner. Disturbance of this mechanism can result in less effective movement of food and liquid boluses from the lips to the stomach. The swallowing mechanism can be divided into four stages for simplification purposes: oral preparatory stage, oral stage, the pharyngeal stage, and the esophageal stage (Dodds, Stewart, & Logemann, 1990).

During the oral preparatory stage, the food bolus is prepared in the oral cavity by chewing in order to manipulate the presented bolus into a consistency suitable for swallowing. Movement patterns and preparation time vary, depending on the volume and consistency of the bolus. From the time the bolus is placed in the oral cavity, labial seal is sustained to avoid anterior spillage. The tongue positions the bolus on the teeth and when the upper and lower teeth meet, the food falls medially toward the tongue, which in turn then moves the bolus back onto the teeth. The tongue moves the food laterally to the molar ridges with repetitive movements of the jaw. This is an almost entirely a voluntary movement pattern. The trigeminal nerve innervates muscles responsible for chewing (masseter, temporalis, and pterygoid muscles) and the facial nerve innervates the muscles of the mandible and the maxillae including the buccinator muscles. The intrinsic muscles of the tongue are innervated by the hypoglossal nerve.

When the bolus propulsion begins posteriorly by the tongue, the oral stage is initiated. The tongue creates a propulsive anterior-to-posterior wave as it presses up and back against the hard palate, moving the bolus to the back of the mouth. The bolus is propelled into the oropharynx and then to hypopharynx at the moment of swallow response.

During the pharyngeal phase, the soft palate rises, the hyoid bone and larynx move upward and forward, the vocal folds move to midline, the epiglottis folds backward to protect the airway, and the tongue pushes backward and downward into the pharynx to propel the bolus. The pharyngeal musculature (superior, middle, and inferior constrictors) contracts to push the bolus through the pharynx in coordination with relaxation of the upper esophageal sphincter (UES), which relaxes and is pulled open by the forward movement of the larynx and hyoid bone. After the bolus passage, the UES closes and the pharyngeal structures return to their reference positions. The pharyngeal swallow response involves the motor and sensory tracts from the trigeminal (V), facial (VII), glossopharyngeal (IX), vagus (X), and hypoglossal (XII) cranial nerves and lasts 1 second (Paik, 2008).

In the esophageal phase, the bolus is propelled downward by peristalsis of circular and longitudinal smooth muscle coordinated by Auerbach's plexus. At the distal end, the lower esophageal sphincter (LES) relaxes, allows the bolus to pass into the stomach, and closes again. This phase can be measured from the point the bolus passes the UES until it enters the stomach. According to studies, normal esophageal transit time varies from 8 to 20 seconds.

Swallowing Evaluation

Dysphagia has been defined as any difficulty moving food or liquid from the mouth to the stomach (Logemann, 1986). It can be considered, therefore, an abnormality of bolus flow (McCullough, Wertz, Rosenbek, & Dinneen, 1999). Food and liquid remaining in the oropharynx (residue) reduces the amount of food and liquid reaching the gut and increases the risk of dehydration and malnutrition. People who aspirate food and liquid increase their risk of developing pneumonia more than seven times compared to nonaspirating individuals (Schmidt, Holas, Halvorson, & Reding, 1994).

To swallow safely and efficiently, muscles of the tongue and pharynx must create sufficient pressures to propel the bolus through the pharynx while maintaining opening of the UES, allowing the bolus to move into the esophagus (Castell & Castell, 1997). Impairment in the timing of oropharyngeal events, the magnitude of pharyngeal propulsive force, or the extent of UES relaxation and opening can lead to varying amounts of pharyngeal residue (material left in the pharynx after the swallow) and aspiration (material that is misdirected into the larynx and passes below the vocal folds into the trachea).

Clinical Swallow Evaluation

Clinical swallow evaluation is the most common examination to diagnose dysphagia in numerous settings but it should not be confused with swallow "screen." It is the first step in obtaining information that helps make the diagnosis of dysphagia and whether additional diagnostic tests are needed, as well as determining which therapeutic interventions that may be helpful. Speech–language pathologists present small volumes of various consistencies to the patient and observe for overt signs of laryngeal penetration, aspiration, or any signs of abnormal swallowing function, such as anterior spillage, facial weakness, reduced hyolaryngeal elevation, coughing/throat clearing, and/or changes in voice quality after swallow. The main limitation of this assessment is that it relies on findings that are subjective and clinician dependent (Singh & Hamdy, 2006). Several investigators have tried to create objective and reliable scoring systems for the bedside assessment. These investigations are still in process to ensure validity and reliability.

Videofluoroscopic Swallow Study

The videofluoroscopic swallow study (VFSS) is the most commonly used technique to evaluate oropharyngeal swallowing (Logemann, 1998). There are various terms that are used for the examination depending on the institution: modified barium swallow (MBS), videofluoroscopic swallow evaluation (VFSE), swallow study. VFSS provides information on bolus flow and the biomechanical movements of oral and laryngopharyngeal structures affecting bolus flow. This procedure enables visualization of the oral activity during chewing and oral bolus propulsion, the triggering of the pharyngeal swallow in relation to position of the bolus, and the biomechanics of the pharyngeal swallow, including movement of the larynx, hyoid, tongue base, pharyngeal walls, and cricopharyngeal region. It also enables the clinician to scan the esophagus in the anterior–posterior plane. In addition to diagnosing dysphagia, VFSS provides a means for examining the effects of various compensatory strategies to improve the efficiency of swallow. The clinician can obtain direct evidence of the efficacy for various methods of bolus presentation, sensory input prior to the swallow, head positioning, and swallow maneuvers.

VFSS has the advantages of clear visualization of barium through the oral cavity, oropharynx, pharynx, and esophagus. It can easily be recorded and played back in slow motion many times if needed to identify laryngeal penetration or aspiration penetration of barium into the airway and below the true vocal cords, respectively.

A disadvantage of VFSS is exposure to radiation. The procedure is carried out in very "controlled" conditions that may not accurately reflect the patient's eating and swallowing habits. Barium's density is different compared to normal liquid and solid consistencies. There is no standard protocol for the volumes tested or the consistencies delivered (Singh & Hamdy, 2006).

Fiberoptic Endoscopic Evaluation of Swallowing

Like the VFSS, fiberoptic endoscopic evaluation of swallowing (FEES) is another instrumental swallow evaluation that provides an objective assessment of swallowing anatomy and physiology. It is a relatively newer examination in the field compared with the VFSS but is steadily gaining greater use in medical centers and nursing homes. It was first described as flexible endoscopic evaluation of swallowing safety (FEESS) by Langmore, Schatz, and Olsen (1988). The FEESS term was recommended by the American Speech-Language-Hearing Association (ASHA) but other terms have been used in the past such as videoendoscopic evaluation of dysphagia (VEED; Bastian, 1991), and flexible endoscopy with sensory testing (FEEST). The purpose of the examination, the materials used, and the process of the evaluations are similar to the videofluoroscopic examination (Crary & Groher, 2010). FEES is indicated when there is need to evaluate nasopharyngeal and oropharyngeal anatomy, alterations in the anatomy of the larynx or pharyngeal symmetry, and the ability of the patient to maintain airway protection during a longer period of time. It is also a useful tool when providing feedback to the patient while using various compensatory strategies.

FEES does require skilled therapists and technical equipment that may not be available in all settings. Limitations of FEES include nonvisualization of the oral and oropharyngeal phase of swallowing and a "white out" as the bolus passes through the pharynx (Singh & Hamdy, 2006). There is about four tenths of a second during the swallow known as "white-out" when the airway cannot be visualized because the pharynx squeezes around the endoscope's camera and causes a white colored reflection on the computer screen

Esophageal Manometry

Esophageal manometry has historically been used to diagnose motility disorders of the esophagus and, specifically, intraluminal pressures and coordination of muscular contractions within the esophagus. Recent technological advances with this procedure, such as solid-state intraluminal transducers capable of rapid data collection, have resulted in renewed interest in manometry (Castell & Castell, 1994). Solid-state manometry has made it possible to obtain accurate manometric profiles of the pressures and durations of events associated with the pharynx and UES, as well as the esophagus (Hatlebakk et al., 1998; Hila, Castell, & Castell, 2001).

The solid-state intraluminal manometry catheter is soft and flexible with microtransducers that are in contact with the pharyngeal or esophageal wall. Unlike the older water-perfused catheters, solid-state intraluminal catheters measure contractions directly and without respect to the relative positions of the patient and the equipment. In this manner, studies can be performed with the participant in an upright position, which allows testing of various food consistencies and volumes as well as different head positions.

Despite advances, the use of manometry in clinical evaluations of pharyngeal dysphagia remains controversial. Malhi-Chowla, Anchem, Stark, and DeVault (2000) argued that UES and pharyngeal manometry should not be included as a routine procedure for patients undergoing esophageal manometry. The authors reviewed 435 complete manometry evaluations and found that only six of the patients were offered an intervention based on abnormal findings of the UES. Only three of the patients presented with dysphagia. However, the authors did not specifically select patients with complaints of dysphagia, which could explain the low incidence of UES and pharyngeal abnormalities.

Xue et al. (2000) examined manometry records for 114 individuals diagnosed with dysphagia and compared the findings with the recordings of 80 patients with complaints of chest pain. In their study, patients with dysphagia demonstrated significantly higher UES residual pressures, weak pharyngeal contractions, and UES/pharyngeal incoordination compared with participants presenting with chest pain. Seventy-one percent of participants with dysphagia had at least one UES and pharyngeal manometric abnormality.

Although, the true incidence of swallowing disorders may not be known, it is apparent that the problem is widespread. The symptomatology produced by dysphagia is broad and matches the variety of etiologies for the deficit. Thus, managing patients with a swallowing impairment has become a daily routine for many health care providers regardless of their specialty. Until the late 1980s, there was minimal literature addressing the diagnosis and treatment of dysphagia. Since then, clinical and basic science research, development of discussion groups, journals, and conferences have helped speech-language pathologists manage and improve the quality of care for patients with dysphagia. Appropriate management and early intervention in patients with dysphagia provide benefits to the patients, their families, and to the physicians, nurses, and other therapists involved in patient care.

Speech, language, voice, and swallowing disorders can adversely affect social interaction of patients and quality of life. Timely swallowing evaluation and treatment can prevent dehydration, weight loss, malnutrition, and pulmonary compromise to patients with dysphagia. Speech–language pathologists are trained to provide interventions that lead to improved swallowing safety, function, and independence and to assist patients to reach their full communicative potential. Speech–language pathology services ensure early management of communication, speech, voice, and swallowing disorders, which in turn enable the maximum social, academic, and professional integration.

REFERENCES

Almore, A., Kempler, D., MacDonanld, M. C., Anderson, E. S., & Tyler, L. K. (1999). Why do Alzheimer Patients have difficulty with pronouns. Working memory, semantics, and reference in comprehension and production in Alzheimer's Disease. *Brain and Language*, *67*, 202–227.

American Speech-Language-Hearing Association. (2007). *Scope of practice in speech-language pathology [Scope of practice]*. Retrieved from http://www.asha.org/docs/html/SP2007-00283.html

Bastian, R. W. (1991). Videoendoscopic evaluation of patients with dysphagia: An adjunct to the modified barium swallow. *Otolaryngology—Head and Neck Surgery, 104*(3), 339–350.

Batty, S. (2009). Communication, swallowing and feeding in the intensive care unit patient. *Nursing in Critical Care*, *14*, 175–179.

Bayles, K. A., & Kaszniak, A. W. (1987). *Communication and cognition in normal aging and dementia*. Austin, TX: Pro-Ed.

Behrman, A. (2013). *Speech and voice*. San Diego, CA: Plural Publishing.

Bless, D., & Hicks, D. (2000). *Organic voice disorders-assessment and treatment* (pp. 49–84). San Diego, CA: Singular Publishing Group.

Borod, J., Obler, J., Erhan, H., Grunwald, I., Cicero, B., Welkowitz, J., . . . Whalen, J. (1983). Right hemisphere emotional perception: Evidence across multiple channels. *Neuropsychology*, *12*(3), 446–458.

Broussolle, E., Bakchine, S., Tommasi, M., Laurent, B., Bazin, B., & Cinotti, L., (1996). Slowly progressive anarthria with late anterior opercular syndrome: A variant form of frontal cortical atrophy syndromes. *Journal of the Neurological Sciences*, *144*(1–2), 44–58.

Brown, W., Vinson, B. & Crary, M. (2000). Organic Voice Disorders. San Diego, CA: Singular Publishing Group.

Burke, D. M., & Shafto, M. A. (2004). Aging and language production. *Current Direction is Psychological Scienc, 1,* 21–24.

Campainha, S., Ribeiro, C., & Guimaraes, M. (2012). Vocal cord dysfunction: A frequently forgotten entity. *Case Reports in Pulmonology, 2012*, 4.

Caruso, A. J., Muellar, P. B., & Shadden, B. B. (1995). Effects of aging on speech and voice. *Physical and Occupational Therapy in Geriatric Journal*, *13*(1–2), 63–79.

Case, J. (1984). *Clinical management of voice disorders*. Rockville, MD: Aspen Systems Corporation.

Castell, J., & Castell, D. (1994). Manometric analysis of the pharyngo-esophageal segment. *Indian Journal Gastroenterology, 13*(2), 58–63.

Chapey, R. (1981). *Intervention strategies in adult aphasia*. Baltimore, MD: Lippincott Williams & Wilkins.

Colton, R. (2000). *Physiology of voice quality*. In W. Brown, B. Vinson, & M. Crary (Eds.), *Organic voice disorders-assessment and treatment* (pp. 49–84). San Diego, CA: Singular Publishing Group.

Crary, M., & Groher, M. (2010). *Adult swallowing disorders*. St. Louis, MO: Elsevier.

Croot, K., Ballard, K., Leyton, C., & Hodges, J. (2012). Apraxia of speech and phonological errors in the diagnosis of nonfluent/agrammatic and logopenic variants of primary progressive aphasia. *Journal of Speech, Language and Hearing Research, 55*, 1562–1572.

Darley, F. L., Aronson, A. E., & Brown, J. R. (1975). *Motor speech disorders*. Philadelphia, PA: W. B. Saunders.

Dodds, W. J., Logemann, J. A., & Stewart, E. T. (1990). Radiologic assessment of abnormal oral and pharyngeal phases of swallowing. *American Journal of Roentgenology, 154*(5), 965–974.

Dronkers, N. F. (1996). A new brain region for coordinating speech articulation. *Nature, 384*, 159–161.

Duffy, J. (2013). *Motor speech disorders* (p. 12). St. Louis, MO: Mosby.

Gardner, H., Brownell, H., & Wapner, W. (1983). Missing the point: The role of the right hemisphere in the processing of complex linguistic materials. In E. Pereman (Ed.), *Cognitive processing in the right hemisphere* (pp. 169–191). New York, NY: Academic Press.

Goodglass, H., & Kaplan, E. (1983). *The assessment of aphasia and other neurological disorders*. Baltimore, MD: Lippincott Williams and Wilkins.

Guitar, B. (2013). *Stuttering: An integrated approach to it nature and treatment*. Baltimore, MD: Lippincott Williams and Wilkins.

Hatlebakk, J., Castell, J., Spiegel, J., Paoletti, V., Katz, P., & Castell, D. (1998). Dilatation therapy for dysphagia in patients with upper esophageal sphincter dysfunction: Manometric and symptomatic response. *Diseases of the Esophagus, 11*(4), 254–259.

Hedge, M. N. (2001). *Pocket guide to assessment in speech-language pathology*. Toronto: Singular Thompson Learning.

Hess, D. R. (2005). Facilitating speech in the patient with a tracheostomy. *Respiratory Care, 50*(4), 519–525.

Hila, A., Castell, J., & Castell, D. (2001). Pharyngeal and upper esophageal sphincter manometry in the evaluation of dysphagia. *Journal of Clinical Gastroenterology, 33*(5), 355–361.

Hillis, A. E., Work, M., Barker, P. B., Jacobs, M. A., Breese, E. L., & Maurer, K. (2007). Re-examing the brain regions crucial for orchestrating speech articulation. *Brain, 127*, 1479–1487.

Hopper, T., & Holland, A. (2005). Aphasia and Learning in Adults: Key Concepts and Clinical Considerations. *Topics in Geriatric Rehabilitation, 21*(4), 315–322.

Langmore, S. E., Schatz, K., & Olsen, N. (1998). Fiberoptic endoscopic examination of swallowing safety: A new procedure. *Dysphagia, 2*(4), 216–219.

Leonard, R., & Kendall, K. (2014). *Dysphagia assessment and treatment planning: A team approach*. San Diego, CA: Plural Publishing.

Logemann, J. (1986). Treatment for aspiration related to dysphagia: An overview. *Dysphagia, 1*(1), 34–38.

Logemann, J. A. (1998). *Evaluation and treatment of swallowing disorders*. Austin, TX: Pro-Ed.

Lubinski, R. (Ed.). (1995). *Dementia and communication*. San Diego, CA: Singular Publishing Group.

Malhi-Chowla, N., Achem, S., Stark, M., & DeVault, K. (2000). Manometry of the upper esophageal sphincter and pharynx is not useful in unselected patients referred for esophageal testing. *The American Journal of Gastroenterology, 95*(6), 1417–1421.

McCullough, G. H., Wertz, R. T., Rosenbek, J. C., & Dinneen, C. (1999). Clinicians' preferences and practices in conducting clinical/bedside and videofluoroscopic swallowing examinations in an adult, neurogenic population. *American Journal of Speech-Language Pathology, 8*(2), 149–163.

McNeil, M. R., Doyle, P., & Wambaugh, J. (2000). Apraxia of speech: A treatable disorder of motor planning and programming. In S. Nadeau, L. J. G. Rothi, & B. Crosson (Eds.), *Aphasia and language: Theory to practice* (pp. 221–266). New York, NY: Guilford.

McNeil, M. R., Robin, D. A., & Schmidt, R. A. (2009). Apraxia of speech: Definition, differentiation, and treatment. In M. R. McNeil (Ed.), *Clinical management of sensorimotor speech disorders* (pp. 249–268). New York, NY: Thieme.

Melfi, R. (2015). Communication disorders: Overview, the normal communication process. Retrieved from http://emedicine.medscape.com/article/317758-overview

Merriam-Webster: Dictionary and Thesaurus. (n.d.). Retrieved from www.merriam-webster.com/dictionary/communication

Muralidhar, K. (2008). Tracheostomy in ICU: An insight into present concerpts. *Indian Journal of Anaesthesia, 52*(1), 28–37.

Nestor, P. J., Graham, N. L., Fryer, T. D., Williams, G. B., Patterson, K., & Hodges, J. R. (2013). Progressive non-fluent aphasia is associated with hypometabolism center on the left anterior insula. *Brain, 126*(11), 2406–2418.

Norman, D. A., & Shallice, T. (1986). Attention to action: Willed and automatic control of behavior. In R. J. Davidson, G. E. Shwartz, & D. Shapiro (Eds.), *Attention to action: Willed and automatic control of behavior* (pp. 1–18). New York, NY: Plenum.

Paik, N. J. (2008). Dysphagia. Retrieved from www.emedicine.medscape.com

Patak, L., Gawlinski, A., Fung, N., Doering, L., Berg, J., & Henneman, E. (2006). Communication boards in critical care: Patients's views. *Applications in Nursing Research, 19*, 182–190.

Peach, R., & Tonkovich, J. (2004). Phonemic characteristics of apraxia of speech resulting from subcortical hemorrhage. *Journal of Communication Disorders, 37*(1), 77–99

Rohrer, J. D., Knight, W. D., Warren, J. E., Fox, N. C., Rossor, M. N., & Warren, J. D. (2008). Word-finding difficulty: A clinical analysis of the progressive aphasias. *Brain, 131*, 8–38.

Rosenbeck, J. C., & LaPointe, L. I. (1985). The dysarthrias: Description and treatment. In D. F. Johns (Ed.), *Clinician management of neurogenic communication disorders* (pp. 97–152). Boston, MA: Little, Brown.

Schmidt, J., Holas, M., Halvorson, K., & Reading, M. (1994). Videofluoroscopic evidence of aspiration predicts pneumonia and death but not dehydration following stroke. *Dysphagia, 9*(1), 7–11.

Singh, S., & Hamdy, S. (2006). Dysphagia in stroke patients. *Postgraduate Medical Journal*, *82*(968), 383–391.

Square, P. A., Roy, A. E., & Martin, R. E. (1997). Apraxia of speech: Another form of praxis disruption. In L. J. G. Rothis & J. M. Heliman (Eds.), *Apraxia: The Neuropsychology of Action* (pp. 173–206). East Sussex: Psychology Press.

Square, P. A., Martin, R. E., & Bose, A. (2001). Nature and treatment of neuromotor speech disorders in aphasia. In R. Chapey (Ed.), *Language intervention strategies in aphasia and related neurogenic communication disorders* (4th ed., pp. 847–882). Philadelphia, PA: Lippincott Williams & Wilkins.

Tompkins, C. A. (2012). Rehabilitation for cognitive–communication disorders in right hemisphere brain damage. *Archives of Physical Medicine and Rehabilitation, 93*(Suppl. 1), S61–S69.

Wambaugh, J. (2006). Treatment guidelines for apraxia of speech: Lessons for future research. *Journal of Medical Speech Language Pathology*, 14(4), 317–321.

Xue, S., Katz, P. O., Castell, J. A., et al. (2000). Upper esophageal sphincter and pharyngeal manometry: Which patients? [Abstract]. *Gastroenterology, 118*, A41.

Yaruss, J. S. (2010). Assessing quality of life in stuttering treatment outcomes research. *Journal of Fluency Disorders 35*, 190–202.

Social Work

Lynn Videka

30

CHAPTER

INTRODUCTION

Social workers play an important role in health care for persons with disabilities from the time of acute illness or injury; through early stabilization; confronting and managing the patient's residual disabilities; aiding and supporting the emotional, financial, and physical aspects of rehabilitation; and helping coordinate and manage the systems of family, financial, emotional, health, and social support that are essential for an optimal rehabilitation and habilitation. Social workers are part of multidisciplinary teams that typically serve people with disabilities. The social worker's roles on the team include linking patient, family, health care and social services, and integrating behavioral and physical health care, all in the service of optimal rehabilitation of the person with a disability.

Disabled people account for a substantial portion of medical costs in the United States (Stanton & Rutherford, 2006). With the introduction of the Patient Protection and Affordable Care Act (ACA) in 2010, populations with disabilities have been the focus of innovation and new and more efficient health services approaches to meet the ACA's "triple aim" standards of better quality care, more efficient care, and better health outcomes for the American public.

In this chapter, social work services will be viewed from public health and boundary spanning perspectives. Social workers work to prevent negative long-term outcomes for persons with disabilities and to optimize the habilitation of the person with residual disabilities.

Social workers are committed to social justice and to advocacy for the rights and optimal outcomes for all people, including those whose rights are abridged by structural and individual discrimination and oppression. Social workers advance the rights of persons with disabilities by ensuring services and supports that fulfill the spirit and the requirements of the Americans with Disabilities Act (ADA), which is discussed later in the chapter.

This chapter is based on a biopsychosocial framework for understanding the broad range of needs of people with disabilities and will present the epidemiology of disability in American adults. Policies that underlie disabilities support and services are discussed. Using an ecological approach, a multilevel, problem-solving approach to social work services is defined, with special attention to services that are delivered within a family-centered perspective, which optimize use of policies, benefits, and financial resources to promote optimal rehabilitation and inclusion of the disabled person, and that integrate physical and behavioral health issues in viewing the whole person in a person-centered care approach.

THE EPIDEMIOLOGY OF DISABILITY IN THE UNITED STATES WITH IMPLICATIONS FOR SOCIAL WORK INTERVENTION

Disability is a very broad term, which is defined in many different ways. Most definitions of disability focus on functional impairments that affect a person's interactions with his or her environments. A disability results from functional limitations of an acute health problem, such as a cerebrovascular accident (stroke) or a spinal cord injury, or of a cumulative impairment of ability to function resulting from chronic health conditions such, as congestive heart failure, chronic obstructive pulmonary disease, dementia, or other mental or cognitive limitation (Altman, 2014). A disability involves problems in basic human functioning such as movement, sensory, emotional, or cognitive actions. These dysfunctions result in limitations in performing necessary, complex human activities such as work, self-care, or social interaction. Disabilities affect a person in all his or her environments, thus the ecological model of human functioning is especially relevant to the disabled person. The concept of disability is as much a social as it is a physical or medical construct. Disabilities are not static over time; nor are they a dichotomous construct. Ability level can ebb and flow over time and there are gradations of disability in different functional areas. But for purposes of operational definition and eligibility for special services or programs for disabled people, it is common for social and health programs to define categories of disability status based on functional impairment resulting from a movement, sensory, emotional, or cognitive ability deficit Altman (2014).

Epidemiology of Disability

The World Health Organization (WHO) estimates that 15% of people worldwide have a disability that compromises their work, social, or emotional functioning. In a landmark study, Nagi found that there were two dimensions of disability, work and independent self-care (WHO, 2011; Nagi, 1976). He found in a probability sample of more than 8,000 households that 14% of his sample reported moderate performance limitations and that 10% of the sample reported substantial or severe limitations in performance. Women were affected more often than men. Those with less education and lower incomes were affected more often than those with higher socioeconomic status. These findings have been largely corroborated in more recent studies (Adams et al., 2009).

The Census Bureau reports that 19% of Americans report living with a disability, with half of them living with a disability they describe as severe (U.S. Census Bureau, 2012). The most common types of disabilities include mobility difficulties requiring assistive devices (30.6 million), being depressed or anxious to the point that it affects daily activities (7.1 million), difficulties in lifting or grasping (19.9 million), Alzheimer's disease or other dementias (2.4 million), blindness or severe visual impairment (2.1 million), and 1.1 million with severe hearing impairments.

Demographic Factors Associated With Disability With Implications for Social Interventions

Disabilities are not distributed across the entire American population, but are concentrated within certain demographic groups. Americans over 80 years of age are eight times more likely to be disabled as compared to Americans under 80, a 71% rate of disability compared to an 8% disability rate for younger Americans (U.S. Census Bureau, 2012).

People with disabilities are less likely to be employed than nondisabled Americans, and, if employed, have lower incomes than Americans without a disability (U.S. Census Bureau, 2013). The median annual income of an adult, age 21 to 64, with a disability is $23,500 compared to a median annual income of $32,700 for 21- to 64-year-olds without a disability (U.S. Census Bureau, 2012). The American Community Survey (ACS) is a census study that estimates information about Americans with disabilities in the workforce. In this study, disability is defined as having serious difficulty with hearing, vision, mobility, or cognition *and* difficulty with bathing, dressing, or performing errands such as shopping. The ACS finds that between 2008 and 2010, Americans with disabilities had employment rates of 32%, one third that of nondisabled Americans; hold lower paying jobs; and earn less than their nondisabled counterparts in the same types of jobs (Erickson, Lee, & vonSchrader, 2014; U.S. Census Bureau, 2013). American adults with a disability have more than double the poverty rates as nondisabled Americans of the same age (28% compared to 13%; U.S. Census Bureau, 2013).

Veterans have a higher disability rate (21% with a service-connected disability) compared to nonveterans (Erickson, Lee, & vonSchrader, 2014). Black Americans and Native Americans have higher disability rates than White, Asian American, or Latino American people (U.S. Census Bureau, 2013).

Many studies demonstrate that having a disability is associated with behavioral health comorbidities including depression, anxiety, and substance abuse (Elliott & Kennedy, 2004; Honey, Emerson, Llewellyn, & Kariuki, 2010; Lucas, 2007; McClure, Teasell, & Salter, 2015; Naylor et al., 2012; Pollard & Kennedy, 2007; Treharne, Lyons, Booth, & Kitas, 2007; Walker & Gonzales, 2007), and that associated behavioral health comorbidities lead to a greater number of disability affected days (Andrews, Henderson, & Hall, 2001; Merikangas et al., 2007). A British study of the added costs of behavioral health disabilities for people with chronic health problems including disabilities found that the comorbid behavioral health conditions added 45% to the cost of the physical condition and accounted for 12% to 18% of National Health Service expenditures for people with chronic and disabling conditions. Research also shows that socioeconomic resources act as buffers to behavioral health difficulties among people who are disabled (Smith, Langa, Kabeto, & Ubel, 2005). People with disabilities with fewer economic resources are at higher risk for mental health or addiction comorbidities. A recent policy brief prepared by the American Hospital Association (AHA) encouraged health care systems to integrate behavioral health with medical care, citing that 29% of patients with medical problems also have a co-occurring behavioral health condition, that the presence of a behavioral health condition raises monthly treatment costs for treating chronic health conditions including disabilities by 65% or $560. The same policy brief showed that providing integrated behavioral and medical health care resulted in more health prevention (screenings and education), and in reducing annual health care costs by 15% or $932 (AHA, 2012; Druss, Rohrbaugh, Levinson, & Rosenheck, 2001; Druss, von Esenwein, Compton, Zhao, & Leslie, 2011).

These statistics paint a clear picture that disability is associated with aging, and that for American adults, aged 18 to 64, disability status is associated with poverty, unemployment, and Black or Native American racial status. The implication is that social workers are likely to encounter disabled Americans in many service contexts. People with disabilities typically present with a complex intersection of social and economic disadvantages and risks for behavioral health comorbidities. Social workers are the health care team members who often deal with these complex social and psychological and behavioral needs as well as how they affect motivation and progress in rehabilitation, family relationships, interaction with health services workers, and other helpers.

This overview shows the broad swath that disabilities cut in American and global society. For this chapter, I focus on people who are identified as disabled in acute care and physical rehabilitation settings.

THE HEALTH POLICY CONTEXT FOR HEALTH SERVICES FOR AMERICANS WITH DISABILITIES

An important social work role is to ensure that patients and families are knowledgeable about and use insurance and other health policies and benefits. Eighty-three percent of people with disabilities are covered by public or private health insurance, leaving 27% uninsured, a rate higher than the national uninsured rate in 2015 (Erickson, Lee, & vonSchrader, 2014). A recent analysis of the ACA's impact on health services for disabled people documents that public insurance programs cover over 61% of the long-term service and support costs for disabled Americans, that Medicaid covers 40% of these costs, and that Medicare postacute care benefits covers 21%. Other public and private insurance covers 18% of health services costs for persons with disabilities; private insurance covers 7%, and out-of-pocket costs covers 15% (Musumeci, 2014). People with disabilities are also eligible for disability income support through the Social Security for Disabled Individuals (SSDI) program and through Veterans Affairs (VA) pension support for veterans with service-connected disabilities. Social workers provide important benefits information to families, patients, and medical care staff. Learn more about the federal government's programs and services for disabled people at its website (Disabilities .gov).

There are two important health and social policy areas that affect people with disabilities today. The first is the 1990 ADA, which is a landmark civil rights legislation that aimed to end the structural exclusions and social isolation that disabled Americans have historically faced. The second is the cluster of health policies that offer financial services for disabled people. These include Medicare, which is the universal health insurance for Americans older than 65 years; Medicaid, the public health insurance entitlement for low-income Americans; VA health care, an integrated health care system for military veterans; and policies that govern private insurance, with the most important new policy being the ACA.

Social workers in physical medicine and rehabilitation should be knowledgeable about basic health benefits and financing, and should develop specialized knowledge about the programs that finance and serve the particular patient population that the health organization serves. Table 30.1 displays basic Internet reference resources to begin to acquaint the rehabilitation social worker with the most important policies and programs.

The Americans With Disabilities Act: Empowerment for People With Disabilities

People with disabilities have long experienced discrimination, stereotyping, societal exclusion, and oppression through broad social acceptance of discrimination toward them. The 1990 ADA is landmark legislation that was hailed by President George H.W. Bush as he signed it into law as "a historic new civil rights act . . . the world's first comprehensive declaration of equality for people with disabilities" (Bush, 1990). The ADA Amendments Act of 2008 restored the inclusion of people with epilepsy, diabetes, and muscular dystrophy, which were removed from the ADA's protections via a series of court challenges to the original act. To find out more about insurance for people with disabilities under the ACA, go to the ACA website (HealthCare.gov, n.d.).

The ADA has had a profound impact on civil rights and societal inclusion for people with disabilities by mandating equal opportunity in employment, and accommodations of the physical structures of public and private environments that are open to the public including public buildings, public transportation, telecommunications, and certain private buildings, including schools, health facilities, hotels, retail establishments, golf courses, health clubs, movie theaters, and sports stadiums (ADA National Network, 2015; Owen, 2012). The

TABLE 30.1

WEB RESOURCES FOR HEALTH AND DISABILITY POLICIES

Policy	Website
Americans with Disabilities Act	An Overview of Americans with Disabilities Act: adata.org/factsheet/ADA-overview The ADA Amendments Act: An Overview of Recent Changes to the ADA: www.law.georgetown.edu/archiveada/documents/benferadaaa.pdf
Medicare	The Official Government Site for Medicare www.medicare.gov Medicare Program: General Information www.cms.gov/medicare/medicare-general-Information/medicareGenInfo/index.html
Medicaid	Medicaid.gov: Keeping America Healthy www.medicaid.gov/medicaid/index.html Medicare-Medicaid General Information www.cms.gov/Medicare-Medicaid-Coordination/Medicare-and-Medicaid-Coordination/Medicare-Medicaid-Coordination-Office/MedicareMedicaidGeneralInformation.html
Veterans Administration	Veterans Benefits Administration www.benefits.va.gov/benefits Veterans Health Administration www.va.gov/health
Affordable Care Act	The ACA: About the Law www.healthcare.gov/health-care-law-protections/rights-and-protections Kaiser Family Foundation: Understanding Health Insurance kff.org/understanding-health-insurance ACA: Health Rights and Protections www.healthcare.gov/health-care-law-protections/rights-and-protections

Act also requires that all state and local public services be accessible to people with disabilities. The law is enforced by the U.S. Department of Justice.

A Disabilities Rights Approach

The history of the passage of the ADA is rooted in the Civil Rights Movement of the 1950s and in grassroots movements of families' advocacy for their children who were disabled and the independent living movement. Powerful advocacy organizations such as the ARC (www.thearc.org), and the National Council on Independent Living (www.ncil.org) were the engines of social reform that led to the inclusion of Section 504 of the 1973 Rehabilitation Act, which banned discrimination on the basis of disability. Eventually this led to the introduction in 1988 of what was to become the 1990 ADA (Mayerson, 1992). The history of advocacy is important to note because discrimination persists against people with disabilities, and the social worker in physical medicine and rehabilitation provides education and advocacy to ensure that the rights of the disabled person are respected (U.S. Department of Justice, 2015).

A thoughtful British book critiques the social work profession for lagging in its advocacy stance for persons with disabilities (Sapey & Oliver, 2006). The profession is criticized for implicitly buying into traditional exclusion and discrimination of people with disabilities by viewing disability in a negative light as opposed to adopting a habilitation perspective, which focuses on providing societal accommodations for people of all abilities. They also criticize social work education for lack of attention to disabilities in the basic social work curriculum and for accepting oppressive policies and structures as the status quo. They advocate for an empowerment approach that entails a "radical shift" in the view of disabilities from an adaptation perspective to a rights and abilities perspective.

The social worker in a physical medicine and rehabilitation setting is in a position to embody the empowerment approach by supporting the patient as he or she tackles the difficult job of accepting the disability and the resulting change in the patient's life; by helping the family to negotiate the resulting changes in the family roles and system; by helping each family member adjust to new role demands and shifting responsibilities; by supporting the decision-making autonomy of the disabled family member while helping the patient think through the consequences of various decision alternatives, especially with respect to motivation for demanding rehabilitation protocols; by educating the patient and family about alternatives in their care and rehabilitation; and by taking a rights perspective in terms of accommodations for the disability.

Patient empowerment can be defined as consisting of four dimensions (Guiterrez, 1994). An empowered person perceives control over his or her life. Regaining a sense of control is a universal task when a person becomes disabled. One of the existential challenges in adapting to disability, which changes people's ability to care for themselves as well as to sense and act on their environments, is to redefine a sense of control in life. In order to regain a sense of control, new behavioral repertoires must be developed. This requires confidence to take risks, to try adaptive devices, to learn new behavioral sequences, and to define and accept areas of dependence and independence. Once the new behavioral repertoire is achieved, the patient and family gain a sense of empowerment. However, rehabilitation is often much more challenging than the patient and family members imagine. It takes a great deal of motivation to see through the physical pain, the strengthening of physical abilities, and the mental and personal challenges of negotiating relationships with providers and family members and friends given the new sets of abilities and disabilities, dependence and autonomy.

Gaining power takes patience, perseverance, and support. And here lies the place for supportive interventions that bolster patients' and families' sense of ability and perseverance. The social worker is certainly an important source of support for the disabled patient who is painstakingly working to build a new set of competencies and power. And, finally, empowerment entails being aware of and having access to make choices. In disability settings, the ability to make choices is important to the rehabilitating person. Making choices is often an area of friction between patient and family. Helping patient and family to negotiate this conflict is a key role for social work intervention in rehabilitation settings.

In order to help patients achieve the greatest sense of empowerment possible, the social worker needs to use a particular set of interventions (Guitierrez, 1994). These include psychoeducation. This approach entails facilitating client learning—about the disability, about the options available to him or her, about the basic medical explanations for why particular treatments and rehabilitation regimes are recommended. Psychoeducation is essential to building motivation and understanding the value of treatment and rehabilitation. It boosts treatment adherence and it supports the grit that is necessary to carry out the rehabilitation course.

Client participation is essential to person-centered rehabilitation, and it is essential to achieve an empowered outlook following the onset of a disabling condition. Consciousness raising is another technique that promotes empowerment. With disabilities, this entails recognition of the reactions of others to the disability, including stares on the street, or comments about being old and unable. Consciousness-raising includes understanding that these excluding and discriminatory microaggressions are not rooted in a response to the individual patient, but are reflections of societal exclusion and discrimination toward differences.

Gaining a historical perspective on disabilities and social response to them may help some patients externalize some of the discriminatory behavior rather than take it as a personal affront. The elements of and the story of the ACA is motivating to many disabled people and it helps them adopt a mindset of rights and inclusion, a very empowering point of view.

Motivational interviewing is an intervention that social workers can use early on to build engagement and participation with disabled clients. Motivational interviewing places priority setting and goal setting squarely in the patient's control, thus it also helps rebuild a sense of control for the patient in rehabilitation (Miller & Rollnick, 2013; Ruffalo, Perron, & Voshel, 2015). Motivational interviewing, which was developed to engage substance abusing clients in treatment, has been found to be an effective approach in many health situations, including orthopedic rehabilitation, where the treatment will not succeed without strong patient commitment to treatment goals. Motivational interviewing skills include adopting a strong empathy-based approach, identifying the patient's ambivalence and discrepancies, supporting patient choice and self-efficacy, and accepting patient resistance and ambivalence to rehabilitation. In motivational interviewing, the social worker communicates strong empathy, uses open-ended questions, affirms the patient's ability to make decisions, reflects the patient's communications and affect, and summarizes what has been said. The social worker then helps the patient identify discrepancies and ambivalence in the situation. The focus is on why the patient is here and what he or she wants to achieve from rehabilitation. A strong, encouraging approach is necessary for the social worker to support self-efficacy and patient empowerment. Finally, the social worker who is using motivational interviewing completely reframes "patient resistance" and "nonadherence." Instead of those pejorative, patient-blaming labels, the social worker accepts ambivalence as a normal human condition, refrains from directly resisting it, and tries a new approach or rationale when resistance to implementing the treatment plan occurs.

American Health Services in Transition: The Impact of the Affordable Care Act on People With Disabilities

The ACA focuses on the "triple aim" of improving the quality and outcomes of health care and reducing costs. Persons with chronic health and disabling conditions figure prominently in improving health services and outcomes in the United States and in reducing costs. When compared to other developed nations, the United States spends more than double the amount per capita on health costs while achieving worse results in key health outcomes such as life expectancy, infant mortality, and disability (Stanhope, Videka, Thorning, & McKay, 2015). The ACA was passed to achieve cost efficiency while improving health outcomes and the quality of services delivered in the American health care system. People with disabilities are an important population focus for the ACA because while only 9% of Americans have a disability, fully 27% of national health care expenditures are spent on people with disabilities (Anderson, Armour, Finklestein, & Wiener, 2010).

In studies of patient satisfaction with health care for their disability, patients were anxious and concerned about insurance coverage eligibility for ongoing services, and dissatisfied with discharge preparation and connection to community-based services. Young, disabled adults complained that services were often targeted to older people. Additional findings included dissatisfaction with the availability of mental health treatment, unaddressed concerns about the help that the family needed in light of the disabling condition, family conflict and readjustment, stigma, and dismissive treatment by some medical providers. It is important to note that many patients also voiced satisfaction with their medical and rehabilitative care, stating that being viewed by medical providers as a "whole person" was especially appreciated. They valued nursing and social work services that helped them adapt to their everyday lives following the onset of a disability (Alaszewski, Alaszewski, Potter, Penhale, & Billins., 2003; McClure, Teasell, & Salter, 2015; Miller, 2012).

ACA Benefits for People With Disabilities

The ACA addresses some of the concerns voiced by disabled patients. The ACA explicitly identifies persons with disabilities as a health disparities population due to lack of access to quality health care services, a status that has been vague in the past. The ACA mandates that persons with disabilities cannot be excluded from obtaining health insurance in eliminating the preexisting conditions clause. Access to insurance is profound and important. Some disabilities advocates predict that the ACA will positively affect employment rates for disabled persons because employment will no longer pose the risk of losing insurance since those who do not qualify for Medicaid when they are working will be able to obtain health insurance privately or through the government insurance marketplace.

Benefits eligibility, including eligibility for private insurance, has increased for persons with disabilities under the ACA. The ACA expanded Medicaid eligibility for low-income persons who earn up to 138% of poverty income ($16,104 for a single individual). Insurance plans must cover 10 essential services including prevention services and behavioral health parity. Many individuals with disabilities are now eligible for Medicaid coverage, or an alternative insurance coverage option on the basis of their low incomes alone if the state has declined Medicaid expansion. If a state has additional benefits based on disability status, once individuals with disabilities meet Medicaid disability eligibility, they are allowed to receive all Medicaid covered services. States are required to make their programs known and accessible to people with disabilities. Insurance marketplaces are prohibited from discriminating against people with disabilities (Musumeci, 2014; Yee, 2015).

Ongoing Challenges to Quality Health Care for People With Disabilities

The ACA does not remove all barriers to quality and cost-effective care for people with disabilities (Yee, 2015). With unstable employment status and income, people with disabilities are more likely to bounce back and forth between Medicaid and private insurance, creating instability in health insurance coverage. As for all Americans, life events such as divorce, marriage, and the birth of a child, can also trigger insurance eligibility disruption.

Ongoing access issues still pose barriers for people with disabilities, despite the law's clear regulations on accessibility. This is due to enforcement lag. The lag in enforcement affects physical facilities of building and equipment, accessibility due to lack of translation of forms and information into formats that people with sensory impairments can take in and comprehend. There also remains a gap in fully addressing the quality of health care services delivered to people with disabilities. This gap is based in ongoing discrimination and exclusion at the service delivery to the individual. Services that are not acceptable to people with disabilities are not changed based on disabled consumers' preferences, and consumers are still blamed for "resistance" and treatment nonadherence. Finally, the institutionally based rather than home-care based orientation of health insurance reimbursement is a serious structural limitation for young and old people with disabilities. People, including those with disabilities, prefer to live in private homes under their own aegis. Living independently is an important aspect of empowerment and independence, yet insurance programs, including Medicaid and Medicare, are resistant to expanding coverage for supportive, home-based services.

Implications for Social Work Services in Physical Medicine and Rehabilitation

Access to health resources, and barriers to health and rehabilitation services are major concerns of persons with disabilities. The social worker should take his or her role very seriously and make it a point to become knowledgeable about disabilities benefits programs and share this information with patients, family members, and interprofessional team members as needed.

In one innovative community-based interprofessional integrated health program for polypharmacy elders with physical disabilities and behavioral health disorders, the "3-Cs program," nurse practitioner–social work–pharmacist teams provide integrated medical and behavioral health services for disabled elders upon discharge from the hospital. Social workers contributed infomation to the program's "tool-kit," concerning entitlement programs and disabilities services. Nurses and pharmacists as well as patients valued this knowledge and found it helpful (Luce, Morton, Spier, & Videka, 2015).

SOCIAL WORK INTERVENTIONS FOR PERSONS WITH DISABILITES

Evidence for Cost Containment and Outcome Effects for Social Work Intervention

Social work intervention has been empirically demonstrated to be effective and to contribute to cost efficiency in serving disabled people. In a review of effectiveness of social work intervention and cost–benefit impact, Steketee, Ross, and Wachman. (2016) conducted a systematic review of 19 studies of social work intervention. Most social interventions were delivered as part of interprofessional teams, a modality that is increasingly common for integrated health services delivery under the ACA. The 19 studies were all randomized controlled trials, but focused on services to a wide array of health populations. Eight studies focused on disabilities-relevant populations including advanced congestive heart failure (CHF), diabetes, and stroke. Other studies focused on a population with disabilities who also are long-term unemployed, and caregivers of disabled elders. In nearly all studies, social work services as part of inter professional teams had positive effects on health outcomes and on reducing per-patient costs. Although this is a diverse sample of studies and precise effects for specific interventions were not replicated, the authors conclude that social work interventions contribute to positive health outcomes and to cost efficiency.

There is a growing set of evidence-based practices in rehabilitation social work. Case management has been shown to modestly improve service utilization and reduce expensive health costs for a variety of disabled populations (Norris et al., 2002; Hickam et al., 2013). Two studies found that for CHF patients, collaborative interprofessional discharge planning, and psychoeducation led to better self-rated health, fewer readmissions, and an average per-person cost saving of $4,300 (Bull, Hansen, & Gross, 2000). This partially replicated findings from an earlier study that found that psychoeducation and early discharge planning with postdischarge follow-up resulted in fewer hospital readmissions and a cost savings of $450 per patient (Rich et al., 1995).

Another study of patients with comorbid advanced diabetes and depression showed that the IMPACT Intervention, which consisted of psychoeducation, behavioral activation, plus the patient's choice of either problem-solving therapy or psychopharmacological treatment reduced depression and decreased per capita health care costs by $1,129 per patient (Katon et al., 2006).

In a study that supported the health of caregivers of disabled elders, Toseland and Smith (2006) found that the Health Education Program (HEP) that included emotion-focused coping support saved $6,307 in caregivers' health costs over 2 years. Claiborne (2006) provided social work care coordination, mental health assessments, crisis intervention, caregiver support, and case management to stroke patients. She found that the intervention was associated with $1,339 in cost savings per patient. Several other studies have found that behavioral health screening and psychopharmacologic, interpersonal, or cognitive behavioral interventions are effective for promoting the rehabilitation of persons with disabilities including strokes, spinal cord injuries, burns, or other disabilities (Carlson, 2014; Hammond et al., 2011; Saulino, 2015; Steketee et al., 2016).

Although not as conclusive as the findings in randomized controlled trials, less controlled studies also point to potentially effective interventions. In a case study of a 90-year-old woman disabled by advanced diabetes and heart disease, Barber, Kogan, Riffenburgh, and Enguidanos (2015) implemented an intervention that consisted of Problem Solving Therapy (Nezu, 2004) and SWIFT (Social Work Interventions Focused on Transitions), an intervention that focuses on transitions from one environment to another—hospital to home or rehabilitation, rehabilitation to home, or home to hospital—and consisted of home safety review, psychosocial assessment, medication review, and implementation of discharge orders, including assistance with follow-up appointments, behavioral health assessments, and psychoeducation on self-management of health conditions.

Thus, a growing number of evidence-based social work interventions in interprofessional team settings positively impact patient health outcomes, quality of life, and hospital costs. Social workers employed in physical and rehabilitation settings should develop competencies in using these models. This tool-box of evidence-based interventions show that social workers can make a true contribution to patient outcomes and to health cost efficiency by careful attention, education, and planning for transitions from environment to environment, review, and psychoeducation for health care self-management, concrete assistance with follow up planning and referrals, medication management, screening for behavioral health problems (mental health and substance use), and medication or talking therapy (cognitive behavioral or interpersonal) for depression and anxiety. The next section of the chapter focuses on a conceptual model as a tool to help the rehabilitation social worker choose and organize the various intervention options that are available depending on the patient's needs and preferences.

The Ecological Context

A distinguishing characteristic of social work on interdisciplinary teams is the ecological framework that a social worker always deploys. Uri Bronfenbrenner was a pioneer in recognizing the importance of human ecologies in human experience and behavior (Bronfenbrenner, 1986). The social worker always thinks about systems: the individual (biological and psychological systems), the family system, the hospital or health service system, the community in which the patient lives, the informal social support system for the patient, the formal supports that the patient needs or will need as rehabilitation progresses, the larger society as an important system in which social policies and programs are determined, as well as cultural, racial, or ethnic subgroups that determine the norms and expectations that govern patient's behavior and desires. The larger societal system is also where the structures that uphold inclusion versus exclusion and discrimination against people with disabilities are located. Figure 30.1 shows the ecological model with special reference to the ecological elements that are of special importance to people undergoing rehabilitation.

Human ecological theoretical models explain the dynamic interactions between people and their environments. Interactions and influences are multidirectional across ecological levels. The patient and health service workers influence the ecological systems that they are part of, and, in turn, their environments influence them. The social worker helps the patient span boundaries across ecological levels. Thus, the social worker's role in health and rehabilitation is to enhance health-promoting interactions among patients, their families, and their health care providers, and to reduce or negotiate conflict that threatens to undermine the patient's successful rehabilitation. The social worker also acts as an agent between the health care systems and the patient's other ecological environments, including family and community, by assessing the patient's home and physical community, by advocating for patient rights to services and support, by helping the patient make connections with other health services and supports for their long-term rehabilitation plan. In advocating for progressive policies and reforms locally (community and health services levels) and nationally through progressive health policy, the social worker acts to influence social inclusion and equity for people with disabilities. Social workers are among the dedicated citizens who made the ADA a reality and who are working every day to implement its provisions and spirit.

Social workers assist a patient by being informed of the patient's physical status, which requires understanding the necessary health concepts about the type of disability that patient presents. Social workers also understand their patient's social psychological status, how family relationships are perceived, the positive and the stressful relationships that are important to the patient, and the mental status and psychological balance of the patient throughout acute treatment and rehabilitation.

It is important for the health care team to understand the importance of the views, values, and actions of other family members and friends who are important to the patient. The social worker should be the expert in this information and should bring it to the interprofessional team

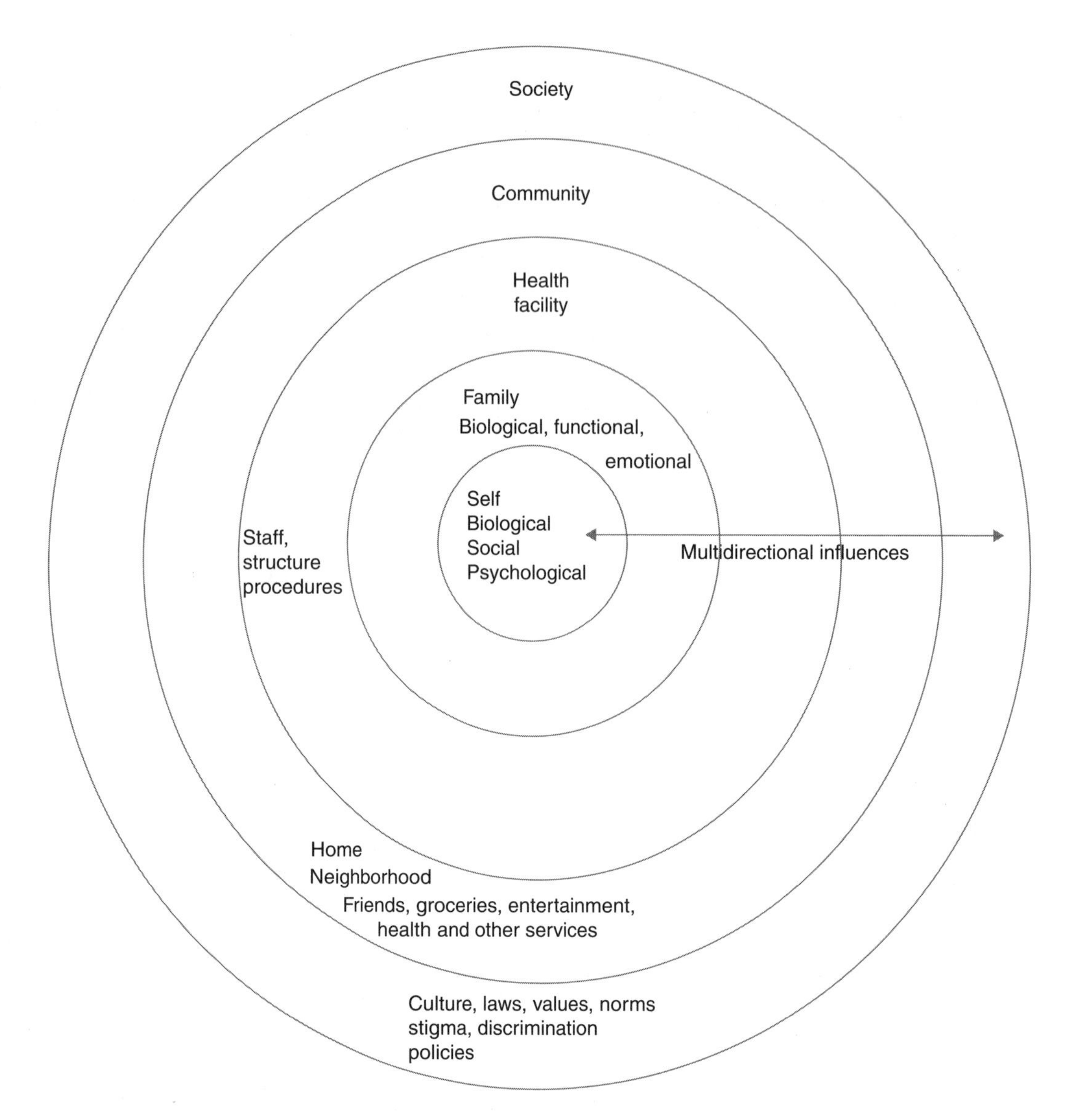

FIGURE 30.1 The ecological model for rehabilitation patients.

as it is relevant to the treatment plan. The people important to the patient will influence the patient's morale and attitude. They can be a source of information and resources, or a drain. They are all under strain and are often adjusting to an unexpected life change as a result of the disabling condition. The social worker often helps navigate relationships as they affect the patient's progress in rehabilitation, helping the parties negotiate conflicts, and building support and resources.

The social worker plays an important role in helping the newly disabled patient and his or her family assess, modify, and adapt their home environment to accommodate the new needs of the patient. They help the patient and family consider how they will function with respect to obtaining daily needs such as groceries, meal planning, laundry, and socialization.

Cultural Competency and Antioppressive Practice

Social groups that patients identify with, including religion, race and ethnicity, identity subcultures such as sexual orientation, age cohorts, special interests, and other matters of identity including gender, are an important part of the patient's social environment. It is part of the social worker's role to learn about the identities that are important to the patient, how the identity reference groups view the disability, and what this means to the patient. Health services and rehabilitation plans have to accommodate the norms and beliefs of the patient's identity reference groups if they are to be effective.

Given that people in marginalized and excluded identity groups (older adults, certain oppressed racial minority groups, lower income persons) are at higher risk for experiencing a disability and are also at higher risk for social exclusion and discrimination on the basis of other aspects of their identity, it is important for the social worker to ensure that this important social and cultural information is part of the treatment and rehabilitation planning for the patient. The social worker is responsible for taking into account all the important ways that multiple identities, such as being a Black man with a disability and a low-income level produces stigma, exclusion, discrimination, and negative expectations for the patient. The social worker must be conscious of these social forces, how they impact the individual, including the rehabilitation plan for the patient. The social forces of racism, exclusion and discrimination are at the roots of health disparities. The social worker must be the champion of anti-oppression by ensuring culturally appropriate services, and relevant and meaningful health education that respects culture and differences, and by ensuring that the patient receives the supports and entitlements for which he or she is eligible. The social worker should be the champion of anti-oppression and respect for culture in the health services setting and on the health care team.

■ Problem-Solving Practice

When working with patients and other health care team members and family members on solving specific problems that the patient is facing, or decisions that the patient must make, a useful and scientifically supported approach to practice is that of problem solving (Nezu, 2004; Perlman, 1957; Reid & Fortune, 2002). Problem solving has been shown to be an effective social intervention approach that can be adapted to many different problems, settings, and people. It is pragmatic and can be used in a short term, rapidly changing context. It is compatible with the ecological framework. It is action oriented and an excellent strategy by which to build a patient's sense of efficacy and empowerment. It is best used with explicit problems that the patient wants to solve or for goals that the patient wants to achieve; thus, it is compatible with person-centered care and health care choice.

Problem solving involves five steps that the patient, social worker, other relevant professionals, and family members of the patient work on collaboratively to identify the problem and its possible solutions. The five steps include: (a) identifying the problem and what goals will be achieved in solving it, (b) developing alternative solutions to the problem, (c) reviewing solution alternatives and selecting the preferred one, (d) implementing the solution, and (e) evaluating whether the solution worked and either accept the outcome or try another alternative (Figure 30.2).

The first step is to identify the problem. While this sounds simple and straightforward, this is often the most difficult step in problem solving because people tend to define their problems in vague and complicated ways. Think of a patient with an amputation who has comorbid advanced diabetes who says, "My problem is losing this leg. I hate not having it." This problem is too vague to work on and not amenable to change—it is not achievable to reverse the amputation. Let's say that this is a patient who has been fitted for a prosthetic limb. The social worker might explore how the limb fits, what progress has been made in physical therapy in using it, and what the patient thinks about the limb. The patient may say that his wife is repulsed by the site of him putting the limb on and that the limb is also uncomfortable. He is not sure he wants to use the prosthetic device at all. With these communications the social worker can begin to focus on potential problem areas, the progress in physical therapy with walking with the prosthesis, the patient's perceptions of his wife's reactions to the limb, and his ambivalent motivation to

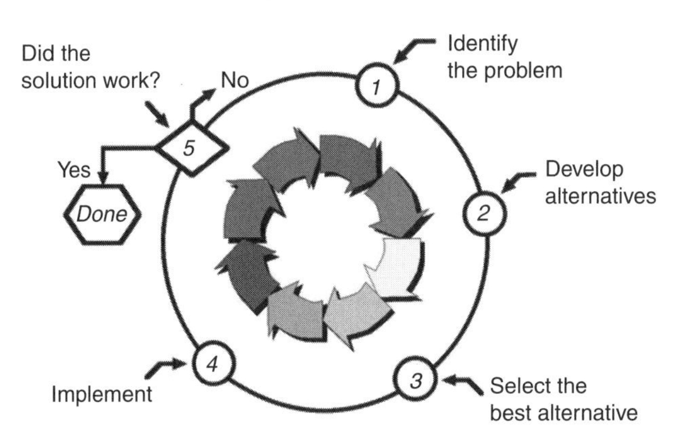

FIGURE 30.2 The problem-solving model of social work intervention.

learn to use the limb. Exploring these more specific areas can help the patient more specifically identify and prioritize aspects of the problem that he wants the social worker's help in solving. A well-defined problem is specific and measurable (Barber et al., 2015). A clear goal should emanate from the problem. It should be obvious when the goal is achieved, or to what extent it is achieved. Let's say that this patient ultimately wants to make a decision about whether he should commit to using the prosthesis. The goal that is important for him to achieve is that he can get around his home to take care of himself and get out to the garden. He does not care about getting out in public. He says he can count on his wife and children to help him in these instances and that he can use a wheelchair as necessary. This is an example of a goal that focuses on resolving ambivalence and making a commitment to a particular path of rehabilitation.

The next step in problem solving is to develop different possible solutions to the problem. The alternatives that the patient identifies is that in order to achieve his mobility goals of moving independently around the house and the garden he can either learn to use the prosthesis for short periods of time or he can use the prosthesis regularly. He decides that not using the prosthesis is not a desirable solution because he will not be able to get out to his garden in the summer. Sometimes the social worker identifies other possible alternatives. The social worker is confident that the patient has identified the alternatives that are plausible and desirable for himself. The garden is the place that he loves and cherishes; it makes him feel great to sit there on a balmy day.

The third step in problem solving is to select the best alternative. The patient has already rejected one alternative, not using the prosthetic leg at all. The patient and social worker will weigh the identified alternatives including approaches to mastery of use of the prosthesis, and how the patient can ask his wife to help support the rehabilitation plan. In helping a patient select the best alternative for himself, it is important that the social worker keep in mind that it is the patient's choice, not the social worker's, to make. The social worker's interventions are geared to bringing the best and most complete set of information to the patient for consideration. In this case, the social worker will consult with the physiatrist and physical therapist about prosthetic limb use and the consequences of the patient's limited goals, both in terms of the skill level and effort it will take to achieve this goal as well as the long-term health implications of different levels of activity and mobility. The social worker may also confer with the patient's wife to assess her reactions to the prosthesis and to help position her to be as strong a support as possible to her husband's goals. Psychoeducational approaches are important for both patient and family members to prepare them for realistic expectations, to help them make choices that will assist the patient achieve his or her goals, and to help prepare for the likely consequences of the chosen problem solutions. Let's say that this patient chooses to use the prosthetic limb some of the time. He wants to become moderately comfortable in using it independently for walking short distances and down and up a few stairs.

The fourth problem-solving step is to implement the intervention. The patient has decided to use the prosthesis. The social worker helps prepare the patient and his wife for the emotional and physical demands of rehabilitation. For this patient, rehabilitation requires maintaining the perseverance required to master the use of the prosthetic limb. For his wife, she must manage her feelings about her husband's disability. The social worker will provide psychoeducation and supportive therapy to her.

The fifth and final step in the problem-solving process is to evaluate the effectiveness of the solution and to either accept its consequences or to choose another alternative. It is possible that the man's motivation may be kindled as he masters the prosthesis and he may decide to strive for greater independence and facility in using the limb. Or the mastery of independent walking with the limb may be slower than he expected and discouraging, requiring a longer rehabilitation period than he expected. The client can choose to extend problem-solving efforts, to change direction in his goal-attainment strategy, or to cease working on this problem. If balance on stairs remains a challenge, the family may decide to build a ramp as an alternative to the stairs. The social worker, other members of the medical team, and the patient will evaluate the success of the problem-solving effort. Another problem may be selected for the next phase of work.

Intervention During Phases of Rehabilitation

It is useful to anticipate some normative challenges that disabled people face in their recovery that social work intervention can address. The final section of this chapter will consider phases of the rehabilitation process and some common concerns and challenges that social workers address. The discussion that follows gives some common areas for social work interventions, but it is not exhaustive in terms of all the challenges entailed in the rehabilitation process or in the particulars of patient situations to which the social worker should respond.

■ The Acute Health Crisis

During the acute health crisis, the patient and the family must adapt to a situation that is often traumatic and unexpected such as a stroke, cardiovascular event, organ failure, spinal cord injury, or orthopedic injury. In some cases, the disability is the result of a progressive disease process such as congestive heart failure, cancer, or end stage renal disease. In these cases, the disabling condition is cumulative until a threshold is crossed in which the patient eventually loses the ability to function independently. During the acute phase, the patient's life-sustaining and physical care needs take priority. The social worker may be available to the family for support and as the prognosis evolves, help them come to grips with the health and residual disability that the patient may endure. This may also be a time to assess medical benefits that can be deployed when the patient's longer term needs can be more accurately assessed.

■ Mourning Loss and Trauma: Coming to Grips With Disability

Following the acute health crisis, the patient and family must confront the trauma or loss associated with the health crisis. Often this manifests as stages of grieving for the lost capacity and independence, moving through phases of shock, denial, bargaining and anger, depression, and acceptance (Kendall & Buys, 1998; Kubler-Ross & Kessler, 2005). Social workers support patients and families through the grief process by providing empathic interviewing, psychoeducation, and supportive counseling.

This is the time when the residual disability becomes known and early planning can take place. Choices have to be made about rehabilitation settings—home, specialized hospital, general hospital rehab unit, outpatient settings, or home care, which is often affected by insurance coverage. The social worker works with the family to plan for an optimal rehabilitation setting given patient's insurance and financial resources and needs including adaptive devices as requested by the patient or health providers and ordered by the physician. Most patients and families do not know what benefits cover and do not cover. The social worker's knowledge of insurance and benefits coverage is an important resource for the patient and family. Psychoeducation about the patient's conditions and needs, and the problem-solving approach, as discussed earlier, are excellent approaches for beginning rehabilitation planning. Empathic interviewing is always important to set the stage for a helping relationship and longer term engagement in the rehabilitation plan. This is the point at which the social worker can contribute to the whole team's work by ensuring that the whole person is respected and viewed as the rehabilitation plan evolves.

In this phase, a careful and thorough assessment is undertaken by the social worker and shared with the patient and interprofessional team in order to make an optimal rehabilitation plan with the family, patient, and health providers. The social worker's assessment plays an important role in the rehabilitation plan. The assessment plan should include a careful psychosocial assessment of the patient and family and social circumstances that will affect the rehabilitation and transition to independence for this patient. Patient history of preexisting behavioral health, family, and social conditions is important. Income resources are important to assess since we know that, on average, patients cover 15% of the cost of rehabilitation themselves. This is also the time to screen the patient for behavioral health needs and to assess the risks for depression, anxiety, and substance misuse disorders. Since the patient and family are working through the grief process during this phase, it is important to separate grief, which is a normative process, from behavioral health disorders. The social worker also assesses family relationships and potential conflicts about rehabilitation choices.

It is important for the social worker to share observations with other interprofessional team members in the team meetings, if these are held, as well as in the electronic medical record, which is quickly evolving to be the communication tool of choice and necessity for health care teams. Communicating succinctly is a key to effective communication in today's health care setting.

Facilitating Rehabilitation

As the patient progresses with the rehabilitation program, the social worker focuses on comorbid behavioral health issues such as depression, anxiety, or drug dependence that pose barriers to rehabilitation progress. During this phase of rehabilitation, the patient typically makes strides in regaining abilities and develops alternate strategies to achieve as much functional independence as possible. The social worker's role is to enhance motivation and to help remove barriers that hinder the best possible rehabilitation.

Screening for behavioral health problems is important. The SAMHSA-HRSA Center for Integrated Health Solutions lists most of the widely used screening tools for problem alcohol and drug use and mental health problems (www.integration.samhsa.gov/clinical-practice/screening-tools). The best screening tools have cut-off scores, indicating a possible clinical condition. If results of screening fall within a clinical-range score, a full behavioral health assessment is in order. This can be done by a licensed social worker or other mental health professional. Full treatment may or may not be the rehabilitation social worker's role, depending on the practices of the program and the time available to engage in treatment.

If the patient has a positive screen for a behavioral health disorder, there are several evidence-based interventions to choose from. Short, Brief Intervention and Referral to Treatment (SBIRT) is a widely tested motivational and referral intervention that is suited for a person with a positive substance use screen. SBIRT relies on the principle of motivational interviewing and it has been shown to decrease the problem of substance use after just one session (Baker et al., 2005; Beich, Thorsin, & Rollnick, 2003; Bernstein et al., 2007). For more information about SBIRT intervention, see the SAMHSA-HRSA Center for Integrated Health Solutions website (www.integration.samhsa.gov/clinical-practice/SBIRT).

Other evidence-based behavioral health intervention approaches include cognitive behavioral treatment (CBT), interpersonal treatment, and the problem-solving model. CBT is a widely used and tested short-term intervention for depression and anxiety and wide range of other mental disorders (Butler, Chapman, Forman, & Beck, 2006). There are several open source manuals that clinicians who want to build CBT skills can use (Cully & Teten, 2008; Muñoz & Miranda, 2000). Interpersonal treatment for depression is another widely used, empirically validated, and efficacious approach to treating depression (Markowitz & Weissman, 2004). This approach focuses on interpersonal relationships as the key to alleviating depression.

The social worker will also focus on barriers to rehabilitation, including household structural modification, care assistance as needed and family friction and conflict. The problem-solving model, discussed in detail earlier in this chapter, is a good practice approach to solve barrier to the rehabilitation process.

Discharge planning is a key role for social workers. Research shows that effective discharge planning reduces hospital readmissions and promotes better health status, especially when community-based supports are arranged and the patient is linked to those supports through referral assistance (Alper, O'Malley, & Greenwald, 2016; McMartin, 2013). Quality evidence-based discharge planning includes the following components: (a) Planning that should begin early in the treatment process. (b) Patients and family members as full partners. (c) Patients should be discharged to environments that meet their support needs. (d) A full functional assessment of relevant patient functioning is made and matched with the resources available in the discharge setting. (e) Plans for support and continued care should be made and the patient should have assistance to actually contact and use these services. (f) A plan for accountability for the patient's care needs must be identified by the discharging health providers and must have the commitment of the health professionals, family members, or friends who will assist the patient in the new environment. (g) Follow-up care should be clearly communicated in writing to the patient, care providers, and supporting family members. There are several specific protocols available for discharge planning at websites of the Institute for Healthcare Improvement (n.d.) and the Centers for Medicare and Medicaid Services (Department of Health and Human Services, 2014).

Integrated Health and Behavioral Health for Long-Term Habilitation

It is ideal to discharge the patient with follow-up services from a coordinated care program in an integrated health service system. These programs have been found to promote independence and positive health outcomes for disabled people (Au et al., 2011). Integrated health systems are those that link payment and services under one umbrella organization, as required in the ACA and, increasingly, in many states' Medicaid programs. A few states, such as Massachusetts, have universal health plans.

Under the ACA, disabled Medicaid populations are required to have "patient-centered medical homes," sometimes also known as "health homes," that coordinate the patient's physical, behavioral, and preventive health care (Stanhope et al., 2015). Accountable care organizations (ACO) are financial structures that coordinate payment for health services by co-locating or contracting services from multiple providers or health organizations. Disabled populations served by the Veterans Administration Health System, Medicare, or Medicaid are likely to receive coordinated care under the health home and ACO system, but some privately insured individuals are still not covered under such systems. It is desirable for the disabled person to have access to coordinated care.

In addition to financial and structural coordination, care coordination with health homes and ACOs is supported by an electronic medical record and by linked specialists (who are sometimes in separate organizations that have a contractual relationship to coordinate care). Care coordination differs from traditional case management in that communication among service providers and patients is emphasized, through the electronic medical record, work relationships, and personal contacts that support treatment plan adherence and ease of coordination of multiple services (Au et al., 2011). Social workers sometimes serve as care coordinators, whose role is defined as follows: The care coordinator is the person responsible for "a person-centered, assessment-based, interdisciplinary approach to integrating health care and social support services in a cost-effective manner in which an individual's needs and preferences are assessed, a comprehensive care plan is developed, and services are managed and monitored" (Stanhope et al., 2015).

CONCLUSION

Social work services in physical medicine and rehabilitation are vital to delivering person-centered services to the whole person in a culturally acceptable way, making use of social resources to advance the patient's rehabilitation and adjustments to independent living. Social workers are integral members of inter professional teams in hospital settings, in rehabilitation settings, and increasingly in coordinated care settings in community-based health care organizations. Social workers focus on an integrated view of patients in their environment, their behavioral health needs, their social situations, and the availability or lack of resources that affect their health and rehabilitation. By using an ecological perspective with evidence-based practices that focus on integrated health promotion and boundary spanning as the patient moves from acute care hospital to rehabilitation setting to independent living or long-term care setting, social work intervention contributes to person-centered care, patient satisfaction, the best possible patient outcomes, and efficiency in health care services.

REFERENCES

Adams, E., Krahn, G. L., Horner-Johnson, W., & Leman, R. (2009). Fundamentals of disability epidemiology. In *Disability and public health* (p. 7). Washington, DC: American Public Health Association.

The Affordable Care Act Helps Persons with Disabilities. (n.d.). Retrieved from https://www.whitehouse.gov/sites/default/files/docs/the_aca_helps_americans_with_disabilities.pdf

Alaszewski, H., Alaszewski, A., Potter, J., Penhale, B., & Billins, J. (2003). *Life after stroke: Reconstructing everyday life*. Report–Nunnery fields trust fund. Project report. Retrieved from http://kar.kent.ac.uk/id/eprint/7745

Alper, E., O'Malley, T. A., & Greenwald, J. (2016). Hospital discharge and readmission. *UpToDate*. Retrieved from https://www.uptodate.com/contents/hospital-discharge-and-readmission

Altman, B. M. (2014). Definitions, concepts, and measures of disability. *Annals of Epidemiology, 24*, 2–7. doi:10.1016/j.annepidem.2013.05.018

American Hospital Associate. (2012). Bringing behavioral health into the care continuum: Opportunities to improve qualities, costs and outcomes. In *Trendwatch*. Washington, DC: Author.

Americans with Disabilities Act National Network. (2015). An overview of the Americans with Disabilities Act. Retrieved from https://adata.org/sites/adata.org/files/files/ADA_Overview_2015%20bitly.pdf

Anderson, W. L., Armour, B. S., Finklestein, E. A., & Wiener, J. M. (2010). Estimates of state-level health-care expenditures associated with disability. *Public Health Reports, 125*, 44–51.

Andrews, G., Henderson, S., & Hall, W. (2001). Prevalence, comorbidity, disability and service utilization: Overview of the Australian National Mental Health Survey. *British Journal of Psychiatry, 178*, 145–153.

Au, M., Simon, S., Chen, A., Lipson, D., Gimm, D., & Rich, E. (2011). *Comparative effectiveness of care coordination for adults with disabilities*. Bethesda, MD: Mathematica Policy Research. Retrieved from http://www.mathematica-mpr.com/~/media/publications/PDFs/hcalth/comparativc_carc_rschbricf.pdf

Baker, A., Lee, N. K., Claire, M., Lewin, T. J., Grant, T., & Pohlman, S. (2005). Brief cognitive behavioral interventions for regular amphetamine users: A step in the right direction. *Addiction, 100*, 367–378.

Barber, R., Kogan, A. C., Riffenburgh, A., & Enguidanos, S. (2015). A role for social workers in improving care setting transitions: A case study. *Social Work in Health Care, 54*(3), 177–192. doi:10.1080/00981389.2015.1005273

Beich, A., Thorsen, T., & Rollnick, S. (2003). Screening in brief intervention trials targeting excessive drinkers in general practice: Systematic review and meta-analysis. *BMJ: British Medical Journal, 327*, 536–542.

Bernstein, E., Bernstein, J., Feldman, J., Fernandez, W., Hagan, M., Mitchell, P., . . . Woolard, R. (2007). An evidence-based alcohol screening, brief intervention, and referral to treatment (SBIRT) curriculum for emergency department (ED) providers improves skills and utilization. *Substance Abuse, 28*(4), 79–92.

Bronfenbrenner, U. (1986). Ecology of the family as a context for human development: Research perspectives. *Developmental Psychology, 22*(6), 723–742.

Bull, M. J., Hansen, H. E., & Gross, C. R. (2000). A professional-patient partnership model of discharge planning with elders hospitalized with heart failure. *Applied Nursing Research, 13*(1), 19–28.

Bush, G. H. W. (1990). Remarks at the signing of the Americans with Disabilities Act of 1990. Retrieved from https://www.eeoc.gov/eeoc/history/35th/videos/ada_signing_text.html

Butler, A. C., Chapman, J. E., Forman, E. M., & Beck, A. T. (2006). The empirical status of cognitive behavioral therapy: A review of meta-analyses. *Clinical Psychology Review, 26*, 17–31.

Carlson, A. (2014). Social worker interventions for patients post-stroke. *Master of social work clinical research papers, paper 300*. Retrieved from http://sophia.stkate.edu/msw_papers/300

Claiborne, N. (2006). Efficiency of a care coordination model: A randomized study with stroke patients. *Research on Social Work Practice, 16*(1), 57–66.

Cully, J. A., & Teten, A. L. (2006). *A therapist's guide to brief cognitive behavioral therapy*. Houston, TX: Department of Veterans Affairs South Central MIRECC. Retrieved from http://www.mirecc.va.gov/visn16/docs/therapists_guide_to_brief_cbtmanual.pdf

Department of Health and Human Services. (2014, October). Discharge planning. Retrieved from https://www.cms.gov/Outreach-and-Education/Medicare-Learning-Network-MLN/MLNProducts/Downloads/Discharge-Planning-Booklet-ICN908184.pdf

Disability.gov. What the Affordable Care Act means for you and your family. Retrieved from https://www.disability.gov/resource/the-affordable-care-act-you-family

Druss, B., Rohrbaugh, R. M., Levinson, C. M., & Rosenheck, R. A. (2001). Integrated medical care for patients with serious psychiatric illness. A randomized trial. *Archives of General Psychiatry, 58*, 861–868.

Druss, B. G., von Esenwein, S. A., Compton, M. T., Zhao, L., & Leslie, D. L. (2011). Budget impact and sustainability of medical care management for persons with serious mental illness. *American Journal of Psychiatry, 168*, 1–8.

Elliott, T. R., & Kennedy, P. (2004). Treatment of depression following spinal cord injury: An evidence-based review. *Rehabilitation Psychology, 49*(2), 134–139.

Erickson, W., Lee, C., & von Schrader, S. (2014). *2013 disability status report: United States*. Ithaca, NY: Cornell University Employment and Disability Institute. Retrieved from http://www.disabilitystatistics.org/StatusReports/2013-PDF/2013-StatusReport_US.pdf

Gutierrez, L. M. (1994). Beyond coping: An empowerment perspective on stressful life events. *Journal of Sociology and Social Welfare, 21*(3), 201–220.

Hammond, F. M., Gassaway, J., Abeyta, N., Freeman, E. S., & Primack, D. (2011). Social work and case management treatment time during inpatient spinal cord injury rehabilitation. *Journal of Spinal Cord Medicine, 34*(2), 216–226. doi:10.1179/107902611X12971826988291

HealthCare.gov. (n.d.). Coverage options for people with disabilities. Retrieved from https://www.healthcare.gov/people-with-disabilities/coverage-options

Hickam, D. H., Weiss, J. W., Guise, J. M., Buckley, D., Motu'apuaka, M., Graham, E., . . . Saha, S. (2013). Outpatient case management for adults with medical illness and complex care needs. *Comparative effectiveness review No. 99* (Prepared by the Oregon Evidence-based Practice Center under Contract No. 290-2007-10057-I, AHRQ Publication No.13- EHC031-EF). Rockville, MD: U.S. Department of Health and Human Services.

Honey, A., Emerson, E., Llewellyn, G., & Kariuki, M. (2010). Mental health and disability. In J. H. Stone & M. Blouin (Eds.), *International encyclopedia of rehabilitation*. Retrieved from http://cirrie.buffalo.edu/encyclopedia/en/article/305

Institute for Healthcare Improvement. (n.d.). SMART discharge protocol. Retrieved from http://www.ihi.org/resources/Pages/Tools/SMARTDischargeProtocol.aspx

Katon, W., Unutzer, K., Fan, M. Y., Williams, J. W., Schoenbaum, M., Lin, E. H., & Hunkeler, E. M. (2006). Cost-effectiveness and net benefit of enhanced treatment of depression for older adults with diabetes and depression. *Diabetes Care, 29*(2), 265–270.

Kendall, E., & Buys, N. (1998). An integrated model of psychosocial adjustment following acquired disability. *Journal of Rehabilitation, 63*(3), 16–20.

Kubler-Ross, E., & Kessler, D. (2005). *On grief and grieving: Finding the meaning of grief through five stages of loss*. New York, NY: Scribner.

Lucas, R. E. (2007). Long-term disability is associated with lasting changes in subjective well-being: Evidence from two nationally representative longitudinal studies. *Journal of Personality and Social Psychology, 92*(4), 717–730.

Luce, V., Morton, P., Spier, S., & Videka, L. (2015). *Social work inter-professional model of health care delivery for polypharmacy, disabled, recently discharged elders*. Presentation at the meeting of American Gerontology Association, Orlando, FL.

Markowitz, J. C., & Weissman, M. M. (2004). Interpersonal pscyhotherapy: Principles and applications. *World Psychiatry, 3*(3), 136–139.

Mayerson, A. (1992). *The history of the Americans with Disabilities Act*. Berkeley, CA: The Disability Rights and Education Defense Fund. Retrieved from http://dredf.org/news/publications/the-history-of-the-ada

McClure, A., Teasell, R., & Salter, K. (2015). Psychosocial issues educational supplement. In R. Teasell, N. Foley, K. Salter, M. Richardson, L. Allen, N. Hussein, . . . M. Speechley (Eds.), *Evidence based review of stroke rehabilitation* (16th ed.). London, Ontario, Canada: Heart and Stroke Foundation, Canadian Partnership for Stroke Recovery. Retrieved from http://www.ebrsr.com/sites/default/files/F_Psychosocial_Issues_(Questions_and_Answers).pdf

McMartin, K. (2013). Discharge planning in chronic conditions: An evidence-based analysis. *Ontario Health Technology Assess Series, 13*(4), 1–72. Retrieved from https://www.ncbi.nlm.nih.gov/pmc/articles/PMC3804053

Merikangas, K. R., Ames, M., Cui, L., Stang, P. E., Ustun, T. B., Von Korff, M., & Kessler, R. C. (2007). The impact of comorbidity of mental and physical conditions on role disability in the U.S. household adult population. *Archives of General Psychiatry, 64*(10), 1180–1188.

Miller, S. R. (2012). A qualitative study of the perspective of individuals with disabilities about their health care experiences: Implications for culturally appropriate health care. *Journal of the National Medical Association, 104*(7&8), 360–365.

Miller, W., & Rollnick, S. (2013). *Motivational interviewing: Helping people to change* (3rd ed.). New York, NY: Guilford Press.

Muñoz, R. F., & Miranda, J. (2000). *Individual therapy manual for cognitive behavioral treatment of depression*. Santa Monica, CA: RAND Corporation.

Musumeci, M. B. (2014). The Affordable Care Act's impact on medicaid eligibility, enrollment and benefits for people with disabilities. *Issue Brief*, April, 2014. The Kaiser Commission on Medicaid and the Uninsured. Retrieved from https://kaiserfamilyfoundation.files.wordpress.com/2014/04/8390-02-the-affordable-care-acts-impact-on-medicaid-eligibility.pdf

Nagi, S. Z. (1976). An epidemiology of disability among adults in the United States. *The Milbank Memorial Fund Quarterly, Health and Society, 54*(4), 439–467. doi:10.2307/3349677

Naylor, C., Parsonage, M., McDaid, D., Knapp, M., Fossey, M., & Galea, A. (2012). *Long-term conditions and mental health: The cost of co-morbidities*. London, England: The Kings Fund and Centre for Mental Health. Retrieved from http://www.kingsfund.org.uk/sites/files/kf/field/field_publication_file/long-term-conditions-mental-health-cost-comorbidities-naylor-feb12.pdf

Nezu, A. M. (2004). Problem solving and behavior therapy revisited. *Behavioral Therapy, 35*, 1–33.

Norris, S. L., Nichols, P. J., Caspersen, C. J., Glasgow, R. E., Engelgau, M. M., Jack L., . . . Task Force on Community Preventive Services. (2002). The effectiveness of disease and case management for people with diabetes: A systematic review. *American Journal of Preventive Medicine, 22*(4S), 15–38.

Owen, J. (2012). The Affordable Care Act and people with disabilities. *Forbes/Entrepreneurs*. Retrieved from https://www.disability.gov/resource/the-affordable-care-act-you-family

Perlman, H. H. (1957). *Social casework: A problem solving process*. Chicago, IL: University of Chicago.

Pollard C., & Kennedy, P. (2007). A longitudinal analysis of emotional impact, coping strategies and post-traumatic psychological growth following spinal cord injury: A 10-year review. *British Journal of Health Psychology, 12*(3), 347–362.

Reid, W. J., & Fortune, A. E. (2002). The task-centered model. In A. R. Roberts & G. J. Greene (Eds.), *Social workers' desk reference* (pp. 101–104). Oxford, England: Oxford University Press.

Rich, M. W., Beckham, V., Wittenberg, C., Leven, C. L., Freedland, K. E., & Carney, R. M. (1995). A multidisciplinary intervention to prevent the readmission of elderly patients with congestive heart failure. *New England Journal of Medicine, 333*(18), 1190–1195.

Ruffalo, M., Perron, B. E., & Voshel, E. H. (2016). *Direct social work practice: Theories and skills for becoming and evidence-based practitioner*. Los Angeles, CA: Sage.

Sapey, B. J., & Oliver, M. (2006). *Social work with disabled people* (3rd ed.). Basingstoke, Hampshire: Palgrave Macmillan.

Saulino, M. F. (2015). Rehabilitation of persons with spinal cord injuries. In J. A. Goldstein (Ed.), *Medscape: Drugs and diseases*. Retrieved from http://emedicine.medscape.com/article/1265209-overview#showall

Smith, D. M., Langa, K. M., Kabeto, M. U., & Ubel, P. A. (2005). Health, wealth, and happiness: Financial resources buffer subjective well-being after the onset of a disability. *Psychological Science, 16*(9), 663–666.

Stanhope, V., Videka, L., Thorning, H., & McKay, M. (2015). Moving toward integrated health: An opportunity for social work. *Social Work in Health Care, 54*(5), 383–407. doi:10.1080/00981389.2015.1025122.

Stanton, M. W., & Rutherford, M. K. (2006). *The high concentration of U.S. health care expenditures*. (Research in Action, 19; AHRQ 06-0060). Rockville, MD: Agency for Healthcare Research and Quality.

Steketee, G., Ross, A. M., & Wachman, M. K. (2016). *Social work services, health outcomes and costs: A systematic review of research findings* (Unpublished manuscript).

Toseland, R., & Smith, T. (2006). The impact of a caregiver health education program on health care costs. *Research on Social Work Practice, 16*(1), 9–19.

Treharne, G. J., Lyons, A. C., Booth, D. A., & Kitas, G. D. (2007). Psychological well-being across 1 year with rheumatoid arthritis: Coping resources as buffers of perceived stress. *British Journal of Health Psychology, 12*, 323–345.

U.S. Census Bureau. (2012). Nearly one in five people have a disability in the U.S. Retrieved from https://www.census.gov/newsroom/releases/archives/miscellaneous/cb12-134.html

U.S. Census Bureau. (2013). Workers with a disability are less likely to be employed, more likely to hold jobs with lower earnings. Retrieved from https://www.census.gov/newsroom/releases/archives/miscellaneous/cb12-134.html

U.S. Department of Justice. (2015). *Twenty five years of progress for Americans with disabilities*. Retrieved from http://www.justice.gov/opa/blog/twenty-five-years-progress-americans-disabilities

Walker, D., & Gonzalez, E. W. (2007). Review of intervention studies on depression in persons with multiple sclerosis. *Issues in Mental Health Nursing, 28*(5), 511–531.

World Health Organization. (2011). *World report on disability*. Retrieved from http://www.who.int/disabilities/world_report/2011/report/en

Yee, S. (2015). The Affordable Care Act and people with disabilities. *GPSolo*. Retrieved from http://www.americanbar.org/publications/gp_solo/2015/march-april/the_affordable_care_act_and_people_disabilities.html

Telerehabilitation: Exercise and Adaptation in Home and Community

Andrew J. Haig and Steven A. Stiens

TELEREHABILITATION: A QUIET TECHNOLOGIC REVOLUTION WITH LIMITLESS OPTIONS

Encumbered. In the era of easy Skype, ubiquitous smart phones, and cheap activity monitors, a chapter on telemedicine should begin with words like "limitless" or "revolution." This chapter begins with the word "encumbered." The fact is that telemedicine remains a token part of health care and that telerehabilitation is even more limited than telemedicine in general. The challenge for the rehabilitation therapist is to decide what is to be accomplished outside the clinic and choose the least encumbered system to meet patients' needs.

Preliminary orientation should include some general guidance on how telerehabilitation fits into the universe of e-medicine. In an ever-expanding use of technology in the care of patients, our terminology attempts to categorize and classify interventions. Around the beginning of the 21st century, the term e-health was used as an all-encompassing word for the combined use of electronic information and communication technology in the care of patients. Telehealth represents a subset that promotes patient health at a distance and may include education, monitoring, and cues for good health and is subdivided into three categories. The first, telemedicine is a more specific subset that requires a heath practitioner to assess patients, provide diagnoses, and treatment at a distance. The second is e-health education. And the third is teleheathcare. Telerehabilitation is within telehealthcare along with telehomecare, telenursing, and telecoaching (Winters, 2002). Telerehabilitation seeks to access and enhance patient function by connecting members of the interdisciplinary team to patients for assessment and therapy using adjunctive equipment in the home or community as needed. Use of these new technologies requires creativity and perseverance, both prevalent in the interdisciplinary team.

It is true that our ideas are limitless, and that the possibilities are endless. Indeed, technical and clinical success stories are increasing, and the research that supports telerehabilitation has grown. However, the very fact that rehabilitation patients—who are uniquely at a disadvantage when it comes to travel—are still showing up in doctors' offices and therapy gyms more than a decade after Skype became ubiquitous tells us that we must focus away from the possibilities and toward pragmatic reality (Aamoth, 2011). Translation of the new clinical capabilities into effective programs and protocols is the challenge for contemporary rehabilitation institutions. A video that reveals interdisciplinary discussions of telerehabilition projects in current utilization and development "How to Establish Telerehabilitation Service" is available at www.youtube.com/watch?v=RU68b6JewBk

Using the vast variety of educational material on the Internet, the therapist can guide patients to material to review and can interact with them by phone as they review it or use it as homework for them to report on later (Manasco, Barone, & Brown, 2010). Patient-specific exercise material can be used to guide exercise sessions or generic material with groups is available for them to work on together with others. Patient-specific education material can be presented to specifically educate the patients and their families or to introduce the educator or clinician. The following videos provide a variety of material to broadly educate on spinal cord injury-related topics: "Dr Spine on Your Health" (www.youtube.com/watch?v=Z-lRR-Ws_jQ&list=PLFBA75D5D7BD755DC and www.christopherreeve.org/site/c.ddJFKRNoFiG/b.5848659/k.5E06/Reeve_Foundation_Videos.htm?bcpid=87913074001&bckey=AQ).

A responsible chapter on telerehabilitation must first focus on the challenge of sustainability. This chapter then reviews programs and concepts from a clinical framework: patient-to-clinician telerehabilitation, clinician-to-clinician telerehabilitation, programmed therapy, and apps.

SUSTAINABILITY: BUSINESS MODELS MAINTAIN PROGRAMS AND PROMOTE REFINEMENTS

"We had a good idea. We got a grant. We proved it works!. . . but, um, we don't do it anymore."

This quote could be a summary of Rashid Bashshur's book, *The History of Telemedicine* (Bashshur & Shannon, 2009). The current status of telemedicine suggests that this unfortunate story has indeed repeated itself over and over across the globe. Failure has resulted due to many reasons. They are all called "money."

Fortunately, we are on the verge of a number of revolutions in society that give advocates of telemedicine the chance to succeed. Telecommunication technology and its integration into lifestyles, substantial and more valid research into the use of telemedicine, and, especially in the United States, the pressures of a revolution in health care all create both crisis and opportunity. Success will come because the people with ideas and clinical goals align their ideas with the resources (money) that will make their ideas survive and grow. This section reviews the factors that must be understood for telerehabilitation to succeed in the long term. A video that shows an interactive lecture discussing the challenges of building and sustaining a telerehabilitation program that started in 2012 out of Caulfield Hospital "How to establish telerehabilitation service" is available at https://www.youtube.com/watch?v=Opzx3uKg4Uo

Telerehabilitation is generally not driven by the idea of making money but rather by the compassion of innovative visionaries who hope they can provide service that is not available elsewhere. Financial models for successful telemedicine do not discount the inspiration and dedication of individuals who would even provide this service for free. Success in telerehabilitation requires that we recognize that even volunteer time is not unlimited. Also a program that is clever enough to attach itself to a good business model may survive, grow, and be emulated by others, and thus multiply its beneficial effect beyond the reach of the original visionaries. The following business models may apply to various telerehabilitation programs:

Government support: Most major telemedicine programs are supported by government. The reasons range from pragmatic (sailors on ships and soldiers in the field are hard to reach), to financial (the U.S. Veterans Affairs, prisons, and others have to pay for expensive travel), to political (some of the most prominent telemedicine programs came from tobacco settlements or other political machinations).

Contracts: Telemedicine may help a health facility adequately care for patients it would otherwise have to transfer. In this scenario, the hospital may pay for the service. It is also valuable to small hospitals to avoid constant referral to larger nearby competitors and instead offer services in house that are provided virtually by a more prestigious (and more distant) center.

Fee-for-service: Until recently, fee-for-service medicine has not been a motive to provide telemedicine. Many states are now requiring that insurers pay for telemedicine just as they do when services are provided in person. Allied health providers are unfortunately often excluded from these laws. Medicare is a federal program that still will not pay except under specific circumstances. This inconsistency in payment policy among insurers makes it difficult for a clinic to offer telemedicine, since it requires that some, not all patients, be offered a covered service.

Capture a new market: By offering online consultations, even free ones, rehabilitation providers can convince patients to seek in-person care.

Out of pocket: When one considers the cost of gas, hotel, and lost work to attend an appointment in person, a telemedicine fee may be cheaper than health care insurance-covered care delivered in person. Patients may pay out of pocket. Workers compensation and litigation case managers who have more liability for nonmedical costs may have the flexibility to cover these nontraditional fees.

Specialized expertise: A heavily overbooked program with specialization in uncommon problems may find that screening out inappropriate distant patients opens up more time for appropriate patients and decreases the frustrations of patients whom they cannot help.

Decreased opportunity cost: The classic case is a surgeon who sees follow-up patients by asynchronous telemedicine, taking maybe a minute per case to determine if they really need to be seen. This frees up the physician to screen more profitable new patients and eliminates cost of space and staff.

Other health service savings: Increasingly, health systems are paid for outcomes, not procedures or hospital days. They may support certain telerehabilitation functions that speed up discharge, decrease readmissions, and limit expensive in-person treatments.

Research grants: Telemedicine can decrease the cost of research by reducing subject travel and the challenge of recruiting enough subjects from a localized geographic area. It provides the opportunity for remote recruitment, screening, and obtaining consent, selected outcome measures and follow-up of research subjects.

Pilot of new technology: Many well-known telemedicine programs are actually driven by income from technology transfer and industry contracts. They may profit as a demonstration site or may be motivated to bring their own devices to market. The clinical programs serve to validate these new market opportunities.

Marketing or partnering: As health systems consolidate and expand geographically, telerehabilitation services can provide a cost-effective link between newly bonded facilities. They may fund telerehabilitation as part of their partnership.

Case management: A large number of patients have separate people managing powers of attorney for finances and medical care. Agencies manage funds in trust and pay for clients' products and services as needed. Telerehabilitation techniques for interaction with the client, caregivers, and therapists in the home centers interventions with the clients where they live and trains those that will sustain the activity. Case managers along with the patients' care team and family carry out life care plans to maximize quality of life, function, longevity, and contributions to family and community for clients. As an extension of the rehabilitation process, problems are listed in a spectrum that goes from active diagnoses under treatment through impairments, activity limitations, and barriers to participation (Stiens, O'Young, & Young, 2008a). Treatment plans are scheduled throughout each day and are prioritized for enjoyment and client participation. Telerehabilitation allows for immediate real-time videoconferencing in the home in any shift or situation.

The Clinical Framework for Telerehabilitation: Person and Environment Interaction

Telemedicine brings clinical care to the patient in his or her own environment. This is a potent tool for the interdisciplinary team to sustain the rehabilitation process in the home and community. Rehabilitation can be defined as the process of development of a person to his or her fullest physical, psychological, social, educational, and vocational potential by eliminating or compensating for any biochemical, pathophysiology, or anatomic impairment, activity limitation or environmental and personal characteristics that make up contextual factors that impact directly on performance (Stiens, 2008b, 2013). Thus, rehabilitation seeks to maximize the greatest personal performance from patients "in vivo" in the environment where they choose to live.

Rehabilitation can be compared to a chemical reaction. If all the reagents are simultaneously present, the reaction is most likely to progress. Patients are typically prepared for telerehabilitation as inpatients or in the clinic. With telerehabilitation extended to the home, the modality acts as a catalyst to facilitate the patient, family, caregivers, and local practitioners to accomplish goals. Telerehabilitation in an environment familiar to the patient supplied with appropriate adaptations and equipment is an ideal and environmentally valid means to achieve skills that will be sustained over time.

For patients with brain injury, cognitive rehabilitation that occurs within the patient's home and community accomplishes greater patient initiation and insight into deficits through self-comparison to past function. Home is where familiar every day interaction occurs along with typical life demands (Ylvisaker, 2003). The prefrontal cortex is very sensitive to the environment and derives the significance of the actions to be performed from the site that links activity directly to person to practical goals (Zampolini et al., 2008). Mirror neurons are sensitive to observing the activity as preformed in context, whether the observation is via video transmission, superimposed with virtual reality (Chinthammit et al., 2014), or robotically generated (Gazzola, Rizzolatti, Wicker, & Keysers, 2007).

In a prosthetic environment such as the hospital, patients can successfully work on impairment reduction but activities that require simulation and learned skills may be more difficult to generalize to the home setting where the skills must be applied. Naturalistic treatment after early discharge to home following inpatient pre-training can shorten length of stay if the patient's home is appropriately modified and sufficiently equipped in advance of discharge. In studies of stroke rehabilitation carried out in the home as compared with the hospital, it was observed that patients take a more active role in the process within their own home environment (Koch, Wootrich, & Holmquist, 1998). In the hospital, the therapist played the role of expert/teacher who instructed patients and communicated goals. Patients were in an unfamiliar environment, which did not invite them to take initiatives. However, in the patient's home, an expanded set of roles were played out in the therapy. The therapist acted in multiple roles: a house guest, friend, and student/layman listening to the patient and family explaining how daily activities are carried out. The patient variously takes the role of the expert/teacher and host and takes initiative in goal setting as the patient recognizes the skills needed to approximate the previous lifestyles. In the familiar environment of the home, the patient takes much more initiative in guiding the therapy and generalizing accomplishments by extending independence to other life demands provided by the environment.

Rehabilitation models help clarify the focus and impact of interventions in planning. A person-centered concentric model of the environment has been designed for consideration in person-centered rehabilitation (Stiens, O'Young, & Young, 2008c). The patient is depicted at the center and pertinent environment sectors surround one another.

The person-centered concentric model is useful to illustrate telerehabilitation in a case of a patient living with C4 ASIA A tetraplegia who was trained in sip and puff controls in the clinic and then coached via two-way communication by radio from the support boat as the patient independently sailed in Chesapeake Bay (Figure 31.1). Telerehabilitation is accomplished with remote communication to the sailor who can act on control and navigation instructions transmitted remotely by the recreation therapist.

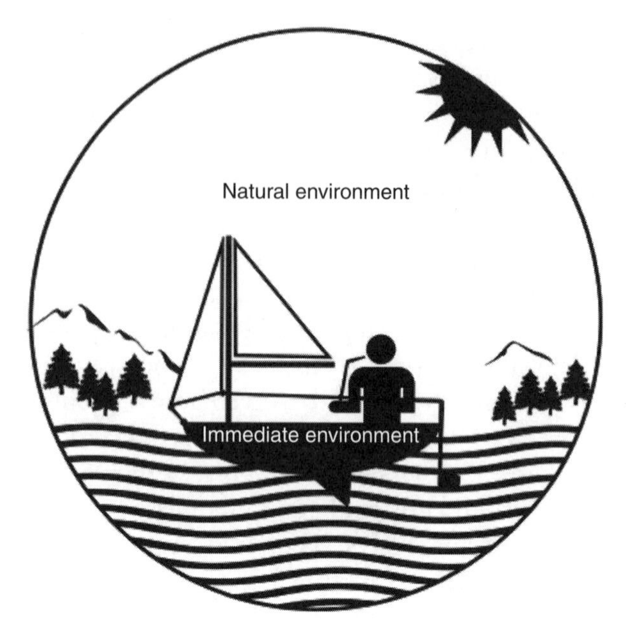

FIGURE 31.1 Person-centered concentric model of the environment. The person sails with C4 tetraplegia. The *immediate environment*, which is in contact with the person and moves with the person is the sailboat with adapted seating and sip and puff controls to tighten jib, sails, and steer with the tiller. Two-way radio communication permits coaching and distress problem solving. The *intermediate environment* (not depicted) is an adapted home or van. The *community environment* (not depicted) surrounds the patient's home and offers public access. The *natural environment* is represented by Chesapeake Bay surrounding the sailboat.

Source: Rojhaui, Stiens, and Recio (2016).

VALIDATION OF THE INTERVENTIONS: RESEARCH COMPARING THE CLINIC TO THE HOME

Rehabilitation interventions are based on treatment theories and what has worked in the very recent past. Therefore, treatment protocols have an intuitive design and are very likely to achieve improvement. Nonetheless, they need to be demonstrated as effective with improvements over standard care. Next, protocols are standardized so they can be delivered uniformly in practice. Thereafter, they need to be validated by comparing outcomes of protocols delivered in the clinic and at home using a telerehabilitation model.

While the idea that patient therapy in the patient's own environment makes sense, one cannot assume that every aspect of video, audio, and mechanical input and output from a distance consistently achieves similar outcomes as conventional therapy in the clinic. Research thus far completed cannot simply validate all of telemedicine or telerehabilitation. In fact, there have been two Cochrane reviews of telerehabilitation. In multiple sclerosis, there was limited evidence that telerehabilitation can improve functional activities, fatigue, and quality of life (Khan, Amatya, Kesselring, & Galea, 2015). There was insufficient evidence to support particular therapies or settings. In stroke, there was insufficient evidence to reach conclusions about greater effectiveness in the home setting versus the clinic. No randomized trials of cost saving from travel are available for review. With literature currently available, review of an array of studies may, however, allow us to extrapolate from one program to another.

In 2003, Jennet et al. performed a monolithic review of 4,646 articles on telehealth (Jennett et al., 2003). They concluded that telemedicine interventions offered

> significant socio-economic benefit, to patients and families, health-care providers and the health-care system. The main benefits identified were: increased access to health services, cost-effectiveness, enhanced educational opportunities, improved health outcomes, better quality of care, better quality of life and enhanced social support. (Jennett et al., 2003)

Van Dijk and Hermens (2004) reviewed quality research studies on rehabilitation interventions. They found that the electromyographic (EMG) biofeedback literature was of relatively good quality, but research on newer concepts like virtual reality was poor, reflecting the immaturity of the concepts. As in every other area of medicine, validation will always lag far behind the technology, leaving the potential user in a vulnerable position of using common sense, rather than good evidence in designing and adopting telerehabilitation techniques.

Just as rehabilitation integrates many other aspects of health care, telerehabilitation can be better understood by dissecting its components and prototypes to begin integration of validation. Using videoconferencing alone, telepsychiatry and telepsychology have shown surprisingly positive effects in reviews (Andersson, 2006). In practice, it is most successful to see the patient in person to ensure and strengthen therapeutic connections through supportive touch, clear mutual recognition of emotion through facial expressions, and mirroring of posture during the interview. After subsequent visits, sufficient rapport is established to sustain a treatment plan at a distance in the environment where the patient actually faces life challenges and achieves successes. A YouTube video that demonstrates how to use iPad-based home exercises with patients "Tele-Rehabilitation in the Home—Clinical examples" is available at www.youtube.com/watch?v=h4EbzgcPO1M

The validity of physical therapy assessment of low back pain via telerehabilitation versus hands-on assessment were compared (Truter, Russel, & Fary, 2014). Video camera placement allowed quantification of the active range of spinal motion and straight leg raise while the remote evaluating therapist guided the assessment and observed the patient. Standing posture was assessed for lordosis and pelvic tilt. Results showed high-level agreement on detecting pain with specific lumbar movements, eliciting symptoms, and sensitizing the straight leg test. Moderate agreement occurred on identification of the direction in which the worst spinal segmental movement occurred, straight leg raise test, range of motion, and active lumbar spine range of motion. These preliminary results demonstrate that rural patients can be triaged for further assessment or generic exercise protocols via telemedicine, leaving open options for reevaluation by telemedicine or in person if results are not adequate.

Telerehabilitation delivered via a virtual reality videogame can be successfully used to improve activities such as gait and balance performance. In a 10-week randomized study of patients with recently stable multiple sclerosis, an experimental group was trained with a specialized set of exercises using the Microsoft Xbox360 with adapted Kinect games that require imitating, throwing, kicking, and avoiding obstacles where the subject is represented by an avatar in the virtual environment (see YouTube video: "Salus: A System for Tele-Rehabilitation Using Kinect" at https://www.youtube.com/watch?v=9ZgK-QLt8M4). The subject controls the avatar with limb movements picked up by infrared sensors to feed into a 3D motion capture system. The software increases the gaming difficulty based on subject performance. Dynamic posturography, sensory organization test, and motor control test showed clinically significant improvement and marginally better performance than the control group getting standard physical therapy (Gutierrez et al., 2013). Gait performance and balance can be improved via telerehabilitation designed and guided by a remote physical therapist as in this YouTube video "REWIRE: Enabling home rehabilitation for stroke patients" is available at www.youtube.com/watch?v=7kGrl3iETug.

Home health care and telehome health comprises a field in the same taxonomic category as telerehabilitation and includes medication compliance, wound management, and patient education (Winters, 2002). Many studies and demonstration projects in home health care have shown improved compliance and understanding, decreased complications, and sometimes decreased cost as compared with standard care. However, evidence is not fully conclusive in telehealth studies. In a comprehensive review of 950 clinical trials, only 24 were felt to be of sufficient quality for a systematic review of telehealth interventions for chronic disease (Garcia-Lizana & Sarria-Santamera, 2007). Topics included monitoring and management of diabetes, hypertension, and heart disease. Among the articles in this review, Hoenig et al. used land-line telephone and video to provide home evaluation and instruction to 13 home-based subjects (Hoenig et al., 2006). There was compliance with 60% of 12 recommendations per subject.

Patients generally respond favorably to telerehabilitation interventions, but it is not known if this is an artifact of the novelty of the intervention or the added attention, rather than actual improvement in quality of care. A survey of 3,329 patients with chronic depression or symptomatic coronary artery disease cared for in practices in England resulted in a 44% response rate. The results revealed that 60% of respondents were interested in telephone and Internet e-mail-based telehealth but only 17% indicated interest in social network-based interactions (Edwards et al., 2014). A demonstration that telemedicine monitoring lowered hemoglobin A1C levels in patients with diabetes provides encouraging objective evidence in favor of this approach. Caregivers on the receiving end of expert advice also are generally delighted with the help received. Rehabilitation impairment measures and changes in activity are not as reliably linked to safe independent function, making it more difficult to demonstrate remarkable outcomes.

Specialists elsewhere in the interdisciplinary circle seem less enthusiastic about telerehabilitation (Rho, Choi, & Lee, 2014). This may be an artifact of technophobia or related to the lack of some cues that the physicians find useful. Smell, touch, and some physical aspects of the interpersonal interactions are not transmitted via cable. Whether these are critical or irrelevant components of the examination or simply hard habits to break is an important consideration. Logan discussed the challenges of videoconferencing between rehabilitation team members who are geographically remote. Physical contact, transfer of physical objects between members, and cultural aspects of care are challenging (Logan & Radcliffe, 2000).

ADOPTION OF TELEMEDICINE: PERMANENT ROLE IN THE INTERDISIPLINARY FAMILY?

Adoption and consistent utilization has been a challenge for telemedicine. A telemedicine service acceptance model was adapted from the technology acceptance model (TAM) and focused on three predictive constructs: accessibility of medical records and clinical use factors, self-efficacy of the physician user, and perceived incentives as regulatory factors. A survey of 183 physicians confirmed the empirical validity of the model and revealed that the major constructs driving physicians to successfully use the modality were perceived usefulness in their practice, and perceived ease of use of the software and equipment. In addition, physicians had concerns about simultaneous access to electronic medical records and the impressions of the patients about usefulness and satisfaction (Logan & Radcliffe, 2000). They concluded that the telemedicine system needs to be linked to the electronic medical record and accessible via secured network connections outside the hospital.

A review of telehealth implementation frameworks included a detailed summary of many articles and 11 frameworks (Van Dyk, 2014). They concluded that successful implementation requires the use of a holistic model that carefully reviews technologic options, organizational structure, clinical and social impacts, economic feasibility, user-friendliness, validation of the application, and successful evidence of use. The needs of the interdisciplinary team in rehabilitation are likely very similar. Implementation should be in a layered approach starting small but thinking big for longevity (Broens et al., 2007).

Developing a telemedicine program is an interdisciplinary activity, deriving the essential information from each discipline to design the program on paper. Then a layered implementation model is used to allow the primary focus on different components to change as the program develops. In the prototype phase, the focus is on wide ease of use and effective technologic support. As use in scale occurs, refinements of the business model will occur. Policy revision and development occurs as the multidisciplinary team reviews aspects of patient availability, quality of service, and success in reimbursement.

THE TECHNOLOGY AND LOGISTICS OF TELEREHABILITATION: PATIENT EQUIPMENT AND CAPABILITIES

The technology and the social use of technology is changing so fast that anything written in this book should be perceived in a historical context by the readers who see it in print. As of 2015, the number of e-mail users has skyrocketed to 2.5 billion people, or one of every three persons in the world (Tschabitscher, 2016). For the last decade, people have networked via Facebook, accessed videos on YouTube, and educated and entertained each other on myriad changing social networking platforms from Twitter to Snapchat. Skype and other web services provide audiovisual communication with easy access at no cost. Unfortunately, computer literacy and health literacy are still barriers, although there are many grandmothers and great-grandfathers who are less socially isolated due to their connectivity.

The hardware has changed, improved, and morphed. The most basic and inexpensive tablets and laptops have capacity for audio recording, video cameras, and wireless broadcasting. Smart phones now duplicate the functions of computers and, as networks now cover most regions, people are dropping their land phone lines altogether. Even the concept of a computer as a separate device is changing as homes, appliances, and vehicles are rapidly becoming an "Internet of things."

The huge storage and logic capacity of many devices has had another effect. Siri and other virtual persons advise smart phone users of the nearest restaurant and the latest sport scores. Likewise, telerehabilitation does not have to involve communication with a real person. In fact, the line drawn between virtual reality and distant communication is somewhat arbitrary and sometimes meaningless. Virtual reality instruction or simulation might involve software contained in the user's computer or web-connection to a server on the other side of the world. Podcasts carried on tablets, smart phones with computer capacity, and global positioning systems blur barriers and definitions. It has become harder to define what is and what is not telerehabilitation. For now, the part of an interaction that is hands-on or face-to-face with a real human being or with physical equipment that is not connected to the Internet is not telerehabilitation. Even that line of distinction will fade away and telerehabilitation as some kind of separate entity may disappear.

There are still technical issues. Many regions of the world are still not connected to the Internet or are connected through slow processes. Some applications require high Internet bandwidth and are affected by delays in transmission. But most rehabilitation interventions are not so time critical. The impact of the nature of technology and the quality of transmission are not clearly understood. For example, Phillips et al. did not find a difference between telephone and video conferencing (Phillips, Vesmarovich, Hauber, Wiggers, & Egner, 2001). Also, Lemaire, Boudrias, and Greene (2001) found low bandwidth video acceptable in transmitting rehabilitation information.

Typing skills remain a barrier to some persons, especially the elderly, who may have little typing or computer training, or persons whose impairment involves the use of the hands. Voice recognition programs are increasingly accurate and accessible to the public. A Japanese group found good success in using a pen-type imaging sensor with home computers to provide social support to elderly clients served by a "home helper" office (Ogawa et al., 2003). This office transferred messages to helpers' mobile phones for timely responses.

Telemedicine was explored decades ago with the transmission of electrocardiographic signals over phone lines. Home-based telerehabilitation has been accomplished via the Internet with validated success as revealed by a systematic review of studies (Neubeck et al., 2009). It was concluded that telerehabilitation of cardiac patients provided effective risk factor reduction and secondary prevention of coronary artery disease and complications. Contemporary analysis of cardiac rehabilitation recognizes that although cardiac rehabilitation is effective, only about one third of eligible patients attend. The home-based telerehabilitation of the future will monitor and report safe risk stratification from computer analysis of the electrocardiogram (EKG). Should there be a change, the system will seek telemedical support and triage to change exercise activity or intervention as required (Piotrowicz & Piotrowicz, 2013).

TELEREHABILITATION HARDWARE: ADAPTATIONS, INNOVATIONS, AND END-USER INTERFACES

Many advances have been made in rehabilitation-related technology. Cognitive and speech therapy are aided by newer software that can measure a patient's ability and provide challenges just at or beyond that ability. Portable devices can act as prosthetic brains, with software and applications available for smartphones for everything from geographical navigation to translation of languages to behavioral reminders.

Distant interventions for speech or cognitive problems is less vulnerable to problems with user devices or bandwidth. Speech and video pictures are well established on the Internet and require less sophistication in terms of devices. Baron et al. views the integration of methodologies; face-to-face speech therapy with family coaching, group therapy, and telerehabilitation communication as optimal (Baron, Hatfield, & Georgeadis, 2005).

Many therapists in the community adapt readily available and fairly inexpensive technology like smartphones and computers/tablets without any rehabilitation-specific software to meet patients' needs for memory and communication. More than a prosthetic memory, portable communication may provide more situation-specific intervention and more timely feedback in the real world. For example, therapists can provide short videos of explanation and instruction on how to communicate with an aphasic patient triggered by an icon on a portable computer. Or an occupational therapist might send a brain-injured person who struggles with social communication alone into a grocery store with a shopping list, and then call to remind the patient to thank the checkout clerk. The efficiencies and timeliness of mobile devices are clear, and the technology is available now, almost everywhere. Once in the community, again there are options for return to work as a visitor as a prelude for development of a vocational rehabilitation plan. With aphasia so prevalent in stroke, use of an iPad or other tablet-based technology provides for a large variety of explanation videos or standardized answers to questions patients may need in the work and community environments (Young, Stiens, & Hirsch, 2015).

Much of rehabilitation involves motion, and advances in technology allows motion capture and feedback. Numerous companies are coming on the market with devices that observe patient exercise and provide instantaneous graphic nonjudgmental feedback. The recording of the patient performance helps the therapist design new routines that will futher challenge the patient to get the fullest most functional recovery. The Rejoyce System for upper extremity exercise includes a wand that is grasped and moved against resistance in a three-dimensional space representing upper extremity range. The articulated mechanical arm provides resistance and records force of effort by the patient as well as position as illustrated in this YouTube video "ReJoyce Hand and Arm Rehabilitation System": www.youtube.com/watch?v=YI8JDGh4Hw8.

Virtual reality games and training are increasingly common. Using strict definitions, a virtual reality rehabilitation exercise that resides on the patient's computer is not telerehabilitation, while one that taps into a distant server or involves interaction with a distant clinician is telerehabilitation (Lemaire & Greene, 2002). Regardless, this is an emerging important technology. Holden's (2005) review of 121 studies in virtual reality has four major conclusions:

> (a) people with disabilities appear capable of motor learning within virtual environments, (b) movements learned by people with disabilities in virtual reality (VR) transfer to real world equivalent motor tasks in most cases, and in some cases even generalize to other untrained tasks, (c) in the few studies that have compared motor learning in real versus virtual environments, some advantage for VR training has been found in all cases, and (d) no occurrences of cyber-sickness in impaired populations have been reported to date in experiments where VR has been used to train motor abilities. (Holden, 2005)

VR techniques can be used to design an augmented reality prototype system for learning called Ghostman, which is a wearable visual augmentation device. The patient has an egocentric view through which users see their own movements overlaid with a "ghost" image of the instructors hand teaching the activity in real-time steps. Patients and therapists are permitted to inhabit the others viewpoint in a technique called inhabiting visual augmentation, allowing the patient to mimic the movement with real-time instructions. Images are generated by two cameras built into the head-mounted display worn by the patient and therapist. The signals can be readily transmitted across the Internet making this modality very valuable for home telerehabilitation. The technique was validated in comparison to face-to-face therapy to train the use of chopsticks with comparable time to completion of the activity and number of errors per session (Chinthammit et al., 2014).

Motor rehabilitation from a distance is difficult as compared with hands-on guidance in clinic. Motor rehabilitation must have preceded watching a simple exercise on the computer or recording the number of repetitions of an exercise day-to-day. Activity-based restorative therapy (ABRT) has been adopted by many clinicians and is a reality for a small but increasing number of patients achieving ongoing recovery from incomplete central nervous system (CNS) injuries that spare at least some sensory or motor function (Dolbow et al., 2015). Intensive regular exercise of upper and lower extremities following CNS injury results in ongoing and functionally significant recovery for many. Telerehabilitation is challenged to provide the kind of immediate force and direction guidance that occurs in hands-on physical therapy. Motion involves force, velocity, and direction, all of which need to be measured and transmitted accurately and rapidly if feedback is to be timely. The feedback loop can be a local resident to the patient device to the Internet, or back to the clinician's workstation for modulation. A blended design approach was used to modify the MusicJacket system designed to teach people to play the violin by guiding the arm to move with the bow on cues of pressure and vibration in the sleeve of the jacket. The designers innovated a gesture-based system to facilitate rehabilitation of people with stroke that included the same vibration motors that provide a haptic feedback mechanism like the touch of the therapist to guide patients in movement of their impaired limb in the patterns depicted on the computer screen (van der Linden & Waights, 2012).

There are a variety of devices that can continuously monitor physical activity that the clinician cannot. EKG can monitor both effort and risk of cardiac danger. Surface EMG can measure tremor, spasm, cocontraction, fatigue, and effort. Force plates can measure effort, speed, strain, and balance. Temperature and EMG biofeedback can measure and train relaxation. These tools are not unique to telerehabilitation but can easily be built into exercise and assessment protocols. Due to the complex nature of most patients' multisystem response to deficits, it is most useful to collect continuous or intermittent data as vital signs. In addition, limb position continuous monitoring, task quality assessment, and activity through the day provide perspective for endurance and generalization of skills.

Wireless devices have been devised to monitor gait and activity at a distance from the home computer. The Smart Cane was designed with pressure sensors in the base and handle to monitor use and safety to prevent falls. Data are transmitted wirelessly for analysis, which is used to warn users of potential dangers. Simultaneously, information can be sent to the remote rehabilitation center, which might be used to modify therapy interventions. A similar product called the Smart Shoe determines fall risk by monitoring walking behavior (Naditz, 2009). Such devices enhance quality of life by permitting patients to use their full gait capabilities in the home and prevent falls with early warning signs (McCue, Fairman, & Pramuka, 2010).

The distant measurement of many physiological parameters is now technologically feasible. Oxygen levels, blood pressure, EKG, pulse, temperature, and numerous other parameters can be measured from a distance and in ambulatory settings (Lymberis, 2004). Monitoring can be synchronous in real time or asychronous with collected data over time available for later analysis of trends.

There have been continuous advances in electronic activity monitors since our early work using devices to monitor walking participation (Yamakawa, Tsai, Haig, Miner, & Harris, 2004). These lightweight devices can be worn for many days at home to measure distances walked and caloric expenditure, among other parameters.

Now, for the first time, instead of surveying the patient regarding integration into the community, clinicians and scientists get an objective measure. For example, we now know that obese people may not only consume more nutrients than other people, they walk less, and thus burn fewer calories during their usual activity at-home. The science of using at home monitoring to determine the real level of activity and the objective effects of treatments ranging from joint replacement to multidisciplinary rehabilitation are just the beginning.

Finally, there must be a reality check on the gimmickry and gee-whiz. The world of telemedicine is strongly influenced by the enthusiasm of inventors who are not clinicians and by industry's motivation to sell their devices. High-resolution, multiscreen dedicated transmission may not be needed where a simple video conference is sufficient. An intelligent and skeptical clinician will realize that there is no need for expensive integrated oxygen monitoring software in cases where the family member can just occasionally point the smartphone camera at the local device's light-emitting diode (LED) readout. Integration with the electronic medical record is an important sales pitch, but offers little efficiency for clinicians who have to type their notes anyway.

As with any new diagnostic tool associated with telerehabilitation, the challenge is to answer the "so what?" question to determine the possible clinical impact. Once patient deficits are identified and goals set, how is that treatment delivered in the home or community and how is outcome measured? Many of the answers come from the ever-expanding range of telerehabilitation treatments.

THE BUREAUCRACY: A CHAIN OF ADMINISTRATIVE, FISCAL, AND LEGAL SUPPORT

Although the basic technology for video conferencing is now intuitive to many in medicine, there are important administrative challenges and technical considerations. The paperwork alone can be overwhelming. Table 31.1 lists the many interests that must be aligned.

The program design, construction, implementation, and evaluation are essential to success. In fact, it is critical that distant care be above reproach in all ways. So when we built the University of Michigan Health System's telemedicine system, the first and most important step was to meet with the administrators in charge of each of these areas and put together an agreed upon set of "pathways" that accommodate each of their rules and regulations. By codifying one acceptable pathway instead of citing many regulatory barriers we provided a way for groups to innovate on their own without harming the patient or the system.

TABLE 31.1

ORGANIZATIONAL PROCESSES THAT MUST BE CONSIDERED FOR A TELEMEDICINE PROGRAM TO FUNCTION WITHIN A HEALTH CARE ORGANIZATION
Scheduling
Registration and scheduling
Informed consent
Privacy
Medical records
Billing
Technical/computer security processes
Credentialing at clinician and patient sites
Licensing in patient's jurisdiction
Risk management
Conflict of interest
Training program regulations
Credentialing agencies (e.g., The Joint Commission, CARF)

CARF, Commission on Accreditation of Rehabilitation Facilities.

PROJECTS IN TELEREHABILITATION: MODELS FOR SUCCESS AND YOUR DESIGN

Invested readers are looking for role models and precedents: what is possible and what has been done. Numerous demonstration projects have shown feasibility of various rehabilitation techniques, but randomized trials are rare, and cost-effectiveness analysis is almost nonexistent. Again it is important to see telerehabilitation as a shifting field where the ideas presented here can only represent a framework and where the best and brightest ideas are more likely on the Internet than in a text.

Telemedicine interventions can be differentiated into clinician–patient interactions (e.g., a distant assessment or treatment of the patient by a therapist or physician) and clinician–clinician interactions (e.g., a therapist consulting with a distant physiatrist) according to Huis, van Dijk, Hermens, and Vollenbroek-Hutten (2006). A therapist–patient consultation after stroke, using a motion-sensitive exoskelton and a visual display to encourage movement, is outlined in the video mentioned in the following. The role of the patient and the attendant for exercise is well demonstrated. The HandTudor successfully quantifies fine movements of the wrist and fingers as patients play games guided by visual imagery on the computer screen, as seen in the YouTube video "Hand Rehabilitation using Hand Tudor": https://www.youtube.com/watch?v=1h1Ucqrqcd0

Pain telerehabilitation has been the subject of some research. One study in chronic pain patients showed that self-regulatory skills can be effectively taught via telephone or closed-circuit television (Appel, Bleiberg, & Noiseux, 2002). On the other hand, Andersson et al. performed a randomized controlled trial of headache sufferers, in which half had frequent contact initiated by the counselor, while the other half initiated contact on a schedule. Dropout rates were about one third regardless of group, and the effectiveness of treatment was not improved upon by therapist-initiated contact (Andersson, 2006).

Using games, exercises, and information, Reinkensmeyer, Pang, Nessler, and Painter (2002) demonstrated the feasibility of a stroke rehabilitation program, including measurement of compliance and improvement. Burdea, Popescu, and Hentz (2000) have designed an orthopedic telerehabilitation system that shows promise, but was only tested in one subject (2000). A monthly pediatric telerehabilitation clinic has been developed to bring interdisciplinary care to medically complex patients in a variety of underserved rural locations. Improvements recognized in care were in family education and inclusion of staff from local agencies that provide care (Conner, 1999).

In some cases, telerehabilitation is best considered in the context of social services changes. For example, in Japan, it has been proposed that the integration of occupational therapy telerehabilitation into community life centers for older patients will help the system to efficiently stretch occupational therapy resources (Tsuchisawa, Ono, Kanda, & Kelly, 2000).

It is quite realistic for persons with severe disability or reduced consciousness to be maintained at home, at great cost savings to society but with substantial stresses on the family (Hauber & Jones, 2002). A few randomized trials support the use of telemedicine to maintain such patients at home. In 111 persons with spinal cord injuries, no difference was noted among those who received 9 weeks of telerehabilitation advice (either video or telephone contact) compared to others in terms of quality of life, but there was a trend toward shorter subsequent hospitalizations in the telerehabilitation group (Phillips et al., 2001). As care plans are more comprehensively designed and careful review of continuous measurement of vital signs continues we will get earlier warnings of infection risks and benefit from immediate care planning in the home with telerehabilitation. A small survey of persons with traumatic brain injury suggested that there was good acceptability for telerehabilitation services, notably for assistance in cognitive areas and activities of daily living (Ricker et al., 2002). For a small group of five persons with traumatic brain injuries at the Ranchos Los Amigos Level of Cognitive Function 1 to 3, video conferencing during the first 2 months after discharge from home resulted in fewer ongoing family needs and more patients remaining at home at 6- to 9-month follow-up, compared to a control group. The Ranchos Los Amigos Level of Cognitive Function scale describes eight levels of cognitive functioning spanning from no response at level 1 to generalized responses at level 2 to localized responses in level 3 when the patient responds consistently to stimuli and may follow a command. At level 8 the patient is oriented but may still exhibit deficits in abstract reasoning (Doble Haig, Anderson, & Katz, 2003).

Because the use of computers for communications involves a machine that is really designed to perform logical functions, it is natural that telemedicine projects often incorporate computer software that could be useful even in a face-to-face situation. One example is a computer-driven hand rehabilitation glove that receives active movement data from electrogoniometers and measures the force and position of the hand in active movement designed by Popescu, Burdea, Bouzit, Girone, and Hentz (1999) and Popescu, Burdea, Bouzit, and Hentz (2000). The device provides guidance tasks for the patient to attempt while the computer records voluntary movement and actively completes individual movements for the patient such as opening the hand. This system may be more valuable for its software and hardware design rather than the fact that it can be used from home versus the clinic. The distinctions between telerehabilitation and computerized rehabilitation are blurred.

Education of practitioners is an important aim of telerehabilitation. Models have ranged from online courses to online peer support. The motivation to share information and the motivation to use it needs to be explored. For example, the University of Michigan's medical school has spent over a million dollars to put its entire curriculum on line for free consumption. The university believes that this information will be available in the future regardless of its effort to contain it, yet if it presents it first and in a very organized and accessible way, the university will gain whatever advantages there are in the global market for education and reputation. Distant education in all areas is becoming more common and in some countries the requirements of professions to show evidence of continued education make telerehabilitation education ideal.

Our group has successfully partnered with a major global employer to develop web-based modular education in rehabilitation and occupational medicine topics for company-employed clinicians throughout the world. The employer is motivated by the savings incurred with improved care. The physicians, often more affluent or in greater leadership positions than independent physicians, become practice leaders for their medical community. The results showed that over half of the company's practitioners anonymously used the program, that they had a statistically significant increase in knowledge, and that simplification and brevity resulted in significant improvement in user satisfaction. Another project is aimed to establish the medical specialty of physical medicine and rehabilitation in countries where there is either a paucity or complete lack of the specialty (Tannor, Haig, Christian, Smith, & Odonkor, 2016). An online, in person pilot involving American experts has been launched and ministries of health are considering whether this kind of training can be stringent enough to establish a recognized specialty.

ORGANIZATIONS INVENTING AND SUSTAINING TELEREHABILITATION: NEED IS THE MOTHER OF INVENTION

The movement toward more telemedicine in general and telerehabilitation in particular is driven by a confluence of expert clinicians, technical innovators, policymakers, health care system leaders, and a growing industry. The various organizations that bring these groups together and lead can be good resources. Among them are the following.

The American Telemedicine Association (ATA) may be the premier telemedicine organization in the world, with very large annual meetings and substantial industry influence. Its Telerehabilitation Special Interest Group is active and effective. They completed and posted A Blueprint for Telemedicine Guidelines, which is essential reading for any group starting a telerehabilitation program. They were built from the ATA's Core Standards for Telemedicine Operations. These documents and a bibliography of research in the field can be found on their web page (www.americantelemed.org).

Numerous regional or international organizations serve a similar purpose including many under the umbrella of the International Society for Telehealth (www.isfteh.org).

The U.S. government's Office of Advancement of Telehealth is a resource in itself, but also funds a number of regional telehealth resource centers, the mission of which is to help establish telehealth programs in their regions (www.telehealthresource center.org).

The World Health Organization (WHO) has been involved in telemedicine development in many areas. Their 2011 report was extensive and included rehabilitation and enabling environments and recommended telerehabilitation. A recent survey and review by the WHO may be useful, although its global survey only captured one telerehabilitation program in Slovenia (www.who.int/goe/publications/goe_telemedicine_2010.pdf).

The U.S. Veterans Administration has a large and well-developed telehealth program and its website has many examples and resources (www.telehealth.va.gov).

Telemedicine is such a dynamic area of intervention that these organizations' websites are a better and more immediate way of keeping up to date on developments in the field. Regular review of these sites, documents issued, and assembled bibliographies will provide a more coherent perspective than individual publications and news releases.

TELEMEDICINE, YOU AND THE FUTURE: POSSIBILITIES?

This review provided definitions for telerehabilitation, examples of equipment for use, demonstration of treatment programs in progress, and suggestions for sustaining programs once started. The mission of rehabilitation clinicians is to know their patient populations and the time segments since initial evaluation that they will continue to cover during the chronic period and provide the best program possible for outcome. As recovery processes and rehabilitation interventions are better understood, models for utilization in outpatient care, home, and the community are being demonstrated to be effective and valid in the home and community as compared with conventional inpatient and outpatient rehabilitative care. The first order of design is use of the telephone with patients in support of their in-home programs. Thereafter, utilization of equipment and protocols already approved and in use in the rehabilitation clinician's department is a further extension of practice. As service is delivered, there needs to be contemplation of other projects or refinement of existing programs to sustain use and provide more options for therapy. Meanwhile, developments in regulation, equipment and programming will continue as needed changes for the future occur.

Academic programs of telemedicine are established and continue to grow. Oregon Health and Science University has been offering telemedicine primarily in the form of physician consultation successfully for the last 9 years (Butcher, 2015). Recent additions of in-home monitoring for chronic patients with congestive heart failure have been clinically successful by anticipating clinical deterioration and guiding appropriate treatments. Telehealth is growing at all the academic medical centers with greater utilization of teleconferencing upon recognition that value would be added to the visit. The University of Pittsburgh is offering 80 subspecialty telemedicine consultations as well as primary care consultations from 70 providers offering virtual primary care. In spite of all this, analytics found that as of early 2014 only 34% of USA hospitals were using telehealth.

The way forward requires focus on the triple aim of reducing costs, improving quality, and improving the patient care experience (Butcher, 2015). With this focus, members of the interdisciplinary rehabilitation team will view telemedicine with a new mindset and continue to innovate, utilize, and improve programs to sustain and expand care options as telemedicine consultations have grown across major academic centers.

Innovations and extensions of current technology and new applications are as vast as the imagination of the interdisciplinary team and innovative patients that tinker at solutions. In the near future, we will see many smart cloth products that can follow temperature, angle of movement, force of heel landing during ambulation as well as the position of the hands as they carry out selected tasks. Robotic end devices used in the home are more haptic in recording and transmitting movement and force meant to be felt back and forth between the therapist and patient along with real time video and audio. With wireless and Bluetooth technologies, devices can be further from the home computer and mobile videocams can be carried about in the house, boat, or yard as needed for therapy and assessment.

Telepresence robots are utilized in schools and in business to bring people in for interactive class tours or test drives. Patients that may have some confinement to the home can get out using avatars in the form of the many robots on the market that can be controlled remotely from a computer or a cell phone with an application. This telepresence allows a patient to explore remote environments, attend social occasions, visit school, or work from home. Most models use an iPad or other tablet for a face-to-face interaction and use teleconferencing software such as Skype for interaction. Remote controls activate the wheels and various joints that position the face to make the best impression or get the best view. A comical video from YouTube dramatizes the experience of the office work environment with a visiting robot with full remote office navigation and face to face conversations at desks: "Meet Robot Boss" (www.youtube.com/watch?v=s1sReQvU1iI).

REFERENCES

Aamoth, D. (2011). A brief history of Skype. Retrieved from http://techland.time.com/2011/05/10/a-brief-history-of-skype

Andersson G. (2006). Internet-based cognitive-behavioral self help for depression. *Expert Review of Neurotherapeutics*, *6*(11), 1637–1642.

Appel, P. R., Bleiberg, J., & Noiseux, J. (2002). Self-regulation training for chronic pain: Can it be done effectively by telemedicine? *Telemedicine Journal & E-Health*, *8*(4), 361–368.

Baron, C., Hatfield, B., & Georgeadis, A. (2005). Management of communication disorders using family member input, group treatment, and telerehabilitation. *Topics in Stroke Rehabilitation, 12*(2), 49–56.

Bashshur, R., & Shannon, G. W. (2009). *History of telemedicine: Evolution, context, and transformation.* New Rochelle, NY: Mary Ann Liebert.

Broens, T. H., Veld, R. M. H., Vollenbroek-Hutten, M. M. R., Hermens, M. J., van Halteren, A. T., & Nieuwenhuis, L. J. M. (2007). Determinants of successful telemedicine implementation: A literature study. *Journal of Telemedicine and Telecare, 13*(6), 303–309.

Burdea, G., Popescu, V., Hentz, V., & Colbert K. (2000). Virtual reality-based orthopedic telerehabilitation. *IEEE Transactions on Rehabilitation Engineering, 8*(3), 430–432.

Butcher, L. (2015). Telehealth and telemedicine today: Physican leaders. Retrieved from http://www.physicianleaders.org

Chinthammit, W., Merritt, T., Petersen, S., Williams, A., Visentin, D., Rowe, R., & Furness, T. (2014). Augmented reality application for telerehabilitation and remote instruction of a novel motor skill. *BioMed Research International, 2014*, 1–7.

Conner, K. (1999). Technology through television: Pediatric telemedicine furthers rehab's continuum of care. *Rehabilitation Management, 12*(2), 72–75.

Doble, J. E., Haig, A. J., Anderson, C., & Katz, R. (2003). Impairment, activity, and participation, life satisfaction and survival in persons with locked in syndrome for over a decade: Follow-up on a previously reported cohort. *Journal of Head Trauma Rehabilitation, 18*(5), 435–444.

Dolbow, D. R., Gorgey, A. S., Recio, A. C., Stiens, S. A., Curry, A. C., Sadowsky, C. L., . . . McDonald, J. W. (2015). Activity-based restorative therapies after spinal cord injury: Inter-institutional conceptions and perceptions. *Aging and Disease, 6*(4), 254.

Edwards, L., Thomas, C., Gregory, A., Yardley, L., O'Cathanijah, A., Montgomery, A., & Salisbury, C. (2014). Are people with chronic diseases interested in using telehealth? A cross section postal survey. *Journal of Medical Internet Research, 16*(5), e123

Garcia-Lizana, F., & Sarria-Santamera, A. (2007). New technologies for chronic disease management and control: A systematic review. *Journal of Telemedicine & Telecare, 13*(2), 62–68.

Gazzola, V., Rizzolatti, G., Wicker, B., & Keysers, C. (2007). The anthropomorphic brain: The mirror neuron system responds to human and robotic actions. *Neuroimage, 35*, 1674–1684.

Gutierrez, R. O., del Rio, F. G., Cano, R., Alguacil-Diego, I. M., González, R. A., & Page, J. C. (2013). A telerehabilitaion program by virtual reality-video games improves balance and postural control in multiple sclerosis patients. *Neurorehabilitation, 33*, 515–554.

Hauber, R. P., & Jones, M. L. (2002). Telerehabilitation support for families at home caring for individuals in prolonged states of reduced consciousness. *Journal of Head Trauma Rehabilitation, 17*(6), 535–541.

Hoenig, H., Sanford, J. A., Butterfield, T., Griffiths, P. C., Richardson, P., & Hargraves, K. (2006). Development of a teletechnology protocol for in-home rehabilitation. *Journal of Rehabilitation Research & Development, 43*(2), 287–298.

Holden, M. K. (2005). Virtual environments for motor rehabilitation: Review. *CyberPsychology & Behavior, 8*(3), 187–211. doi:10.1089/cpb.2005.8.187

Huis in't Veld, M. H., van Dijk, H., Hermens, H. J., & Vollenbroek-Hutten, M. M. (2006). A systematic review of the methodology of telemedicine evaluation in patients with postural and movement disorders. *Journal of Telemedicine & Telecare, 12*(6), 289–297.

Jennett, P. A., Affleck, H. L., Hailey, D., Ohinmaa, A., Anderson, C., Thomas, R., . . . Scott, R. E. (2003). The socio-economic impact of telehealth: A systematic review. *Journal of Telemedicine & Telecare, 9*(6), 311–320.

Khan, F., Amatya, B., Kesselring, J., & Galea, M. (2015). Telerehabilitation for persons with multiple sclerosis. *Cochrane Database of Systematic Reviews, 4*, CD010508. doi:10.1002/14651858.CD010508.pub2

Koch, L. V., Wootrich, W., & Holmquist, L. W. (1998). Rehabilitation in the home versus the hospital: The importance of context. *Disability and Rehabilitation, 20*(10), 367–372.

Lemaire, E. D., Boudrias, Y., & Greene, G. (2001). Low-bandwidth, Internet-based videoconferencing for physical rehabilitation consultations. *Journal of Telemedicine & Telecare, 7*(2), 82–89.

Lemaire, E. D., & Greene, G. (2002). Continuing education in physical rehabilitation using Internet-based modules. *Journal of Telemedicine & Telecare, 8*(1), 19–24.

Logan, G. D., & Radcliffe, D. F. (2000, Summer). Supporting communication in rehabilitation engineering teams. *Telemedicine Journal, 6*(2), 225–236.

Lymberis, A. (2004). Research and development of smart wearable health applications: The challenge ahead. *Studies in Health Technology & Informatics, 108*, 155–161.

Manasco, H. M., Barone, N., & Brown, A. (2010). A role for youtube in telerehabilitation. *International Journal of Telerehabilitation, 7*(2), 15–18.

McCue, M., Fairman, A., & Pramuka, M. (2010). Enhancing quality of life through telerehabilitation. *Physical Medicine and Rehabilitation Clinics of North America, 21*, 195–205.

Naditz, A. (2009). Telenursing: Front-line applications of telehealthcare delivery. *Telemedicine and e-Health, 15*(9), 825–829. doi:10.1089/tmj.2009.9938

Neubeck, L., Redfern, J., Fernandez, R., Briffa, T., Bauman, A., & Freedman, S. B. (2009). Telehealth interventions for the secondary prevention of coronary heart disease: A systematic review. *European Journal of Cardiovascular Prevention & Rehabilitation*, *16*(3), 281–289. doi:10.1097/HJR.0b013e32832a4e7a

Ogawa, H., Yonezawa, Y., Maki, H., Sato, H., Hahn, A. W., & Caldwell, W. M. (2003). A Web-based home welfare and care services support system using a pen type image sensor. *Biomedical Sciences Instrumentation*, *39*, 199–203.

Phillips, V. L., Vesmarovich, S., Hauber, R., Wiggers, E., & Egner, A. (2001). Telehealth: Reaching out to newly injured spinal cord patients. *Public Health Reports*, *116*(Suppl. 1), 94–102.

Piotrowicz, E., & Piotrowicz, R. (2013). Cardiac telerehabilitation: Current situation and future challenges. *European Journal of Preventive Cardiology*, *20*(Suppl. 2), 12–16. doi:10.1177/2047487313487483c

Popescu, V., Burdea, G., Bouzit, M., Girone, M., & Hentz, V. (1999). PC-based telerehabilitation system with force feedback. *Studies in Health Technology & Informatics*, *62*, 261–267.

Popescu, V. G., Burdea, G. C., Bouzit, M., & Hentz, V. R. (2000). A virtual-reality-based telerehabilitation system with force feedback. *IEEE Transactions on Information Technology in Biomedicine*, *4*(1), 45–51.

Reinkensmeyer, D. J., Pang, C. T., Nessler, J. A., & Painter, C. C. (2002). Web-based telerehabilitation for the upper extremity after stroke. *IEEE Transactions on Neural Systems & Rehabilitation Engineering*, *10*(2), 102–108.

Rho, M. J., Choi, I. Y., & Lee, J. (2014). Predictive factors of telemedicine service acceptance and behavioral intentions of physicians. *International Journal of Medical Informatics*, *83*(8), 559–571.

Ricker, J. H., Rosenthal, M., Garay, E., DeLuca, J., Germain, A., Abraham-Fuchs, K., & Schmidt, K. U. (2002). Telerehabilitation needs: A survey of persons with acquired brain injury. *Journal of Head Trauma Rehabilitation*, *17*(3), 242–250.

Rojhani, S. N., Stiens, S. A., & Recio, A. C. (2016). Independent sailing with high tetraplegia using sip and puff controls: Integration into a community sailing center. *The Journal of Spinal Cord Medicine*, 1–10.

Stiens, S. A., Farber, H., & Yuhas, S. (2013). The person with spinal cord injury: An evolving prototype for life care planning. *Physical Medicine and Rehabilitation Clinics of North America*, *24*(3), 419–444.

Stiens, S. A., O'Young, B. J., & Young, M. A. (2008a). Methods and models for mastering physical medicine and rehabilitation. In *Physical medicine and rehabilitation secrets* (3rd ed., pp. xli–xlvi). Maryland Heights, MO: Elsevier

Stiens, S. A., O'Young, B. J., & Young, M. A. (2008b). Person-centered rehabilitation: Interdisciplinary intervention to enhance patient enablement. In *Physical medicine and rehabilitation secrets* (3rd ed., pp. 118–125). Maryland Heights, MO: Elsevier.

Stiens, S. A., Shamberg, S., & Shamberg, A. (2008c). Environmental barriers: Solutions for participation, collaboration, and togetherness. In *Physical medicine and rehabilitation secrets* (3rd ed., pp. 76–86). Maryland Heights, MO: Elsevier.

Tannor, A. Y., Haig, A. J., Christian, A., Smith, S., & Odonkor, C. (2016, May 29–June 2). *Online/in-person 1 year fellowship in PRM: A sustainable beginning for rehabilitation medicine in Sub-Saharan Africa*. Paper presented at ISPRM 2016, Kuala Lumpur, Malaysia. Retrieved from http://www.isprm2016.com/Documents/Suppl55KualaLumpur.pdf

Truter, P., Russel, T., & Fary, R. (2014). The validity of physical therapy assessment of low back pain via telerehabilitation in a clinical setting. *Telemedicine and E-Health*, *20*(1), 161–168

Tschabitscher, H. (2016). How many email addresses are there? *About Tech*. Retrieved from http://email.about.com/od/emailtrivia/f/how_many_email.htm

Tsuchisawa, K., Ono, K., Kanda, T., & Kelly, G. (2000). Japanese occupational therapy in community mental health and telehealth. *Journal of Telemedicine & Telecare*, *6*(Suppl. 2), S79–S80.

van der Linden, J., & Waights, V. (2012). A blended design approach for pervasive healthcare: Bringing together users, experts and technology. *Health Informatics Journal*, *18*(3), 212–218.

van Dijk, H., & Hermens, H. J. (2004). Distance training for the restoration of motor function. *Journal of Telemedicine & Telecare*, *10*(2), 63–71.

Van Dyk, L. (2014). A review of telehealth service implementation fromeworks. *International Journal of Environmental Research and Public Health*, *11*(2), 1279–1298.

Winters, J. M. (2002). Telemedicine research: Emerging opportunities. *Annual Review of Biomedical Engineering*, *17*(3), 242–250

Yamakawa, K., Tsai, C. K., Haig, A. J., Miner, J. A., & Harris, M. J. (2004). Relationship between ambulation and obesity in older persons with and without low back pain. *International Journal of Obesity*, *28*(1), 137–143.

Ylvisaker, M. (2003). Context-sensitive cognitive rehabilitation after brain injury: Theory and practice. *Brain Impairment*, *4*(1), 1–16.

Young, M., Stiens, S. A., & Hirsch, A. (2015). Vocational rehabilitation after stroke: Matching capability and contributions In J. Stein, R. L. Harley, C. J. Winstein, & C. J. Wittenberg (Eds.), *Stroke recovery and rehabilitation* (2nd ed.). New York, NY: Demos Medical.

Zampolini, M., Todechini, E., Guitart, M. B., Hermens, H., Ilsbroukx, S., Macellari, V., . . . Giacomozzi, C. (2008). Tele-rehabilitation: Present and future. *Annali dellIstituto Superiore di Sanità*, *44*(2), 125–134.

32

CHAPTER

Assistive Technology: Adaptive Tools of Enablement for Multiple Disabilities

Mark Young, Steven A. Stiens, Bryan O'Young, Raymona Baldwin, and Bryn N. Thatcher

Assistive technology enables dreams.
—Mathew Lee (personal communication)

Assistive technology (AT) provides powerful tools used to diminish disability, enable activities of daily living (ADLs), and promote recreational and vocational pursuits (Grott, 2015; Stiens, 1998). Persons with disabilities benefit from AT in a variety of ways: within their own bodies, such as through cochlear transplantation to enhance hearing; within the immediate environment, such as with a scooter to improve mobility; and within an extended environment, such as a wheelchair-adapted van (Boninger et al., 2008). This chapter serves as an introduction to AT tools, patient assessment, person-centered application of AT, and resources for patients and clinicians alike.

INTRODUCTION: DEFINITIONS AND VARIETIES OF INTERVENTIONS

Although the terms assistive technology, accessible technology, and adaptive technology are often used synonymously, there are semantic differences (Figure 32.1). Hersh and Johnson (2008) define *assistive technology* as

> . . . a generic or umbrella term that covers technologies, equipment, devices, apparatus, services, systems, processes, and environmental modifications used by disabled and/or elderly people to overcome the social, infrastructural, and other barriers to independence, full participation in society, and carrying out activities safely and easily. (p. 196)

Accessible technology is a general term used to describe "any item, piece of equipment or system, whether acquired commercially, modified or customized, that is utilized to increase, maintain or improve functional capabilities of individuals with disability" (Assistive Technology Act of 1998). Accessible technology may incorporate principles of universal design, and is either directly available and usable by people with a wide range of abilities and disabilities, or is compatible with assistive technology (AccessibleTech.org, 2014). *Adaptive technology* is a product created specifically to aid those who cannot use a regular version of a product. Adaptive technology is a subset of assistive technology and is almost solely used by persons with disabilities.

Nearly 8.5% of the U.S. civilian noninstitutionalized population is considered to have disability status, including hearing difficulty (6.2%), vision difficulty (6.5%), cognitive difficulty (7.0%), ambulatory difficulty (7.1%), self-care difficulty (7.1%), and independent living difficulty (6.9%; U.S. Census Bureau, 2014). AT has emerged as an essential tool in the rehabilitation and functional self-sufficiency in this growing and often underserved population. AT tools can improve cognitive, mental, and physical functioning by allowing persons with disabilities to compensate for impairments. As such, AT has become one

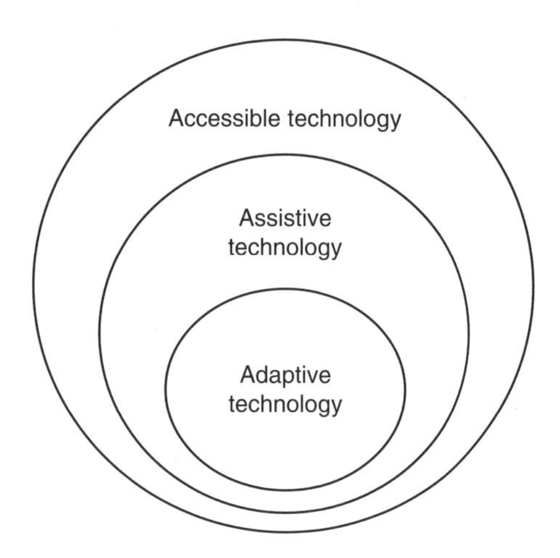

FIGURE 32.1 Hierarchy of technology categorizations from most inclusive to most specific.

of the most powerful tools in assisting persons with disabilities achieve social equality (Santiago-Pintor, Hernández-Maldonado, Correa-Colón, & Méndez-Fernández, 2009).

AT solutions are diverse in form, function, technology, and cost. Not all AT is sophisticated and high cost. Simple, low-tech solutions designed to address a particular impairment are often very effective and accessible to a broad range of consumers. A sticky note may aid a patient with a traumatic brain injury to compensate for memory deficits. A thicker spoon handle may aid a person with a dexterity impairment eat more easily. AT can increase independence, improve quality of life, and aid persons with disabilities in accomplishing educational and vocational pursuits.

The physical medicine and rehabilitation (PM&R) and neurorehabilitation fields have seen a dramatic increase in academic attention and scientific activities devoted to AT and innovation promoting equality among persons with disabilities. Many regional and international conferences focus on the expanding role of AT solutions. A recent learning colloquium focused on AT took place in 2012 at Johns Hopkins Hospital and the Workforce & Technology Center AT laboratory in Baltimore, Maryland. This teaching session served as a learning experience and informational session for health care providers in PM&R to acquaint them with strategies for incorporating AT into treatment arenas. Emphasis was placed on enabling people with disabilities or age-related impairments to reenter or competitively remain in the workforce (Young, Tumanon, & Sokal, 2000). On an international level, there have also been several seminal meetings, such as the 2009 International Neurorehabilitation Symposium, which have focused on emerging technologies and the critically important role of technology-assisted neurorehabilitation.

Although there are an increasing number of commercial technology and fee-based "add-on" programs available to meet the needs of persons with disabilities, this chapter emphasizes emerging technologies and basic complementary computer-based commercial applications, which are commonly found as part of standard operating systems. Computer technology, including Internet applications, serves as an indispensable tool to enhance vocational reentry and personal satisfaction. This chapter has a major emphasis on profiling specific AT solutions that enhance prognostic efficacy of vocational rehabilitation programs. Job descriptions and the series of steps a patient may need to complete in-work tasks need to be sequential, simple, adaptive interventions, introduced to produce efficiency and ease of work. This simply entails users turning functions on or off, or adjusting intensities or other such settings for optimal personal use on their electronic devices.

Enhancing quality of life for people with disabilities is an overarching goal of rehabilitation, and health care providers treating people with disabilities must be well versed in AT solutions to better serve patients (Stiens, Biener-Bergman, & Formal, 1997). When physical limitations and impairments hamper ADLs and functional skills, health care providers must serve as vital intermediaries to suggest solutions.

DISABILITY RIGHTS LAWS: ENTITLEMENT TO ASSISTIVE TECHNOLOGY AND REHABILITATION SERVICES

In 1989, the Office of Special Education and Rehabilitative Services in the U.S. Department of Education issued a statement saying, ". . . for some individuals with disabilities, assistive technology is a necessity that enables them to engage in or perform many tasks." Since this declaration, many laws addressing AT have been passed. The Technology Related Assistance for Individuals with Disabilities Act of 1988 (P.L. 100-407) provided federal funding to states to develop training and delivery systems for AT. The Assistive Technology Act of 1998 (P.L. 105-394) was an amendment to the previous Tech Act that extended the funding to develop "permanent, comprehensive, statewide programs of technology-related assistance." The Americans with Disabilities Act (ADA) of 1990 (and amendments of 2008) prohibits discrimination against individuals with disabilities in employment, transportation, public accommodation, communications, and governmental activities, often satisfied utilizing AT. The Individuals with Disabilities Education Act (IDEA), 1990 (P.L. 101-476) and 1997 (P.L. 105-17) outlined the responsibilities of school districts to provide AT to students with disabilities. AT must be "considered" on all individualized education plans (IEPs) to determine which AT devices or services are needed in order for the district to provide the student with a free and appropriate public education (FAPE). The 21st Century Communications and Video Accessibility Act of 2010 (P.L. 111-260) updated the nation's telecommunications protections for people with disabilities, including access to broadband, digital, and mobile innovations. The Workforce Innovation Opportunity Act (WIOA) was reauthorized in July 2014 and took effect in July 2015. This law mandates that AT devices and services be utilized with vocational training and in transition to employment. Education, vocation, and rehabilitation services are increasing major sources for funding of AT.

ASSISTIVE TECHNOLOGY TOOLS: PERSON-CENTERED, UNIQUE APPLICATIONS, AND UNIVERSAL INSTALLATIONS

Assistive technology tools span a large range, from simple machines to some of the most cutting-edge technology on the market today. Because of the expansive range of types and complexities of AT available, it is important for health care professionals to keep up-to-date with what can be utilized by their patients, and ways to adapt the tools for individual use.

AT must be considered in context, with the patients as developing individuals within their environments of choice. Each clinician must develop their concept of each patient within their environment in order to develop a consistent routine for assessment, AT intervention, and evaluation of outcome. A concentric model of the environment (see Figure 32.2) has been designed to relate the spaces spanning from inside a person out to the natural environment, which is not altered by adaptations for personal use. Within the environment, AT acts as a catalyst for function at various interfaces between environmental sectors. A series of examples includes a heart valve within the heart guiding blood flow; a pacemaker on the surface of the heart sequencing contraction of heart chambers; and an ankle foot orthosis fitted over the calf and across the ankle levering the person up as he or she leans forward for push off in gait. In the community environment, there may be ramps for access to higher surfaces, and synthetic voices and light signals to guide pedestrians safely across the street. This constellation of AT, either applied individually and prescriptively in person-centered rehabilitation of individuals, or governmental innovations to make cities more universally accessible, work synergistically to maximize independence of persons, and create potential for participation through collaboration to contribute to society.

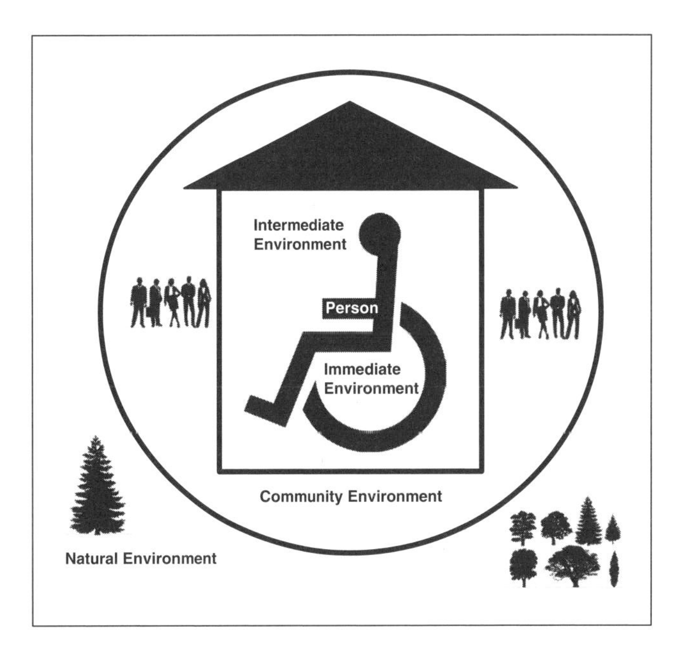

FIGURE 32.2 Individual person living in disablement. The sector inside the person is called the internal environment; the immediate environment is in contact with the person and travels with the person (i.e., clothes, braces, mobility devices, and communication devices); the intermediate environment includes the areas adapted for and used by the person (i.e., home and adapted vehicle); the community environment is managed by the local government and is as accessible as mandated by local law; the natural environment is unaltered and accessed as adaptive mobility solutions or trails will allow.
Source: Reprinted with permission from Stiens (1998).

The variety of conceptual models constructed to provide a big-picture understanding of AT intervention and outcomes are available for contemplation and comparison. Each clinician should explore descriptions of a subset of these models in order to construct his or her working model for clinical practice in order to have a vocabulary for interaction with institutions, interdisciplinary colleagues, patients, and families. Rehabilitation models illustrate relationships among measures of human performance, task completion, and societal impact. They depict relationships among current knowledge and provide a framework for consideration of new interventions, patient outcomes, and interdisciplinary strategies. Lenker and Paquet (2003) compared conceptual models examining the impact of AT. They considered models' descriptive characteristics, validation by literature, predictive characteristics, and utility to clinicians, developers, consumers, and payers.

Lewin published *Principles of Topological Psychology* in 1936 and articulated the roots of person–environmental models by suggesting individual's thoughts and behaviors result from the interaction between the person and the environment, and the best convergence produces the best outcomes. AT was categorized in an original, comprehensive text by Cook and Hessey published in 2002. They utilized a human activity and assistive technology (HAAT) model, including three components: human, activity, and assistive technology. They included the physical environment but added social and cultural influences to define "context." The human component includes innate capabilities and acquired skills at various levels of proficiency. Activity includes tasks in three principal life roles: self-care, work and school, and play and leisure. The AT device has a human–technology interface, a processor, and mechanical linkages to produce activity output. The activity output impacts the environment and is played out in the environment, including physical and social contexts. This model successfully accounts for variance in user, skill acquisition, AT device efficiency, and the influence of the environment and culture on task performance. The multiple variables considered provide the option of attempted standardization for case analysis and research.

The World Health Organization's (WHO) International Classification of Functioning, Disability and Health (ICF), revised in 2001, is a very useful model. Individuals are viewed from six perspectives: body structure and function, activity, perception of activity, and participation with awareness of environmental and personal factors. Activities and participation are carried out in the environment, which includes physical and sociocultural contexts. AT devices fit in the environment as indicated to improve activity and participation. The model provides a structure to classify AT devices. This model has transformed medical, and now rehabilitation research, from a problem-in-person perspective to consideration of an entire conceptual framework with multiple variables as foci for intervention and assessment (WHO, 2001). Such models provide an abstraction of the actual system providing variables that remind us to assess when planning AT intervention and to watch as AT implementation progresses in order to expect, facilitate, and recognize improvement in patients' participation, for example.

Universal Design: Adaptations to Maximize Function in Community Use

Global application of AT can be achieved through universal design, which is the process of designing products and spaces in a way that is accessible to the widest range of people possible (Rogers, 2015). Ronald Mace coined the term in 1997, and collaborated with architects, product designers, engineers, and environmental designers to develop the seven principles of universal design: equitable use, flexibility in use, simple and intuitive use, perceptible information, tolerance for error, low physical effort, and size and space for approachable use. This differs from mandates set forth by the ADA in that the ADA standards are the bare minimum design adjustments required to curb discrimination against people with disabilities, whereas universal design strives to make things safer, easier, and more convenient for everyone, regardless of disability status. For example, a ramp constructed next to a set of stairs may make a business ADA compliant, while a universally designed business might not have stairs at all, but rather a smooth, wide ramp entrance. Everything can be universally designed, from door handles to smartphones, and even teaching methods.

Everyone benefits from universal design because it takes into account the full range of human diversity, including physical, cognitive, and perceptual differences, as well as differences in body shapes and sizes (Rogers, 2015). In 2012, Steinfeld and Maisel created a list of goals to complement the principles of universal design, including body fit, comfort, awareness, understanding, wellness, social integration, personalization, and cultural appropriateness.

Simple Machines: Low Tech, High Impact

Not all AT is brand new and high or complicated tech. The greater goal of AT—to promote greater independence through enabling people to perform tasks that they were previously unable to do—can often be handled quite well with simple machines. Wedges, for instance, can be great positioning aids. Wedges are also utilized in the form of ramps, to lift people who cannot navigate steps or uneven surfaces. Wheels are another example of important AT, particularly for people who may need mobility assistance or aid in moving objects that would otherwise be too heavy. Levers are used as door handles and as joysticks, which are easily manipulated and can give input to other devices. Pulleys are often utilized for positioning or to complete strengthening exercises. Simple machines were some of the earliest tools utilized by humans. Many contain components of universal design, and are still extremely helpful in aiding people with disabilities and able-bodied people alike.

The Computer Age: A Renaissance in Enablement

This chapter would not be complete without a brief discussion of new frontiers and novel horizons in the field of AT. Undoubtedly, the emergence of new and unique computer, Internet, cyberspace technology, and program applications has revolutionized accessibility for people with all types of disabilities.

It is estimated that more than 277 million Americans (87%) currently use the Internet (Internet World Stats, 2014). The computer revolution resulted in a growing commitment of rehabilitation providers and their patients to successfully deploy technology to creatively accommodate impairments (Young et al., 2000). The global proliferation of desktops, laptops, notebooks, tablets, E-readers, personal digital assistants (PDAs), smartphones, and various other forms of technology has been met with a simultaneous increase in the number of persons with disabilities who use these devices for a wide range of purposes. Some of these include social (establishing friendships, relationships, and support); medical (providing data and information about conditions and treatment options, and telehealth, which is the act of seeing a clinician for a visit entirely on a computer screen); personal and household (accomplishing daily activities, such as shopping and ordering meals); psychological (providing access to resources); and vocational (optimizing employment outcomes and possibly securing home-based work) purposes (National Council on Disability, 1993). Microsoft, Apple, Google, and other manufacturers have web pages dedicated to accessibility for their operating systems and devices (see Microsoft Accessibility: www.microsoft.com/enable; Apple Accessibility: www.apple.com/accessibility; Google Accessibility: www.google.com/accessibility).

With the maturation of cyberspace, cell phone technology, and the introduction of new services and innovative applications, many new programs and imaginative products originally intended for the general public have proven to serve as a viable means of accommodation for persons with disabilities. Voice dictation is now widely available on Android, iPhone, and iPad. Users speak what they want dictated, including punctuation, and the device converts it to text. Voice dictation is also available for languages other than English. Composing and sending text messages, e-mails, and files by voice may be of benefit for persons with physical impairments of the upper extremities or visual impairments (see www.howtogeek.com/177387/use-voice-dictation-to-save-time-on-android-iphone-and-ipad for voice dictation instructions for your device).

Built-in "personal assistants" on smartphones are also a beneficial form of AT, sending messages, placing calls, searching the web, adding appointments, finding directions, and much more, all through voice command interactions with the user (see support.apple.com/en-us/HT204389 for Apple's Siri; windows.microsoft.com/en-us/windows-10/getstarted-what-is-cortana for Windows' Cortana; or www.google.com/landing/now/#howtogetit for Google Now). In addition to the built-in personal assistants, many apps provide alternative options that differ in settings and interface. With so many options and settings available through operating systems and apps, it really comes down to user preference and frequency of upgrade path possible for the individual and his or her budget.

Cutting-edge research developments recently spawned the growth of a new generation of AT, which successfully deploys robotics controlled by a neural–computer interface. Neural interface systems (NISs) have garnered much attention in the past few decades and represent a unique approach to restoring function and to managing nervous system disorders. NISs are devices placed into neurological tissue, such as the brain, which record and/or stimulate the tissue through electrode sites. Unfortunately, there are several issues with the current NISs, including poor reliability and degradation of the implant over time, and tissue trauma at the implant site (Anderson et al., 2015). Examples of currently used NISs include cochlear implants (CIs) for restoration of hearing, which came about in 1984, and deep brain stimulators (DBS), which began to be used in 2000, to attenuate tremor in patients with Parkinson's and other movement disorders (Peña et al., 2007). Motor cortex–based NISs that produce robotic motor movements in patients with tetraplegia and other paralytic states are in the early stages of development, and show tremendous promise as a new neurotechnology (Donoghue et al., 2006). Chou et al. (2015) have been working with a closed-loop neural interface to enable bidirectional communication between the biological and artificial parts of a hybrid system. This technology holds promise for increased performance of future NISs.

Another piece of cutting-edge AT being developed is brain–machine interface (BMI). BMI systems are able to infer user intent from neural data and transform it into output to control screen cursors, prosthetics, orthotic devices, and so forth, in real time (Venkatakrishnan, Francisco, & Contreras-Vidal, 2014). Important methods that need further development include training users to produce consistent electroencephalogram (EEG) signals and providing accurate EEG signals under subject-specific conditions. Signals are processed including incorporation of context and language information designs, and as with all AT, tailored to individual users (Akcakaya et al., 2014).

■ Social Media: An Environment That Neutralizes Disabilities

Since its inception in the late 1990s, use of social media has exploded. People of all ages from all over the world are utilizing social media. Some easy guidelines to remember are to use styles that help screen readers navigate content in the correct order, refrain from setting type in smaller than 12-point font, and make sure every picture has a caption that accompanies it and adequately describes it. Several accessibility checkers exist on the World Wide Web.

In 2011, Dr. Scott Hollier, a researcher with Media Access Australia and The Australian Communications Consumer Action Network (ACCAN), set out to analyze the accessibility of social media and provide practical guides for social media use and how to overcome accessibility issues for some of the major forms of social media (Facebook, LinkedIn, YouTube, Twitter, blogging, and Skype). Major themes include the benefits of persons with disabilities to have access to personal, social, professional, educational, and entertainment resources without having to navigate difficult physical or social terrains. Overviews of practical tips and tricks users have used to make the different platforms more acces sible are provided. Hollier's full report can be downloaded here: www.mediaaccess.org.au/web/social-media-for-people-with-a-disability

■ The Virtual Self: Living Other Lives Independent of Impairments

Recent attention has been drawn to the experiences of people with lifelong disabilities and their presence in virtual worlds as avatars. Such experiences provide out of body lives in separate prosthetic environments. Avatars can be created with and without visible disability, allowing people to disclose as much or as little as they choose about their disability status as they interact with others embodied in the environment. In 1998, Witmer and Singer created a presence questionnaire (PQ) to measure presence in virtual environments and an immersive tendencies questionnaire (ITQ) to measure different tendencies in the experience of presence. Stendal, Molka-Danielsen, Munkvold, and Balandin (2012) looked at this phenomenon through the lens of embodied social presence (ESP) theory and found users felt a sense of connectedness with others, and experienced users felt a strong connection with their avatars and had an understanding that other humans are represented by their avatars as means for visual and simulated physical encounters for communication. This form of interaction allows people with disabilities to present themselves in ways that may avoid their insecurities and the biases present in the real world.

ASSESSMENT OF THE PATIENT: PERSON-CENTERED APPLICATIONS

AT can be useless if it is not adapted for the use of the specific individual (Stiens, Shamberg, & Shamberg, 2008). Prosthetics need to fit appropriately, technological innovations need to be understood and easily managed by the user and hearing aids need to be adjusted to the perceptual needs of the user. Even if a similar device is being used with multiple patients, the specific user's personal needs and life aspirations are of the utmost importance in the choice and customization of AT. Fit and settings vary widely from one user to another. Person-centered application plays a vital role in the utilization of AT.

There are a number of interventions and strategies that may be used to aid in the successful application of AT. Physicians, occupational therapists, and biomedical engineers can work with individuals to ensure appropriate fit or settings on prosthetics and perceptual aids. Physical and occupational therapists can aid in the proper utilization of AT devices for clinical purposes and make referrals to other providers for topics outside the clinic's scope. Psychologists, counselors, social workers, and palliative care teams work with patients and families to elicit values, develop goals, and seek resources for procuring and paying for AT devices (some pertinent resources can be found at resnaprojects.org/statewide/resources.html and www.rmmor.org). It is extremely important for these health care professionals to work together and with the patient to provide the most efficient care possible and have the best practical outcomes.

In the past two decades, shared decision making (SDM) has become an important model for patients, families, and health care providers to communicate and determine the best treatment plan for the individual. The provider brings clinical evidence, the patient and family bring personal values, and a discussion of clinical risks and benefits, quality-of-life considerations and ethical considerations allows for informed, collaborative decisions to be made (Nelson & Mahant, 2014). It is important to remember that these discussions may need to be repeated and adjusted as treatment progresses, and that other health care professionals that the family trusts can be added to the decision-making team. Counselors, social workers, or palliative care teams may help the family consider hopes and concerns around both daily living and the broader picture; understand family structure, support and finances; and possibly even be able to link patient families to other families and resources, such as listservs, blogs, or online support groups, for support and discussion. SDM lends itself well to overall patient and family satisfaction, and can be particularly useful with elderly, pediatric, or incapacitated patients whose families may have a larger role in the decision-making process.

AT evaluation and implementation are subcomponents of the process of rehabilitation. Rehabilitation is the process of development of a person to his or her fullest physical, psychological, social, educational, and vocational potential by eliminating or compensating for any biochemistry/pathophysiology, systemic impairment, activity limitation, or environmental barrier (Stiens, O'Young, & Young, 2008). The purpose of the AT assessment is to determine the specific equipment and services needed to help the patient meet health and functional life goals. The process can begin the first phase with a consult from a physiatrist, or by recognition of need by an allied health clinician. Assessment should be driven by the therapist or clinician most familiar with the problem (impairment, disability, or participation barrier). Patient and family interviews provide sufficient information for identification of impairments, task limitations, and participation barriers that prevent essential life roles and personal passions. Specific target activities are identified, such as attendance at school when at home or on required bed rest. Specifications are defined, such as computer keyboard control, adjustable gaze in the classroom, and sufficient voice volume to be heard in class. The second phase begins with device trial and training. The patient, family, and attendants trial screen options for telepresence starting with Skype and Facetime, and continuing to robotic options that can be driven through the classroom. The clinician must carefully match and adapt each device for ideal trial, and provide a perspective for the amount of training or practice required to achieve best proficiency. The aim is to design a match that will achieve training to acceptance and efficient functions used to meet person-centered life goals.

Abandonment can be prevented with attention to patient characteristics, environmental factors, and AT device technology (Galvin & Scherer, 1996). Environmental factors need to be addressed with intensive training in environment of use, minimization of obstacles, and establishment of a sound financial plan. AT device specifications need to meet functional performance. There must be compatibility with user capabilities, sufficient training, dependability, usability, and aesthetics. Patient-centered characteristics must include minimal needs, activity prioritized by high motivation, fluctuation in strength, daily schedule, and lifestyle, assistance available to sustain device use, self-esteem, status, and independence associated with device use.

IMPAIRMENT-SPECIFIC ASSISTIVE TECHNOLOGY: UNIQUE APPLICATIONS

Motor and Dexterity: The Human Path of Ambulation and Manipulation

According to the U.S. Census Bureau (2014), 7.1 % of the population has ambulatory difficulty. Increased motor impairment in the aging population, and returning war veterans who have experienced traumatic injury, are two populations increasingly utilizing mobility AT. Although voice-recognition technology is often useful in helping motor- and dexterity-impaired patients meet their needs, many of these patients prefer to initially use whatever residual dexterity and motor functioning they have. In addition, patients with quadriplegia, stroke, amyotrophic lateral sclerosis, amputations or cerebral palsy can benefit from using environmental control units (ECUs), more broadly described as electronic aids to daily living (EADLs). ECUs are apparatuses that control household systems and devices, such as lamps, televisions, telephones, and alarm systems. Similar to television remote controls, they are typically switches manipulated by the lips, chin, eyes, or other body or muscular movements. One such method, sip-and-puff (SNP), sends signals to a device using air pressure: "sipping" (inhaling) or "puffing" (exhaling) on a straw, tube, or wand. Examples of such ECUs using SNP include doors equipped with electronic openers, electronic locks, coffee makers, lights, call buttons, and TV sets controlled by switch control. It is common for these ECUs to be in place in the home setting, and workplaces can also utilize them to appropriately accommodate employees with motor or dexterity impairments.

Persons with disabilities or elderly persons with mobility issues can often benefit from AT that assists with ADLs. AT devices like the Roomba, Scooba, and Braava, which use sensors to navigate floor space and vacuum, scrub floors and mop with the push of a button, provide accessible cleaning options. A similar device, the Mirra, cleans pools. This robotic technology doesn't just assist, but actually completes tasks independently, allowing people to save valuable time and complete other tasks.

■ Computer Use

Dexterity impairment and difficulty with coordination are caused by a number of neurological and musculoskeletal conditions, including stroke, carpal tunnel syndrome, arthritis, cerebral palsy, Parkinson's disease, multiple sclerosis, loss of limbs or digits, spinal cord injuries, and repetitive stress injury, among others. In their book, *Physical Disabilities and Computing Technologies: An Analysis of Impairments*, Sears and Young (2003) comprehensively survey health conditions that induce impairments affecting computer use.

A new and evolving generation of AT has facilitated the use of computers by people with motor or dexterity impairments. The Microsoft and Apple accessibility web pages have sections that specifically address dexterity and mobility impairments. These highlight settings that can be adjusted on devices, such as keyboard shortcuts and mouse keys.

People with motor or dexterity impairments often encounter difficulty using standard "hands-on" input items such as the keyboard, mouse, or track pad. Several hardware and software alternatives or enhancements are available. A chin mouse, a headset that generates a radio signal, an eye-gaze unit, a mouth stick, or other hands-free signaling units can aid users with independent computer access. There are also frames that fit over a keyboard that help reduce errant keystrokes. Other physical interventions include adjusting settings on a programmable mouse or keyboard guard to best suit the user. Individuals who have little or no use of their hands need on-screen keyboards with user-selectable functions. The user selects the keys with a mouse, touch screen, trackball, joystick, switch, or electronic pointing device that allows the user to control his or her computer entirely without a keyboard. Keyboard filters include typing aids such as word prediction utilities and add-on spell-checkers. This technology reduces the minimum number of keystrokes and enables users to quickly access letters and avoid selecting the wrong keys.

Touch screens are devices placed on the computer monitor (or built into it) that allow direct selection or activation of the computer by touching the screen and completely eliminate the need for a mouse. Brain–machine interfaces are also being explored for this medium (for a comparison of hands-on versus hands-free modes of computer-related AT for people with motor impairments, see Table 32.1).

Software-Based (Operating System) Adaptations: Keystroke Modifications

In addition to input devices, there are various software-based adaptations to help people with motor impairments operate computers more easily. For instance, the Microsoft filter key feature blocks repeated keystrokes, ignores rapid or extraneous keystrokes, and slows down repeated key rates. This enables quick access to letters and helps users avoid inadvertently selecting the wrong keys. The filter key feature can help patients suffering from chronic neurological disorders such as parkinsonism or other conditions that manifest symptoms such as tremors, stiffness, or poor coordination. Voice-to-text software, such as Dragon Naturally Speaking, also assists these users, especially in initial stages of progression. Individuals who are mobile and lucid, but experiencing significant tremor or varying levels of speech acuity, are good candidates for this technology. They want to make the most of the functional capacity they have at any given moment.

TABLE 32.1

HANDS-ON VS. HANDS-FREE ASSISTIVE TECHNOLOGY AT INPUT MODES

Hands-On	Hands-Free
Keyboard	Sips and puffs (SNP)
Mouse	Head movement
Joystick	Eye movement
Trackball	Foot movement
Touch pads	Switches manipulated by other body parts
Touchscreen	Brain–machine interfaces (BMI)

Spelling-prediction software is a good example of universally designed AT, making things like texting quick and convenient for users of all abilities. When using spelling-prediction software, a list of predicted words appears as each key is typed, in the hope of finishing user words in the least amount of keystrokes. The software also predicts the next word (word prediction) and offers abbreviation expansion and speech output. Spell check is another feature of spelling prediction software, reducing the number of keys typed and improving word accuracy.

Visual: Acuity Enhancement, Auditory Cues, and Tactile Compensations

Auditory stimuli are often valuable for persons with vision impairments. Listening to audiobooks or to radio stations that broadcast readings are two viable forms of AT. Various read-aloud devices, including watches, clocks, thermostats, calculators, microwave ovens, money identifiers, compasses, toys, dictionaries, e-readers, and medical devices such as thermometers, scales, sphygmomanometers, and glucometers, are all valuable tools that aid in ADLs, medical, recreational, vocational, and educational activities.

For people with low vision, many magnification options, including handheld optics and monocular glasses, are available. For greater magnification, closed circuit television (CCTV) or software may be used to magnify and enhance images and text for those with residual vision. CCTVs are readily available in a variety of formats, including smaller handheld cameras, self-contained units with folding flat screens, and virtual-reality helmets.

Braille technology combined with voice applications promotes self-sufficiency in ADLs, such as walking and wayfinding. A new AT system has been designed to aid vision-impaired people in wayfinding through the use of a camera cell phone, to find and read aloud specially designed signs in the environment. These signs are wayfinding barcodes marked with simple color patterns (targets) that can be quickly and reliably identified using image-processing algorithms running on the camera cell phone (Coughlan & Manduchi, 2007). Another approach is the application of Braille or other tactile markings on items such as thermostats, telephones, rulers, clocks, calendars, ATM machines, and keyboards.

Computer Use

Persons with visual impairments using a computer with a QWERTY keyboard layout can obtain output through the use of screen-reader software, which provides computer-synthesized voice output. For those who prefer to obtain Braille output, refreshable Braille displays are available. This display, which is hardware that is attached to a computer, receives messages from the computer through screen translator software and presents these messages to the user in Braille. The Braille display updates as the user moves the cursor on the computer screen.

Screen color configurations, screen magnification, and cursor enhancements can also be altered and utilized to match the requirements of computer users with vision impairments. Several screen magnification programs, most significantly Zoom Text, offer a connected speech component that supplements the visible text with voice interpretation. Persons who are blind or visually impaired often benefit from using text-to-speech software, such as JAWS or NVDIA, which read aloud the text that is on a computer screen. A host of solutions are also available to make a keyboard and mouse easier to use, or completely eliminate their use for those who are completely blind. A user can dispense with mouse and keyboard altogether by typing on screen and by using speech recognition software. A growing number of Certified Vocational Rehabilitation Programs throughout the United States, including the Workforce & Technology Center in Baltimore, Maryland, have pioneered technology programs for blind patients seeking to mainstream back into the workplace using these technologies and strategies (Young, Desai, & Young, 2009).

Considerations for Patients With Diabetes

In the acute inpatient rehabilitation setting and in the subacute and outpatient arenas, diabetes-related visual impairments often become obvious to the clinician. For those diabetic patients identified in the rehabilitation setting who do not have visual disturbances or other forms of secondary diabetic complications, the rehabilitation team can play an essential preventive and educational role in averting the long-term consequences of the disease.

However, if the disease has progressed such that a diabetic patient experiences serious visual impairment, the job of the physicians becomes much more challenging, and disease management becomes more complicated. The blind diabetic patient poses a special rehabilitation challenge because of the critically important goals of balancing optimal management of glycemic control (maintaining sugars at a normal level) and increasing the ability to perform essential ADLs, thus improving overall functional status.

Blind diabetic patients who live alone often encounter problems reading standard glucose meters. This may lead to worsening of complications of many diabetes-related conditions. It is important to understand the relevance of vision-related problems in diabetic patients and the respective challenges they pose for physicians and caregivers alike. A better understanding on the part of physicians can enhance their ability to provide better care and more thorough chronic disease management for this population. Devices like talking glucometers "speak" blood glucose concentrations, time, date, and historical blood glucose levels. Use of this device has revolutionized the lives of diabetic patients with vision impairments and other disabilities. For a vision-impaired diabetic patient who does not have access to help from others to monitor blood glucose, a talking glucometer can provide essential assistance. The talking glucometer is one type of AT that should be introduced as part of comprehensive management of diabetes-related vision impairment.

Auditory: Amplification, Translation to Text and Visual Cues

According to Blackwell, Lucas, and Clarke (2014), in their research for the National Center for Health Statistics, over 15% of U.S adults have some sort of hearing trouble without the assistance of a hearing aid. Hearing impairments, represented by a wide range of conditions from mild hearing loss to deafness, are often discovered on the rehabilitation unit or in the outpatient PM&R setting. Although the incidence of hearing impairments is higher among older individuals, no age range is excluded. Presence of auditory impairment may impede the rehabilitation process, and can severely decrease work productivity and efficiency in the occupational setting if unaddressed.

Deafness is broadly defined as "a hearing impairment that impairs the processing of linguistic information through hearing, with or without amplification." Deafness can be viewed as a sensory state that prevents an individual from receiving sound in all or most of its forms. In contrast, "hearing loss" implies an impaired ability to sense sound but with some level of responsiveness to auditory stimuli, including speech.

Amplification devices, such as hearing aids and amplification telephones, have long been the mainstay for people with hearing impairments (Ross, 2008). However, hearing aids can be incapable of providing adequate assistance in certain situations, like noisy environments. In such situations, hearing impairment may instead be remedied by use of directional microphones or devices based on induction loops, infrared, or frequency modulation. These devices make events such as watching movies, meetings, and seminars more accessible. An alternative AT solution is TV monitor closed captioning, which is mandated by the Federal Communications Commission for TV programs from video programming distributors, and can be utilized by other media as needed.

Many AT devices are available to aid deaf people in common daily activities. These include signals that utilize senses other than hearing, such as flashing lights and vibrations, to alert of ringing phones, doorbells, smoke detectors, and alarm clocks. Vibrating watch alarms and pagers are other valuable assistive technologies for those with hearing impairments. Some people with hearing impairments, while unable to hear spoken words, may still be able to hear sounds. This should be taken into account when recommending appropriate AT.

Computer Use

With the prevalence of technology in modern society, it is important to understand the various challenges computers present for people with hearing impairments, and what clinicians, caregivers, and patients can do to overcome these challenges. Add-on software, allowing users to adjust volume and other sound options, enables computer users with hearing impairments to set settings that fit their individual needs, or receive information visually.

Various software companies, including Microsoft and Apple, manufacture products that enhance computer accessibility for hearing-impaired and deaf people. Audio alerts can be replaced with visual alerts. Physicians and therapy teams can suggest some of these features to facilitate smoother use of computer operating systems for patients with hearing impairments. Some patients, particularly older individuals, may benefit from a referral to occupational therapy or community-based services for assistance in setup and use of newer technological interventions.

Telecommunications

State or federal funds support telecommunications relay service (TRS) for persons with hearing or speech disabilities. Some common forms of TRS are text-to-voice (TTY), voice carryover, and video relay service (VRS). Communication assistants (CAs) are intermediaries who facilitate the calls. TTY is the "traditional" form of TRS in which a person with a hearing disability communicates by text to the CA, who voices the messages to a hearing recipient and then responds what was said in response via text. However, with advancements in technology, this medium is becoming used far less frequently. Voice carryover allows a person with a hearing disability to vocalize outgoing messages while receiving responses via text from a CA. VRS allows persons who communicate in sign language to communicate with a CA in ASL who speaks what is signed to the called party and then signs back to the caller what was said. Persons who cannot speak may benefit from using synthetic speech software, which generates speech produced by an electronic synthesizer activated by a keyboard. Currently, programs such as Facetime and Skype enable people who communicate in sign language to communicate through video stream. Many of these programs are free and Internet-based, making them convenient and highly utilized forms of communication.

Hearing With Visual: Utilizing Hybridized AT and Tactile Cues

People with both hearing and vision impairments are sometimes referred to as being deaf–blind. Many of the technologies helpful to people with individual sensory impairments also apply to the deaf–blind population. However, adaptations are necessary. For example, telephone access can be optimized through the use of TTYs with large print capability. Amplification phones equipped with Braille markings may assist people with partial residual hearing (Fellbaum & Koroupetroglou, 2008). Computer operating systems can be adapted to enable those with visual or auditory impairments to enjoy unconstrained computer usage. Apple, Google, Microsoft, and others provide resources for this rich and varied area.

Devices in the home and workplace can attract the attention of people who are deaf–blind to inform them of particular environmental circumstances. Alarm clocks equipped with crystal and tactile markings or pillow alarm shakers alert users who would otherwise be unable to hear or see standard alarms. Devices can use assertive vibration, scents or fan-driven air to alert of a telephone ringing or a smoke detector sounding.

Given the prevalence of visual and hearing impairments of patients treated with rehabilitation, it is critical for clinicians to understand the impact these disabilities have on the long-term well-being of their patients. With the goal of promoting better case management, clinicians can use AT as the instrument to assist in improving the quality of life of a deaf–blind patient.

Cognitive: Multimodal Learning Methods, Cueing for Productivity, and Monitoring for Safety

Approximately 7.0% of the U.S. civilian noninstitutionalized population has cognitive difficulty (U.S. Census Bureau, 2014). People with cognitive impairments include but are not limited to those with learning disabilities, psychiatric disabilities, Alzheimer's disease and other dementias, and traumatic brain injury. Cognitive impairments are often overlooked in the evaluation for AT; however, AT proves quite beneficial in providing aid and independence for patients experiencing difficulty with abstract thinking, decision making, long- or short-term memory, learning skills, perception, coordination, or concentration (Disability Rights New Jersey, 2015). AT utilizes the skills patients with cognitive disabilities have in order to offset skills they do not possess (Iowa Center for Assistive Technology Education and Research, 2015).

AT is being highly utilized with student populations with cognitive impairments in the educational setting. Low tech AT, such as color-coding systems, can be used as organizational tools. Higher-tech solutions, such as speech recognition software and scan-and-read programs, can aid students with dyslexia and a host of other learning disabilities. Universal design for learning (UDL) consists of instructional approaches that incorporate multiple forms of materials, content, tools, context, and supports that allow students choices and alternatives that best suit their learning needs (Izzo & Bauer, 2013). Apps for tablets, speech-to-text programs, and other technologies are being integrated into IEPs (an "IEP" is an individualized educational plan customized and designed to meet the educational needs of persons with disability), 504 plans (a 504 is a civil rights safeguard that seeks to remove barriers from participation and facilitates students with disabilities to pursue educational opportunities no different than an able-bodied person). UDL methods often meet IEP objectives and also provide many benefits for the general education population.

An estimated 5.3 million Americans had Alzheimer's disease in 2015, including one in nine people aged 65 and older (Alzheimer's Association, 2015). AT can be very beneficial for this population, supplementing human caregiving and fostering independence. Three pertinent goals of AT for cognition include providing assurance an elder is safe and performing ADLs, and if not, alerting caregivers; assisting with ADLs and providing compensation for impairments; and assessing an elder's cognitive status (Pollack, 2005). Assurance systems, such as sensors and monitoring systems, are currently available as commercial products; compensation systems, including navigational systems and schedule management, continue to be researched; and cognitive assessment systems that can be performed outside the clinical setting are emerging.

Performance of ADLs within the home environment of aged persons (with and without Alzheimer's) is an essential requisite for independence. Home environmental skills and tasks, often taken for granted during earlier life, now frequently become an impediment to independent living. An example of this is home environmental maintenance, including custodial and cleaning tasks. The advent of robotic technology has mitigated this potential impediment. Service robots are a distinct category of functional automated technology that is designed to perform a precise task. Robotic cleaning products, such as the Roomba, provide automated robotic assistance to elderly people living alone. The Roomba is an example of a service robot in a domestic environment that vacuums the floor automatically (Forlizzi & DiSalvo, 2006).

Improving socialization skills among Alzheimer's patients can also be optimized with AT and robotic technology. PARO is an advanced interactive robot that advances the benefits of animal therapy with aged patients in environments such as hospitals and extended care facilities. PARO is an example of a robotic animal (panda), which promotes interaction and social discourse among citizens with Alzheimer's disease. Burton (2013) examines the benefits and disadvantages of animal treatment modalities for persons with neurologic disorders.

CONCLUSION: IDENTIFYING IMPAIRMENTS, PRESCRIBING INDIVIDUALIZED AT, AND RECOGNIZING EMERGING USEFUL TECHNOLOGIES

The coming of the computer age and the revolutionary array of Internet technologies have enabled persons with disabilities to optimize quality of life now more than ever through creative accommodation (Young et al., 2000). While the practice of medicine and the domain of PM&R have traditionally emphasized healing and rehabilitation through physical, pharmacological, and psychological interventions, the rehabilitation process often requires another critical, yet overlooked component—evaluation for and provision of assistive technology.

This chapter has attempted to provide a comprehensive overview of available and emerging technologies that provide persons with disabilities the opportunity to further their rehabilitation process through accessibility and accommodation. After reading this chapter, we hope you have gained an understanding of the breadth of AT available for a variety of disabilities, and will seek out further and more specific knowledge as it applies to your own patients. AT has the potential to help people with disabilities function personally and professionally, and as health care providers, it is vital to be informed about different modalities, and assist patients in choosing, procuring, and funding AT that will benefit them the most.

RESOURCES

AbleData: http://abledata.squarespace.com
Accessibility Apple: http://www.apple.com/accessibility
Accessibility Microsoft: http://www.microsoft.com/enable
Center for Inclusive Design and Environmental Access (IDeA): http://idea.ap.buffalo.edu//Home/index.asp
Cortana (Windows): http://windows.microsoft.com/en-us/windows-10/getstarted-what-is-cortana
FCC TRS: https://www.fcc.gov/guides/telecommunications-relay-service-trs
GoodHealthwill: http://www.rmmor.org
Google Now: https://www.google.com/landing/now
National Assistive Technology Technical Assistance Partnership (NATTAP): http://resnaprojects.org/statewide/resources.html
Siri (Apple): https://support.apple.com/en-us/HT204389
Social Media for People with a Disability: http://www.mediaaccess.org.au/web/social-media-for-people-with-a-disability
UniversalDesign.com: http://www.universaldesign.com
Voice Dictation: http://www.howtogeek.com/177387/use-voice-dictation-to-save-time-on-android-iphone-and-ipad

YouTube Videos:

What is Assistive Technology: https://www.youtube.com/watch?v=SIm2MuJUCTE&feature=youtu.be

Assistive Technology: Enabling Dreams: https://www.youtube.com/watch?v=rXxdxck8Gic&feature=youtu.be

Ellen—Using Assistive Technology:
https://www.youtube.com/watch?v=fAdEOXD9Tvk&feature=youtu.be

Assistive Technology in Action—Meet Jared: https://www.youtube.com/watch?v=Bhj5vs9P5cw&feature=youtu.be

I Love Assistive Technology!: https://www.youtube.com/watch?v=l_P8OG04wqc&feature=youtu.be

REFERENCES

AccessibleTech.org. (2014). What is accessible electronic and information technology? Retrieved from http://accessibletech.org/access_articles/general/whatIsAccessibleEIT.php

Anderson, D., Kipke, D. R., Hetke, J., Vetter, R. J., Kong, K., & Seymour, J. (2015). *U.S. patent No. 8954144 B2*. Washington, DC: U.S. Patent and Trademark Office.

Akcakaya, M., Peters, B., Moghadamfalahi, M., Mooney, A. R., Orhan, U., Oken, B., . . . Fried-Oken, M. (2014). Noninvasive brain-computer interfaces for augmentative and alternative communication. *IEEE Reviews in Biomedical Engineering, 7*, 31–49.

Alzheimer's Association. (2015). 2015 Alzheimer's disease facts and figures. *Alzheimer's & Dementia, 11*(3), 1–83.

Assistive Technology Act of 1998. (1998). Retrieved from http://www.section508.gov/docs/AT1998.html

Blackwell, D. L., Lucas, J. W., & Clarke, T. C. (2014). Summary health statistics for U.S. adults: National health interview survey, 2012. National center for health statistics. *VitalHealth Statistics, 10*(260), 1–161.

Boninger, M. L., Choi, H., Johnson, K., Young, M. A., Stiens, S. A., & Sears, A. (2008). Assistive technologies: Catalysts for adaptive function. In B. O'Young, M. Young, & S. Stiens (Eds.), *Physical medicine & rehabilitation secrets* (3rd ed., pp. 201–206). Philadelphia, PA: Mosby Elsevier.

Burton, A. (2013). Dolphins, dogs, and robot seals for the treatment of neurological disease. *The Lancet Neurology, 12*(9), 851–852.

Chou, Z., Lim, J., Brown, S., Keller, M., Bugbee, J., Broccard, F. D., . . . Cauwenberghs, G. (2015). Bidirectional neural interface: Closed-loop feedback control for hybrid neural systems. *Engineering in Medicine and Biology Society (EMBC), 2015 37th Annual International Conference of the IEEE, 10*, 3949–3952.

Coughlan, J., & Manduchi, R. (2007, April). *Functional assessment of a camera phone-based wayfinding system operated by blind users*. The Conference on IEEE Computer Society and the Biological and Artificial Intelligence Society (IEEE-BAIS). Research on Assistive Technologies Symposium (RAT '07), Dayton, OH.

Disability Rights New Jersey. (2015). Assistive technology for individuals with cognitive andpsychiatric disabilities. Retrieved from http://www.drnj.org/atac/?p=66

Donoghue, J. P., Friehs, G. M., Caplan, A. H., Stein, J., Mukand, J. A., Chen, D., . . . Hochberg, L. R. (2006). BrainGate neuromotor prosthesis: First experience by a person with brainstem stroke. *Society for Neuroscience Abstracts, 256*, 10.

Fellbaum, K., & Koroupetroglou, G. (2008). Principles of electronic speech processing withapplications for people with disabilities. *Technology and Disability, 20*, 55–85.

Forlizzi, J., & DiSalvo, C. (2006). Service robots in the domestic environment: A study of the Roomba vacuum in the home. *Proceedings of the 1st ACM SIGCHI/SIGART conference on human-robot interaction (HRI '06)*, 258–265.

Galvin, J. C., & Scherer, M. J (Eds.). (1996). *Evaluating, selecting and using appropriate assistive technology*. Gaithersburg, MD: Aspen.

Grott, R. (2015). Maximizing employment outcomes through the use of "lower-tech" assistivetechnology & rehabilitation engineering. *Studies in Health Technology and Informatics, 217*, 241–246.

Hersh, M. A., & Johnson, M. A. (2008). On modeling assistive technology systems-Part I: Modeling framework. *Technology and Disability, 20*, 193–215.

Internet World Stats. (2014). *United States of America internet usage and broadband usage report*. Retrieved from http://www.internetworldstats.com/am/us.htm

Iowa Center for Assistive Technology Education and Research. (2015). Module 6: Overview of assistive technology for people with various disabilities. Retrieved from http://www.continuetolearn.uiowa.edu/nas1/07c187/Begin%20Here.htm

Izzo, M. V., & Bauer, W. M. (2013). Universal design for learning: Enhancing achievement and employment of STEM students with disabilities. *Universal Access in the Information Society, 14*, 17–27.

Lenker, J. A., & Paquet, V. L. (2003). A review of conceptual models for assistivetechnology outcomes research and practice. *Assistive Technology, 15*(1), 1–15.

National Council on Disability. (1993). *Study on the financing of assistive technology devices and services for individuals with disabilities: Report to the President and the Congress of the United States*. Washington, DC: Author.

Nelson, K. E., & Mahant, S. (2014). Shared decision-making about assistive technology for thechild with severe neurological impairment. *Pediatric Clinics of North America, 61*(4), 641–652.

Peña, C., Bowsher, K., Costello, A., DeLuca, R., Doll, S., Li, K., . . . Stevens, T. (2007). An overview of FDA medical device regulation as it relates to deep brain stimulation devices. *IEEE Transactions on Neural Systems & Rehabilitation Engineering, 15*(3), 421–424.

Pollack, M. E. (2005). Intelligent technology for an aging population: The use of AI to assist elders with cognitive impairment. *AI Magazine, 26*(2), 9–24.

Rogers, D. (Ed.). (2015). What is universal design? Retrieved from http://www.universaldesign.com/what-is-ud/

Ross, M. (2008). What did you expect? Hearing aids: Expectation and aural rehabilitation. *Hearing Loss, 29*, 20–24.

Santiago-Pintor, J., Hernández-Maldonado, M., Correa-Colón, A., & Méndez-Fernández, H. L. (2009). Assistive technology: A health care reform for people with disabilities. *Puerto Rico Health Sciences Journal, 28*, 44–47.

Sears, A., & Young, M. (2003). *Physical disabilities and computing technologies: An analysis of impairments.* Hillsdale, NJ: L. Erlbaum Associates.

Stiens, S. A. (1998). Personhood, disablement, and mobility technology. In D. B. Gray, L. A. Quatrano, & M. Lieberman (Eds.), *Designing and using assistive technology: The human perspective* (pp. 29–49). Towson, MD: Paul Brookes.

Stiens, S. A., Biener-Bergman, S., & Formal, C. S. (1997). Spinal cord injury rehabilitation: Individual experience, personal adaptation, and social perspectives. *Archives of Physical Medicine and Rehabilitation, 78*, S65–S72.

Stiens, S. A., O'Young, B. J., & Young, M. A. (2008). Person-Centered rehabilitation: Interdisciplinary intervention to enhance patient enablement. In B. J. O'Young, M. A. Young, & S. A. Stiens (Eds.), *Physical medicine and rehabilitation secrets* (3rd ed., pp. 118–125). Maryland Heights, MO: Mosby.

Stiens, S. A., Shamberg, S., & Shamberg, A. (2008). Environmental barriers: Solutionsfor participation, collaboration, and togetherness. In B. J. O'Young, M. A. Young, & S. A. Stiens (Eds.), *Physical medicine and rehabilitation secrets* (3rd ed., pp. 76–86). Maryland Heights, MO: Mosby.

Steinfeld, E., & Maisel, J. (2012). *Universal design: Creating inclusive environments.* Hoboken, NJ: Wiley.

Stendal, K., Molka-Danielsen, J., Munkvold, B. E., & Balandin, S. (2012). Virtual worlds and people with lifelong disability: Exploring the relationship with virtual self and others. *ECIS2012 Proceedings, Paper 156*, 156–179.

U.S. Census Bureau. (2014). 2014 American community survey 1-year estimates. Retrieved from http://factfinder.census.gov/faces/tableservices/jsf/pages/productview.xhtml?pid=ACS_12_1YR_S1810&prodType=table

Venkatakrishnan, A., Francisco, G. E., & Contreras-Vidal, J. L. (2014). Applications of brain-machine interface systems in stroke recovery and rehabilitation. *Current Physical Medicine and Rehabilitation Reports, 2*, 93–105.

Witmer, B. G., & Singer, M. J. (1998). Measuring presence in virtual environments: A presencequestionnaire. *Presence: Teleoperators and Virtual Environments, 7*(3), 225–240.

World Health Organization. (2001). *International classification of functioning, disability and health.* Geneva, Switzerland: Author.

Young, M. A., Desai, M., & Young, M. J. (2009, March). The eyes have it: Diabetes-related vision impairment is a growing concern. *ADVANCE for Directors in Rehabilitation, 18*(3), 29–31.

Young, M. A., Tumanon, R. C., & Sokal, J. O. (2000). Independence for people with disabilities: A physician's primer on assistive technology. *Maryland Medical Journal, 1*, 28–32.

33

CHAPTER

Trends in Medical Rehabilitation Delivery and Payment Systems

Geoffrey W. Hall, Kirk S. Roden, and Matthew B. Huish

THE HISTORY AND EVOLUTION OF THE U.S. CARE SYSTEM

The history of the health care system in the United States is a long study, although fascinating in its roots and progression. Like the country itself, the health care industry has evolved proportional to the advances in science and technology. Health care has been transforming since its inception when public health issues were not understood, through epidemics and a plethora of infectious diseases, to today's sophisticated medicine with its myriad levels of subspecialization.

Historically, as environmental conditions became understood and controlled, a swing occurred away from epidemics of the masses to acute and chronic conditions of individuals, including heart disease, pneumonia, tuberculosis, and cancer. Hospitals began to specialize and be more sophisticated in their treatment regimes. Significant advancement across the field of medicine has occurred, including safer surgical techniques solving many historical medical conditions.

As the impact of illnesses transformed over time, so did the medical professions, the health care facilities, and the concept of insurance to assist in covering the rising cost of care. With World War II, the role of government in health care became more prominent, not only for the active military personnel, but for the veterans through the Veterans Affairs system. Society's views were simultaneously evolving, from every individual taking responsibility for financing his or her own health care to an interest in taking advantage of third-party or fiscal intermediaries that pooled individuals into insurance risk classes for the common group objective of protection from potential financial disasters.

To have a discussion about health insurance, it is important to begin with some definitions. What was historically termed *insurance* is very different than what one would find in today's marketplace, otherwise known as a third-party payer. Insurance is defined as "a practice or arrangement by which a company or government agency provides a guarantee of compensation for specified loss, damage, illness, or death in return for payment of a premium, or a thing providing protection against a possible eventuality." So insurance was supposedly designed and intended to pay for unexpected losses and out-of-the-ordinary, unavoidable, and financially devastating events. Yet, today's health insurance companies have taken on a very different role—primarily as a payment mechanism for everything and anything related to one's health, including routine preventive care. To do this, health insurers have become actuarial specialists in determining the percentage of a population that will experience certain health care costs over a variety of conditions, from simple colds, to accidents or emergencies, to complex chronic diseases. They then determine a premium price required to cover the costs for such medical expenses, including the related administrative overhead. So, in today's world, health insurance is not so much about covering the costs of an unavoidable risk as it is a mechanism to pay for coverage of most health-related care, including physician, hospital, dental, therapies, pharmaceuticals, diagnostics, labs, and so forth. The term is used interchangeably with health benefits and health care coverage.

The history of health insurance corresponds to the development of an industrial nation and its wars. Early health care in the United States was provided in most people's homes, including surgical procedures. Costs associated with such were nominal and could be covered by barter or individual payment to the visiting country doctor. The costs of health as a percentage of one's total household expenditures were small, so no one felt a need to pay a premium to an intermediary insurance company to cover such insignificant costs. Sickness insurance plans were some of the first formal insurances, because the cost of being sick, out of work, and not able to bring home a paycheck was a bigger cost to a household than the costs to the providers for the provision of their care. However, in 1847, Massachusetts Health Insurance of Boston became the first group policy to issue individual disability and illness insurance.

Unions were also partially responsible for promoting the concept of insurance due to the dreadful conditions in many of the early factories and the resultant high employee injury and death rates. Hence, burial insurance was created to cover the costs of funeral expenses. Gradually, the shift from care in the home to care in a hospital occurred as medical advances were realized in medicines, and the understanding of bacteria related to surgical procedures became known. As hospitals took on the role of treatment centers, there was a growing acceptance of medicine as a science, and physician training became more sophisticated with stricter entrance requirements and tougher standards.

Williams (1980) writes, "However, the real beginning of modern health insurance took place in 1929, when a group of teachers made a contract with Baylor Hospital in Dallas, Texas, to provide coverage against certain hospital expenses," effectively starting the first Blue Cross plan. Over the next several decades, the number of individuals insured and the types of coverage offered grew slowly. But, during the 1940s and 1950s, because employers were incented to provide coverage to their employees as a way to retain them and because of the tax deduction upside, the number of "insured" began to dramatically increase.

MEDICARE

In July 1965, Congress passed Title XVIII of the Social Security Act, creating Medicare, the first national social insurance program. With 35% of the adults over 65 years old uninsured and unable to afford the high cost of medical care, or secure insurance coverage due to their age, the American government created a statutory health insurance that was affordable to those who qualified, either by age, unemployment, or disability. Medicare is financed by individuals during their younger working years through a payroll tax to both the employer and the employee and differs from private insurance in that Medicare cannot change their eligibility or covered benefits by trying to manage their "risk pool." Rather, Medicare is legally obliged to provide a guaranteed benefit package.

Medicare has several benefit parts. See Figure 33.1. Part A provides insurance coverage for inpatient hospitalization costs (care, tests, labs, food, etc.), as well as brief stays in rehabilitation units, skilled nursing facilities (SNFs), and hospice care. As with any insurance product, there are copays, coinsurance, deductibles, length of stay criteria, and related policies.

Part B covers some costs that Part A does not (outpatient hospital procedures) and generally covers all outpatient services, including physician office visits, nursing, diagnostic tests, laboratory, medications if administered by a physician's office, durable medical equipment (DME), prosthetic devices, and one pair of corrective lenses for vision problems each year.

Part C, a newer component of Medicare (1997 and 2003) provides Medicare beneficiaries an opt-out option from the traditional Medicare fee-for-service (FFS) model, instead receiving their coverage through private insurers in what has been called Medicare Advantage Plans. Medicare, in essence, pays the private insurer a capitated (per member per month) rate, transferring the responsibility of care of the Medicare beneficiaries to the private insurer. Medicare Advantage Plans typically have a restricted network of providers that the beneficiaries must use, and often, they can pay a small supplemental premium to get "extended" benefits not typically covered under traditional Medicare, that is, vision care, dental care, fitness club memberships, prescription coverage, and more. The

Part	Coverage	Description/Explanation
Part A	Hospital insurance	Part A covers most medically necessary hospital, skilled nursing facility, home health, and hospice care. It is free if the individual has worked and paid Social Security taxes for at least 40 calendar quarters (10 years); individuals will pay a monthly premium if they have worked and paid taxes for less time.
Part B	Medical insurance	Part B covers most medically necessary doctors' services, preventive care, durable medical equipment, hospital outpatient services, laboratory tests, x-rays, mental health care, and some home health and ambulance services. Individuals pay a monthly premium for this coverage.
Part C	Not a separate benefit	Part C is the part of Medicare policy that allows private health insurance companies to provide Medicare benefits. These Medicare private health plans, such as HMOs and PPOs, are known as *Medicare Advantage Plans*. Individuals can choose to get Medicare coverage through a Medicare Advantage Plan instead of original Medicare. Medicare Advantage Plans must offer at least the same benefits as original Medicare (those covered under Parts A and B) but can do so with different rules, costs, and coverage restrictions. Individuals can also get Part D as part of the benefits package if they wish. Many different kinds of Medicare Advantage plans are available. Individuals may pay a monthly premium for this coverage, in addition to their Part B premium.
Part D	Outpatient prescription drug insurance	Part D is the part of Medicare that provides outpatient prescription drug coverage. Part D is provided only through private insurance companies that have contracts with the government—it is never provided directly by the government (like original Medicare is). If individuals want Part D, they must choose Part D coverage that works with their Medicare health benefits. If individuals have original Medicare, they can choose a stand-alone Part D plan.

FIGURE 33.1 Medicare coverage table—part coverage and explanation.
Source: Your Medicare Benefits (2015).

Medicare Advantage Plans function much like health maintenance organizations (HMOs), requiring the beneficiary to select a primary care physician as a gatekeeper for coordinating the care.

Part D, the most recent part of Medicare, went into effect on January 1, 2006. Part D was designed to help cover the often unaffordable costs of prescription drugs, which seem to escalate with age. To receive this benefit, the Medicare-eligible beneficiary must enroll in the Prescription Drug Plan (PDP) or a Medicare Advantage Plan that offers the prescription benefit. Part D is unlike Part A and Part B in that the exact coverage is not legislated or mandated. Rather, those insurance plans that offer this coverage can select what drugs they wish to cover, or exclude, so it is important that the beneficiaries research the details and coverage of each plan.

Although Medicare remains the largest health insurance payer in the United States, it is important to note that the Medicare payment systems vary per the setting where care is delivered, that is, inpatient rehabilitation facilities (IRF), SNFs, home health agencies (HHAs), long-term care hospitals (LTCHs), and outpatient services.

With the creation of the inpatient prospective payment system (IPPS) for acute care, Medicare created a payment model that eliminated payments for additional inpatient services with the exception of select diagnosis-related groups (DRGs). DRGs established a per-episode payment model that helped to curtail inflation with respect to inpatient hospital charges. The difference in marginal payments helped to shift patients from acute care and into postacute facilities, which created significant cost increases in postacute care (Sood, Huckfeldt, Escarce, Grabowski, & Newhouse, 2011).

The 1997 Balanced Budget Act tried to address this disparity by mandating prospective payment systems for postacute providers, but reimbursement was based on the provider's average costs, which differ greatly by location. This resulted in different levels of reimbursement for similar services for the same patient, which served as an incentive for health care providers to send patients to the setting with the highest reimbursement, not necessarily the setting with the highest value. To further explain this problem between acute inpatient and postacute settings, IRFs and HHAs are paid a fixed episode price. These settings do not receive a marginal reimbursement as a postacute setting would, so there is an incentive to discharge patients early even if they would benefit from a longer stay (Sood et al., 2011). The Medicare Payment Commission (2006) explains the contrast for SNFs, which are reimbursed on a per-diem basis, thereby creating incentives to place long-term patients into nursing facilities and patients into short-term rehabilitation facilities regardless of clinical appropriateness.

As patients were discharged from acute and postacute systems, Medicare established a third payment system for outpatient services. FFS payment models were used to pay for hospital outpatient visits, dental services, medical equipment, supplies, and medications. Jencks, Williams, and Coleman (2009) noted that nearly 20% of Medicare FFS patients were readmitted to a hospital within 30 days of discharge, and nearly half did not see a physician before the readmission, indicating poor care coordination between systems (2009). Mor, Intrator, Feng, and Grabowski (2010) indicated a similar trend for patients discharged from hospitals to SNFs, with 24% requiring readmission within 30 days, resulting in more than $4 billion in costs.

MEDICAID

Authorized by Title XIX of the Social Security Act, Medicaid was signed into law in 1965. It represents a cooperative program between the federal and state governments. Medicaid was developed and designed to pay the costs of medical services for certain low-income persons in the United States. The federal government mandates certain medical services be provided (mandatory eligibility groups) while granting the states flexibility to cover other benefits and population groups (optional eligibility groups). The states administer their own Medicaid programs, that is, determining applicant eligibility, which health services to cover, setting provider reimbursement rates, paying for a portion of the total program, and processing claims, whereas the Centers for Medicare & Medicaid Services (CMS) is charged with administering Medicaid for the federal government. States pay providers or managed care organizations for Medicaid costs and then report these payments to CMS. The federal government pays a percentage of the costs of medical services by reimbursing each state. This percentage is known as the Federal Medical Assistance Percentage (FMAP). The Affordable Care Act (ACA) specifies FMAPs for adult beneficiaries who are newly eligible as a result of the Medicaid expansion that began in 2014 (in states that implement the expansion). Additionally, the federal government pays a portion of each state's administration costs.

In contrast to the federal Medicare program, Medicaid's financial operations are not financed through trust funds. Other than a very small amount of premium revenue from enrollees, as noted earlier, and other sources of state revenue such as provider taxes, there are no dedicated revenue sources comparable to the Medicare hospital insurance payroll tax. Federal and state revenues primarily cover Medicaid costs on an as-needed basis. The states may also rely on local government revenues to finance a portion of their share of Medicaid costs, which is federally financed through an annual appropriation by Congress.

Beginning January 2014, the ACA provides the states the authority under their state plan to expand Medicaid eligibility to almost all individuals under age 65 years who are living in families with income below 138% of the Federal Poverty Level (FPL), with the federal government paying 100% of the costs.

Services usually covered by Medicaid include hospital care, physician services, laboratory and other diagnostic tests, prescription drugs, dental care, and many long-term care services. The states also have the options to use managed care plans to provide and coordinate benefits and to apply for waivers that allow the states more flexibility in developing specialized benefit packages for specific populations. With limited exceptions, states must provide the same benefit package to all Medicaid enrollees. However, there may be limited benefits provided for individuals who are eligible based only on medical need, through Medicare savings programs or through special family planning groups. Additionally, states must extend eligibility to all mandatory populations and cover all mandatory services defined by Title XIX in order to receive federal matching funds for their Medicaid programs.

The joint federal–state Medicaid program is one of the largest payers for health care in the United States. Medicaid and the Children's Health Insurance Program (CHIP) serve as a safety net for the nation's most vulnerable populations by providing health coverage to nearly 60 million Americans. The Medicaid program is critically important, representing one sixth of the national health economy.

Some important facts regarding the size, costs, and the growth of inflation rates regarding Medicaid can be seen in the following:

In 2013:

- Total Medicaid spending was $457.8 billion; $265.4 billion (58%) in federal and $192.5 billion (42%) in state funds.
- Between 2012 and 2013, Medicaid payments increased by 6.1%, whereas enrollment increased by 1.6%.
- Nearly one of every five persons in the United States was enrolled in Medicaid for at least 1 month.
- Per-enrollee spending was $6,897 for health goods and services, with $2,807 for children, $4,391 for adults, $15,483 for the aged, and $17,352 for disabled beneficiaries.

In 2014:

- Medicaid expenditures increased 9.4% to $498.9 billion, which includes the expenditures for newly eligible enrollees.
- Because the federal government paid 100% of the costs of newly eligible enrollees, the federal share of all Medicaid expenditures is estimated to have increased 60%.

FUNDING OF HEALTH CARE FOR CHILDREN

Beginning with Medicaid expansion starting in 1984, the Deficit Reduction Act marked the first movement by the United States to create mandatory coverage for uninsured children in families with incomes up to 133% of the FPL. Following a series of reforms, Congress enacted changes that enabled states to provide supplemental Medicaid to low- and moderate-income families who had children with disabilities that had insufficient private health insurance coverage (Rosenbaum & Kenney, 2014).

With the recognition that millions of children were falling through the cracks as their family incomes were too high to qualify for Medicaid, yet too low to pay for other forms of insurance, CHIP was created in 1997, and by 1999, all states had implemented the program (Jarlenski, 2015). CHIP coverage levels are benchmarked to an approximate level of what a family may be offered by an employer (Rosenbaum & Kenney, 2014).

By 2012, the number of uninsured children had fallen from 15% in 1989 to just over 6%. In fiscal year 2011, more than 30 million children representing 38% of children under the age of 19 were enrolled in Medicaid or CHIP. Several states were able to achieve near universal coverage of all children, and one study suggests that the transition from private to public coverage yielded $1,500 in annual cash equivalent per family through reduced premiums and cost sharing (Shaefer, Grogan, & Pollack, 2011).

The ACA was structured to align with Medicaid and CHIP programs for children. Specifically, Congress directed the development of comprehensive guidelines for children and adolescents to receive "evidence informed preventive care and screenings" that go beyond the earlier requirements for well-baby and well-child standards and include both oral and vision care (U.S.C. Sect. 300gg-13).

Although programs like Medicaid and CHIP have extended health insurance for millions of children, there remain a number of gaps that impact children with disabilities. Plans that focus on the provision of essential benefits can impose limits on the utilization of treatment and may not always account for the provision of additional treatments that may be medically necessary for individual children. Rosenbaum and Kenney note that plans may use "treatment exclusions" denying services otherwise covered, including speech and physical therapies, on the basis that treatments are "educational," which is contrary to developmental disability research advocating for early intervention. Consideration of the adequacy of coverage also differs from that for adults, in that children may not always follow a recovery model but may have conditions in need of covered treatment to foster healthy development (Rosenbaum & Kenney, 2014).

MANAGED CARE

Private insurance is in contrast to public health insurance programs such as the government-supported and/or social programs of Medicaid, Medicare, and Federal Employees Health Benefits Program, Indian Health Services, Veterans Health Administration, CHIP, and others. Managed care commercial payers include companies such as AETNA, CIGNA, United Health, and thousands of other local, regional, or national health insurers. Private health insurance is accessed in most cases on a group basis through an employer-sponsored program, with the employer paying for their employees. Individual consumers can also purchase private insurance, although it is usually quite costly. Figure 33.2 shows the cost and percentage of total health care costs under private versus public programs.

Managed care systems in the United States were initially developed in the 1980s as HMOs with the primary goal of providing health care coverage to a large population, while at the same time aggressively attempting to control costs. HMO plans were initially administered by health insurance companies that sold policies to businesses and individuals at a lower cost than their traditional FFS policies.

The HMO model was designed to place primary care physicians as the gatekeepers of care by providing them economic incentives to limit the amount and type of care allowed, especially referrals to specialists, and by requiring preauthorization of all diagnostics and otherwise traditionally expensive treatment options. It was believed that this provider gatekeeper approach would maintain good health for the patient population while controlling costs by limiting unnecessary health care services. Common practices included the use of preferred networks of providers, wherein the

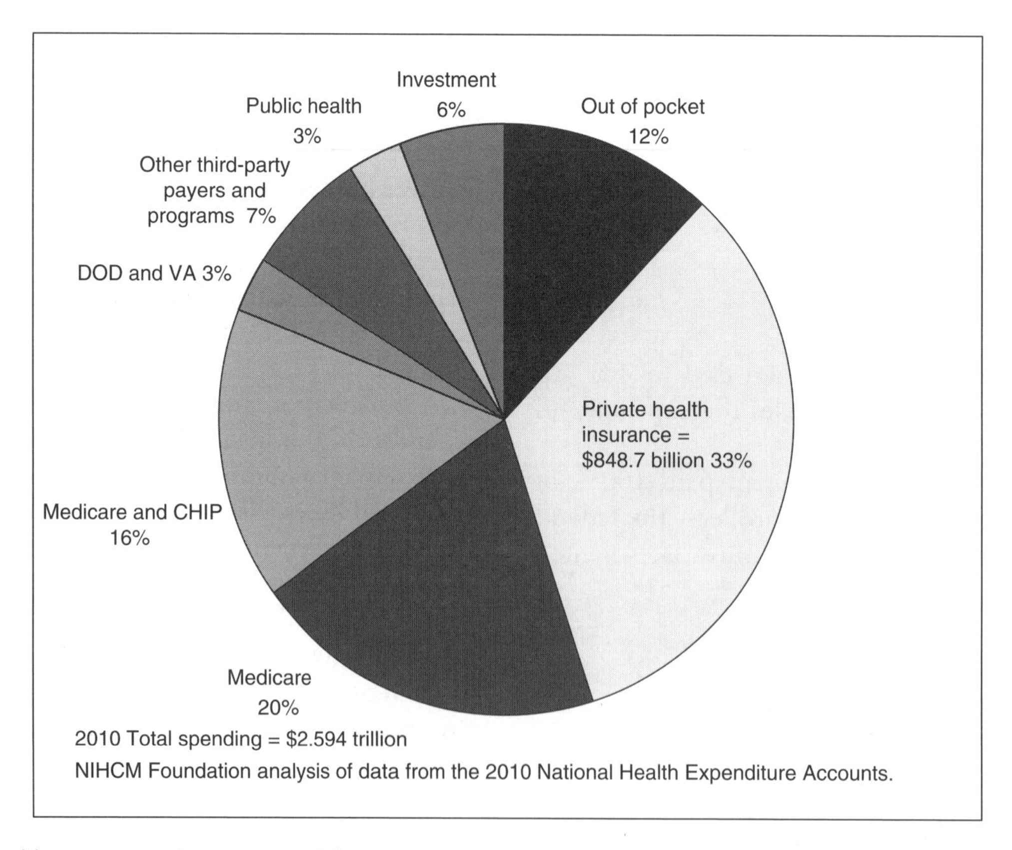

FIGURE 33.2 Health care costs: private versus public programs.

CHIP, Children's Health Insurance Program; DOD, Department of Defense; NICHM, National Institute for Health Care Management; VA, Veterans Affairs.

Source: NIHCM Foundation analysis of data from the 2010 National Health Expenditure Accounts, The National Institute for Health Care Management (NIHCM) Foundation.

insurer contracted with providers (physicians and hospitals) to provide care at a discounted cost with the promise of increased patient volume.

These efforts were mostly unsuccessful and most HMO plans failed financially. One of the exceptions was Kaiser Permanente, which is still a very successful HMO in that it owned all of its facilities and employed its own physicians. In this way, the organization was able to truly control costs and provide quality health care, ensuring good outcomes by implementing excellent management systems and processes. Today this model still works.

It has been years since the HMO experiment. Since then, U.S. health care spending has continued to escalate with a corresponding increasing percentage related to the United States' gross domestic product (GDP). The financial pressure is at an all-time high because the current system is inefficient, expensive, and unsustainable. In recent years, as health care costs continue to climb, either the employer or the private managed care plan has changed the patient's benefit by increasing the copay amount or annual deductibles to manage access to care.

ACCOUNTABLE CARE ORGANIZATIONS

The U.S. government is using the CMS to implement the next phase of managed care organizations, called accountable care organizations (ACOs). ACOs are systems for providing health care to a large population base. The health care providers and health care organizations receive annual financing to provide effective health care to a specific population. The providers and health care organizations assume the financial risk to provide the necessary care for their selected population. In order for these organizations to mitigate risk successfully, they require sophisticated systems to collect and analyze large amounts of health care data to predict their costs. The use of complex information systems and analytical tools to mine data and report detailed information is paramount to an ACO's success. (Berkowitz & Miller, 2015)

FLEXIBLE SPENDING ACCOUNTS

Flexible spending accounts (FSAs), or medical savings accounts (MSAs), serve as another tool to offset health care costs. With an FSA, individuals can direct money to pay for certain out-of-pocket health care costs. Money directed into an FSA is not included in an individual's payroll tax and can be used as payment of copays, deductibles, prescription drugs, medical equipment, and some dental expenses. FSAs are only available through employer-based health plans and generally have to be used within the same plan year.

AN UNSUSTAINABLE SYSTEM

The fact that many employers are assuming responsibility to provide insurance coverage for their employees has served to significantly increase the number of individuals covered by health insurance. As insurance plans have taken on the responsibility of most health care costs, utilization of services has skyrocketed. Because the insurance premium paid by employers is directly tied to the costs that the insurance carriers pay out to health care providers and facilities as reimbursement, employers have experienced double-digit percentage increases in their insurance premiums. This situation has been compounded because insurance companies have paid providers on an FFS basis, incenting treatment churning (more provider income for more patient visits). This made for a spiraling cycle of volume-based care. As patients sought more and more care, because it was paid for by their employer's premiums and not out of their pocket, insurance companies increased their premiums to the employers to cover the costs to the providers and facilities. In the end, employers were left holding the financial burden as the responsible party covering the cost of health care across America. Finally, in an attempt to manage this, all companies, both small and large, pushed to sell more of their products and services, which often was not possible. It is easy to see how such a cycle became unsustainable after decades (Brown & Jared, 2015).

Clearly, the marketplace is shifting as more and more large self-funded employers are seeking their own solutions. Many strategies being implemented include in-house employee health and wellness clinics, healthy lifestyle incentives, use of preferred and integrated provider networks with a proven value history, care coordination, bundled payments around high cost conditions, annual health risk assessments, disease management programs, and health coaching.

In 2014, the United States' total national spending on health care was $3 trillion. According to the Organization for Economic Cooperation and Development (OECD), the health care costs per capita in the United States were $9,523, representing 17.5% of the GDP. The United States pays almost twice as much per capita on health care as other advanced nations, yet the quality in the United States trails these nations. With this level of health care expenditure, one would predict that the quality of health care in the United States would be equal to or proportionally higher than that of other OECD nations, when in fact, the opposite is true. Cost outlay has not translated to quality as the United States has a lower life expectancy and a lower infant survival, and is lower in most quality metrics (access, readmissions, infections) than most developed nations. The Commonwealth Fund ranked the United States last in quality care compared to 10 other developed countries (see Figure 33.3).

VALUE, RISK, AND BUNDLING

As a way to begin addressing the unsustainable financial model, gaps in care coordination, and poor health outcomes, Medicare recently committed to a bundled payment model. In a bundled payment, one payment is provided for an entire episode of care, which could include both acute and postacute care services. The entity that receives the bundled payment accepts the financial risk of any costs that occur in that episode of care, including hospital readmission and the cost throughout the postacute continuum (PAC). Because the cost is fixed, the expectation is that this will foster better communication, care coordination, and improved outcomes.

Bundled payments clearly shift financial risk from payers to providers. Although physicians are primarily focused on their clinical duty to their patients, payment methods clearly have an effect on care delivery. Examples of this, relative to bundled payments, could include the utilization of diagnostic imaging, frequency of physician office visits, inpatient length

Country rankings

Top 2*

Middle

Bottom 2*

	AUS	CAN	FRA	GER	NETH	NZ	NOR	SWE	SWIZ	UK	US
Overall ranking (2013)	4	10	9	5	5	7	7	3	2	1	11
Quality care	2	9	8	7	5	4	11	10	3	1	5
Effective care	4	7	9	6	5	2	11	10	8	1	3
Safe care	3	10	2	6	7	9	11	5	4	1	7
Coordinated care	4	8	9	10	5	2	7	11	3	1	6
Patient-centered care	5	8	10	7	3	6	11	9	2	1	4
Access	8	9	11	2	4	7	6	4	2	1	9
Cost-related problem	9	5	10	4	8	6	3	1	7	1	11
Timeliness of care	6	11	10	4	2	7	8	9	1	3	5
Efficiency	4	10	8	9	7	3	4	2	6	1	11
Equity	5	9	7	4	8	10	6	1	2	2	11
Healthy lives	4	8	1	7	5	9	6	2	3	10	11
Healthy expenditures/capita, 2011**	$3,800	$4,522	$4,118	$4,495	$5,099	$3,182	$5,669	$3,925	$5,643	$3,405	$8,508

FIGURE 33.3 Health care costs per capita by country.

*Includes ties.

**Expenditures shown in $US PPP (purchasing power parity); Australian $ data are from 2010.

Source: Calculated by the 2011 Commonwealth Fund International Health Policy Survey of Sicker Adults; 2012 International Health Policy Survey of Primary Care Physicians; 2013 International Health Policy Survey; Commonwealth Fund *National Scorecard 2011;* WHO; and Organization for Economic Cooperation and Development (OECD) Health Data, 2013 (Paris: OECD, November, 2013).

of stay, and the number of follow-up visits between hospitals and physicians. These health care payment reforms are an attempt to find the balance between risk and incentives across payers and providers. Recent initiatives to include value-based purchasing, ACOs, medical homes, and cost-sharing programs aim to help consumers receive more health for the health care dollar (Quinn, 2010).

History has demonstrated that health care payment reform can have both positive and negative effects. In 1983, when Medicare changed from paying according to hospital costs to paying for DRGs, there was a significant decrease in hospital costs, shorter inpatient stays, and even improved hospital margins as hospitals became increasingly more efficient. Although this change also helped to develop outpatient and postacute services, these changes may have also contributed to the fragmentation in health care (Quinn, 2010). In 1992, Medicare converted physician payment from per dollar of charges to per service, which helped to protect Medicare against charge inflation but opened it up to significant volume increases. As a result, physician services and FFS payments grew more than twice the rate of other services, given the large growth in volume (Duchovny & Nelson, 2007). Similarly, in 2000, Medicare shifted home health care payments from per dollar of cost to per episode, which resulted in 17% fewer visits and increased efficiency but also improved patient outcomes (Schlenker, Powell, & Goodrich, 2005). It is important to note that although many payment methods are negotiated between providers and commercial payers, any reforms in Medicare have broad influence as many payers follows Medicare (Quinn, 2010).

Why is it important to balance the risk between payer and provider? Consider one of the most important statistics that influence health care policy: Five percent of patients cared for account for more than 50% of the health care spending (Cohen & Uberoi, 2013). Payers are attempting to protect themselves against unnecessary and inefficient care, which has a direct impact on charges (Mullen, Frank, & Rosenthal, 2010). As noted by Quinn, although payers are taking an increasing role toward improving the overall quality and value of care, providers remain the best judges of determining the right care, at the right time for patients. This tension between payers and providers helps to create case mix adjustments in payment for case mix so that the highest payments are assigned to patients who are thought to be the most costly, because statistics show that 5% of patients account for 50% of total health care spending (Cohen & Uberio, 2013).

So, in an attempt to control costs while simultaneously improving quality, there is a transition from volume-based payment and care to quality-based payment and care, linking reimbursement to quality outcome metrics. Value-based payments include a series of models that step away from FFS toward shared risk models of gradual intensity (see Figure 33.4).

Such alternative value-based payment models consist of the following steps and range:

1. FFS, with links tied to quality
2. Hospital- and physician-integrated case rates
3. Episodic specific bundling, with links to include the PAC of care
4. FFS/case rates or bundling, with gain sharing on the savings achieved, between providers and payers
5. Capitation, on a per member per month, around specified populations

The U.S. Secretary of Health and Human Services has indicated that by 2018, CMS will have transitioned 90% of their traditional FFS care to a quality- or value-based system, and 50% of all reimbursement will be in an alternative payment model (APM). Other public and private insurance plans are planning to follow CMS's lead by also transitioning into these value-based and APMs. As this change is rapidly being implemented, providers and hospitals are entering a transition period as their revenues are changing from volume to value. As shown in Figure 33.5, the "revenue transition period" is now underway.

This shift in revenue mix is a new and challenging transition for most health systems and providers and requires sophisticated IT and billing systems to track various patient reimbursement methodologies.

PAY FOR PERFORMANCE

Pay for performance (or "P4P") is part of the new model for reimbursing hospitals and physicians. By definition, and as previously mentioned, P4P consists of financial rewards to those who achieve

Unit of Payment	Common Term	Examples (Common Classification Systems)	Comment
1. Per time period	Budget and salary	Salaried physicians and government hospitals	Typically but not necessarily per year
2. Per beneficiary	Capitation	Managed care organizations (ACG, COPS, CMS-HCC, CRG, and DxCG)	More commonly used to pay health plans than to pay individual providers
3. Per recipient†	Contact capitation	Physician specialist services	Not common; an example is a cardiologist accepting financial risk for treatment of cardiac patients
4. Per episode	Case rates, payment per stay, and bundled payments	Hospital inpatient (DRG), physician surgeries (RBRVS), home health care (HHRG), and multiple providers (ECR, ETG, MEG, and PFE)	Defined here as related clinical services across multiple days
5. Per day	Per diem and per visit	Nursing facilities (RUG), hospital outpatient (EAPG), and ambulatory surgical centers (APC)‡	An outpatient visit may be defined as all services on 1 day
6. Per service	Fee for service	Physician services (RBRVS), hospital outpatient (APC)‡, dentists, medical equipment and supplies, and drugs	Separate payments are often made for multiple services per day
7. Per dollar of cost	Cost reimbursement	Critical access hospitals, government-owned providers, and nursing facilities	Payers typically pay a percentage of cost as allowed by the payer
8. Per dollar of charges	Percentage of charges	Any provider type	Based on charges as billed by the provider

FIGURE 33.4 The 8 basic payment methods in health care. Shown in decreasing order of financial risk borne by the provider or, alternatively, in increasing order of financial risk borne by the payer. The units of payment correspond to financial risk factors within the health care spending identity, as shown in Figure 33.2.

† A beneficiary is eligible for care, where as a recipient he or she has received at least one service.

‡ In practice, the incentives of the Medicare APC-based method align most closely with payment per day for ambulatory surgical centers and with payment per service for hospital outpatient care.

ACG, adjusted clinical group; APC, ambulatory payment classification; COPS, chronic illness and disability payment system; CMS-HCC, Centers for Medicare & Medicaid Services—hierarchical condition category; CRG, clinical risk group; DRG, diagnosis-related group; EAPG, enhanced ambulatory patient group; ECR, evidence-informed case rate; ETG, episode treatment group; HHRG, home health resource group; MEG, medical episode group; PFE, patient-focused episode; RBRVS, resource-based relative value scale; RUG, resource utilization group.

or exceed predefined metrics, typically consisting of improving quality or decreasing costs relative to historical nationally established benchmarks. As such, P4P consists of a performance target or measurement, an incentive, and data transparency. New levels of transparency will be part of the "consumerism" that is beginning to take place in health care, similar to the retail marketplace, where "shoppers" of products, and now services, can compare costs and associated results/outcomes across providers.

MEDICARE ACCESS AND CHIP REAUTHORIZATION ACT

With the final repeal of the sustainable growth rate (SGR), Medicare will begin paying providers under one of the two components that make up Medicare Access and CHIP Reauthorization Act of 2015 (MACRA). Merit-based incentive pay (MIPS) will replace FFS with fee for value and can affect reimbursement +/- 9% based on attaining

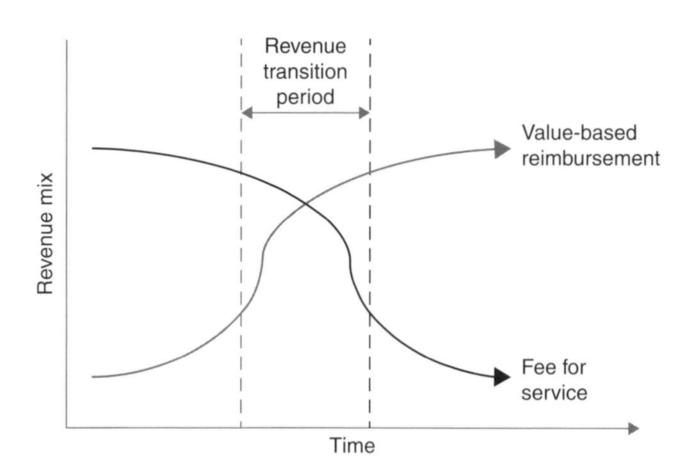

FIGURE 33.5 Transitioning from fee for service to value-based reimbursement.

quality measures. MIPS is an aggregate of previous CMS initiatives including physician quality reports (PQRSs), meaningful use (MU), and value-based modifier. Based on data collected in 2016 and on, CMS will begin to pay all eligible providers in 2019 under this new methodology. The APMs growing out of CMS's demonstration projects including bundled payments are continuing to be defined. Quality metrics that are considered to be measured include timely access to care, use of electronic medical records by providers, and the patients' perception of the care provided to them. Incentive pay up to 5% to providers for meeting certain performance measures is new to the financing and reimbursement of care. Large national public insurance entities besides CMS are migrating to this model. Although the incentive amount or percentage of compensation can change, the target benchmark will be attainable and clear, with real-time data provided throughout the process, as providers are held accountable for their performance. Clearly, as physicians modify their clinical behavior, the challenge is to ensure that the incentive is commensurate with the incremental costs made by the providers to achieve the targeted benchmarks.

Payment methods will not be neutral on quality, but they also need to curtail over- and underuse based on skewed financial incentives. These mechanisms often include utilization review, credentialing, peer review, licensure and certification, prohibition of self-referral, and even disciplinary actions.

Success of these new initiatives depends on providers having sufficient incentive to provide care for the patients who require the most care and physicians not avoiding the costliest of patients. Additionally, success will depend on minimizing the administrative burden and clinical oversight on physicians providing the care, who have referred to the current climate as a "regulatory nightmare." Finally, the notable outcome of health care transformation will be the number of provider and hospital mergers that will occur. Many of the recent reform initiatives encourage providers to align or integrate for care coordination and quality outcomes (Ginsburg & Pawlson, 2014).

As payments begin to be tied to value, the analytical capabilities of the hospital and physician's billing and quality tracking systems will be critical. The ability to hone in on any problematic patient conditions that could adversely impact payments will be important. No other industry has undergone such a total transformation in the way it is financed as the health care industry is currently experiencing.

POSTACUTE CONTINUUM

The PAC consists of LTCHs, IRFs, SNFs, HHAs, and outpatient therapy (OPT) centers. There is a clear focus on the PAC by CMS and others because 43% of Medicare patients discharged from a hospital enter at least one PAC level of service. Twenty-three percent of Medicare dollars are spent on postacute care and there has been a 90% increase per capita in PAC spending by Medicare since 2000 (8% increase per year) (Lansky, Nwachukwu, & Bozic, 2012).

Sood et al. (2011) explain that although bundling and other alternate payment models do create new incentives to avoid readmissions, it may not allow for other valuable services that improve a patient's health, and it does not have safeguards for a health system that may minimize care because bundled payments do not include payment for additional services outside of the bundle. To encourage larger participation in bundling payment models, it may be necessary to reduce risks to health providers and ensure that quality care is delivered through the use of outlier payments to cover costs incurred beyond set price thresholds. Another option to reduce these risks is to use loss and gain sharing. In this system, Medicare would cover some provider spending in excess of set payment targets and the health system would share with Medicare any profit achieved if spending was less than the set payment target. By combining P4P with bundled payments, Medicare can help ensure that the overall quality of care improves while minimizing the risk of compromising on care. Due to the need to tightly coordinate care across all settings to make a bundled payment successful, hospital systems may exert greater control influence on the postacute care network continuum. Hospitals may even expand their own postacute services and/or contract the size of their postacute network in order to manage the quality of care (Sood et al., 2011). The Impact Act of 2014 was passed into law with the objective of standardizing postacute care assessment data for quality, payment, and discharge planning. It includes provisions that affect delivery of care and operations across the full continuum of care. Once fully operational, it will change and standardize patient assessment and related documentation requirements, quality reporting measures, hospital discharge planning, and payment reform initiatives (Buntin et al., 2005).

THE PATIENT PROTECTION AND AFFORDABLE CARE ACT (ACA)

The ACA, signed into law by President Obama in 2010, aims to expand health insurance coverage, improve quality, and reduce health care costs. This law created mandates for individual and employer health coverage; created new regulations for insurance providers; changed Medicare's payment systems; expanded Medicaid; and established a number of demonstration projects across the health care industry. Specifically, individuals other than the very poor are required to purchase health insurance or pay an Internal Revenue Service (IRS) tax, and employers with more than 50 employees are required to provide insurance or face penalties (Sood et al., 2011).

The ACA also created health insurance exchanges (HIXs) to increase competition in the health insurance market, thus driving down costs. These exchanges, which are not insurers, served to regulate and monitor compliance, expand health care coverage for individuals and families not eligible for Medicaid yet with income 138% over the federal poverty limit, and created tax subsidies for individuals under 139% to 400% of the federal poverty limit.

The ACA law also eliminated lifetime or annual limits for individual health-related expenditures and eliminated insurance limitations for preexisting conditions. The law created minimum essential health benefits that included 10 categories of care. Physical medicine and rehabilitation (PM&R) is one of the 10 categories covered, with minimal coverage levels determined by each state (Chan, 2015).

Since the ACA went into effect, there has been a significant reduction in national health expenditures, and health insurance coverage has been expanded to more than 30 million individuals in the United States. Undocumented immigrants (approximately 12 million individuals) are not covered by the ACA, so this group will continue to have an impact on health costs, as they will still require health care services, as shown in Figure 33.6.

It is estimated that hospitals under the ACA will save more than $5 billion in uncompensated care in 2015.

PLANNING FOR THE FUTURE

To accommodate expected demand while remaining fiscally solvent, health care organizations must prioritize among the array of compelling facility, equipment, and infrastructure investments. Disruptive innovations will continue to present at an even more rapid pace, which will challenge and impact investment decisions. Clinical technological advances are threatening to rewrite the rules of traditional service line economics, yet it is impossible to forecast with any certainty when, how, or which of these innovations will fully affect the market.

Although demographics are driving across-the-board inpatient growth, technological advances are poised to change the mix of cases. A wave of new implantable medical devices is greatly expanding the market relative to surgical interventions.

Although acute inpatient care will always remain an important part of the health care delivery system, care will continue to be driven into the ambulatory environment. Outpatient services, including surgery, will continue to see robust growth propelled by the rise of "lifestyle-enhancing" procedures—technological advances creating an arsenal of effective, minimally invasive interventions for common ailments and medical conditions.

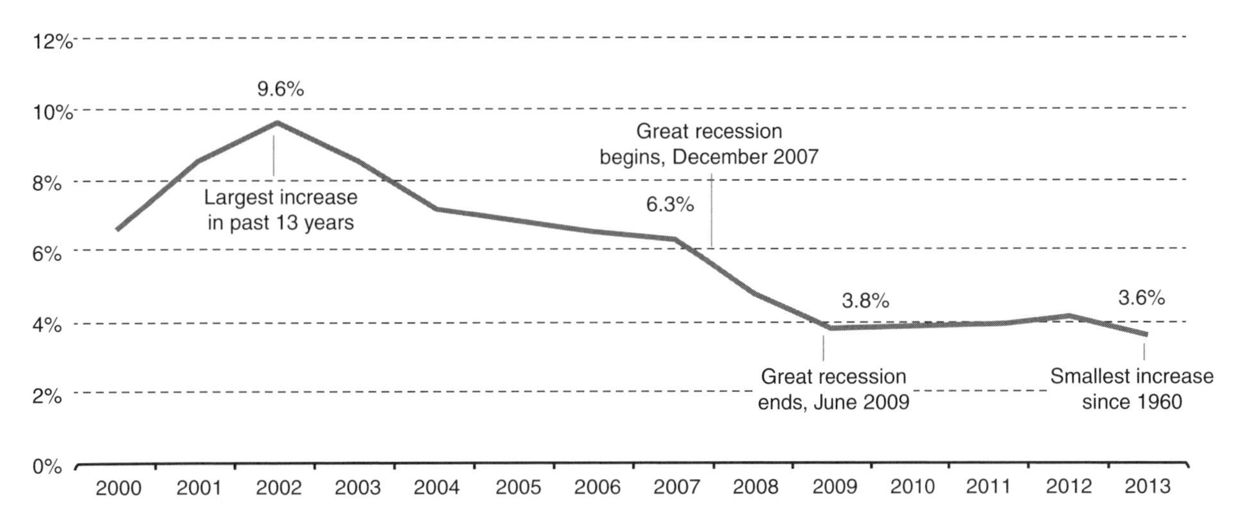

FIGURE 33.6 Total national health expenditures (NHE), annual percent change from previous year, 2000–2013.
Source: Centers for Medicare & Medicaid Services, National Bureau of Economic Research.

Diagnostic imaging will also experience high-volume growth, as refinements in imaging technology will expand and become an integral part of medicine leading to more accurate and timely diagnosis.

Telehealth and Telerehabilitation

Some argue that modern health care has been slow to embrace technology to leverage patient care and provide economic advantage, even though most of these potentially beneficial technologies have been around for many years. The majority of medical health care technology has been primarily focused on techniques to diagnose and treat patients. The use of technology to augment and enhance patient care has been limited to telemedicine or telehealth. Telemedicine or telehealth was defined by the IOM in 1996 as "the use of electronic information and communications technologies to provide and support health care when distance separates participants" (Donaldson, Yordy, Lohr, & Vanselow, 1996). As technology and clinical experience have developed, telehealth effectiveness has increased significantly. Telehealth has the potential to dramatically disrupt the current form or method of delivering health care to individuals by connecting the highest qualified providers with the patients who need specialized care, irrespective of geographic distances.

As a subset of telehealth, telerehabilitation has become a viable option for providers and payers to effectively manage rehabilitation care in the postacute environment. The three main pillars of effective telerehabilitation services are (a) remote monitoring, (b) provider-to-patient interaction, and (c) provider-to-provider consultation with remote control of external devices (Bashshur, Shannon, Krupinski, & Grigsby, 2013).

The remote monitoring of patients provides the provider with visual observation, measuring physiological activity by location and physical activity, and collecting continuous data over extended periods of time, which provides valuable information.

Provider-to-provider consultations can in real-time provide effective multidisciplinary patient care. Provider-to-provider consultations can leverage the access of multispecialty experts and teams to provide an integrated patient care experience (MacRae, 2012).

The importance of telehealth and rehabilitation continuity during the postacute phase has shown effectiveness in reducing patient readmission to acute care facilities and improving the patient's overall functioning and continued improvement. As telerehabilitation technology continues to develop and improve, future applications such as continuous monitoring and feedback for patients in treatment will provide an excellent mechanism to provide quality patient care at a reduced cost.

A current challenge for providers in health care organizations to provide telerehabilitation services is the ability to get reimbursed for their services and licensure to practice across state lines. These challenges will need to be addressed on a national scale in order to take full advantage of telerehabilitation.

Wearable Technology for Patient Monitoring

With the introduction of newer technologies, such as wearable devices, providers will have enhanced clinical tools available to effectively interact and treat rehabilitation patients. With the enhanced reach to provide patient care over a wide geographical area, this technology creates an opportunity to provide care by the specialty physicians directly to the patients who need it the most.

This technology also creates clinical research opportunities using mobile technologies to enroll trial patients from much larger geographical areas and diverse populations. This will allow new areas for researchers to explore and implement.

The opportunity to collect important patient care data will improve the level of patient care. To perform data analysis and transform it into knowledgeable information will allow for intelligent decision making, assisting in improved patient outcomes and potential for cost reduction.

Health care providers are used to new medical and technological advances that require flexibility and adaptation. Use of data for decision making is second nature by training. To achieve the triple aim in health care, health care providers will need to demonstrate both creativity and flexibility. Health care delivery systems will need to include new efficiencies and align incentive models to provide the right level of care, to the right patient, at the right time, in the right setting, with the right utilization of resources, for the best outcomes.

Health insurance plans and health systems will find it important to work closely with PM&R providers to ensure cost-effective care and outcomes for their patient populations in the PAC. Traditionally, rehabilitation providers were consulted toward the end of acute care, limiting opportunities to restore patient's function and independence. Early intervention from the rehabilitation team can help to reduce patient recovery time; restore higher levels of patient functioning; and improve patient outcomes while significantly reducing costs. Examples of this can be found in the early mobilization of patients in critical care settings, which has significantly lowered length of stay while improving outcomes.

In summary, rehabilitation medicine has the potential to provide critical services to help lead and drive health care reforms. In providing early rehabilitation services and providing high-quality interventions across the acute and postacute continuums of care, rehabilitation can be instrumental in improving patient outcomes and lowering overall health care costs.

Although no country or health system in the world has patented the perfect health care delivery system or financing model, there are key metrics of success that warrant attention. Developing and implementing incentives that move the United States closer to the triple aim of (a) improving the patient experience to include both quality and satisfaction, (b) improving the health of the population, and (c) reducing the per capita cost are critical.

Health systems, hospitals, and providers are facing an unparalleled requirement to change. Industry experts project that multiple, intersecting pressures will continue to drive the transformation of health care delivery and financing over the next decade.

The majority of strategists conclude the need for a transformative change in order to address the problems of the number of uninsured and the runaway unsustainable costs bankrupting this nation. The actual costs of care need to be understood and managed by those who provide the care. Quality outcomes need to be tracked and made transparent to the health care consumers—either employers or individuals. Reimbursements need to move from volume based to value based. Risk needs to be shared by those participating in the provision of care. Duplicative services and perverse special interest groups need to be managed. Expanded integrated delivery systems need to be promulgated for leveraging scale. Use of technology for cost-saving efficiencies needs to be incentivized and implemented. Sophisticated analytics and related data need to be at the center of all decision making. Patient-centered integrated specialty-specific clinical care models need to be developed and become the norm. Clinical outcomes and patient perceptions of care received need to be transparent and readily available.

An American Hospital Association Performance Improvement report (2011) should identify must-do, priority strategies and core organizational competencies organizations to remain successful during this time of sweeping transitional change.

Transformational strategies to succeed in the future include:

1. Aligning hospitals, physicians, and other providers across the care continuum
2. Utilizing evidence-based practices to improve quality and patient safety
3. Improving efficiency through productivity and financial management
4. Developing integrated information systems
5. Joining and growing integrated provider networks and care systems
6. Educating and engaging employees and physicians to create leaders
7. Strengthening finances to facilitate reinvestment and innovation
8. Partnering with payers
9. Advancing scenario-based strategic, financial, and operational planning
10. Seeking population health improvement through pursuit of the "triple aim"

It will be important that organizations that implement such strategies must also achieve competency in efficient care delivery and organizational management to be intrinsically connected clinically and aligned managerially.

Core competencies include:

1. Design and implementation of patient-centered, integrated care
2. Creation of accountable governance and leadership
3. Strategic planning in an unstable environment
4. Internal and external collaboration
5. Financial stewardship and enterprise risk management
6. Engagement of full employee potential
7. Collection and utilization of electronic data for performance improvement

As the saying goes, "The only constant is change"—and change is happening. It is up to each organization to plan its unique path to embrace the opportunities that lie ahead.

REFERENCES

American hospital association performance improvement report. (2011). Hospitals and care systems of the future. *Journal of Interprofessional Care*, *26*, 162–163.

Bashshur, R. L., Shannon, G., Krupinski, E. A., & Grigsby, J. (2013). Sustaining and realizing the promise of telemedicine. *Telemedicine and e-Health, 19*(5), 339–345. doi:10.1089/tmj.2012.0282

Berkowitz, S. A., & Miller, E. D. (2015). Accountable care at academic medical centers: Lessons from Johns Hopkins. *New England Journal of Medicine, 364*, e12. Retrieved from http://www.hopkinsmedicine.org/news/media/releases/accountable_care_at_academic_medical_centers_lessons_learned

Brown, B., & Jared, C. (2015). The key to transitioning from fee-for-service to value-based reimbursement. Retrieved from https://www.healthcatalyst.com/hospital-transitioning-fee-for-service-value-based-reimbursements

Buntin, M. B., Garten, A. D., Paddock, S., Saliba, D., Totten, M., & Escarce, J. J. (2005). How much is postacute care use affected by its availability? *Health Services Research, 40*(2), 413–434. doi:10.1111/j.1475-6773.2005.00365.x

Chan, L. M. (2015). *The Patient Protection & Affordable Care Act.* Paper presented at the Association of Academic Physiatrists Annual Meeting 2015, San Antonio, TX.

Cohen, S. B., & Uberoi, N. (2013). Statistical brief #421: Differentials in the concentration of health expenditures across population subgroups in the U.S. 2010. *Medical expenditure panel survey.* Retrieved from http://meps.ahrq.gov/mepsweb/data_files/publications/st421/stat421.shtml

Donaldson, M. S., Yordy, K. D., Lohr, K. N., & Vanselow, N. A. (Eds.). (1996). *Primary care: America's health in a new era.* Washington, DC: National Academies Press.

Duchovny, N., & Nelson, L. (2007). *The state children's health insurance program* (A CBO Paper 2970). Retrieved from https://www.cbo.gov/sites/default/files/110th-congress-2007-2008/reports/05-10-schip.pdf

Ginsburg, P. B., & Pawlson, L. G. (2014). Seeking lower prices where providers are consolidated: An examination of market and policy strategies. *Health Affairs, 33*(6), 1067–1075. doi:10.1377/hlthaff.2013.0810

Jarlenski, M. (2015). Evidence, politics, and the future of the children's health insurance program. *JAMA Pediatrics, 169*(8), 711–712. doi:10.1001/jamapediatrics.2015.0915

Jencks, S. F., Williams, M. V., & Coleman, E. A. (2009). Rehospitalizations among patients in the medicare fee-for-service program. *The New England Journal of Medicine, 360*(14), 1418–1428. doi:10.1056/NEJMsa0803563

Lansky, D., Nwachukwu, B. U., & Bozic, K. J. (2012). Using financial incentives to improve value in orthopaedics. *Clinical Orthopaedics and Related Research, 470*(4), 1027–1037. doi:10.1007/s11999-011-2127-0

MacRae, M. (2012). The robo-doctor will see you now. Retrieved from https://www.asme.org/engineering-topics/articles/robotics/robo-doctor-will-see-you-now

Mor, V., Intrator, O., Feng, Z., & Grabowski, D. C. (2010). The revolving door of rehospitalization from skilled nursing facilities. *Health Affairs, 29*(1), 57–64. doi:10.1377/hlthaff.2009.0629

Mullen, K. J., Frank, R. G., & Rosenthal, M. B. (2010). Can you get what you pay for? Pay-for-performance and the quality of healthcare providers. *The RAND Journal of Economics, 41*, 64–91. doi:10.1111/j.1756-2171.2009.00090.x

Quinn, K. (2010). Achieving cost control, care coordination, and quality improvement in the medicaid program. *Journal of Ambulatory Care Management, 33*(1), 38–49, discussion 69–70. doi:10.1097/JAC.0b013e3181cfc12a

Rosenbaum, S., & Kenney, G. M. (2014). The search for a national child health coverage policy. *Health Affairs, 33*(12), 2125–2135. doi:10.1377/hlthaff.2014.0906

Schlenker, R. E., Powell, M. C., & Goodrich, G. K. (2005). Initial home health outcomes under prospective payment. *Health Services Research, 40*(1), 177–193. doi:10.1111/j.1475-6773.2005.00348.x

Shaefer, H. L., Grogan, C. M., & Pollack, H. A. (2011). Transitions from private to public health coverage among children: Estimating effects on out-of-pocket medical costs and health insurance premium costs. *Health Services Research, 46*(3), 840–858. doi:10.1111/j.1475-6773.2010.01238.x

Sood, N., Huckfeldt, P. J., Escarce, J. J., Grabowski, D. C., & Newhouse, J. P. (2011). Medicare's bundled payment pilot for acute and postacute care: Analysis and recommendations on where to begin. *Health Affairs, 30*(9), 1708–1717. doi:10.1377/hlthaff.2010.0394

Using a Flexible Spending Account. (2015). Retrieved from https://www.healthcare.gov/flexible-spending-accounts

Williams, S. J. (1980). *Introduction to health services* (4th ed.). Albany, NY: Delmar.

34

CHAPTER

Disability Legislation Considerations for Rehabilitation Practitioners

Thomas P. Golden, Matt Saleh, and Susanne M. Bruyère

Over the course of the past decades, the field of rehabilitation has seen sweeping changes, as laws have been enacted to support the rights of individuals with disabilities, and the efforts of the professionals who provide services to these people have also changed in response. These legislative mandates have granted rights to persons with disabilities in the accessibility of goods and services, transportation, telecommunications, housing, and employment (U.S. Department of Justice, 2002).[1] Although each of these areas is vital for accessing a full life as an American citizen, it is the area of employment that is the center of attention in this chapter. Economic self-sufficiency and the ability to use one's talents and abilities in meaningful work are key to a person's financial independence and experience of personal well-being (Fujiura, Yamaki, & Czechowicz, 1998; Stapleton, O'Day, Livermore, & Imparato, 2006; Saunders & Nedelec, 2014). To provide the broadest possible perspective on employment issues that may affect the functioning of rehabilitation professionals, we focus not only on rehabilitation legislation and legislation specifically targeted to persons with disabilities, but also on other pieces of employment legislation that provide protection for persons with disabilities. For the purposes of this discussion, the laws that are focused on are presented as follows: Titles I (Vocational Rehabilitation Services) and V (Rights and Advocacy) of the Rehabilitation Act of 1973 as amended, the employment provisions of the Americans with Disabilities Act of 1990 (ADA) as amended, the Ticket to Work and Work Incentives Improvement Act of 1999 (TWWIIA), the Workforce Innovation and Opportunity Act of 2014 (WIOA) and its predecessor the Workforce Investment Act of 1998 (WIA), the Family Medical Leave Act (FMLA), the Occupational Safety and Health Act (OSHA), the National Labor Relations Act (NLRA), the Patient Protection and Affordable Care Act of 2010 (ACA), and state workers' compensation laws. Table 34.1 provides an overview of key components of these laws as well as a list of acronyms used to refer to them.

This chapter provides a brief overview of each law with an explanation of issues, concerns, or critical areas in service delivery that may arise from it. These are issues that have caused much consternation to employers who attempt to fulfill their responsibilities under several—at times seemingly conflicting—pieces of disability and employment legislation (Gault & Kinnane, 1996). They are therefore of concern to the individual with a disability who is trying to either gain or maintain employment, as well as to rehabilitation professionals who serve people with disabilities. The intent of this chapter is to contribute to the ability of rehabilitation professionals to assist employers and individuals with disabilities in navigating this maze. The authors offer a summary of some key strategies for operating effectively within the regulatory environment, which rehabilitation professionals can use either for coaching individuals about their rights or for providing consultation to employers about their responsibilities to persons with disabilities to lessen or eliminate discrimination in the employment process.

More broadly, an understanding of the legislative environment that affects an employer's receptivity to hiring and retaining individuals with disabilities is important not only for rehabilitation professionals who are providing direct services, but also

TABLE 34.1

KEY COMPONENTS OF DISABILITY LEGISLATION			
Legislation	**Acronym**	**Year**	**Key Components for Rehabilitation Professionals**
Rehabilitation Act, as amended (1992, 1998, 2014)	–	1973	Provides for employment and related support services available to persons with disabilities as provided by the state–federal vocational rehabilitation system (Title I). Prohibits discrimination on the basis of disability in programs conducted by federal agencies, in programs receiving federal financial assistance, in federal employment, and in the employment practices of federal contractors (Title V).
Americans with Disabilities Act	ADA	1990	Protects qualified individuals with disabilities from employment discrimination (Title I). Outlines reasonable accommodation requirements for employers so that a qualified individual with a disability can participate in the application process, perform the essential functions of a job, and enjoy the benefits and privileges of employment (Title I).
ADA Amendments Act	ADAAA	2008	Rejects narrow judicial constructions of the definition of disability in favor of broader coverage that was the original intent of the ADA. Clarifies that a condition that is episodic or in remission can still be a disability if it would be considered a disability when active.
Ticket to Work and Work Incentives Improvement Act	TWWIIA	1999	Provides incentives and supports to beneficiaries and recipients of Supplemental Security Income (SSI) and Social Security Disability Insurance needed to prepare for, achieve, maintain, and advance in work. Expands vocational services options for persons with disabilities. Ticket to Work and Self-Sufficiency Program supplements Social Security Administration's (SSA's) existing traditional cost reimbursement vocational rehabilitation program with an outcomes-based program (Title I). Attempts to reduce disincentives to employment for people with disabilities posed by the threat of loss of health care benefits by encouraging states to improve access to health care coverage available under Medicaid (Title II).
Workforce Investment Act	WIA	1998	Aims to consolidate workforce preparation and employment services into a unified system of support that is responsive to the needs of job seekers, employers, and communities. Develops a framework for the delivery of workforce investment activities at the state and local level to provide services in an effective and meaningful way to all consumers, including persons with disabilities (Title I). Creates a workforce development system that encourages one-stop service delivery, an employment and training system intended to serve every job seeker through a central location that provides access to numerous workforce development programs. Reauthorizes the VR program under the Rehabilitation Act (Title IV).
Workforce Innovation and Opportunity Act	WIOA	2014	Supersedes WIA (including amendments to the Rehabilitation Act), with the professed aim of helping job seekers access the educational, training, and support services necessary for success in the 21st century labor market, while matching employers with skilled workers. Seeks to further align state VR programs with other core programs of the workforce development system, through unified strategic planning, common performance accountability measures, and one-stop delivery. Increases services to youth with disabilities by increasing opportunities for this population to practice workplace skills, exercise self-determination in career interests, and obtain work-based experience.

(*continued*)

TABLE 34.1 (*continued*)

KEY COMPONENTS OF DISABILITY LEGISLATION			
Legislation	**Acronym**	**Year**	**Key Components for Rehabilitation Professionals**
Family Medical Leave Act, as Amended (2008)	FMLA	1993	Establishes minimum labor standard with regard to leaves of absence for family or medical reasons. Specifies that during family medical leave, an employer must maintain the employee's existing level of coverage under a group health plan. At the end of family medical leave, an employer must take an employee back into the same or an equivalent job. 2008 amendments specifically incorporate additional military family leave entitlements.
Occupational Safety and Health Act	OSHA	1970	Recognizes that every worker has a right to a workplace that is free from hazardous conditions. Section 18 of OSHA encourages states to develop and operate their own job safety and health programs. Requires certain employers to develop and maintain a written emergency action plan. The ADA requires that any such plan created in compliance with OSHA standards must include people with disabilities.
National Labor Relations Act	NLRA	1935	Establishes framework for labor relations in the United States, covering union–management relations. Protects workers from the effects of unfair labor practices by employers and requires employers to recognize and bargain collectively with a union that the workers elect to represent them. Incorporates principles such as exclusivity of representation, a policy against direct dealing, and the duty to provide information.
Patient Protection and Affordable Care Act	ACA	2010	Aims to improve health care coverage and security for the U.S. population by expanding coverage, holding insurance companies accountable, lowering health care costs, increasing consumer choice, and enhancing quality of care. Increases access to private health insurance, removes preexisting conditions from insurance eligibility determinations, and expands the population of individuals eligible to receive health care through Medicaid programs, depending on states' willingness to participate. Provides, on an optional basis, for the expansion of community-based services such as vocational supports and case management, allowing participating states to offer such services through their regular state Medicaid plans without seeking a waiver, for individuals with incomes up to 300% of the maximum SSI payment and a high level of need.

for service administrators and those in state and national leadership positions contributing to public policy evolution. Since the institution of many of these laws, significant changes have occurred in the U.S. economic, political, and social contexts. As two examples, the return of veterans with disabilities in the aftermath of the U.S. involvement in wars overseas and the unprecedented weakening of the American economic infrastructure necessitate an informed rehabilitation professional who can be vigilant in advocating for the inclusion of people with disabilities in all facets of new public policy initiatives. Knowledge of the legislative roots of specific public policy proposals, as well as of our country's response to contemporary challenges in the public policy arena, is imperative for the rehabilitation professional's maximal effectiveness.

EMPLOYMENT LEGISLATION AFFECTING REHABILITATION SERVICE DELIVERY

The Rehabilitation Act of 1973 as Amended

Two titles of the Rehabilitation Act are discussed here. Title I deals with employment and related support services available to persons with disabilities as provided by the state–federal vocational rehabilitation (VR) system. Title V prohibits discrimination on the basis of disability in programs conducted by federal agencies, in programs receiving federal financial assistance, in federal employment, and in the employment practices of federal contractors.

Title I of the Vocational Rehabilitation Act of 1973, as modified by the Rehabilitation Act Amendments of 1992 and 1998 and then again by the WIOA of 2014, has the following as its purpose:

> To assist States in operating statewide comprehensive, coordinated, effective, efficient, and accountable programs of vocational rehabilitation, each of which is (A) an integral part of a statewide workforce development system; and (B) designed to assess, plan, develop, and provide vocational rehabilitation services for individuals with disabilities, consistent with their strengths, resources, priorities, concerns, abilities, capabilities, interests, and informed choice, and economic self-sufficiency, so that such individuals may prepare for and engage in competitive integrated employment. (Sec. 100(a)(2))[2]

It should be noted that the WIOA legislation, which we discuss later in this chapter, recently amended the purpose of the Rehabilitation Act. Most notably, the preference for preparing people with disabilities for "gainful employment" was replaced with "competitive integrated employment," as seen in the preceding text. Among the significant amendments included in WIOA are specific language requiring further integration of VR programs and workforce development systems, new focus on "transition" VR services for youth with disabilities, and a shift toward allocating program funds for "21st century" work-based learning needs.

Some of the earliest legislative seeds for the VR service delivery system as we know it today were sown almost 100 years ago with the 1920 Civilian Rehabilitation (Smith-Fess) Act, Public Law 66–236 (Wright, 1980). The Rehabilitation Act has provided funds to states on a formula basis since that time. In the years following the passage of this legislation, VR services have evolved and greatly expanded to provide an extensive array of both public sector and private sector services to address the employment and independent living needs of persons with disabilities.

The federal funding appropriation for the VR service delivery system during fiscal year 2015 was over $3.4 billion (U.S. Department of Education, 2015). The state VR system is made up of 80 agencies in 56 states and territories. Twenty-four states have two agencies: one designed for specific services to the blind and visually impaired and the other providing VR services to all other individuals with disabilities. The remaining 32 agencies offer combined services.[3] Services that can be provided to persons with disabilities, as authorized under the legislation, may include vocational assessment, career counseling, vocational training, job development and job placement, assistive technology, supported employment, and follow-along services. The legislative mandate requires that the order of selection for the provision of VR services shall be determined on the basis of first serving those individuals with the most significant disabilities. Individuals with disabilities, including individuals with the most significant disabilities, are generally presumed to be capable of engaging in competitive integrated employment, and the provision of individualized rehabilitation services is designed to improve their ability to become gainfully employed. A successful outcome is considered to be placement in an integrated employment setting at a prevailing wage for a minimum of 90 days. The state and federal VR program serves approximately 1.2 million individuals with disabilities a year, placing close to a quarter of a million consumers into competitive employment (Council of State Administrators of Vocational Rehabilitation, n.d.).

Until recently, certain other uncompensated vocational outcomes, such as homemaker and unpaid family worker, were accepted as legitimate VR closures for certain individuals who were deemed unable to seek competitive employment. However, proposed regulations for the recently enacted WIOA have indicated that uncompensated employment will no longer be deemed a successful outcome for state VR systems (U.S. Department of Labor [U.S. DOL], Employment and Training Administration [ETA], 2015). The notice of proposed rulemaking (NPRM) does propose adding new outcomes targeting customized and supported employment outcomes.

Title V of the Rehabilitation Act prohibits discrimination against persons with disabilities.

Section 501 requires affirmative action and nondiscrimination in employment by federal agencies of the executive branch.[4] Section 503 requires affirmative action and prohibits employment discrimination by federal government contractors and subcontractors with contracts of more than $10,000.[5] Under Section 503, any federal contractor or subcontractor with 50 or more employees and a contract of $50,000 or more must develop and implement a compliant affirmative action program.

Section 504 of the Rehabilitation Act states that "no qualified individual with a disability in the United States shall, solely by reason of her or his disability, be excluded from, denied the benefits of, or be subjected to discrimination under" any program or activity that either receives federal financial assistance or is conducted by any executive agency or the U.S. Postal Service. Requirements include reasonable accommodation for employees with disabilities, program accessibility, effective communication with people who have hearing or vision disabilities, and accessible new construction and alterations.[6] Although the ADA does not apply to workplaces with fewer than 15 employees, the Tenth Circuit has ruled that that limit does not apply to claims brought under the Rehabilitation Act against entities that receive federal funds (Hellwege, 2002).

Section 508 of the Rehabilitation Act applies to all federal agencies when they develop, procure, maintain, or use electronic and information technology. Section 508 was added to the Rehabilitation Act in 1986, but lacked teeth until 1998, when Congress amended the Rehabilitation Act to require federal agencies to make their electronic and information technology accessible to people with disabilities and pushed the Executive branch to develop accessibility standards. Those standards were developed by the Architectural and Transportation Barriers Compliance Board (Access Board)[7] and served to advance the development of new accessible technologies. Federal web designers also have to make their sites accessible to users with disabilities, and anyone in government who develops or maintains technology products has to make sure that those technologies are accessible (Jaeger, 2006).

In August of 2013, the U.S. DOL (U.S. DOL, Office of Federal Contract Compliance, 2013), OFCCP published new regulations for Section 503. The new regulations have potentially large implications for the employment and recruitment practices of the approximately 200,000 federal contractors in the United States (Shiu, 2013). Most significantly, the new regulations establish a new nationwide 7% "aspirational goal" for federal contractors and subcontractors hiring people with disabilities. Although not technically a quota, the new utilization goal requires "appropriate outreach and positive recruitment activities" as well as accountability measures for demonstrating effective outreach activities and new data collection and reporting requirements for contractors overviewing several quantitative comparisons for job applications, hires, and outreach and recruitment efforts targeted at people with disabilities.

In addition, contractors must now invite applicants to self-identify as individuals with disabilities during the pre- and postoffer phases of the job application process, using a standardized OFCCP form, in order to support affirmative action efforts. To address concerns that such invitations to self-identify may violate the ADA's proscription of preemployment inquiries, OFCCP published a letter from the U.S. Equal Employment Opportunity Commission (EEOC) Office of Legal Counsel affirming its position that preoffer invitations to self-identify do not violate the ADA or accompanying regulations.

The Section 503 self-identification process must be voluntary, meaning that employers may not impose a penalty for nondisclosure, and all record of disclosure must remain confidential and separate from other personnel records (EEOC, 2013). Where an applicant or employee discloses, that information may not be used for hiring, promotion, or termination decisions; such data should be used only for aggregate assessments of employers' efforts to improve outreach, recruitment, employment, and inclusivity in their workplace in compliance with the new regulations (EEOC, 2013).

Despite reassurances, disability disclosure remains a complex issue for both employers and employees, and recent analyses have indicated that individuals with disabilities perceive or experience certain trade-offs when they make the decision to disclose. A recent study by von Schrader, Malzer, and Bruyère (2013) assessed common barriers to self-identification for people with disabilities in the workplace, finding that among surveyed respondents, barriers such as the risk of being fired or not hired, loss of health care benefits, limited promotion opportunities, unsupportive supervisors, and being treated or viewed differently by supervisors and coworkers remain very real concerns for employees with disabilities who are facing the decision to disclose.

Concurrent with the new 503 regulations, OFCCP published new rules for the Veterans Era Veterans Readjustment Assistance Act (VEVRAA). For veterans in a protected disability category, the OFCCP set an annual hiring benchmark of 8%, similar to the Section 503 "aspirational goal" and reflecting metrics for regional and industry-specific workforce availability.

The standards for determining employment discrimination under the Rehabilitation Act are the same as those used in Title I of the ADA, and therefore the issues for rehabilitation professionals in dealing with how these rights play out in the workplace are similar. The implications for rehabilitation professionals are discussed in greater detail under the presentation of issues around implementation of Title I of the ADA.

The ADA of 1990

The ADA is a landmark piece of civil rights legislation that extends the prohibitions against discrimination on the basis of race, sex, religion, and national origin to persons with disabilities.[8] Individuals may have both rights and responsibilities under the law, depending on the roles they assume: as employers or consultants to employers, as practitioners providing health services to the public, or as individuals who today or in the future may be protected by the Act (O'Keeffe, 1994). Title I, which contains the employment provisions of the ADA, applies to private employers with at least 15 employees and to state and local government employers. The ADA protects qualified individuals with disabilities from discrimination. A qualified individual with a disability is a person who meets the necessary prerequisites for a job and can perform the essential functions with or without reasonable accommodation. A reasonable accommodation is any modification or adjustment to a job, an employment practice, or the work environment that makes it possible for a qualified individual with a disability to participate in the job application process, perform the essential functions of a job, and/or enjoy benefits and privileges of employment equal to those enjoyed by employees without disabilities (EEOC, 1992).[9]

The ADA employment provisions make it unlawful to discriminate on the basis of disability in a wide range of employment-related actions, including recruitment, job application, hiring, advancement, compensation, benefits, training, and discharge. Title I prohibits both intentional discrimination and employment practices with discriminatory effect. Additionally, Title I limits the use of both preemployment and postemployment medical examinations and inquiries. An individual with a disability may be subjected to a preemployment medical examination and inquiry only after a conditional offer of employment has been made and only if all entering employees in the job category, regardless of disability, are subjected to such an examination. Postemployment medical examinations and inquiries must be job related and consistent with business necessity. Employee medical information is to be maintained separately from other personnel information, treated in a confidential manner, and shared only with supervisors and managers who need to know about necessary restrictions on the work duties of the employee and necessary accommodations. First aid and safety personnel can also be given selected information if the disability might require emergency medical treatment, as can government officials investigating compliance with the ADA.

The reasonable accommodation requirement is central to the mandate of nondiscrimination against people with disabilities. The concept of reasonable accommodation was not introduced by the ADA. Reasonable accommodation is required under the Rehabilitation Act regarding the employment and participation of individuals with disabilities under federal contracts and programs and under Title VII of the Civil Rights Act with respect to religious observances of employees. In contrast to fears expressed by many employers about the cost and burden associated with reasonable accommodation requests under the ADA and Rehabilitation Act, national estimates suggest that the vast majority of workplace accommodation requests (about 95%) actually come from employees without disabilities (von Schrader, Xu, & Bruyère, 2014). The ADA provides the following examples of reasonable accommodations: job restructuring; part-time or modified work hours; reassignment to a vacant position; acquisition or modification of equipment or services; appropriate adjustment or modifications of examinations, training materials, or policies; and provision of qualified readers or interpreters.

Employers are not, under the ADA, required to hire employees who may pose a "direct threat" to the workplace safety or health environment (EEOC, 1992). The statutory definition of the term "direct threat" is "a significant risk to the health or safety of others that cannot be eliminated by reasonable accommodation." Employers may use the direct threat defense only in cases where risk is significantly increased, and standards for determining how severe a risk is must be applied to all employees—both with and without disabilities (EEOC, 1997).

Despite these landmark civil rights employment protections for people with disabilities, enforcement of the law as originally intended has been problematic. The U.S. EEOC holds responsibility for receiving and investigating reports of disability-related employment discrimination. An ongoing concern is that the EEOC has had significant difficulty handling complaints that it receives in a timely fashion (Moss & Johnsen, 1997; Percy, 2001). Initially, the Supreme Court had also issued a number of opinions that dramatically changed the way the ADA is interpreted (National Council on Disability, 2004). Decisions on the definition of disability, who can be considered "disabled," and the applicability of the statute to state governments limited the application of the ADA in many cases (National Council on Disability, 2007). As discussed in the following text, the ADA Amendments Act (ADAAA) largely rectified these issues of court interpretation, although concerns about EEOC enforcement persist (Greenberg, 2014).

A number of employers, and their legal representatives, have raised questions and concerns about accommodations for persons with psychiatric disabilities (Billitteri, 1997; Pechman, 1995), and employer surveys have found that the majority still hold patronizing or potentially discriminating attitudes (Kosyluk, Corrigan, & Landis, 2014; Scheid, 1998). In response to these concerns, the EEOC issued enforcement guidance on the ADA as it applies to persons with psychiatric disabilities (EEOC, 1997). This publication provides useful information to persons with disabilities as well as to rehabilitation practitioners who provide services to them, about the rights of persons with disabilities to accommodation and disclosure of disability under the ADA. However, this area continues to warrant further attention, as a study by Ullman, Johnson, Moss, and Burris (2001) of disability discrimination claims to the EEOC found that psychiatric illnesses were significantly less likely to be classified as Category A claims and fully investigated than were other disabilities. Category A claims are those that the EEOC offices prioritize in investigation, litigation, and settlement efforts. A study by Goldberg, Killeen, and O'Day (2005) found lingering issues surrounding disclosure of disability status on the part of people with psychiatric disabilities, and Hsieh (2013) notes continued challenges pertaining to ADA enforcement, disclosure, and dispute resolution for individuals with psychiatric disabilities.

When the ADA employment provisions first became effective, some industries were more concerned about their hiring practices and restraints than being able to ask questions about prior injuries (Setzer, 1992); other employers responded with concerns about additional facets of employment that would be affected, such as the implications for insurance benefits and compensation (Huss, 1993; Nobile, 1996; Zolkos, 1994). Over the more than two and a half decades since the law's passage, employers also have become aware of the importance of examining how they treat job incumbents with disabilities. According to statistics kept by the U.S. EEOC, the federal agency that oversees compliance with the ADA employment provisions, more than half (55%) of the charges filed from 1993 to 2007 were related to alleged unlawful discharge, twice as many as were filed for the next most common issue, reasonable accommodation (25%; Bjelland, Bruyère, Houtenville, Ruiz-Quintanilla, & Webber, 2009).[10] Thus, it appears that employers need assistance in navigating requirements for nondiscrimination across all phases of the employment process. Informed rehabilitation professionals can be of great assistance in this process both to these employers and to job applicants and job incumbents with disabilities.

The ADA Amendments Act of 2008

The ADA definition of disability, intended by legislators to be broad and open-ended, was so contentious and limited by subsequent court rulings that, in 2008, Congress passed the ADAAA. The intent of the ADAAA was to reject the increasingly narrow judicial constructions of the ADA in favor of the broad coverage that was the original intent of the Act (EEOC, 2008). The ADAAA specifically overturned Supreme Court rulings on the definition of disability and the effect of mitigating measures such as medications or assistive devices.

It should be noted that in subsequent regulations, the EEOC clarified that the ADAAA's prohibition on assessing mitigating measures applies only to the determinations of whether an individual meets the definition of having a disability under the Act; the EEOC noted that the positive and negative effects of mitigating measures may still be considered in reasonable accommodations and direct threat considerations (EEOC, 2011). The ADAAA and final regulations provide a nonexhaustive list of mitigating measures.

The ADAAA retained the basic definition of disability but provided clearer definitions of terms, expanding on the description of other terms and providing nonexhaustive lists of examples. It also clarified that a condition that is episodic or in remission (such as bipolar disorder or depression) can still be a disability if it would be considered a disability when active (EEOC, 2008). The definition of reasonable accommodation was also retained from the ADA, although the ADAAA and final regulations reaffirmed that the duty to accommodate applies to only two of the three qualifying "prongs" for meeting the definition of disability ("actual" or "record of" disability but not "regarded as" having a disability; EEOC, 2011). It was clarified that the "regarded as" prong, where an employee is *perceived* by the employer as having a disability but where there is no actual qualifying impairment or "record of" disability, applies primarily to issues of discrimination (e.g., disqualification or termination from employment, failure to promote, harassment). An employee who is covered under the "regarded as" prong is not entitled to a reasonable accommodation but is protected from other forms of workplace discrimination (EEOC, 2011).

A subsequent empirical analysis of ADAAA litigation outcomes by Befort (2013) found that summary judgments for employers on the basis of a lack of disability status were down significantly since the passage of the ADAAA. However, the author also found that post-ADAAA case outcomes showed an increased tendency by judges to rule that an individual is not "qualified for" employment in ADAAA cases, suggesting that judicial unease with disability discrimination claims, and with reasonable accommodation requests more specifically, persists even after the passage of the ADAAA (Befort, 2013).

Ticket to Work and Work Incentives Improvement Act of 1999

The TWWIIA, signed into law on December 17, 1999, was intended to provide beneficiaries and recipients of either Supplemental Security Income (SSI) or Social Security Disability Insurance (SSDI), or both, the incentives and supports needed to either prepare for, achieve, maintain, or advance in work.[11] TWWIIA attempted to reduce and remove certain barriers to employment for individuals who receive SSI and SSDI and to encourage beneficiaries and recipients to access the services and supports needed to assist them in their pursuit of employment. At the heart of the Act was a desire by Congress to increase options available to beneficiaries of the SSA's disability programs by expanding upon the existing network of service providers available and creating a more comprehensive set of supports for people with disabilities considering work.[12]

The TWWIIA includes three important titles: Ticket to Work and Self-Sufficiency, Expansion of Health Care, and Demonstration Projects/Studies. Title I expands vocational services options for persons with disabilities. The Ticket to Work and Self-Sufficiency Program is an important provision of Title I. This program supplements the SSA's existing traditional cost reimbursement VR program with an outcomes-based and market-driven program.

All SSI recipients and SSDI beneficiaries who have been determined to be disabled under SSA's adult definition of disability, are more than 18 years of age, and receive benefits will receive a Ticket to Work. The SSA administers the provisions of Title I.[13]

The Ticket Program permits the individual beneficiary or recipient to choose from an array of service providers (called Employment Networks [ENs]), placing control over provider selection in the hands of the consumer. The Ticket Program is purely voluntary and beneficiaries and recipients can choose whether to use their Ticket or not, decide who to deposit their Ticket with, and decide at any point to retract their Ticket from a provider if they feel the services they are receiving are inadequate.

The EN, an approved service provider under the Ticket Program, can be a private organization or public agency that agrees to work with SSA to provide VR, employment, and/or other support services to assist an SSA beneficiary/recipient to prepare for, obtain, and remain at work. Under the Ticket Program, a service provider can elect to become an EN, become a service provider under another EN, or both. An EN that agrees to provide services can decide to receive either outcome payments for months in which a beneficiary does not receive benefits due to work activity (up to 60 months) or reduced outcome payments in addition to payments for assisting the beneficiary to achieve phased milestones connected with employment. In addition, state VR agencies can also elect to receive payment as they have in the past under the cost reimbursement option. This special status is in recognition of the fact that under the Rehabilitation Act of 1973 as amended, state VR agencies cannot deny services and supports to a consumer who is eligible. State VR agencies differ from other ENs in that the other ENs can make a decision to not accept someone's Ticket.

Despite SSA's efforts to promote the Ticket Program from its outset, initial studies have found that participation rates have remained low and that most beneficiaries have remained in the traditional payment system. Thus, SSA has attempted to strengthen the Ticket with revisions to the regulations, including increased financial incentives for service providers to participate in the program (milestone payments earlier in the employment process, milestone payments for lower paying and part-time work outcomes, and payments based on gross earnings at Substantial Gainful Activity rather than reducing earnings by the value of SSA work incentives received by the beneficiary). In addition, the regulations established the Partnership Plus option, allowing Ticket to Work participants who are served under the traditional cost reimbursement program with state VR programs to continue access to individualized employment services through an EN, following their case closure with the state VR program under the Ticket to Work program. Partnership Plus was enacted in recognition of the fact that many disability beneficiaries require long-term employment supports as they progress toward greater economic self-sufficiency and independence. This option allows individuals to benefit from more intensive employment preparation services offered by the state VR program, which may not be available through some ENs, but still allow them to continue to gain additional employment experience, earn more money, continue to access critical employment supports such as benefits counseling, and advance in their careers under the Ticket to Work program once their case has been closed with the state VR program. These revisions took effect in late 2008.

Initial analyses have found only limited evidence of changes in participant-level outcomes after revision (Livermore, Hoffman, & Bardos, 2012). The numbers of EN providers and participants have increased following the revisions, as have certain benchmark data for benefits forgone and termination of benefits for work. However, such benchmarks pertain to both Ticket to Work participants and nonparticipants, and participant-level outcomes resulting from the program have yet to be demonstrated (Schimmel, Stapleton, Mann, & Phelps, 2013).

Title II of TWWIIA governs the provision of health care services to workers with disabilities. This section of the law attempted to reduce the disincentives to employment for people with disabilities posed by the threat of loss of health care benefits by encouraging states to improve access to health care coverage available under Medicaid (Goodman & Livermore, 2004). Under this provision, new optional eligibility groups are established, creating two new Medicaid Buy-In eligibility categories and also extending the period of premium-free Medicare Part A eligibility and requiring protection for certain individuals with Medigap. The Department of Health and Human Services, through the Centers for Medicare & Medicaid Services (CMS), administers the health care provisions.[14]

Workforce Investment Act of 1998 and Workforce Innovation and Opportunity Act of 2014

The WIA of 1998[15] was intended to consolidate workforce preparation and employment services into a unified system of support that is responsive to the needs of job seekers, employers, and communities (Public Law 105–220). Title I of the Act developed a framework for the delivery of workforce investment activities at the state and local levels to provide services in an effective and meaningful way to all consumers, including persons with disabilities. The law was positioned not only to empower consumers but also to provide opportunities for business and human resource professionals to focus public programs on marketplace needs. In 2014, WIA was superseded by WIOA, which retains most of the statutory language from the previous iteration but implements key changes discussed later in this chapter.

WIA created a workforce development system that encourages and facilitates one-stop service delivery (WIA of 1998, August 7, 1998). This employment and training system was intended to serve every job seeker through a central location that provides access to numerous workforce development programs. Core services—including assessment, basic job readiness, and help with job searches—are open to a universal population. For those who require further assistance finding employment, intensive services and job training are also available. The one-stop system is based on four principles: (1) universal access—making core services available to all people; (2) consumer choice—allowing consumers to select services based on their needs; (3) service integration—consolidation of all workforce development services into one-stop centers; and (4) accountability—centers are evaluated on the basis of measurable outcomes with future funding linked to the results of services provided to customers (Imel, 1999). These principles are not only retained but also strengthened in WIOA.

Title IV of the WIA reauthorized the VR program under the Rehabilitation Act. WIA stated that "linkages between the VR program and other components of the statewide workforce investment system are critical to ensure effective and meaningful participation by individuals with disabilities in workforce investment activities." Collaboration between the state units administering the VR program and generic workforce development services (Departments of Labor) is intended to produce better information, more comprehensive services, easier access to services, and improved long-term employment outcomes (WIA of 1998, Title IV, Section 403: 2; see also WIOA of 2014, Title IV, Section 433).

To ensure such participation, WIA and the U.S. DOL's ETA stressed the need for access and partnership when addressing the needs of people with disabilities. Universal access to one-stop services was a central component of WIA.[16] In a notice published in April 2000, the ETA stated: "The Department of Labor is committed to ensuring that the programs, services, and facilities of each One-Stop delivery system are accessible to all of America's workers, including individuals with disabilities" (U.S. DOL, 2000). Every job seeker should have access to the core services available at their local one-stop center. Federal law mandates that all WIA activities, from core to intensive services, must be accessible to individuals with disabilities. Although physical access to the one-stop center is important, access to all tools and services offered by the center—including virtual and computer-based resources—is critical if job seekers with disabilities are to benefit fully from the one-stop system.

WIA mandated a series of partnerships in the one-stop system, including VR. VR has a seat on state and local workforce investment boards and, ideally, is involved in the design of the workforce development system. States and local areas also can bring other disability organizations into the system as partners. The U.S. DOL encourages state and local policy makers to develop partnerships with disability-specific organizations to create an effective and universal workforce investment system.

Although VR's involvement in the workforce development system is critically important and the Rehabilitation Act of 1973 as amended was incorporated into Title IV of both WIA and WIOA, it does not appear that the two systems have yet become completely integrated. This is evidenced in the fact that both systems maintain separate administrations and in some states, the systems are housed in entirely separate state agencies. As discussed in the following, WIA was recently replaced by the WIOA of 2014, which aimed, in part, to address concerns about integrating VR and workforce investment systems. The challenge of integrating a specialized field (VR) into the broader workforce development system presented an opportunity for the development of articulation agreements established to provide clarity regarding who provides what types of services and supports within the one-stop infrastructure (Golden, Zeitzer, & Bruyère,

2014). Articulation of these roles and responsibilities was further reinforced by the 2002 launch of the Disability Program Navigator (DPN) position within the DOL, jointly sponsored by the SSA and the U.S. DOL's ETA. The DPN pilot was administered through the state DOL infrastructure, and in some cases, states actually expanded resources beyond the federal appropriation to ensure that individuals with disabilities who wanted to go to work have assistance accessing and maneuvering the one-stop system.

On July 22, 2014, President Obama signed into law the WIOA, and the law took effect on July 1, 2015. WIOA supersedes the WIA of 1998 (including amendments to the Rehabilitation Act), with the professed aim of helping job seekers access the educational, training, and support services necessary for success in the 21st century labor market, while matching employers with skilled workers needed for global economic competition (U.S. DOL, ETA, 2014). One purpose of WIOA is to further align state VR programs with other core programs of the workforce development system, through unified strategic planning, common performance accountability measures, and one-stop delivery. Under the new law, state governors are required to submit "unified state plans" pertaining to workforce investment programs, adult education, and VR to the secretary of the U.S. DOL by March 1, 2016.

The Act seeks to streamline the workforce development system through (a) common outcome measures for federal workforce programs, including six performance indicators for adults and six for youth served under the Rehabilitation Act; (b) smaller, more strategic state/local workforce development boards; (c) integration of intake, case management, evaluation and reporting systems; and (d) elimination of the sequence of services to allow local boards to meet unique individual's needs (Employer Assistance and Resource Network, 2014). WIOA empowers local boards to tailor services to regional workforce needs and supports access to real-world education and workforce development opportunities for job seekers in the system (e.g., work-based learning, incumbent worker, customized training, pay-for-performance contracts; Employer Assistance and Resource Network, 2014).

WIOA will similarly increase services to youth with disabilities by increasing opportunities for this population to practice workplace skills, exercise self-determination in career interests, and obtain work-based experience. State VR agencies will now be required to offer preemployment transition services to students with disabilities, setting aside at least 15% of federal VR program funds for such purposes. WIOA encourages agencies to prioritize serving youth with disabilities, supports advanced training in science, technology, engineering, and mathematics (STEM fields), and emphasizes competitive integrated employment in supported and customized employment programs (U.S. Department of Education, 2014).

WIOA's job-driven programs emphasize employer engagement in matching employers with skilled individuals, with more opportunities, under the VR program, to help employers provide work-based learning for people with disabilities (e.g., apprenticeships and internships; Employer Assistance and Resource Network, 2014). An NPRM for WIOA was released by the U.S. DOL's, ETA in April 2015, and final rules will be published by January 2016. The NPRM, in part, indicates possible changes to Title IV of the Act, which covers VR programs authorized by the Rehabilitation Act. The NPRM proposes changing regulatory language to reflect WIOA's shift from "gainful employment" to "competitive integrated employment" for people with disabilities and to specify that "customized employment" constitutes an employment outcome under the VR program. The change in terminology from "gainful" to "competitive integrated" employment apparently reflects the shift in definition toward pay for employment, which is commensurate with the income received by other individuals without disabilities, in similar occupations, and with similar training, experience, and skills (WIOA of 2014, Title IV, Section 404(5)). The NPRM also proposes eliminating uncompensated and subminimum wage work from the scope of VR outcomes under the Act (U.S. DOL, ETA, 2015). The final regulations will also specify common performance accountability measures for core state workforce development systems.

Finally, commentators have noted that WIOA was "enacted against the backdrop of a proliferation of state Employment First initiatives" by state VR systems during the preceding decade (Kiernan, Hoff, Freeze, & Mank, 2011; Novak, 2015, p. 101). The state-level Employment First movement, as described in a U.S. DOL, Office of Disability

Employment Policy (ODEP) Memorandum, was characterized by states

> mov[ing] forward to implement policies that focus on integrated, community-based employment earning at or above the minimum wage as the first option for individuals with intellectual and other developmental disabilities. . . . [In] employment first states, sheltered employment with sub-minimum wages and non-work "day activities" are no longer acceptable employment outcomes. (U.S. Department of Education, ODEP, 2009)

Although the "Employment First" terminology is not directly utilized in WIOA, even U.S. DOL officials have noted the influence of this initiative, which is characterized by a commitment among state VR systems to align policies, services, and funding to promote paid, integrated employment as a preferred outcome for both youth and adults with significant disabilities (U.S. Department of Education, 2009).

Family Medical Leave Act of 1993

The FMLA (Public Law 103–3) went into effect on August 5, 1993.[17] It established, for employers with 50 or more employees, a minimum labor standard with regard to leaves of absence for family or medical reasons.

Under the FMLA, an eligible employee may take up to 12 workweeks of leave during any 12-month period for one or more of the following reasons: the birth of a child and to care for the newborn child; the placement of a child with the employee through adoption or foster care and to care for the child; to care for the employee's spouse, son, daughter, or parent with a serious health condition; and a serious health condition of the employee that makes the employee unable to perform one or more of the essential functions of his or her job.[18] An FMLA serious health condition is an illness, injury, impairment, or physical or mental condition that involves inpatient care or continuing treatment by a health care provider. During the FMLA leave, the employer must maintain the employee's existing level of coverage under a group health plan. At the end of FMLA leave, an employer must take an employee back into the same or an equivalent job. The FMLA does not require an employer to let an employee who is medically unable to do his job return to work, nor does it require modification of the job or reassignment to a new position.

In 2008, the FMLA was amended to clarify the rights of military personnel and their families to take and use FMLA leave (U.S. DOL, 2009c). The new regulations specifically incorporated additional military family leave entitlements, including up to 26 weeks of leave during a 12-month period to care for a covered service member recovering from a serious injury or illness incurred in the line of active duty (U.S. DOL, 2009c). In 2013, additional regulations were issued clarifying that the definition of a "serious injury or illness" was expanded to include injuries or illnesses existing before the beginning of active duty, which aggravated during military service (U.S. DOL, Wage and Hour Division 2013).

Some of the questions relating to the use of the FMLA by rehabilitation professionals arise from the interplay of FMLA leave with accommodation and return-to-work efforts (Geaney, 2004; Scott, 1996; Shalowitz, 1993). The interaction between FMLA, the ADA, and workers' compensation has been dubbed "the Bermuda Triangle of employment law" by some writers (Postol, 2002). In some cases, FMLA leave itself can be an accommodation (FMLA Leave Can Be ADA Accommodation, 2002). In other situations, the FMLA may create difficulties for an employer attempting to get injured workers back to work and off benefits. Many employers have used "light duty" to bring an injured worker back to work within his or her medical restrictions. Light duty jobs typically are very different from the job an employee was doing at the time of injury. Because the FMLA requires that a worker be restored to the same or an equivalent position on return from leave, an employer may not compel an injured worker to accept light duty work in lieu of exercising his or her FMLA entitlement. Likewise, the DOL has taken the position that an employer may not require an FMLA-eligible employee to accept reasonable accommodation instead of FMLA leave.

An employer may offer accommodation or light duty but may not compel it. On the other hand, if an employee rejects an offer of employment that is within his or her medical restrictions, an employer may contest the employee's entitlement to workers' compensation indemnity benefits. In addition, if an employee voluntarily accepts light duty, an employer may not designate time on light duty as FMLA leave, as the employee is working. However, time spent on light duty does not lessen an employee's right to be restored to the same or an equivalent position held at the time leave commenced.

The issue of FMLA employee notice provisions and ADA prohibitions on medical inquiries has raised many questions for employers (Geaney, 2004). FMLA allows employers to ask for certification of a serious health condition, whereas the ADA places restrictions on disability-related inquiries by employees. The EEOC issued a fact sheet to address some of these questions most often asked about the ADA and FMLA interaction (EEOC Answers, 1997).[19] This publication clarifies the point that when an employee requests leave under the FMLA for a serious health condition, employers will not violate the ADA by asking for the information specified in the FMLA certification form. The ADA allows medical inquiries that are "job related" and consistent with business necessity. However, employers continue to note that differences between FMLA and the ADA cause difficulties when leave requests trigger obligations under each statute (Lipnic & DeCamp, 2007). After amendments to the FMLA in 2008 that clarified the definition of "serious health condition" and required that employees follow their employer's usual sick leave call-in requirements immediately upon the start of their health condition, the DOL published revised rules and guidance for employers and employees (U.S. DOL, 2009a).

The FMLA form requests only information relating to the particular serious health condition for which the person is seeking leave. An employer is entitled to know why an employee, who otherwise should be at work, is requesting time off under the FMLA. Medical inquiries that are strictly limited in this fashion are therefore not ADA violations (EEOC, 2000).

Occupational Safety and Health Act of 1970

The OSHA of 1970 represents the culmination of nearly a century of Congress's growing concern for workplace safety (Rothstein, 1990). Throughout the 20th century, laws were passed in response to specific workplace health issues, but no piece of legislation covered all safety and health issues in every workplace for every employee until the passage of OSHA in 1970. Unlike some other employment regulation, OSHA is applied universally to all employers, regardless of the volume of business they conduct or the number of people they employ (Rothstein, 1990).

At OSHA's core is the recognition that every worker has a right to a workplace that is free from recognized hazards. Therefore, when a potential hazard is identified, the OSH Administration, through the DOL, develops a standard against which workplace practices or conditions should be measured (Bureau of National Affairs, 1997).

After the implementation of a standard, the DOL can determine which workplaces will be inspected—either by the request of an employee in the particular workplace or at the OSH Administration's discretion. Inspections are conducted with the permission of the employer and according to OSHA guidelines. Violations of a standard are punishable by government-ordered abatement and monetary fines, set according to the size of the business, the seriousness of the violation, the good faith of the employer, and the record of prior violations. Violations that result in the death of an employee can be punished by criminal law (Bureau of National Affairs, 1997).

Section 18 of OSHA encourages states to develop and operate their own job safety and health programs. These state plans must be approved and monitored by the federal government. As of 2015, there were 22 states and territories operating complete state plans, whereas an additional four states had OSH plans covering only public employees. States must set job safety and health standards that are at least as affective as comparable federal standards but have the option of promulgating standards covering hazards not addressed by the federal regulations (U.S. DOL, 2009b).

A major way in which this law may affect the functioning of rehabilitation professionals is its interplay with ADA requirements regarding employment-screening prohibitions, medical confidentiality of records, and required accommodations. The ADA's limitations on employee testing can be in conflict with OSHA's need for testing in furtherance of workplace safety goals.

The ADA places significant restrictions on an employer's right to require preemployment physicals, to make medical inquiries of employees and applicants, and to require that employees submit to physical examinations, and it restricts access to such information in an effort to prevent potential discrimination. OSHA, in contrast, affirmatively requires employers to conduct testing in various situations to ensure safety. For example, employees exposed to high noise levels are required to be included within an audiometric testing program, which includes, among other things, annual hearing tests (Taylor, 1995; U.S. DOL, 2001). The ADA requires strict confidentiality of medical records. OSHA, on the other hand, requires employers to provide employees, and their representatives, with signed authorizations, and OSHA personnel access to such records in the interest of exposing potential hazards and their causes. By having the employee sign an information release, the employer can better ensure that the information being released stays in the appropriate hands and that the ADA confidentiality requirements are not violated. The EEOC has stated that the ADA does not override health and safety requirements established under other federal laws, such that if certain standards are required by another law, an employer does not have to show that it is job related and consistent with business necessity (EEOC, 1992; Occupational Injury and Illness Recording and Reporting Requirements, 2001).

OSHA requires certain employers to develop and maintain a written emergency action plan. Although the ADA does not require emergency planning, it does require that any plan created in compliance with OSHA standards must include people with disabilities (U.S. DOL, 2005).

Although OSHA requirements can often take precedence over the ADA requirements to ensure adherence to health and safety requirements, the reasonable accommodation element of the ADA can still be applied to OSHA-mandated policies and modifications. For example, an eyewash station, which may be required by OSHA for certain positions, must be installed in such a way that a wheelchair user would have access to it.

The lines are not always so clear, however, particularly in terms of the direct threat defense to ADA claims. Take, for example, the case of an employee with epilepsy working on an assembly line. The way an employer handles the situation is largely contingent on which legislation he or she believes is more likely to be invoked. Removal of the employee, satisfying the general duty clause of OSHA, may violate the ADA. The direct threat defense is so difficult to prove that employers are likely to avoid the ADA claim at all costs, often leaving themselves in violation of OSHA standards. The complications arise when OSHA does not explicitly call for an action such as removal of an employee who has seizures. As a general rule, OSHA standards "trump" the ADA's duty to accommodate, but employers cannot rely on using OSHA as a defense to ADA claims unless the employment action in question was specifically called for by OSHA (Skoning & McGlothlen, 1994).

National Labor Relations Act of 1935

The NLRA, also called the Wagner Act, was passed in 1935. It stands as the established framework for labor relations in the United States, covering union–management relations in almost every private firm in operation. The law protects workers from the effects of unfair labor practices by employers and requires employers to recognize and bargain collectively with a union that the workers elect to represent them (Gold, 1998).

Among the main principles of the NLRA are the idea of exclusivity of representation, a policy against direct dealing, and the duty to provide information. Seniority rights gained through collective bargaining are also among the most valued benefits of having a unionized workplace (Gold, 1998). All of these areas may yield conflict for individuals seeking to invoke protection from laws such as the ADA, FMLA, or the Rehabilitation Act. These laws rely on making exceptions to or changes in terms and conditions of employment on an individual basis, whereas collective bargaining agreements under the NLRA make the union the broker of employment rights for all its members (Schwab, 2009). Compliance with these laws may include dealing with the employer to discuss and secure those agreements that may fall outside the scope of the union's normal interactions, the unilateral implementation of an accommodation for an employee, and often the security of medical information, which the union may feel it has the right to access under the NLRA (Evans, 1992).

Reasonable accommodations for individuals with disabilities may present an especially problematic situation for employers and unions alike. Both parties are required by law to operate in a nondiscriminatory manner: The employer must accommodate a worker so that his or her essential job functions may be performed regardless of disability and must provide terms and conditions of employment that are free of discriminatory intent. The union must represent its constituency equally and consistently, as well as allow accommodations for people with disabilities to be implemented without unreasonable opposition (President's Committee of People with Disabilities, 1994).

Whenever a modification in the terms or conditions of employment is required, a review of the collective bargaining agreement would be advisable, as well as some kind of communication between the employer and the union concerning the accommodation and the potential effects it may have on the lives of other workers (President's Committee of People with Disabilities, 1994). An effective way to approach this is the use of joint labor–management teams (Bruyère, Gomez, & Handelmann, 1996).

In a unionized workplace, the rehabilitation professional can contribute to an injured worker's effective return to the workplace, taking into the account the interests of the employee, the employer, and the union to effect a successful reintegration. Organized labor has been an important part of the history of fighting for worker rights and against job discrimination, and these social issues are very important to workers with disabilities. Yet many employment professionals have little experience with unions and little knowledge of their purpose and structure (Bruyère, 1996). Adopting a position that favors both the person with a disability and the union will go a long way in the service delivery process to minimize conflict and maximize union support in the accommodation process.

A 2002 Supreme Court decision (*U.S. Airways, Inc. v. Barnett*) ruled that employees with disabilities are not always entitled to reassignment to a job intended for workers with more seniority. The Supreme Court held that, in situations involving a conflict between a requested accommodation and an employer-created seniority system, the "seniority system will prevail in the run of cases." However, the court left open the possibility of an employee showing that reassignment would be a reasonable accommodation in a particular case despite the existence of a seniority system. Lower courts, such as the Third Circuit Court of Appeals have held that, even subsequent to Barnett, if an employee can demonstrate that a "feasible reassignment" exists within a seniority or best qualified system, then the burden shifts to the employer to demonstrate that the reassignment would cause an undue hardship (Conway, 2014). Thus, questions remain about the legalities of accommodating workers with disabilities within a collective bargaining agreement (Flores, 2008).

Patient Protection and Affordable Care Act of 2010

The Patient Protection and Affordable Care Act (ACA), effective in 2010, refers to two separate pieces of legislation: the Patient Protection and Affordable Care Act (Public Law 111–148) and the Health Care and Education Reconciliation Act (Public Law 111–152). Together, these statutes aim to improve health care coverage and security for the U.S. population by expanding coverage, holding insurance companies accountable, lowering health care costs, increasing consumer choice, and enhancing quality of care (U.S. Department of Health and Human Services, 2010). The ACA ushered in the most far-reaching regulatory and legal changes to the U.S. health care system since the passage of Medicare and Medicaid in 1965 (Manchikanti, Caraway, Parr, Fellows, & Martinez, 2013).

In June 2012, the U.S. Supreme Court upheld all provisions of the ACA except for those mandating expansion of Medicaid eligibility for low-income adults by state governments. The Court held that a state opting not to participate in the Medicaid expansion of Medicaid eligibility may not be penalized by a loss of federal funding to its existing Medicaid program. Nevertheless, many states have opted into the Medicaid expansion, with significant implications for VR services and professionals.

One of the main issues affecting the administration of VR by state VR agencies involves managing and maximizing federal and state funding to pay for VR services and supports, including health-related services and supports, and the ACA includes significant new potential funding sources for such services (Silverstein, 2012). The ACA increases access to private health insurance, removes preexisting conditions from insurance eligibility determinations, and also expands the population of individuals eligible to receive health care through Medicaid programs, although this now depends on states' willingness to participate (Silverstein, 2012). As of July 2015, 31 states had adopted the Medicaid expansion (Kaiser Family Foundation, 2015). Essential health benefits, including rehabilitative and habilitative services, may therefore be more readily available to individuals receiving VR services following passage of the ACA.

Issues pertaining to health care and insurance are important in the VR context, because people with disabilities often have lower employment rates and therefore experience less access to employer-sponsored health insurance as a population (Croft & Parish, 2012). The ACA directly impacts issues of integration of care and access to care, including by expanding the criteria for Medicaid eligibility, and important issues for many under- and unemployed individuals with disabilities. The ACA provides additional federal funding for states opting to expand their Medicaid programs to cover adults under 65 years with income up to 133% of the federal poverty level, as well as children at that income level (U.S. Centers for Medicare and Medicaid Services, 2015).

As a result, in states with expanded Medicaid, free or low-cost health coverage is available to people with incomes below a certain level, regardless of disability, family status, financial resources, and other designations usually factoring into Medicaid eligibility determinations (U.S. Centers for Medicare and Medicaid Services, 2015). The ACA also provides, on an optional basis, for the expansion of community-based services such as vocational supports and case management, allowing participating states to offer such services through their regular state Medicaid plans without seeking a waiver, for individuals with incomes up to 300% of the maximum SSI payment and with a high level of need (Croft & Parish, 2012; Kaiser Family Foundation, 2010).

Workers' Compensation

Workers' compensation programs are government-sponsored, employer-financed systems for compensating employees who incur an injury or illness in connection with their employment. They are designed to ensure that employees who are injured on the job receive timely compensation for their losses without proof of fault. Workers' compensation laws allow employees or their survivors to file claims for economic losses resulting from work-related injuries or occupational diseases. Benefits provided under workers' compensation laws include medical care, disability payments, rehabilitation services, survivor benefits, and funeral expenses. Employers who participate in workers' compensation programs usually are protected against tort actions that employees might otherwise pursue to redress their losses.

State workers' compensation statutes generally provide benefits to employees for job-related injuries, whether or not the injury is permanently disabling. In addition to medical care and treatment for job-related injuries, these statutes typically also provide benefits for temporary incapacity, scarring, and permanent impairment of specific parts of the body. Workers' compensation laws are maintained by all 50 states, the District of Columbia, American Samoa, Guam, the Virgin Islands, and Puerto Rico. In addition, the federal government administers workers' compensation programs authorized by the Federal Coal Mine Health and Safety Act, the Longshore and Harbor Workers' Compensation Act, and the Federal Employers' Liability Act. Rehabilitation professionals working in private sector rehabilitation and in the return-to-work process for persons with disabilities must interact with this system and its regulations regularly.

Although much attention was paid immediately after the passage of the ADA to disability nondiscrimination and the hiring process, some employers were already focusing on its effect on job incumbents with disabilities (Walworth, Damon, & Wilder, 1993). Now, even more attention is being paid to the ADA's effect on job retention aspects of the employment process. Of the ADA charges filed with the EEOC between 1992 and 2007, 12.2% were cited as being related to a back impairment (Bjelland et al., 2009), which is a disability or injury often seen in the workers' compensation system. It is inevitable that the rehabilitation practitioner will deal with some persons for whom there will be an interplay of these two pieces of legislation.

Some authors have pointed out that disability nondiscrimination legislation such as the ADA appears to rest on very different principles than the workers' compensation system (Bell, 1994; Geaney, 2004). The ADA is predicated on the premise that disability does not necessarily mean inability to work, and it focuses on how accommodation can assist in removing barriers to employment caused by the interaction between functional limitations and the workplace. Workers' compensation legislation, however, focuses on the apparently contrasting premise that impairments are the cause of work limitations, and employees must prove loss of earning capacity because of injury.

For workers' compensation purposes, it is often necessary for an employee to emphasize the limitations caused by a disability, but these statements can be detrimental to requests for reinstatement and accommodation under the ADA (Geaney, 2004). Further highlighting this juxtaposition, an analysis by Burkhauser, Schmeiser, and Weathers (2012) found that employers seemingly engage in cost–benefit considerations related to experience ratings for workers' compensation programs when determining whether they will provide reasonable accommodations under the ADA. Employers are more likely to provide reasonable accommodations to employees who are eligible for workers' compensation, likely because they are balancing the cost of accommodation and the cost of compensation benefits (Burkhauser et al., 2012).

Rehabilitation professionals in this area will need to concern themselves with clarifying for individuals with disabilities and for employers the significant aspects of workers' compensation legislation as they relate to protections provided by the ADA and FMLA. These include issues of the injured worker as a protected person under the ADA, queries by an employer about a worker's prior workers' compensation claims, hiring persons with a prior history of an occupational injury and application of the direct threat standard, reasonable accommodation for persons with disability-related occupational injuries, light duty, and exclusive remedy provisions in workers' compensation laws. In response to a need for clarification of these issues, the EEOC issued enforcement guidance concerning the interaction between Title I of the ADA and state workers' compensation laws that can greatly assist rehabilitation professionals in responding to many of these employer questions (EEOC, 1996; Welch, 1996).

IMPLICATIONS FOR REHABILITATION SERVICE DELIVERY

To prepare persons with disabilities appropriately for initial entry or reentry into the workplace and to provide effective consultation to employers on disability nondiscrimination and equal access in the workplace, rehabilitation professionals must be apprised of state and federal legislation that affects both safety and equity practices in the workplace. The issues presented here in the implementation of specific pieces of legislation, and more specifically as they interrelate with disability nondiscrimination legislation, such as the ADA, and workforce preparation and benefits support, such as the Ticket legislation and WIOA, point to areas where rehabilitation professionals need more knowledge and expertise and also where they can provide effective service. A list of specific skills and knowledge needed by rehabilitation professionals in implementing the ADA as consultants were identified by Pape and Tarvydas (1994) as cutting across the following three distinct areas: core rehabilitation principles, knowledge, and functions; disability concepts, functions, and knowledge; and ADA knowledge and functions.

The implications of disability nondiscrimination legislation specifically for the role of psychologists were addressed by Crewe (1994), who encourages specialized pre- or postdoctoral preparation in disability and rehabilitation for psychologists who are planning to apply their clinical or counseling psychology training to services for people with disabilities. The implications of disability nondiscrimination legislation such as the ADA for preparation of rehabilitation undergraduate and graduate professionals are discussed by Stude (1994), who encourages rehabilitation educators to include this information in existing course work rather than isolating it into a specialized course. The importance of examining the gap between existing employment and disability policy and desired employment outcomes for persons with disabilities was the focus of a recent conference and resulting publication sponsored by the American Psychological Association and the National Institute of Disability and Rehabilitation Research (Bruyère et al., 2003).

The ADA has afforded rehabilitation professionals, who contribute to employment opportunities for persons with disabilities, a tool to more effectively combat discrimination in the recruitment, hiring, retention, and termination processes. Under the ADA, a significant service that VR counselors might provide is assisting employers with job analyses, writing job descriptions, and helping develop or design the reasonable accommodations that will make initial hiring or return to work feasible for workers with disabilities (Walker & Heffner, 1992). Employers need assistance in the development of policies and procedures that do not discriminate against people with disabilities in the recruitment, hiring, health and other employment benefits, promotion and training, and termination processes.

The workers' compensation system is cited as being particularly difficult for both employees and employers to navigate, seemingly fanning the fires for a contentious and litigious relationship. One of the most important things rehabilitation professionals can do is to facilitate communication between the employer and the employee (Commerce Clearing House, 1997). Rehabilitation professionals can either make themselves that bridge with employers or serve as consultants to encourage supervisors and others in the workplace to address the employees' questions and provide supportive follow-up during disability leave. Rehabilitation professionals also can play a role in bringing human resource, safety, and health professionals within a given organization together to develop a unified approach to the ADA and workers' compensation (Walker & Heffner, 1992).

Across all facets of this legislation, working with both individuals with disabilities and employers and teaching them how to communicate their respective needs effectively is imperative. Often, when coached appropriately, both employees with disabilities and their supervisors or the human resources staff in a given organization can effectively address accommodation requests and resolve any conflicts that arise in negotiating final decisions on accommodations. Problems arise when there has been a prior history of poor performance, of poor relationship between supervisor and employee, or of general discord or conflict in a unit or workplace environment, creating a culture of mistrust in responding to employee needs.

Increasingly, federal law and regulatory guidance encourages employers to partner with employment service providers, rehabilitation professionals, and others. The new Section 503 regulations, for example, call for federal contractors to "engage in appropriate outreach and recruitment," which the DOL defines as giving such employers "the flexibility to choose the specific resources they believe will be most helpful in identifying and attracting qualified individuals with disabilities," including linkages to rehabilitation professionals in the community (U.S. DOL, Office of Federal Contract Compliance, 2013). Many employers with federal contracts looking to comply with this outreach mandate will likely be seeking these linkages to the valuable insights of rehabilitation professionals in their communities (Rudstam et al., 2014).

Importantly, disability employment–focused legislation and policy has slowly come around toward acknowledging the importance of "demand side" issues affecting employer practices—or how employer workforce *needs* impact employment outcomes for people with disabilities (Bruyère, VanLooy, von Schrader, & Barrington, in press). Recent research has indicated that even decades after the passage of landmark legislation such as the ADA, employers and HR representatives continue to experience difficulties not only in navigating legal requirements but also in perceiving the potential positive impact that inclusive hiring can have on their labor needs, such as finding and retaining qualified talent (Bruyère, in press; Chan et al., 2010). Rehabilitation professionals can play a vital role in informing both clients and employers, identifying opportunities where job seeker skills align with employer needs.

SUMMARY

The purpose of this chapter has been to provide rehabilitation professionals with a basic overview of some of the pieces of disability and employment legislation that may affect their functioning in the rehabilitation and return-to-work process. Several of these laws, such as the NLRA and the OSHA, are designed to protect workers' rights before injury occurs and to emphasize employer responsibilities in the safety and equitable treatment of workers in all terms and conditions of employment. Regulatory requirements such as the FMLA, short-term disability leave requirements as dictated by state regulations, and workers' compensation legislation are designed to deal with the rights of employees once an injury or illness has occurred. These laws protect the right to a medical leave that gives the worker the time needed for the rehabilitation process and they ensure the security of benefits to cover part of the medical costs and salary lost to time off work due to illness or injury, as well as a job upon their return. Legislation, such as the Rehabilitation Act of 1973 as amended and the ADA and ADAAA, focuses more specifically on the rights of workers with disabilities. These laws require equal access in the seeking and securing of employment as well as retention and equitable access to other terms and conditions of employment. Regulatory requirements such as confidentiality of medical information also serve a role here, in terms of providing requirements for employers to keep confidential any medical diagnostic information on employees that they may gain access to. New regulations pertaining to voluntary self-disclosure add wrinkles to the traditional prohibition on disability and medical inquiry under the ADA and Rehabilitation Act. Legislation such as the TWWIIA and the WIOA provide needed supports and services to remove barriers to employment and to the employment-seeking process. The ACA, although not immediately obvious in its application to rehabilitation providers, offers new funding streams for both community and health-based services through the Medicaid expansion.

Assisting the individual through the rehabilitation process to return to productive functioning in the community and in the workplace is the core of the rehabilitation professional's job. When employment outcomes are part of the rehabilitation goal, knowledge of the regulatory requirements that surround the workplace and have an effect on employer and employee behavior is vital for the rehabilitation professional to function effectively. This chapter has pointed out some of the possible areas of conflict or concern that may influence both worker and employer behaviors and has provided a basic introduction for practitioners to pursue further information, given the nature of their services and interventions for persons with disabilities.

ACKNOWLEDGMENTS

The contents of this chapter have been developed under a grant from the National Institute on Disability, Independent Living, and Rehabilitation Research (NIDILRR grant number 90RT5010-01-00). NIDILRR is a center within the Administration for Community Living (ACL), Department of Health and Human Services (HHS). The contents of this chapter do not necessarily represent the policy of NIDILRR, ACL, HHS, and you should not assume endorsement by the federal government.

The authors would also like to acknowledge the work of Rebecca DeMarinis and Sara VanLooy, coauthors of prior versions of this chapter, and Erin Sullivan, Fordham University law student, and Sara Furguson, Cornell University of International and Labor Relations (ILR) student, who also have assisted in the review of literature for related chapters in previous editions.

ENDNOTES

1. A brief publication discussing these pieces of legislation, entitled *A Guide to Disability Rights Laws*, is available from the U.S. Department of Justice Civil Rights Division, Disability Rights Section, P.O. 66738, Washington, DC 20035–6738; call (800) 514–0301 (voice) or (800) 514–0383 (TTY), or go to www.usdoj.gov/crt/ada/cguide.pdf to download the full publication.
2. See www2.ed.gov/policy/speced/leg/rehabact.doc for complete text of the Rehabilitation Act, as amended.
3. For further information, visit the Council for State Administrators in Vocational Rehabilitation (CSAVR) at www.rehabnetwork.org or contact the Executive Office: 1 Research Court, Suite 450, Rockville, MD 20850; call (301) 519-8023 (voice), 771 (TTY).
4. To obtain more information or to file a complaint, employees should contact their agency's Equal Employment Opportunity Office; call (800) 669–4000 (voice) or (800) 669–6820 (TTY), or visit www.eeoc.gov
5. For more information on Section 503, contact Office of Federal Contract Compliance Programs (OFCCP), U.S. DOL, 200 Constitution Ave., NW, Washington, DC 20210; (202) 693–0101. Visit https://www.dol.gov/ofccp for a list of regional offices, Section 503 information, and instructions for filing complaints.
6. For information on how to file complaints under Section 504 with the appropriate agency, contact U.S. Department of Justice, 950 Pennsylvania Avenue, NW, Civil Rights Division, Disability Rights Section—NYAV, Washington, DC 20530; (800) 514–0301 (voice), (800) 514–0383 (TTY), or see http://www.ada.gov
7. Information about these standards can be found at the Access Board website at www.access-board.gov/news/508.htm

8. Cornell University has developed an online guide to the ADA and reasonable accommodations for people with specific disabilities. See www.hrtips.org for more information
9. A modification or adjustment is "reasonable" if it seems reasonable on its face, that is, ordinarily or in the run of cases; this means it is "reasonable" if it appears to be "feasible" or "plausible." A deeper discussion of what is "reasonable" accommodation can be found in U.S. EEOC (2003).
10. For more information on common issues, charge rates, and employee discrimination areas in EEOC complaints, see the EEOC Charge Data provided at Cornell University's Disability Statistics website www.disabilitystatistics.org
11. For more information on the TWWIIA, see the Social Security Administration (SSA) website at www.ssa.gov/work/overview.html
12. Cornell University has developed a series of Policy and Practice Briefs on Social Security issues, including one on the Ticket Program. They can be found at www.edi.cornell.edu/s-PPBriefs.cfm
13. Further information about the Ticket Program is available through the SSA on their toll-free number at 1–800-772–1213 or on the SSA website at www.ssa.gov/work
14. Further information about the Medicaid Buy-In program can be found at the CMS website at https://www.medicaid.gov/medicaid/ltss/employmment/index.html
15. For further information about the WIA, see https://www.doleta.gov/wioa. For information on the WIOA, which recently superseded WIA, see www.doleta.gov/wioa
16. The U.S. DOL has developed an online toolkit (www.onestoptoolkit.org) for one-stops to help grantees ensure access for people with disabilities.
17. See https://www.gpo.gov/fdsys/pkg/FR-2016-08-19/pdf/2016-15975.pdf for the complete text of this law.
18. For additional information about the FMLA or to file an FMLA complaint, individuals should contact the nearest office of the Wage and Hour Division, Employment Standards Administration, U.S. DOL. The Wage and Hour Division is listed in most directories under U.S. Government, Department of Labor, or you can visit their website at www.dol.gov/whd/america2.htm
19. The EEOC fact sheet, the *Family and Medical Leave Act, the Americans with Disabilities Act, and Title VII of the Civil Rights Act of 1964* can be ordered by writing or calling the EEOC's Office of Communications and Legislative Affairs at 1801 L St., NW, Washington, DC 20507; telephone (202) 663–4900, TTY (202) 663–4494, or visit the EEOC website at www.eeoc.gov/policy/docs/fmlaada.html

REFERENCES

Befort, S. F. (2013). An empirical analysis of case outcomes under the ADA Amendments Act. *Washington and Lee Law Review, 70*, 2027–2071.

Bell, C. (1994). The Americans with Disabilities Act and injured workers: Implications for rehabilitation professionals and the workers compensation system. In S. Bruyère & J. O'Keeffe (Eds.), *Implications of the Americans with Disabilities Act for psychology* (pp. 137–149). New York, NY: Springer Publishing.

Billitteri, T. (1997). Mental health policy: The issues. *CQ Researcher, Congressional Quarterly Inc, 7*, 795–797.

Bjelland, M., Bruyère, S., Houtenville, A., Ruiz-Quintanilla, A., & Webber, D. (2009). *Trends in disability employment discrimination claims: Implications for rehabilitation counseling practice, administration, training, and research.* Ithaca, NY: Cornell University Employment and Disability Institute.

Bjelland, M., Bruyère, S., von Schrader, S., Houtenville, A., Ruiz-Quintanilla, A., & Webber, D. (2009). Age and disability employment discrimination: Occupational rehabilitation implications. *Journal of Occupational Rehabilitation, 20*, 456–471. doi:10.1007/s10926–009-9194-z

Bruyère, S (Ed.). (1996). *A job developer's guide to working with unions: Obtaining the support of organized labor for the hiring of employees with disabilities.* St. Augustine, FL: Training Resource Network.

Bruyère, S. M (Ed.). (in press). *Disability and employer practices: Research across the disciplines.* Ithaca, NY: Cornell University Press.

Bruyère, S. M., Erickson, W., VanLooy, S., Sitaras, E., Cook, J., Burke, J., . . . Morris, J. (2003). Employment and disability policy: Recommendations for a social sciences research agenda. In F. E. Menz & D. F. Thomas (Eds.), *Bridging gaps: Refining the disability research agenda for rehabilitation and the social sciences—Conference proceedings.* Menomonie, WI: University of Wisconsin-Stout, Stout Vocational Rehabilitation Institute, Research and Training Centers.

Bruyère, S. M., Gomez, S., & Handelmann, G. (1996). The reasonable accommodation process in unionized environments. *Labor Law Journal, 48*, 629–647.

Bruyère, S. M., VanLooy, S., von Schrader, S., & Barrington, L. (in press). Disability and employment: Framing the problem and our approach. In S. M. Bruyère (Ed.), *Disability and employer practices: Research across the disciplines*. Ithaca, NY: Cornell University Press.

Bureau of National Affairs, Inc. (1997). Job safety and health (No. 228). In *The laws in brief: OSHA*. Washington, DC: Author.

Burkhauser, R. V., Schmeiser, M. D., & Weathers, R. R. (2012). The importance of anti-discrimination and workers' compensation laws on the provision of workplace accommodations following the onset of a disability. *Industrial and Labor Relations Review, 65*, 161–180.

Chan, F., Strauser, D., Maher, P., Lee, E., Jones, R., & Johnson, E. T. (2010). Demand-side factors related to employment of people with disabilities: A survey of employers in the midwest region of the United States. *Journal of Occupational Rehabilitation, 20*, 412–419.

Commerce Clearing House. (1997). Communication and concern help workers return to work. In *Workers' compensation business management guide* (pp. 299–301). Chicago, IL: Author.

Conway, C. (2014). Ordinarily reasonable: Using the supreme court's barnett analysis to clarify preferential treatment under the Americans with Disabilities Act. *Journal of Gender, Social Policy, and Law, 22*, 721–748.

Council of State Administrators of Vocational Rehabilitation. (n.d.). Public vocational rehabilitation program fact sheet. Retrieved from www2.ed.gov/policy/speced/guid/rsa/im/1999/im-99-21.doc

Crewe, N. (1994). Implications of the Americans with Disabilities Act for the training of psychologists. *Rehabilitation Education, 8*, 9–16.

Croft, B., & Parish, S. L. (2012). Care integration in the Patient Protection and Affordable Care Act: Implications for behavioral health. *Administration and Policy in Mental Health and Mental Health Services Research, 40*, 258–263.

Employer Assistance and Resource Network. (2014). Workforce Innovation and Opportunity Act of 2014 (WIOA). Retrieved from http://askearn.org/refdesk/Disability_Laws/WIOA

Evans, B. (1992). Will employers and unions cooperate? *Human Resource Magazine, 37*, 59–63.

Flores, C. (2008). A disability is not a trump card: The Americans with Disabilities Act does not entitle disabled employees to automatic reassignment. *Valparaiso University Law Review, 43*, 195–260.

FMLA Leave can be ADA Accommodation. (2002, September). *HR Focus, 79*, 2.

Fujiura, G., Yamaki, K., & Czechowicz, S. (1998). Disability among ethnic and racial minorities in the United States. *Journal of Disability Policy Studies, 9*, 111–130.

Gault, R., & Kinnane, A. (1996). Navigating the maze of employment law. *Management Review, 85*, 9–11.

Geaney, J. (2004). The relationship of workers' compensation to the Americans with Disabilities Act and Family and Medical Leave Act. *Clinics in Occupational and Environmental Medicine, 4*, 273–293.

Gold, M. (1998). *An introduction to labor law*. Ithaca, NY: Cornell University/ILR Press.

Goldberg, S., Killeen, M., & O'Day, B. (2005). The disclosure conundrum: How people with psychiatric disabilities navigate employment. *Psychology, Public Policy, and Law, 11*, 463–500.

Golden, T., Zeitzer, I., & Bruyère, S. (2014). New approaches to disability in social policy: The case of the United States. In T. Guloglu (Ed.), *Social policy in a changing world*. Munster: MV Wissenschaft Publishing.

Goodman, N., & Livermore, G. (2004, July 28). *The effectiveness of medicaid buy-in programs in promoting the employment of people with disabilities*. Briefing paper prepared for the ticket to work and work incentives advisory panel of the social security administration. Retrieved from https://www.scribd.com/document/1947561/Social-Security-Buy-in-20paper-20Goodman-Livermore-20072804r

Greenberg, J. (2014). Not a 'second class' agency: Applying chevron step zero to EEOC interpretations of the ADA and ADAAA. *George Mason University Civil Rights Law Journal, 3*, 297–323.

Hellwege, J. (2002). Tenth circuit blocks attempt to narrow Rehabilitation Act in disability cases. *Trial, 38*, 88–90.

Hsieh, A. (2013). Catch-22 of ADA title I remedies for psychiatric disabilities. *McGeorge Law Review, 44*, 989–1036.

Huss, A. (1993). ADA, insurance, and employee benefits. *Journal of the American Society of CLU & ChFC, 47*, 82–89.

Imel, S. (1999). *One stop career centers* (*ERIC Digest No. 208*). Columbus, OH: ERIC Clearinghouse on Adult, Career, and Vocational Education (ERIC Document Reproduction Service No. ED434244).

Jaeger, P. (2006). Assessing section 508 compliance on federal e-government web sites: A multi-method, user-centered evaluation of accessibility for persons with disabilities. *Government Information Quarterly, 23*, 169–190.

Kaiser Family Foundation. (2010). *Summary of new health reform law*. Menlo Park, CA: Henry J. Kaiser Family Foundation.

Kaiser Family Foundation. (2015). *Status of state action on the medicaid expansion decision*. Retrieved from http://kff.org/health-reform/state-indicator/state-activity-around-expanding-medicaid-under-the-affordable-care-act

Kiernan, W. E., Hoff, D., Freeze, S., & Mank, D. M. (2011). Employment first: A beginning not an end. *Intellectual and Developmental Disabilities, 49*, 300–304.

Kosyluk, K. A., Corrigan, P. W., & Landis, R. S. (2014). Employer stigma as a mediator between past and future hiring behavior. *Rehabilitation Counseling Bulletin, 57*, 102–108.

Lipnic, S., & DeCamp, P. (2007). *Family and Medical Leave Act regulations: A report on the department of labor's request for information.* Washington, DC: U.S. Department of Labor. Retrieved from http://digitalcommons.ilr.cornell.edu/key-workplace/315

Livermore, G. A., Hoffman, D., & Bardos, M. (2012, September). *Ticket to work participant characteristics and outcomes under the revised regulations.* Washington, DC: Mathematica Policy Research Institute.

Manchikanti, L., Caraway, D., Parr, A. T., Fellows, B., & Martinez, K. (2013). Integrated employment, employment first, and U.S. federal policy. *Journal of Vocational Rehabilitation, 38*, 165–168.

Moss, K., & Johnsen, M. (1997). Employment discrimination and the ADA: A study of the administrative complaint process. *Psychiatric Rehabilitation Journal, 21*, 111–121.

National Council on Disability. (2004). *Righting the ADA.* Washington, DC: Author. Retrieved http://www.ncd.gov/newsroom/publications/2004/pdf/righting_ada.pdf

National Council on Disability. (2007). *Implementation of the Americans with Disabilities Act: Challenges, best practices, and new opportunities for success.* Washington, DC: Author. Retrieved from http://www.ncd.gov/newsroom/publications/2007/pdf/implementation_07-26-07.pdf

Nobile, R. (1996). How discrimination laws affect compensation. *Compensation & Benefits Review, 28*, 38–42.

Novak, J. (2015). Raising expectations for U.S. youth with disabilities. Federal disability policy advances integrated employment. *Center for Educational Policy Studies Journal, 5*, 91–110.

O'Keeffe, J. (1994). Disability, discrimination, and the Americans with Disabilities Act. In S. Bruyère & J. O'Keeffe (Eds.), *Implications of the Americans with Disabilities Act for psychology* (pp. 1–14). New York, NY: Springer Publishing.

Occupational Injury and Illness Recording and Reporting Requirements (2001, January). Retrieved from http://www.osha.gov/pls/oshaweb/owadisp.show_document?p_table=FEDERAL_REGISTER&p_id=16312

Pape, D., & Tarvydas, V. (1994). Responsible and responsive rehabilitation consultation on the ADA: The importance of training for psychologists. In S. Bruyère & J. O'Keeffe (Eds.), *Implications of the Americans with Disabilities Act for psychology* (pp. 169–186). New York, NY: Springer Publishing.

Pechman, L. (1995). Coping with mental disabilities in the workplace. *New York State Bar Journal, 67*, 22, 24–26, 49.

Percy, S. (2001). Challenges and dilemmas in implementing the Americans with Disabilities Act: Lessons from the first decade. *Policy Studies Journal, 29*, 633–640.

Postol, L. (2002). Sailing the employment law bermuda triangle. *The Labor Lawyer, 18*, 165–192.

President's Committee on Employment of People with Disabilities. (1994). *Seniority and collective bargaining issues and the Americans with Disabilities Act—A strategy for implementation.* Final Report of the seniority/collective bargaining agreement work group. Washington, DC: Author.

Rothstein, M. A. (1990). *Occupational safety and health law* (3rd ed.). St. Paul, MN: West Publishing Co.

Rudstam, H., Golden, T. P., Gower, W. S., Switzer, E., Bruyère, S., & Van Looy, S. (2014). Leveraging new rules to advance new opportunities: Implications of the Rehabilitation Act section 503 new rules for employment service providers. *Journal of Vocational Rehabilitation, 41*, 193–208.

Saunders, S. L., & Nedelec, B. (2014). What work means to people with work disability: A scoping review. *Journal of Occupational Rehabilitation, 24*, 100–110.

Scheid, T. (1998). The Americans with Disabilities Act, mental disability, and employment practices. *Journal of Behavioral Health Sciences and Research, 25*, 312–324.

Schimmel, J., Stapleton, D., Mann, D. R., & Phelps, D. (2013, July 25). *Participant and provider outcomes since the inception of ticket to work and the effects of the 2008 regulatory changes.* Washington, DC: Mathematica Policy Research Institute.

Schwab, S. (2009). *The union as broker of employment rights.* Cornell law faculty working papers. Retrieved from http://scholarship.law.cornell.edu/clsops_papers/55

Scott, M. (1996). Compliance with ADA, FMLA, workers' compensation, and other laws requires road map. *Ehmployee Benefit Plan Review, 50*, 20–30.

Setzer, S. (1992, February 24). Hiring restraints loom in disability law. *ENR News*, 8–9.

Shalowitz, D. (1993, December 6). Return to work obstacle. *Business Insurance, 53*, 2.

Shiu, P. (2013, October 22). *Innovative research on employer practices: Improving employment for people with disabilities.* Presentation at the cornell university school of industrial relations employment and disability institute state-of-the-Science conference, Arlington, VA.

Silverstein, B. (2012). *Funding health-related VR services: The potential impact of the Affordable Care Act on the use of private health insurance and medicaid to pay for health-related VR services.* Boston, MA: Institute for Community Inclusion.

Skoning, G., & Mc Glothlen, C. (1994). Other laws shape ADA policies. *Personnel Journal, 73*, 116.

Stapleton, D., O'Day, B., Livermore, G., & Imparato, A. (2006). Dismantling the poverty trap: Disability policy for the twenty-first century. *The Milbank Quarterly, 84*, 701–732.

Stude, E. (1994). Implications of the ADA for master's and bachelor's level rehabilitation counseling and rehabilitation services professionals. *Rehabilitation Education, 8*, 17–25.

Taylor, R. W. (1995). Medical examinations under the ADA and OSH Act: A dilemma for employers. *Employment in the Mainstream, 20*, 23–25.

Ullman, M., Johnson, M., Moss, K., & Burris, S. (2001). The EEOC charge priority policy and claimants with psychiatric disabilities. *Psychiatric Services, 52*, 642–649.

U.S. Centers for Medicare & Medicaid Services. (2015). Medicaid expansion & what it means for you. Retrieved from https://www.healthcare.gov/medicaid-chip/medicaid-expansion-and-you

U.S. Department of Education. (2014, July 24). *Workforce Innovation and Opportunity Act: Amendments to the Rehabilitation Act of 1973*. Washington, DC: Author.

U.S. Department of Education. (2015, February 2). Fiscal year 2016 budget: Summary and background information. Retrieved from http://www2.ed.gov/about/overview/budget/budget16/index.html

U.S. Department of Education. (2009). American Recovery and Reinvestment Act of 2009: Vocational rehabilitation recovery funds. Retrieved from http://www.ed.gov/policy/gen/leg/recovery/factsheet/vr.html

U.S. Department of Health and Human Services. (2010). Patient Protection and Affordable Care Act: Requirements for group health plans and health insurance issuers under the Patient Protection and Affordable Care Act relating to preexisting condition exclusions, lifetime and annual limits, rescissions, and patient protections. *Federal Register, 75*, 37187–37241.

U.S. Department of Justice. (2002). *A guide to disability rights laws*. Washington, DC: Author. Retrieved from http://www.usdoj.gov/crt/ada/cguide.pdf

U.S. Department of Labor, Employment and Training Administration. (2014). Workforce Innovation and Opportunity Act. Retrieved from http://www.doleta.gov/wioa

U.S. Department of Labor, Employment and Training Administration. (2015). Workforce Innovation and Opportunity Act; Notice of proposed rulemaking; Proposed rules. *Federal Register, 80*, 20689–21150.

U.S. Department of Labor, Office of Disability Employment Policy. (2009, January 15). *Memorandum of neil romano, assistant secretary of the U.S. department of labor, office of disability employment policy*. Washington DC: U.S. Department of Labor.

U.S. Department of Labor, Office of Federal Contract Compliance (2013). Frequently asked questions: New section 503 regulations. Retrieved from http://www.dol.gov/ofccp/regs/compliance/faqs/503_faq.htm

U.S. Department of Labor, Wage and Hour Division. (2013). Side-by-side comparison of current/final regulations. Retrieved from http://www.dol.gov/whd/fmla/2013rule/comparison.htm

U.S. Department of Labor. (2000, April 12). Training and employment information notice no. 16–99. Retrieved from https://wdr.doleta.gov/directives/corr_doc.cfm?DOCN=1206

U.S. Department of Labor. (2001). Frequently asked questions: Various topics: What if an employee declines an audiometric test? Retrieved from http://www.osha.gov/html/faq-various.html

U.S. Department of Labor. (2005). *Innovative workplace safety accommodations for hearing impaired workers* (Safety and health information bulletin SHIB 07–22-2005). Retrieved from http://www.osha.gov/dts/shib/shib072205.html

U.S. Department of Labor. (2009a). *Frequently asked questions and answers about the revisions to the Family and Medical Leave Act*. Washington, DC: Author. Retrieved from http://www.dol.gov/whd/fmla/finalrule/NonMilitaryFAQs.pdf

U.S. Department of Labor. (2009b). Frequently asked questions about state occupational safety and health plans. Retrieved from https://www.dol.gov/agencies/ebsa/about-ebsa/our-activities/resource-center/faqs

U.S. Department of Labor. (2009c). *Military family leave provisions of the FMLA (Family and Medical Leave Act): Frequently asked questions and answers*. Washington, DC: Author. Retrieved from http://www.dol.gov/whd/fmla/finalrule/MilitaryFAQs.pdf

U.S. EEOC answers biggest FMLA/ADA questions. (1997). *Disability leave and absence reporter, 104*, 4.

U.S. Equal Employment Opportunity Commission. (1992). *A technical assistance manual on the employment provisions (Title I) of the Americans with Disabilities Act*. Washington, DC: Author.

U.S. Equal Employment Opportunity Commission. (1996). *EEOC enforcement guidance: workers' compensation and the ADA*. Washington, DC: Author.

U.S. Equal Employment Opportunity Commission. (1997, March 25). *EEOC enforcement guidance on the Americans with Disabilities Act and psychiatric disabilities* (No. 915.002). Washington, DC: Author.

U.S. Equal Employment Opportunity Commission. (2000). The Family and Medical Leave Act, the Americans with Disabilities Act, and Title VII of the Civil Rights Act of 1964. Retrieved from https://www.eeoc.gov/policy/docs/fmlaada.html

U.S. Equal Employment Opportunity Commission. (2003). *Annual report, fiscal year 2002*. Retrieved from https://www.eeoc.gov/federal/reports/fsp2003/part1.html

U.S. Equal Employment Opportunity Commission. (2008). Notice concerning the Americans with Disabilities Act (ADA) Amendments Act of 2008. Retrieved from http://www.eeoc.gov/ada/amendments_notice.html

U.S. Equal Employment Opportunity Commission. (2011). Questions and answers on the final rule implementing the ADA Amendments Act of 2008. Retrieved http://www.eeoc.gov/laws/regulations/ada_qa_final_rule.cfm

U.S. Equal Employment Opportunity Commission. (2013). Informal letter to patricia shiu, director OFCCP, August 8, 2013. Retrieved from https://www.dol.gov/ofccp/regs/compliance/sec503/Self_ID_Forms/OLC_letter_to_OFCCP_8-8-2013_508c.pdf

von Schrader, S., Malzer, V., & Bruyère, S. (2013). Perspectives on disability disclosure: The importance of employer practices and workplace climate. *Employee Responsibilities and Rights Journal, 26*, 237–255. Retrieved from http://link.springer.com/article/10.1007/s10672-013-9227-9#page-1

von Schrader, S., Xu, X. & Bruyère, S. (2014). Accommodation requests: Who is asking for what? *Rehabilitation Research, Policy, and Education, 28*, 329–344. Retrieved from http://www.ingentaconnect.com/content/springer/rrpe/2014/00000028/00000004/art00008

Walker, J., & Heffner, F. (1992). The Americans with Disabilities Act and workers compensation. *Chartered Property Casualty Underwrite Journal, 45*, 151–152.

Walworth, C., Damon, L., & Wilder, C. (1993). Walking a fine line: Managing the conflicting obligations of the Americans with Disabilities Act and workers' compensation laws. *Employee Relations, 19*, 221–232.

Welch, E. (1996). The EEOC, the ADA, and WC. *Ed Welch on Workers' Compensation, 6*, 178–179.

Wright, G. (1980). *Total rehabilitation.* Boston, MA: Little, Brown.

Zolkos, R. (1994). Avoiding charges of bias. *Business Insurance, 28*(29), 85.

35 CHAPTER

Accreditation—A Quality Framework in the Consumer-Centric Era

Brian J. Boon

Arguably, health care stands out as the most complex of service industries. As a sector within this industry, medical rehabilitation struggles with its many unique challenges. Downstream from acute care services, medical rehabilitation is now confronted with the task of demonstrating its value in a reimbursement environment that is directed toward more services for less money. Payment systems have not kept up to changes in service demand driven by the patient's need and the rising requirement for specialized rehabilitation services.

In response to the many challenges in the rehabilitation industry, leadership is intensely focused on efforts to improve quality to demonstrate value to their many constituents. Although the use of formalized quality frameworks have been the norm in the manufacturing industry, such as total quality control or management, it is only in the past 20 years that the rehabilitation industry has employed with vigor the many quality frameworks available. Because practitioners in rehabilitation are key participants in quality improvement efforts conducted by organizations, it is a professional obligation that they critically understand features of the quality framework to be used, and where possible, influence decisions regarding which framework to embrace. Often an administrator or business leader in an organization will lean toward a quality framework employed in other industries, such as manufacturing, and extend it to health care because of their familiarity with quality programs or awards in terms of consumer products or services. For the rehabilitation industry, it is suggested that a rehabilitation-focused accreditation quality model is the best fit as a quality framework for advancing the performance of organizations that provide medical rehabilitation services. In an era where health care expenditures are so significant, value-based rehabilitation in a pay-for-performance environment may be the only way to competitively lower care costs, improve care quality, and drive better patient outcomes. The accreditation model provides the blueprint to cost containment through outcomes.

To be comparable with other quality management alternatives, an accreditation model must include quality standards that reflect sound business practices and address the systematization of continuous improvement efforts. However, to become a best fit quality model in medical rehabilitation, quality standards must also include a prominent place for the person served and, by extension, specific quality standards directed to advancing service to unique rehabilitation populations, such as persons with brain injury, spinal cord injury, and chronic pain. It is these population-specific standards that differentiate rehabilitation accreditation as a quality framework from other frameworks as the best fit.

To understand and appreciate the value of accreditation for medical rehabilitation as a quality framework, it is important that accreditation be considered within its evolutionary context in relation to the dynamics of the broader health care industry. Accreditation as a quality framework was constructed by the rehabilitation industry in response to environmental pressures to demonstrate a commitment to quality. Since its inception in 1966, as the only rehabilitation-specific accreditor, the Commission on Accreditation of Rehabilitation Facilities (CARF) has been setting quality standards for the broad rehabilitation industry, including medical rehabilitation. As the primary rehabilitation accreditor, CARF's quality standards have changed to meet the demands of the broader health care environment. Since 1966, many new quality management approaches have been trialed by the industry. It is again argued by the author that a rehabilitation-specific quality framework will continue to serve both the rehabilitation industry and its patients in that industry well into the future of consumer-directed and value-based care. Further, the CARF quality model of accreditation will be compared and then differentiated through its unique focus on persons served, which is an orientation different from other "product" or "service to the consumer" quality management models. The other highly reputable and respected quality management frameworks include the Malcolm Baldrige National Quality Program (Baldrige), the International Organization for Standardization (ISO), and the European Foundation for Quality Management (EFQM).

EVOLUTIONARY PHASES IN ACCREDITATION

The evolutionary phases of accreditation as a rehabilitation industry–specific quality management framework can be illustrated against the dynamic characteristics of the broader health care environment (Figure 35.1). One characteristic is the degree to which the environment is closed or exclusive. In contrast, an inclusive environment would purposefully engage and optimize the involvement

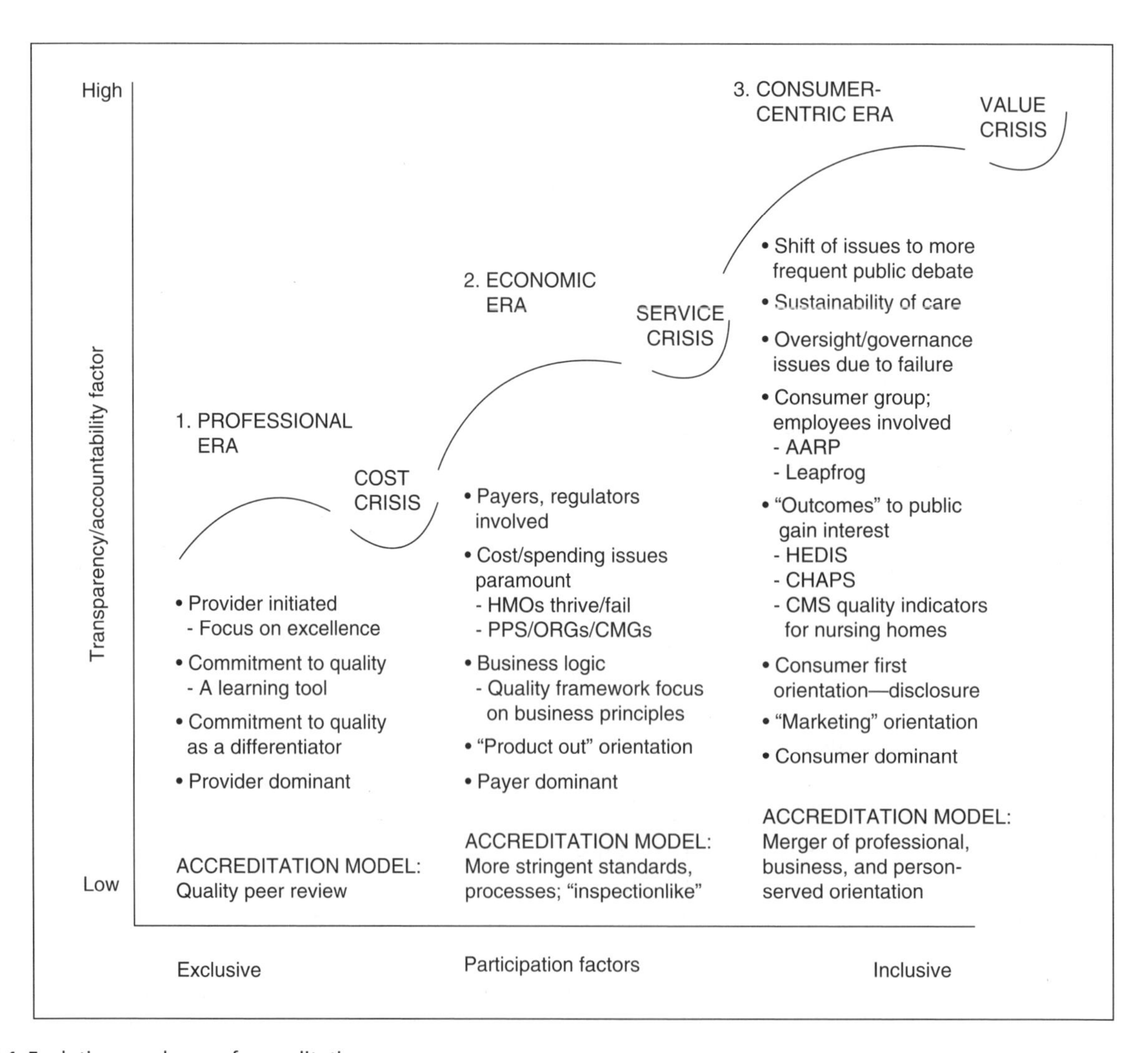

FIGURE 35.1 Evolutionary phases of accreditation.

CAHPS, Consumer Assessment of Healthcare Providers and Systems; CMS, Centers for Medicare & Medicaid Services; HMO, health maintenance organization; HEDIS, Healthcare Effectiveness Data and Information Set.

of diverse stakeholders or participants in its processes. Another characteristic is the degree to which an environment is transparent and therefore provides for an enhanced public accountability. A transparent environment often evolves in response to demands for greater accountability. As these environmental factors change, so do characteristics of the quality management framework. The continuum of these factors (exclusiveness to inclusiveness and low to high degrees of transparency) acts as reference points to the evolution of accreditation. Accreditation, as described through various eras, is influenced by environmental dynamics concurrent to the period of time or era. The described eras are not mutually exclusive and the features of one, in fact, can carry over to future eras. Over time, accreditation evolves to satisfy the demands of quality. As a unique quality framework and business orientation, accreditation is greatly positioned to optimize its effect on enhancing services to improve the lives of persons served (Stavert & Boon, 2003). Each of the following eras illustrates accreditation's evolutionary paths with specific reference to rehabilitation.

The Professions Era (1960–1980)

In its early evolutionary steps, accreditation began as the result of the exclusive activity of the rehabilitation professions seeking to provide a quality template and to pursue excellence in the delivery of service and care. Although certification, licensure, and various forms of regulation and/or "professional oversight" existed regarding the practice of care, these administrative requirements were not seen by rehabilitation professionals or regulators as guides to improving services or programs. As there existed no external benchmark for excellence, accreditation in the United States was sponsored in rehabilitation as a guide to excellence from a supporting grant from the Vocational Rehabilitation Administration in 1966 (Galvin, 1999). Many of the professional rehabilitation and health care associations supported and promoted accreditation as an industry-based quality initiative. Until recently, CARF's governance model was comprised of a large board of trustees of sponsoring members who represented many of the major professional organizations in the rehabilitation industry. The CARF Board can be traced back to these early days sourcing its board from the professions in health care.

During this era, quality standards were developed collegially, via expert consensus-based panels, and then endorsed by the community of providers. Accreditation processes took the form of on-site review visits or surveys of organizations to determine the degree of compliance/conformance to required standards. The act of preparing for and successfully completing accreditation demonstrated that an organization was committed to demonstrating its conformance to quality standards and continuous improvement for the benefit of consumers. This distinction was used to differentiate organizations from one another, sometimes allowing for those organizations that were accredited to claim specialty status. Being accredited by a neutral third party gave organizations the opportunity to proclaim that their organization met the standard of a quality-based organization. Accreditation was promoted as a voluntary initiative in rehabilitation, although it was also used as a supplement to regulation or rule requirements to receive certain payments. Peer-based accreditation maintained and advanced the privilege of the professions "regulating" themselves through this commitment to quality via accreditation.

The process of quality accreditation review by peers maintained provider autonomy and "control" over quality for a significant period of time. To some extent, during this period of provider dominance, consumers were, as a group, less organized or active and, to a degree, individually "passive" recipients of service or treatment. However, this apparent era of professional autonomy was soon challenged by the era of economics as costs began to challenge the collective system. Advances in the use of medical technology and pharmaceuticals, and a growing demand for more health care and specialized rehabilitation services, resulted in rising costs. The challenges associated with these trends shifted the dynamics of the system from one predominated by professional direction and influence to one in which economics became a predominant factor in a changing and dynamic environment.

The Economic Era (1980–Present)

Cost Containment Tactics

As health care costs dramatically increased, discussions and concerns regarding the long-term affordability of health care and its effect on the delivery of quality service became a paramount industry and public policy concern. Although the rehabilitation industry continued to support accreditation, emerging environmental factors provided the opportunity for new management philosophies to be considered in the industry as it responded to the crisis in the "business" of health care. It was during this period that regulators and payers became more involved, as service concerns and rapidly rising costs, specifically in rehabilitation, became more transparent to the public. Managed care approaches evolved to control costs during this period while trying to maintain access to appropriate care (Eccleston, 1995). In response to economic crisis, health care leadership shifted to employing and adopting business logic to its health industry problems. Payers looked to alternative payment schemes and contract management approaches to control costs. Providers experienced lower reimbursement rates or deep discount contracts, which resulted in fewer dollars per case and was part of the "rehabilitation carve-out" cost–management effort. The mantra of "doing more with less" was and remains a predominant theme in health care, much like the oft-heard phrase "Funding dictates form." With an increasing sensitivity to costs, accreditation was used as a vendor prequalification step in the procurement of services by some payers. Some insurers used accreditation as a contract management risk tool to ensure that quality rehabilitation service was embedded in their extended specialty service provider networks (e.g., brain injury services). Insurers would only reimburse providers if they received third-party accreditation for their claimed specialty in rehabilitation. Insurers used accreditation to confirm that those claiming to provide specialty rehabilitation services were qualified and ran programs to known quality standards. Similar logic was employed by regulators and policy makers who may have passed rules, declarations, mandates, or directives regarding the requirements of accreditation for reimbursement and "quality" oversight purposes.

Employees Enter as New Participants

In response to the cost crisis and the new business logic being employed, accreditation quality standards adjusted accordingly. Standards became longer, more stringent, and, at times, definitive or prescriptive. New programs/standards were added as outpatient rehabilitation or specialty services grew. By way of example, in response to the cost crisis in the workers compensation industry, CARF created "work-hardening" standards to focus the provider, payer, and injured worker on the importance of return to work as an outcome of rehabilitation. The typical goals in rehabilitation, such as "improved strength" of the worker, included the demands to ensure the worker's return to work and ultimately contain costs. Quality rehabilitation standards relating to performance were also added, referencing measures of effectiveness, efficiency, or satisfaction. In an era of rising costs, results for dollars spent on quality standards relating to safety also became more of a priority with the increasing transparency of reported safety errors in the general health care system (Institute of Medicine, 1999). In partial response to the public safety crisis, the accreditation process became a more rigorous or "inspectionlike" quality assurance exercise for organizations. The large, fragmented U.S. health care system, its structures and processes, led to disrupted service delivery experiences, poor information flows, and misaligned incentives that degraded the quality and safety of care (Cebul, Rebitzer, Taylor, & Votruba, 2008). Cost containment strategies, less sophisticated and based on "managed practices" with less evidence, resulted in a safety and service crisis for patients and a collective frustrated and disillusioned provider community.

It was also during this era that the employer community became a more vocal and influential participant in the industry, even a proxy representative of their employees' health care quality concerns. Examples of this include the National Business Group on Health (NBGH), formerly known as the Washington Business Group on Health, and The Leapfrog Group. The NBGH is a not-for-profit organization whose members are primarily Fortune 500 companies dedicated to fostering the development of a safe, high-quality health care delivery system and treatments based on scientific evidence of effectiveness (NBGH, 2015). It has most recently established a number of initiatives and institutes to advance its cause to improve outcomes, enhance quality and patient safety, manage cost challenges, and educate policy makers and lawmakers how these issues impact employer-sponsored care. The Leapfrog Group (2015) is also a not-for-profit coalition of large employers and other purchasers whose publicized priority tasks include improving quality and safety of patient care or "saving lives," mobilizing employer purchasing power, recognizing and rewarding excellence in care through market-based incentives, and giving consumers information to make good choices about which hospital to use. Specifically, the Leapfrog Hospital Survey collects and reports, in a public and transparent manner, hospital safety performance information via a Hospital Safety Score to protect patients/consumers from errors, injuries, and infection. The stated motivations of both of these groups are to advance safer health care practice, manage costs, and extend the value of service for the benefit of the employer and employees. For some employers, health care benefit expenses are a cause for concern as they increase infrastructure costs. Higher health benefits result in a higher cost of goods or services delivered, placing in jeopardy an employer's competitive position in a cost-conscious global environment.

It is also during this era that cost concerns and the effect of cost containment strategies on quality led to public discussions and debates. The cost crisis therefore creates greater transparency in various forms, such as commissions, agencies, institutes, and "think tanks" to consider potential remedies and changes to improve the system. As one example, the President's Advisory Commission on Consumer Protection and Quality in the Health Care Industry (1998), established by President Clinton, studied health care quality and recommended improvement strategies to enhance the health system's responsiveness and effectiveness. Patient's rights legislation was one option considered from the report, the other being the established agency known as the National Quality Forum—an agency directed to establish common set performance indicators for the health system, such as public reporting of quality in systems of care (e.g., Nursing Home Compare). As a further illustration, other U.S.-based entities that developed during this era include the Institute for Healthcare Improvement (2015), an outcome of a national demonstration project on quality improvement, which focused on the identification and spread of best practices to reduce defects and errors, and this has since evolved to innovation, research, and a current formulation of health care as a complete social, geopolitical enterprise optimizing performance, experience of patient care, and per capita cost of care. In a specific example of a cost management strategy, even the Centers for Medicare & Medicaid Services (CMS) are trying to manage and control costs related to reimbursement of intensive rehabilitation services provided to patients in inpatient rehabilitation hospital units—known as the "75% rule" (now 60%). All payers of services try to define and manage the cost parameters of health care, whether they are private insurance companies or "government"-reimbursed services. An apparent universal truth in health care exists—demand always exceeds supply, a trend likely to continue. Significant public domain efforts signal collective unrest and potential changes in the environment, ultimately leading to a new era of health care delivery.

As the dynamics of the environment became more inclusive and open, and as issues related to cost-effectiveness, customer satisfaction, and safety became more prominent, the health care industry concurrently borrowed other industries' lessons and logic concerning quality. Health care/rehabilitation organizations began to employ quality frameworks (Counte & Meurer, 2001) such as ISO 9000, Baldrige, total quality management (TQM), continuous quality improvement (CQI), quality control circles, statistical process control (SPC), balanced scorecards/reports, process reengineering, management by results, and outcome management. The Disney Institute (2015) even provides various seminars for health care organizations that wish to advance their customer service approach. A good organization will always challenge itself to discover cost-effective methods of delivering quality rehabilitation service balance with "good service." All of the quality techniques noted earlier, if implemented effectively, help organizations "to do more with less."

Cost containment is a predominant theme within the economic era, and the resulting service reality for the rehabilitation field was to "do more with less." An employed business logic that embraced quality frameworks from other industries created a gap between leadership and those who provided direct services to persons served. Essentially, a gap of cultures was created between management and practitioners in relation to the methods of delivering high-quality care in a reducing reimbursement environment.

A prevailing countertrend to the economically driven cost containment era was a more vigilant, autonomous, and empowered collective of consumer groups. Consumers fought the apparent restrictions to access and care practices imposed by managed care techniques. Employers, too, continued to be concerned by rising health benefit costs with no end in sight. Over time, as more costs shift to employers and their employees, and, overall, there is less access to services for the masses, the public debate will continue regarding the value for dollars spent in the emerging, "to be dominant" consumer-centric marketplace. The "crisis of value" will challenge the industry to once again reorient and adjust to a new circumstance of environment dynamics. Payers, regulators, and providers will need to embrace the shifting influence that persons served will have in reshaping the future delivery of health care and rehabilitation.

Consumer-Centric Era (2000 and Beyond)

The health and human services industry is experiencing a fundamental change in its environment. Consumers or persons served are beginning to exercise choice, control, and, with greater frequency, bear the financial cost for services received. This period, referenced as the consumer-centric era, is that time when the economic and service challenges in the health care system are so great that the apparent sustainability of the health service system is at stake. The current federal and state fiscal crises, an aging population with growing health demands, and other industry factors will likely conspire to create a service crisis. Costs will remain a critical variable for ongoing management. The crisis of service, cost, and sustainability will shift the debate from the private boardrooms of companies to the broader and transparent public arena, where concerns regarding accountability for quality are at the forefront of that debate.

It is during this period that the Internet savvy consumer will demonstrate unprecedented influence and create new demands and channels (e.g., Facebook, Twitter) in the health care system. Consumers are transitioning from relatively uninformed, passive recipients of service to engaged and informed participants in their care and service plans. Consumers will be vigilant about timely access to affordable, high-quality service with expected outcomes commensurate with experienced risk. Informed consumers will begin to advocate for improvements in the dimensions of rehabilitation, such as timely and friendly access to care, practice patterns consistent with established guidelines, and outstanding clinical and functional outcomes (Goonan, 1994). This social shift in influence already can be observed in the growing number of consumer-directed health plans, spending accounts, and service options that have become instituted with greater frequency in the marketplace. Pharmaceutical companies have also recognized the power of consumer authority as they begin marketing directly to consumers.

In an era of greater transparency, consumers will want access to information with respect to quality indicators of rehabilitation service. They will also demand more information over time in the form of "public report cards." Signs of increasing transparency and, by extension, public accountability already exist, which are illustrated in a set of first-generation public reports. Examples of these public reports include, to name a few, the Healthcare Effectiveness Data and Information Set (HEDIS), which is the tool used by the National Committee on Quality Assurance (2003, 2015) and which comprises a group of measures designed to evaluate health plans' key processes; the Consumer Assessment of Healthcare Providers and Systems (CAHPS) developed and managed by a consortium of organizations (Agency for Healthcare Research and Quality, American Institutes for Research, Harvard Medical School, the RAND Corporation, and Westat); the CMS Nursing Home Compare; and general satisfaction questionnaires that contribute to Healthgrades data on patient satisfaction and hospital quality. Clearly, insurers/payers, regulators, and health organizations are focused on indices of quality as they relate to the consumer. Outcomes for services rendered will drive consumers and payers to select and reinforce the high-performance providers. Further, with the growing influence of consumers and greater health care costs being paid directly by consumers (Organization for Economic Cooperation and Development [OECD], 2015), the dominant social forces that have an effect on human service systems will be consumer collectives. According to the OECD, 19% of health spending in 2013 was directly financed by private households (OECD, 2015). Consumer enclaves, in the traditional sense (e.g., AARP) or via Internet swarms (virtual collectives with common values and purpose) will create powerful social forces of significant magnitude to affect public policy, influence purchase trends, review quality, and ultimately assess the value of care via cost, service, and outcomes.

It is during this period of response to crises that key participants will reaffirm their primary focus on the task at hand—to organize systems, organizations, and services around persons served. If the explicit value of the system is to serve an engaged consumer, then services should be organized around the person served. In August 2014, the National Quality Forum released its report *Priority Setting for Healthcare Performance Measurement: Addressing Performance Measure Gaps in Person-Centered Care and Outcomes*. The report recognizes that higher quality care needs to be organized around the requirements of individuals and their families and that emerging evidence demonstrates that outcomes and cost are positively impacted by collaborative partnerships between persons, families, and health care providers (NQF, 2014). A quality framework specific to rehabilitation should both support and advance this orientation. To be of value, quality frameworks must be inclusive and transparent to key participants in the system—provider, payer, and person served. With inclusive participation from key participants in the development of standards, rehabilitation accreditors can enhance their quality framework by importing the valuable knowledge from the rehabilitation field and including input from persons served—the consumer.

Industries outside of human services incorporate the customer requirement in their production or manufacturing process, to meet the customers' specifications. Quality is built into the design of the product. In an inclusive environment, a rehabilitation accreditor must also incorporate multiple-party input into the process of designing and promoting quality standards. Providers, payers, regulators, and persons served should be "at the table" when accreditors develop quality standards and establish the process to assess quality. They all participate in the rehabilitation system. This approach is inclusive, transparent, and leads to advancing accountability in the system. In turn, quality rehabilitation standards should also prominently recognize the unique role that the person served plays in the design, delivery, and output of care. The emerging consumer-centric environment will require that organizational practices be consistent with the values in rehabilitation to fully and meaningfully engage persons served. Further, this quality framework should reestablish the link between process and outcome, which recognizes the important role that both clinicians and persons served play in contributing to a quality result. Accreditation will provide the architecture for organizational service design and quality assessment and will create an integrated, transparent, and value-based organization. In the consumer-driven era, a rehabilitation-specific accreditation quality framework will position organizations to shift their orientation by transitioning from pure business quality templates to accreditation quality templates to serve individuals better.

TRANSITION FROM A BUSINESS QUALITY MODEL TO AN ACCREDITATION QUALITY MODEL

Health care as an industry is a "big and complex business" in most developing countries. Internationally, health care spending continues to outpace economic growth in most industrialized countries, and in response, each country struggles with its own unique way to fund services through public, private, or variant hybrid payment systems. The magnitude of dollars spent on health care is poignantly reflected as a percentage of a country's gross domestic product (GDP). Utilizing data from OECD (2015), the proportion of GDP spent on health care in the United States reached 16.4% compared to the OECD average of 8.9%. In other countries, the numbers are almost as high: France at 10.9%, 11.1% for Switzerland, 11.1% for Germany, Canada and Belgium each with 10.2%, and Australia at 8.8%. In the United States, costs continue to escalate and outstrip other countries on many factors. In particular, total health spending per capita was $8,713, almost 2.5 times greater than the OECD average of $3,453 and nearly 40% more than Switzerland, the next biggest spender. In the United States, health care spending reached $2.75 trillion in 2013, with a growth rate of 1.5% in 2013 (OECD, 2015). Health care is big business, and the cost and ability to access care for Americans was a priority for the Obama administration. With the passing of the Patient Protection and Affordable Care Act (PPACA), commonly referred to as the Affordable Care Act (ACA) or colloquially as ObamaCare, CMS forecasts even higher growth in spending as more Americans gain health insurance coverage (OECD, 2015). In order to address costs, provisions of the ACA include bundled payment pilot programs or the Bundled Payments for Care Improvement (BPCI) initiative. Composed of four broadly defined care models, payments are bundled for multiple services that beneficiaries receive during episodes of care. Payment arrangements include financial and performance accountability for an entire episode. The intent of these pilot programs is to create higher quality and better coordinated care at a lower cost (CMS, 2015).

As previously noted, the overall environment of health care has recently and predominantly focused on cost relative to service. In an attempt to deal with the cost-to-quality issue, regulators, payers, and health care leaders in charge of health care plans or systems of care, including hospitals and rehabilitation settings, have tried to address the business complexity of health care by employing the logic necessary to survive in such a demanding environment. As a consequence, health care has employed and adapted a multitude of business-based quality tools, techniques, and principles. There exists some evidence that utilizing quality tools or techniques is perceived by management or organizational leadership as contributing to an organization's strategic or business goals (Yasin, Zimmerer, Miller, & Zimmerer, 2002). It is also interesting to note that the business-based quality frameworks are predated by accreditation-based quality framework methods (e.g., CARF accreditation—1966, ISO 9000—1987, Baldrige—1988). However, evolving quality management approaches found their way as, at times, competing alternatives or supplements to accreditation. It is plausible that accreditation of business standards had not kept up with the business needs of organizations via its standards and therefore was no longer felt to be relevant or of value. An equally plausible reason is that the accreditation process was seen as a professional validation effort by clinicians to affirm that their processes were of high quality, resulting in clinical/functional gains. However, during an "economic squeeze" cycle, pure functional gains appear to be less relevant to cost-focused administrators and payers. Perhaps accreditation was really never perceived by administrators as a "true quality framework," but rather as a requirement for payment or a clinically focused exercise. Further, in larger human service systems, the accreditation of a rehabilitation program was rarely elevated to the attention of the president/CEO or executive director. In fact, if successful accreditation was realized repeatedly, it may have lost significance over time. Finally, as the business challenges in health care grew, executives employed to lead health plans and hospitals had other management, industry, and educational experiences and were more familiar with other quality models to advance the performance of their organization.

Because industry-based quality programs were known to help the competitiveness of industry globally, it was reasoned that these quality programs could help the health care industry to address its concerns. Industry quality frameworks were innovative, prestigious, and something new to many organizations. As a by-product of adopting the business quality techniques, it was hoped that these programs would create organizational spirit, trust, and renewal with staff. Undoubtedly, the opportunity for the clinician to become empowered in an organization to identify, discuss, and provide solutions to work problems can create a better service and work environment. However, although these quality programs were being introduced and business logic was employed, the greatest long-term result of these organizational efforts, even if it was not appropriately implemented, was to create organizations comprised of leadership and practitioners that were "two minded and culturally disintegrated" (Goldsmith, 1998). In essence, the leadership and staff became disengaged from one another. This gap relates to an "orientation gap" in which the actions of the business-based quality framework, such as business process improvement teams, at times are disengaged from the reality of day-to-day interactions between clinicians and the treatment complexities of their patients. Often-heard statements from clinicians during such sessions were "But my patients are not like those identified"; hence the tensions created by a lopsided business-only quality management approach.

In the human services industry and particularly in rehabilitation, there are unique issues that are foreign to the typical manufacturing or service environments in which quality frameworks operate. As an illustration (Figure 35.2), in the manufacturing industry quality is a function of many causal

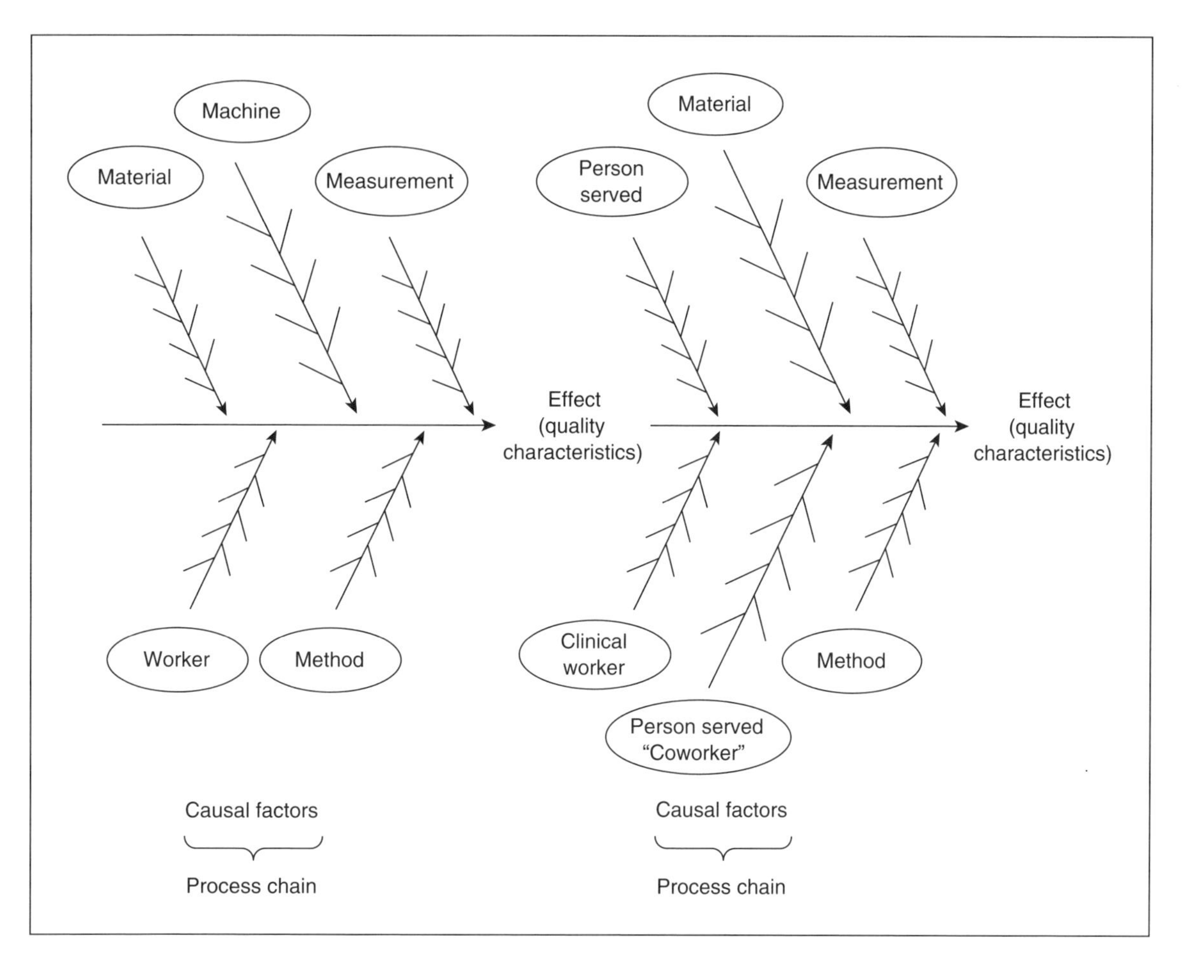

FIGURE 35.2 Cause–effect diagram.

factors, including worker, material, method, measurement, and machine (Ishikawa, 1985). These collectives of causal factors constitute a process that can be controlled via standardization to create a quality effect. In manufacturing, the effect is targeted quality—a certain level of design quality. Quality of conformance is an indication of how far the actual product conforms to its quality target or design. Let us translate this quality formula to the human services industry and, specifically, to rehabilitation. The worker providing the services is the clinician. The method employed is his or her clinical intervention and/or process. The material is the person served, and the machine could be pharmaceutical or a technology that helps with functional restoration (e.g., a weight machine for strengthening exercise). However, the formula is even more complex in rehabilitation because an engaged consumer, or person served, is both the material *and* part worker or producer of an outcome. This is a unique factor that differentiates an accreditation quality framework from that employed in business where customer needs or requirements are defined and a product is produced or service generated to meet those desired needs and features. In the case of rehabilitation, the person served is both the coproducer of service and the recipient of service with an associated outcome. The rehabilitation process makes accommodations for this complex variable in the equation, and therefore a quality framework must emphasize this distinct point if it is to be relevant and of value. It is this distinction that those who provide direct services in the health and rehabilitation environment recognize and the reason that most business-based quality programs employed in health care are perceived as "foreign" or force-fitted into the health and rehabilitation industry.

As an interesting note, despite the business philosophy employed during the economic era, health care and its delivery continued to remain fragmented, and escalating cost factors often outstripped inflation at a rate two or three times that of the consumer price index rate.

THE IMPORTANCE OF PROCESS MEASURES AND PERSONS SERVED

Leaders in health and rehabilitation want to ensure that human service systems meet the highest standards with respect to both business and clinical service excellence. Much study that is specific to assessing quality in health care has already been conducted. One well-known approach is to assess quality via its structure, processes, and outcomes (Donabedian, 1978, 1996). Structural assumptions of quality identify the necessary and enabling conditions that must be present in the provision of care or service, such as infrastructure and staff. Structural elements are necessary conditions but alone do not ensure quality. Process measures focus on the activities delivered according to accepted and predetermined standards, that is, those standards related to care and the delivery of care within a program or organizational unit of analysis. Outcomes refer to the attainment of desired goals for the individual (e.g., return to work), at the level of the organization (e.g., reduced medical errors, patient satisfaction), or at a systems level (e.g., measures of community health, social participation). For organizational leadership, structure and outcomes factors are of more relevance and interest because they are more tangible for deliberation and debate. Administrative staff see "aggregate numbers"; therefore, they understand structure and outcome data such as unit costs, total paid staff time, profit margins, and patient satisfaction. Process measures typically fall under the primary domain of interest for providers of health services. Clinicians treat patients one person at a time and need to manage all the service intersect processes that occur during the rehabilitation continuum. This insight into the service continuum is a gap for some administrators. When outcomes can be linked to process, certainly providers are as engaged as other parties in an evidence-based or a promising practice approach. Persons served are also concerned with outcomes and the processes that they must participate in as well as their risks and consequences.

The advantages and disadvantages of process measures relative to outcome measures have been well articulated in other articles (Mant, 2001; Rubin, Provonost, & Diette, 2001). Outcome measures are of relevance to persons served. However, quality frameworks again fail to recognize the role of persons served in producing an outcome, and therefore process measures are also relevant to persons served. Process measures have immediate appeal to clinicians in the health and rehabilitation environment. These measures identify exactly which processes are followed that are believed to result in an effective output or outcome. Measures that relate to process, the "science and art of doing," provide information that is observable and therefore function as a frame of reference for what needs to be changed to improve outcomes. Process measures utilized as standards of quality also reflect the care of service delivered, and therefore clinicians feel accountable for them because they have face validity—"It is what we do." Although outcomes are the desired goals of any rehabilitation process, it is recognized that many factors affect health care outcomes beyond the control of the provider, such as patient involvement and commitment to treatment regimens, as well as many other external factors. There exists clinical comfort in using process measures. The challenge to a processes-only approach is confirming evidence that supports the relationship between a clinical process and outcome, which then puts the clinician and, by extension, the persons served at risk in an environment where economics alone begins to influence the method, timing, and appropriateness of services. Where these links have been determined, all parties will focus on good processes for expected outcomes. However, it is difficult to link the processes to outcomes because of the necessity to provide for risk-adjusted outcomes to incorporate unique features of complex rehabilitation patient populations. Much research is needed to advance promising practices or the practice of evidence-based care and to advance the role of the person served as a critical resource in that process–outcome linkage analysis.

For an accreditation model to provide a robust quality framework, it must appeal to the various key participants in the delivery system. Governance and executive leadership want a framework that is a template for the system of business (structure/process) and service performance (outcomes) of the organization that the excellence award programs typically provide. Clinical staff members desire a template to judge their care processes (process) and results (outcomes) achieved with respect to some standard or benchmark. Persons served want input, participation (process), and assurances of quality (outcomes) results. The drive of the collective then is to ensure that organizations are assessed against the framework of structure, process, and outcomes. In relation to these dimensions, accreditation will be assessed in reference to three other respected business quality frameworks (Baldrige, ISO, and EFQM) and then will be differentiated against these frameworks to demonstrate the best fit within the rehabilitation industry and in the consumer-centric era.

QUALITY IMPROVEMENT FRAMEWORKS AND THE ACCREDITATION MODEL OF QUALITY

Clearly, the success of any business enterprise depends upon how an organization manages its resources to create effective and efficient delivery systems of service. In an effort to meet this challenge, health care organizations have implemented various respected quality frameworks referenced previously. Further, many organizations simultaneously pursue accreditation for purposes of "deemed status," mandates, or the extended philosophy of continuous improvement in the rehabilitation setting. The CARF accreditation model of quality is compared to three predominant and respected business-quality frameworks: Baldrige—Health Care Criteria for Performance Excellence (2015/2016), ISO—ISO 9000: 2015 Quality Management Principles (2015), and EFQM—Excellence Model (2013). The accreditation model used is CARF—Medical Rehabilitation Standards (2015). In September 2015, the ISO 9001:2015 version of the certification process was released, and EFQM also released major revisions to their model in 2013. CARF releases updates every year on its standards, with a major review every 3 years. The comparison approach has been adapted from an international review of business excellence and award programs (Calingo, 2002). All of these models are excellent for organizations that wish to advance their business and service practices. Further, all of these frameworks are complementary and can be employed as a holistic stepwise model to enhance business and service improvement.

All of the selected quality frameworks have a directional purpose, which is to advance the success of the organization employing the respective framework (Table 35.1). The Baldrige and

TABLE 35.1

PURPOSE OF QUALITY IMPROVEMENT FRAMEWORKS

Framework	Inception (Revisions)	Orientation	Percentage of Applicant Sites Visited	Outcome
Baldrige	1988, health in 1999 (annual revisions)	Recognition of organizational excellence and best practice promotion	15–20	Award
ISO 9000	1987, 1994, 2000, 2008, 2015 (originated in 1947)	Requirements for quality management systems and guidance for performance improvement	100	Certification, follow-up surveillance audits on corrective actions, option for scheduled audits
EFQM	1991 (many)	Recognition of organizational excellence and best practice promotion	20	Award
CARF	1966 (many)	Recognition that an organization demonstrates quality, value, and optimal outcomes of services through continuous improvement focused on enhancing lives of persons served	100	Accreditation, follow-up quality improvement plan, and ongoing annual conformance to quality reports

CARF, Commission on Accreditation of Rehabilitation Facilities; EFQM, European Foundation for Quality Management; ISO, International Organization for Standardization.

EFQM models evolved in response to industry concerns regarding quality in an increasingly competitive national and global economy. The Baldrige approach was extended to health care in 1999, and the EFQM has been employed as a guide in the health industry via the EFQM International Health Sector Group. Since its inception, the oldest of the quality models, namely the CARF model, has been directed to "enhancing the lives of persons served" as a quality framework in the human services. To provide a sense of CARF's extended reach, CARF accredits more than 51,000 programs at more than 24,000 sites, all attributable to its 50-year history of valued accreditation. ISO, like other quality frameworks, has been equally utilized in health along with many other industry sectors (Table 35.2). The orientations of these programs also differ. Both Baldrige and EFQM focus on advancing an organization's practices, capabilities, and results. The award process, which includes self-assessment and external scoring, could include a site visit if the potential of finalist status exists. An ISO outcome is the status of certification that demonstrates compliance with quality management system principles via specific 9001 requirements, and thus requires that all organizations be assessed via a site visit. In CARF accreditation, organizations must demonstrate their conformance to business and service/care standards, confirmed by a site visit to receive an accreditation outcome. CARF requires ongoing conformance—the sustainability of quality. By far, ISO is the largest of the quality framework models comprising 165 national standards bodies and 3,511 technical bodies, reflecting the scope of this organization. As of December 2014, 1,138,155 ISO 9001:2008 conformity certificates were issued by more than 750 certification bodies in 162 countries (ISO, 2015).

Each of the quality frameworks also recognizes that there exist many pathways to performance improvement and operational excellence. The excellence benchmarks in Baldrige and EFQM are found

TABLE 35.2

ADAPTATION OF QUALITY IMPROVEMENT FRAMEWORKS TO SECTORS		
Framework	**Adaptation**	**Number of Sectors**
Baldrige	Unique but equal criteria (process/results) for sectors: businesses—manufacturing, service, and small organizations—education, health care, and nonprofit	6
ISO 9000	Multiple industries and increased depth (example: ISO 9001 criteria is applied)	Multiple industries
EFQM	Unique but nine equal criteria for sectors: large commercial, subsidiary operating units, small to medium enterprise, public sector	4
CARF	Equal business criteria, multiple sector–specific criteria—aging services, children and youth, employment and community, behavioral health, medical rehabilitation, and increased depth by program within sector	Medical rehabilitation subsector programs: Comprehensive integrated inpatient Spinal cord system of care Interdisciplinary pain Brain injury Outpatient medical Home and community Case management Health enhancement Pediatric family centered Occupational rehabilitation Residential Vocational Amputation specialty Stroke specialty Rehabilitation process for persons served

TABLE 35.3

LEVELS OF QUALITY RECOGNITION OF KEY ACCREDITATON FRAMEWORKS

Framework	Number of Levels	Description
Baldrige	1	1,000 points; >600 points usually trigger site visit
ISO 9000	1	Certification of compliance
EFQM	3	Commitment to excellence, recognition of excellence (300 points), European quality award (>600 points)
CARF	3	Time based—3 years, 1 year, or nonaccreditation

TABLE 35.4

EVALUATION DIMENSIONS OF KEY ACCREDITATON FRAMEWORKS

Framework	Dimension Structure
Baldrige	Process: approach, deployment, learning, and integration. Results: levels, trends, comparisons, and integration
ISO 9000	Compliance/noncompliance: plan–do–check–act process improvement approach is endorsed
EFQM	For Enablers and Results criteria: results, approach, deployment, assessment, and review
CARF	Conformance rating: nonconformance, partial conformance, substantial conformance, exemplary conformance

both in their scoring structure and evaluative dimensions. A points system is employed in Baldrige and EFQM. Those exceeding a cumulative 600 points in Baldrige or a 600–cumulative point threshold in EFQM are typically eligible as finalists to receive a quality award (Brown 2013; Table 35.3). The EFQM Excellence Model also provides gradients in the evolution of excellence via its stepwise approach: commitment to excellence, recognition of excellence status, and award status. In order to be considered for the EFQM award, an organization must have a current 5-Star EFQM Recognized for Excellence status issued within the previous 2 years. The EFQM Excellence Award signifies the best of excellent performing organizations. Similarly, although Baldrige does not provide a gradient in the evolution to excellence, it encourages organizations to begin their process at state or local award recognition programs through the Alliance for Performance Excellence before applying for the Baldrige award. Seventy percent of Baldrige award winners started at the state or local levels (Baldrige, 2015). ISO 9000 compliance is audited on-site via a checklist guide reflecting the audit 9001 criteria. Compliance is either met or not met—the resulting outcome leading to a certificate of compliance that extends to 3 years. CARF accreditation has two determined outcomes, accreditation or nonaccreditation. The accreditation outcome is based on the degree of conformance (Table 35.4) to standards as determined by surveyor via checklist. However, there are levels of accreditation that are time based.

A 1-year level of accreditation outcome signifies that there is organizational conformance to many standards; however, deficiencies are noted requiring correction, and therefore a return site visit in 1 year. A 3-year outcome is awarded if the organization exemplifies substantial conformance to standards—both in policy and in practice. Both Baldrige and EFQM review their respective criteria of quality along the evaluative dimensions of whether an organization plans and deploys improvement strategies in the organizations, links the results to action, and learns and integrates information to further improve organizational performance. The notion of this "approach, deployment, results, learning, and integration" sequence is embedded within the structure of CARF's Aspire to Excellence standards that are scorable because of their unidimensional and measurable design. In all four quality frameworks, the "review" is conducted by a third party or neutral agent to the organization seeking an award, certification, or accreditation (Table 35.5). In the case of Baldrige, EFQM, and CARF, award or accreditation is provided by the quality organization that conducts and manages the review/accreditation process. In contrast, ISO utilizes its 165 national standard body organizations to accredit registration bodies that employ auditors to determine ISO compliance and certification. ISO does not directly certify ISO compliance.

TABLE 35.5

REVIEWER CATEGORIES OF KEY ACCREDITATON FRAMEWORKS			
Framework	**Title of Reviewers**	**Number of Reviewers**	**Training Time**
Baldrige	Examiner	≈450	3–4 days, inclusive of 40–60 hours pretraining
ISO 9000	Registrar—auditor	–	–
EFQM	Assessor	≈500	3 days, 10–15 hours pretraining
CARF	Surveyor	1,400	3.0 days, 20 hours pretraining and intern program

Finally, each quality framework also employs set criteria or standards. Although the scope of the chapter is not to review the details of each framework's criteria, there exist both notable high-level similarities and differences (Table 35.6). All frameworks recognize the importance of leadership, focus on customer, involvement of staff/human resources, continuous improvement utilizing information, and performance. The Baldrige, EFQM, and CARF frameworks have well-formulated leadership/strategic planning standards that reinforce the need to set short-/long-term direction, and the deployment of plans with follow-up, comparison, and revision. Key organizational performance results are also well emphasized in Baldrige/EFQM, including results for patients, financial results, staff, and operating results. Baldrige, EFQM, and ISO focus on higher order system measures (e.g., financial results, market share measures). EFQM also includes results for society, extending the notion of social responsibility to an outcome for the organization. The other quality frameworks also address results in similar ways. Again, Baldrige includes results for patient and stakeholder (e.g., payers), financial, and marketplace performance results.

CARF also has a well-defined organizational performance section that requires an organization to focus on the metrics of efficiency, effectiveness, service access, and satisfaction from the perspective of persons served and other stakeholders. CARF's accreditation focus looks at the business components of an organization and drills down to the organizational unit (program) delivering rehabilitation to persons served. CARF requires that effectiveness (e.g., work status at 1 month after discharge) to persons served also be measured at a point in time following service to measure true long-term effectiveness or the specific organizational outcomes related to persons served. CARF's other accreditation criteria, such as input from persons served, accessibility, and rights of persons served, also differentiate CARF from the other quality frameworks.

Other quality frameworks typically lack standards that detail the quality standards to protect the rights of persons served, such as requirements to demonstrate a commitment to recognize diversity (culture), to exceed policies to ensure confidentiality and privacy, and to provide access to information and ensure informed choice. The key stakeholders who have contributed to CARF's medical rehabilitation standards development have placed the persons served at the center of an organization's quality assessment. It has been this way since its inception 50 years ago. This approach affirms that, in rehabilitation, quality is influenced by the inclusiveness of persons served as key participants in the output or outcome of the process. Hence, service or treatment planning includes shared responsibility and commitment between provider and persons served. As an example of a measured substandard, treatment goals are to be written in the words of persons served in order that the person is engaged and understands the purpose and goals of service. Further, the rehabilitation practitioner is aware of why the person is seeking services, what goals he or she wants to achieve, and the activities in which he or she wishes to participate.

The person-centric theme or approach has been similarly referenced in a publication written by the Institute of Medicine (2001), which identified that one of the aims for health care improvement is to include a patient-centered approach that is customized to patient needs/values, where the patient is

TABLE 35.6

CRITERIA OF QUALITY FRAMEWORKS

Baldrige: 2015/2016	ISO 9000: 2015	EFQM—Excellence Model 2013	CARF—Aspire to Excellence Model
Organizational profile	Customer focus	Leadership	Assess the environment
Leadership	Leadership	People	Set strategy
Strategy Customers	Engagement of people	Policy and strategy	Persons served and other stakeholders—obtain input
Measurement, analysis, knowledge, and management	Process approach	Customers	Implement the plan Legal Finance Risk Technology Rights of persons served Accessibility Health and safety Human resources
Workforce	Improvement	Processes	Review results
Operations	Continued improvement	People results	Effect change
Results	Evidence-based decision making Relationship Management	Customer results Society results Business results	Rehabilitation process for persons served

the source of control and in a system that is transparent in its efforts. In the behavioral health sector of rehabilitation, a similar theme has also emerged in the final report of the U.S. President's New Freedom Commission on Mental Health (2003), which also affirmed that mental health services and treatment should be consumer and family centered to promote and ensure that individualized care plans are directed to enhancing full community participation. Social responsibility and value of rehabilitation also come to the forefront via CARF's focus on accessibility. Accessibility standards are directed to promoting access to services and removing barriers for persons with disability, such as attitudinal or environmental barriers, to effect a positive outcome for persons served as active participants in society. This single feature differentiates CARF and its rehabilitation industry values from the other reputable and noteworthy quality frameworks.

To further instill the person-served orientation, the organization and its leadership must also demonstrate that they promote and protect the rights of persons served as part of their business/service focus. The accreditation-based quality framework emphasizes that enhanced communication efforts to the consumer, the creation of programs and services appropriate to the diversity of the population served, and a demonstration of cultural competency will differentiate providers in the future. Accreditation standards focused on consumer input go beyond mere assessment of input forums of persons served, satisfaction surveys, or market analysis of customer requirements. These are all excellent exercises to better serve customers. Quality frameworks in rehabilitation should advance the orientation to persons served within the organizational business context to organizations that seek to provide high-quality service to people in an era where there will be no alternative to the benchmark of assessed value. Rehabilitation organizations of the future must embrace their responsibility to persons served to ensure value and quality in their privileged position of service. Those organizations, the leadership and staff, that embrace this orientation will be well prepared for the consumer-centric era.

The last differentiator in the CARF quality framework is the standard related to the rehabilitation process—specific "process-based" standards often defined by the person-served population (e.g., persons with brain injury). A quality framework in rehabilitation must outline process standards that are directed to effecting positive change in the functional ability of persons served. On the basis of the specific rehabilitation population served, the composition of the rehabilitation team, scope of services, program goals, assessment or diagnostic services rendered, establishing treatment plans and goals, and community reintegration planning all vary dramatically. CARF's accreditation quality model outlines specific quality protocols for such processes that do not exist in other quality frameworks (see Table 35.2).

A quality framework that also provides rehabilitation-relevant consensus standards creates an additional point of reference for organizations to design new rehabilitation programs or to offer more services in their community. Further, a quality framework can serve as a reference point to experiment and assess outcomes when deviating from the designed rehabilitation standard or targeted quality. Standards can act as blueprints for design, as process controls, and as benchmarks for internal or external comparison. These kinds of standards have "face validity" for clinicians and persons served and/or their families in the rehabilitation community not offered by other quality frameworks. It is the accreditation-based quality framework with its unique orientation to persons served and sector specificity that differentiates it from other quality frameworks.

THE EXTENDED VALUE OF ACCREDITATION

All of the previously referenced quality frameworks, techniques, and philosophies offer the discipline of thought and action necessary to improve the performance of an organization. Accreditation, with its unique history, depth of rehabilitation-specific standards, and persons-served orientation, offers an extended value beyond the accreditation site visit to the benefit of key participants in the system. The extended value of accreditation can be seen in the benefits to persons served, organizations, payers, regulators, and society (Table 35.7).

TABLE 35.7

EXTENDED VALUE IN ACCREDITATION
Society
General • Maintains the importance of quality in "human services" in a world of competing interests • Quality and excellence in systems lead to greater access for people • Systems focused on people, perform well, create participation opportunities for persons with disabilities; these outcomes contribute to thriving communities/nations • A well-performing rehabilitation sector reduces stigma of disability, enhances participation for persons • Congruence with laws (e.g., Americans with Disabilities Act [ADA], Olmstead decision)
Regulators—Government • Allows experts and public to determine quality indicators in "specialty" areas; done by a third-party accreditor • Highest priority risks can be focus of quality oversight by regulator • Accreditation template provides systems with quality benchmarks across a continuum of services • Accreditation, with specificity built into programs, sets service standards expectation regardless of location, size, etc. All people deserve high-quality care regardless of location/site (standardized quality) • Supports public's demand for enhanced quality
Payers • Requirement that providers be accredited demonstrates commitment to quality on behalf of accounts/lives covered • Accreditation standards can be used for service protocols/ management practices/cost models, etc. • Accreditation used as external confirmation of declared specialty, ensuring best care/outcome/service expectation for all stakeholders • Accreditation requirement of all providers to establish information and outcome management system could be leveraged to establish system improvement efforts; contribute to provider report cards, contract management of providers, and individual outcomes of patients • Standards used to create a quality continuum of service to better serve accounts/lives concerned • Standards guide, as a "blueprint" for the development and evolution of a network of services to address rehabilitation needs, and, therefore, services through a continuum • Helps payers understand the socioeconomic value of rehabilitation as an important part of holistic health, e.g., accountable care organizations, medical or health home services • Congruent with value-based purchasing principles and practices

(*continued*)

TABLE 35.7 (*continued*)

EXTENDED VALUE IN ACCREDITATION
Organization
Governance/executive • Third-party review enhances accountability disclosure/quality assurance/risk management function • Snapshot of human service/business competencies • Maintains corporate vigilance to society/persons served • Public demonstration of commitment to quality; can be used as promotional tool • Bridges "the business with the care" to learn and improve • May fulfill legal and regulatory requirements • Balances long-term/short-term business and care priorities
Clinician • Maintains prominence of persons served as cocreators of outcomes, helps to focus on person-based outcomes • Program standards act as process templates (validity), expedite program/service development • Standards represent embedded knowledge of profession and service of those who participate, at different levels, in the service system • Standards can be used to appropriately minimize or extinguish undesirable variations in service; enhance learning • Standards can be translated to technology platform to enhance practice
Person served • Reasonable assurance of quality, focus on person orientation • Expectation of individualized approach, participation, that rights and dignity will be maintained • In rehabilitation, designation of specialty states if program accredited (e.g., spinal cord injury)

To persons served, accreditation offers a reasonable assurance that the services they are to receive meet "current industry standards" with respect to quality and that they will be engaged in care processes and decisions that affect them. Organizations benefit by knowing that they practice their trade against known standards, endorsed by experts and consumers alike. Accreditation creates and confirms the "business and service to person served" alignment. Organizations that maintain their commitment to quality via third-party accreditation, specifically designed and conducted for their rehabilitation-specific business, commit to an accountability framework—both internal and external. In an era of transparency, post-Enron, public trust can be further fortified by organizations that undergo additional third-party review. The accreditation process also bridges the business with the clinical care of components of rehabilitation service delivery. Payers can participate in quality systems by endorsing the requirement of quality service via accreditation as part of their extended service strategy, rebuilding public confidence to well-run and well-intended health service organizations. The opportunity also extends beyond a public relations exercise if accreditation is used to employ service protocols and aid in contract management practices inclusive of incentives for performance and the collection of data for system improvement opportunities.

Persons served, providers, and payers must integrate their efforts in the long run if the system is to achieve a desired state of sustained performance and enhanced access. Regulators who utilize accreditation as a partial oversight function are also afforded the opportunity to focus on their highest priorities, relieving providers of administrative review processes that are duplicative to accreditation and outside their area of expertise. Most importantly, a hallmark differentiator of the value of accreditation specific to rehabilitation is confirmed in its social responsibility function, which links results for the individual served to that of the greater society. As one of many available quality frameworks, only accreditation maintains the importance of rehabilitation to broader society. With its intense focus on persons served, accreditation standards act as "reference grids" to create effective systems of service and set goals focused on enhancing community participation opportunities for persons with disabilities (e.g., work) to minimize the stigma and barriers associated with disabilities. This clarity of purpose afforded by accreditation is the extended thread of value from persons served to society as a whole.

CONCLUSIONS

Accreditation has evolved over many years in response to different trends in the health and rehabilitation industry. Many indicators suggest discontinuous change in the health care and rehabilitation field. The engaged and informed consumer will continue to challenge the entire service delivery system—its leadership and skilled health professionals. The Internet will grow to be of greater use to consumers as they make decisions about care and service options. Report cards will be accessed by the masses. Payers and employers are likely to facilitate the development of incentives to reward providers for quality and excellence. Excellence awards and accreditation models, in principle, will remain focused on their similar intent to improve and guide organizations to performance excellence. Quality frameworks utilized by organizations will be required to embrace the changing and unique features specific to the business of delivering health care and rehabilitation services. Valued quality frameworks will need to recognize the importance and role of persons served both as contributors to the health and rehabilitation process and as recipients of the output or outcomes. This factor requires a unique quality framework that accreditation alone can provide. Further, the accreditor who builds a model of quality and standards through an inclusive process will create greater face validity and value within the broader community served—the community of citizenship.

To be of value and relevant, accreditation must also evolve to the needs of its customers. Accreditors are in a unique position of having many beneficiaries, such as accredited organizations, state agencies that mandate third-party accreditation, payers, and, to some extent, the general public. The general public will insist that accountability be created in the health system. One "check and balance" process that employs the necessary integrity is the accreditation process and the outcome or "seal of quality." As not-for-profit entities, accreditors must serve a higher purpose in view of the direct recipients of service, the persons served. That higher order purpose is a moral obligation. In the collective sense, persons served are the community, the country, and the nation served. Because the wealth of any nation is no greater than its health, creating efficient and effective quality-based delivery systems is the ultimate for the benefit of society. Efficiency, effectiveness, and satisfaction, regardless of the quality framework employed, create capacity in the human services system for greater access to those who may not be privileged to receive the best of care. It also stands to reason that the health of any nation and the quality of its health care is no greater than its access to that care. A commitment to quality, therefore, is a commitment to all persons served.

ACKNOWLEDGMENT

The author would like to thank Ms. Lori Rogers, MPA, for technical assistance in completing this chapter.

REFERENCES

Baldrige National Quality Program. (2015/2016). *Health care criteria for performance excellence*. Gaithersburg, MD: National Institute of Standards and Technology.

Brown, M. G. (2013). *Baldrige award winning quality—18th Edition: How to interpret the baldrige criteria for performance excellence*. Boca Raton, FL: CRC Press.

Calingo, L. M. R. (2002). National quality and business excellence awards: Mapping the field and prospects for Asia. In L. M. R. Calingo (Ed.), *The quest for global competitiveness through national quality and business excellence awards* (pp. 21–40). Tokyo, Japan: Asia Productivity Organization.

Cebul, R. D., Rebitzer, J. B., Taylor, L. J., & Votruba, M. (2008). Organizational fragmentation and care quality in the U.S. healthcare system. *Journal of Economic Perspectives, 22*, 93–113.

Centers for Medicare & Medicaid Services. (2015). Bundled payments for care improvement initiative (BPCI) fact sheet. Retrieved from https://www.cms.gov/Newsroom/MediaReleaseDatabase/Fact-sheets/2015-Fact-sheets-items/2015-08-13-2.html

Commission on Accreditation of Rehabilitation Facilities. (2015). *Medical rehabilitation standards manual*. Tucson, AZ: Author.

Counte, M. A., & Meurer, S. (2001). Issues in the assessment of continuous quality improvement implementation in health care organizations. *International Journal for Quality Health Care, 13*, 197–207.

Disney Institute. (2015). Retrieved from http://www.disneyinstitute.com

Donabedian, A. (1978). The quality of medical care. *Science, 200*, 856–864.

Donabedian, A. (1996). Evaluating quality of medical care. *Millbank Quarterly, 44*, 166–206.

Eccleston, S. M. (1995). *Managed care and medical cost containment in workers' compensation: A national inventory 1995–1996*. Cambridge, MA: Workers' Compensation Research Institute.

European Foundation for Quality Management. (2015). *The EFQM excellence model 2013*. Tilburg, Netherlands: Pabo Prestige Press.

Galvin, D. (1999). Accreditation as an accountability strategy. In L. R. McConnell (Ed.), *Accountability from several perspectives: A report on the 20th Mary E. Switzer memorial seminar* (pp. 44–51). Alexandria, VA: National Rehabilitation Association.

Goldsmith, J. (1998). Integration reconsidered: Five strategies for improved performance. *Health Care Strategist*, 1–8.

Goonan, K. J. (1994). Using quality assurance systems to change behaviour. In T. W. Granneman (Ed.), *Review, regulate or reform? What works to control workers' compensation medical costs* (pp. 247–267). Cambridge, MA: Workers' Compensation Research Institute.

Institute for Healthcare Improvement. (2015). Retrieved from http://www.ihi.org/Pages/default.aspx

Institute of Medicine. (1999). *To err is human*. Washington, DC: National Academies Press.

Institute of Medicine. (2001). *Crossing the quality chasm. A new health system for the 21st century*. Washington, DC: National Academies Press.

International Organization for Standardization (ISO). (2015). *ISO 9000—2015 (E)*. Geneva, Switzerland: Author.

Ishikawa, K. (1985). *What is total quality control. The Japanese way*. Englewood Cliffs, NJ: Prentice-Hall.

The Leapfrog Group. (2015). Retrieved from http://www.leapfroggroup.org

Mant, J. (2001). Process versus outcome indicators in the assessment of quality of health care. *International Journal of Quality Health Care*, *13*, 475–480.

National Business Group on Health. (2015). Retrieved from http://www.businessgrouphealth.org

National Committee on Quality Assurance. (2003). *Achieving the promise: Transforming mental health care in America. Final Report*. Rockville, MD: Department of Health and Human Services.

National Committee on Quality Assurance. (2015). Retrieved from http://www.ncqa.org

National Quality Forum. (2014). Priority setting for healthcare performance measurement: Addressing performance measure gaps in person-centered care and outcomes. Retrieved from http://www.qualityforum.org/Publications/2014/08/Priority_Setting_for_Healthcare_Performance_Measurement__Addressing_Performance_Measure_Gaps_in_Person-Centered_Care_and_Outcomes.aspx

Organization for Economic Cooperation and Development. (2015). Health at a glance 2015. Retrieved from http://www.oecd-ilibrary.org/social-issues-migration-health/health-at-a-glance-2015_health_glance-2015-en

President's Advisory Commission on Consumer Protection and Quality in the Health Care Industry. (1998). *Quality first: Better care for all Americans*. Washington, DC: U.S. Government Printing Office.

Rubin, H. R., Provonost, P., & Diette, G. B. (2001). The advantages and disadvantages of process-based measures of health care quality. *International Journal for Quality in Health Care*, *13*, 469–474.

Stavert, D., & Boon, B. J. (2003). Listening to consumers . . . Canada opens. *International Journal of Heath Care Quality Assurance Incorporating Leadership in Health Service*, *16*, 1–9.

Yasin, M. M., Zimmerer, L. W., Miller, P., & Zimmerer, T. W. (2002). An empirical investigation of the effectiveness of contemporary management philosophies in a hospital operational setting. *International Journal of Health Care Quality Assurance*, *15*, 268–276.

36

CHAPTER

Quality and Quality Improvement in Rehabilitation

Dale C. Strasser

INTRODUCTION

Quality in health care refers to a systems approach to evaluating and improving the health of the individuals served and is closely linked to quality improvement (QI) as an ongoing process of problem identification, intervention, evaluation, and further refinements in service delivery (Deming, 1986; Plsek, 1999; Taylor et al., 2014). QI strives for measureable improvements in services and health status of targeted patient groups (U.S. Department of Health and Human Services, Health Resources and Services Administration [DHHS, HRSA], 2011). In defining quality, the Institute of Medicine (IOM) emphasizes the linkage between improved services and desired health outcomes of individuals and populations (IOM, 2015). The systems approach highlights the complex interplay of the diverse components of service delivery and strives for solutions at the systems and organizational levels with a corresponding de-emphasis on a punitive approach directed at specific individuals.

The quality movement arose with the awareness of wide variations in clinical outcomes, alarming rates of medical errors, and inappropriate and costly care and was spurred by two influential reports from the IOM—*To Err Is Human: Building a Safer Health System* (IOM, 1999) and *Crossing the Quality Chasm: A New Health System for the 21st Century* (IOM, 2001). Significant variations in health care services have been well documented in various areas including stroke rehabilitation, brain injury outcomes, and the management of acute myocardial infarctions, hip fractures, colon cancer, diabetes, and depression, along with surgical procedures such as coronary artery bypass graft, hysterectomies, and spinal procedures. To update the earlier IOM findings, James (2013) conducted a comprehensive review of current findings and concluded that medical errors result in at least 210,000 deaths per year and possibly as many as 400,000 deaths per year. Furthermore, he finds that serious, but not fatal, harm from medical errors is even 10 to 20 times higher. Clearly, there is more room for improvement.

Variations in rehabilitation outcomes have been well documented and are summarized in a recent publication (Centers for Medicare & Medicaid Services [CMS], 2015; CMS, Center for Clinical Standards and Quality [CCSQ], 2015, p. 30). Risk-adjusted rehabilitation functional outcomes vary by insurance type, geographic region, and race/ethnicity (Reistetter et al., 2014). Our work in the Veterans Affairs (VA) Rehabilitation Teams Project found that characteristics of team functioning, such as team cohesiveness, physician engagement, and patient-centered goals all correlated with stroke rehabilitation outcomes (Strasser et al., 2005). The variations in patient outcomes, high rates of medical errors, and heath care costs imply that changes in service delivery could lessen these disparities and improve the overall quality of care.

Issues of communication, care coordination, resource utilization, and the provision of patient-centered care have emerged as common themes across areas in quality (e.g., medical errors, patient satisfaction, poor outcomes, and inappropriate care). A team approach to QI is recommended to address such complex issues along with a plea for a *health care culture* to promote communication and care coordination. These themes should not be foreign to rehabilitation providers, given the similarities to core rehabilitation principles of function, a biopsychosocial model and interdisciplinary team treatment.

KEY CONCEPT—QUALITY AND HEALTH CARE SYSTEMS

Health care quality is a difficult topic for health professionals and their patients to grasp. At one level, it seems fairly straightforward. Issues of medical errors, significant variations in patient outcomes, and inappropriate and costly care demand attention. The challenges to utilize these insights and improve health quality arise from the complexities and contradictions within health care delivery and the competing perspectives of what constitutes quality. Although QI is touted as a less punitive method than earlier approaches, which tended to focus blame on individuals, many rehabilitation professionals experience quality as heavy-handed and threatening. With the increasing linkage of quality indicators to funding and accreditation, it is easy to see how clinicians and hospital leaders also experience quality as punitive. "Quality" is further complicated by differing usages of the word in usual conversation and its connotation in health care and engineering. This section provides an overview of health care quality and QI and offers a framework for quality in rehabilitation medicine.

In contrast to the usual connotation of quality as a trait or attribute (e.g., "red" shirt, "fertile" soil) or as a judgement on this attribute (e.g., "high-quality" product, "low-quality" construction), health care quality refers to a systems approach to improving health care outcomes. Early proponents of health care quality built on successes in engineering and manufacturing, including those associated with W. Edwards Deming. Principles of systems engineering were credited with dramatic improvements in airline and automobile safety in the 1960s and 1970s, with an emphasis on the flow of manufacturing processes. Steps in the process amenable to change were articulated (e.g., manufacturing design and human–machine interface); changes were implemented (e.g., construction design and safety belts); results analyzed (e.g., automobile fatalities and airplane crashes); and interventions refined in an ongoing process of continuous QI.

The "Plan, Do, Study, Act" cycle of Deming and Shewhart (Figure 36.1; Deming, 1986; Plsek, 1999; Taylor et al., 2014) is commonly applied to a host of health care service delivery issues including medication errors, hospital falls, pressure sores, and adherence to post-myocardial infarction treatment recommendations. Interventions depend on

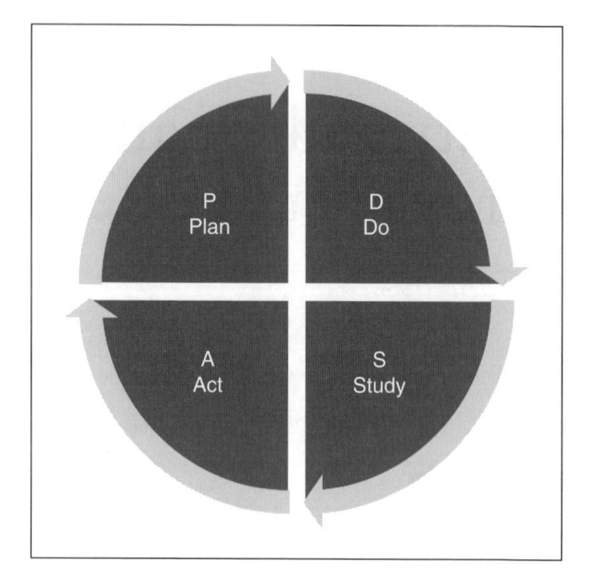

FIGURE 36.1 "Plan, Do, Study, Act" (PDSA) wheel.
Source: Adapted from Deming (1986).

the particular issues addressed and the specific settings. Interventions to address medication errors, for example, may include adoption of a standardized patient handoff system across shifts and services, refinements to the medical reconciliation process, and scanner technologies for patient identification. Initiatives to reduce hospital falls could include bed alarms, call button response time, and fall risk assessment tools. The process repeats itself, following each cycle at least until the desired goals are achieved. The iterative nature of QI resembles the feedback and feed-forward systems familiar to clinicians through physiology.

Pivotal in the development of quality and QI in health care is the Structure–Process–Outcomes (SPO) model (Figure 36.2; Donabedian, 1980, 1988). Structure encompasses the organizational and physical characteristics of services such as staffing levels, academic affiliations, for-profit status, dedicated disease-specific units, urban versus rural location, and so forth. Process is the what and how of services such as the adherence to recommended guidelines, the appropriate use of antibiotics, and swallowing evaluations for stroke patients. Outcomes are customarily thought of in terms of patient outcomes (survival, functional status, postacute hospital services, etc.) and resource utilization. The Donabedian model provides a useful framework for understanding and measuring the components of health care service delivery. Jesus and Hoeing (2015) and others have adapted

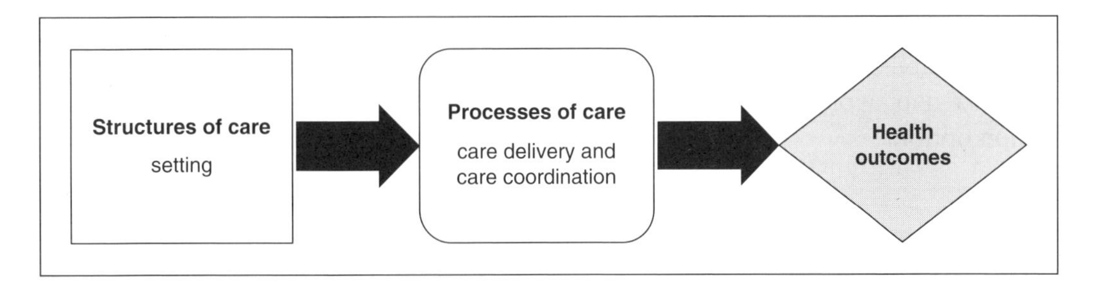

FIGURE 36.2 Donabedian model (SPO): Structure–Process–Outcomes.
Note: See Jesus and Hoenig (2015) for contemporary insights of how this model can inform postacute rehabilitation quality of care.
Source: Donabedian (1988).

and expanded upon this model to rehabilitation in postacute care (PAC) settings.

Structure: I prefer Structure as bolded and/or italized given its' role in the tripartite Donabedian Model. Structural characteristics of rehabilitation services affect outcomes. For example, the degree to which the physical facility and organizational structure promote functional independence of patients, family and caregiver education, discharge planning, and the interdisciplinary collaboration is a potential quality measure. Examination of the influences of space and design on rehabilitation process and outcomes brings valuable insights on potential and modifiable determinants of stroke rehabilitation effectiveness (Connell, 1997). Likewise, the organization of clinical services such as discipline-specific units (e.g., occupational therapists [OTs], speech-language pathologists) versus patient diagnostic categories (e.g., stroke or spinal cord injury unit) influences interdisciplinary collaboration among health care professionals. Generally, discrete, measureable structural variables have proven more difficult to link to changes in patient outcomes than process measures.

Process: I prefer Process as bolded and/or italized given its' role in the tripartite Donabedian Model. The process of rehabilitation refers to how services are delivered and include the "active ingredients of care." An interdisciplinary team of rehabilitation professionals deliver coordinated care to address the multifaceted determinants of function. In this respect, rehabilitation units resemble educational environments as much as they do traditional medical settings. As in a school setting, positive outcomes occur when a patient and his or her family demonstrate new skills and functional abilities. Outcomes are measured through the demonstration of specific actions performed by the patient. In other health care settings, positive outcomes are seen in more passive terms such as recovery from an infection or survival of a myocardial infarction. Recent work by Jesus and Hoenig (2015) offers an innovative and thought-provoking view on rehabilitation quality of care. Their work integrates key attributes of rehabilitation, such as interdisciplinary team treatments and a biopsychosocial orientation, with the Donabedian SPO framework to offer a rehabilitation-specific conceptual model and framework for rehabilitation quality of care across the postacute rehabilitation continuum.

Outcomes: I prefer Outcomes as bolded and/or italized given its' role in the tripartite Donabedian Model. Outcomes of medical rehabilitation are commonly thought of in terms of functional improvement, rehabilitation hospital discharge destination, and resource utilization. The primary outcome of function is customarily subdivided into categories. Activities of daily living (ADL) include basic hygiene, dressing, toileting, and self-care and are closely associated with bowel and bladder continence. Mobility includes the type (e.g., walking, wheelchair), the level of assistance (e.g., minimal, moderate), endurance, and terrain (e.g., stairs, uneven surfaces), cognition (including safety), communication, and swallowing. Rehabilitation hospital discharge is usually framed in terms of community settings (with or without additional support), skilled nursing facilities (SNFs or subacute rehabilitation), or acute hospital transfer. In an era of increasing concerns on the health care cost, resource utilization is a closely monitored quality measure, commonly defined as value or costs divided by patient outcomes. Rehabilitation length of stay (LOS) is a useful surrogate for resource utilization as costs of services correlate closely with LOS. Clinicians are familiar with the Functional Independence Measure (FIM®) efficiency measures (FIM change divided by LOS; Granger, Deutsch, Russell, Black, & Ottenbacher, 2007; Granger &

Fiedler, 1997). In addition, criteria for admission to an acute inpatient rehabilitation facility (IRF) have become more restricted in favor of the less expensive SNF rehabilitation option.

FEDERAL STANDARDS AND THE MANDATED QUALITY REPORTING PROGRAM

With the passage of the Affordable Care Act (ACA) in 2011, interest in health care QI continues to grow across a spectrum of stakeholders—payors, clinicians, consumers, and regulatory agencies. As reported by the *National Healthcare Quality and Disparities Report* (*NHQDR*), there has been significant progress in health care quality as evidenced by documented progress in each of the six of the priority areas of the Agency for Healthcare Research and Quality (AHRQ, 2015; Berger, n.d.). Still, major deficiencies exist.

CMS declares, "Driving quality is a core function of CMS" (CMS, 2016). CMS links quality to payments. Specifically, CMS proposes to tie Medicare payments to quality or value through alternative payment models—30% by the end of 2016; 50% by the end of 2018; and 85% of all Medicare Fee-for-Service (FFS) payments tied to quality or value by the end of 2016 and 90% by the end of 2018.

As part of the ACA, the AHRQ created the National Strategy for Quality Improvement in Health Care (National Strategy; Berger, n.d.). Established in March 2011, the National Strategy has three key aims and six priorities to guide QI efforts at the local, regional, and national levels (AHRQ NQS, 2011; 2014). The three key aims can be summarized as:

1. Making health care more patient centered, reliable, accessible, and safe
2. Addressing behavioral, social, and environmental determinants of health through proven interventions
3. Reducing the health care costs for individuals, families, employers, and government

The six priorities of the National Strategy are

1. Reducing harm in the delivery of care
2. Promoting patient and family engagement in care
3. Improving effective communication and care coordination
4. Achieving effective prevention and treatment for the leading causes of mortality, starting with cardiovascular
5. Promoting best practices to enable healthy living
6. Promoting health care delivery models for more affordable services

In January 2002, the CMS implemented a congressional mandate that fundamentally changed the funding of inpatient rehabilitation services from a cost-based system to a prospective payment system (PPS) supported by Medicare Part A. Although the earlier system paid hospitals proportional to their reported cost, the PPS reimbursed hospitals based on severity-adjusted averages. With the newer PPS, there were clear incentives for hospitals to deliver comparable services at lower costs. The most obvious methods to reduce costs are to lower acute inpatient rehabilitation LOS or provide services in lower intensity subacute rehabilitation settings in SNFs. Physician reimbursement under Medicare Part B did not undergo such a dramatic shift. One can speculate whether the differing payment approaches (hospitals [part A] vs. physicians [part B]) affects the intensity of responses among different rehabilitation providers and entities.

The ACA directed the Secretary of DHHS to establish the IRF Quality Reporting Program (QRP), which is a component of the Standardized Post-Acute (PAC) Assessment Data for Quality, Payment, and Discharge Planning report (CMS; CCSQ, 2015). This report details the specific measures across the three PAC settings providing inpatient services (SNFs, IRFs; and long-term acute care hospitals or LTACHs; CMS; CCSQ, 2015). Note, the term LTACH is sometimes used in reference to LTCH. Quality measures adopted by the Final Rule: IRF FY 2016 applicable to acute inpatient rehabilitation services are:

1. Unplanned readmissions—30 days after discharge from IRFs
2. New or worsened pressure ulcers
3. Functional outcome—change and discharge score in self-care
4. Functional outcome—change and discharge score in mobility

The IRF QRP occurs within the broader context of PAC services, which also includes inpatient care provided in SNFs and LTCHs. Home Health Services (HH), outpatient rehabilitation services, and durable medical equipment (DME) are also within the PAC grouping. To address the stated quality aims and priorities within medical rehabilitation, patient outcomes must be analyzed across settings of rehabilitation services to guide service delivery changes in a rational and effective manner. Risk-adjusted measures of costs, value, functional gains, and the impact on quality of life are required to address quality concerns. The need for standardized terminology and assessment items lead to the Continuity Assessment Record and Evaluation (CARE) Item Set to allow comparisons across the PAC settings (Table 36.1; CMS, 2015).

Developed under contract from CMS and based on findings of a Medicare-sponsored clinical demonstration project, the CARE Item Set targets a range of measures that document variations in a patient's level of care needs including factors related to treatment and staffing patterns such as predictors of physician, nursing, and therapy intensity. This tool is designed to measure outcomes in physical and medical treatments while controlling for factors that affect outcomes, such as cognitive impairments and social and environmental factors. Four of the 25-page CARE Item Set measure function and are grouped into *Self Care* (6 items), *Functional Mobility* (6 items), and, for patients needing further PAC services, *Supplemental*

TABLE 36.1

THE CONTINUITY ASSESSMENT RECORD AND EVALUATION (CARE) FUNCTIONAL MEASURES	
A. Core self-care (all patients) A1. Eating A2. Tube feeding A3. Oral hygiene A4. Toilet hygiene A5. Upper body dressing A6. Lower body dressing B. Core functional mobility (all patients) B1. Lying to sitting on side of bed B2. Sit to stand B3. Chair-/bed-to-chair transfer B4. Toilet transfer B5. Primary mobility wheelchair vs. walk (Subcategories on distance) C. Supplemental functional ability (further postacute care services anticipated C1. Wash upper body C2. Shower/bathe self C3. Roll left and right C4. Sit to lying C5. Picking up object C6. Putting on/taking off footwear C7. Primary mobility wheelchair vs. walk (Subcategories on distance) C8. Telephone—answering C9. Telephone—placing call C10. Medication management—oral C11. Medication management—inhalant/mist C12. Medication management—injectable C13. Make light meal C14. Wipe down surface C15. Light shopping C16. Laundry C17. Use public transportation	Safety and quality of performance 6. Independent 5. Set-up or clean-up assistance 4. Supervisions or touching assistance 3. Partial/moderate assistance 2. Substantial/maximal assistance 1. Dependent Reasons for not assessing M. Medical S. Safety concerns A. Attempted, but not completed N. Not applicable P. Patient refused

Source: Care Tool Institutional Admission, Centers for Medicare and Medicaid Services.

Activities (17 items). Although many of the items or similar information is already collected in the PAC settings, the required new CMS reporting items came online in 2016 (LTACHs—4/1/2016; IRFs and SNFs—10/1/2016).

PAC services account for not only a significant portion of health care expenditures in the United States, but perhaps more importantly, an even higher amount of increases in health care costs (Strasser, in press). PAC accounts for 40% of the growth of CMS expenses, which explains the close scrutiny of all PAC services. Medicare payments to PAC providers reached $59 billion in 2013, more than doubling the costs since 2001. Proposed solutions include bundling of services and payment neutrality across PAC sites (SNFs, IRFs, LTCHs). A predetermined amount of funds per event (e.g., hip fracture, stroke, pneumonia) is allocated (or bundled), and a health care system has the flexibility to utilize the resources as it deems best. Comparable payments across settings (e.g., SNF vs. IRF) characterize payment neutrality.

There is widespread acknowledgment that costs must be contained and there are correspondingly divergent perspectives on how to accomplish the goal. Payors, health care service industries, professional organizations, patient advocates, and regulators have valid, unique, and biased perspectives. Although the issue of unintended consequences of well-intentioned QI efforts is discussed later in this chapter, one suspects that an underlying theme of these missteps arises when QI efforts from one stakeholder are initiated, which do not adequately account for other factors.

The dizzying array of quality concepts and acronyms baffle many providers (see Table 36.2). A common and understandable response is to ignore or deny the process and concentrate on the immediate issues that impact your work. Health care professionals and others should be reminded that these CMS and related activities will profoundly impact the who, what, where, and how of resource allocation. Furthermore, these CMS changes will likely succeed in improving the quality of rehabilitation services, at least as it is currently measured. Although acknowledging a possible self-interest, rehabilitation providers are encouraged to understand, critique, and participate in the process.

"It does not count if it isn't counted." Variations of this mantra abound in health care and in rehabilitation. The idea behind this sentiment is sobering, given the challenges to understanding and measuring the inner workings of rehabilitation. Some fear that our inability to measure the determinants of rehabilitation quality may relegate the field to the proverbial trash can. And clearly as health care resources become more constrained, rehabilitation professionals must justify their interventions. For busy clinicians, gathering current findings to support care improvements, along with conducting

TABLE 36.2

ABBREVIATIONS
ACA—Affordable Care Act
AHRQ—Agency for Healthcare Research and Quality
AMRPA—American Medical Rehabilitation Providers Association
ARA—Applied Research Associates, an affiliate of AMRPA
BPCI—Bundled Payments for Care Improvement Initiative
CARE—Continuity Assessment Record and Evaluation
DHHS—Department of Health and Human Services (Federal Department)
CMS—Centers for Medicare & Medicaid Services
DME—durable medical equipment
HH—home health services
IRF—inpatient rehabilitation facility
LTCH—Long Term Care Hospitals.
MDS—Minimum Data Set (used in nursing homes and SNFs),
NHQDR—National Healthcare Quality and Disparities Report
NQF—National Quality Forum
OASIS—Outcome and Assessment Information Set (used in home health)
PAC—postacute care
PAI—Patient Assessment Instrument (for use in IRFs)
PM&R—Physical Medicine and Rehabilitation
PPS—prospective payment system
RTE—rehabilitation team effectiveness
RTI—Research Triangle Institute (under CMS contract)
SNF—skilled nursing facility (also called subacute rehab)
TEP—Technical Expert Panel

primary research in treatment effectiveness, is a daunting task.

As "beauty lies in the eyes of the beholder," so are the values and objectives of quality. Inherent within this orientation is the fact that individual players within the system such as payors, regulators, individual providers, and professional groups have valid and distinct insights, but they rarely have a comprehensive grasp of the entire system. The image of blindfolded individuals touching a large elephant captures a fundamental challenge of achieving high-quality health services.

ACUTE (IRF) VERSUS SUBACUTE (SNF)—GROUND ZERO IN A "REHAB QUALITY" DEBATE?

Rehabilitation professionals and other stakeholders are concerned about the potential deleterious effects of either of the two main CMS proposals discussed—bundling or payment neutrality—as they could precipitate an inappropriate shift from IRFs to SNFs. Patients treated in SNFs stay longer with lower intensity of professional services and per diem costs than patients treated in IRF settings. Geriatricians or other primary care physicians provide medical oversight in SNFs with a minimum of a monthly visit. In contrast, physicians with documented rehabilitation expertise, usually in physical medicine and rehabilitation (PM&R), provide medical management in IRFs, which includes daily physician visits and weekly team conferences. Comparisons of outcomes have been challenging because of the different but overlapping types of patients served and the lack of common functional outcome measures between the two settings. In addition, influential trade organizations for the respective entities advocate for their constituencies, creating added challenges to meaningful outcome comparisons. Organizations representing SNFs versus IRFs can draw very different conclusions from the same data set. The primary impetus for the CARE Item Set described earlier is the standardization of key measurements for more accurate comparisons.

IRFs and SNFs serve different populations with distinct services. The criterion for admission to an SNF is a need for skilled level of services, which can be provided by either nursing, physical therapists (PTs), or OTs. The per diem cost of SNFs is approximately one third to half of that of IRFs, and the use of skilled rehabilitation therapies is not required for SNF services. In contrast, IRF admission criteria include the patient's ability to participate in a minimum of 3 hours of therapy services a day, justification for two of three rehabilitation therapies (i.e., PT, OT, Speech Language Pathology [SLP]), and the need for ongoing medical and nursing services. Furthermore, CMS stipulates that a minimum of 60% of the patients fall into 1 of 13 diagnostic categories (such as stroke, Parkinson's disease, or brain injury). Hence, services provided in IRF settings are more intensive (medical, nursing, and therapies), more focused on specific diagnostic categories, and with more effort devoted to care coordination. IRFs have shorter LOS at significantly higher per diem costs and total costs.

As clinicians are all too familiar, the dichotomy of SNFs and IRFs can be problematic for individual patients who do not fit well into either category. For example, a medically complex patient may benefit from daily physician and nursing monitoring along with the proximity to other medical specialists in IRFs but lack the physical endurance for this level of therapies. A medically tenuous patient may not be accepted in SNF or IRF settings and still not meet the criteria for LTACH. Also even within particular settings, the interpretation of admission criteria varies. The wide variations in services and outcomes found particularly in SNFs, but also across other PAC settings, further complicate acute care hospital discharge planning. SNF bed availability seems to be inversely related to the perceived quality and reputation of a particular facility; better SNFs have fewer available beds! With pressure to take the first available opening, acute hospital discharge planners are placed in an uncomfortable situation. Likewise, IRFs vary in their knowledge and skills in managing the frail, elderly patient. And finally, there are patients who would likely benefit from IRF service intensity after a period of convalesce with an SNF level of exercise and mobilization. However, planned transitions from SNF to IRF are uncommon and reflect the financial disincentives for the SNF.

The evidence, which does exist, supports the superiority of IRFs versus SNFs for stroke, hip fracture, and other patient groups in the 13 diagnostic group categories mandated by CMS (Deutsch et al., 2006; Strasser, in press, p. 13). In a study commissioned by the ARA Research Institute, an affiliate of AMRPA, Dobson DaVanzo & Associates, LLC, examined the outcomes of comparable patients treated in IRFs and SNFs (Dobson DaVanzo & Associates, July 10, 2014; Dobson DaVanzo & Associates, 2014). As an industry-sponsored study, which has not been published in peer-reviewed journals, readers are advised to examine the methods closely (see URL in reference). Still, given the methodological rigor and consistency with findings from other published work, the study merits a discussion.

Cross-sectional and longitudinal analyses were applied to over 100,000 matched pairs of patients treated between 2005 and 2009 (89.6% of IRF patients and 19.6% of SNF patients). The study documented a proportional shift of elective joint replacement patients from IRFs to SNFs. During this time period, the cross-sectional analyses found a shift to IRFs for patients with stroke, brain injury, major medical complexity, and neurological disorder. Compared to the SNF patients, IRF patients had better clinical outcomes in five of six measures in the longitudinal analysis. The sixth measure was hospital readmission, and IRF patients had fewer hospital readmissions than SNF patients for amputation, brain injury, hip fracture, major medical complexity, and pain syndrome (see Table 36.3 for one subgroup analysis—hip fracture).

The process of rehabilitation has been called a black box because of the limited knowledge on how processes influence outcomes. Nevertheless, extensive evidence exists to support the team approach in rehabilitation (Langhorne & Dennis, 2004). Over the past 25 years, Judy Falconer and I have developed and tested a model of rehabilitation team effectiveness (RTE) and have shown that team functioning can be measured in a valid and reliable manner and that measured attributes of team functioning predict clinically relevant outcomes (Smits, Bowden, Falconer, & Strasser, 2014; Strasser et al., 2005). Furthermore, rehabilitation providers are responsive to staff training interventions to improve team function (Stevens, Strasser, Uomoto, Bowen, & Falconer, 2007), and in a cluster randomized clinical trial, the staff training and improved team functioning were associated with improved patient outcomes (Strasser et al., 2008). Subsequent exploratory analysis revealed that measures of team functioning correlated with patient outcomes consistent with the Team Effectiveness Model (TEM) over a 1-year period (Strasser, Burridge, Falconer, Uomoto, & Herrin, 2014). Specifically, increases in team functioning measures correlated with gains in the proportion of patients discharged to the community (teamness and team effectiveness) and decreased in the patients' LOS (physician engagement). Although this work was exploratory and merits further confirmation, it suggests that measures of team functioning could be used as process and performance measures in QI.

The TEM is a systems model of rehabilitation treatment effectiveness. In this model, rehabilitation team functioning consists of inputs, transformational processes, and outcomes (Smits et al., 2014; Strasser & Falconer, 1997a, 1997b). The system inputs include organizational characteristics (such as hospital culture), treatment/technology (specifics of therapy), and participants (patients, families, and staff). The model postulates that team functioning plays a central role as a transformational variable between inputs (structural elements) and patient outcomes. Team functioning consists of team relations (social climate and professional networks) and team actions (team leadership and managerial practices). The primary outcomes are functional gain, discharge destination, and LOS. This model guided the comprehensive study of stroke rehabilitation outcomes and VA rehabilitation teams referenced earlier (Strasser et al., 2005, 2008). In addition, other research supports the use of process measures to understand rehabilitation outcomes (DeJong, Horn, Conroy, Nichols, & Healton, 2005; Duncan et al., 2002).

Smits et al. (2014) examined this body of work in the context of contemporary ideas of medical

TABLE 36.3

ACUTE (IRF) VERSUS SUBACUTE (SNF) HIP FRACTURE PATIENT OUTCOMES OVER A 2-YEAR PERIOD ($P < .0001$; $N = 20,970$)
• 13.3 vs. 32.7 days' length of stay
• 8.3 % lower mortality rate
• 55.1-day increase in average days alive
• 53.1 fewer hospital readmissions per 1,000 patients per year
• 52.8 more days residing at home
• Cost $9.77 more per day (2-year period)

Source: Dobson DaVanco & Associates (2014).

leadership and rehabilitation teams. Four practical observations emerged from this work: (a) Models depicting the patient care–teamwork nexus provide a mental map, a common language, a structure to facilitate the collection and interpretation of data, and a decision framework for the continuous improvement of services; (b) team functioning focuses the shared experience and multiple perspectives of a rehab team; (c) leadership integrates and focuses team expertise; and (d) performance feedback is essential for learning and iterative improvements. In terms of leadership development and team functioning improvement interventions, they offer three observations: (a) Expectations and preparations matter; (b) an intervention should model the model; and (c) reinforcements of information gained and actions taken promote successful interventions. Hence, the conclusion by Smits et al. (2014) provides helpful insights on how to incorporate the team service delivery model into medical leadership development and into rehabilitation QI.

THE QUALITY PARADOX—GETTING BEYOND MISHAPS AND UNINTENDED CONSEQUENCES

Clinicians experience a paradox about quality and QI efforts. We endorse the idea but see organizational efforts to improve quality as a distraction from our own clinical experience (Casalino, 1999). Quality issues are presented at the macrolevel of medical errors and appropriateness of services. Clinicians treat individual patients at the microlevel, where patient-specific issues dominate in the context of community norms and financial considerations.

Many clinicians use the term "quality" in reference to a particular trait or characteristic of an entity (such as a restaurant) or a person. In contrast, its use in health service research refers to the extent to which health services can be associated with patient outcomes. Operationally, quality is linked to system issues of process improvement where hospital leadership identifies a problem, implements intervention, monitors the effect, and modifies the intervention based on the data collected. Clinicians may view the specific issue selected as tangential to their concerns with individual patients. Hence, the health care approach to quality, the relevance of the identified issue, and the associated terminology may not resonate with busy clinicians treating individual patients. Clinicians have multiple and diverse demands on their time. When presented with yet another time request, many of us will look for ways to minimize the perceived intrusion on our work.

Quality initiatives can have unintended consequences of worsening of quality of care (Casalino, 1999; Walter, Davidowitz, Heineken, & Covinsky, 2004; Werner & Asch, 2005; Werner & Asch, 2007). An emerging literature, both research and expert commentary, reveals evidence of mishaps and unintended consequences associated with QI efforts. In a randomized trial comparing the implementation of electronic health records and quality information feedback, with and without financial incentives, Ryan et al. (2014) found that although physicians performed higher on incentivized measures, they performed lower on the unincentivized measures. In a similar vein, Ganz et al. (2007) used masked conditions (conditions not targeted by the intervention) to determine whether a practice redesign, which improved care for the targeted areas of falls, incontinence, and cognitive impairment, also effected the quality of care in nine masked conditions. Although two of the three targeted interventions showed improvement, none of the masked conditions in either study arm showed significant changes. These studies and others reinforce concerns about unintended consequences and the common lack of generalizability, particularly from mandated QI initiatives.

Much goes on in a patient–physician encounter and quality measures only capture a small fraction of the variables. By directing attention to a few easily measurable aspects, the subtext is that the rest of the patient encounter is not important. The proverbial baby is thrown out with the bathwater.

A disconnect between how issues are defined at the organizational level and how they are experienced by hands-on providers hampers QI. The diverging perspectives of hands-on clinicians versus regulatory agencies typify this paradox. On the one hand, clinician arrogance and naïveté inhibits the recognition of the contribution of one's own actions to the problem, whereas on the other hand, directives from regulatory agencies and hospital leadership can be out of step with what is feasible in given situations, leading to "chart" compliance without substantive change. As a clinician, if I see limited utility of quality measures in patient care activities, I am not likely to devote much effort into the accuracy of data collection or the use of the reports generated from the data.

The resolution of this quality paradox will involve a multipronged effort among clinicians, hospital organizations, and accrediting and regulatory agencies. Quality initiatives should be relevant to the day-to-day experience of clinicians and framed such that clinicians see their clinical work as more effective when merged with quality. Physicians and other rehabilitation professionals will adopt quality approaches more readily if the approach produces better outcomes or makes it easier to do their job. Hands-on clinician engagement in developing quality initiatives is more likely to produce feasible programs. Likewise, by avoiding or at least limiting "unfunded mandates," regulatory agencies and hospital leadership improve the chances that effective interventions will be adopted. A clinician-centered cost–benefit analysis of proposed quality programs should produce more effective initiatives.

In a national study of process improvement, we asked rehabilitation team leaders at 16 Veterans Affairs hospitals to learn the basics of team functioning and to utilize this knowledge in clinical practice (Stevens et al., 2007). In general, we found that clinicians incorporate new approaches in their busy clinical practice if they experience the effort as improving patient outcomes or in making them more effective clinicians. The crucial issue is whether the quality initiative improves the patient outcomes of individual providers. Effective QI initiatives should be woven into the fabric of clinical care.

SUGGESTED ACTIVITIES TO IMPROVE QUALITY

Quality initiatives most likely to succeed are those generated by the hands-on clinical staff, which directly address local barriers to optimal care and for which there is sufficient administration support to carry the project to fruition. Based on the author's own clinical experience and a review of the literature, examples of relevant areas are offered in Tables 36.4 and 36.5. Table 36.4 highlights interdisciplinary topics in the categories of specific patient issues (e.g., bladder management and sleep hygiene), processes of care (e.g., team conference attendance by direct clinical providers), and staff training–information feedback (e.g., use of a patient-centered structure for team conference such as the Siebens Domain Management Model [SDMM]®). Table 36.5 offers examples that are more likely to be physician driven in the categories of medication management (rational prescribing) and patient safety (e.g., optimal arrival time on unit). Common recommendations among quality specialists are regular case discussions among peers, as such discussions improve quality. In

TABLE 36.4

QUALITY IMPROVEMENT—EXAMPLES OF INTERDISCIPLINARY TEAM ACTIVITIES
Patient-specific areas • Sleep hygiene • Patient and family engagement in goal setting • Pain management (nonpharmacological) • Bowel and bladder management
Processes of care areas • Team conference attendance • Regular case discussions among peers • Nursing involvement in rehabilitation process • Therapy involvement in medical and nursing issues
Staff training and information feedback • Staff training to improve team effectiveness* • A patient-centered structure to rehabilitation team meetings** • Processes of care and outcomes information feedback • Use of conceptual model and systems framework***

*Stevens et al. (2007); Strasser et al. (2008).

**Kushner, Peters, and Johnson-Greene (2015a, 2015b, 2015c). Also, SDMM Communication Card at www.siebenspcc.com.

***Smits et al. (2014); Siebens (2011).

TABLE 36.5

QUALITY IMPROVEMENT—EXAMPLES OF PHYSICIAN-INITIATED ACTIVITIES
Medication management • Rational prescribing and polypharmacy* • Reduction of opioid medication • Medical reconciliation—admission and postacute care
Patient safety • Preadmission evaluations and medical stability • Optimization of arrival time and day of week for patient care • Postdischarge care coordination

Source: Zhukalin, Williams, Reed, and Strasser (2016);
*Geller, Nopkhun, Dows-Martinez, and Strasser (2012).

rehabilitation, clinical experience suggests that the role of nursing is less clearly defined and demonstrates wider variations than other core disciplines on rehabilitation teams. Activities to integrate nursing into the rehabilitation treatment process should improve quality, including carryover of skills learned in therapy to the nursing unit, and engagement of the patient and caregivers.

CONCLUSIONS

QI is an iterative process of "plan, do, check, act" to address shortcomings in health services delivery (Deming, 1986; Plsek, 1999; Taylor et al., 2014). Although this systems approach shares attributes with the physiological feedback loops familiar to health care professionals, quality and QI can seem foreign to busy clinicians providing services to individual patients. We have a hard time looking at ourselves and at the impact of the services we deliver. For example, in prescribing an antibiotic, a clinician can forget that he or she may be contributing to the emergence of resistant bacteria, or that an aggressive approach to rehabilitation therapy services in one setting may limit the availability of services in another. Frankly, it is hard to know the downstream impact and unintended consequences of specific actions. Clinicians need to stay abreast of these messy issues so they can incorporate new insights, change practices when indicated, advocate in those areas they know best, and perhaps most importantly, participate in the dialogue.

ACKNOWLEDGMENT

Special thanks to Ms. Regina B. Bell, MPH, Emory University Department of Rehabilitation Medicine, Atlanta, Georgia, for her invaluable assistance with manuscript preparation.

REFERENCES

Agency for Healthcare Research and Quality, National Quality Strategy. (2014, September). The national quality strategy: Fact sheet. Retrieved from http://www.ahrq.gov/workingforquality/nqs/nqsfactsheet.htm

Agency for Healthcare Research and Quality, National Quality Strategy. (2011, March). *2011 Report to congress: National strategy for quality improvement in health care*. Retrieved from http://www.ahrq.gov/workingforquality/nqs/nqs2011annlrpt.htm

Agency for Healthcare Research and Quality. (2015, May). *2014 national healthcare quality and disparities report* (AHRQ Pub No. 15-0007). Retrieved from http://www.ahrq.gov/sites/default/files/wysiwyg/research/findings/nhqrdr/nhqdr14/2014nhqdr.pdf

Berger, K. (n.d.). An update on United States healthcare quality improvement efforts. Retrieved from https://ecpe.sph.harvard.edu/newsstory.cfm?story=healthcare-quality-improvement-efforts-in-united-states

Casalino, L. P. (1999). The unintended consequences of measuring quality on the quality of medical care. *New England Journal of Medicine*, *341*(15), 1147–1150.

Centers for Medicare & Medicaid Services, Center for Clinical Standards and Quality. (2015, August). *Inpatient rehabilitation facility quality reporting program: Specifications for the quality measures adopted through fiscal year 2016 final rule* (CMS Contract No. HHSM-500-2013-130151 (HHSM-500-T0001). Retrieved from https://www.cms.gov/Medicare/Quality-Initiatives-Patient-Assessment-Instruments/IRF-Quality-Reporting/Downloads/IRF_Final_Rule_Quality_Measure_Specifications_7-29-2015.pdf

Centers for Medicare & Medicaid Services. (2015, January 13). CARE item set and B-CARE. Retrieved from https://www.cms.gov/Medicare/Quality-Initiatives-Patient-Assessment-Instruments/Post-Acute-Care-Quality-Initiatives/CARE-Item-Set-and-B-CARE.html

Centers for Medicare & Medicaid Services. (2016). CMS quality strategy 2016. Retrieved from https://www.cms.gov/Medicare/Quality-Initiatives-Patient-Assessment-Instruments/QualityInitiativesGenInfo/Downloads/CMS-Quality-Strategy.pdf

Connell, B. R. (1997). The physical environment of inpatient stroke rehabilitation settings. *Topics in Stroke Rehabilitation*, *4*(2), 40–58. doi:10.1310/BYJT-HTHY-DV6R-QX6A

DeJong, G., Horn, S. D., Conroy, R., Nichols, D., & Healton, E. B. (2005). Opening the black box of poststroke rehabilitation: Stroke rehabilitation patients, processes, and outcomes. *Archives of Physical Medicine and Rehabilitation*, *86*(12, Suppl. 2), S1–S7.

Deming, W. E. (1986). *Out of crisis*. Cambridge, MA: MIT-CAES.

Deutsch, A., Granger, C. V., Heinemann, A. W., Fiedler, R. C., DeJong, G., Kane, R. L., . . . Trevisan, M. (2006). Poststroke rehabilitation: Outcomes and reimbursement of inpatient rehabilitation facilities and subacute rehabilitation programs. *Stroke*, *37*(6), 1477–1482.

Dobson DaVanzo & Associates, LLC. (2014). Assessment of patient outcomes of rehabilitative care provided in inpatient rehabilitation facilities (IRFs) and after discharge: Study highlights for hip fracture patients. Retrieved from https://www.amrpa.org/newsroom/HipFractureSummary.pdf

Dobson DaVanzo & Associates, LLC. (2014, July 10). Assessment of patient outcomes of rehabilitative care provided in inpatient rehabilitation facilities (IRFs) and after discharge. Retrieved from https://www.amrpa.org/newsroom/Dobson%20DaVanzo%20Final%20Report%20-%20Patient%20Outcomes%20of%20IRF%20v%20%20SNF%20-%207%2010%2014%20redated.pdf

Donabedian, A. (1980). *Explorations on quality assessment and monitoring: The definition of quality and approaches to its assessment* (Vol. 1). Ann Arbor, MI: Health Administration Press.

Donabedian, A. (1988). Quality assessment and assurance: Unity of purpose, diversity of means. *Inquiry*, *25*(1), 173–192.

Duncan, P. W., Horner, R. D., Reker, D. M., Samsa, G. P., Hoenig, H., Hamilton, B. B., . . . Dudley, T. K. (2002). Adherence to postacute rehabilitation guidelines is associated with functional recovery in stroke. *Stroke*, *33*(1), 167–177.

Ganz, D. A., Wenger, N. S., Roth, C. P., Kamberg, C. J., Chang, J. T., MacLean, C. H., . . . Shekelle, P. G. (2007). The effect of a quality improvement initiative on the quality of other aspects of health care: The law of unintended consequences? *Medical Care, 45*(1), 8–18.

Geller, A. I., Nopkhun, W., Dows-Martinez, M. N., Strasser, D. C. (2012). Polypharmacy and the role of physical medicine and rehabilitation. *Physical Medicine and Rehabilitation*, *4*(3), 198–219.

Granger, C. V., Deutsch, A., Russell, C., Black, T., & Ottenbacher, K. J. (2007). Modifications of the FIM instrument under the inpatient rehabilitation facility prospective payment system. *American Journal of Physical Medicine & Rehabilitation*, *86*(11), 883–892.

Granger, C. V., & Fiedler, R. C. (1997). The measurement of disability. In M. J. Fuhrer (Ed.), *Assessing medical rehabilitation practices: The promise of outcomes research* (pp. 103–126). Baltimore, MD: Paul Bowles Publishing.

Institute of Medicine. (1999). *To err is human: Building a safer health system*. In L. Kohn, J. Corrigan, & M. Donaldson (Eds.). Washington, DC: National Academies Press.

Institute of Medicine. (2001). *Crossing the quality chasm: A new health system for the 21st century*. Washington, DC: National Academies Press.

Institute of Medicine. (2015). *Vital signs: Core metrics for health and health care progress*. Washington, DC: National Academies Press.

James, J. T. (2013). A new, evidence-based estimate of patient harms associated with hospital care. *Journal of Patient Safety, 9*(3), 122–128.

Jesus, T. S., & Hoenig, H. (2015). Postacute rehabilitation quality of care: Toward a shared conceptual framework. *Archives of Physical Medicine and Rehabilitation, 96*(5), 960–969. doi:10.1016/j.apmr.2014.12.007

Kushner, D. S., Peters, K. M., & Johnson-Greene, D. (2015a). Evaluating siebens domain management model for inpatient rehabilitation to increase functional independence and discharge rate to home in geriatric patients. *Archives of Physical Medicine and Rehabilitation, 96*(7), 1310–1318. doi:10.1016/j.apmr.2015.03.011

Kushner, D. S., Peters, K. M., & Johnson-Greene, D. (2015b). Evaluating the siebens model in geriatric-stroke inpatient rehabilitation to reduce institutionalization and acute-care readmissions. *Journal of Stroke and Cerebrovascular Diseases, 25*(2), 317–326. doi:10.1016/j.jstrokecerebrovasdis.2015.09.036

Kushner, D. S., Peters, K. M., & Johnson-Greene, D. (2015c). Evaluating use of the siebens domain management model during inpatient rehabilitation to increase functional independence and discharge rate to home in stroke patients. *Physical Medicine and Rehabilitation, 7*(4), 354–364. doi:10.1016/j.pmrj.2014.10.010

Langhorne, P., & Dennis, M. S. (2004). Stroke units: The next 10 years. *The Lancet, 363*(9412), 834–835.

Plsek, P. E. (1999). Quality improvement methods in clinical medicine. *Pediatrics*, *103*(1, Suppl E), 203–214.

Reistetter, T. A., Karmarkar, A. M., Graham, J. E., Eschbach, K., Kuo, Y. F., Granger, C. V., . . . Ottenbacher, K. J. (2014). Regional variation in stroke rehabilitation outcomes. *Archives of Physical Medicine and Rehabilitation*, *95*(1), 29–38. doi:10.1016/j.apmr.2013.07.018

Ryan, A. M., McCullough, C. M., Shih, S. C., Wang, J. J., Ryan, M. S., & Casalino, L. P. (2014). The intended and unintended consequences of quality improvement interventions for small practices in a community-based electronic health record implementation project. *Medical Care, 52*(9), 826–832. doi:10.1097/MLR.0000000000000186

Siebens, H. (2011). Proposing a practical clinical model. *Topics in Stroke Rehabilitation,18*, 60–65.

Smits, S. J., Bowden, D. E., Falconer, J. A., & Strasser, D. C. (2014). Improving medical leadership and teamwork: An iterative process. *Leadership in Health Services*, *27*(4), 299–315. doi:10.1108/LHS-02-2014-0010

Stevens, A. B., Strasser, D. C., Uomoto, J., Bowen, S. E., & Falconer, J. A. (2007). Utility of treatment implementation methods in a clinical trial with rehabilitation teams. *Journal of Rehabilitation Research and Development*, *44*(4), 537–546.

Strasser, D. C. (in press). Rehabilitation. In J. R. Burton, A. G. Lee, & J. F. Potter (Eds.), *Geriatrics for specialists* (pp. 189–196). New York, NY: Springer Publishing.

Strasser, D. C., Burridge, A. B., Falconer, J. A., Uomoto, J. M., & Herrin, J. (2014). Toward spanning the quality chasm: An examination of team functioning measures. *Archives of Physical Medicine and Rehabilitation, 95*(11), 2220–2223. doi:10.1016/j.apmr.2014.06.013

Strasser, D. C., & Falconer, J. A. (1997a). Linking treatment to outcomes through teams: Building a conceptual model of rehabilitation effectiveness. *Topics in Stroke Rehabilitation, 4*(1), 15–27.

Strasser, D. C., & Falconer, J. A. (1997b). Rehabilitation team process. *Topics in Stroke Rehabilitation, 4*(2), 34–39.

Strasser, D. C., Falconer, J. A., Herrin, J. S., Bowen, S. E., Stevens, A. B., & Uomoto, J. (2005). Team functioning and patient outcomes in stroke rehabilitation. *Archives of Physical Medicine and Rehabilitation, 86*(3), 403–409.

Strasser, D. C., Falconer, J. A., Stevens, A. B., Uomoto, J. M., Herrin, J., Bowen, S. E., & Burridge, A. B. (2008). Team training and stroke rehabilitation outcomes: A cluster randomized trial. *Archives of Physical Medicine and Rehabilitation, 89*(1), 10–15.

Taylor, M. J., McNicholas, C., Nicolay, C., Darzi, A., Bell, D., & Reed, J. E. (2014). Systematic review of the application of the plan-do-study-act method to improve quality in healthcare. *BMJ Quality & Safety, 23*(4), 290–298. doi:10.1136/bmjqs-2013-001862

U.S. Department of Health & Human Services, Health Resources and Services Administration. (2011, April). Quality improvement. Retrieved from http://www.hrsa.gov/quality/toolbox/508pdfs/qualityimprovement.pdf

Walter, L. C., Davidowitz, N. P., Heineken, P. A., & Covinsky, K. E. (2004). Pitfalls of converting practice guidelines into quality measures: Lessons learned from a VA performance measure. *Journal of the American Medical Association, 291*(20), 2466–2470.

Werner, R. M., & Asch, D. A. (2005). The unintended consequences of publicly reporting quality information. *Journal of the American Medical Association, 293*(10), 1239–1244.

Werner, R. M., & Asch, D. A. (2007). Clinical concerns about clinical performance measurement. *Annals of Family Medicine, 5*(2), 159–163.

Zhukalin, M. A., Williams, C. J., Reed, M., & Strasser, D. (2016). Polypharmacy and rational prescribing: Finding the "Golden Mean" for the "Silver Tsunami", In K. Poduri (Ed.), *Geriatric Rehabilitation.* Boca Raton, FL: Taylor and Frances.

SELECTED BIBLIOGRAPHY

Centers for Medicare & Medicaid Services, Department of Health & Human Services. (2015, July 24). *IRF patient assessment instrument* (OMB No. 0938-0842). Retrieved from https://www.cms.gov/Medicare/Quality-Initiatives-Patient-Assessment-Instruments/IRF-Quality-Reporting/Downloads/Final_IRF-PAI_V_1_4_07-24-15.pdf

Chen, T. T., Chung, K. P., Lin, I. C., & Lai, M. S. (2011). The unintended consequence of diabetes mellitus pay-for-performance (P4P) program in Taiwan: Are patients with more comorbidities or more severe conditions likely to be excluded from the P4P program? *Health Services Research, 46*(1, Pt. 1), 47–60. doi:10.1111/j.1475-6773.2010.01182.x

Deutsch, A., Kline, T., Kelleher, C., Lines, L. M., Coots, L., & Garfinkel, D. (2012, November). *Analysis of crosscutting medicare functional status quality metrics using the continuity and assessment record and evaluation (CARE) item set* (RTI Project Number 0212050.022.000.001). Washington, DC: RTI International.

Eldar, R. (1999). Quality of care in rehabilitation medicine. *International Journal for Quality in Health Care, 11*(1), 73–79. Retrieved from http://intqhc.oxfordjournals.org/cgi/reprint/11/1/81.pdf

Gage, B., Constantine, R., Aggarwal, J., Morley, M., Kurlantzick, V. G., Bernard, S., . . . Barch, D. (2012, August). *The development and testing of the continuity assessment record and evaluation (CARE) item set: Final report on the development of the CARE item set* (Vol. 1 of 3, RTI Project Number 0209853.004). Washington, DC: RTI International.

Khot, U. N. (2012). Exploring the risk of unintended consequences of quality improvement efforts. *Journal of the American College of Cardiology, 60*(9), 812–813. doi:10.1016/j.jacc.2012.04.039

Kim, W., Charchian, B., Chang, E. Y., Liang, L. J., Dumas, A. J., Perez M., . . . Kim, H. S. (2013). Strengthening information capture in rehabilitation discharge summaries: An application of the Siebens Domain Management Model. *Physical Medicine and Rehabilitation, 5*(3), 182–188. doi:10.1016/j.pmrj.2013.01.003

O'Brien, S. R., Xue, Y., Ingersoll, G., & Kelly, A. (2013). Shorter length of stay is associated with worse functional outcomes for Medicare beneficiaries with stroke. *Physical Therapy, 93*(12), 1592–1602.

Reker, D. M., Duncan, P. W., Horner, R. D., Hoenig, H., Samsa, G. P., Hamilton, B. B., & Dudley T. K. (2002). Post stroke guideline compliance is associated with greater patient satisfaction. *Archives of Physical Medicine and Rehabilitation, 83*(6), 750–756.

Strasser, D. C. (Ed.). (2010). Quality and quality improvement. *Topics in Stroke Rehabilitation, 17*(4). (Special Issue on Rehabilitation Quality and QI; Nine Articles)

Strasser, D. C., Smits, S. J., Falconer, J. A., Herrin, J. S., & Bowen, S. E. (2002). The influence of hospital culture on rehabilitation team functioning in VA hospitals. *Journal of Rehabilitation Research and Development, 39*(1), 115–125

37

CHAPTER

Future Directions of Rehabilitation Research

Tamara Bushnik

The ultimate purpose of rehabilitation research is to improve clinical and community-based practice and service delivery to maximize the function and quality of life of individuals with disabilities. A myriad of external factors have created an environment where rehabilitation research must become more rigorous in order to provide the evidence base for treatments and interventions to best benefit people with disabilities. This chapter begins with a brief history of rehabilitation and rehabilitation research, describes the key values that should be included in conducting rehabilitation research, introduces some common frameworks that can assist researchers in designing and describing their studies, describes the current status of rehabilitation research, discusses the need for knowledge translation at all stages of the research process, and concludes with future directions.

HISTORY OF REHABILITATION RESEARCH

It was not until the 20th century that modern-day rehabilitation centers were established to provide not only care for individuals with disabilities but also education and training to maximize the physical and mental functional abilities of those individuals to participate in society. Physical, occupational, and vocational therapies were the first to develop into recognized fields to provide for the needs of those in federal service, primarily veterans in the armed services, to return to work following injury. By the 1940s, federal law had established the Veterans Administration and the Social Security Act to provide vocational and other services for military and civilian populations. In 1946, the first rehabilitation service in the United States with dedicated personnel and beds serving the civilian population was established by Dr. Howard Rusk at Bellevue Medical Center in New York City. The term *rehabilitation* was added to the physical medicine medical specialty in 1947 in response to two events: individuals returning from World War II and those who had contracted poliomyelitis during the 1945 to 1952 poliomyelitis epidemic.

Rehabilitation has continued to evolve to meet the needs of those with disabilities. The very nature of rehabilitation is to involve multiple disciplines working together to address the unique physical, mental, and psychosocial needs of each individual to optimize the ability of that person to function maximally within society. As centers and programs dedicated to rehabilitation were established, there was a concomitant growing pressure to document the benefits of specialized rehabilitation programs for the purposes of reimbursement, as well as to develop new interventions and strategies to balance the need to better serve the individual and to minimize costs. Rehabilitation is, by no means, the only specialty that has needed to provide evidence to support its practices; all of medicine is facing these requirements to provide better services and outcomes in the most cost-effective manner.

As a result, rehabilitation research has also evolved to meet these requirements and has followed other medical fields in adopting the premise of evidence-based medicine (EBM). EBM is defined as "the conscientious, explicit, and judicious use of current best evidence in making decisions about the care of individual patients" (Sackett, Rosenberg, Gray, Haynes, & Richardson, 1996). The goal of EBM is to produce standardized practice guidelines that are created from a well-constructed body of evidence to support those guidelines. As is discussed later, there are particular challenges to the rehabilitation field in producing the kinds of evidence that are found in other medical specialties. Regardless, rehabilitation research is the essential bedrock on which rehabilitation clinical practice must rest, and researchers must be aware of the unique aspects of rehabilitation in designing and implementing research studies.

KEY VALUES GUIDING REHABILITATION RESEARCH

The very nature of rehabilitation is to involve multiple disciplines—physiatry; physical, occupational, and recreational therapies; speech language pathology; (neuro)psychology; social work; nursing; and other medical disciplines as required—that work together as an interdisciplinary team to address all of the physical and cognitive needs of the individual with a disability. Consequently, rehabilitation must embrace this interdisciplinary approach when conducting research.

Other key tenets for conducting rehabilitation research are as follows:

- Importance of theory
- Inclusion of clients and families in planning
- Incorporation of cultural context in planning
- Incorporation of the perspectives of all stakeholders—practitioners, payers, policy makers, and researchers, in addition to service recipients and families in research
- Investigation of all components of the International Classification of Functioning, Disability and Health (ICF) (World Health Organization [WHO], 2001) in research designs
- Use of a broad range of research designs and analytical methods that provide alternatives to randomized controlled trials—these include practice-based evidence studies (Horn, DeJong, & Deutscher, 2012), small-sample research designs (Graham, Karmarkar, & Ottenbacher, 2012), and point-of-care clinical trials (Hart & Bagiella, 2012)

EBM: COMMON FRAMEWORKS FOR RESEARCH

International Classification of Functioning, Disability, and Health

In 2001, the WHO endorsed the ICF as the international standard to describe and measure health and disability, and it has won increasing endorsement as the overarching framework in rehabilitation. It was developed to measure health and disability both at the individual and the population level and uses a common metric that can facilitate investigations into the rehabilitation process and recovery. It makes the assumption that anyone can experience a decrease in health that will result in some level of disability and shifts the emphasis away from "fixing the problem" to assessing the impact of the disability on the individual and trying to accommodate to maximize function. The ICF contains three major interacting areas: body functions and structures, activities, and participation. Disability can result from any of these areas being impacted: impairment of body functions and structures, restriction of activities, and limitation in participation. Moderating these three major areas are environmental factors such as the physical, social, and attitudinal milieus in which the individual lives and personal factors such as unique features of the individual and his or her background. By using the structure and language of the ICF, rehabilitation researchers can ensure that all aspects of disability are investigated.

As an example, a study may choose to examine an intervention to mitigate the disability experienced after a motor and sensory complete cervical level 5 traumatic spinal cord injury (SCI). At the level of body function and structure, the study may address the effectiveness of injecting a compound into the spinal cord at the level of injury to decrease glial scarring, promote axonal growth across the injury, and lower the functional level of injury one level, thereby increasing upper extremity function. At the level of activities, the study may seek to investigate how to improve the individual's independence in eating through the use of a novel orthotic device. At the level of participation, the study may investigate methods to decrease the individual's exclusion from social situations such as dining out. The moderating factors would include investigating environmental factors such as the attitudes of other people and personal factors such as the age of the individual with SCI.

Grading the Levels of Evidence

■ Cochrane Collaboration and American Academy of Neurology

There are a number of classification systems that exist to provide grading algorithms of individual studies and facilitate the synthesis of research results. The Cochrane Collaboration (Higgins & Green, 2011) and the American Academy of Neurology (AAN, 2011) are two of the more widely used systems for grading evidence based solely on research design. The Cochrane system only allows evidence from randomized clinical trials of interventions to be considered; if these studies are lacking, then no practice guideline is created and "more research needed" is recommended. In the AAN system, minimum requirements for the number of studies of a particular design are set before a practice recommendation is created; if these requirements are not met, again no recommendation is made (AAN, 2011).

For use in rehabilitation research, however, both of these systems are difficult. In many cases, it is difficult to design a randomized controlled trial (RCT) of the highest quality; for example, in a hypothetical study of a range of motion therapy, it is virtually impossible to "blind" the participant as to the therapy that he or she is receiving. Similarly, the therapist administering the therapy cannot be practically "blinded" either. In addition, the typical high-quality RCT compares an intervention against a control or placebo condition. In rehabilitation, it is not ethical to withhold treatment to create a true control condition; therefore, comparisons must be made between standard of care therapy and a novel intervention. Finally, interventions of interest in rehabilitation are not typically a single well-defined entity, such as a medication, but interventions that are rather difficult to define, such as patient education and advocacy training, which do not lend themselves to a simple RCT framework. These natural constraints within the practice of rehabilitation medicine make it exceedingly difficult to meet the "gold standard" of RCTs to build an evidence base for rehabilitation practice.

Grades of Recommendation, Assessment, Development and Evaluation

A more helpful example of a system of grading evidence that is appropriate for rehabilitation is the Grades of Recommendation, Assessment, Development and Evaluation (GRADE; GRADE Working Group, 2004; Guyatt, Oxman, Kunz, et al., 2008; Guyatt, Oxman, Vist, et al., 2008). The GRADE approach specifies four levels of quality of the evidence: high, moderate, low, and very low. At the simplest level, the research design dictates the level, similar to Cochrane and AAN; randomized trials are high, observational trials are low, and case series/case reports are very low. However, the level of a study may be upgraded or downgraded because of the presence of factors that impact the quality of the evidence. The moderating factors that could increase the quality level of a study include a large magnitude of effect, demonstration of a dose–response gradient, or confounding factors would be expected to decrease the reported effect size. Factors that could decrease a study's quality level include limitations in the design and implementation of the study suggesting a high probability of bias, indirectness of the evidence, unexplained heterogeneity or inconsistency of results, imprecision of results, and high probability of publication bias. These factors are more subjective in nature and require an expert consensus of the reliability of the evidence among the reviewers to accurately classify each study. With these moderating factors, the GRADE levels of quality are as follows:

- *High:* Sufficient confidence in the estimate of the effect that it is unlikely that further research will change the conclusion. Typical studies that support this level of evidence are randomized trials without serious limitations and/or observational studies with very large effects.
- *Moderate:* The current estimate of the effect will probably be impacted by further research. Typical studies are randomized trials with serious limitations and/or observational studies with large effects.
- *Low:* There is a high likelihood that further research will change the estimate of the effect; therefore, confidence is low. Typical studies are randomized trials with very serious limitations and/or observational studies with important limitations.
- *Very low:* The estimate of effect is very uncertain. Typical studies are randomized trials with very serious limitations and inconsistent results, observational studies with serious limitations, and/or unsystematic clinical observations such as case series or case reports (Brozek, Akl, Alonso-Coello, et al., 2009; Brozek, Akl, Jaeschke, et al., 2009).

As can be seen, this type of classification system allows for non-RCTs to be considered as a basis for making practice recommendations. Indeed, the Task Force on Systematic Reviews and Guidelines, convened by the National Center for the Dissemination of Disability Research (NCDDR), published a position paper that strongly cautioned against the absolute reliance on RCTs (Dijkers et al., 2009a, 2009b) and recommended that, for rehabilitation researchers, the most appropriate approach is to select a study design that will best answer the research question and not be forced into the often unnatural constraint of conducting an RCT. This idea was expanded upon in 2012 by Whyte and Barrett who suggested that the development of effective rehabilitation treatments should be viewed as a phased approach with specific goals and research methodologies attached to each phase: idea inception, natural history and measurement, proof of concept, evaluation of efficacy, and evaluation of effectiveness (Whyte & Barrett, 2012).

Indeed, if a number of very well designed, large-sample, nonrandomized trials with concurrent controls all point to the same conclusion that an intervention is effective, should it matter that an RCT has not been conducted? Many rehabilitation researchers would argue “no” and that it is more than sufficient to accept the evidence of all well-designed studies addressing the issue. As such, the GRADE system is far more appropriate for rehabilitation research and the construction of evidence-based recommendations for rehabilitation. For further reading, please see Brozek, Akl, Alonso-Coello, et al. (2009), Brozek, Akl, Jaeschke, (2009), and Dijkers et al. (2009b).

■ Reporting Guidelines

To ensure that the highest quality of research is published and to facilitate the assessment of peer-reviewed research, in 2014, 28 rehabilitation journals agreed to require the use of reporting guidelines when manuscripts are submitted to the peer review process (Chan & Heinemann, 2014). The reporting guidelines are templates that can be used to assist the reporting of research findings in a consistent manner. Reporting guidelines exist for nearly every study design. This effort will serve to improve the understanding of how a study was conducted by ensuring that all relevant details are included and will, thereby, also facilitate the compilation of original research studies into systematic reviews. Ultimately, these templates can be used to assist during the design phase of the study, the intention being to raise the level of rehabilitation research that is being conducted.

Current State of Rehabilitation Research

Recently, a number of new initiatives have begun in response to the growing realization that isolationism, be it one agency or one institution, cannot effectively and efficiently conduct the caliber of research that is needed to advance the field. No one agency has the funding and no one institution has the participant pool and infrastructure to conduct the large-scale trials that are required to provide the basis for evidence-based guidelines for rehabilitation clinical practice. The continued support and funding of research networks, not only within the civilian and military realms but also between them, is a critical component that will ensure that rehabilitation research continues to advance the field and improve the lives of individuals with disabilities and their families.

■ Model Systems of Care

The National Institute on Disability, Independent Living, and Rehabilitation Research (NIDILRR) Model Systems of research were the first large-scale collaborative projects that were tasked with developing a comprehensive system of care extending from the time of injury throughout the life span of the individual. The Spinal Cord Injury Model Systems of Care (SCIMS), in fact, were authorized by Congress in 1970 and funded in 1973, preceding the creation of the National Institute of Disability and Rehabilitation Research (NIDILRR). The Traumatic Brain Injury Model Systems of Care (TBIMS) was funded in 1987, followed by the Burn Injury Rehabilitation Model Systems of Care (BIRMS) in 1994. The uniqueness and strength of the Model Systems (MS) programs are twofold. First, each program has established a national database, with set inclusion and exclusion criteria, into which information about individuals with the disability of interest is entered. This information has changed over the years but can be categorized into the following main groups: premorbid history, demographic characteristics, causes and severity of injury, nature of diagnoses, types of treatment/services, costs of treatment/services, and measurement and prediction of outcomes including impairment, disability, and participation. Both the SCIMS and TBIMS follow individuals longitudinally until the person withdraws, is lost to follow-up, or expires; thus, the SCIMS and TBIMS have information on individuals who are at least 35 years post-SCI and 25 years post-TBI, respectively, at the time of the writing of this chapter. The BIRMS is slightly different in that outcomes are captured up until 2 years after injury. The richness of the information contained within the national databases has resulted in numerous seminal papers that have impacted and will continue to impact the rehabilitation field over the years. Second, the MS structure, bringing together rehabilitation programs with similar levels of clinical and research expertise, permits a level of collaboration that is extremely difficult to attain without explicit support from funding agencies. This has allowed monetary, intellectual, and, crucially, participant resources to be combined in such a way that research questions could be posed, which could not have been answered in a single-site project.

National Research Action Plan

On August 31, 2012, the President issued an executive order calling for the Department of Defense (DoD), Veterans Affairs (VA), Department of Health and Human Services (DHHS), and the Department of Education (DoE) to develop the National Research Action Plan (NRAP) focused on three conditions: posttraumatic stress disorder (PTSD); other mental health conditions including suicide; and TBI. The NRAP was developed in August 2013 and contains a 10-year research framework moving along the translational research continuum from foundational science to services research (NRAP, 2013). One of the important aspects of NRAP is the call for cooperation and sharing of resources among the identified agencies with respect to:

- Standardizing, integrating, and sharing data
- Innovative ways to increase scarce research resources to facilitate access for research
- Building upon current large-scale research initiatives to maximize impact

Although NRAP is focused upon three specific areas of inquiry, the NRAP research framework and timelines for advancing research can be applied to all areas of disability.

Brain Research Through Advancing Innovative Neurotechnologies

In April 2013, the President announced the Brain Research Through Advancing Innovative Neurotechnologies (BRAIN) Initiative, which is hoped to foster significant and quick advances to understanding brain function in a manner similar to what occurred with the Human Genome Project and the field of genomics (www.whitehouse.gov/share/brain-initiative). The aim is to create collaborations among federal, public, and private sector agencies and companies to discover new ways to treat, prevent, and cure brain disorders. As of the end of September 2014, five participating federal agencies—National Institutes of Health, National Science Foundation, Defense Advanced Research Projects Agency, Food and Drug Administration, and Intelligence Advanced Research Projects Agency—have been joined by a growing number of private sector companies, universities, and philanthropists to align their funding priorities with the BRAIN Initiative.

Knowledge Translation

The last consideration in this section is the concept of knowledge translation as another framework that rehabilitation researchers should use when conducting research. The term *knowledge translation* was first defined by the Canadian Institutes of Health Research (CIHR) in 2000 as

> the exchange, synthesis and ethically-sound application of knowledge—within a complex system of interactions among researchers and users—to accelerate the capture of the benefits of research for Canadians through improved health, more effective services and products, and a strengthened health care system. (CIHR, 2005, para. 2)

More recently, NIDILRR created a working definition of knowledge translation as a framework that "promotes the use of research-based knowledge to support the ability of individuals to live successfully in society" (NIDRR, 2013).

The CIHR model details six opportunities during the research process where activities to foster and facilitate knowledge translation should occur (CIHR, 2005). The first two opportunities are in the process of defining the research question/methodology and conducting the research. Of particular importance for EBM are the remaining four opportunities: making the research results accessible in terms of format and language appropriate to the audience; placing the results in the context of other knowledge and sociocultural norms; using the results to make decisions; and influencing future research based on how the knowledge is used. What this effectively means is that conducting research without a plan to disseminate the results to the appropriate audience is no longer acceptable. Researchers must consider how the research may be used a priori when designing either a single research project or a research program. Although EBM calls for practice decisions being made using a body of research for justification, there continue to be significant impediments to this interactive process (Bennett et al., 2003; Meline & Paradiso, 2003).

How can knowledge translation be facilitated? Jacobson, Butterill, and Goering (2003) proposed five domains that should be considered when planning for this interaction: the user group; the issue; the research; the researcher–user relationship; and the dissemination strategies. Essentially, each domain needs to be examined and characterized to better frame how the information should be presented. For example, the Model Systems Knowledge Translation Center (MSKTC) has partnered with a number of professional organizations, including the NIDILRR-funded TBIMS, SCIMS, and BIRMS, to produce consumer versions of professional peer-reviewed abstracts relevant to these diagnoses (see www.msktc.org).

The interaction between the professional who produced the original research and consumers and other professionals is an iterative process whereby information is made accessible to individuals and their family members in an appropriate format. Throughout rehabilitation research, knowledge translation needs to be implemented so that decisions informing practice and future research can be made on a solid evidence base. For a more in-depth examination of knowledge translation, refer to Sudsawad (2007).

FUTURE DIRECTIONS FOR REHABILITATION RESEARCH

The multidisciplinary nature of rehabilitation must extend to the conduct of research as well. Rehabilitation is a complex process that involves all aspects of the physical, cognitive, and psychosocial characteristics of the individual; the research that is required to address this complex interplay of factors is not contained within any one federal and/or state agency that currently funds rehabilitation research programs. As described earlier, initiatives continue at the federal level to facilitate interagency collaboration, including increased dialogue among civilian and military organizations that fund rehabilitation research. An excellent example of just such collaboration is the interagency agreement between NIDILRR and VA in which the TBIMS National Datacenter is providing expert advice and assistance in helping VA polytrauma research centers that have been so designated to develop and maintain a compatible longitudinal database to track long-term outcomes of soldiers who have incurred TBI. Hopefully, such efforts will continue to expand to the betterment of rehabilitation research and ultimately to the provision of the most effective rehabilitation services.

The recognized need for interagency collaboration has also brought to light the wide range of outcome and assessment tools and measures that are used. It is frequently very difficult to compare a body of work in a particular area because the studies use different metrics for assessment and outcome. There are several initiatives that have begun to address this problem and to try and create a common measurement compendium that researchers can use. The Patient Reported Outcomes Measurement Information System (PROMIS; Cella et al., 2007) and the Quality of Life in Neurological Disorders (Neuro-QoL; Cella et al., 2011) initiatives are both federally funded efforts to create scales that will be used in clinical trials and clinical practice and provide the crosswalk that is needed to compare and contrast interventions and treatment results across studies. In addition, researchers are working with the PROMIS and Neuro-QOL items as a basis for developing disability-specific scales, such as for TBI and SCI, which will not only provide information that is relevant to the disability, because original PROMIS and Neuro-QOL items are included, but also allow for comparison with other populations who have taken the PROMIS and/or Neuro-QOL (Tulsky et al., 2015; Tulsky et al., 2016).

Another example of such an effort is the work conducted by the interagency TBI and Psychological Health work groups that were convened by the

National Institute of Neurological Disorders and Stroke, Department of Veterans Affairs, DoD, and NIDILRR to create recommendations for common data elements (CDEs) to support TBI and Psychological Health research studies (Thurmond et al., 2010). The intent is to facilitate the selection of assessment and outcome tools by researchers in the field through the provision of recommendations for "core" measures that must be included if appropriate, "supplemental" measures that should be included for specific topics or populations, and "emerging" measures, which are currently under development and may prove to be superior to current "core" or "supplemental" measures.

All of these laudable efforts have the potential to create a common platform from which researchers and clinicians can "speak the same language." Indeed, the NRAP calls for efforts similar to the TBI/Psychological Health CDEs initiative within PTSD and other mental health disorders. Within the next few years, it is hoped that the current lack of standardization of metrics will be a historical curiosity; the increase in knowledge generated by rehabilitation research should then be able to grow at a much greater rate.

As has been described earlier, rehabilitation research has started to embrace a number of common frameworks—interagency cooperation, collaborative research networks and consortia, and the development of common metrics—by which investigators can facilitate the establishment of a body of research on which practice can be based. However, these initiatives must continue to grow and expand. Rehabilitation research needs to involve *all persons* to whom that research may pertain—this must include individuals with disabilities and their families, as well as the community at large, all allied health care professionals, policy makers, and others—at every stage of the research cycle. When this process is effective, the resultant research is focused and has the greatest likelihood of addressing questions that are important to the intended recipient—irrespective of whether he or she is a researcher, clinician, or an individual with a disability.

REFERENCES

American Academy of Neurology. (2011). *Clinical practice guideline process manual, 2011*. St. Paul, MN: Author.

Bennett, S., Tooth, L., McKenna, K., Rodger, S., Strong, J., Ziviani, J., . . . Gibson, L. (2003). Perceptions of evidence based practice: A survey of Australian occupational therapists. *Australian Occupational Therapy Journal, 50*, 13–22.

Brozek, J. L., Akl, E. A., Alonso-Coello, P., Lang, D., Jaeschke, R., Williams, J. W., . . . GRADE Working Group. (2009). Grading quality of evidence and strength of recommendations in clinical practice guidelines (Part 1 of 3): An overview of the GRADE approach and grading quality of evidence about interventions. *Allergy, 64*, 669–677.

Brozek, J. L., Akl, E. A., Jaeschke, R., Lang, D. M., Bossuyt, P., Glasziou, P., . . . GRADE Working Group. (2009). Grading quality of evidence and strength of recommendations in clinical practice guidelines (Part 2 of 3): The GRADE approach to grading quality of evidence about diagnostic tests and strategies. *Allergy, 64*, 1109–1116.

Canadian Institutes of Health Research. (2005). About knowledge translation. Retrieved from http://www.cihr-irsc.gc.ca/e/29418.html

Cella, D., Nowinski, C., Peterman, A., Victorson, D., Miller, D., Lai, J. S., & Moy, C. (2011). The neurology quality-of-life measurement initiative. *Archives of Physical Medicine and Rehabilitation, 92*(Suppl. 10), S28–S36.

Cella, D., Yount, S., Rothrock, N., Gershon, R., Cook, K., Reeve, B., . . . PROMIS Cooperative Group. (2007). The patient-reported outcomes measurement information system (PROMIS): Progress of an NIH roadmap cooperative group during its first two years. *Medical Care, 45*(Suppl. 1), S3–S11.

Chan, L., & Heinemann, A. W. (2014). Elevating the quality of disability and rehabilitation research: Mandatory use of the reporting guidelines. *Annals of Physical and Rehabilitation Medicine, 57*, 558–560.

Dijkers, M. P. J. M., & the NCDDR Task Force on Systematic Review and Guidelines. (2009a). *When the best is the enemy of the good: The nature of research evidence used in systematic reviews and guidelines*. Austin, TX: SEDL.

Dijkers, M. P. J. M., & The Task Force on Systematic Reviews and Guidelines. (2009b). The value of "traditional" reviews in the era of systematic reviewing. *American Journal of Physical Medicine and Rehabilitation, 88*, 423–430.

GRADE Working Group. (2004). Grading quality of evidence and strength of recommendations. *British Medical Journal, 328*, 1490–1494.

Graham, J. E., Karmarkar, A. M., & Ottenbacher, K. J. (2012). Small sample research designs for evidence-based rehabilitaton: Issues and methods. *Archives of Physical Medicine and Rehabilitation, 93*(Suppl. 2), S111–S116.

Guyatt, G. H., Oxman, A. D., Kunz, R., Vist, G. E., Falck-Ytter, Y., & Schunemann, H. J. (2008). What is 'quality of evidence' and why is it important to clinicians? *British Medical Journal, 26*, 995–998.

Guyatt, G. H., Oxman, A. D., Vist, G. E., Kunz, R., Falck-Ytter, Y., Alonso-Coello, P., . . . GRADE Working Group. (2008). GRADE: An emerging consensus on rating quality of evidence and strength of recommendations. *British Medical Journal, 26*, 924–926.

Hart, T., & Bagiella, E. (2012). Design and implementation of clinical trials in rehabilitation research. *Archives of Physical Medicine and Rehabilitation, 93*(Suppl. 2), S117–S126.

Higgins, J. P. T., & Green, S. (Eds.). (2011). *Cochrane handbook for systematic reviews of interventions 5.1.0* [updated March 2011]. The Cochrane Collaboration. Retrieved from www.cochrane-handbook.org

Horn, S. D., DeJong, G., & Deutscher, D. (2012). Practice-based evidence research in rehabilitation: An alternative to randomized controlled trials and traditional observational studies. *Archives of Physical Medicine and Rehabilitation, 93*(Suppl. 2), S127–S137.

Jacobson, N., Butterill, D., & Goering, P. (2003). Development of a framework for knowledge translation: Understanding user context. *Journal of Health Services Research Policy, 8*, 94–99.

Meline, T., & Paradiso, T. (2003). Evidence-based practice in schools: Evaluation research and reducing barriers. *Language, Speech, and Hearing Services in Schools, 34*, 273–283.

National Institute on Disability and Rehabilitation Research. (2013). *Long-range plan for fiscal years 2013–2017*. Retrieved from https://www.gpo.gov/fdsys/pkg/FR-2013-04-04/html/2013-07879.htm

National Research Action Plan. (2013). *Responding to the executive order: Improving access to mental health services for veterans, service members, and military families*. Retrieved from www.whitehouse.gov/sites/default/files/uploads/nrap_for_eo_on_mental_health_august_2013.pdf

Sackett, D. L., Rosenberg, W. M., Gray, J. A., Haynes, R. B., & Richardson, W. S. (1996). Evidence-based medicine: What it is and what it isn't. *British Medical Journal, 312*, 71–72.

Sudsawad, P. (2007). *Knowledge translation: Introduction to models, strategies, and measures*. Austin, TX: SEDL. Retrieved from ktdrr.org/ktlibrary/articles_pubs/ktmodels/index.html

Thurmond, V. A., Hicks, R., Gleason, T., Miller, A. C., Szuflita, N., Orman, J., & Schwab, K. (2010). Advancing integrated research in psychological health and traumatic brain injury: Common data elements. *Archives of Physical Medicine and Rehabilitation, 91*, 1633–1636.

Tulsky, D. S., Kisala, P. A., Victorson, D., Carlozzi, N., Bushnik, T., Sherer, M., . . . Cella, D. (2016). TBI-QOL: Development and calibration of item banks to measure patient reported outcomes following traumatic brain injury. *Journal of Head Trauma Rehabilitation, 31*, 40–51.

Tulsky, D. S., Kisala, P. A., Victorson, D., Tate, D. G., Heinemann, A. W., Charlifue, S., . . . Cella, D. (2015). Overview of the spinal cord injury-quality of life (SCI-QOL) measurement system. *Journal of Spinal Cord Medicine, 38*, 257–269.

World Health Organization. (2001). *International classification of functioning, disability and health (ICF)*. Geneva, Switzerland: Author.

Whyte, J., & Barrett, A. M. (2012). Advancing the evidence base of rehabilitation treatments: A developmental approach. *Archives of Physical Medicine and Rehabilitation, 93*(Suppl. 2), S101–110.

Index